Fourth Edition

Evidence-Based Practice in Nursing & Healthcare

A Guide to Best Practice

Bernadette Mazurek Melnyk

PhD, RN, APRN-CNP, FAANP, FNAP, FAAN

Vice President for Health Promotion
University Chief Wellness Officer
Dean and Professor, College of Nursing
Professor of Pediatrics and Psychiatry, College of Medicine
Executive Director, Helene Fuld Health Trust National Institute for
     Evidence-based Practice in Nursing and Healthcare
The Ohio State University
Columbus, Ohio
Editor, Worldviews on Evidence-Based Nursing

Ellen Fineout-Overholt

PhD, RN, FNAP, FAAN

Mary Coulter Dowdy Distinguished Professor of Nursing
College of Nursing and Health Sciences
Gallup Certified Strengths Coach for the School of Nursing
University of Texas at Tyler
Tyler, Texas
Editorial Board, Worldviews on Evidence-Based Nursing
Editorial Board, Research in Nursing & Health

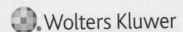
. Wolters Kluwer

Philadelphia • Baltimore • New York • London
Buenos Aires • Hong Kong • Sydney • Tokyo

Not authorised for sale in United States, Canada, Australia, New Zealand, Puerto Rico, and U.S. Virgin Islands.

Acquisitions Editor: Mark Foss
Director of Product Development: Jennifer K. Forestieri
Development Editor: Roxanne Ward
Editorial Coordinator: Lindsay Ries
Marketing Manager: Katie Schlesinger
Production Project Manager: Marian Bellus
Design Coordinator: Joan Wendt
Manufacturing Coordinator: Kathleen Brown
Prepress Vendor: S4Carlisle Publishing Services

Fourth edition

Library of Congress Cataloging-in-Publication Data

Names: Melnyk, Bernadette Mazurek, author.
Title: Evidence-based practice in nursing & healthcare: a guide to best
  practice / Bernadette Mazurek Melnyk, PhD, RN, APRN-CNP, FAANP, FNAP,
  FAAN, Vice President for Health Promotion, University Chief Wellness
  Officer, Dean and Professor, College of Nursing, Professor of Pediatrics &
  Psychiatry, College of Medicine, The Ohio State University, Editor,
  Worldviews on Evidence-Based Nursing, Ellen Fineout-Overholt, PhD, RN,
  FNAP, FAAN, Mary Coulter Dowdy Distinguished Professor of Nursing, College
  of Nursing & Health Sciences, University of Texas at Tyler, Editorial
  Board, Worldviews on Evidence-Based Nursing, Editorial Board, Research in
  Nursing & Health.
Other titles: Evidence-based practice in nursing and healthcare
Description: Fourth edition. | Philadelphia: Wolters Kluwer Health, [2019] |
  Includes bibliographical references.
Identifiers: LCCN 2018032178 | ISBN 9781496384539
Subjects: LCSH: Evidence-based nursing—Practice. | Nurse
  practitioners—Practice.
Classification: LCC RT42 .M44 2019 | DDC 610.73—dc23
LC record available at https://lccn.loc.gov/2018032178

CCS1018

I dedicate this book to my loving family, who has provided tremendous support to me in pursuing my dreams and passions: my husband, John; and my three daughters, Kaylin, Angela, and Megan; as well as to my father, who always taught me that anything can be accomplished with a spirit of enthusiasm and determination, and my sister Chris, who taught me to "just get out there and do it!" It is also dedicated to all of the committed healthcare providers and clinicians who strive every day to deliver the highest quality of evidence-based care.

Bernadette Mazurek Melnyk

For Rachael and Ruth, my precious daughters who are my daily inspiration. May you have the kind of healthcare you deserve—evidence-based with demonstrated reliable outcomes that is delivered by conscientious care providers who intentionally incorporate your preferences into your care. For my dear husband, Wayne, and my sweet Mom, Virginia Fineout, from whom I learn so much about how healthcare could/should be. Finally, this edition is dedicated to all care providers in primary care, community/public health, and at point of care in acute and long-term care who diligently seek to consistently deliver evidence-based care.

Ellen Fineout-Overholt

Contributors

Anne W. Alexandrov, PhD, RN,
AGACNP-BC, CNS, ANVP-BC,
NVRN-BC, CCRN, FAAN
Professor of Nursing and Neurology
Acute, Critical Care and Department of
Neurology
Chief Nurse Practitioner
UTHSC Memphis Mobile Stroke Unit
University of Tennessee Health Science
Center at Memphis
Memphis, Tennessee

Karen Balakas, PhD, RN, CNE
Retired Director of Research & EBP
St. Louis Children's Hospital & Missouri
Baptist Medical Center
St. Louis, Missouri

Cecily L. Betz, PhD, RN, FAAN
Professor
Department of Pediatrics
University of Southern California Keck
School of Medicine
General Pediatrics
Children's Hospital Los Angeles
Los Angeles, California

Cheryl L. Boyd, PhD, MSN, RN
Adjunct Assistant Professor
College of Nursing
The Ohio State University
Director
Professional Development
Nationwide Children's Hospital
Columbus, Ohio

Barbara B. Brewer, PhD, RN, MALS,
MBA, FAAN
Associate Professor
College of Nursing
The University of Arizona
Tucson, Arizona

Tracy L. Brewer, DNP, RNC-OB, CLC
Clinical Professor
College of Nursing
University of Tennessee-Knoxville
Knoxville, Tennessee

Terri L. Brown, MSN, RN, CPN
Clinical Specialist
Quality and Safety
Texas Children's Hospital
Houston, Texas

Jacalyn S. Buck, PhD, RN, NEA-BC
Administrator Health System Nursing
ACNO Medical Surgical and Women and
Infants Nursing
Health System Nursing
Medical Surgical and Women and Infants
Nursing
The Ohio State University Wexner Medical
Center
Columbus, Ohio

Emily Caldwell, MS
Media Relations Manager
University Communications/Office of the
President
The Ohio State University
Columbus, Ohio

Katie Choy, DNP, RN, CNS, NEA-BC,
RN-BC
Consultant
Nursing Practice and Education
San Jose, California

Denise Cote-Arsenault, PhD, RN, CPLC,
FNAP, FAAN
Eloise R. Lewis Excellence Professor
School of Nursing
University of North Carolina
Greensboro
Greensboro, North Carolina

John F. Cox III, MD
Associate Professor of Clinical
Medicine
Department of Medicine
Primary Care Physicians
School of Medicine & Dentistry
University of Rochester
Internist, Clinton Medical Associates
Rochester, New York

Laura Cullen, DNP, RN, FAAN
Adjunct Faculty
University of Iowa College of Nursing
University of Iowa
EBP Scientist
Office of Nursing Research, EBP and Quality
Department of Nursing and Patient Care
    Services
University of Iowa Hospitals and Clinics
Iowa City, Iowa

Maria Cvach, DNP, RN, FAAN
Assistant Director
Nursing, Clinical Standards
The Johns Hopkins Hospital
Baltimore, Maryland

Deborah Dang, PhD, RN, NEA-BC
Graduate School of Nursing
Johns Hopkins University
Director of Nursing, Practice, Education, &
    Research
Central Nursing Administration
The Johns Hopkins Hospital
Baltimore, Maryland

Lynn Gallagher-Ford, PhD, RN, DPFNAP,
    NE-BC, FAAN
Senior Director
Director, Clinical Core
The Helene Fuld Institute for Evidence-based
    Practice in Nursing and Healthcare
College of Nursing
The Ohio State University
Columbus, Ohio

Martha J. Giggleman, RN, DNP
Consultant
Evidence-based Practice
Livermore, California

Doris Grinspun, RN, MSN, PhD,
    LLD (hon), Dr (hc), O.ONT
Adjunct Professor
Lawrence S. Bloomberg Faculty of Nursing
University of Toronto
Chief Executive Officer
Registered Nurses' Association of Ontario
    (RNAO)
Toronto, Ontario

Tami A. Hartzell, MLS
Senior Librarian
Werner Medical Library
Rochester General Hospital
Rochester, New York

Marilyn J. Hockenberry, PhD, RN,
    PPCNP-BC, FAAN
Associate Dean for Research Affairs
Bessie Baker Professor of Nursing
Center for Nursing Research
Duke University School of Nursing
Durham, North Carolina

Robin Kretschman, HC-MBA, MSN, RN,
    NEA-BC
Vice President Clinical Business Strategic
    Operations
Nursing Administration
OSF HealthCare
Peoria, Illinois

June H. Larabee, PhD, RN
Professor Emeritus
West Virginia University and West Virginia
    University Hospitals
Charleston, West Virginia

Lisa English Long, PhD, RN
Consultant
Evidence-based Practice
Cincinnati, Ohio

Jacqueline M. Loversidge, PhD,
    RNC-AWHC
Associate Professor of Clinical
    Nursing
College of Nursing
The Ohio State University
Columbus, Ohio

Pamela Lusk, DNP, RN, PMHNP-BC,
    FAANP, FNAP
Associate Professor of Clinical Practice
College of Nursing
The Ohio State University
Columbus, Ohio
Psychiatric/Mental Health Nurse
    Practitioner
Pediatrics Yavapai Regional Medical Center
Prescott, Arizona

Tina L. Magers, PhD, MSN, RN-BC
Nursing Excellence and Research
    Coordinator
Mississippi Baptist Medical Center
Jackson, Mississippi

Kathy Malloch, PhD, MBA, RN, FAAN
Clinical Professor
College of Nursing
Ohio State University
Columbus, Ohio

Mikki Meadows-Oliver, PhD, RN, FAAN
Associate Professor
Department of Nursing
Quinnipiac University School of Nursing
North Haven, Connecticut

Dianne Morrison-Beedy, PhD, RN, WHNP,
    FNAP, FAANP, FAAN
Chief Talent & Global Strategy Officer
Centennial Professor of Nursing
College of Nursing
The Ohio State University
Columbus, Ohio

Dónal P. O'Mathúna, PhD
Associate Professor
Fuld Institute for Evidence-based Practice
    College of Nursing
The Ohio State University
Columbus, Ohio
Associate Professor
School of Nursing & Human Sciences
Dublin City University
Glasnevin, Dublin 9, Ireland

Tim Porter-O'Grady, DM, EdD, APRN,
    FAAN, FACCWS
Clinical Professor
School of Nursing
Emory University
Clinical Wound Specialist
Street Medicine Program/Clinic
Mercy Care of Atlanta
Atlanta, Georgia

Cheryl C. Rodgers, PhD, MSN, BSN
Associate Professor
Duke University School of Nursing
Durham, North Carolina

Jo Rycroft-Malone, PhD, MSc,
    BSc(Hons), RN
Professor and Pro Vice-Chancellor Research
    & Impact
School of Health Sciences
Bangor University
Bangor, United Kingdom

Alyce A. Schultz, RN, PhD, FAAN
Consultant
Clinical Research and Evidence-based
    Practice
Bozeman, Montana

Kathryn A. Smith, RN, MN, DrPH
Associate Professor of Clinical Pediatrics
Department of Pediatrics
Keck School of Medicine
General Pediatrics
Children's Hospital Los Angeles
Los Angeles, California

Cheryl B. Stetler, RN, PhD, FAAN
Retired Consultant

Kathleen R. Stevens, RN, MS, EdD,
    ANEF, FAAN
Castella Endowed Distinguished Professor
School of Nursing
University of Texas Health Science Center
    San Antonio
San Antonio, Texas

Susan B. Stillwell, DNP, RN ANEF,
    FAAN
EBP Expert Mentor and Independent
    Consultant
Vancouver, Washington

Timothy Tassa, MPS
Network for Excellence in Health
    Innovation
Washington, District of Columbia

Amanda Thier, RN, MSN
Staff Nurse
Specialty Care Unit
Baylor University Medical Center
Dallas, Texas

Kathleen M. Williamson, RN, PhD
Professor, Chair
Wilson School of Nursing
Midwestern State University
Wichita Falls, Texas

Jennifer Yost, PhD, RN
Associate Professor
M. Louise Fitzpatrick College of Nursing
Villanova University
Villanova, Pennsylvania

Cindy Zellefrow, DNP, MSEd, RN
Director, Academic Core and Assistant
  Professor of Practice
The Helene Fuld Health Trust
National Institute for Evidence-based
  Practice in Nursing and Healthcare at
  The Ohio State University College of
  Nursing
The Ohio State University
Reynoldsburg, Ohio

Reviewers

Ashley Leak Bryant, PhD, RN-BC, OCN
Assistant Professor
School of Nursing
The University of North Carolina at Chapel Hill
Clinical Nurse
North Carolina Cancer Hospital
UNC Healthcare
UNC Lineberger Comprehensive Cancer Center
Chapel Hill, North Carolina

Lynne E. Bryant, EdD, MSN, RN, CNE
Professor
Ron and Kathy Assaf College of Nursing
Nova Southeastern University
Fort Lauderdale, Florida

Mary Mites-Campbell, PhD
Assistant Professor
College of Nursing
Nova Southeastern University
Fort Lauderdale, Florida

Lisa Chaplin, RN, NP-C, DNP
Assistant Professor
Department of Advanced Practice Nursing
School of Nursing and Health Studies
Georgetown University
Washington, District of Columbia

Karyn E. Holt, RN, PhD
Director of Online Quality and Faculty
    Development and Clinical Professor
College of Nursing and Health Professions
Drexel University
Philadelphia, Pennsylvania

Kathy James, DNSc
Associate Professor of Nursing
Department of Nursing
University of San Diego
San Diego, California

Lynette Landry, PhD, RN
Professor and Chair, Nursing and Health Science
Nursing Program
California State University, Channel Islands
Camarillo, California

Susan Mullaney, EdD
Professor and Chair
Department of Nursing
Framingham State University
Framingham, Massachusetts

Mary Ann Notarianni, PhD, RN
Professor
School of Nursing
Sentara College of Health Sciences
Chesapeake, Virginia

Doreen Radjenovic, PhD, ARNP
Associate Professor
School of Nursing, Brooks College
    of Health
University of North Florida
Jacksonville, Florida

Theresa Skybo, PhD, RN, CPNP
Associate Professor
Mt. Carmel College of Nursing
Columbus, Ohio

Margaret (Peggy) Slota, DNP, RN, FAAN
Associate Professor
Director, DNP Graduate Studies
School of Nursing and Health Studies
Georgetown University
Washington, District of Columbia

Ida L. Slusher, PhD (RN, PhD, CNE)
Professor
Baccalaureate & Graduate Nursing
Eastern Kentucky University
Richmond, Kentucky

Debbie Stayer, PhD, RN-BC, CCRN-K
Assistant Professor
Department of Nursing
Bloomsburg University
Bloomsburg, Pennsylvania

Ann Bernadette Tritak, RN, EdD, MA, BSN
Professor and Associate Dean
Department of Graduate Nursing
Felician University
Lodi, New Jersey

Supakit Wongwiwatthananukit, PharmD,
    MS, PhD
Professor
Pharmacy Practice
The Daniel K. Inouye College of Pharmacy
University of Hawai'i at Hilo
Hilo, Hawaii

Like many of you, I have appreciated healthcare through a range of experiences and perspectives. As someone who has delivered healthcare as a combat medic, paramedic, nurse, and trauma surgeon, the value of evidence-based practice is clear to me. Knowing what questions to ask, how to carefully evaluate the responses, maximize the knowledge and use of empirical evidence, and provide the most effective clinical assessments and interventions are important assets for every healthcare professional. The quality of U.S. and global healthcare depends on clinicians being able to deliver on these and other best practices.

The Institute of Medicine (now the National Academy of Medicine) calls for all healthcare professionals to be educated to deliver patient-centered care as members of an interdisciplinary team, emphasizing evidence-based practice, quality improvement approaches, and informatics. Although many practitioners support the use of evidence-based practice, and there are indications that our patients are better served when we apply evidence-based practice, there are challenges to successful implementation. One barrier is knowledge. Do we share a standard understanding of evidence-based practice and how such evidence can best be used? We need more textbooks and other references that clearly define and provide a standard approach to evidence-based practice.

Another significant challenge is the time between the publication of research findings and the translation of such information into practice. This challenge exists throughout public health. Determining the means of more rapidly moving from the brilliance that is our national medical research to applications that blend new science and compassionate care in our clinical systems is of interest to us all.

As healthcare professionals who currently use evidence-based practice, you recognize these challenges and others. Our patients benefit because we adopt, investigate, teach, and evaluate evidence-based practice. I encourage you to continue the excellent work to bring about greater understanding and a more generalizable approach to evidence-based practice.

Richard H. Carmona, MD, MPH, FACS
17th Surgeon General of the United States

Preface

OVERVIEW OF THIS BOOK

The evidence is irrefutable: evidence-based practice (EBP) is key to meeting the quadruple aim in healthcare. It improves the patient experience through providing quality care, enhances patient outcomes, reduces costs, and empowers clinicians, leading to higher job satisfaction. Although there are many published interventions/treatments that have resulted in positive outcomes for patients and healthcare systems, they are not being implemented in clinical practice. In addition, qualitative evidence is not readily incorporated into care. We wrote this book to address these issues and many others as well. We recommend that learners read this book, then read it again, engage in the online resources, the appendices, the glossary . . . then read it again. It is chock-full of information that can help learners of all disciplines, roles and educational levels discover how to be the best clinicians. We hope you find that EBP pearl that is just the right information you need to take the next step in your EBP journey to deliver the best care!

Purpose

The purpose of *Evidence-Based Practice in Nursing and Healthcare* has never changed. The purpose of this edition, as with the last three, is to incorporate what we have learned across the years to provide resources and information that can facilitate clinicians' ready translation of research findings into practice, as well as their use of practice data to improve care and document important outcomes, no matter the clinician's healthcare role. Each edition has provided additional features and resources for readers to use in their journey to become evidence-based clinicians. Since the first book was published, there has been some progress in the adoption of EBP as the standard of care; however, there is still much work to be done for EBP to *the* paradigm used in daily clinical decision making by point-of-care providers. Clinicians' commitment to excellence in healthcare through the intentional integration of research findings into practice while including patients in decisions remains a daunting endeavor that will take anywhere from years to decades. Therefore, increased efforts across the healthcare industry are required to provide a culture that fosters empowered point-of-care clinicians with the knowledge, skills, attitudes, and resources they need to deliver care that demonstrates improved healthcare system, clinician, and patient outcomes.

We will always believe that anything is possible when you have a big dream and believe in your ability to accomplish that dream. It was the vision of transforming healthcare with EBP, in any setting, with one client–clinician encounter at a time and the belief that this can be the daily experience of both patients and care providers, along with our sheer persistence through many "character-building" experiences during the writing and editing of the book, that culminated in this user-friendly guide that aims to assist all healthcare professionals in the delivery of the highest quality, evidence-based care.

The fourth edition of this book has been revised to assist healthcare providers with implementing and sustaining EBP in their daily practices and to foster a deeper understanding of the principles of the EBP paradigm and process. In working with healthcare systems and clinicians throughout the nation and globe and conducting research on EBP, we have learned more about successful strategies to advance and sustain evidence-based care. The new material throughout the book, including new chapter material, a unit-by-unit EBP example, new chapters, EBP competencies, and tools to advance EBP, are included so that clinicians can use them to help with daily evidence-based decision making.

Worldview

A solid understanding of the EBP paradigm, or worldview, is the first mastery milestone for readers of this EBP book. The next milestone is using the paradigm as the foundation for making clinical decisions with patients. This worldview frames why rigorously following the steps of the EBP process is essential, clarifies misperceptions about implementing evidence-based care, and underpins practical action strategies that lead to sustainable evidence implementation at the point of care. It is our dream that the knowledge and understanding gained from thoughtfully and intentionally engaging the contents of this book will help clinicians across the country and globe accelerate adoption of the EBP paradigm until evidence-based care is the lived experience for clinicians, patients, and health professions students across various healthcare settings and educational institutions.

NEW FEATURES AND RESOURCES FOR THIS EDITION

The book contains vital, usable, and relatable content for all levels of practitioners and learners, with key exemplars that bring to life the concepts within the chapters. Each unit now begins with "Making Connections: An EBP Exemplar." This unfolding case study serves as a model or example of EBP in real-life practice. We recommend that learners read each unit exemplar before they engage in that unit's content; the characters in the healthcare team in the exemplar use the information within the unit's chapters to carry out the steps of EBP, leading to a real evidence-based change to improve the quality and safety of care. These characters may be fictional, but the exemplar is based on an important quality indicator (i.e., hospital falls) and an actual synthesis of published research that offers the opportunity for readers to better understand how they can use EBP in their clinical practice or educational setting to improve outcomes. Readers may wish to refer back to the exemplar as they are reading through the chapters to see how the healthcare team used the information they are learning. Furthermore, it is recommended that readers follow the team as they make evidence-based decisions across the units within the book. There are online resources as well as resources within the appendices of the book that will be used in the exemplar, offering readers the opportunity to see how the team uses these resources in evidence-based decision making.

Our unit-ending feature, "Making EBP Real: A Success Story," has been updated and continues to provide real-life examples that help readers to see the principles of EBP applied. Readers can explore a variety of ways that the steps of the EBP process were used in real EBP implementations. Clinicians who desire to stimulate or lead change to a culture of EBP in their practice sites can discover in both of these unit-level features how functional models and practical strategies to introduce a change to EBP can occur, including overcoming barriers in implementing change, evaluating outcomes of change, and moving change to sustainability through making it standard of care.

To help recognize that knowledge and understanding of EBP terms and language is essential to adopting the EBP paradigm, in this edition, we added *EBP Terms to Learn* that features key terms at the beginning of each unit and chapter. Readers can review terms in the glossary before reading the chapters so that they can readily assimilate content. Furthermore, we have provided learning objectives at the unit and chapter level to continue to reinforce important concepts and offer the opportunity for readers to quickly identify key chapter content. When readers come across bolded terms within the chapter, they are encouraged to go to the glossary at back of the book to further explore that concept. EBP Fast Facts is an important feature at the end of each chapter that we retained for this edition, offering readers some of the most important pearls of wisdom from the chapter. These elements in our fourth edition will help learners master the terminology of EBP and identify important content for developing EBP competence.

Finally, for faculty, there is new content in the chapter on teaching EBP in academic settings that can help educators to parse teaching EBP across academic learning degrees. Educators are encouraged to review the online resources that can facilitate teaching EBP in both academic and clinical settings.

Further resources for all readers of the book include appendices that help learners master the process of evidence-based change, such as rapid critical appraisal checklists (be sure to check online on thePoint° for Word versions of RCA checklists for readers to use), sample instruments to evaluate EBP in both educational and clinical settings, a template for asking PICOT questions, and more. Some appendices appear online only on thePoint°, including an appraisal guide for qualitative evidence, an ARCC model EBP mentor role description, and examples of a health policy brief, a press release, and an approved consent form for a study. More details about the great resources available online can be found below.

ORGANIZATION OF THE BOOK

As in prior editions, the Table of Contents is structured to follow the steps of EBP:

- Chapters 1 to 3 in **Unit 1** encompass steps 0, 1, and 2 of the EBP process. This unit gets learners started by building a strong foundation and has significant content updates in this new edition.
- Chapters 4 to 8 in **Unit 2** delve deeply into step 3 of the EBP process, the four-phased critical appraisal of evidence. In this edition, Chapters 7 and 8 were moved into Unit 2 to better align the steps of the EBP process with the chapters, including the important consideration of patient concerns, choices, clinical judgment, and clinical practice guidelines in the recommendation phase of critical appraisal.
- In **Unit 3**, Chapters 9 to 12 move the reader from recommendation to implementation of sustainable practice change. To facilitate understanding how to implement evidence-based change, Chapter 11 was added to describe the context, content, and outcome of implementing EBP competencies in clinical and academic settings.
- **Unit 4** promotes creating and sustaining a culture of EBP. In this unit, we included new content and resources in the chapters on teaching EBP in educational and healthcare settings (Chapters 16 and 17, respectively). Educators can be most successful as they make the EBP paradigm and process understandable for their learners.
- **Unit 5** features a new Chapter 19 on health policy. In today's political climate, nurses and healthcare professionals need to understand how to ensure sustainable change through influencing the formulation of policies governing healthcare, fully supported by the latest and best evidence. This new chapter joins Chapter 20 on disseminating evidence.
- In **Unit 6**, Chapter 21 now combines two previous chapters' content on generating evidence through qualitative and quantitative research, greatly streamlining the material for enhanced understanding of important concepts and making the information more accessible to learners. Chapter 23 provides updated information on ethics in EBP and research generation.
- The glossary is one of the best resources within this book. Readers are encouraged to use it liberally to understand and master EBP language, and thereby enhance their fluency.

Often, educators teach by following chapters in a textbook through their exact sequence; however, we recommend using chapters of this fourth edition that are appropriate for the level of the learner (e.g., associate degree, baccalaureate, master's, doctoral). For example, we would recommend that associate degree students benefit from Units 1, 3, and 4. Curriculum for baccalaureate learners can integrate all units; however, we recommend primarily using Units 1 to 4, with Unit 5 as a resource for understanding more about research terminology and methods as readers learn to critical appraise evidence. Master's and doctoral programs can incorporate all units into their curricula. Advanced practice clinicians and doctorally-prepared clinical experts will be able to lead in implementing evidence in practice, thoughtfully evaluate outcomes of practice, and move to sustainable change, whereas those learning to become researchers will understand how to best build on existing evidence to fill gaps in knowledge with valid, reliable research that is clinically meaningful.

An important resource for educators to use as a supplement to this EBP book is the *American Journal of Nursing* EBP Step-by-Step series, which provides a real-world example of the EBP process from step 0 through 6. We recommend this series as a supplement because the series was written to expose readers to the EBP process in story form, but used alone it does not provide the level of learning to establish competence in evidence-based care. In the series, a team of healthcare providers encounters a challenging issue and uses the EBP process to find a sustainable solution that improves healthcare outcomes. If educators choose to use this series, we caution on using it as the sole source for learning about EBP. Rather, assigning the articles to be read before a course begins or in tandem with readings from this book that match the article being read provides a complete learning opportunity, including context and adequate content for competence—the goal of learning about EBP, regardless of the learner's level of education or clinical practice. For example, the first three chapters of the book could be assigned along with the first four articles, in an academic or clinical setting. The learners could use discussion boards or face-to-face group conference-type settings to discuss how the team used the content the learners studied within the chapter, allowing educators opportunity for evaluation of content mastery (see suggested curriculum strategy at this book's companion website on thePoint®, http://thepoint.lww.com/Melnyk4e). Multiple approaches are offered for educators and learners to engage EBP content, and, in doing so, we believe that this book continues to facilitate changes in how research concepts and critical appraisal are being taught in clinical and academic professional programs throughout the country.

UPDATED FEATURES

This edition of *Evidence-Based Practice in Nursing & Healthcare* includes many features that readers have come to expect. These features are designed to benefit both learners and educators:

- **Quotes:** As proponents of cognitive-behavioral theory, which contends that how people think directly influences how they feel and behave, we firmly believe that how an individual thinks is the first step toward or away from success. Therefore, **inspirational quotes** are intertwined throughout our book to encourage readers to build their beliefs and abilities as they actively engage in increasing their knowledge and skills in EBP to accomplish their desired learning goals.
- **Clinical Scenarios** describe a clinical case or a supervisory decision clinicians could encounter in clinical practice, prompting readers to seek out best evidence and determine a reasonable course of action.
- **Web Tips:** With the rapid delivery of information available to us, **web tips** direct readers to helpful Internet resources and sites that can be used to further develop EBP knowledge and skills.
- **EBP Fast Facts** act as a chapter-closing feature, highlighting important points from each chapter. Reviewing these pearls can help readers know if they retained the important concepts presented within the chapter.
- **Making EBP Real:** A successful real-world case story emphasizing applied content from each unit.
- **NEW: Learning Objectives:** Each unit and chapter now begins with learning objectives, to help learners focus on key concepts.
- **NEW: EBP Terms to Learn:** Each unit and chapter also now includes a list of the key terms discussed or defined in the chapter that are to help students build familiarity with the language and terminology of EBP.
- **NEW: Making Connections: An EBP Exemplar:** Opening each unit, this new feature walks the learner through the EBP process in an unfolding case study that is applicable to a real-time important practice issue.

ADDITIONAL RESOURCES ON thePoint®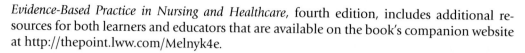

Evidence-Based Practice in Nursing and Healthcare, fourth edition, includes additional resources for both learners and educators that are available on the book's companion website at http://thepoint.lww.com/Melnyk4e.

Learner Resources Available on thePoint®

Learners who have purchased *Evidence-Based Practice in Nursing and Healthcare,* fourth edition, have access to the following additional online resources:

- Appendices D, E, F, G, H from the book
- Learning Objectives for each chapter
- **Checklists and templates** in MS Word format include checklists for rapid critical appraisal, conducting an evidence review, or holding a journal club; sample templates for PICOT questions and for evaluation and synthesis tables; an ARCC model EBP mentor role description; and more.
- **A searching exercise** to help develop mastery of systematic searching.
- **Journal articles** corresponding to book chapters to offer access to current research available in Wolters Kluwer journals.
- The *American Journal of Nursing* **EBP Step-by-Step Series,** which provides a real-world example of the EBP process as a supplement to learning within the EBP book.
- An example of a poster (to accompany Chapter 20).
- A **Spanish–English audio glossary** and **Nursing Professional Roles and Responsibilities**

See the inside front cover of this book for more details, including the passcode you will need to gain access to the website.

Educator Resources Available on thePoint®

Approved adopting instructors will be given access to the following additional resources:
- An **eBook** allows access to the book's full text and images online.
- **Test generator** with updated NCLEX-style questions. Test questions link to chapter learning objectives.
- Additional **application case studies and examples** for select chapters.
- **PowerPoint presentations,** including multiple choice questions for use with interactive clicker technology.
- An **image bank,** containing figures and tables from the text in formats suitable for printing, projecting, and incorporating into websites.
- **Strategies for Effective Teaching** offer creative approaches.
- **Learning management system cartridges.**
- Access to all learner resources.

COMPREHENSIVE, INTEGRATED DIGITAL LEARNING SOLUTIONS

We are delighted to introduce digital solutions to support educators and learners using *Evidence-Based Practice in Nursing & Healthcare,* Fourth Edition. Now for the first time, our textbook is embedded into an integrated digital learning solution that builds on the features of the text with proven instructional design strategies. To learn more about this solution, visit http://nursingeducation.lww.com/, or contact your local Wolters Kluwer representative.

Lippincott CoursePoint

Lippincott CoursePoint is a rich learning environment that drives academic course and curriculum success to prepare learners for practice. Lippincott CoursePoint is designed for the way students learn. The solution connects learning to real-life application by integrating content from *Evidence-Based Practice in Nursing & Healthcare* with video cases, interactive modules, and evidence-based journal articles. Ideal for active, case-based learning, this powerful solution helps students develop higher-level cognitive skills and asks them to make decisions related to simple-to-complex scenarios.

Lippincott CoursePoint for Evidence-Based Practice features:

- **Leading content in context:** Digital content from *Evidence-Based Practice in Nursing & Healthcare* is embedded in our Powerful Tools, engaging students and encouraging interaction and learning on a deeper level.
  - The complete interactive eBook features annual content updates with the latest evidence-based practices and provides students with anytime, anywhere access on multiple devices.
  - Full online access to *Stedman's Medical Dictionary for the Health Professions and Nursing* ensures students work with the best medical dictionary available.
- **Powerful tools to maximize class performance:** Additional course-specific tools provide case-based learning for every student:
  - **Video Cases** help students anticipate what to expect as a nurse, with detailed scenarios that capture their attention and integrate clinical knowledge with EBP concepts that are critical to real-world nursing practice. By watching the videos and completing related activities, students will flex their problem-solving, prioritizing, analyzing, and application skills to aid both in NCLEX preparation and in preparation for practice.
  - **Interactive Modules** help students quickly identify what they do and do not understand so they can study smartly. With exceptional instructional design that prompts students to discover, reflect, synthesize, and apply, students actively learn. Remediation links to the eBook are integrated throughout.

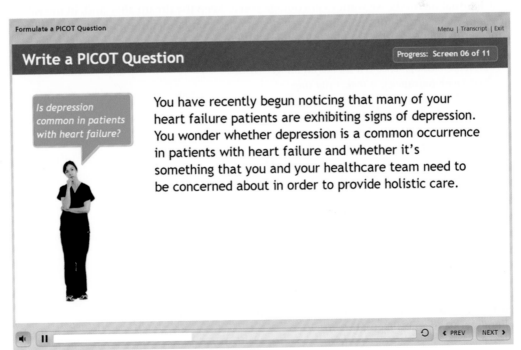

- **Curated collections of journal articles** are provided via *Lippincott NursingCenter*, Wolters Kluwer's premier destination for peer-reviewed nursing journals. Through integration of CoursePoint and NursingCenter, students will engage in how nursing research influences practice.
- **Data to measure students' progress:** Student performance data provided in an intuitive display lets instructors quickly assess whether students have viewed interactive modules and video cases outside of class, as well as see students' performance on related NCLEX-style quizzes, ensuring students are coming to the classroom ready and prepared to learn.

To learn more about Lippincott CoursePoint, please visit: http://nursingeducation .lww.com/our-solutions/course-solutions/lippincott-coursepoint.html

A FINAL WORD FROM THE AUTHORS

As we have the privilege of meeting and working with clinicians, educators, and researchers across the globe to advance and sustain EBP, we realize how important our unified effort is to world health. We want to thank each reader for your investment of time and energy to learn and use the information contained within this book to foster your best practice. Furthermore, we so appreciate the information that you have shared with us regarding the benefits and challenges you have had in learning about and applying knowledge of EBP. That feedback has been instrumental to improving the fourth edition of our book. We value constructive feedback and welcome any ideas that you have about content, tools, and resources that would help us to improve a future edition. The spirit of inquiry and life-long learning are foundational principles of the EBP paradigm and underpin the EBP process so that this problem-solving approach to practice can cultivate an excitement for implementing the highest quality of care. As you engage in your EBP journey, remember that it takes time and that it becomes easier when the principles of this book are placed into action with enthusiasm on a consistent daily basis.

As you make a positive impact at the point of care, whether you are first learning about the EBP paradigm, the steps of the EBP process, leading a successful, sustainable evidence-based change effort, or generating evidence to fill a knowledge gap or implement translational methods, we want to encourage you to keep the dream alive and, in the words of Les Brown, "Shoot for the moon. Even if you miss, you land among the stars." We hope you are inspired by and enjoy the following EBP rap.

> *Evidence-based practice is a wonderful thing,*
> *Done with consistency, it makes you sing.*
> *PICOT questions and learning search skills;*
> *Appraising evidence can give you thrills.*
> *Medline, CINAHL, PsycInfo are fine,*
> *But for Level I evidence, Cochrane's divine!*
> *Though you may want to practice the same old way*
> *"Oh no, that's not how I will do it," you say.*
> *When you launch EBP in your practice site,*
> *Remember to eat the chocolate elephant, bite by bite.*
> *So dream big and persist in order to achieve and*
> *Know that EBP can be done when you believe!*

© **2004 Bernadette Melnyk**
Bernadette Mazurek Melnyk and Ellen Fineout-Overholt

Note: You may contact the authors at bernmelnyk@gmail.com
ellen.fineout.overholt@gmail.com

Acknowledgments

This book could not have been accomplished without the support, understanding, and assistance of many wonderful colleagues, staff, family, and friends. I would first like to acknowledge the outstanding work of my coeditor and cherished friend, Ellen—thank you for all of your efforts, our wonderful friendship, attention to detail, and ongoing support throughout this process; I could not have accomplished this revised edition without you. Since the first edition of this book, I have grown personally and professionally through the many opportunities that I have had to teach and mentor others in evidence-based practice across the globe—the lessons I have learned from all of you have been incorporated into this book. I thank all of my mentees for their valuable feedback and all of the authors who contributed their time and valuable expertise to this book. Along with my wonderful husband John and my three daughters, Kaylin, Angela, and Megan, I am appreciative for the ongoing love and support that I receive from my mother, Anna May Mazurek, my brother and sister-in-law, Fred and Sue Mazurek, and my sister, Christine Warmuth, whose inspirational words to me "Just get out there and do it!" have been a key to many of my successful endeavors. I would also like to thank my wonderful colleagues and staff at The Ohio State University for their support, understanding, and ongoing commitment to our projects and their roles throughout this process, especially Dr. Margaret Graham and Kathy York. Finally, I would like to acknowledge the team at Wolters Kluwer for their assistance with and dedication to keeping this project on track.

Bernadette Mazurek Melnyk

Now is the time to join together to ensure that EBP is *the* paradigm for clinical decision making. Healthcare providers and educators have made tremendous strides across the years to establish that EBP is an expectation of providers, educators, and systems. I am grateful to the American Nurses Credentialing Center (ANCC) for the impact of the Magnet movement as well as educational accrediting agencies (e.g., Commission on Collegiate Nursing Education [CCNE], National League for Nurses Accreditation Commission [NLNAC], Liaison Committee on Medical Education [LCME], Accreditation Council of Pharmacy Education [ACPE]) for putting forward standards that have had an impact on adoption of the EBP paradigm and process in education, practice, and policy. As a result, all of us across the wonderful diversity of providers who make up the healthcare team are supported as we choose the EBP paradigm as the foundation for daily clinical decisions. Thank you to the students, clinicians, healthcare leadership, clinical educators, faculty, and researchers for demonstrating the ownership of practice that is the key to placing EBP at the center of healthcare transformation. We are at a tipping point . . . let's see it through to fruition!

To those of you who have shared with me personally the difference this book has made in your practice, educational endeavors, and teaching, I heartily extend my deepest thanks. The value of our work is measured by the impact it has on advancing best practice in healthcare and how it helps point-of-care providers and educators make a difference in patients' and students' lives and health experiences. You help us know that we are making progress on achieving our dream of transforming healthcare—one client–clinician/learner–educator relationship at a time. Bern, almost 30 years ago, we started our work together—not knowing where our path would take us. Thank you for seeing the potential and taking the chance—I have enjoyed the wonderful privilege to work alongside you to bring our dream to life. To my colleagues at University of Texas at Tyler, thank you for the privilege of joining the family—you are the best!!

With the writing of this fourth edition, my life experiences, and those of contributors to the book, have helped me recognize more completely how blessed I am to have the support of my precious family and friends and to have wonderful people in my life who are committed to this often-arduous journey toward best care for all patients. My sweet family has trekked with me across these four editions. With the first edition, our eldest daughter wasn't yet one year old; now, she is a senior in high school. Our youngest daughter was a dream who is now is in eighth grade. Every day, these sweet young ladies inspire me to continue to strive to achieve the goal of evidence-based care as the standard for healthcare. Their gift of love and laughter delivered in packages of hugs is invaluable—Thank You, Rachael and Ruth! Thank you to my steadfast husband, Wayne, who faithfully offers perspective and balance that are so important to me—your support for this work is invaluable! Thank you to my mother, Virginia (Grandginny), who continues to help me see the best and not best in healthcare as she experiences it as an older old adult (now 87). Her encounters remain a reminder that advocating for evidence-based consumers is an imperative. Thank you to my brother John, and his family, Angela, Ashton, and Aubrey—your music lifts my spirits; your healthcare experiences serve as fodder for this work. To those of you who have prayed for me during this writing adventure—thank you so very much! During my extenuating health issues that have flavored this fourth edition, my Savior and Friend's continual care for me has been profound. I am eternally grateful. Healthcare should serve all of us well. Let us all strive to ensure that every encounter is an experience in excellent care.

Finally, I am grateful to each of you who choose to read this book, take the knowledge contained in its pages, and make the EBP paradigm and process come alive in your work. You make our dream of healthcare transformation through EBP live! The Wolters Kluwer team with whom we have had the privilege to work has been so helpful to make this fourth edition the best yet!! Thank you so much! This book is not written by one person—or even two. It is written by many people who give of their expertise and wisdom so that readers can have such a wonderful resource. I am very grateful for each of the faithful contributors to this work and their decision to join us in advancing EBP as the solution for improving healthcare.

Ellen Fineout-Overholt

Contents

UNIT 4 Creating and Sustaining a Culture and Environment for Evidence-Based Practice 349

UNIT 5

Step Six: Disseminating Evidence and Evidence-Based Practice Implementation Outcomes   531

UNIT 6

Generating External Evidence and Writing Successful Grant Proposals   603

APPENDICES AVAILABLE ON thePoint®

Steps Zero, One, Two: Getting Started

> To accomplish great things, we must not only act, but also dream; not only plan, but also believe.
> —Anatole France

EBP Terms to Learn
Background questions
Bibliographic database
Body of evidence
Boolean connectors
Clinical inquiry
Critical appraisal
EBP competencies
Evidence-based practice
  (EBP)
Evidence-based quality
  improvement (EBPI)
External evidence
Foreground questions
Grey literature
Internal evidence
Keywords
Meta-analysis
Outcomes management
PICOT format
Point-of-care resources
Preappraised literature
Proximity searching
Randomized controlled trials
  (RCTs)
Reference managers
Search strategy
Subject headings
Yield

UNIT OBJECTIVES

Upon completion of this unit, learners will be able to:

1. Identify the seven steps of evidence-based practice (EBP).

2. Describe the differences among EBP, research, and quality improvement.

3. Explain the components of a PICOT question: population, issue or intervention of interest, comparison of interest, outcome, and time for intervention to achieve the outcome.

4. Discuss basic and advanced strategies for conducting a systematic search based on the PICOT question.

5. Describe a body of evidence based on the evidence hierarchy for specific types of clinical questions.

MAKING CONNECTIONS: AN EBP EXEMPLAR

On the orthopedic unit of a tertiary hospital in the Eastern United States, a nurse manager, Danielle, and the unit EBP Council representative, Betsy, were discussing recent quality improvement (QI) reports in the staff lounge. Danielle noted that the unit's patient satisfaction rates had dropped as their fall rates had increased.

To help provide context, Betsy, who has a passion for fall prevention (*Step 0: Spirit of Inquiry*), shared the story of Sam, an elderly patient who sustained a fall with injury during the last quarter, despite the fact that he was not a high fall risk. As Sam's primary nurse, Betsy had initiated universal fall prevention precautions as recommended by the Agency for Healthcare Research & Quality in their Falls Prevention Toolkit (AHRQ; https://www.ahrq.gov/sites/default/files/publications/files/fallpxtoolkit.pdf). Betsy hoped that Sam's story would help illuminate some of the issues that surround falls that are more challenging to predict.

Sam had awakened from a deep sleep and needed to void. He was oriented when he went to bed, but upon waking he became confused and couldn't locate his call light because, although it was placed close to him, it had been covered by his pillow. In an interview after he fell, Sam told Betsy that he had to go so badly that he just didn't think about looking under the pillow. He also forgot that there was a urinal on the bedside table. He simply focused on getting to the bathroom, and when he tried to get out of bed with the rails up, he pinched his wrist, causing a hematoma and soft tissue injury.

Danielle had more information that shed light on the rising fall rates. All of the falls during the past quarter occurred during the night shift. Over a period of several weeks, a number of the night nurses had been ill, leading to per-diem and float staff covering those positions. Staff had documented rounding, but Betsy and Danielle wondered whether introducing regularly scheduled rounding could prevent future falls like Sam's.

Danielle and Betsy discussed some tools that they had heard could help structure regular rounding; both agreed that staff would need more than just their recommendation for the implementation of any tool to be successful. They gathered a group of interested staff who had reviewed the fall data to ask about their current regular rounding habits. The nurses indicated that they rounded on a regular basis, but sometimes up to three hours might pass between check-ins with more "stable" patients like Sam, particularly if there were other urgent needs on the unit. One of the newer nurses, Boqin, mentioned that in nursing school he had written a paper on hourly rounding and perhaps that may be a solution.

All of the unit nurses agreed that the outcome of a rising fall rate required evaluation and that hourly rounding may help, so Betsy guided the group in crafting a properly formatted PICOT question (P: population; I: intervention or issue of interest; C: comparison intervention or condition; O: outcome to see changed; T: time for the intervention to achieve the outcome or issue to be addressed). After reviewing the QI data, discussing the context of the clinical issue, and looking at case studies for clues about why the outcome was occurring, the question that the group posed was, *In elderly patients with low risk for falls with universal precautions in place, how does hourly rounding at night compared to no hourly rounding affect preventable fall rates within 3 months of initiation? (Step 1: Ask a Clinical Question in PICOT Format).*

The nurses became excited about answering the question and asked Betsy about the next steps in the EBP process. Betsy already had a great relationship with their hospital librarian, Scott, who was well versed in EBP and had demonstrated his expertise at systematic searching when helping with previous EBP Council projects. Betsy e-mailed the group's PICOT question to Scott and asked him to conduct a systematic search

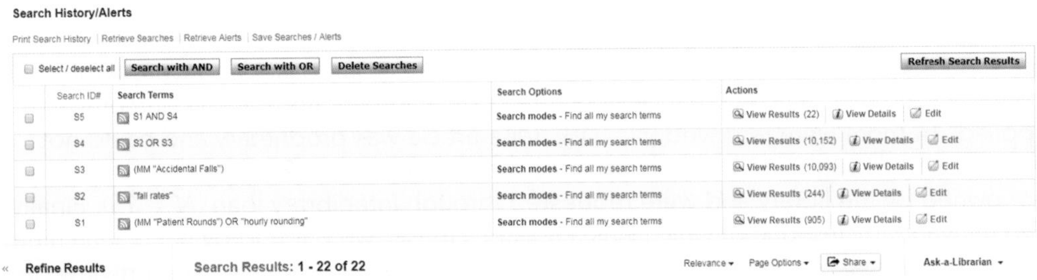

Search History/Alerts

Print Search History | Retrieve Searches | Retrieve Alerts | Save Searches / Alerts

	Search ID#	Search Terms		Search Options	Actions		
☐	S5	🔊 S1 AND S4		Search modes - Find all my search terms	🔍 View Results (22)	ℹ️ View Details	✏️ Edit
☐	S4	🔊 S2 OR S3		Search modes - Find all my search terms	🔍 View Results (10,152)	ℹ️ View Details	✏️ Edit
☐	S3	🔊 (MM "Accidental Falls")		Search modes - Find all my search terms	🔍 View Results (10,093)	ℹ️ View Details	✏️ Edit
☐	S2	🔊 "fall rates"		Search modes - Find all my search terms	🔍 View Results (244)	ℹ️ View Details	✏️ Edit
☐	S1	🔊 (MM "Patient Rounds") OR "hourly rounding"		Search modes - Find all my search terms	🔍 View Results (905)	ℹ️ View Details	✏️ Edit

☐ Select / deselect all   **Search with AND**   **Search with OR**   **Delete Searches**   **Refresh Search Results**

« **Refine Results**   Search Results: 1 - 22 of 22   Relevance ▾   Page Options ▾   ⬆ Share ▾   Ask-a-Librarian ▾

Figure 1: Systematic search of Comprehensive Index of Nursing and Allied Health Literature (CINAHL) database. (Source: EBSCO Information Services)

(Step 2: Systematic Searching). Scott knew that his initial search terms had to come from the PICOT question, so he carefully considered what the nurses had asked. He knew a great start would be finding a systematic review that contained multiple studies about the impact of hourly rounding on fall rates within elderly patients who were at low risk for falls, so he began his search with the O: fall rates. In addition, all studies Scott would consider including in his body of evidence would need to have the outcome of preventable fall rates; otherwise, the studies could not answer to the clinical question.

A systematic search using the advance search interface of the Cochrane Library to find systematic reviews that included the terms *hourly rounding* AND *falls* yielded no hits. The term *hourly rounding* yielded one hit, a systematic review focused on the impact of hourly rounding on patient satisfaction. Scott decided to keep that review, since Betsy had mentioned that their patient satisfaction had varied at the same time as their fall rates. Using the same approach, Scott continued the systematic search in the Comprehensive Index of Nursing and Allied Health Literature (CINAHL) database, beginning with the same terms, *hourly rounding* and *falls* and their associated subject headings. Scott used the focus feature in CINAHL for each subject heading to make sure the topic was the major point of the article. This search yielded 22 articles. A systematic search of PubMed with the same approach yielded 12 studies (see Figures 1 and 2 for details of these searches).

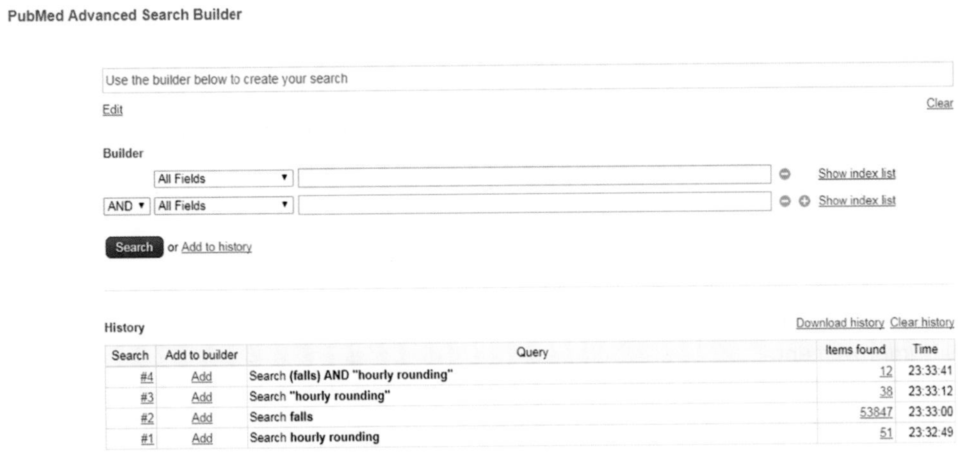

PubMed Advanced Search Builder

Use the builder below to create your search

Edit   Clear

Builder

| All Fields ▾ | | ⊖ | Show index list |
| AND ▾ | All Fields ▾ | | ⊖ ⊕ | Show index list |

Search or Add to history

History   Download history Clear history

Search	Add to builder	Query	Items found	Time
#4	Add	Search **(falls) AND "hourly rounding"**	12	23:33:41
#3	Add	Search **"hourly rounding"**	38	23:33:12
#2	Add	Search **falls**	53847	23:33:00
#1	Add	Search **hourly rounding**	51	23:32:49

Figure 2: Systematic search of PubMed database. (From National Library of Medicine, www.pubmed.gov)

Now that all three databases had been searched, the total yield of 35 studies were available for Scott's review to see if they were keeper studies to answer the PICOT question. Eight hits were found to be redundant among databases and were removed from the yield ($N = 27$). When inclusion criteria of fall preventions as the outcome was applied, 14 more were removed ($N = 13$). One article was proprietary and could not be accessed through interlibrary loan or via the Internet ($N = 12$). Three articles were not owned by the library and were requested through interlibrary loan ($N = 15$). Finally, two relevant articles, one of which was a master's thesis, were found by hand searching, which resulted in 17 articles to enter into the critical appraisal process. After review of the study designs, the final cohort of studies that Scott currently had (i.e., the body of evidence) included one systematic review, no single randomized controlled trials, four quasi-experimental studies, eight evidence-based or quality improvement projects, and one expert opinion article (see Table 1). He knew he had three more articles to add to the body of evidence when they came in from interlibrary loan; however, Scott thought it was important to discuss the current body of evidence with Betsy and Danielle, who decided to take the current articles to the EBP Council.

Join the group at the beginning of Unit 2 as they continue their EBP journey.

TABLE 1

Synthesis: Levels of Evidence

Level of Evidence for Intervention Questions	1	2	3	4	5	6	7	8	9	10	11	12	13	14
I. Systematic review/meta-analysis of randomized controlled trials									X					
II. Single randomized controlled trial														
III. Quasi-experimental studies/nonrandomized controlled trials	X					X				X		X		
IV. Cohort or case–control studies														
V. Systematic review/meta-synthesis of qualitative studies														
VI. Single qualitative or descriptive studies/evidence implementation and quality improvement projects		X	X	X			X	X			X		X	X
VII. Expert opinion					X									

1, Brown; 2, Callahan; 3, Dyck; 4, Goldsack; 5, Hicks; 6, Krepper; 7, Leone; 8, Lowe; 9, Mitchell; 10, Olrich; 11, Stefancyk; 12, Tucker; 13, Waszynski; 14, Weisgram.

References

Brown, C. H. (2016). The effect of purposeful hourly rounding on the incidence of patient falls. *Nursing Theses and Capstone Projects.* Retrieved from http://digitalcommons.gardner-webb.edu/nursing_etd/246

Callahan, L., McDonald, S., Voit, D., McDonnell, A., Delgado-Flores, J., & Stanghellini, E. (2009). Medication review and hourly nursing rounds: An evidence-based approach reduces falls on oncology inpatient units. *Oncology Nursing Forum, 36*(3), 72.

Daniels, J. F. (2016). Purposeful and timely nursing rounds: A best practice implementation project. *JBI Database of Systematic Reviews and Implementation Reports, 14*(1), 248–267. doi:10.11124/jbisrir-2016-2537.*

Dyck, D., Thiele, T., Kebicz, R., Klassen, M., & Erenberg, C. (2013). Hourly rounding for falls prevention: A change initiative. *Creative Nursing, 19*(3), 153–158.

Goldsack, J., Bergey, M., Mascioli, S., & Cunningham, J. (2015). Hourly rounding and patient falls: What factors boost success? *Nursing, 45*(2), 25–30.

Hicks, D. (2015). Can rounding reduce patient falls in acute care? An integrative literature review. *MEDSURG Nursing, 24*(1), 51–55.

Jackson, K. (2016). Improving nursing home falls management program by enhancing standard of care with collaborative care multi-interventional protocol focused on fall prevention. *Journal of Nursing Education and Practice, 6*(6), 85–96.*

Krepper, R., Vallejo, B., Smith, C., Lindy, C., Fullmer, C., Messimer, S., . . . Myers, K. (2014). Evaluation of a standardized hourly rounding process (SHaRP). *Journal for Healthcare Quality, 36*(2), 62–69. doi:10.1111/j.1945-1474.2012.00222.x

Leone, R. M., & Adams, R. J. (2016). Safety standards: Implementing fall prevention interventions and sustaining lower fall rates by promoting the culture of safety on an inpatient rehabilitation unit. *Rehabilitation Nursing, 41*(1), 26–32.

Lowe, L., & Hodgson, G. (2012). Hourly rounding in a high dependency unit. *Nursing Standard, 27*(8), 35–40.

Mitchell, M. D., Lavenberg, J. G., Trotta, R. L., & Umscheid, C. A. (2014). Hourly rounding to improve nursing responsiveness: A systematic review. *The Journal of Nursing Administration, 44*(9), 462–472. doi:10.1097/NNA.0000000000000101

Morgan, L., Flynn, L., Robertson, E., New, S., Forde-Johnston, C., & McCulloch, P. (2017). Intentional rounding: A staff-led quality improvement intervention in the prevention of patient falls. *Journal of Clinical Nursing, 26*(1/2), 115–124.*

Olrich, T., Kalman, M., & Nigolian, C. (2012). Hourly rounding: A replication study. *MEDSURG Nursing, 21*(1), 23–36.

Stefancyk, A. L. (2009). Safe and reliable care: Addressing one of the four focus areas of the TCAB initiative. *American Journal of Nursing, 109*(7), 70–71.

Tucker, S. J., Bieber, P. L., Attlesey-Pries, J. M., Olson, M. E., & Dierkhising, R. A. (2012). Outcomes and challenges in implementing hourly rounds to reduce falls in orthopedic units. *Worldviews on Evidence-Based Nursing, 9*(1), 18–29.

Waszynski, C. (2012). More rounding means better fall compliance. *Healthcare Risk Management, 34*(2), 21.

Weisgram, B., & Raymond, S. (2008). Military nursing. Using evidence-based nursing rounds to improve patient outcomes. *MEDSURG Nursing, 17*(6), 429–430.

---

*Waiting for interlibrary loan.

1 Making the Case for Evidence-Based Practice and Cultivating a Spirit of Inquiry

Bernadette Mazurek Melnyk and Ellen Fineout-Overholt

Believe you can and you're half-way there
—*Theodore Roosevelt*

EBP Terms to Learn

Critical appraisal
EBP competencies
Evidence-based practice (EBP)
Evidence-based quality improvement
Evidence-based quality improvement projects
Evidence-based theories
External evidence
Internal evidence
Meta-analyses
Outcome management
Predictive studies
Quadruple aim in healthcare
Quality improvement (QI)
Randomized controlled trials (RCTs)
Randomly assigned
Rapid critical appraisal
Research
Research utilization
"so-what" outcomes
Spirit of inquiry
Synthesis
Systematic reviews
Translational research

Learning Objectives

After studying this chapter, learners will be able to:

1. Discuss how evidence-based practice (EBP) assists hospitals and healthcare systems achieve the quadruple aim.

2. Describe the differences among EBP, research, and quality improvement.

3. Identify the seven steps of EBP.

4. Discuss barriers to EBP and key elements of cultures that support the implementation of EBP.

The evidence is irrefutable. **Evidence-based practice (EBP)** enhances healthcare quality, improves patient outcomes, reduces costs, and empowers clinicians; this is known as the **quadruple aim in healthcare** (Bodenheimer & Sinsky, 2014; Melnyk & Fineout-Overholt, 2015; Tucker, 2014). Hospitals and healthcare systems across the United States are continually striving to reach the quadruple aim and improve the safety of care. However, problems with quality persist; for example, preventable medical errors are the third leading cause of death in the United States, and clinician burnout is a public health epidemic (Johnson et al., 2017; Makary & Daniel, 2016; Melnyk, 2016a; Shanafelt et al., 2015). Although EBP is a key strategy for reaching the quadruple aim, it is not the standard of care in many healthcare systems because practices steeped in tradition and organizations that foster a culture of "this is the way we do it here" continue to thrive across the United States and the world.

Recently, there has been an explosion of scientific evidence available to guide health professionals in their clinical decision making. Even though this evidence is readily available, the implementation of evidence-based care is still not the norm in many healthcare systems across the United States and the globe because clinicians across the United States lack competency in EBP and cultures are still steeped in tradition (Melnyk et al., 2017). The translation of research evidence into clinical practice remains painfully slow, often spanning from years to decades. However, when clinicians are asked whether they would personally like to receive evidence-based care themselves, the answer is a resounding "yes!" For example,

- If you were diagnosed with a brain tumor today, would you want your oncologist to share with you the best and latest evidence regarding the risks and benefits of each type of chemotherapy and radiation treatment available so that you could make the best collaborative decision about your care?
- If your child was in a motor vehicle accident and sustained a severe head injury, would you want his neurologist to know and use the most effective research-supported treatment established from **randomized controlled trials (RCTs)** to decrease his intracranial pressure and prevent him from dying?
- If your mother were diagnosed with Alzheimer's disease, would you want her healthcare provider to give you information about how other family caregivers of patients with this disease have coped with the illness, based on evidence from well-designed studies?

If your answer to the above three questions is yes, how can we as healthcare professionals deliver anything less than EBP?

DEFINITION AND EVOLUTION OF EVIDENCE-BASED PRACTICE

In 2000, Sackett et al. defined EBP as the conscientious use of current best evidence in making decisions about patient care. Since then, the definition of EBP has broadened in scope and is referred to as a lifelong problem-solving approach to clinical practice that integrates the following:
- A systematic search for and **critical appraisal** of the most relevant and best research (i.e., **external evidence**) to answer a burning clinical question;
- One's own clinical expertise, including use of **internal evidence** generated from **outcomes management** or **evidence-based quality improvement projects**, a thorough patient assessment, and evaluation and use of available resources necessary to achieve desired patient outcomes;
- Patient/family preferences and values (Figure 1.1).

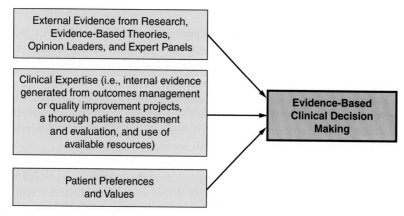

Figure 1.1: The components of evidence-based practice. (From Melnyk, B. M., & Fineout-Overholt, E. [2011]. *Evidence-based practice in nursing & healthcare. A guide to best practice.* Philadelphia, PA: Wolters Kluwer/Lippincott Williams & Wilkins.)

DIFFERENCES AMONG EBP, RESEARCH, AND QUALITY IMPROVEMENT

Unlike **research** that uses a scientific process to generate new knowledge/external evidence and **research utilization**, which has been frequently operationalized as the use of knowledge typically based on a single study, the EBP process involves rigorous critical appraisal, including **synthesis** and recommendations for practice, of a body of evidence comprised of multiple studies and combines it with the expertise of the clinician as well as patient/family preferences and values to make the best decisions about patient care (Melnyk & Fineout-Overholt, 2015). **Quality improvement (QI)**, a systematic process that often uses the plan, do, study, act (PDSA) model, is used by healthcare systems to improve their processes or outcomes for a specific population once a problem is identified and is often confused with EBP (Shirey et al., 2011). An example of a QI initiative would be triggered by a sudden increase in ventilator-associated pneumonia that, when practice data were evaluated, indicated that an oral care protocol was not being implemented on a regular basis. The PDSA cycle culminated in an educational booster for the staff about the oral care protocol and further monitoring of the process to reduce a high rate of ventilator-associated pneumonia in critically ill patients. The difference between QI and **evidence-based QI** is that the former relies primarily on internal evidence and often does not involve a systematic search for and critical appraisal of evidence, whereas the latter must include both internal and external evidence in decision making about a practice change to be implemented to improve an important clinical outcome (Melnyk, Buck, & Gallagher-Ford, 2015). The goal is for all QI to become evidence-based.

Another process intended to improve healthcare is outcomes management, which is very similar to evidence-based QI. Outcomes management typically uses a four-step process to (1) define a clinical problem and outcome that need to be improved (e.g., falls, hospital readmissions); (2) establish how the outcome will be measured; (3) identify practices supported by evidence that need to be implemented to improve the outcome; and (4) measure the impact of implementing the best practice on the targeted outcome (Brewer & Alexandrov, 2015). **Translational research** is also often confused with EBP. However, translational research is rigorous research that studies how evidence-based interventions are translated to real-world clinical settings.

WHAT IS EVIDENCE?

Evidence is a collection of facts that are believed to be true. External evidence is generated through rigorous research (e.g., RCTs or **predictive studies**) and is intended to be generalized and used in other settings. An important question when implementing external evidence is whether clinicians can achieve the same results with their patients that were obtained in the studies they reviewed (i.e., can the findings from research be translated to the real-world clinical setting with the same outcomes?). This question of transferability is why measurement of key outcomes is necessary when implementing practice changes based on evidence. In contrast, internal evidence is typically generated through practice initiatives, such as outcomes management or evidence-based QI projects. Researchers generate new knowledge through rigorous research (i.e., external evidence), and EBP provides clinicians the process and tools to translate the external evidence into clinical practice and integrate it with internal evidence to improve quality of healthcare, patient outcomes, and cost reductions.

Unfortunately, there are many interventions (i.e., treatments) with substantial evidence to support their use in clinical practice to improve patient outcomes that are not routinely used. For example, findings from a series of RCTs testing the efficacy of the Creating Opportunities for Parent Empowerment (COPE) program for parents of critically ill/hospitalized and premature infants support that when parents receive COPE (i.e., an educational–behavioral skills-building intervention delivered by clinicians to parents at the point of care through a series of brief CDs, written information, and activity workbooks) versus an attention control program, COPE parents (a) report less stress, anxiety, and depressive symptoms during hospitalization; (b) participate more in their children's care; (c) interact in more developmentally sensitive ways; and (d) report less depression and posttraumatic stress disorder symptoms up to a year following their children's discharge from the hospital (Gonya, Martin, McClead, Nelin, & Shepher, 2014; Melnyk & Feinstein, 2009; Melnyk et al., 2004, 2006). In addition, the premature infants and children of parents who receive COPE have better behavioral and developmental outcomes as well as shorter hospital stays and readmission rates versus those whose parents who receive an attention control program, which could result in billions of dollars of healthcare savings for the healthcare system if the program is routinely implemented by hospitals across the United States (Melnyk & Feinstein, 2009). Despite this strong body of evidence generated in multiple studies spanning two decades of research, including the important **"so-what" outcomes** of decreased length of stay and reduced hospital costs, COPE is still not the standard of practice in many healthcare systems throughout the nation.

In contrast, many practices are being implemented in healthcare that have no or little evidence to support their use (e.g., double-checking pediatric medications, routine assessment of vital signs every 2 or 4 hours in hospitalized patients, use of a plastic tongue patch for weight loss). Further more, some practices in which evidence has shown adverse outcomes have prevailed (e.g., 12-hour shifts for nurses). Unless we know what interventions are most effective for a variety of populations through the generation of evidence from research and practice data (e.g., outcomes management, evidence-based QI projects) and how to rapidly translate this evidence into clinical practice through EBP, substantial sustainable improvement in the quality and safety of care received by U.S. residents is not likely (Melnyk, 2012; Melnyk & Fineout-Overholt, 2015).

COMPONENTS OF EVIDENCE-BASED PRACTICE

Although evidence from **systematic reviews** of RCTs has been regarded as the strongest level of evidence (i.e., level 1 evidence) on which to base practice decisions about treatments to achieve a desired outcome, evidence from descriptive and qualitative studies as well as from opinion leaders should be factored into clinical decisions as part of the body of evidence. These lower level studies should be compared in their findings with higher level studies. When RCTs are not available, these lower level studies may be the best knowledge available for clinical decision making (Melnyk & Fineout-Overholt, 2015). **Evidence-based theories** (i.e., theories that are empirically supported through well-designed studies) also should be included as evidence. In addition, patient/family preferences, values, and concerns should be incorporated into the evidence-based approach to decision making along with a clinician's expertise, which includes (a) clinical judgment (i.e., the ability to think about, understand, and use research evidence and to assess a patient's condition through subjective history taking, thorough physical examination findings, and laboratory reports); (b) internal evidence generated from evidence-based QI or outcomes management projects; (c) clinical reasoning (i.e., the ability to apply the above information to a clinical issue); and (d) evaluation and use of available healthcare resources needed to implement the chosen treatment(s) and achieve the expected outcome (Figure 1.2).

Clinicians often ask how much and what type of evidence is needed to change practice. A good rule of thumb to answer this question is that there needs to be strong enough evidence to make a practice change. Specifically, the level of evidence plus the quality of evidence

EBP Organizational Culture and Environment

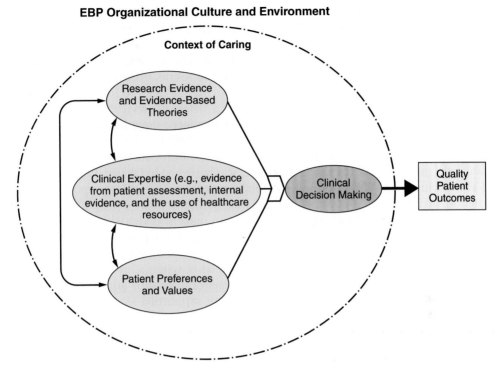

Figure 1.2: The merging of science and art: Evidence-based practice (EBP) within a context of caring and an EBP culture and environment result in the highest quality of healthcare and patient outcomes. © Melnyk & Fineout-Overholt, 2017.

equals the strength of the evidence, which provides clinicians the confidence needed to change clinical practice (Box 1.1).

ORIGINS OF THE EVIDENCE-BASED PRACTICE MOVEMENT

The EBP movement was founded by Dr. Archie Cochrane, a British epidemiologist, who struggled with the effectiveness of healthcare and challenged the public to pay only for care that had been empirically supported as effective (Enkin, 1992). In 1972, Cochrane published a landmark book criticizing the medical profession for not providing rigorous reviews of evidence so that policy makers and organizations could make the best decisions about healthcare. Cochrane was a strong proponent of using evidence from RCTs, because he believed that this was the strongest evidence on which to base clinical practice treatment

BOX 1.1

Rule of Thumb to Determine Whether a Practice Change Should Be Made

The level of the evidence + quality of the evidence = strength of the evidence → *Confidence to act upon the evidence and change practice!*

decisions. He asserted that reviews of research evidence across all specialty areas need to be prepared systematically through a rigorous process, and that they should be maintained to consider the generation of new evidence (The Cochrane Collaboration, 2001).

In an exemplar case, Cochrane noted that thousands of premature infants with low birth weight died needlessly. He emphasized that the results of several RCTs supporting the effectiveness of corticosteroid therapy to halt premature labor in high-risk women had never been analyzed and compiled in the form of a systematic review. The data from that systematic review showed that corticosteroid therapy reduced the odds of premature infant death from 50% to 30% (The Cochrane Collaboration, 2001).

Dr. Cochrane died in 1988. However, owing to his influence and call for updates of systematic reviews of RCTs, the Cochrane Center was launched in Oxford, England, in 1992, and The Cochrane Collaboration was founded a year later. The major purpose of the collaboration, an international network of more than 37,000 dedicated people from over 130 countries, is to assist healthcare practitioners, policy makers, patients, and their advocates to make evidence-informed decisions about healthcare by developing, maintaining, and updating systematic reviews of healthcare interventions (i.e., Cochrane Reviews) and ensuring that these reviews are accessible to the public. Examples of systematic reviews housed on the Cochrane website include vaccines to prevent influenza in healthy adults, steroids for the treatment of influenza, psychosocial interventions for supporting women to stop smoking in pregnancy, and gabapentin for chronic neuropathic pain and fibromyalgia in adults.

 Further information about the Cochrane Collaboration, including a complete listing of systematic reviews, can be accessed at http://www.cochrane.org/

WHY EVIDENCE-BASED PRACTICE?

The most important reason for consistently implementing EBP is that it leads to the highest quality of care and the best patient outcomes (Melnyk, 2017). In addition, EBP reduces healthcare costs and geographic variation in the delivery of care (Dotson et al., 2014). Findings from studies also indicate that clinicians report feeling more empowered and have higher job satisfaction when they engage in EBP (Fridman & Frederickson, 2014; Kim et al., 2016, 2017). With recent reports of pervasive "burnout" and depression among healthcare professionals and the pressure that many influential healthcare organizations exert on clinicians to deliver high-quality, safe care under increasingly heavy patient loads, the use and teaching of EBP may be key not only to providing outstanding care to patients and saving healthcare dollars, but also to reducing the escalating turnover rate in certain healthcare professions (Melnyk, Fineout-Overholt, Giggleman, & Cruz, 2010; Melnyk, Orsolini, Tan et al., 2017).

Despite the multitude of positive outcomes associated with EBP and the strong desire of healthcare providers to be the recipients of evidence-based care, an alarming number of healthcare systems and clinicians do not consistently implement EBP or follow evidence-based clinical practice guidelines (Dotson et al., 2014; Melnyk, Grossman et al., 2012; Vlada et al., 2013). Findings from a national survey of more than 1,000 randomly selected nurses from the American Nurses Association indicated that major barriers to EBP continue to persist in healthcare systems, including lack of EBP knowledge and skills, time, and organizational culture (Melnyk, Fineout-Overholt, Gallagher-Ford, & Kaplan, 2012). In addition, the nurses who responded to this national survey reported that, along with peer and physician resistance, a major barrier to their implementation of EBP was nurse leader/manager resistance. Therefore, a national survey with 276 chief nurse executives was conducted to learn more about this issue from nurse leaders as well as to describe their own implementation of EBP and the portion of their budgets they invested in equipping their clinicians with the skills needed to deliver evidence-based care. Results of this survey indicated that, although the chief nurses believed in the value of EBP, their own implementation was low, with over 50% reporting that they were uncertain about how to measure the outcomes of care being delivered in their hospitals (Melnyk et al., 2016). Most chief nurses also reported that they did not have a critical mass of nurses in their hospital who were skilled in EBP and that they only invested 0% to 10% of their budgets in equipping their staff with EBP knowledge, skills, and resources. Although the chief nurses reported that their top two priorities were quality and safety of care being delivered in their hospitals, EBP was listed as their lowest priority, which indicated their lack of understanding that EBP was a direct pathway to achieving quality and safety. Therefore, it was not surprising that one third of hospitals from this survey were not meeting the National Database of Nursing Quality Indicators metrics, and almost one third of the hospitals were above national core performance measure benchmarks, including falls and pressure ulcers (Melnyk et al., 2016). Recent findings from the first U.S. study on the **EBP competencies** also revealed that practicing nurses reported not being qualified in any of the 24 EBP competencies (Melnyk et al., 2017). Knowledge, beliefs about the value of EBP, mentorship in EBP, and a culture that supports EBP were all associated with reports of EBP competency.

On a daily basis, nurse practitioners, physicians, pharmacists, nurses, occupational and physical therapists, and other healthcare professionals seek answers to numerous clinical questions. (Examples: In postoperative surgical patients, how does relaxation breathing compared with cognitive behavioral skills building affect anxiety during recovery? In adults with dementia, how does a warm bath during the 30 minutes prior to bedtime improve sleep compared with music therapy? In depressed adolescents, how does cognitive behavioral therapy combined with Prozac compared with Prozac alone reduce depressive symptoms within the first year of diagnosis?) An evidence-based approach to care allows healthcare providers to access the best evidence to answer these pressing clinical questions in a timely fashion and to translate that evidence into clinical practice to improve patient care and outcomes.

Without current best evidence, practice is rapidly outdated, often to the detriment of patients. As a classic example, for years, pediatric primary care providers advised parents to place their infants in a prone position while sleeping, with the underlying reasoning that this was the best position to prevent aspiration in the event of vomiting. With evidence indicating that prone positioning increases the risk of sudden infant death syndrome (SIDS), the American Academy of Pediatrics released a clinical practice guideline recommending a supine position for infant sleep that resulted in a decline in infant mortality caused by SIDS in the years following this recommendation (Task Force on Sudden Infant Death Syndrome, 2016). As a second example, despite strong evidence that the vaccination against human papilloma virus is safe and effective, vaccination rates by healthcare providers are low (Jin, Lipold, Sikon, & Rome, 2013). Yet another study indicated that adherence to evidence-based guidelines in the treatment of severe acute pancreatitis is poor (Vlada et al., 2013). Therefore, the critical question that all healthcare providers need to ask themselves is whether they can continue to implement practices that are not based on sound evidence, and, if so, at what cost (e.g., physical, emotional, and financial) to our patients and their family members.

Even if healthcare professionals answer this question negatively and remain resistant to implementing EBP, now third-party payers often provide reimbursement only for healthcare practices whose effectiveness is supported by scientific evidence (i.e., pay for performance). Furthermore, hospitals are now being denied payment for patient complications that develop when evidence-based guidelines are not followed. In addition to pressure from third-party payers, a growing number of patients and family members are seeking the latest evidence posted on websites about the most effective treatments for their health conditions. This is likely to exert even greater pressure on healthcare providers to provide the most up-to-date practices and health-related information. Therefore, despite continued resistance from some clinicians who refuse to learn EBP, the EBP movement continues to forge ahead full steam.

Another important reason for clinicians to include the latest evidence in their daily decision making is that evidence evolves on a continual basis. As a classic example, an RCT was funded by the National Institutes of Health to compare the use of the medication metformin, standard care, and lifestyle changes (e.g., activity, diet, and weight loss) to prevent type 2 diabetes in high-risk individuals. The trial was stopped early because the evidence was so strong for the benefits of the lifestyle intervention. The intervention from this trial was translated into practice within a year by the Federally Qualified Health Centers participating in the Health Disparities Collaborative, which is a national effort to improve health outcomes for all medically underserved individuals (Talsma, Grady, Feetham, Heinrich, & Steinwachs, 2008). This rapid translation of research findings into practice is what needs to become the norm instead of the rarity.

KEY INITIATIVES UNDERWAY TO ADVANCE EVIDENCE-BASED PRACTICE

The gap between the publishing of research evidence and its translation into practice to improve patient care often takes decades (Melnyk & Fineout-Overholt, 2015) and continues to be a major concern for healthcare organizations as well as federal agencies. To address this research–practice time gap, major initiatives such as the federal funding of EBP centers and the creation of formal task forces that critically appraise evidence to develop screening and manage clinical practice guidelines have been established.

The Institute of Medicine's Roundtable on Evidence-Based Medicine helped to transform the manner in which evidence on clinical effectiveness is generated and used to improve healthcare and the health of Americans. The goal set by this Roundtable is that, by 2020, 90% of clinical decisions will be supported by accurate, timely, and up-to-date information based on the best available evidence (McClellan, McGinnis, Nabel, & Olsen, 2007). The Roundtable convened senior leadership from multiple sectors (e.g., patients, healthcare professionals, third-party payers, policy makers, and researchers) to determine how evidence can be better generated and applied to improve the effectiveness and efficiency of healthcare in the United States (Institute of Medicine of the National Academies, n.d.). It stressed the need for better and timelier evidence concerning which interventions work best, for whom, and under what types of circumstances so that sound clinical decisions can be made. The Roundtable placed its emphasis on three areas:

1. Accelerating the progress toward a learning healthcare system, in which evidence is applied and developed as a product of patient care;
2. Generating evidence to support which healthcare strategies are most effective and produce the greatest value;
3. Improving public awareness and understanding about the nature of evidence, and its importance for their healthcare (Institute of Medicine of the National Academies, n.d.).

Among other key initiatives to advance EBP is the U.S. Preventive Services Task Force (USPSTF), which is an independent panel of 16 experts in primary care and prevention who systematically review the evidence of effectiveness and develop evidence-based recommendations for clinical preventive services, including screening, counseling, and preventive medications. Which preventive services should be incorporated by healthcare providers in primary care and for which populations are emphasized. The USPSTF is sponsored by the Agency for Healthcare Research and Quality (AHRQ), and its recommendations are considered the gold standard for clinical preventive services. Evidence-based centers, funded by AHRQ, conduct systematic reviews for the USPSTF and are the basis on which it makes its recommendations. The USPSTF reviews the evidence presented by the EBP centers and estimates the magnitude of benefits and harms for each preventive service. Consensus about the net benefit for each preventive service is garnered, and the USPSTF then issues a graded recommendation for clinical practice. If the preventive service receives an A or B grade, which indicates the net benefit is substantial or moderate, clinicians should provide this service. A C recommendation indicates the net benefit is small and clinicians should provide the service to selected people based on individual circumstances. A D recommendation indicates the service has no benefit or harm outweighs the benefit, and, therefore, clinicians are discouraged from implementing it. When the USPSTF issues an I statement, it means that the evidence is insufficient to assess the balance of benefits and harms. If there is insufficient evidence on a particular topic, the USPSTF recommends a research agenda for primary care for the generation of evidence needed to guide practice (Melnyk, Grossman et al., 2012).

 All of the USPSTF evidence-based recommendations are freely available and updated routinely at https://www.uspreventiveservicestaskforce.org/.

Examples of the USPSTF recommendations include breast cancer screening, visual screening, colorectal screening, and depression screening as well as preventive medication topics. Clinical considerations for each topic are also discussed with each recommendation. The USPSTF recommendations provide general practitioners, internists, pediatricians, nurse practitioners, nurses, and family practitioners with an authoritative source for evidence to make decisions about the delivery of preventive services in primary care. In 2010, the Patient Protection and Affordable Care Act created a link between the USPSTF recommendations and various coverage requirements (Siu, Bibbins-Domingo, & Grossman, 2015). The Affordable Care Act mandates that commercial and individual plans must at minimum provide coverage and not impose cost sharing on any preventive services that receive an A or B grade from the USPSTF. Medicare and Medicaid are excluded from this provision.

 An app, the Electronic Preventive Services Selector (ePSS), is also available for free to help healthcare providers implement the USPSTF recommendations at https://epss.ahrq .gov/PDA/index.jsp

Similar to the USPSTF, a panel of national experts who comprise the Community Services Task Force uses a rigorous systematic review process to determine the best evidence-based programs and policies to promote health and prevent disease in communities. Systemic reviews by this panel answer the following questions: (a) Which program and policy interventions have been shown to be effective? (b) Are there effective interventions that are right for my community? (c) What might effective interventions cost and what is the likely return on investment?

 These evidence-based recommendations for communities are available in a free evidence-based resource entitled *The Guide to Community Preventive Services* (http:// www.thecommunityguide.org/)

Another funded federal initiative is the Patient-Centered Outcomes Research Institute (PCORI), which is authorized by Congress to conduct research to provide information about the best available evidence to help patients and their healthcare providers make more informed decisions. PCORI's studies are intended to provide patients with a better understanding of the prevention, treatment, and care options available, and the science that supports those options.

 Find the PCORI online at www.pcori.org.

The Magnet Recognition Program by the American Nurses Credentialing Center has facilitated the advancement of EBP in hospitals throughout the United States. The program was started to recognize healthcare institutions for quality patient care, nursing excellence, and innovations in professional nursing practice. Magnet-designated hospitals reflect a high quality of care. The program evaluates quality indicators and standards of nursing practice as defined in the American Nurses Association's (2009) *Scope and Standards for Nurse Administrators (3rd edition)*. Conducting research and using EBP are critical for attaining Magnet status. Hospitals are appraised on evidence-based quality indicators, which are referred to as Forces of Magnetism. The Magnet program is based on a model with five key components: (1) transformational leadership; (2) structural empowerment; (3) exemplary professional practice; (4) new knowledge, innovation, and improvements, which emphasize new models of care, application of existing evidence, new evidence, and visible contributions to the science of nursing; and (5) empirical quality results, which focus on measuring outcomes to demonstrate the benefits of high-quality care (American Nurses Credentialing Center [ANCC], 2017). ANCC (2017) requires that Magnet organizations produce data that their nurses incorporate as new evidence into practice. Findings from research indicate that nurses employed by Magnet facilities report fewer barriers to EBP than those in non-Magnet facilities (Wilson et al., 2015).

With a $6.5 million gift, the Helene Fuld Health Trust National Institute for Evidence-based Practice in Nursing and Healthcare was founded by Bernadette Melnyk and launched at The Ohio State University College of Nursing in 2017. The Fuld National Institute for EBP (a) works with nursing and transdisciplinary faculty across the nation to integrate EBP throughout their curricula to produce the highest caliber of evidence-based graduates; (b) educates nursing and transdisciplinary students at all levels on how to access the latest gold standards of care and implement as well as sustain EBP; (c) assists nurses and other health professionals to advance evidence-based care to improve the safety and quality of care; (d) conducts national webinars on the best and latest evidence to guide high-quality practice; (e) serves as a clearinghouse for best evidence on a variety of healthcare practices and health conditions for the public; and (f) conducts research to advance the body of knowledge regarding EBP and how to accelerate the translation of research findings into practice at a more rapid rate to improve outcomes. A National EBP Expert Forum was held on October 18, 2017, that brought over 40 leaders from national professional organizations and federal agencies together to determine best strategies for advancing EBP. The top action tactics from this expert panel included the following: (1) enhanced reimbursement for EBP; (2) more interprofessional education and skills building in EBP; and (3) leaders to prioritize EBP and fuel it with resources (Melnyk et al., 2017). These entities have formed an action collaborative to advance EBP throughout the United States.

   See https://fuld.nursing.osu.edu/

THE SEVEN STEPS OF EVIDENCE-BASED PRACTICE

The seven critical steps of EBP are summarized in Box 1.2 and are described in more detail in this section. These steps must be implemented in sequence and be rigorously engaged to accomplish the end goal of improved patient, provider, and system outcomes.

Step 0: Cultivate a Spirit of Inquiry Within an EBP Culture and Environment

Before embarking on the well-known steps of EBP, it is critical to cultivate a **spirit of inquiry** (i.e., a consistently questioning attitude toward practice) so that clinicians are comfortable with and excited about asking questions regarding their patients' care as well as challenging current

---

BOX 1.2	*The Steps of the Evidence-Based Practice Process*

0. Cultivate a spirit of inquiry within an evidence-based practice (EBP) culture and environment.
1. Ask the burning clinical question in PICOT format.
2. Search for and collect the most relevant best evidence.
3. Critically appraise the evidence (i.e., rapid critical appraisal, evaluation, and synthesis).
4. Integrate the best evidence with one's clinical expertise and patient/family preferences and values in making a practice decision or change.
5. Evaluate outcomes of the practice decision or change based on evidence.
6. Disseminate the outcomes of the EBP decision or change.

---

institutional or unit-based practices. Without a culture and environment that is supportive of a spirit of inquiry and EBP, individual and organizational EBP change efforts are not likely to succeed and be sustained (Melnyk, 2016a). A culture that fosters EBP promotes this spirit of inquiry and makes it visible to clinicians by embedding it in its philosophy and mission of the institution.

Key elements of an EBP culture and environment include the following:

- A spirit of inquiry where all health professionals are encouraged to question their current practices;
- A philosophy, mission, clinical promotion system, and evaluation process that incorporate EBP and the EBP competencies;
- A cadre of EBP mentors, who have in-depth knowledge and skills in EBP, mentor others, and overcome barriers to individual and organizational change;
- An infrastructure that provides tools to enhance EBP (e.g., computers for searching at the point of care, access to key databases and librarians, ongoing EBP educational and skills-building sessions, EBP rounds and journal clubs);
- Administrative support and leadership that values and models EBP as well as provides the needed resources to sustain it;
- Regular recognition of individuals and groups who consistently implement EBP.

Step 1: Formulate the Burning Clinical PICOT Question

In step 1 of EBP, clinical questions are asked in **PICOT** format (i.e., *patient population, intervention* or *issue* of interest, *comparison* intervention or group, *outcome*, and *time frame*) to yield the most relevant and best evidence from a search of the existing literature. For example, a well-designed PICOT question would be as follows: In teenagers (the patient population), how does cognitive behavioral skills building (the experimental intervention) compared with yoga (the comparison intervention) affect anxiety (the outcome) after 6 weeks of treatment (the time taken for the interventions to achieve the outcome)? Questions asked in a PICOT format result in an effective search that yields the best, relevant information and saves an inordinate amount of time (Melnyk & Fineout-Overholt, 2015). In contrast, an inappropriately formed question (e.g., What is the best type of intervention to use with anxious teenagers?) would lead to an unfocused search and an outcome that would likely include hundreds of nonusable abstracts and irrelevant information.

For other clinical questions that are not focused on intervention, the meaning of the letter *I* can be "issue of interest" instead of "intervention." An example of a nonintervention PICOT question would be the following: How do new mothers (the patient population) who have breast-related complications (the issue of interest) perceive their ability to breastfeed (the outcome) past the first 3 months after their infants' birth (the timeframe in which their perception matters)? In this question, there is no appropriate comparison group, so the PIOT is appropriate; however, it is still referred to as a PICOT question.

When a clinical problem generates multiple clinical questions, priority should be given to those questions with the most important consequences or those that occur most frequently (i.e., those clinical problems that occur in high volume and/or those that carry high risk for negative outcomes to the patient). For example, nurses and physicians on a surgical unit routinely encounter the question, "In postoperative adult patients, how does morphine compared with hydromorphone affect pain relief within the first half hour after administration?" Another question might be "In postoperative mobile patients, how does daily walking compared with no daily walking prevent pressure sores during hospitalization?" The clinical priority would be answering the question of pain relief first because pain is a daily occurrence in this population, versus prioritizing seeking an answer to the second question because pressure ulcers rarely occur in postoperative adult patients. Chapter 2 provides more in-depth information about formulating PICOT questions.

Step 2: Search for the Best Evidence

The search for best evidence should first begin by considering the elements of the PICOT question. Each of the keywords from the PICOT question should be used to begin the systematic search. The type of study that would provide the best answer to an intervention or treatment question would be systematic reviews or meta-analyses, which are regarded as the strongest level of evidence on which to base treatment decisions (i.e., level 1) (Melnyk & Fineout-Overholt, 2015). There are different levels of evidence for each kind of PICOT question (see Chapter 2 for more in-depth discussion). Although there are many hierarchies of evidence available in the literature to answer intervention PICOT questions, we have chosen to present a hierarchy of evidence to address questions that encompass a broad range of evidence, including systematic reviews of qualitative evidence, also referred to as metasyntheses (Box 1.3). Chapter 3 has more in-depth information on conducting a systematic search of the literature based on the PICOT question.

BOX 1.3

Rating System for the Hierarchy of Evidence for Intervention/Treatment Questions

Level I: Evidence from a systematic review or meta-analysis of all relevant randomized controlled trials (RCTs)

Level II: Evidence obtained from well-designed RCTs

Level III: Evidence obtained from well-designed controlled trials without randomization

Level IV: Evidence from well-designed case-control and cohort studies

Level V: Evidence from systematic reviews of descriptive and qualitative studies

Level VI: Evidence from a single descriptive or qualitative study

Level VII: Evidence from the opinion of authorities and/or reports of expert committees

---

Modified from Guyatt, G., & Rennie, D. (2002). *Users' guides to the medical literature*. Chicago, IL: American Medical Association; Harris, R. P., Hefland, M., Woolf, S. H., Lohr, K. N., Mulrow, C. D., Teutsch, S. M., & Atkins, D. (2001). Current methods of the U.S. Preventive Services Task Force: A review of the process. *American Journal of Preventive Medicine, 20,* 21–35.

There are many study designs within a body of evidence; however, it is important to first look for the best quality and highest level of evidence. A systematic review is a synthesis of evidence on a particular topic, typically conducted by an expert or expert panel that uses a rigorous process for identifying, appraising, and synthesizing studies, to answer a specific clinical question. Conclusions are then drawn about the data gathered through this process. Examples of clinical questions that could be answered through a systematic review include the following: (1) In adult women with arthritis, how does massage compare with pharmacologic agents to reduce pain after 2 weeks of treatment? and (2) In women, how does an early lifestyle adoption of a healthy diet and exercise predict heart disease in older adulthood? Using a rigorous process of well-defined, preset criteria to select studies for inclusion in the review as well as stringent criteria to assess quality, bias is overcome and results are more credible. Population health can be improved by making the best evidence available in the form of policy briefs to influence the decisions of policy makers.

Many systematic reviews incorporate quantitative methods to compare the results from multiple studies. These reviews are called **meta-analyses**. A meta-analysis generates an overall summary statistic that represents the effect of the intervention across multiple studies. When a meta-analysis can combine the samples of each study included in the review to create one larger study, the summary statistic is more precise than the individual findings from any one of the contributing studies alone (Melnyk & Fineout-Overholt, 2015). Thus, systematic reviews and meta-analyses yield the strongest level of evidence on which to base practice decisions. Caution must be used when searching for systematic reviews because some evidence reviews or narrative reviews may be labeled systematic reviews; however, they lack the rigorous process that is required of true systematic reviews. Although studies are compared and contrasted in narrative and integrative reviews, a rigorous methodology with explicit criteria for reviewing the studies is often not used, and a summary statistic is not generated. Therefore, conclusions and recommendations by authors of narrative and integrative reviews may be biased.

 In addition to the Cochrane Database of Systematic Reviews, the journals *Worldviews on Evidence-Based Nursing* and *Nursing Research* frequently provide systematic reviews to guide nursing practice across many topic areas. More information on *Worldviews* and *Nursing Research* can be found at http://onlinelibrary.wiley.com/journal/10.1111/(ISSN)1741-6787 and http://www.nursingresearchonline.com/. Chapters 5 and 6 have more in-depth information on understanding types of research study designs and how they contribute to a body of evidence.

Evidence-based clinical practice guidelines are specific practice recommendations grouped together, which have been derived from a methodologically rigorous review of the best evidence on a specific topic. Guidelines usually do not answer a single specific clinical question, but rather a group of questions about care. As such, they have tremendous potential as tools for clinicians to improve the quality of care, the process of care, and patient outcomes as well as reduce variation in care and unnecessary healthcare expenditures (Institute of Medicine [US] Committee on Standards for Developing Trustworthy Clinical Practice Guidelines, 2011). It is imperative for clinicians to seek out evidence-based guidelines to inform decisions.

The following are examples of two evidence-based clinical practice guidelines:

1. *Management of chronic pain in survivors of adult cancers: American Society of Clinical Oncology clinical practice guideline*: available online at http://ascopubs.org/doi/abs/10.1200/JOP.2016.014837.
2. *Prevention of dental caries in children from birth through age 5 years: USPSTF recommendation statement*: available online at http://pediatrics.aappublications.org/content/early/2014/04/29/peds.2014-0483.

The Guidelines International Network (G-I-N) houses another comprehensive database of clinical practice guidelines. The mission of G-I-N is to lead, strengthen, and support collaboration in guideline, adaptation, and implementation. G-I-N facilitates networking, promotes excellence, and helps members create high-quality clinical practice guidelines that foster safe and effective patient care. It is comprised of 99 organizations representing 47 countries.

 G-I-N is online at http://www.g-i-n.net/home.

It is important to note the latest publication date of clinical practice guidelines because many guidelines need updating so that the latest evidence is included in making practice recommendations. It also is important to note the process through which the guidelines were created, because there are many guidelines created by professional organizations that have not followed rigorous processes for development (e.g., systematic reviews; Melnyk, Grossman et al., 2012). Although clinical practice guidelines have tremendous potential to improve the quality of care and outcomes for patients as well as reduce healthcare variation and costs, their success depends on a highly rigorous guideline development process and the incorporation of the latest best evidence. Guideline success also depends on implementation by healthcare providers because their dissemination does not equate to implementation.

 A toolkit to enhance the use of clinical practice guidelines is available from the Registered Nurses' Association of Ontario and can be downloaded from its website at http://ltctoolkit.rnao.ca/clinical-topics. More information about guideline development and implementation can be found in Chapter 8.

If syntheses (e.g., systematic reviews, meta-analyses) are not available to answer a clinical practice treatment question, the next step should be a search for original RCTs found in databases such as MEDLINE or the Cumulative Index of Nursing and Allied Health Literature. If RCTs are not available, the search process should then include other types of studies that generate evidence to guide clinical decision making (e.g., nonrandomized, descriptive, or qualitative studies) to determine the best available body of evidence.

Other searchable databases helpful to clinicians in deciding what evidence-based interventions to implement in their practices are the Research Tested Intervention Programs (RTIPs) by the National Cancer Institute and the AHRQ's Health Care Innovations Exchange.

 RTIPs is a database of over 175 evidence-based cancer control interventions and program materials designed to provide practitioners with easy and immediate access to research-tested materials (https://rtips.cancer.gov/rtips/index.do).

Programs listed have undergone rigorous reviews before their inclusion on this website. The Innovations Exchange was created to speed the implementation of new and better ways of delivering healthcare by sharing, learning about, and adopting evidence-based innovations and tools appropriate for a range of healthcare settings and populations.

The Innovations Exchange is online at https://innovations.ahrq.gov/about-us.

Step 3: Critical Appraisal of Evidence

Step 3 in the EBP process is vital in that it involves critical appraisal of the evidence obtained from the search process. Although healthcare professionals may view critical appraisal as an exhaustive, time-consuming process, the first steps of critical appraisal can be efficiently accomplished by answering three key questions as part of a **rapid critical appraisal** process in which studies are evaluated for their validity, reliability, and applicability to answer the posed clinical question (summarized in Box 1.4):

1. **Are the results of the study valid? (Validity)** Are the results as close to the truth as possible? Did the researchers conduct the study using the best research methods possible? For example, in intervention trials, it would be important to determine whether the subjects were **randomly assigned** to treatment or control groups and whether they were equal on key characteristics prior to the treatment.
2. **What are the results? (Reliability)** For example, in an intervention trial, this includes (a) whether the intervention worked; (b) how large a treatment effect was obtained; and (c) whether clinicians could expect similar results if they implemented the intervention in their own clinical practice setting (i.e., the preciseness of the intervention effect). In qualitative studies, this includes evaluating whether the research approach fits the purpose of the study, along with evaluating other aspects of the study.
3. **Will the results help me in caring for my patients? (Applicability)** This third rapid critical appraisal question includes asking whether (a) the subjects in the study are similar to the patients for whom care is being delivered; (b) the benefits are greater than the risks of treatment (i.e., potential for harm); (c) the treatment is feasible to implement in the practice setting; and (d) the patient desires the treatment.

The answers to these questions ensure relevance and transferability of the evidence to the specific population for whom the clinician provides care. For example, if a systematic review provided evidence to support the positive effects of using distraction to alleviate pain in postsurgical patients between the ages of 20 and 40 years, those same results may not be relevant for postsurgical patients who are 65 years or older. In addition, even if an RCT supported the effectiveness of a specific intervention with a patient population, the risks and benefits of that intervention must be carefully considered before its implementation. Critically appraising a body of evidence to guide practice decisions begins with rapid critical appraisal of the studies found in the search, and also includes evaluation of the studies in the form of an evidence synthesis to determine whether the findings from the studies are in agreement or not. A synthesis of the study findings is important to draw a conclusion about the body of evidence on a particular clinical issue and make subsequent recommendations for practice. Unit 2 in this book contains in-depth information on critical appraisal of all types of evidence, from expert opinion and qualitative studies to RCTs and systematic reviews.

BOX 1.4	*Key General Critical Appraisal Questions*

1. Are the results of the study valid? (Validity)
2. What are the results? (Reliability)
3. Will the results help me in caring for my patients? (Applicability)

Step 4: Integrate the Evidence With Clinical Expertise and Patient/Family Preferences to Make the Best Clinical Decision

The next key step in EBP is integrating the best evidence found from the literature with the healthcare provider's expertise and patient/family preferences and values to implement a decision (i.e., putting evidence into action). Clinical expertise includes how clinicians understand the given population for whom they care and known sequelae of clinical issues, the available healthcare resources, their personal experiences with healthcare decision making, and their competence in critical appraisal. In addition, consumers of healthcare services want to participate in the clinical decisionmaking process, and it is the ethical responsibility of the healthcare provider to involve patients in treatment decisions. Even if the evidence from a rigorous search and critical appraisal strongly supports that a certain treatment is beneficial (e.g., hormone replacement therapy [HRT] to prevent osteoporosis in a very high-risk woman), a discussion with the patient may reveal her intense fear of developing breast cancer while taking HRT or other reasons that the treatment is not acceptable. Moreover, as part of the history-taking process or physical examination, a comorbidity or contraindication may be found that increases the risks of HRT (e.g., prior history of stroke). Therefore, despite compelling evidence to support the benefits of HRT in preventing osteoporosis in high-risk women, a decision against its use may be made after a thorough assessment of the individual patient and a discussion of the risks and benefits of treatment.

Similarly, a clinician's assessment of healthcare resources that are available to implement a treatment decision is a critical part of the EBP decisionmaking process. For example, on follow-up evaluation, a clinician notes that the first-line treatment of acute otitis media in a 3-year-old patient was not effective. The latest evidence indicates that antibiotic A has greater efficacy than antibiotic B as the second-line treatment for acute otitis media in young children. However, because antibiotic A is far more expensive than antibiotic B and the family of the child does not have prescription insurance coverage, the practitioner and parents together may decide to use the less expensive antibiotic to treat the child's unresolved ear infection. Organizational culture is another important consideration when implementing evidence into practice. Unit 4 has in-depth information on strategies to implement evidence into practice.

Step 5: Evaluate the Outcomes of the Practice Change Based on Evidence

Step 5 in EBP is evaluating the evidence-based initiative in terms of how the change affected patient outcomes or how effective the clinical decision was with a particular patient or practice setting. This type of evaluation is essential to determine whether the change based on evidence resulted in the expected outcomes when implemented in the real-world clinical practice setting. Measurement of outcomes, especially "so-what" outcomes that are important to today's healthcare system (e.g., length of stay, readmission rates, patient complications, turnover of staff, costs), is important to determine and document the impact of the EBP change on healthcare quality and/or patient outcomes (Melnyk & Morrison-Beedy, 2012). If a change in practice based on evidence did not produce the same findings as demonstrated in rigorous research, clinicians should ask themselves a variety of questions (Was the intervention administered in exactly the same way that it was delivered in the study? Were the patients in the clinical setting similar to those in the studies?). Chapter 10 contains information on how to evaluate outcomes of practice changes based on evidence. See Figure 1.3 for the key steps of EBP to improve quality healthcare.

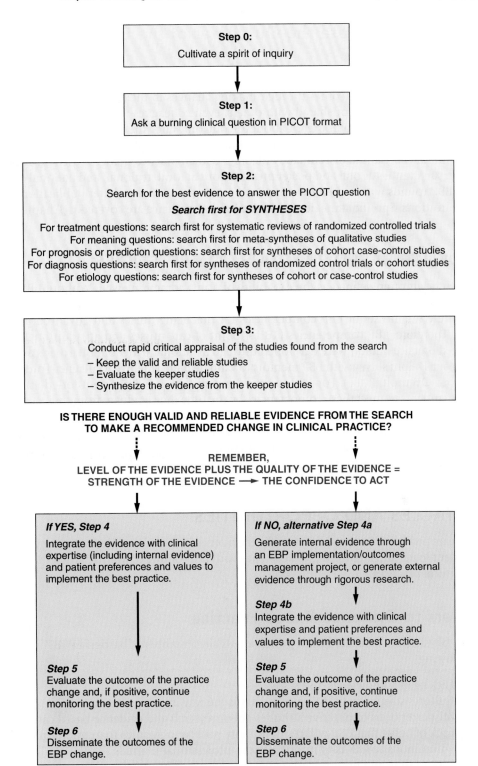

Step 0:

Cultivate a spirit of inquiry

Step 1:

Ask a burning clinical question in PICOT format

Step 2:

Search for the best evidence to answer the PICOT question

Search first for SYNTHESES

For treatment questions: search first for systematic reviews of randomized controlled trials
For meaning questions: search first for meta-syntheses of qualitative studies
For prognosis or prediction questions: search first for syntheses of cohort case-control studies
For diagnosis questions: search first for syntheses of randomized control trials or cohort studies
For etiology questions: search first for syntheses of cohort or case-control studies

Step 3:

Conduct rapid critical appraisal of the studies found from the search
  – Keep the valid and reliable studies
  – Evaluate the keeper studies
  – Synthesize the evidence from the keeper studies

**IS THERE ENOUGH VALID AND RELIABLE EVIDENCE FROM THE SEARCH
TO MAKE A RECOMMENDED CHANGE IN CLINICAL PRACTICE?**

REMEMBER,
**LEVEL OF THE EVIDENCE PLUS THE QUALITY OF THE EVIDENCE =
STRENGTH OF THE EVIDENCE ⟶ THE CONFIDENCE TO ACT**

If YES, Step 4

Integrate the evidence with clinical expertise (including internal evidence) and patient preferences and values to implement the best practice.

Step 5
Evaluate the outcome of the practice change and, if positive, continue monitoring the best practice.

Step 6
Disseminate the outcomes of the EBP change.

If NO, alternative Step 4a

Generate internal evidence through an EBP implementation/outcomes management project, or generate external evidence through rigorous research.

Step 4b
Integrate the evidence with clinical expertise and patient preferences and values to implement the best practice.

Step 5
Evaluate the outcome of the practice change and, if positive, continue monitoring the best practice.

Step 6
Disseminate the outcomes of the EBP change.

Figure 1.3: Steps of the evidence-based practice (EBP) process leading to high-quality healthcare and best patient outcomes. © Melnyk & Fineout-Overholt, 2017.

Step 6: Disseminate the Outcomes of the Evidence-Based Practice Change

The last step in EBP is disseminating the outcomes of the EBP change. All too often, clinicians achieve many positive outcomes through making changes in their care based on evidence, but those outcomes are not shared with others, even colleagues within their same institution. As a result, others do not learn about the outcomes nor the process that led to them, and clinicians as well as patients in other settings do not benefit from that knowledge. It is important for clinicians to disseminate outcomes of their practice changes based on evidence through such venues as oral and poster presentations at local, regional, and national conferences; EBP rounds within their own institutions; journal and newsletter publications; and lay publications. Specific strategies for disseminating evidence are covered in Chapter 20.

EVIDENCE-BASED PRACTICE COMPETENCIES

Competency is often defined as the capability of doing something well. Without EBP competencies, expectations for the implementation of evidence-based care are unclear. Until 2014, there was no set of EBP competencies for practicing nurses and advanced practice nurses. Therefore, EBP competencies (13 for point of care nurses and an additional 11 for advanced practice nurses) were developed through a national panel of EBP experts and two rounds of a Delphi survey with EBP mentors to validate them (Melnyk, Gallagher-Ford, Long, & Fineout-Overholt, 2014). For EBP to thrive and sustain, it is important for educators to prepare students to meet these competencies by the time they graduate from their academic programs. Healthcare systems also should require their clinicians to demonstrate these competencies and provide education and skills building for those who do not yet meet them. Chapter 11 covers specific details about these competencies, and how to integrate them into clinical practice settings to improve healthcare quality, safety, and outcomes.

OBSTACLES AND OPPORTUNITIES

Healthcare providers are struggling to deliver evidence-based care while managing demanding patient loads and attempting to keep pace with the volume of journal articles related to their clinical practices.

Barriers to Evidence-Based Practice

Nurses, physicians, and other health professionals cite a number of barriers to EBP including the following:

- Lack of EBP knowledge and skills;
- Cultures steeped in tradition (e.g., that is the way it is done here);
- Misperceptions or negative attitudes about research and evidence-based care;
- Lack of belief that EBP will result in more positive outcomes than traditional care;
- Voluminous amounts of information in professional journals;
- Lack of time and resources to search for and critically appraise evidence;
- Overwhelming patient loads;
- Organizational constraints, such as lack of administrative support or incentives;
- Lack of EBP mentors;
- Demands from patients for a certain type of treatment (e.g., patients who demand antibiotics for their viral upper respiratory infections when they are not indicated);

- Peer pressure to continue with practices steeped in tradition;
- Resistance to change;
- Lack of consequences for not implementing EBP;
- Peer and leader/manager resistance;
- Lack of autonomy and power to change practice;
- Inadequate EBP content and behavioral skills building in educational programs along with the continued teaching of how to conduct rigorous research in baccalaureate and master's programs instead of teaching an evidence-based approach to care.

(Melnyk, Fineout-Overholt et al., 2012; Melnyk, 2016a; Squires, Estabrooks, Gustavsson, & Wallen, 2011; Wilson et al., 2015)

Facilitators of Evidence-Based Practice

To overcome the barriers in implementing EBP, there must be champions at all levels of practice (i.e., clinicians who believe so strongly in the EBP paradigm that they will do what it takes to facilitate it in their daily practice and their organizational culture) and an EBP culture and environment with mechanisms to support the cause (Melnyk, 2016a). For healthcare professionals to advance the use of EBP, misconceptions about how to implement practice based on the best available evidence need to be corrected, and knowledge and skills in this area must be enhanced. It must also be realized that changing behavior is complex and influenced by multiple factors, including beliefs, attitudes, resources, and the availability of evidence to change practice.

The following facilitating conditions have been found to enhance EBP:

- Support and encouragement from leadership/administration that foster an EBP culture with expectations for EBP;
- Alignment of stakeholders;
- Time to critically appraise studies and implement their findings;
- Clearly written research reports;
- EBP mentors with excellent EBP skills as well as knowledge and proficiency in individual and organizational change strategies;
- Proper tools to assist with EBP at the point of care (e.g., computers dedicated to EBP; computer-based educational programs);
- Integrating EBP into health professions curricula;
- Clinical promotion systems and performance evaluations that incorporate the EBP competencies;
- Evidence-based clinical practice policies and procedures;
- EBP models that can guide implementation and sustainability of EBP (see Chapter 14);
- Journal clubs and EBP rounds;
- A certification credential and high level of education.

(Gallagher-Ford, 2014; Melnyk, 2016a; Melnyk & Fineout-Overholt, 2015; Ten Ham, Minnie, & van der Walt, 2015; Stetler, Ritchie, Rycroft-Malone, & Charns, 2014)

OVERCOMING BARRIERS TO EVIDENCE-BASED PRACTICE

For evidence-based care to become the gold standard of practice, EBP barriers must be overcome and facilitators maximized. Federal agencies, healthcare organizations and systems, health insurers, policy makers, and regulatory bodies must advocate for and require its use.

Funding agencies must continue to establish translational research (i.e., how findings from research can best be transported into clinical practice to improve care and patient outcomes) as a high priority. Interdisciplinary professionals must work together in a collaborative team spirit to advance EBP. In addition, healthcare organizations must build a culture and environment of EBP and devise clinical promotion ladders and performance evaluations that incorporate its use.

As an initial step, barriers and facilitators to EBP along with organizational culture and readiness for system-wide implementation of EBP must be assessed within an organization. Surveys or focus groups should first be conducted with healthcare providers to assess their baseline knowledge, beliefs, and behaviors regarding EBP (Melnyk, Fineout-Overholt, & Mays, 2008). Objective documentation of the status of EBP is essential to demonstrate a change in outcomes, even when there is a subjective consensus of the leaders regarding the state of EBP in their agency. An additional benefit of conducting surveys or focus groups at the outset of any new EBP initiative is that research shows that these strategies also are effective in raising awareness and stimulating a change to evidence-based care.

As part of the survey or focus group, clinicians should be asked about their baseline knowledge of EBP as well as to what extent they believe that implementing EBP will result in improved care and better patient outcomes. This is a critical question because knowledge alone usually does not change behavior. Although healthcare providers must possess basic knowledge and skills about EBP, it is essential for them to believe that EBP will produce better outcomes in order for changes in their practices to occur (Melnyk et al., 2008).

❝

Belief at the beginning of any successful undertaking is the one ingredient that will ensure success.

WILLIAM JAMES

Healthcare providers who do not believe that EBP results in improved care and patient outcomes need to be exposed to real-case scenarios in which evidence-based care resulted in better outcomes than care steeped in traditional practices. For example, many primary care providers continue to prescribe antidepressants as the sole treatment for depressed adolescents when RCTs have indicated that medication in combination with cognitive behavioral therapy is better than medication alone in reducing depressive symptoms (Melnyk & Jensen, 2013).

Correcting Misperceptions

Because misperceptions about EBP constitute another barrier to its implementation, clarifying these perceptions and teaching the basics of EBP are critical to advancing evidence-based care. For example, many practitioners believe that searching for and critically appraising research articles is an overwhelming, time-consuming process. However, practitioners who have this belief frequently do not have skills in systematic searching and have not had exposure to databases such as the Cochrane Library and the Guidelines International Network, which can provide them with quick, easily retrievable systematic reviews and evidence-based guidelines to inform their practices. In addition, because many educational curricula continue to teach the in-depth critique of a single study versus time-efficient approaches to the gathering and critical appraisal of a body of empirical studies, clinicians may have the misperception that the EBP process is not feasible in the context of their current practice environments. Therefore, the basics of EBP (e.g., how to formulate a searchable question that will yield the best evidence, how to systematically search for and rapidly critically appraise studies, how to synthesize the evidence) must be taught first to create baseline knowledge and skills.

The teaching of EBP can and should be accomplished with multiple strategies, including continuing education conferences with skills-building activities; interactive workshops; and dissemination of educational materials, such as journal articles, textbooks, and informational handouts. The best learning method incorporates the teaching of didactic information with interactive behavioral skills building. Helping clinicians put the educational content into practice is especially important for long-time clinicians, because the conversion from traditional practice to delivering evidence-based care involves behavior change and takes time. Therefore, creating opportunities for clinicians to practice the skills that they learn in didactic sessions is superior to didactic sessions alone. Chapters 16 and 17 contain more detailed information about teaching EBP.

 Three active EBP centers in the United States can also serve as resources for the teaching and implementation of EBP.

1. The Helene Fuld Health Trust National Institute for Evidence-based Practice in Nursing and Healthcare at The Ohio State University College of Nursing: www.fuld.nursing.osu.edu
2. The Sarah Cole Hirsh Institute for Evidence Based Practice at Case Western Reserve School of Nursing: https://nursing.case.edu/hirsh/
3. The Johns Hopkins Nursing Center for Evidence-based Practice at Johns Hopkins University: https://www.ijhn-education.org/content/evidence-based-practice

---

The Fuld National Institute for EBP offers national and international EBP continuing education conferences for nurses and other interdisciplinary healthcare professionals. It also offers 5-day EBP mentorship immersion programs for clinicians and faculty along with an online EBP fellowship program. In addition, it sponsors EBP national expert forums that gather leaders from national professional organizations, federal agencies, and healthcare institutions to make recommendations for future directions for EBP, and biennial EBP summits that highlight the best current evidence. The Sarah Cole Hirsh Institute focuses on annual training and research in EBP for graduate students, leaders, and current clinicians. The Johns Hopkins Nursing Center for Evidence-based Practice also offers 5-day EBP workshops.

Centers for EBP have also been established internationally in countries such as Australia, New Zealand, Hong Kong, Germany, the United Kingdom, and Canada. The mission of most of these centers is to educate clinicians through workshops or formal courses on EBP or to conduct systematic reviews.

Other reputable sources of information about EBP are from abstraction journals, such as *Evidence-Based Medicine, Evidence-Based Nursing, Evidence-Based Mental Health*, and *Evidence-Based Health Policy and Management*, through which professionals can find evidence to guide their practice. These journals summarize high-quality studies that have important clinical implications and provide a commentary by an expert in the field. The commentary addresses strengths and limitations of the research reviewed.

Questioning Clinical Practices, Changing Practice With Evidence, and Evaluating Impact

After basic EBP knowledge and skills are attained, it is important for healthcare professionals to actively ask questions about their current clinical practices, such as the following: In neonates, how does the use of pacifiers compared with no pacifiers reduce pain

> **"**
> Never stop questioning!
>
> **SUSAN L. HENDRIX**

during intrusive procedures? In adult surgical patients, how does heparin compared with antiembolic stockings prevent deep vein thrombosis within the first 2 months after surgery? Efforts also should be made to prioritize practice problems within an organization or practice setting. Once high-priority areas are recognized, it is helpful to identify colleagues who have an interest in the same clinical question so that a collaboration can be formed to search for and critically appraise the evidence found. The results of this search and appraisal should be shared with colleagues through a variety of mechanisms (e.g., journal clubs, EBP practice rounds, or informational handouts). If a current practice guideline does not exist, one can be developed and implemented. However, guideline development is a rigorous endeavor, and adequate time must be allotted for individuals to complete the work. Chapter 8 describes useful processes for developing and implementing clinical practice guidelines. To complete the EBP process, evaluation of the key outcomes of evidence implementation is essential to determine its effects on the process and outcomes of care.

Change to EBP within an organization or practice requires a clear vision, a written strategic plan, a culture and environment in which EBP is valued and expected, and persistence to make it happen. In addition, the chance to succeed in making a change to EBP and sustaining it will be greater where there is administrative support, encouragement, and recognition, EBP mentors, expectations for EBP as contained in clinical promotion criteria and evaluations, interprofessional collaboration, and allocated resources. It is often best to start with a small evidence-based change with high impact, especially when there is skepticism about EBP and elevated levels of stress or complacency within a system, rather than to expect a complete change to EBP to happen within a short time. For example, finding a mechanism for routinely discussing evidence-based literature, such as journal clubs or EBP rounds that can spark interest and enhance "buy-in" from colleagues and administration, may be a wonderful start to facilitating a change to EBP.

❝

I don't think there is any other quality so essential to
success of any kind as the quality of perseverance.
It overcomes almost everything,
even nature.

JOHN D. ROCKEFELLER

Chapters 9 through 14 provide further information on how to infuse EBP into clinical settings and review a variety of specific EBP strategies and implementation models. Chapter 15 outlines assessment strategies for determining an organization's stage of change. It also provides multiple suggestions for motivating a vision for change to best practice, based primarily on evidence-based organizational change principles. The section at the end of each unit entitled Making EBP Real: A Success Story provides case examples on how evidence-based care can positively impact patient outcomes. These examples highlight how EBP can improve both the process and outcomes of patient care. Countless examples similar to these can be found in the literature. Evidence-based success stories stem from first asking compelling clinical questions, which emphasizes the need to cultivate a never-ending spirit of inquiry within our colleagues, our students, and ourselves. These case examples teach a valuable lesson: Never stop questioning because providers need to take evidence-based responsibility for clinical decisions and stay up to date with data that can further support or dramatically change their practice standards. Once that spirit of inquiry is cultivated within us and our clinical settings, the journey toward a change to EBP will begin.

We have come to a time when the credibility of the health professions will be judged by which of its practices are based on the best and latest evidence from sound scientific studies, in combination with clinical expertise, astute assessment, and respect for patient values and preferences. The chance to influence health policy also rests on the ability to provide policy makers with the best evidence based on which they can make important decisions. However, it is important to remember that high-quality healthcare also depends on the ability to deliver EBP within a context of caring, which is the merging of science and art.

For EBP to evolve more quickly, commitments to advancing evidence-based care must be made by individuals, leaders, and organizations. Basic and graduate professional programs must teach the value and processes of EBP, leveled appropriately (see Chapter 16). Doctor of Philosophy (PhD) programs must prepare researchers and leaders who advance EBP through building on existing bodies of evidence to generate new knowledge from research to support the most effective practices, as well as testing of established and new models of EBP implementation to determine which models are most effective on both staff and patient outcomes. Doctor of Nursing Practice (DNP) programs must prepare advanced practice nurses, who are experts at translating evidence generated from research into clinical practice to improve care and outcomes (Melnyk, 2013; Melnyk, 2016b). Researchers and practitioners across disciplines must also unite to produce evidence on the effectiveness of numerous practices and to answer high-priority, compelling clinical questions, as well as to determine how best those initiatives or interventions can be translated into practice.

It is time for practitioners from all healthcare professions to embrace EBP and quickly move from practices steeped in tradition or based on outdated policies to those supported by sound evidence from well-designed studies. In doing so, patients, healthcare professionals, and healthcare systems will be more confident about the care that is being delivered and know that the best outcomes for patients and their families are being achieved.

> ❝
> Knowing is not enough; we must apply. Willing is not enough; we must do.
>
> **GOETHE**

EBP FAST FACTS

- Research supports that EBP improves healthcare quality and safety, patient outcomes, and healthcare costs as well as empowers clinicians, leading to higher job satisfaction.
- EBP is a problem-solving approach to the delivery of healthcare that integrates the best evidence from research with a clinician's expertise, including internal evidence from patient data, and a patient's/family's preferences and values.
- The level of evidence plus the quality of a body of evidence will determine whether a practice change should be made.
- Without EBP, it often takes decades to translate findings from research into real-world clinical practice settings.
- There are seven steps to EBP, which should be consistently implemented by clinicians to improve healthcare quality and patient outcomes (see Box 1.2).
- All clinicians should be expected to meet the EBP competencies.
- An EBP culture and environment must be created within an organization for EBP to sustain.

> ### WANT TO KNOW MORE?
>
> A variety of resources is available to enhance your learning and understanding of this chapter.
>
> - Visit thePoint® to access
>   - Articles from the AJN EBP Step-By-Step Series;
>   - Journal articles;
>   - Checklists for rapid critical appraisal and more.
>
> - Lippincott CoursePoint combines digital text content with video case studies and interactive modules for a fully integrated course solution that works the way you study and learn.

References

American Nurses Association. (2009). *Scope and standards for nurse administrators* (3rd ed.). Silver Spring, MD: Author.

American Nurses Credentialing Center. (2017). A new model for ANCC's Magnet Recognition Program. Retrieved from https://www.nursingworld.org/organizational-programs/magnet/magnet-model/

Bodenheimer, T., & Sinsky, C. (2014). From triple to quadruple aim. Care of the patient requires care of the provider. *Annals of Family Medicine, 12*(6), 573–576.

Brewer, B., & Alexandrov, A. W. (2015). The role of outcomes and quality improvement in enhancing and evaluating practice changes. In B. M. Melnyk & E. Fineout-Overholt, *Evidence-based practice in nursing & healthcare. A guide to best practice* (3rd ed.). Philadelphia, PA: Wolters Kluwer.

Cochrane, A. L. (1972). *Effectiveness and efficiency: Random reflections on health services.* London, UK: Nuffield Provincial Hospitals Trust.

Dotson, J. A., Roll, J. M., Packer, R. R., Lewis, J. M., McPherson, S., & Howell, D. (2014). Urban and rural utilization of evidence-based practices for substance use and mental health disorders. *Journal of Rural Health, 30*(3), 292–299.

Enkin, M. (1992). Current overviews of research evidence from controlled trials in midwifery obstetrics. *Journal of the Society of Obstetricians and Gynecologists of Canada, 9,* 23–33.

Fridman, M., & Frederickson, K. (2014). Oncology nurses and the experience of participation in an evidence-based practice project. *Oncology Nursing Forum, 41*(4), 382–388.

Gallagher-Ford, L. (2014). Implementing and sustaining EBP in real world healthcare settings: A leader's role in creating a strong context for EBP. *Worldviews on Evidence-based Nursing, 11*(1), 72–74.

Gonya, J., Martin, E., McClead, R., Nelin, L., Shepherd, E. (2014). Empowerment programme for parents of extremely premature infants significantly reduced length of stay and readmission rates. *Acta Paediatrics, 103*(7), 727–731.

Institute of Medicine (US) Committee on Standards for Developing Trustworthy Clinical Practice Guidelines. (2011). In R. Graham, M. Mancher, D. Miller Wolman, S. Greenfield, & E. Steinberg (Eds.), *Clinical practice guidelines we can trust.* Washington, DC: National Academies Press.

Institute of Medicine of the National Academies. (n.d.). *Roundtable on evidence-based medicine.* Retrieved from https://www.nap.edu/initiative/roundtable-on-evidence-based-medicine

Jin, X. W., Lipold, L., Sikon, A., & Rome, E. (2013). Human papillomavirus vaccine: Safe, effective, underused. *Cleveland Clinic Journal of Medicine, 80*(2), 49–60.

Johnson, J., Louch, G., Dunning, A., Johnson, O., Grange, A., Reynolds, C., . . . O'Hara, J. (2017). Burnout mediates the association between depression and patient safety perceptions: A cross-sectional study in hospital nurses. *Journal of Advanced Nursing, 73*(7), 1667–1680.

Kim, S. C., Ecoff, L., Brown, C. E., Gallo, A. M., Stichler, J. F., & Davidson, J. E. (2017). Benefits of a regional evidence-based practice fellowship program: A test of the ARCC Model. *Worldviews on Evidence-based Nursing, 14*(2), 90–98.

Kim, S. C., Stichler, J. F., Ecoff, L., Brown, C. E., Gallo, A. M., & Davidson, J. E. (2016). Predictors of evidence-based practice implementation, job satisfaction, and group cohesion among regional fellowship program participants. *Worldviews on Evidence-based Nursing, 13*(5), 340–348.

Makary, M., & Daniel, M. (2016). Medical error—the third leading cause of death in the U.S. *British Medical Journal, 353,* i2139. doi:10.1136/bmj.i2139

McClellan, M. B., McGinnis, M., Nabel, E. G., & Olsen, L. M. (2007). *Evidence-based medicine and the changing nature of healthcare.* Washington, DC: The National Academies Press.

Melnyk, B. M. (2012). Achieving a high-reliability organization through implementation of the ARCC model for systemwide sustainability of evidence-based practice. *Nursing Administration Quarterly, 36*(2), 127–135.

Melnyk, B. M. (2013). Distinguishing the preparation and roles of the PhD and DNP graduate: National implications for academic curricula and healthcare systems. *Journal of Nursing Education, 52*(8), 442–448.

Melnyk, B. M. (2016a). Culture eats strategy every time: What works in building and sustaining an evidence-based practice culture in healthcare systems. *Worldviews on Evidence-based Nursing, 13*(2), 99–101.

Melnyk, B. M. (2016b). The Doctor of Nursing Practice degree = Evidence-based practice expert. *Worldviews on Evidence-based Nursing, 13*(3), 183–184.

Melnyk, B. M. (2017). The foundation for improving healthcare quality, patient outcomes, & costs with evidence-based practice. In B. M. Melnyk, L. Gallagher-Ford, & E. Fineout-Overholt (Eds.), *Implementing the evidence-based practice competencies in healthcare. A practice guide for improving quality, safety & outcomes* (pp. 3–18). Indianapolis, IN: Sigma Theta Tau International.

Melnyk, B. M., Alpert-Gillis, L., Feinstein, N. F., Crean, H., Johnson, J., Fairbanks, E., Corbo-Richert, B. (2004). Creating opportunities for parent empowerment (COPE): Program effects on the mental health/coping outcomes of critically ill young children and their mothers. *Pediatrics, 113*(6), e597–e607.

Melnyk, B. M., Buck, J., & Gallagher-Ford, L. (2015). Transforming quality improvement into evidence-based quality improvement: A key solution to improve healthcare outcomes. *Worldviews on Evidence-based Nursing, 12*(5), 251–252.

Melnyk, B. M., & Feinstein, N. F. (2009). Reducing hospital expenditures with the COPE (Creating Opportunities for Parent Empowerment) program for parents and premature infants: An analysis of direct healthcare neonatal intensive care unit costs and savings. *Nursing Administrative Quarterly, 33*(1), 32–37.

Melnyk, B. M., Feinstein, N. F., Alpert-Gillis, L., Fairbanks, E., Crean, H. F., Sinkin, R., Gross, S. J. (2006). Reducing premature infants' length of stay and improving parents' mental health outcomes with the COPE NICU program: A randomized clinical trial. *Pediatrics, 118*(5), 1414–1427.

Melnyk, B. M., & Fineout-Overholt, E. (2015). *Evidence-based practice in nursing & healthcare. A guide to best practice* (3rd ed.). Philadelphia, PA: Wolters Kluwer.

Melnyk, B. M., Fineout-Overholt, E., Gallagher-Ford, L., & Kaplan, L. (2012). The state of evidence-based practice in US nurses: Critical implications for nurse leaders and educators. *Journal of Nursing Administration, 42*(9), 410–417.

Melnyk, B. M., Fineout-Overholt, E., Giggleman, M., & Cruz, R. (2010). Correlates among cognitive beliefs, EBP implementation, organizational culture, cohesion and job satisfaction in evidence-based practice mentors from a community hospital system. *Nursing Outlook, 58*(6), 301–308.

Melnyk, B. M., Fineout-Overholt, E., & Mays, M. (2008). The evidence-based practice beliefs and implementation scales: Psychometric properties of two new instruments. *Worldviews on Evidence-Based Nursing, 5*(4), 208–216.

Melnyk, B. M., Gallagher-Ford, L., Long, L. E., & Fineout-Overholt, E. (2014). The establishment of evidence-based practice competencies for practicing registered nurses and advanced practice nurses in real-world clinical settings: Proficiencies to improve healthcare quality, reliability, patient outcomes, and costs. *Worldviews on Evidence-based Nursing, 11*(1), 5–15.

Melnyk, B. M., Gallagher-Ford, L., Thomas, B., Troseth, M., Wyngarden, K., & Szalacha, L. (2016). A study of chief nurse executives indicates low prioritization of evidence-based practice and shortcomings in hospital performance metrics across the United States. *Worldviews on Evidence-based Nursing, 13*(1), 6–14.

Melnyk, B. M., Gallagher-Ford, L., Zellefrow, C., Tucker, S., Thomas, B., Sinnott, L. T., & Tan, A. (2017). The first U.S. study on nurses' evidence-based practice competencies indicates major deficits that threaten healthcare quality, safety, and patient outcomes. *Worldviews on Evidence-based Nursing, 15*(1), 16–25.

Melnyk, B. M., Grossman, D. C., Chou, R., Mabry-Hernandez, I., Nicholson, W., Dewitt, T. G.; US Preventive Services Task Force. (2012). USPSTF perspective on evidence-based preventive recommendations for children. *Pediatrics, 130*(2), 399–407.

Melnyk, B. M., & Jensen, Z. (2013). *A practical guide to child and adolescent mental health screening, early intervention and health promotion.* New York, NY: NAPNAP.

Melnyk, B. M., & Morrison-Beedy, D. (2012). Setting the stage for intervention research: The "so what," "what exists" and "what's next" factors. In B. M. Melnyk & D. Morrison-Beedy (Eds.), *Designing, conducting, analyzing and funding intervention research. A practical guide for success.* New York, NY: Springer Publishing.

Melnyk, B. M., Orsolini, L., Tan, A., Arslanian-Engoren, C., Melkus, G. D., Dunbar-Jacob., . . . Lewis, L. M. (2017). A National Study Links Nurses' Physical and Mental Health to Medical Errors and Perceived Worksite Wellness. *Journal of Occupational & Environmental Medicine, 60*(2), 126-131.

Sackett, D. L., Straus, S. E., Richardson, W. S., Rosenberg, W., & Haynes, R. B. (2000). *Evidence-based medicine: How to practice and teach EBM.* London, UK: Churchill Livingstone.

Shanafelt, T. D., Hasan, O., Dyrbye, L. N., Sinsky, C., Satele, D., Sloan, J., & West, C. P. (2015). Changes in burnout and satisfaction with work-life balance in physicians and the general U.S. working population between 2011 and 2014. *Mayo Clinic Proceedings, 90*(12), 1600–1613.

Shirey, M., Hauck, S., Embree, J., Kinner, T., Schaar, G., Phillips, L., & McCool, I. (2011). Showcasing differences between quality improvement, evidence-based practice, and research. *Journal of Continuing Education in Nursing, 42*(2), 57–68.

Siu, A. L., Bibbins-Domingo, K., & Grossman, D. (2015). Evidence-based clinical prevention in the era of the patient protection and affordable care act. *Journal of the American Medical Association, 314*(19), 2021–2022.

Squires, J. E., Estabrooks C. A., Gustavsson, P., & Wallin, L. (2011). Individual determinants of research utilization by nurses: A systematic review update. *Implementation Science, 6*, 1–20.

Stetler, C. B., Ritchie, J. A., Rycroft-Malone, J., & Charns, M. P. (2014). Leadership for evidence-based practice: Strategic and functional behaviors for institutionalizing EBP. *Worldviews on Evidence-Based Nursing, 11*(4), 219–226.

Talsma, A., Grady, P. A., Feetham, S., Heinrich, J., & Steinwachs, D. M. (2008). The perfect storm: Patient safety and nursing shortages within the context of health policy and evidence-based practice. *Nursing Research, 57*(1 Suppl), S15–S21.

Task Force on Sudden Infant Death Syndrome. (2016). SIDS and other sleep-related infant deaths: Updated 2016 recommendations for a safe infant sleeping environment. *Pediatrics, 138*(5). doi:10.1542/peds.2016-2938

Ten Ham, W., Minnie, K., & van der Walt, C. (2015). Integrative review of benefit levers' characteristics for system-wide spread of best healthcare practices. *Journal of Advanced Nursing, 72*(1), 33–49.

Tucker, S. (2014). Determining the return on investment for evidence-based practice: An essential skill for all clinicians. *Worldviews on Evidence-based Nursing, 11*(5), 271–273.

The Cochrane Collaboration. (2001). *The Cochrane Collaboration—Informational leaflets.* Retrieved from http://www.cochrane.org/cochrane/cc-broch.htm#cc

Vlada, A. C., Schmit, B., Perry, A., Trevino, J. G., Behms, K. E., & Hughes, S. J. (2013). Failure to follow evidence-based best practice guidelines in the treatment of severe acute pancreatitis. *HPB (Oxford), 15*(10), 822–827.

Wilson, M., Sleutel, M., Newcomb, P., Behan, D., Walsh, J., Wells, J. N., & Baldwin, K. M. (2015). Empowering nurses with evidence-based practice environments: Surveying Magnet˜ Pathway to Excellence, and non-Magnet facilities in one healthcare system. *Worldviews on Evidence-Based Nursing, 12*(1), 12–21.

2 Asking Compelling Clinical Questions

Ellen Fineout-Overholt and Susan B. Stillwell

The important thing is not to stop questioning. Curiosity has its own reason for existing.

—*Albert Einstein*

EBP Terms to Learn
Background question
Body of evidence
Clinical inquiry
Foreground question
PICOT format

Learning Objectives

After studying this chapter, learners will be able to:

1. Explain the components of a PICOT question: population, issue or intervention of interest, comparison of interest, outcome, and time for intervention to achieve the outcome.

2. Discuss the purpose of the PICOT format.

3. Describe the difference among clinical questions, quality improvement questions, and research questions.

4. Describe the difference between background and foreground questions.

5. Craft a clinical question using proper PICOT format.

With ever present technology such as the Internet, patient portals, electronic health records with evidence-based clinical decision support systems, and mobile health applications, seeking and using health information has changed over the past several decades, not only for healthcare professionals, but also for patients, who are increasingly accessing health information via multiple sources (Butler, 2017; Ferran-Ferrer, Minguillón, & Pérez-Montoro, 2013; Shaikh & Shaikh, 2012). Over the past few years, significant strides have been made to make digital health information even more readily available, thus leading to informed evidenced-based clinical decisions (Elias, Polancich, Jones, & Convoy, 2017; Institute of Medicine, 2011) with the aim of improving the patient's experience, population health, and healthcare costs (Butler, 2017; Whittington, Nolan, Lewis, & Torres, 2015). Furthermore, the growing complexity of patient illness has required clinicians to become increasingly proficient at obtaining information they need *when* they need it. Access to reliable information is necessary to this endeavor (Kosteniuk, Morgan, & D'Arcy, 2013), as well as clinicians definitively identifying what they want to know and what they need to access (Fineout-Overholt & Johnston, 2005; Melnyk, Fineout-Overholt, Stillwell, & Williamson, 2010). Resources (e.g., computers, databases, libraries, and digital applications) exist to ensure clinicians can retrieve needed information to perform the best patient care possible, and there is expressed need by policy makers for all patients to receive evidence-based care (Altman, Butler, & Shern, 2015); yet the barrier remains that not all practice environments have or allow unrestricted access to necessary resources. Scantlebury, Booth, and Hanley (2017) found that clinicians continue to have challenges with information access due to fees, time constraints, and quality of computers.

Although many variables influence clinicians' capacity to gather information quickly (e.g., financial ability to purchase a computer, availability of Internet service providers), at minimum, every clinician must be able to articulate the clinical issue in such a way that information retrieval is maximized with the least amount of time investment. Hence, the first step in getting to the right information is to determine the "real" clinical issue and describe it in an answerable fashion, which is the focus of this chapter—a searchable, answerable question. However, skill level in formulating an answerable question can be a barrier to getting the best evidence to apply to practice (Gray, 2010; Green & Ruff, 2005; Rice, 2010). Clinicians continue to ask questions that are not in the proper format—often with directional outcomes (e.g., improved, reduced)—or begin with "what is the effect of," both of which are not clinical questions, rather they are elements to formulating research questions. Furthermore, articles on clinical questions can be confusing with some indicating that the clinical question **PICOT format** (i.e., *P*: population of interest; *I*: intervention or issue of interest; *C*: comparison of interest; *O*: outcome expected; and *T*: time for the intervention to achieve the outcome) is the best approach to developing a research question (Carman, Wolf Henderson, Kamienski, Koziol-McLain, Manton, & Moon, 2013; Riva, Malik, Burnie, Endicott, & Busse, 2012). Elias, Polancich, Jones, and Convoy (2015) advocated that a D be added to PICOT to represent digital data; however, the PICOT question describes the clinical issue about which clinicians will systematically search, not the sources of data or the project; therefore, adding a D would not be beneficial.

This kind of confusion about how to properly write a clinical question can lead to a confusing question and a poorly articulated search for literature to answer it. It is essential for clinical questions to be written well for the rigor of the evidence-based practice (EBP) process to be maintained. The search for evidence depends on a well-written question. This chapter provides clinicians with strategies to hone skills in properly formulating clinical questions to clarify the clinical issue and to minimize the time spent searching for relevant, valid evidence to answer them. To help with mastery of constructing PICOT questions, review Competencies 1 to 3 in Chapter 11.

FINDING THE RIGHT INFORMATION AT THE RIGHT TIME BEGINS WITH A GOOD QUESTION: HOW TO FIND A NEEDLE IN A HAYSTACK

The key to successful patient care for any healthcare professional is to stay informed and as up to date as possible on the latest best practices. *External* pressure to be up to date on clinical issues increasingly comes from patients, employers, certifying organizations, insurers, and healthcare reforms (American Nurses Credentialing Center, 2014; Centers for Medicare and Medicaid Services, 2016; Greiner & Knebel, 2003; Joint Commission, 2017; Rice, 2010). Clinicians' personal desire to provide the best, most up-to-date care possible along with expectations from healthcare consumers that practice will be based on the latest and best evidence fosters EBP (Carman et al., 2016). However, the desire to gather the right information in the right way at the right time is not sufficient. Mastering practical, lifelong learning skills (e.g., asking focused questions, learning to systematically search) is required to negotiate the information-rich environment that clinicians encounter. With the amount of information that clinicians have at their disposal today, finding the right information at the right time is much like weeding through the haystack to find the proverbial needle. If one has any hope of finding the needle, there must be some sense of the needle's characteristics (i.e., a clear understanding of what is the clinical issue). Clinical questions arise from inquiry, which is the initial step of the EBP process. Clinicians become curious about a clinical issue that they then turn into a question. In recent years, patients or laypersons are also engaging inquiry and asking clinical questions along with clinicians. Whoever initiates the question, it is important to carefully consider how to ask it so that it is reasonable to answer. Formulating the clinical question is much like identifying the characteristics of the needle. Question components guide the searching strategies undertaken to find answers. Yet, clinicians are not always equipped to formulate searchable questions (Melnyk, Fineout-Overholt, Feinstein, Sadler, & Green-Hernandez, 2008), which often can result in irrelevant results and inefficient use of clinicians' time (Rice, 2010). Once the needle's characteristics are well understood (i.e., the PICOT question), knowing how to sift through the haystack (i.e., the evidence) becomes easier (see Chapter 3 for information on mastering systematic searching).

A Cumulative Index of Nursing and Allied Health Literature (CINAHL) search for evidence to determine how clinicians use the PICOT format in asking clinical questions revealed 14 results with four hits describing the PICOT question as a research question. None spoke of examining how clinicians have mastered using the PICOT format in asking clinical questions. Though some of these studies were conducted over 10 years ago, they offer insight into continuing challenges for clinicians in using the PICOT format to ask clinical questions. Huang, Lin, and Demnar-Fushman (2006) found in a study examining the utility of asking clinical questions in PICOT format that when clinicians asked clinical questions for their patient's clinical issues, their format almost always fell short of addressing all the aspects needed to clearly identify the clinical issue. Two of 59 questions contained an intervention (*I*) and outcome (*O*), but no other components (*P, C,* or *T*), although these aspects were appropriate. Currie et al. (2003) indicated that approximately two thirds of clinicians' questions are either not pursued or answers are not found even though pursued. However, if properly formulated, the question could lead to a more effective search. Price and Christenson (2013) concur with these researchers' findings, indicating that getting the question right determines the success of the entire EBP process. In addition, in a randomized controlled trial (RCT) examining the effect of a consulting service that provides up-to-date information to clinicians, Mulvaney et al. (2008) found that such a knowledge broker improves the use of evidence and subsequent care and outcomes. However, without having a well-built question to communicate what clinicians genuinely want to know, efforts to search for or provide appraised evidence will likely be less than profitable. Hoogendam, de Vries Robbé, and Overbeke (2012) determined that the PICO(T) format was not helpful in guiding efficient searches; however, their report did not indicate how they measured the proficiency of the participants in writing PICOT questions or how they were taught question formulation. How a question is written makes a difference in how the search is conducted. Writing a research question will lead searchers in a different direction—often yielding biased results focused only on studies that demonstrated improvement in desired outcomes. How searchers learn to use PICOT questions to drive a systematic search compared with traditional searching also is key to successful searching. Understanding how to properly formulate a clinical question in PICOT format and using it systematically in your search is essential to effectively begin the EBP process.

The Haystack: Too Much Information

Although there is a plethora of information available and increasingly new modalities to access it, news of clinical advances can diffuse rather slowly through the literature. Additionally, for years, only a small percentage of clinicians have been known to access and use the information in a timely fashion (Cobban, Edgington, & Clovis, 2008; Estabrooks, O'Leary, Ricker, & Humphrey, 2003; MacIntosh-Murray & Choo, 2005; McCloskey, 2008; Melnyk, Fineout-Overholt, Gallagher-Ford, & Kaplan, 2012; Pravikoff, Tanner, & Pierce, 2005).

Clinicians are challenged with the task of effectively, proactively, and rapidly sifting through the haystack of scientific information to find the right needle with the best applicable information for a patient or practice. Scott, Estabrooks, Allen, and Pollock (2008) found that uncertainty in clinicians' work environment promoted a disregard for research as relevant to practice. In a 2012 study of over 1,000 nurses, Melnyk and colleagues reinforced these researchers' finding with their participants indicating that lack of access to information was one of the top five deterrents to implementing EBP in daily practice. To reduce uncertainty and facilitate getting the right information at the right time, EBP emphasizes first asking a well-built question, then searching the literature for an answer to the question. This will better prepare all clinicians to actively discuss the best available evidence with colleagues and their patients.

The EBP process focuses on incorporating good information-seeking habits into a daily routine. Pravikoff et al. (2005) indicated that not all nurses were engaged in daily information seeking, supporting the notion that, in a busy clinical setting, there is seldom time to seek out information, a finding reinforced in the study by Melnyk et al. (2012). The purchase of a good medical text and regular perusal of the top journals in a specialty were once considered adequate for keeping up with new information, but scientific information is expanding faster than anyone could have foreseen. The result is that significant clinical advances occur so rapidly that they can easily be overlooked. Reading every issue of the top three or four journals in a particular field from cover to cover does not guarantee that clinicians' professional and clinical knowledge is current. With the increase in biomedical knowledge (especially information about clinical advances), it is clear that the traditional notion of "keeping up with the literature" is no longer practical. Before the knowledge explosion as we know it today, Haynes (1993) indicated that a clinician would have to read 17 to 19 journal articles a day, 365 days a year to remain current. This compels every clinician to move toward an emphasis on more proactive information-seeking skills, starting with formulating an answerable, patient-specific question.

Digitization and the Internet have improved accessibility to information, regardless of space and time; however, these innovations have not resolved the issue of finding the right information at the right time. It is important to become friendly with and proficient at utilizing information technology, including the Internet and other electronic information resources, which means that clinicians must be skilled at using a computer. Access to computers and other sources of digital data at the point of care also is essential (Elias, Polancich, Jones, & Convoy, 2017). It bears repeating that though this access is paramount and germane to searching for evidence, to add a D to the PICOT format to represent digital data is not helpful and has the potential to add confusion to the clinicians' understanding of the purpose of the PICOT question. That said, it is essential that clinicians consider digital data as a primary source of evidence for their systematic search. The information needed cannot be obtained if the clinician has to leave the unit or seek an office to locate a computer to retrieve evidence. Proficient use and access to computers are essential to EBP and best practice. In addition, the same barriers have been described by nurses and other healthcare professionals to getting the right information at the right time for some time, including (a) access to information; (b) a low comfort level with library and search techniques; (c) access to electronic resources; and (d) a lack of time to search for the best evidence (Melnyk & Fineout-Overholt, 2002; Melnyk et al., 2012; Pravikoff et al., 2005; Sackett, Straus, Richardson, Rosenberg, & Haynes, 2000; Ubbink, Guyatt, & Vermeulen, 2013; Warren et al., 2016). Mastering how to construct a properly formatted, well-thought-out clinical question will lead to an efficient search process. Other barriers to finding the necessary evidence to improve patient outcomes can be adequately addressed through clinicians first learning to ask a searchable, answerable question.

> **"**
> A prudent question is one-half of wisdom.
>
> **FRANCIS BACON**

ASKING SEARCHABLE, ANSWERABLE QUESTIONS

Finding the right information in a timely way amid an overwhelming amount of information is imperative. The first step to accomplish this goal is to formulate the clinical issue into a searchable, answerable question. It is important to distinguish between the two types of questions that clinicians might ask: **background questions** and **foreground questions**.

Background Questions

Background questions are those that need to be answered as a foundation for asking the searchable, answerable foreground question (Fineout-Overholt & Johnston, 2005; Spek, Waard, Lucas, & van Dijk, 2013; Stillwell, Fineout-Overholt, Melnyk, & Williamson, 2010; Straus, Richardson, Glasziou, & Haynes, 2011). These questions ask for general information about a clinical issue. This type of question usually has two components: the starting place of the question (e.g., what, where, when, why, and how) and the outcome of interest (e.g., the clinical diagnosis). The following is an example of a background question: How does the drug acetaminophen work to affect fever? The answer to this question can be found in a drug pharmacokinetics text. Another example of a background question is "How does hemodynamics differ with positioning?" This answer can be found in textbooks as well.

Often, background questions are far broader in scope than foreground questions. Clinicians often want to know the best method to prevent a clinically undesirable outcome: "What is the best method to prevent pressure ulcers during hospitalization?" This question will lead to a foreground question, but background knowledge is necessary before the foreground question can be asked (i.e., not all the PICOT components are known). In this example, the clinician must know what methods of pressure ulcer prevention are being used. Generally, this information comes from knowledge of what is currently being used in clinicians' practices and what viable alternatives are available to improve patient outcomes, or the information may come from descriptive research, such as survey research. Once the methods most supported are identified, clinicians can formulate the foreground question and compare the two most effective methods of pressure ulcer prevention by asking the following foreground PICOT question: In my population, how does the alternative intervention compared with the current intervention affect the outcome that I am concerned is not meeting expectations? The time frame would differ with specific interventions. If a clinician does not realize the difference between a foreground and a background question, time may be lost in searching for an answer in the wrong haystack (e.g., electronic evidence databases vs. a textbook).

Foreground Questions

Foreground questions are those that can be answered from scientific evidence about diagnosing, treating, or assisting patients in understanding their prognosis or their health experience. These questions focus on specific knowledge. In the first two background question examples, the subsequent foreground questions could be as follows: In children, how does acetaminophen affect fever within 30 minutes of administration compared with ibuprofen? In patients with acute respiratory distress syndrome, how does the prone position compared with the supine position affect heart rate, cardiac output, oxygen saturation, and blood pressure after position change? The first question builds on the background knowledge of how acetaminophen works but can be answered only by a group of studies (i.e., **body of evidence**) that compare the two listed medications. The second question requires the knowledge of how positioning changes hemodynamics (i.e., the background question) and in particular the outcomes listed, but the two types of positioning must be compared in a body of evidence focused on a specific population of patients to best answer it. The foreground question generated from the third background question example could be as follows: In patients at high risk for pressure ulcers, how do pressure mattresses compared with pressure overlays affect the incidence of pressure ulcers within a week of application? The answer provided by the body of evidence would indicate whether pressure mattresses or overlays are more effective in preventing pressure ulcers in the high-risk population. The most effective method established by the body of evidence will become the standard of care that will be delivered to all patients in the given population. Recognizing the difference between the two types of questions is the challenge. To help gain mastery of understanding the difference between background and foreground questions, review more examples in Table 2.1.

Straus, Richardson, Glasziou, and Haynes (2011) stated that a novice might need to ask primarily background questions. As one gains experience, the background knowledge grows, and the focus changes to foreground questions. Although background questions are essential and must be asked, the foreground questions are the searchable, answerable questions that, when answered, drive practice and are the focus of this chapter.

Clinical Inquiry and Uncertainty in Generating Clinical Questions

Where clinical questions come from (i.e., their origin) is an important consideration. On a daily basis, most clinicians encounter situations for which they do not have all the information they need (i.e., uncertainty) to care for their patients as they would like (Kamhi, 2011; Nelson, 2011; Scott et al., 2008). The role of uncertainty is to spawn **clinical inquiry**, which can be defined as a process in which clinicians gather data using narrowly defined clinical parameters to appraise the available choices of treatment to find the most appropriate choice of action (Horowitz, Singer, Makuch, & Viscoli, 1996).

Clinical inquiry must be cultivated in the work environment. To foster clinical inquiry, one must have a level of comfort with uncertainty. Uncertainty is the inability to predict what an experience will mean or what outcome will occur when encountering ambiguity (Cranley, Doran, Tourangeau, Kushniruk, & Nagle, 2009; Scott et al., 2008). Although uncertainty may be uncomfortable, uncertainty is imperative to good practice (Carman et al., 2016;

TABLE 2.1	Comparing Background and Foreground Questions

Background Question	Foreground Question
(General Approach—"I Was Just Wondering")	(Want to Find a Body of Evidence [Studies] to Answer It)
What is the best approach to new nurse retention?	In newly graduated licensed nurses, how does a nurse residency program compared with traditional precepted orientation affect retention rates after 1 year?
How does a clinical decision support system (CDSS) help clinicians provide best care?	In acute care clinicians, how does an electronic health record (EHR) with a CDSS compared with an EHR without a CDSS affect a clinician's adherence to clinical pathway choices, documentation of care, and completion of documentation within his or her given shift?
How do parents cope with their hospitalized children's illness?	How do parents with ill children perceive their coping skills during hospitalization?

Kamhi, 2011), and is a means to inquiry and clinical reasoning (Engebretsen, Heggen, Wieringa, & Greenhalgh, 2016) needed for developing focused foreground questions (Nelson, 2011).

Clinicians live in a rather uncertain world. Although seeking information to resolve uncertainty may be beneficial, the outcome may not be realized or may even be harmful (Hsee & Ruan, 2016). What works for one patient may not work for another or the same patient in a different setting. The latest product on the market claims that it is the solution to wound healing, but is it? Collaborating partners in caring for complex patients have their own ways of providing care. Formulating clinical questions in a structured, specific way, such as in PICOT format, assists clinicians to find the right evidence to answer those questions and to decrease uncertainty. This approach to asking clinical questions facilitates a well-constructed systematic search. Experienced evidence-based clinicians would agree with Price and Christenson (2013), who indicated that the PICOT question is the key to the entire EBP process. Success with PICOT question formation fosters further clinical inquiry.

> "
> ### By doubting we are led to question, by questioning we arrive at the truth.
>
> **PETER ABELARD**

Formatting Foreground Questions to Drive the Search

Clinical circumstances, such as interpretation of patient assessment data (e.g., clinical findings from a physical examination or laboratory data), a desire to determine the most likely cause of the patient's problem among the many it could be (i.e., differential diagnosis), or simply wanting to improve one's clinical skills in a specific area, can prompt the following five types of foreground questions:

1. Intervention questions that ask what intervention most effectively leads to an outcome;
2. Prognosis/prediction questions that ask what indicators are most predictive of or carry the most associated risk for an outcome;
3. Diagnosis questions that ask what mechanism or test most accurately diagnoses an outcome;
4. Etiology questions that ask to what extent a factor, process, or condition is highly associated with an outcome, usually undesirable;
5. Meaning questions that ask how an experience influences an outcome, the scope of a phenomenon, or perhaps the influence of culture on healthcare.

Whatever the reason for the question, the components of the question need to be considered and formulated carefully using the proper format to efficiently find relevant evidence to answer the question.

Posing the Question Using PICOT

Focused foreground questions are essential to judiciously finding the right evidence to answer them (Hartzell & Fineout-Overholt, 2017; Schardt, Adams, Owens, Keitz, & Fontelo, 2007). Foreground questions posed using PICOT format offer a sound framework to construct the systematic search required to gather the body of evidence needed to guide practice (Hartzell & Fineout-Overholt, 2017). Thoughtful consideration of each PICOT component can provide a clearly articulated question. Using a consistent approach to writing the PICOT question assists the clinician to systematically identify the clinical issue (Stillwell et al., 2010). Table 2.2 provides a quick overview of the PICOT question components. Well-built, focused clinical questions drive the subsequent steps of the EBP process (Hartzell & Fineout-Overholt, 2017; O'Connor, Green,

TABLE
2.2
PICOT: Components of an Answerable, Searchable Question

PICOT Component	Description
Patient population/disease	The patient population or disease of interest, for example: • Age • Gender • Ethnicity • With certain disorder (e.g., hepatitis)
Intervention or Issue of interest	The intervention or range of issues of interest: • Therapy • Exposure to disease • Prognostic factor A • Risk behavior (e.g., smoking)
Comparison intervention or issue of interest	What you want to compare the intervention or issue against: • Alternative therapy, placebo, or no intervention/therapy • No disease • Prognostic factor B • Absence of risk factor (e.g., nonsmoking)
Outcome	Outcome of interest: • Outcome expected from therapy (e.g., pressure ulcers) • Risk of disease • Accuracy of diagnosis • Rate of occurrence of adverse outcome (e.g., death)
Time	The time involved to demonstrate an outcome: • The time it takes for the intervention to achieve the outcome • The time over which populations are observed for the outcome (e.g., quality of life) to occur, given a certain condition (e.g., prostate cancer)

& Higgins, 2011). As a result, clinicians, faculty, or leaders who do not invest in understanding the proper use for the PICOT format are likely not equipped to teach or guide clinicians or students how to best construct a well-written clinical question.

The purpose of the PICOT question is to guide the systematic search of healthcare databases to find the best available evidence to answer the question. It is important to remember that the PICOT question is NOT an EBP project.

DR. ELLEN FINEOUT-OVERHOLT

The patient population (**P**) may seem easy to identify. However, without explicit description of who the population is, the clinician can get off on the wrong foot in searching. The *Cochrane Handbook for Systematic Reviews of Interventions* (O'Connor et al., 2011) suggests careful consideration of the patient and the setting of interest. Limiting the population to those in a certain age group or other special subgroups (e.g., young adult females with lung cancer) is a good idea if there is a valid reason for doing so. Arbitrary designations for the patient population will not help the clinician retrieve the most relevant evidence.

The intervention or issue of interest (*I*) may include but is not limited to any exposure, treatment, diagnostic test, condition, or predictor/prognostic factor, or it may be an issue that the clinician is interested in, such as fibromyalgia or a new diagnosis of cancer. For example, if the (*I*) is an intervention, it is what clinicians determine from background information that may be a reasonable alternative to current practice. The more specifically the intervention or issue of interest is defined, the more focused the search will be.

The comparison (*C*) needs special consideration, because it is sometimes appropriate to include in a question and not needed at other times. If the (*I*) is an intervention, the comparison should be the usual standard of care. Some clinicians use "usual care" in their PICOT question; however, this does not provide reliable information for the systematic search, and, therefore, identifying the current treatment falling short of achieving the desired outcome is necessary. For example, a clinician wants to ask the question, in disabled, older adult patients (*P*), how does the use of level-access showers (*I*) compared with bed bathing (*C*) affect patient satisfaction with hygiene (*O*)? The intervention of interest is level-access showers, and the comparison is the usual care of bed bathing. In a meaning question, the (*I*) is an issue of interest. For example, a meaning question may be, "How do parents (*P*) with children who have been newly diagnosed with cancer (*I*) perceive their parent role (*O*) within the first month after diagnosis (*T*)?" In this question, there is no appropriate comparison to the issue of interest, and, therefore, *C* is not found in the question.

The outcome (*O*) in the intervention example above is patient satisfaction with their hygiene and the outcome of the meaning question above is the parental role. Specifically identifying the outcome in a question enables the searcher to find evidence that examined the same outcome variable, although the variable may be measured in various ways.

In some questions, there may be more than one outcome of interest found in a study, but all of these outcomes are affected by the intervention or issue. For example, the question may be, "In preschool-age children (*P*), how does a flavored electrolyte drink (*I*) compared with water alone (*C*) affect symptoms of dry mouth (*O1*), tachycardia (*O2*), fever (*O3*), and irritability (*O4*) during playtime?" An alternate way to format the question may be to use the umbrella term *dehydration* for all these listed symptoms; however, clinicians would keep in mind each of the outcomes that they desire to change. The question would then be, "In preschool-age children, how does a flavored electrolyte drink compared with water alone affect dehydration (e.g., dry mouth, tachycardia, fever, irritability) during playtime?" Specifying the outcome will assist the clinician to focus the search for relevant evidence.

Considering whether a time frame (*T*) is associated with the outcome is also part of asking a PICOT question. For example, "In family members who have a relative undergoing cardiopulmonary resuscitation (*P*), how does presence during the resuscitation (*I*) compared with no presence (*C*) affect family anxiety (*O*) during the resuscitation period (*T*)?" In the intervention example given earlier, there is no specific time identified for bathing or showering to achieve patient satisfaction with hygiene, because it is immediately on completion of these interventions. Although this is understood, it would not be incorrect to use "immediately after intervention" as the *T* for this question. However, for the meaning question example, it would be important to consider that the first month after diagnosis may be a critical time for parental role to be actualized for this population; therefore, it is essential to include a specific time in the question. To answer this meaning question, studies that collected data to evaluate parental role for at least 1 month after diagnosis would be sought; studies with evaluation of parental role with less than 1 month would not be an acceptable answer to the question. *T* and *C* are not always appropriate for every question; however, *P*, *I*, and *O* must always be present. Finally, it is important to note that *T* does not mean "therapy" or the "type" of PICOT question. *T* means *time* and is critical to the PICOT question when the outcome requires time to manifest. For example, "In patients who are mechanically ventilated (*P*), how does oral care colistin mouthwashes (*I*) compared with oral care with chlorhexidine buccal swabs (*C*) affect ventilator-associated pneumonia (*O*) during the ICU stay (*T*)?"

Distinguishing Between PICOT, Research, and Quality Improvement Questions

Different question types have different purposes. Three common types of questions used in healthcare—PICOT questions, research questions, and quality improvement (QI) questions—may appear similar but have different purposes and formats (Table 2.3). Standardized language within different types of question is reflected in how the question is formatted, which offers insight into understanding the intent of the question and type of evidence that can be produced by the question. Consider that research questions have a directional outcome (i.e., to reduce or improve). Clinical questions want to gather all of the evidence—the body of evidence—so there is no distinction about the outcome. QI questions are focused on processes that influence outcomes, so they often contain "why." To help gain mastery in understanding the difference between clinical, research, and QI questions, see if you can distinguish which kind of question is needed to get the team the answer they need within the scenario in Box 2.1.

Three Ps of Proficient Questioning: Practice, Practice, Practice

The best way to become proficient in formulating searchable, answerable questions is to practice. This section includes five clinical scenarios that offer you the opportunity to practice formulating a searchable, answerable question. Read each scenario and try to formulate the question using the appropriate template for the type of question required (see Box 2.2 for

TABLE 2.3 *Differentiating Clinical, Research, and Quality Improvement Questions*

	Clinical Question	Research Question	Quality Improvement Question
Purpose	To guide the systematic search for evidence to determine the best intervention to affect the outcome	To generate new knowledge/external evidence	To identify and fix the processes leading to a problem that is internal to the clinical setting
Evidence type	Best available evidence	External evidence	Internal evidence
Example	In postoperative kidney transplant patients (P), how does a health coach (I) compared with no health coaching (i.e., current practice) (C) affect hospital readmission rates (O1) and patient satisfaction (O2) within 90 days of discharge (T)? PICOT format required	What is the effect of a health coach on kidney transplant patients' satisfaction with hospitalization? What is the effect of health coaching on kidney transplant patients' readmission rates?	Why is hospital readmission rate in our post-kidney transplant patient population so high? On our Press Ganey reports, why are our patient satisfaction scores not meeting benchmarks for our kidney transplant patients?

Test Yourself: Can You Find the Right Question?

Quality Improvement (QI)

The intensive care unit evidence-based practice (EBP) team consisting of critical care nurses, physicians, and respiratory therapists have noticed an increase in ventilator-associated pneumonia in trauma patients who are intubated and on ventilators. This is a surprising outcome for the EBP team.

Select the relevant QI question:

a) Does oral care with chlorhexidine reduce ventilator-associated pneumonia in patients receiving mechanical ventilation?
b) Why are ventilator-associated pneumonia rates so high in our trauma patients?
c) In trauma patients who are mechanically ventilated, how do chlorhexidine mouthwashes compared with probiotics affect ventilator-associated pneumonia development?

Research

The EBP team is frustrated with this pulmonary complication and is wondering how to reduce it. They wonder if they would need to do a research study.

Select the relevant research question:

a) Does oral care with chlorhexidine improve ventilator-associated pneumonia rates in patients receiving mechanical ventilation?
b) Why are ventilator-associated pneumonia rates so high in our trauma patients?
c) In trauma patients who are mechanically ventilated, how do probiotics compared with no probiotics affect ventilator-associated pneumonia development while on the ventilator?

Intervention Clinical Question

In their brainstorming session, they discuss several options that members of the team have heard other agencies are doing and consider two interventions they feel will work in their organization: (1) starting a chlorhexidine mouthwash protocol and (2) probiotics for their mechanically ventilated patients. The EBP mentor acknowledges their frustration and desire for a quick fix, guides the group to understand that formulating a clinical question is a better choice to consider when the goal is to improve patient outcomes, and the team moves forward with the EBP process.

Select the intervention clinical question:

a) Why are ventilator-associated pneumonia rates so high in our trauma patients?
b) Which is more effective in reducing ventilator-associated pneumonia in patients receiving mechanical ventilation, chlorhexidine, or probiotics?
c) In trauma patients who are mechanically ventilated, how do chlorhexidine mouthwashes compared with probiotics affect ventilator-associated pneumonia development while on the ventilator?

Answer QI: b; Research: a; Clinical Question: c

| BOX 2.2 | *Question Templates for Asking PICOT Questions* |

Intervention

In _____ (*P*), how does _____ (*I*) compared with _____ (*C*) affect _____ (*O*) within _____ (*T*)?

Prognosis/Prediction

In _____ (*P*), how does _____ (*I*) compared with _____ (*C*) influence/predict _____ (*O*) over _____ (*T*)?

Diagnosis or Diagnostic Test

In _____ (*P*) are/is _____ (*I*) compared with _____ (*C*) more accurate in diagnosing _____ (*O*)?

Etiology

Are _____ (*P*), who have _____ (*I*) compared with those without _____ (*C*) at _____ risk for/of _____ (*O*) over _____ (*T*)?

Meaning

How do _____ (*P*) with _____ (*I*) perceive _____ (*O*) during _____ (*T*)?

---

a list of all question types and templates; see Appendix A). You may be tempted to ask the question in any format you choose. It is highly recommended that you use the templates to formulate each question to ensure that components of the question (i.e., PICOT) are not missed. Furthermore, the templates offer the proper standardized language to ensure that the question is a clinical question versus a directional research question, a QI question, or a background question. Once you craft your questions, read the discussion section that follows to determine the success of your question formulation.

All of these examples and templates are intended to help you master formulating a well-constructed clinical question. There may be various ways in which to ask a certain type of question; however, all the appropriate components must be present in the question. Clinicians, whether novice or expert, who use the PICOT format to construct a clinical question ensure that no component is missed and increase the likelihood that the question is answered (Huang et al., 2006; Price & Christenson, 2013). Consider your clinical scenario and try to identify the PICOT components specifically. Then formulate the clinical question, complete with question mark. Carefully consider which template may work for the clinical situation driving your question; it is not wise to try to form cookie-cutter questions (e.g., applying the intervention template to every situation), because some important component(s) most assuredly will be missed.

When evaluating the appropriateness of each question that arises from clinical issues you are most concerned about, consider the harm, cost, feasibility, and availability of the intervention, diagnostic test, or condition, because these can preclude the ability to apply the evidence to clinical practice. These issues also influence ethical considerations for implementing the best evidence (see Chapter 23).

Clinical Scenario 2.1 Intervention Example

Scenario

Glenda, a 45-year-old Caucasian woman, 5'6" weighing 250 lb, presented to her primary care provider (PCP) with complaints of malaise and "pressure in her head." The physical examination revealed that she was hypertensive (blood pressure [BP] 160/98 mm Hg). Her PCP asked her about her lifestyle. After gathering data, Glenda and her PCP agreed that she had an excessive amount of stress in her life. Her weight, sedentary job, and stressful lifestyle were discussed as they decided on her treatment plan. Her PCP recommended first putting her on an angiotensin converting enzyme (ACE) inhibitor for 6 months; however, Glenda was concerned about its effects because she had an aunt who did not tolerate an ACE inhibitor. Also, she wondered how adding exercise and dietary alterations to promote weight loss would affect her BP. She had heard on the evening news that for every 10 lb of weight loss, BP was reduced by 5 mm Hg. As Glenda's PCP, you want to make sure that she is safe, so you inform her that you are going to do a little homework to find out the latest evidence.

Intervention Clinical Question Template

This clinical scenario is about an intervention. Given the PICOT format below for an intervention question, fill in the blanks with information from the clinical scenario.

In _____ (**P**), how does _____ (**I**) compared with _____ (**C**) affect _____ (**O**) within _____ (**T**)?

Discussion

Remember that a well-formulated question is the key to a successful search. The question could be, "In middle-aged Caucasian obese females (body mass index [BMI] > 30 kg/m^2) (**P**), how do lifestyle interventions (e.g., healthy diet, exercise, and stress reduction) (**I**) compared with daily administration of ACE inhibitors (**C**) affect BP (**O**) over 6 months (**T**)?" A more general background question might read, "In overweight women, what is the best method for reducing high BP?" Background knowledge would be necessary to know the lifestyle interventions that may reduce BP in this population. Intervention questions are about what clinicians do; therefore, it is important to be able to determine the *best* intervention to achieve an outcome. Once the question has been answered with confidence (i.e., a body of evidence filled with well-done studies that agree on the best intervention to achieve the outcome), the next step would be implementing the interventions in practice, evaluating their outcomes, and establishing them as the standard of care.

In this example, the patient's concern is about her recognition of the impact of lifestyle change on hypertension and her prior experience with a family member who did not have successful results with ACE inhibitors. She is asking the clinician to provide her with information about how successful she can be with what she prefers to engage versus what may be the accepted practice. Therefore, the *I* is the intervention that is most desired (e.g., lifestyle interventions) and the *C* is what is the current standard of care or usual practice (e.g., ACE inhibitors).

The evidence to answer this type of question requires substantiated cause-and-effect relationships. The research design that best provides this cause-and-effect information is an RCT. An RCT is defined as having three key elements:

continued on the following page

(1) an intervention or treatment group that receives the intervention; (2) a comparison or control group that has a comparison or control intervention; and (3) random assignment to either group (i.e., assignment of patients to either the experimental or comparison/control group by using chance, such as a flip of a coin). The groups are evaluated on whether or not an expected outcome is achieved. In the example, we would look for studies with a defined sample (e.g., overweight women) with common characteristics (e.g., BMI > 30 kg/m^2) that were randomly assigned to the intervention (i.e., lifestyle interventions) and the comparison (i.e., daily ACE inhibitors) and evaluated if the desired outcome was achieved (i.e., reduction in BP values). Ideally, we would search for a synthesis, or compilation of studies, that compared how daily administration of ACE inhibitors and weight loss affected BP. A synthesis of these RCTs is considered Level 1 evidence to answer this type of question.

TABLE 2.4	Examples of Different Types of Clinical Questions in PICOT Format and Their Associated Levels of Evidence Hierarchy
Types of Clinical Questions With PICOT Example	**Levels of Evidence to Answer This Type of Question**
Intervention: In patients living in a long-term care facility who are at risk for pressure ulcers (**P**), how does a pressure ulcer prevention program (**I**) compared with the standard of care (e.g., turning every 2 hours) (**C**) affect signs of emerging pressure ulcers (**O**)? **OR** **Diagnosis or diagnostic test:** In patients with suspected deep vein thrombosis (**P**) is D-dimer assay (**I**) compared with ultrasound (**C**) more accurate in diagnosing deep vein thrombosis (**O**)?	1. Systematic review/metaanalysis (i.e., synthesis) of RCTs 2. RCTs 3. Non-RCTs 4. Cohort study or case–control studies 5. Metasynthesis of qualitative or descriptive studies 6. Qualitative or descriptive single studies 7. Expert opinion
Prognosis/prediction: In patients who have a family history of obesity (BMI > 30 kg/m^2) (**P**), how does dietary carbohydrate intake (**I**) predict healthy weight maintenance (BMI < 25 kg/m^2) (**O**) over 6 months (**T**)? **OR** **Etiology:** Are fair-skinned women (**P**) who have prolonged unprotected UV ray exposure (>1 hour) (**I**) compared with darker-skinned women without prolonged unprotected UV ray exposure (**C**) at increased risk of melanoma (**O**)?	1. Synthesis of cohort study or case–control studies 2. Single cohort study or case–control studies 3. Metasynthesis of qualitative or descriptive studies 4. Single qualitative or descriptive studies 5. Expert opinion
Meaning: How do middle-aged women (**P**) with fibromyalgia (**I**) perceive loss of motor function (**O**)?	1. Metasynthesis of qualitative studies 2. Single qualitative studies 3. Synthesis of descriptive studies 4. Single descriptive studies 5. Expert opinion

BMI, body mass index; RCTs, randomized controlled trials.

Keep in mind that syntheses are always Level 1 evidence, no matter what kind of question you may ask. Table 2.4 provides an example of a clinical question and the levels of evidence that would answer that question. The Level 1 evidence is listed first. If well done (i.e., bias is minimized through rigorous research methods), this type of research would provide the valid information that would enable us to have confidence in using the findings in clinical practice. With each drop in the level of evidence and/or drop in the quality of evidence, the confidence in using the findings drops. Hence, it is best to search for Level 1 evidence first. It is important to keep in mind that the type of the clinical question will indicate the study design that would be synthesized as Level 1 evidence for that question (e.g., intervention questions require a synthesis of RCTs as Level 1 evidence).

In the desired RCTs found in our example, the BP values for both groups would be evaluated after they received either what is called the experimental intervention (i.e., lifestyle interventions) or the comparison intervention (i.e., ACE inhibitor). It is important that the evaluation of the outcome occurs after the individuals receive the intervention; otherwise, causality is in question. Also, it is important that all other factors (e.g., age, comorbidities, genetic predisposition to high BP) that may influence the outcome (e.g., BP) be considered and key factors be accounted for (i.e., data are collected about these key factors that may influence outcome - also called controlled for, hence the name ran-domized *controlled* trial). When these factors are controlled for, and if it is shown that weight loss does just as good a job as or a better job than ACE inhibitors in reducing BP, clinicians can confidently prescribe weight loss as an alternative intervention to manage high BP for those who prefer it.

Clinical Scenario 2.2 Prognosis Example

Scenario

Shawn is a 63-year-old man diagnosed with prostate cancer. He has been married to his wife, Laura, for 40 years and is greatly concerned about his ability to be physically intimate with her should he pursue surgery as a treatment method. He mentions that he is most interested in living his life fully with as much normality as he can for as long as he can. He requests information about whether or not having surgery will be the best plan for him.

Prognosis Clinical Question Template

This clinical scenario concerns prognosis. The following is the format for prognosis questions. Fill in the blanks with information from the clinical scenario.

In ＿＿＿＿＿ (**P**), how does ＿＿＿＿＿ (**I**) compared with ＿＿＿＿＿(**C**) influence or predict ＿＿＿＿＿ (**O**)?

Discussion

The prognosis/prediction question for this example could read as follows: In older adult patients with prostate cancer (**P**), how does choosing to undergo surgery (**I**) compared with choosing not to undergo surgery (**C**) influence lifespan and quality of life (**O**)?

continued on the following page

Prognosis/prediction questions assist the clinician to estimate a patient's clinical course across time. This type of question allows inference about the likelihood that certain outcomes will occur. Clinical issues that may lend themselves to be addressed with a prognosis/predictive question could involve patients' choices and future outcomes. The difference in prognosis or prediction questions and intervention questions is that the conditions (*I* and *C*) cannot be randomized owing to the potential for harm (i.e., this would be unethical). In these questions, the *I* is the issue of interest (e.g., choice to have surgery) and the *C* is the counter to the issue of interest (i.e., the negative case; e.g., choice not to have surgery).

This is an important distinction for prognosis/predictive questions. Therefore, an answer to a prognosis/prediction question would require a study that examined a group of people with an identified condition (e.g., prostate cancer) that self-selected the issue of interest and counter issue (e.g., choosing surgery or not) and was observed over time to evaluate the likelihood of an outcome occurring or not. In the example, we would look for studies that followed a group of older adults with prostate cancer (a *cohort*) who chose to have surgery (*I*) or not (*C*), and then evaluated how the older adults reported their quality of life and how long they lived. This is called a *cohort study*. A single cohort study (i.e., not a synthesis) would be considered Level 2 evidence for prognosis/prediction questions (see Table 2.4). If there was a synthesis of cohort studies examining older adults with prostate cancer who had surgery or not and their relationship between their choice, their quality of life, and how long they lived, then that would be Level 1 evidence. Case–control studies, further discussed in Chapter 5, are another study design that can be used to answer this kind of question.

Clinical Scenario 2.3 Diagnosis Example

Scenario

Renada, a 58-year-old woman, is having increased gastroesophageal reflux, clay-colored stools, and overall malaise. She is greatly concerned, because her brother had so many gallstones that they adhered to his liver and his gallbladder completely ceased to function; she has also heard that gallstones can be extremely painful, even dangerous. She asks you what is the best way to diagnose dysfunction in the gallbladder. You usually order an ultrasound as the first diagnostic for this population, but wonder with Renada's history if a hepatobiliary iminodiacetic acid (HIDA) scan may be a better choice. Both offer visual representations of the liver, gallbladder, biliary tract, and small intestine, but you decide to explore the literature to see what the evidence tells you about which diagnostic tool will get the best outcomes.

Diagnosis Clinical Question Template

This clinical scenario is about diagnosis. Given the format for diagnosis questions, fill in the blanks with information from the clinical scenario.

In _____ (*P*) are/is _____ (*I*) compared with _____ (*C*) more accurate in diagnosing _____ (*O*)?

Discussion

Questions about diagnosis are focused on determining how reliable a test is for clinical practice (i.e., will the test correctly identify the outcome each time it is used?). Risks of the test, likelihood of misdiagnosis of a high-risk outcome, and cost of the test are some of the considerations for how such questions would be answered. Benefit of the test to patients is the overall goal of these kinds of questions. In the clinical example, the question could read as follows: In patients at high risk for gallbladder dysfunction (signs and symptoms plus family history) (**P**), is a HIDA scan (**I**) compared with an ultrasound (**C**) more accurate in diagnosing eminent gallbladder dysfunction (**O**)?

The evidence to answer this type of question requires substantiated certainty that the diagnostic test will reliably provide a true positive (i.e., the outcome does exist and is diagnosed accurately by the test) or true negative (i.e., the outcome does not exist and is accurately diagnosed as such by the test). The research design that best provides this information (Level 1) is a synthesis of RCTs; this design involves groups that randomly (i.e., by chance) receive a diagnostic test and a comparison diagnostic test and are then evaluated based on the presence or absence of the expected outcome (i.e., diagnosis). Sometimes, however, it would be unethical to randomly assign a diagnostic test to some patients and not others because the risks for the diagnostic test or misdiagnosing the outcome are too high. In this situation, the best research design to answer the question would be a cohort study (see Table 2.4). In our example, this is the not case, because it would not be unethical to randomly assign ultrasound and HIDA scan to participants in an RCT; so we would look for either a systematic review of RCTs or single studies. Most commonly, the comparison is the test considered the gold standard for the industry.

Clinical Scenario 2.4 Etiology Example

Scenario

An 18-year-old college freshman agreed to be a patient in the School of Nursing simulation exercises. She picked the bariatric case situation because her mother was obese and died at the age of 55. She realizes that she does not have her mother's family history because she is adopted, but is still concerned whether her mother's obesity will affect her lifelong. When she asks this question in the simulation, you tell her that though this is not part of the scenario for the exercise, you are very interested in her question and will help her discover the answer after the exercise is completed.

Etiology Clinical Question Template

This clinical scenario is an etiology scenario. Given the format for etiology questions, fill in the blanks with information from the clinical scenario.

Are _____ (**P**), who have _____ (**I**) compared with those without _____ (**C**) at _____ risk for/of _____ (**O**) over _____ (**T**)?

Discussion

In the example, the question could read, "Are adopted children (**P**), who have parents with elevated BMI (**I**) compared with those with parents with normal BMI (**C**) at increased

continued on the following page

risk for obesity (**O**) after age 18?" Because the freshman is interested in the impact life-long, the **T** would be necessary, but it may not be in all etiology questions.

Etiology questions help clinicians address potential causality and harm. These questions can be answered by cohort or case–control studies that indicate what outcomes may occur in groups over time; however, it requires an abundance of longitudinal studies that consistently demonstrate these relationships to generate confidence in the potential causality. For example, it is commonly believed that smoking causes lung cancer; however, there are people who defy this conviction by smoking all of their adult lives and yet have no diagnosis of lung cancer. Potential causality from case–control or cohort studies must be carefully interpreted. RCTs are the only design that establishes with confidence a cause-and-effect relationship between an intervention and an outcome. However, the difference in an etiology/harm question and an intervention question is that the conditions (**I** and **C**) cannot be randomized owing to the potential for harm, which is often the reason for the question.

In the clinical scenario, potential causality is the focus of the question. As always, it is preferable to search for syntheses first. To answer this type of question, the desired research design would be cohort or case–control studies in which groups of people with a given condition (e.g., adopted children) were prescribed either the intervention of interest (i.e., **I**, e.g., parents with elevated BMI) or the comparison of interest (e.g., parents with normal BMI) by their healthcare providers and were observed over time to evaluate the likelihood of a suspected outcome (e.g., obesity; see Table 2.4). In the example, we would look for studies that followed a group of adopted children whose parents had elevated and normal BMIs to determine how many were obese after age 18.

Clinical Scenario 2.5 Meaning Example

Scenario

You are caring for Brandon, an 85-year-old man, who has been on the orthopedic rehabilitation floor for 3 weeks after complications from a fall and subsequent hip replacement. He is not progressing as expected, and the healthcare team can find no physiological reason for his lack of progress. You notice that Brandon has had no visitors for the entire 3 weeks on your unit, despite numerous calls by staff to his family. You ask Brandon what he misses most about his home and find out that he has a pet cat named Fluffy that "means the world" to him. You wonder how missing Fluffy has affected Brandon's recovery progress. To facilitate the best outcomes, you determine to find evidence to inform decision making.

Meaning Clinical Question Template

This clinical scenario is about meaning. The following is the format for meaning questions. Fill in the blanks with the information from the clinical scenario.

How do _____ (**P**) with _____ (**I**) perceive _____ (**O**) during _____ (**T**)?

Discussion

In this example, the question could read: How do elderly patients in orthopedic rehabilitation (**P**) with separation from significant other pets (**I**) perceive their motivation to progress (**O**) during their recovery (**T**)?

This question is remarkably different from the others that we have discussed. You may notice that a **C** is not present in this question. It is not required because there is no comparison with "separation from significant other pets" (**I**) in regard to patients' motivation to progress (**O**). The emphasis is on how elderly patients with extended stays (rehabilitation) experience separation from their significant other pets, particularly in regard to their motivation to progress during their recovery. The best evidence to answer this type of question would be qualitative research. A synthesis of qualitative studies would be considered Level 1 evidence (see Table 2.4). Research designs such as an RCT, cohort, or case–control study would not be able to provide the data required to answer this question. Therefore, we would look for qualitative studies, such as a phenomenological study (see Chapter 6), to answer this question.

WHY WORK HARD AT FORMULATING THE CLINICAL QUESTION?

Remember that a clinical question is not a research question or a QI question (see Table 2.3); these questions differ primarily in their approach to the evidence in the literature. Research questions usually have directional outcomes (i.e., improved or reduced) and bring with them a sense of expectation of what will be found in the literature. Researchers have a vested interest in the intervention working. In contrast, clinical questions come with no expectations of what will be found in the literature. These questions ask about how an issue or intervention affects an outcome, which includes answers from studies that may be positive, negative, or neutral (i.e., no effect). Furthermore, well-formulated clinical questions guide clinicians away from "as-you-like-it" searches that usually result in incorrect, too much, or irrelevant information to systematic searches that quickly result in relevant answers. A QI question is formulated when a concern or problem is exposed and processes are evaluated to establish steps in a plan that is rapidly implemented and evaluated.

Honing one's skills in formulating a well-built question can provide confidence that the clinical issue is well defined and the search will be more systematic, successful, and timely. There are different types of PICOT questions that are formulated based on the clinical encounter/situation. PICOT questions are not clinical projects, but in fact they are key to the EBP process of finding evidence, appraising and evaluating it, and synthesizing it for practice. From their vast experience, Straus et al. (2011) identified that formulating a searchable, answerable question is the most difficult step in the EBP process. However, they also suggested several other benefits from constructing good questions, including clearly communicating patient information with colleagues, helping learners more clearly understand content taught, and furthering the initiative to become better clinicians through the positive experience of asking a good question, finding the best evidence, and making a difference. A caveat about library guides for understanding how to construct good clinical questions: some have questions that are in the required templates and others have research or QI questions. Be discerning when looking for a library guide (for example, LibGuides) to help with understanding how to ask a PICOT question. To help in mastery of understanding how to formulate searchable, answerable questions, review the various web-based resources given here.

Find web-based information on formulating searchable, answerable questions at the following websites:

- Centre for Evidence-Based Medicine: http://www.cebm.net/asking-focused-questions/
- The Center for Transdisciplinary Evidence-Based Practice at The Ohio State University: https://ctep-ebp.com/online-modular-ebp-program
- Library Guide at Georgia Gwinnett College: http://libguides.ggc.edu/c. php?g=362349&p=2447296

Formulating a well-built question is worth the time and effort it takes. It is step 1—and as some have said, the most challenging—toward providing evidence-based care to patients (Schlosser, Koul, & Costello, 2007; Straus et al., 2011).

Reason and free inquiry are the only effectual agents against error.

THOMAS JEFFERSON

EBP FAST FACTS

- **What are background questions?** Background questions ask what, where, when, why, and how. These questions are important as a starting place to learn more about the clinical issue to develop a PICOT question. These questions ask information to which the answers can generally be found in textbooks. Examples: What is the normal BP range? How do you measure BP? When is BP considered abnormal?
- **What is a PICOT question?** A PICOT question, also known as a foreground question, is critical to finding evidence to answer that question. *P* refers to the population of interest, *I* is the intervention or area of interest, *C* is the comparison intervention or area of interest, and is generally the "usual standard of care" (the C does not mean "control" group). *O* is the outcome of interest, and *T* is the time it takes for the intervention or issue to achieve the outcome. Not all of the components may be appropriate for a clinical question; however, the essential components of a PICOT question include a *P*, *I*, and *O*.
- **What is the purpose of a PICOT question?** Once the PICOT question is formulated, the components of the question are the basis for the keywords used to search databases such as CINAHL and MEDLINE to find the evidence to answer the question.
- **What are the kinds of PICOT questions?** There are five types of PICOT questions: meaning, diagnosis, intervention, prediction/prognosis, and etiology. The PICOT question guides the systematic search to find the best evidence to answer the question. Remember that the PICOT question is NOT a research or QI question and it is NOT what will be done in an EBP project!

References

Altman, S. H., Butler, A. S., & Shern, L. (2015). *Assessing progress on the Institute of Medicine Report the Future of Nursing Committee for assessing progress on implementing the recommendations of the Institute of Medicine Report the future of nursing: Leading change, advancing health.* Washington, DC: The National Academies Press.

American Nurses Credentialing Center. (2014). *2014 Magnet® application manual.* Silver Spring, MD: Author.

Butler, M. (2017). Making HIPAA work for consumers. *Journal of American Health Information Management Association, 88*(3), 14–17.

Carman, K. L., Maurer, M., Mangrum, R., Yang, M., Ginsburg, M., Sofaer, S., . . . Siegel, J. (2016). Understanding an informed public's views on the role of evidence in making health care decisions. *Health Affairs, 35*(4), 566–574.

Carman, M. J., Wolf, L. A., Henderson, D., Kamienski, M., Koziol-McLain, J., Manton, A., Moon, M. D. (2013). Developing your clinical question: The key to successful research. *Journal of Emergency Nursing, 39*(3), 299–301.

Centers for Medicare and Medicaid Services. (2016). *Quality initiatives.* Retrieved from https://www.cms.gov/Medicare/Quality-Initiatives-Patient-Assessment-Instruments/QualityInitiativesGenInfo/index.html

Cobban, S. J., Edgington, E. M., & Clovis, J. B. (2008). Moving research knowledge into dental hygiene practice. *Journal of Dental Hygiene, 82*, 21.

Cranley, L., Doran, D., Tourangeau, A., Kushniruk, A., & Nagle, L. (2009). Nurses' uncertainty in decision-making: A literature review. *Worldviews on Evidence-Based Nursing, 6*(1), 3–15.

Currie, L. M., Graham, M., Allen, M., Bakken, S., Patel, V., & Cimino, J. J. (2003). Clinical information needs in context: An observational study of clinicians while using a clinical information system. *American Medical Informatics Association Annual Symposium Proceedings/AMIA Symposium*, 190–194.

Elias, B. L, Polancich, S., Jones, C., & Convoy, S. (2015). Evolving the PICOT method for the digital age: The PICOT-D. *Journal of Nursing Education, 54*(10), 594–599.

Elias, B. L., Polancich, S., Jones, C., & Convoy, S. (2017). Evolving the PICOT method for the digital age: The PICOT-D. *Journal of Nursing Education, 54*(10), 594–599.

Engebretsen, E., Heggen, K., Wieringa, S., & Greenhalgh, T. (2016). Uncertainty and objectivity in clinical decision making: A clinical case in emergency medicine. *Medical Health Care and Philosophy, 19*, 595–603.

Estabrooks, C., O'Leary, K., Ricker, K., & Humphrey, C. (2003). The internet and access to evidence: How are nurses positioned? *Journal of Advanced Nursing, 42*, 73–81.

Ferran-Ferrer, N., Minguillón, J., & Pérez-Montoro, M. (2013). Key factors in the transfer of information-related competencies between academic, workplace, and daily life contexts. *Journal of the American Society for Information Science and Technology, 64*(6), 1112–1121.

Fineout-Overholt, E., & Johnston, L. (2005). Teaching EBP: Asking searchable, answerable clinical questions. *Worldviews on Evidence-Based Nursing, 2*(3), 157–160.

Gray, G. E. (2010). Asking answerable questions. In C. B. Taylor (Ed.), *How to practice evidence-based psychiatry: Basic principles and case studies* (pp. 17–19). Arlington, VA: American Psychiatric Publishing.

Green, M. L., & Ruff, T. R. (2005). Why do residents fail to answer their clinical questions? A qualitative study of barriers to practicing evidence-based medicine. *Academic Medicine, 80*, 176–182.

Greiner, A., & Knebel, E. (2003). *Health professions education: A bridge to quality.* Washington, DC: Institute of Medicine and National Academy Press.

Hartzell, T. & Fineout-Overholt, E. (2017). The Evidence-based Practice Competencies related to Searching for Best Evidence. In Melnyk, Gallagher-Ford, & Fineout-Overholt's *Implementing the Evidence-Based Practice (EBP) Competencies in Healthcare: A Practical Guide for Improving Quality, Safety, and Outcomes.* Sigma Theta Tau International: Indianapolis, IN (pp. 55–76).

Haynes, R. (1993). Where's the meat in clinical journals? *ACP Journal Club, 119*, A23–A24.

Hoogendam, A., de Vries Robbé, P., & Overbeke, A. J. (2012). Comparing patient characteristics, type of intervention, control, and outcome (PICO) queries with unguided searching: A randomized controlled crossover trial. *Journal Medical Library Association, 100*(2), 120–126.

Horowitz, R., Singer, B., Makuch, R., & Viscoli, C. (1996). Can treatment that is helpful on average be harmful to some patients? A study of the conflicting information needs of clinical inquiry and drug regulation. *Journal of Clinical Epidemiology, 49*, 395–400.

Hsee, C., & Ruan, B. (2016). The Pandora effect: The power and peril of curiosity. *Psychological Science, 27*(5), 659–666.

Huang, X., Lin, J., & Demnar-Fushman, D. (2006). Evaluation of PICO as a knowledge representation for clinical questions. *American Medical Informatics Association Annual Symposium Proceedings/AMIA Symposium*, 359–363.

Institute of Medicine. (2011). Digital infrastructure for the learning health system: The foundation for continuous improvement in health and health care—Workshop series summary. Washington, DC: The National Academies Press.

Joint Commission. (2017). *National patient safety goals effective January 2017.* Retrieved from https://www.jointcommission.org/assets/1/6/NPSG_Chapter_NCC_Jan2017.pdf

Kamhi, A. (2011). Balancing certainty and uncertainty in clinical practice. *Language, Speech and Hearing Services in Schools, 42*, 88–93.

Kosteniuk, J. G., Morgan, D. G., & D'Arcy, C. K. (2013). Use and perceptions of information among family physicians: Sources considered accessible, relevant, and reliable. *Journal of the Medical Library Association, 101*(1), 32–37.

MacIntosh-Murray, A., & Choo, C. W. (2005). Information behavior in the context of improving patient safety. *Journal of the American Society of Information Science and Technology, 56*, 1332–1345.

McCloskey, D. J. (2008). Nurses' perceptions of research utilization in a corporate health care system. *Journal of Nursing Scholarship, 40*, 39–45.

Melnyk, B. M., & Fineout-Overholt, E. (2002). Putting research into practice. *Reflections on Nursing Leadership, 28*(2), 22–25, 45.

Melnyk, B. M., Fineout-Overholt E., Feinstein N. F., Sadler L. S., Green-Hernandez C. (2008). Nurse practitioner educators' perceived knowledge, beliefs, and teaching strategies regarding evidence-based practice: implications for accelerating the integration of evidence-based practice into graduate programs. *Journal of Professional Nursing, 24*(1), 7–13.

Melnyk, B. M., Fineout-Overholt, E., Gallagher-Ford, L., & Kaplan, L. (2012). The state of evidence-based practice in US nurses: Critical implications for nurse leaders and educators. *Journal of Nursing Administration, 42*(9), 410–417.

Melnyk, B. M., Fineout-Overholt, E., Stillwell, S. B., & Williamson, K. M. (2010). Evidence-based practice: Step by step: The seven steps of evidence-based practice. *American Journal of Nursing, 110*(1), 51–53.

Mulvaney, S., Bickman, L., Giuse, N., Lambert, E., Sathe, N., & Jerome, R. (2008). A randomized effectiveness trial of a clinical informatics consult service: Impact on evidence-based decision-making and knowledge implementation. *Journal of the American Medical Informatics Association, 15*, 203–211.

Nelson, N. (2011). Questions about certainty and uncertainty in clinical practice. *Language, Speech and Hearing Services in Schools, 42*, 81–87.

O'Connor, D., Green, S., & Higgins, J. (2011). Chapter 5: Defining the review question and developing criteria for including studies. In J. P. T. Higgins & S. Green (Eds.), *Handbook for systematic reviews of interventions.* Retrieved from http://handbook.cochrane.org

Pravikoff, D., Tanner, A., & Pierce, S. (2005). Readiness of U.S. nurses for evidence-based practice. *American Journal of Nursing, 105*, 40–50.

Price, C. & Christenson, R. (2013). Ask the right question: A critical step for practicing evidence-based laboratory medicine. *Annals of Clinical Biochemistry, 50*(4), 306–314.

Rice, M. J. (2010) Evidence-based practice problems: Form and focus. *Journal of the American Psychiatric Nurses Association, 16*(5), 307–314.

Riva, J. J.; Malik, K. M. P.; Burnie, S. J.; Endicott, A. R.; Busse, J. W. (2012). What is your research question? An introduction to the PICOT format for clinicians. *Journal of the Canadian Chiropractic Association, 56*(3), 167–171.

Sackett, D. L., Straus, S. E., Richardson, W. S., Rosenberg, W., & Haynes, R. B. (2000). *Evidence-based medicine: How to practice and teach EBM.* Edinburgh, Scotland: Churchill Livingstone.

Scantlebury, A., Booth, A., & Hanley, B. (2017). Experiences, practices and barriers to accessing health information: A qualitative study. *International Journal of Medical Informatics, 103*, 103–108.

Schardt, C., Adams, M. B., Owens, T., Keitz, S., & Fontelo, P. (2007). Utilization of the PICO framework to improve searching PubMed for clinical questions. *BMC Medical Informatics and Decision Making, 7*(16), 1–6.

Schlosser, R., Koul, R., & Costello, J. (2007). Asking well-built questions for evidence-based practice in augmentative and alternative communication. *Journal of Communication Disorders, 40*, 225–238.

Scott, S., Estabrooks, C., Allen, M., & Pollock, C. (2008). A context of uncertainty: How context shapes nurses' research utilization behaviors. *Qualitative Health Research, 18*, 347–357.

Shaikh, M. H., & Shaikh, M. A. (2012). A prelude stride in praxis & usages of healthcare informatics. *International Journal of Computer Sciences Issues, 9*(6), 85–89.

Spek, B. Waard, M. W., Lucas, C., & van Dijk, N. (2013).Teaching evidence-based practice (EBP) to speech–language therapy students: Are students competent and confident EBP users? *International Journal of Language and Communication Disorders, 48*(4), 444–452.

Stillwell, S. B., Fineout-Overholt, E., Melnyk, B. M., & Williamson, K. (2010). Evidence-based practice, step by step: Asking the clinical question: A key step in evidence-based practice. *American Journal of Nursing, 110*(3), 58–61.

Straus, S. E., Richardson, W. S., Glasziou, P., & Haynes, R. B. (2011). *Evidence-based medicine: How to teach and practice it* (4th ed.). Edinburgh, Scotland: Churchill Livingstone.

Ubbink, D., Guyatt, G., & Vermeulen, H. (2013). Framework of policy recommendations for implementation of evidence-based practice: A systematic scoping review. *British Medical Journal Open, 3*(1), 1–12.

Warren, J. I., McLaughlin, M., Bardsley, J., Eich, J., Esche, C. A., Kropkowski, L., Risch, S. (2016). The strengths and challenges of implementing EBP in healthcare systems, *Worldviews on Evidence-Based Nursing, 13*(1), 15–24.

Whittington, J. W., Nolan, K., Lewis, N., & Torres, T. (2015). Pursuing the triple aim: The first seven years. *Milbank Quarterly, 93*(2), 263–300.

Finding Relevant Evidence to Answer Clinical Questions

Tami A. Hartzell and Ellen Fineout-Overholt

> The two words "information" and "communication" are often used interchangeably, but they signify quite different things. Information is giving out; communication is getting through.
>
> —Sydney J. Harris

EBP Terms to Learn

Adjacency searching
Ancestry method
Bibliographic database
Boolean connector
Citations
Discussion board
Explode feature
Filters
Full text
Grey literature
Handsearch
Hits
Keyword
Limit
Listserv
MeSH

Open access
Point-of-care resources
Preappraised literature
Primary source
Proximity searching
Reference managers

Search history
Search strategy
Secondary source
Subject headings
Truncation
Yield

Learning Objectives

After studying this chapter, learners will be able to:

1. Describe the role of the PICOT question in guiding a systematic search.
2. Describe sources of evidence.
3. Discuss basic and advanced strategies with which to conduct a systematic search.
4. Discuss what constitutes a search yield.

In any clinical setting, there are numerous sources of information (e.g., journal literature, practice-based data, patient information, textbooks) to answer a variety of questions about how to improve patient care or update clinical procedures and protocols. You can find the best information available (i.e., evidence) by using the PICOT question to guide you as you conduct a systematic, efficient, and thorough search (Stillwell, Fineout-Overholt, Melnyk, & Williamson, 2010). For example, a patient in the medical surgical unit is recovering from a myocardial infarction (MI) and now must undergo cardiac rehabilitation classes. The patient's anxiety about a recurring MI has thwarted her engagement in rehabilitation activities, and therefore her success. After hearing about a new study on music therapy on the evening news, the patient asks whether listening to music on her iPhone during rehab exercises might reduce her anxiety. While other members of the healthcare team discuss pharmaceutical options to help the patient engage in the rehabilitation process, you wonder if music may help. With this inquiry, you formulate the following PICOT question to address the patient's anxiety: In hospitalized adult patients with recent MI undergoing rehabilitation (P), how does listening to music (I) compared with pharmacological interventions (C) affect anxiety (O) while engaging in rehabilitation activities (T)? Your PICOT question-guided, systematic search produces several recent **randomized controlled trials (RCTs)** that report positive benefits of music therapy, including reducing anxiety. You share the evidence with the healthcare team and collaborate with the music therapist to initiate music therapy and arrange for additional music for your patient.

In this chapter, you will find several key features to assist you in gaining mastery of systematic searching strategies. Be sure to carefully engage all of the boxes, figures, and tables as supports for mastery. Competencies for systematic searching are helpful in ensuring that clinicians have the knowledge and skills to find relevant evidence to answer clinical questions (Hartzell & Fineout-Overholt, 2017). The first key feature is Figure 3.1, which highlights specific basic and advanced behaviors that clinicians would use to competently search **bibliographic databases**, such as the Cumulative Index to Nursing and Allied Health Literature (CINAHL) and *MEDLINE*. Competency 3H (Figure 3.1) indicates that finding the right information to answer a given question often requires using more than one source of evidence. Table 3.1 provides a select list of information sources that a clinician may wish to search. When clinicians explore only one source and find no evidence, they may incorrectly conclude that there is no evidence to answer their question. For example, if clinicians are searching for a systematic review to answer an intervention question and decide to search only a web-based search engine (e.g., Google), they may not find any recent systematic reviews. Instead, they may find a case study that was published in a journal about 5 years ago. Not having found any systematic reviews, they may be tempted to ignore the case study and conclude that there is no evidence to answer the question. But, because a body of evidence answers the clinical question, discarding the case study would be inadvisable. Although the case study may not be able to answer the clinical question fully or support a practice change, a case study can inform clinical care. When searching for answers to clinical questions, all evidence should be considered (i.e., the body of evidence from multiple sources). However, clinicians must exercise caution when deciding about practice changes that are based solely on evidence that may have substantial bias (e.g., descriptive designs such as case studies). To help gain mastery of the categories of clinical questions and the corresponding research designs (i.e., external evidence), review Table 3.2.

Clinicians need to quickly find answers to clinical questions; therefore, searching for evidence that has already been appraised for the quality of the study methodology and the reliability of its findings is desirable. This **preappraised literature** can range from integrative **systematic reviews** to **meta-analyses** (see Chapter 5) and **meta-syntheses** (see Chapter 6) to synopses of single studies. By using preappraised literature, clinicians can cut down on the amount of time they spend in determining whether they have reliable information, which reduces the time between finding suitable evidence and providing best care. Systematic reviews have long been referred to as the type of preappraised syntheses of studies that form the heart of evidence-based practice (Stevens, 2001). However, there is often not enough quality research to address all clinical issues with a synthesis, and sometimes there may only be a handful of primary studies that exist, which is another reason to systematically search more than one source when looking for evidence to answer a clinical question (Competency 3H, Figure 3.1).

Systematic reviews (not a narrative review, see Chapter 5), primary studies, and guidelines may contain the answers—the challenge is how to efficiently and effectively find them. Often, the process may seem like finding the proverbial needle in a haystack. To ensure that reliable evidence is found, clinicians must move beyond unsystematic search techniques (e.g., searching any word that comes to mind and searching only one source of evidence instead of multiple sources) toward using available supports (healthcare librarians) and strategies (systematic searching approach, multiple sources, and well-practiced techniques) that help them find the needle in the haystack, the essential evidence to answer their clinical question.

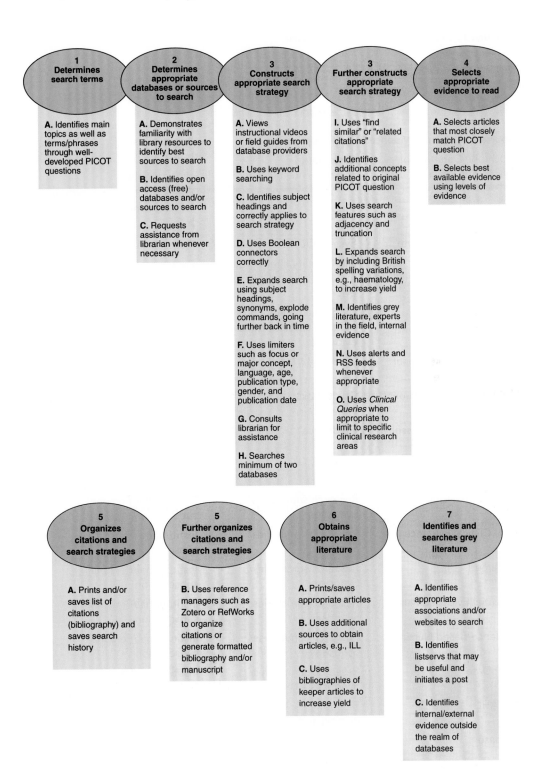

Figure 3.1: Suggested basic and advanced searching competencies. Blue-shaded areas are basic competencies, and orange-shaded areas are advanced competencies. (Adapted from Hartzell, T. A., & Fineout-Overholt, E. [2016]. The evidence-based practice competencies related to searching for best evidence. In B. M. Melnyk, L. Gallagher-Ford, & E. Fineout-Overholt (Eds.), *Implementing the evidence-based competencies in healthcare: A practical guide for improving quality, safety, and outcomes.* Indianapolis, IN: Sigma Theta Tau International. © Hartzell & Fineout-Overholt, 2017.)

TABLE 3.1 *Sources of External Evidence by Type/Application and Access/Cost*

Source of External Evidence	Type/Application	Access/Cost*
Cochrane Database of Systematic Reviews	Systematic reviews—healthcare	Institutional/personal subscriptions Free website access with restricted content Pay-per-view with registration
Joanna Briggs Institute	Systematic reviews—nursing	Institutional subscription
National Institute for Health and Care Excellence (NICE) Evidence Search	High-quality filtering of multiple types of clinical evidence	Free
Trip Database	High-quality filtering of multiple types of clinical evidence	Free; low-cost premium version
Guidelines International Network (G-I-N)	Guidelines**	Free; membership required for some materials
Professional Associations/ Organizations	Guidelines**	Free; content may be available only to members
Registered Nurses Association of Ontario	Guidelines**	Free
Scottish Intercollegiate Guideline Network (SIGN)	Guidelines**	Free
ACP Journal Club	Research summaries/ Synopses	Institutional/Personal subscription
BMJ Clinical Evidence	Research summaries/ Synopses	Institutional/Personal subscription
Dynamed	Research summaries/ Synopses	Institutional/Personal subscription
Essential Evidence Plus	Research summaries/ Synopses	Institutional/Personal subscription
Evidence-Based Nursing	Research summaries/ Synopses	Institutional/Personal subscription
UpToDate	Research summaries/ Synopses	Institutional/Personal subscription
CINAHL	Bibliographic database— nursing and allied health	Institutional subscription
Embase	Bibliographic database—healthcare	Institutional subscription
ERIC	Bibliographic database—education	Free or institutional subscription
MEDLINE	Bibliographic database—healthcare	Free via PubMed Institutional subscription through other vendors
PubMed	Bibliographic database—healthcare	Free

TABLE 3.1 — Sources of External Evidence by Type/Application and Access/Cost (continued)

PsycINFO	Bibliographic database—psychology	Institutional subscription
ClinicalTrials.gov	Clinical trials	Free
Cochrane Central	Clinical trials	Institutional subscription Free website access with restricted content Pay-per-view with registration
Google Scholar	Internet search engine	Free
Google	Internet search engine	Free

* May be a fee for full text of articles.

** Check the ECRI Institute website for updates on another source of evidence-based guidelines: https://www.ecri.org/Pages/default.aspx

TABLE 3.2 — Best Evidence to Answer Different Clinical Questions

Type of Clinical Question: Examples	Best Evidence Design to Answer the Question (Levels of Evidence)
Intervention Questions: Example 1: In patients with acute respiratory distress syndrome (P), how does prone positioning (I) compared with supine positioning (C) affect weaning parameters (O) during weaning protocol (T)? Example 2: In pregnant women (P), how does prenatal care (I) compared with no prenatal care (C) affect complications (e.g., bleeding, fetal distress) (O1) and a healthy baby (O2) during delivery (T)?	Systematic reviews and meta-analyses Single RCTs Well-controlled, nonrandomized experimental studies
Prognosis Questions: In college students (P), how does past experience with group studying (I) compared with past experience with individual studying (C) influence/predict success in standardized testing (O) at the end of a degree program (T)?	Case-control or cohort studies
Meaning Question: How do spouses with a loved one (P) who has Alzheimer's disease (I) perceive their ability to provide care (O) during the course of the disease (T)?	Meta-analyses or single qualitative studies
Background Question*: What are the coping mechanisms of parents who have lost a child to AIDS?	Descriptive studies
Background Question*: What is my professional organization's theoretical/conceptual framework said to underpin excellence in clinical practice?	Opinion reports of experts and professional organizations
Multiple Intervention Questions in One Question*: What are the national standards for the prevention and management of wandering in patients with Alzheimer's disease who live in long-term care facilities?	Evidence-based clinical practice guidelines

*PICOT format not appropriate.

SUPPORTS AND STRATEGIES FOR FINDING THE NEEDLE IN THE HAYSTACK

Given the consistent need for current information in healthcare, frequently updated databases that hold the latest studies reported in journals are the best choices for finding relevant evidence to answer compelling clinical questions. To help gain mastery of systematic searching strategies, we will follow Clinical Scenario 3.1 throughout the chapter.

The use of a standardized format, such as PICOT (Fineout-Overholt & Stillwell, 2015; Richardson, Wilson, Nishikawa, & Hayword, 1995; see Chapter 2) to guide and clarify the important elements of the clinical question is an essential first step toward finding the right information to answer it. Often, in searching for the best evidence to answer a PICOT question, clinicians use databases that have their own specific database language that helps eliminate or minimize searching errors such as spelling or missing a synonym of a **keyword** (Competency 3B, Figure 3.1). Learning how to competently navigate through different databases will increase clinicians' abilities to quickly find relevant evidence. Novices to this type of searching are wise to consult a healthcare librarian who can assist them in this process (Competency 2C, Figure 3.1). Many hospitals employ healthcare librarians who are able to help clinicians find their needle in the haystack either through one-on-one training or by searching on behalf of clinicians. If you are in an academic setting, you may have many healthcare librarians available for a consult. However, if you do not have one, be creative in your partnerships and resource sharing. For example, this kind of partnership can enable universities and healthcare agencies the opportunity to shore up access to the evidence within their healthcare delivery systems as well as healthcare education to ensure that their communities have best practice. It is imperative that all clinicians have some connection with librarians and access to databases.

After formulating a well-built PICOT question (Competency 1A, Figure 3.1), your next step is to determine the sources most likely to contain the best evidence (Competency 2A, Figure 3.1). Clinicians need **peer-reviewed** research to answer their questions, and most often

---

Clinical Scenario 3.1

A nurse manager has been noticing that the newly licensed nurses she has hired haven't stayed on the unit more than a year or two. Although primarily a medical unit, their patient acuity level has been steadily rising, and her staff does not feel confident to care for the ever expanding patient mix and populations. Having read an article on compassion fatigue recently, the manager wonders if her newest nurses are experiencing compassion fatigue. The nurse manager realizes that there could be several clinical questions she could ask to help her understand how to best assist the new graduates on her unit with their potential compassion fatigue. She considers the current orientation program and wonders whether adding a mentorship component might reduce compassion fatigue and increase her new nurses' resilience. She also considers whether including a writing journal or participating in a focus group may reduce compassion fatigue. The nurse manager wants to be thorough in her EBP process and simplifies her inquiry into two clinical questions. She decides that she will formulate her first PICOT question, namely—"*In new graduates hired into acute care settings (P), how does mentorship in orientation (I) compared with traditional orientation (C) affect compassion fatigue (O1) and resilience (O2) during the first 3 years of employment (T)?*"—and systematically search the literature that evening.

the source of that evidence will be a database of published studies. These databases contain references to the healthcare literature, including conference proceedings, books, or journal publications. Although these databases may be discipline specific (i.e., allied health, nursing, medicine, psychology), clinicians need to choose the right databases that will help them get to the evidence that can answer their question (Competency 2B, Figure 3.1). Knowing how to systematically search these databases is essential to a quick, successful retrieval of answers to a clinical question.

Busy clinicians may not have the time or resources to systematically search indexed databases. There are additional resources that save clinicians time, such as critically appraised topics (CAT). Some CATs are well done and reliable, whereas others may not be. Although these resources offer efficiency, clinicians still need to know how the appraisal process was performed to ensure that the preappraised evidence is trustworthy.

 One example of a CAT is the evidence posted by BestBets (**B**est **E**vidence **T**opics):
http://www.bestbets.org/

Knowledge and skill in asking the PICOT question, searching for the best type of evidence to answer it, and **critically appraising** the body of evidence are essential for clinicians to know which sources of evidence (i.e., the haystack) are the best to search for the desired information.

Support and Strategy 1: Sources of External Evidence—Description of the Haystack

Answers to clinical questions may be found in a variety of evidence sources, ranging from practice data found in the healthcare record (i.e., **internal evidence**) to research articles in journals (i.e., **external evidence**), all of which have been moving from print to digital format. The transition of evidence to electronic format has enabled clinicians to gain more immediate access to external evidence through the use of **point-of-care resources** that integrate almost seamlessly into the **electronic health record (EHR)**. These sources of evidence contain timely clinical topic summaries and are designed to provide both background information and the best available external evidence to improve patient care.

Types of Evidence Sources

Various types of evidence sources exist, including textbooks, journals and consolidated sources, which are discussed below.

Textbooks. Healthcare professionals can consult a good textbook to refresh or gain new knowledge. This background information may be all that is necessary in certain situations (see Chapter 2). At other times, consulting a textbook may help clinicians better understand the context for the PICOT question they are asking. Once clinicians have gathered their background information, they can begin to formulate their PICOT questions. When clinicians are trying to answer a specific question that requires more specialized knowledge (i.e., PICOT), textbooks are insufficient because the information may be incomplete or out of date. At this point, clinicians need to seek out research studies to answer their foreground (PICOT) questions (see Chapter 2).

Journals. A journal article is the typical source from which to find an answer to a foreground question (see Chapter 2), if one is to be found. The journal literature is an entry point, the place where all new ideas first enter the healthcare knowledge base and where clinicians first go to look for answers to their clinical questions. Journals contain a number of publication types, including systematic reviews, article synopses, research articles, narrative reviews, discussion articles, news items, editorials, and letters to the editor (listed from most to least useful in answering foreground questions).

Consolidated Sources and Beyond. In a landmark article, Haynes (2007) characterized and organized the new genre of consolidated information sources in a pyramid framework, which is presented in a simplified version in Figure 3.2. The pyramid is a hierarchy in which the most useful, easily accessible evidence is at the top. The pyramid's top layer, *Decision Support in Medical Record*, describes the ideal situation, a **clinical decision support system** integrated into the EHR. Here, data on a specific patient are automatically linked to the current best evidence available in the system that matches that patient's specific circumstances. Upon matching the evidence with patient data, the clinical decision support system assists clinicians with evidence-based interventions for that patient. This technology is important to healthcare decision making; therefore, it is important to determine whether the information contained within these systems is evidence based and current (Haynes, 2007; Wright et al., 2011). Effective use of this source of evidence requires that practitioners value the use of evidence in daily practice and have the knowledge and skills to use the given information.

The middle level of the pyramid is called *Reviews of Evidence* and contains preappraised literature, which, when done well, may be considered one of the needles in the evidence haystack. These reviews are considered consolidated sources of evidence (e.g., Clinical Evidence, Dynamed, Essential Evidence Plus) and have been designed to answer both background and foreground questions. They include comprehensive disease summaries that are formatted with sections and subcategories that are easily expanded. These summaries include hyperlinks to electronic journal articles or practice guidelines. They combine a textbook-like resource with easy access to the evidence contained in the journal literature—a format that is easy for busy clinicians to use. These sources can contain many types of evidence, ranging from systematic reviews, **clinical practice guidelines**, **health topic summaries**, to **article synopses**. Reviews within these evidence sources are written by individuals or panels of experts who

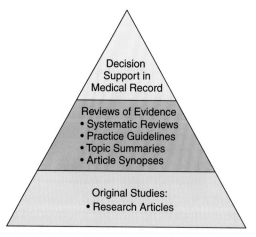

Figure 3.2: Pyramid framework for making evidence-based decisions. (Adapted from Haynes, B. [2007]. Of studies, syntheses, synopses, summaries, and systems: The "5S" evolution of information services for evidence-based healthcare decisions. *Evidence-Based Nursing, 10*(1), 6–7. With permission from BMJ Publishing Group Ltd.)

have evaluated the available evidence, determined its worth to practice, and made recommendations about how to apply it to a particular clinical issue. These evidence sources are updated frequently. Guideline revisions frequently will trigger an update. Although these sources of evidence are preappraised, it is important that clinicians understand the appraisal process used to produce each of the sources of evidence to determine whether the information contained within the product is reliable for clinical decision making. Documentation of the appraisal process is sometimes difficult to find. Terms like editorial policy or evidence-based methodology are frequently used to describe the appraisal process in the *About Us* section. Despite these vague terms, reading the editorial policy or methodology can give clinicians an idea of the appraisal process that is used.

The pyramid's base reflects original research articles that form the foundation on which the rest of the pyramid is built. Databases where these original research articles are indexed (e.g., MEDLINE or CINAHL) are the gateways for finding a **body of evidence**. These databases contain the largest number and widest variation of articles reporting on clinical research. Clinicians who look for evidence within the base of the pyramid need specialized knowledge and skill both in finding the evidence and in appraising its worth (Lefebvre, Manheimer, & Glanville, 2011a; Stillwell et al., 2010).

The shape of the pyramid reflects the number of sources of evidence available. For example, there are millions of original research articles on the bottom layer; however, the number of highly functioning computerized decision support systems is far fewer. The number of evidence reviews is somewhere in between. One reason for this disparity in sources of evidence is the time and money it takes to develop highly sophisticated EHR systems with integrated current evidence, systematic reviews, practice guidelines, summaries, and synopses—all requiring updating on a regular basis.

The names of specific information sources that fall into the bottom two sections of the pyramid can be found in Table 3.1. Several sources are available at no cost to all healthcare providers, no matter where they practice (e.g., PubMed, National Institute for Health and Care Excellence [NICE], Cochrane Databases, and Guidelines International Network [G-I-N]). Several of these databases are government-sponsored databases, which is why they are free. Other sources of evidence are available to institutions through a subscription. It is important to note that MEDLINE is produced by the National Library of Medicine (NLM) and is available free of charge through PubMed but can also be obtained for a cost via commercial vendors (e.g., Ovid, EBSCOhost). Commercial vendors offer their own search interfaces along with a limited number of **full-text** articles/journals. Figure 3.3 illustrates the relationship between the MEDLINE database and various vendors. Each healthcare institution may have a different array of database offerings, depending on the institution size, professions it serves, and library budget.

Support and Strategy 2: Gathering the Right Evidence From the Right Source

Healthcare professionals, faculty, librarians, and students are all very busy in their roles and need reliable, efficient sources for evidence. The key is to know how to match the sources of evidence with the question to be answered.

Which Evidence Source or Database Is a Good Match?

Reliable, accurate evidence is needed to reduce the risk, uncertainty, and time involved in clinical decision making that will lead to desired patient outcomes. With all of the sources of evidence potentially available to clinicians, the first step in finding answers to their clinical questions is to search for evidence in synthesized, preappraised sources (e.g., Cochrane

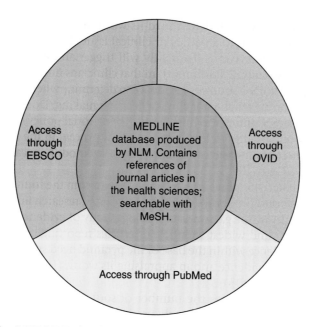

Figure 3.3: The MEDLINE database can be accessed through a variety of vendors. Each vendor offers a variety of features and functions to search the same MEDLINE records. MeSH, medical subject headings; NLM, National Library of Medicine.

Database of Systematic Reviews [CDSR], American College of Physicians [ACP] Journal Club, and the journal, *Evidence-Based Nursing* [EBN]). Refer back to Table 3.1 for more information on these sources. Finding the evidence in **full text** (i.e., electronic copies of articles available online) can promote timely decision making. Open-source full-text articles are available (i.e., no fee), but a subscription is required to access most full-text journals. For example, in the CDSR, only an abstract of the systematic review can be obtained without a subscription. To obtain the full systematic review, a subscription is required or a fee may be paid per article.

For point-of-care decisions, clinicians may choose to consult one of the preappraised summaries or synopsized sources listed earlier. However, when making practice changes, it is important to either find a synthesis that has conducted an exhaustive search (i.e., found all that we know on the topic) or get as close to that as possible by searching multiple databases to try to ensure that studies are not missed (Competency 3H, Figure 3.1). Searching subject-specific databases that index peer-reviewed research is the next step for finding best available evidence. For example, searching MEDLINE, which contains thousands of articles in hundreds of journals that cut across disciplines, enables clinicians to find a large chunk of the evidence that exists on a topic. However, searching only MEDLINE would be a limitation, because other databases that index journals not covered in MEDLINE and studies in those journals would not be discovered. Key knowledge that might impact outcomes could be missed. As mentioned, clinicians need to routinely search more than one database to find answers to their clinical questions (Competency 3H, Figure 3.1). Healthcare covers a wide range of topics, which is a good reason to consider searching other healthcare databases, such as CINAHL and PsycINFO.

In addition, clinicians should think about which organizations or professional associations might produce evidence (e.g., guidelines, standards) and search their websites (Competency 7A, Figure 3.1). Furthermore, when searches in mainstream databases do not lead to sufficient quality evidence, a healthcare librarian can recommend other databases (Competency 2C, Figure 3.1) that provide evidence to answer a PICOT question (e.g., ERIC for education literature, Web of Science, Social Sciences Citation Index [SSCI], or Health Business Elite).

Sources of evidence located through such search engines as Google or Google Scholar can provide value for background information; however, caution should be used and careful evaluation of the evidence retrieved from these sources is required. Clinicians should follow an appraisal process to ensure the information is reliable. Although major search engines may help clinicians get started in finding literature, it is important to remember that Google may find older evidence, and older evidence may not be relevant for answering clinical questions. In addition, many journals appear in Google Scholar that may not be found while searching in Google. When choosing between Google and Google Scholar, busy clinicians need to keep in mind that Google Scholar searches across evidence that is found primarily in academic publications and will therefore find mostly peer-reviewed evidence although the publications will vary in quality. In a small study, Nourbakhsh, Nugent, Wang, Cevik, and Nugent (2012) reported that using both PubMed and Google Scholar could retrieve different evidence. Google Scholar tended to find more articles, and the articles it found were more likely to be classified as relevant, and were more likely to be written in journals with higher impact factors than those in Google (Nourbakhsh et al., 2012). Web-based search engines such as Google and Google Scholar are insufficient as sole sources of evidence, but using Google Scholar in conjunction with PubMed and other databases may result in clinicians finding more evidence to answer their clinical question.

 For more on evaluating evidence sources for credibility, visit this site by University of Kansas Librarians: https://www.youtube.com/watch?v=NYI1FK7xbHY

Finding Evidence Requires Collaboration With Healthcare Librarians

An essential step in achieving success is knowing the extent of one's sources of evidence (Competency 2A, Figure 3.1). Collaboration with librarians who are knowledgeable about evidence-based practice (EBP) is essential to finding efficient answers to clinical questions (Competency 3G, Figure 3.1). The first step, however, is for clinicians to become familiar with sources of evidence that can help answer their PICOT question. These sources may be provided by a hospital or university library, but clinicians in private practice may need to turn to their local public library for sources of evidence. Although all clinicians may not be expert searchers, each one should have the skills to be able to search and find answers as there are time and resources to do so. Librarians, with their specialized knowledge in the organization of information, can be helpful at any point in the search; however, librarians shine when clinicians have attempted to search multiple databases and other sources but not found the evidence they seek. Often, librarians are able to find evidence to answer a clinical question when clinicians cannot. Don't hesitate to enlist the help of a librarian when time is short and patient care requires evidence. Involve healthcare librarians in your organization's efforts to promote and sustain EBP. They are the knowledge brokers and knowledge miners of healthcare information. Without their involvement in establishing an EBP culture, important pieces will be missed. As you formulate your PICOT question, consider some advice and "take your librarian to lunch."

Get to know what sources of evidence are available in your organization to help you hone your systematic searching skills. Take time to watch the short tutorials that most databases provide (Competency 3A, Figure 3.1). Get to know your healthcare librarian, and share your areas of interest so they can notify you when recent studies come to their attention. Furthermore, ask them to set up alerts for you that target areas of interest you need to stay on top of (Competency 3N, Figure 3.1). This collaboration enables you to become aware of other evidence in real time. By staying current, you are able to respond more quickly when new evidence seems to suggest a practice change. Key aspects that contribute to clinician–librarian collaboration are dialogue, role delineation, and purpose. Talk about how PICOT questions are the drivers of searches. Explore the most effective way for clinicians to get the data now.

Currently, some healthcare professionals are finding evidence at the bedside. By 2020, it is expected that all healthcare professionals will be evidence-based clinicians, conducting rapid, efficient searches *at the bedside*, often in sources of evidence that will not be primary databases (Institute of Medicine, 2009). For this to happen, clinicians will need to master systematic searching. Furthermore, collaboration between librarians and clinicians will be instrumental in exploring how to access information rapidly and efficiently. As information experts, librarians are partners with clinicians in achieving the mission of transforming healthcare from the inside out. The desired effect of the clinician–librarian collaboration is synergy that leads to consistent best practices by clinicians to achieve optimal outcomes for healthcare consumers.

Support and Strategy 3: Mastering Database Searching

When searching databases for evidence, clinicians need to be aware of features common to most databases. Understanding the structure and content of a particular information source before attempting to search it is critical (Competency 3A, Figure 3.1). Without this background, the search terms and strategies used may not **yield** the desired information, or the chosen database may not contain the information sought. It is important to note the fundamental difference between licensed databases, such as MEDLINE or CINAHL, and search engines, such as Google. Licensed databases list the journals they index, so it's easy for searchers to know which journals they are searching in a given database. This decreases the likelihood of missing an important journal because searchers know from the start whether or not they are searching key journals. The database vendor also makes available a field guide that instructs searchers in sound searching techniques and provides a description of the contents of the database. This transparency isn't available from Google or other search engines. Searchers may be searching the Internet, but have no idea what is being searched.

Types of Databases

Databases today are likely to contain records (i.e., article **citations**) as well as the full text of many types of documents. Records might include **subject headings** (i.e., terms that act as an umbrella for other related terms—search subject headings and capture more than one term), the author name(s), title of the article, and other details. MEDLINE, CINAHL, and PsycINFO are bibliographic databases whose primary content is made up of published journal records.

Full-text databases that contain whole articles or books, including the text, charts, graphs, and other illustrations, are often referred to as point-of-care sources of evidence. These sources may be enhanced by supplemental data (i.e., in spreadsheets), by multimedia content, and/or by hypertext links to other articles and supporting references and frequently contain patient care recommendations supported by links to general patient care information, evidence-based articles, or guidelines. Examples of point-of-care sources of evidence would be Dynamed and Nursing Reference Center. Examples of other full-text sources of evidence would be online journals or books (e.g., *Evidence-Based Nursing* or *Harrison's Online*).

Content of Databases

A clinician must be familiar with what databases and other information sources are available and what they contain before determining the value of searching it for answers to particular clinical questions (Competencies 2A and 2B, Figure 3.1). Databases can contain references to articles, the full text of the articles, entire books, dissertations, drug and pharmaceutical information, and other resources (e.g., news items, clinical calculators). To determine which databases to search, clinicians must consider the clinical question and which databases might contain relevant evidence. Competent searchers search a minimum of two databases to lessen the chance of missing relevant evidence (Competency 3H, Figure 3.1). Searching only one database or only in one's discipline will limit clinicians in retrieving the best evidence to answer their questions. Therefore, evidence must come from multiple databases that primarily serve healthcare disciplines (e.g., nursing and allied health, medicine, biomedicine, psychology).

Searching Databases

To effectively find answers to questions, clinicians need to understand a few details about the databases they are searching, for example, (1) Is the evidence current? (2) Will subject headings and/or keywords be more effective in getting to the best evidence quickly? (3) How frequently is the database updated?

Often, clinicians wonder how many years back they should search. Although some consider searching back 5 years as sufficient, this may not be adequate to discover evidence that can address the clinical issue. While there is no rule for how far back to search for evidence, clinicians should search until they can confidently indicate that there is little or no evidence to answer their clinical question or they feel confident that the evidence they have found represents the body of evidence that exists (Competency 3E, Figure 3.1). An interesting example is Dr. Priscilla Worral of SUNY Upstate Health System, who, when engaging clinicians in the emergency department (ED) who were using salt pork to prevent rebleeding from epistaxis, had to search for articles dating back to the late 1800s to find relevant evidence to address her clinical question (P. S. Worral, personal communication, 2001). To accomplish the goal of finding *all that we know* about a topic, we must use databases that include older published evidence as well as the newer evidence. This enables clinicians to search over a large span of time to find the best answer to their question. For example, MEDLINE offers citations ranging from the late 1940s to the present. If clinicians want to search farther back than 1946, they will need to search older indexes in print format.

To know if evidence is current, clinicians must be aware of the years covered in a database. The CDSR, for instance, always states the date of the most recent update. Other sources of evidence also require investigating when they were last updated. For example, textbooks are updated much less frequently than point-of-care sources of evidence. Most point-of-care sources follow an update protocol that might dictate a yearly or biannual review. Additionally, point-of-care sources of evidence will be updated as soon as the reviewers become aware that guidelines or other evidence have been revised. If there is no known date for evidence (e.g., Internet sources of evidence), it may be outdated, making it difficult for clinicians to determine its applicability.

Keyword, Subject Heading, and Title Search Strategies

Searchers should use three major search strategies across multiple bibliographic databases to increase the certainty that best evidence is not missed. These major strategies are (1) keyword searching (Competency 3B, Figure 3.1), (2) subject heading searching (Competency 3C, Figure 3.1), and (3) title searching. Because each of the three major search strategies has strengths and weaknesses, all three should be used in combination to provide high levels of certainty that best evidence is not missed. To gain mastery in understanding the strengths and weaknesses of these major search strategies, review Table 3.3. Systematic searching involves following the same **search strategy** or sequence of strategies as closely as possible to ensure the same approach across multiple databases. This consistency in approach will minimize the chance of missing important steps within the strategy and ensures that the same search is being conducted in each database. To support this consistency in approach, searchers can print out or take screenshots of their **search history** (i.e., how you searched) within the first database they search so that they can replicate it in other databases they will search. If searchers add new keywords or subject headings to their search strategy as they

TABLE
3.3

Strengths and Weaknesses of Three Search Strategies

Search Strategy	Strengths	Weaknesses
Keyword search	• Provides quick snapshot of resource's relevance to PICOT question • Identifies records when keyword appears with and without major relevance • Included in three most powerful search strategies	• Misses studies when authors' choices of keywords differ • Requires advanced search skills to quickly sort for relevance among too many citations • Requires combined subject headings search • Requires all three strategies to achieve certainty that nothing was missed
Subject heading search	• Provides quick snapshot of evidence's relevance to PICOT question • Retrieves only citations when topic is deemed by reviewers as at least 25% relevant to the topic is being searched • Increases chances that best citations will not be missed when authors and searchers use different synonyms because of database • Maps all synonyms to one assigned subject heading • Retrieves citations searched using related and narrower MeSH terms associated with searchers' MeSH • Increases chances that MeSH's broader terms identifying fields, environments, settings, industries can be combined with a very specific common keyword to target relevant citations • Included in the three most powerful search strategies	• Not always assigned for every keyword (i.e., new cutting edge terminology, coined phrases, acronyms) may not yet be assigned MeSH or be a successful match for auto mapping • Requires combining three major search strategies to avoid missing something • Not available across all major databases, search engines
Title search	• Provides quick snapshot to evidence's relevance to topic • Increases chances that keywords appearing in title are major topics • Increases chances that the P & I are related as required for PICOT question • Increases chances assigned subject headings are precise and best for a subject heading search • Effective in quickly targeting highly relevant articles within all search strategies • Included in three most powerful search strategies	• Misses studies when author's choices of title words differ • Requires all three major strategies to achieve certainty nothing missed • Not available across all major databases, search engines. Note: Google Scholar provides title search mode

search, they should go back to the databases they have searched previously and complete the search strategy sequence (including all keywords or subject headings) as well. Maintaining uniformity in the searching approach will assure searchers that all identified keywords and subject headings have been consistently used across databases as much as possible.

Where to start with the three major strategies described above is decided on by the PICOT question (Competency 1A, Figure 3.1). After the PICOT question has been formulated, there are several approaches to the search. The Cochrane Handbook (Higgins & Green, 2011) recommends that the search begin with the terms for the population (P) and intervention (I). Others recommend beginning with the outcome (O) and intervention (I) (Stillwell et al., 2010). All approaches recommend using as many synonyms for the keywords and related subject headings as possible (Competencies 3B and 3C, Figure 3.1).

The Cochrane Handbook is currently being updated. Please check the url for updates http://training.cochrane.org/handbook.

Once an initial approach is decided, searchers must determine whether to search all keywords and subject headings in one search or to conduct individual searches of each of the keywords and subject headings. Individual searches are recommended so that the number of **hits** is known for a certain term (i.e., keyword and synonyms or subject headings). The searches of synonyms should then be combined with what is called the **Boolean connector** "OR" (also known as a Boolean operator). The individual subject heading searches and combined synonym searches should then be combined with the Boolean connector "AND" to determine what the final number of viable hits will be within the database. Combining searches will be described in more depth later in the chapter.

Keywords. The first major search strategy is KEYWORD searching (Competency 3B, Figure 3.1). Keywords are generated from the PICOT question. Using keywords is the most common search strategy used across databases, search engines (e.g., Google), and other online sources. With this strategy, searchers enter all appropriate keywords, including common terms, synonyms, acronyms, phrases, coined phrases, and brand names. Searchers scan the citations found with this search strategy, continuing to note the alternate terms and synonyms that are found and use these terms as searching continues. Keyword searching attempts to locate the keyword entered in the title, abstract, or other searchable fields in the digital record. The citations that are found will only be records that contain the keyword(s) used in the search strategy. The strength of the keyword search strategy is that it provides a quick snapshot of how helpful the database is in finding relevant evidence to answer the PICOT question.

Sometimes, it may be challenging to consider all of the synonyms for a keyword, or yields may be low for those used. In these circumstances, advanced searchers should use **truncation** (Competency 3K, Figure 3.1). Truncation uses special symbols to locate additional letters beyond the root that is identified. Truncation is indicated by using an asterisk (*) or other symbol immediately after a word or part of a word. For example, in PubMed and CINAHL, adolescen* would retrieve *adolescent, adolescents,* or *adolescence*. Again, a librarian and the help section of individual databases can offer guidance to determine relevant symbols to apply when truncating (Competencies 3A and 3G, Figure 3.1)

The inherent challenge to keyword searching is that all synonyms, plurals, and alternate spellings of each keyword must be included in the search, or evidence will be missed. Advanced searchers understand that entering the keyword *behavior,* for example, will find any citations containing the word *behavior* in either the title or the abstract of that citation. However, all records with the alternative spelling *behaviour* in the title or abstract would be missed. In addition, different spellings of singulars and plurals (e.g., *mouse* and *mice*) must be included, or evidence will be missed. Therefore, competent advanced searchers have knowledge and skill in increasing the search yield (i.e., results) through expanding the strategy by including spelling variations, e.g., British spellings like *fibre* for *fiber* (Competency 3L, Figure 3.1).

Using keywords can be ambiguous and jargon laden. Consider the following question: *In people diagnosed with AIDS, how does age compared with being in the community influence pneumonia rates in the fall?* An example of a keyword search for this question might start with the word *AIDS*. This search would include articles on other types of aids, such as visual or hearing aids. In addition, this search would retrieve only articles containing the word *AIDS*. Those articles that used *acquired immune deficiency syndrome* or *acquired immunodeficiency syndrome* would be missed. When a topic is so recent that there is likely to be very little available in the journal literature, using keywords may be the best way to find relevant evidence because a subject heading for the topic is unlikely. Searching with keywords can be helpful, especially when no subject heading exists to adequately describe the topic searched. For this reason, the importance of carefully formulating the PICOT question cannot be overemphasized. Using any term(s) that will describe the PICOT components of the clinical question will assist in obtaining the best search in the shortest time.

Another weakness of the keyword strategy is that even though your keywords appear in the document's searchable fields, it does not mean that the article has these concepts as major topics. Also, the author may not have used the keywords you chose to search, so you may have missed best evidence. Yet another weakness with keyword searching is that you can potentially find a large yield. With only keyword searching, searchers may not have the skills to quickly target the most relevant results and can waste time scanning and sorting articles for relevance. This keyword approach weakness is mitigated when used in combination with two additional strategies, subject heading and title searching.

Subject Headings. The second major search strategy that can quickly identify articles to answer your clinical question is the SUBJECT HEADINGS search (Competency 3C, Figure 3.1). Searchers will use a standardized set of terms known as subject headings to locate all material that is available on a particular topic. Subject headings may be referred to as controlled vocabulary, subject terms, thesaurus, descriptors, or taxonomies. The content of an article will determine which subject headings it falls under (e.g., fibromyalgia or fatigue). Subject headings are used to help searchers find information on a particular topic, no matter what words the author may use to refer to a concept in the article. If a database has the capacity to incorporate subject headings with keyword searching, regardless of what words the author used in the article, when searchers type their words into the search box of the database, the database can "map" or find the subject headings that best matches the keyword. Using subject headings, searchers can broaden their searches without having to consider every synonym for the chosen keyword. An example of subject headings is Medical Subject Headings (**MeSH**), which is the set of terms used by the NLM to describe the content of articles indexed in MEDLINE. If the MeSH term *acquired immunodeficiency syndrome* was searched, all of these articles would contain information about it regardless of what terms the author(s) chose to use when writing, including HIV, HIV-positive, acquired immune deficiency syndrome, STI, STD, sexually transmitted disease, and sexually transmitted infection.

Many subject heading systems also have a hierarchical structure that helps searchers retrieve the more specific terms that fall under a general term. In searching a general MeSH term such as *heart diseases*, the PubMed search engine will automatically map keywords to subject headings and retrieve every term listed under it in the hierarchical "tree structure." This search retrieves articles ranging from MI to familial hypertrophic cardiomyopathy and everything in between—all at one time. Some search engines, rather than doing it automatically, offer the user the option of including or not including all of the specifics under a general term (e.g., Ovid and CINAHL present the option to "explode" the subject heading, which means to include all the specific terms listed under a more general heading). Exploding the search term when using subject headings is recommended, although it may yield irrelevant studies (Competency 3E, Figure 3.1). When clinicians use the **explode feature** and retrieve irrelevant articles, they can eliminate many of them by setting appropriate **limits** and combining subject heading searches using the PICOT question as the guide. Some search systems enable searchers to click on the subject heading and see the other narrower headings in the controlled vocabulary tree structure. This option helps searchers create the most relevant search by making a decision about whether to explode terms in the search.

An example of the usefulness of the explode function (Competency 3E, Figure 3.1) is a search to find information on food poisoning. In MEDLINE, the MeSH term *food poisoning* is the broad subject heading that describes various types of food poisoning, including botulism, ciguatera poisoning, favism, mushroom poisoning, salmonella poisoning, and staphylococcal poisoning. Using this heading to initiate the search and then exploding it means that the name of each of those types of food poisoning is a part of the search without needing to enter each one into the search strategy, saving valuable search time. In a PubMed search, the term you enter is automatically exploded. In the search, you have to instruct PubMed NOT to explode the term. For busy clinicians, exploding the subject heading is a wise choice, and irrelevant hits can then be removed through relevant combinations and limits.

Bibliographic databases, such as MEDLINE, CINAHL, and PsycINFO, use subject headings to describe the content of the items they index. Most databases will attempt to map the keyword entered in the search box to a subject heading. This assists searchers in finding relevant evidence without needing to know the subject heading up front. For example, in most search engines, the term *Tylenol* is mapped to the generic term *acetaminophen*, as is the European term *paracetamol*, or any of the following that are acetaminophen types of pain relievers: *Tempra, Panadol*, and *Datril*. As the system searches the subject heading *acetaminophen*, any article using the term *Tylenol* or any of the other words noted earlier will be retrieved because an indexer cataloged it under that heading, regardless of the term used in the article.

There is a caveat to subject headings searching: This mapping process may not be efficient with very current topics that have only recently entered the literature. In these cases, a subject heading is likely not available; therefore, keyword searching, using synonyms or variant forms of the word, may yield more relevant results. For example, the MeSH term, *resistance training*, did not become a subject heading until 2009. The only way a searcher could retrieve relevant evidence was to use the keywords *weight training, strength training, weight bearing*, or additional keywords.

To help with mastering how to find other subject headings to help further your search that are contained in the MEDLINE format in PubMed, review Figure 3.4. You will have to choose the MEDLINE format, because the format that is first shown in PubMed is typically the abstract. Also, it is important to note that not all vendors display all subject headings found in the MEDLINE record; therefore, searchers must consider use of subject headings in each database.

Some evidence sources do not have subject headings, or they rely on searchers to be familiar with existing subject headings. For example, any of the Cochrane databases can be searched using MeSH or keywords. To search using the MeSH option, you have to know the MeSH term you want to search. If you use MeSH often, you may know the term you want to search and can easily make use of this feature. If you want to find the appropriate subject headings, you may search MeSH independently through PubMed. *A cautionary note:* don't rely on MeSH alone when searching the Cochrane databases because you will exclude relevant, unique citations that are indexed in other databases whose records Cochrane includes. Nevertheless, keyword searching requires some creativity; searchers must think of all the different ways that an author could have referred to a particular concept. To maximize your search, keep in mind the caveats about keyword searching that were described earlier in this chapter.

Title Search. The TITLE search is the final major search strategy. Searching your P, I, and O terms in the title increases the chance of finding relevant citations, and it can help you identify relevant subject headings. The keyword is the mechanism for title searching and

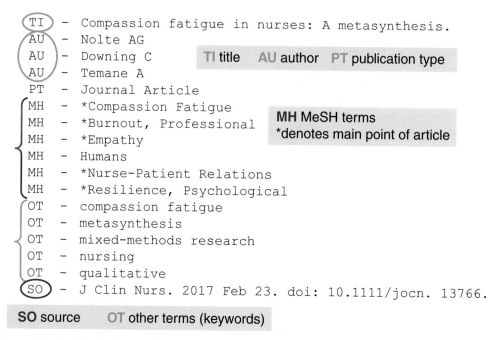

TI – Compassion fatigue in nurses: A metasynthesis.
AU – Nolte AG
AU – Downing C   TI title   AU author   PT publication type
AU – Temane A
PT – Journal Article
MH – *Compassion Fatigue   MH MeSH terms
MH – *Burnout, Professional   *denotes main point of article
MH – *Empathy
MH – Humans
MH – *Nurse-Patient Relations
MH – *Resilience, Psychological
OT – compassion fatigue
OT – metasynthesis
OT – mixed-methods research
OT – nursing
OT – qualitative
SO – J Clin Nurs. 2017 Feb 23. doi: 10.1111/jocn. 13766.

SO source   OT other terms (keywords)

Figure 3.4: MEDLINE record in PubMed.

should not be attempted until you know the keywords that are most frequently used. The weakness of the title search is that if authors do not use your terms in their title, you likely missed best evidence. Your vigilance at listing all the synonyms that an author could use for your PICOT question is essential to refining your title search and increasing your certainty that best evidence is not missed. When using this method, scan the subject headings of the relevant citations you have discovered to identify additional subject headings you may not have used earlier in your search.

Combining and Limiting Searches

In a focused search for a clinical topic using the PICOT question as the framework for the search, clinicians have the option to enter multiple concepts simultaneously into the search system. The disadvantage of this method is that there is no way to determine which concept has the most evidence available. To see how many **hits** (i.e., articles or studies that contain the searched word) that each term retrieves, clinicians can enter the terms from the PICOT question into the search box one at a time. By entering them one at a time, especially in very large databases (e.g., MEDLINE, CINAHL), you can discover the number of hits for each individual term searched. For example, searching MEDLINE for the keywords *Tylenol* and *pain* separately yielded 173 and 535,185 hits, respectively; however, when searching them together, *Tylenol AND pain*, the yield was 62. There is clearly more evidence about pain than Tylenol. It is important to consider that out of a possible 173 studies, only 62 were found that contained both terms. To enter each PICOT term individually may not be possible with every search because of competing clinical priorities; however, it is the best method to fully understand what evidence exists to answer the clinical question.

When combining subject headings or keywords, the Boolean connectors *AND* or *OR* are used (Competency 3D, Figure 3.1). The *AND* connector is useful when attempting to link different concepts together (e.g., PICOT question components). Using *AND* is appropriate when clinicians wish to narrow their search by having both of the combined terms required in the retrieved articles. Because *AND* is a restrictive word (i.e., both words must appear in the article), it will reduce the number of articles retrieved, which serves well with a finely honed PICOT question. Conversely, the *OR* Boolean connector is generally used to expand a search because either one or both of the search terms will be included in the results list. When concepts using synonyms are searched for, *OR* should be used. To gain mastery in understanding the concepts of the Boolean connector *AND* and *OR*, review Figure 3.5. Each search system has its own unique way of combining terms. For example, one system may require typing in the word *AND* or *OR*, whereas another may offer the ease of clicking on a "combine" option and specifying the correct connector. The same is true for how to best search databases. In PubMed, clinicians often enter their keywords and use Boolean connectors to search all the terms at once. However, searchers can search individual terms in PubMed by using the advanced search option and choosing "add to history" instead of "search" with each term. This will enable searchers to know the yield for each term, much like the results of using *AND* and *OR* in Figure 3.6. Consulting the databases' help documents can assist in determining the unique ways to conduct a search using Boolean connectors within that database (Competency 3D, Figure 3.1). To dig deeper and build your searching skills, follow the searching example found in the Examples on this book's companion website thePoint˚.

Here is a further example that illustrates the principle of combining search terms in a basic and advanced search. Clinicians begin searching for articles to answer the following diagnosis question:

In patients with suspected schizophrenia, is magnetic resonance imaging (MRI) compared with computed tomography (CT scan) more accurate in diagnosing the disorder?

For mastering using the PICOT question and incorporating Boolean connectors in searching, review Figures 3.6 and 3.7. The basic searcher would use the keywords *magnetic resonance imaging, MRI, computed tomography, CT scan, schizophrenia,* and *diagnosing* to search each term individually (s1, s2, s3, s4, s5, and s6) whereas the advanced searcher would add the truncated keyword *diagnos** (s12), which would allow the searchers to capture diagnose, diagnosis, diagnoses, or diagnosing with one search term. If the use of subject headings is an option, both searchers would use that option. Beginning with the basic searcher, the terms *magnetic resonance imaging OR MRI* as well as *computed tomography OR CT scan* would be searched separately (*magnetic resonance imaging* [s1] *OR MRI* [s2]; *computed tomography* [s3] *OR CT scan* [s4]), forming the first two combined search statements (s7 and s8). Next, these *OR*-combined searches would be combined using the *AND* connector (s7 *AND* s8), forming the third combined search statement (s9). These results would then be combined with the terms *schizophrenia* (s5) and *diagnosing* (s6) using *AND* (i.e., s5 *AND* s6 *AND* s9) because this search would theoretically yield the best answer to the question (see s10). However, if few results were found, the yield (0 in this example) could be increased by combining s7 and s8 with the connector *OR* (s7 *OR* s8), which will create s11. The basic searcher would combine

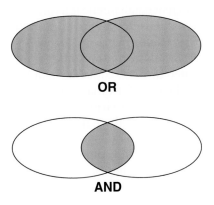

OR

AND

Figure 3.5: Boolean connectors *OR, AND.*

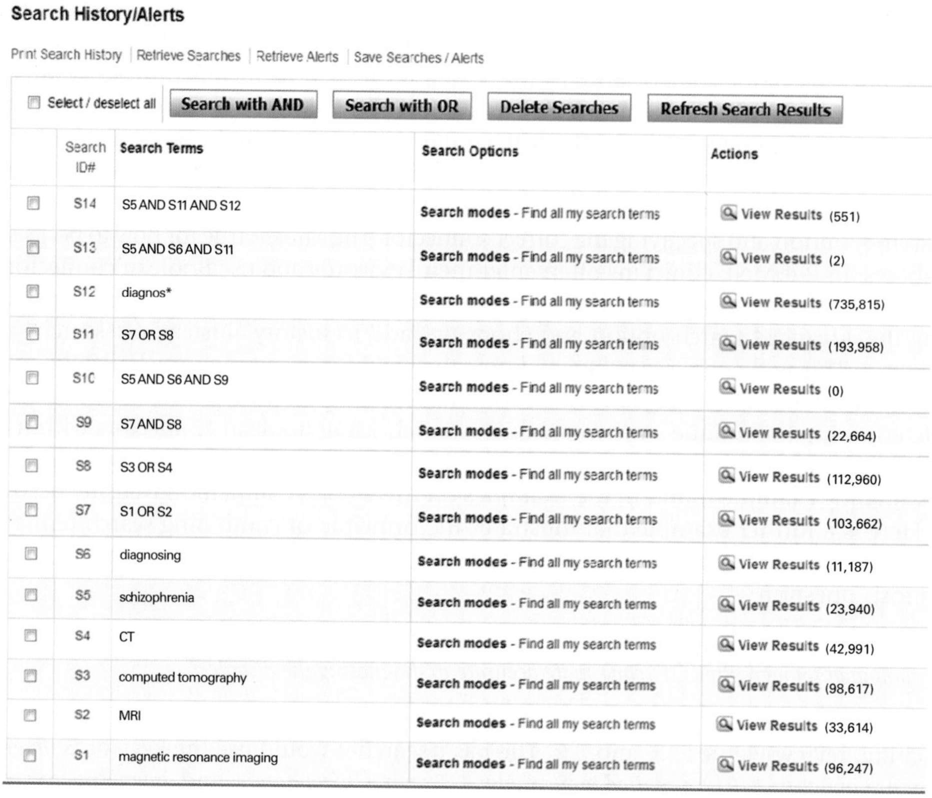

Search History/Alerts

Print Search History | Retrieve Searches | Retrieve Alerts | Save Searches / Alerts

	Search ID#	Search Terms	Search Options	Actions
	S14	S5 AND S11 AND S12	Search modes - Find all my search terms	🔍 View Results (551)
	S13	S5 AND S6 AND S11	Search modes - Find all my search terms	🔍 View Results (2)
	S12	diagnos*	Search modes - Find all my search terms	🔍 View Results (735,815)
	S11	S7 OR S8	Search modes - Find all my search terms	🔍 View Results (193,958)
	S1C	S5 AND S6 AND S9	Search modes - Find all my search terms	🔍 View Results (0)
	S9	S7 AND S8	Search modes - Find all my search terms	🔍 View Results (22,664)
	S8	S3 OR S4	Search modes - Find all my search terms	🔍 View Results (112,960)
	S7	S1 OR S2	Search modes - Find all my search terms	🔍 View Results (103,662)
	S6	diagnosing	Search modes - Find all my search terms	🔍 View Results (11,187)
	S5	schizophrenia	Search modes - Find all my search terms	🔍 View Results (23,940)
	S4	CT	Search modes - Find all my search terms	🔍 View Results (42,991)
	S3	computed tomography	Search modes - Find all my search terms	🔍 View Results (98,617)
	S2	MRI	Search modes - Find all my search terms	🔍 View Results (33,614)
	S1	magnetic resonance imaging	Search modes - Find all my search terms	🔍 View Results (96,247)

Select / deselect all | **Search with AND** | **Search with OR** | **Delete Searches** | **Refresh Search Results**

Figure 3.6: Example of a basic and advanced search using Boolean connectors *OR* and *AND*.

s11 with the terms *schizophrenia* (s5) and *diagnosing* (s6) using the Boolean connector *AND* (i.e., s5 *AND* s6 *AND* s11). The yield in our example is two articles, which is not sufficient. Therefore, the basic searcher would seek out an advanced searcher who would combine s11 with the terms *schizophrenia* (s5) and the advanced searchers truncated term *diagnos** (s12) using the Boolean connector *AND* (i.e., s5 *AND* s11 *AND* s12) in hopes of a higher yield, which is realized in our example with 551 hits. The advanced searching strategy of truncation made a difference in this search strategy. It is important to keep in mind that this search provides some insight into the answer to the question, although it won't answer it completely because it has only the (I) *OR* the (C).

Different databases treat terms entered in the search box in different ways; therefore, it is wise to use the tutorials provided in the database to fully understand how to search various databases (Competency 3A, Figure 3.1). Although it is important to enter and combine the same keywords in the same order, as much as possible, when searching in different databases, each database may require a slight variation to the search strategy. You should be able to explain the need for variations and recognize that different combinations of keywords will result in a different yield. It is not easy to know how a database will search the keywords you enter because there may be unique aspects of databases that are automatic and not clearly evident. Some Internet search engines may look for the keywords entered together as a phrase first, while other search systems automatically put the Boolean connector *OR* or *AND* between the terms. As you are learning to search a database, take the time to consult help documents that can help you become familiar with how the database searches terms

(Competency 3A, Figure 3.1). Systematic searching must become a habit, or your search becomes a disorganized approach to seeking evidence.

Limiting Searches. Databases can be very large, and even with the best search strategies, there are often more citations retrieved than clinicians can review to determine whether they are relevant to a clinical question. Limit functions are designed to help searchers pare down a large list of citations to the most relevant studies (Competency 3F, Figure 3.1). In PubMed, limit functions are referred to as **filters**, whereas Ovid MEDLINE uses Limiters and CINAHL uses "Limit to." Choosing the limit function leads searchers to a set of options for limiting the results by various parameters (e.g., study design [called publication type], language, human studies, publication year, age, gender, full text). For example, limiting the results of a search to a type of study design (e.g., RCTs or meta-analysis) can help searchers know how many of the articles in that yield are higher-level evidence to answer the clinical question (see Chapter 2). Higher-level evidence helps searchers answer the clinical question with relevant, stronger studies, thereby increasing confidence that the clinical outcome can be achieved (Competency 4B, Figure 3.1).

Another limit option, full text, narrows the search to "e-documents," in which the entire article is available electronically. The ease of limiting a search to full-text retrieval can be tempting; however, clinicians can miss evidence by limiting their search to only those articles whose full text is readily available. Keep in mind that the answer to a clinical question comes from a body of evidence, not just a few articles; therefore, it is important to seek all relevant articles to answer the clinical question.

There are times when searchers would like the full text of an article but the library does not have a subscription to the journal or the publisher offers the full text for a fee. If you don't want to pay the publisher for the article, find out if the library you are affiliated with

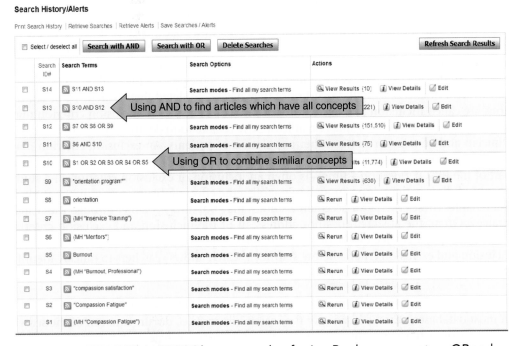

Figure 3.7: MEDLINE via EBSCOhost example of using Boolean connectors *OR* and *AND.*

can get a copy through *interlibrary loan* (ILL). Interlibrary loan is a network of libraries that collaborate to supply articles or books to other libraries that either don't subscribe to the journal or don't own the book (Competency 6B, Figure 3.1). Some libraries offer this service at no charge and others charge a fee. Contact your librarian to request the article or, if there is no librarian to partner with regarding the evidence you need, contact your local public library. Also, many local college libraries, state libraries, or hospital libraries will allow unaffiliated healthcare providers to use their resources. Be aware that there may be policies in place that restrict library staff from assisting unaffiliated users in their searches, and you may be unable to borrow from their resources. Copying articles in the library's collection is generally available for a fee. Another solution may be to register to use the document delivery service through the NLM called Loansome Doc. This service requires you to establish a relationship with a nearby library, and there may be a fee for each document, depending on that library's policies.

An important limiting option in a database that uses subject headings is to designate the subject headings as the main point of the article. This option does not fall within the limits list but can be found as searchers are designating which subject headings to search.

 Instructions for Loansome Doc may be found at https://www.nlm.nih.gov/pubs/factsheets/ loansome_doc.html

---

When indexers assign subject headings for MEDLINE, CINAHL, and PsycINFO, they will index the subject headings as either a major or a minor concept for each article. In the sample MEDLINE record in Figure 3.4, the asterisk (*) beside some MeSH terms indicates the subject headings the indexer considered to be the main points of the article. Many search systems permit searchers to limit the search to articles where a particular concept is the main focus of the article. For example, Ovid provides the "focus" option to the right of the subject heading and CINAHL provides the option "major concept." Limiting a subject heading to the main point will increase the relevance of the retrieved articles (Competency 3C, Figure 3.1).

The final method for limiting the number of relevant citations is used when reviewing studies that might be appraised (i.e., after the search strategy in the database is complete), not within the search of the database. Before a search strategy is begun, clinicians identify specific conditions that will assist in determining which evidence they will keep (keepers) and which evidence they will discard once they have completed their search. These conditions are called **inclusion** and **exclusion criteria**. For example, an inclusion criterion may be that a sample for a study must be at least 50% female to make the studies useful to the clinician and be relevant to his or her population of patients. An exclusion criterion may be that clinicians will not accept studies that compare three different medications. The fifth part of the PICOT question—time—is often an inclusion or exclusion criterion. If a study does not follow patients long enough to establish the effect of the intervention, the study is not reliable. These criteria for acceptable studies may not always be met through the search strategy. Often, the abstract does not address all of the inclusion and exclusion criteria. The entire study may need to be obtained to determine whether it is a keeper. Establishing inclusion and exclusion criteria before starting a search allows searchers to quickly identify the most relevant evidence to appraise.

Saving, Printing, or Capturing Screenshot Search Histories: Why and How

In most databases, searchers can save the search history (i.e., documentation of the search strategy; Competency 5A, Figure 3.1). The search history consists of the steps you used to complete the search. This is also referred to as saving a search. There are two reasons to save the search history: (1) repeating the search in other compatible databases or (2) rerunning the search strategy at a later time in the same database without having to retype the entire search history again. This is particularly true if you need to keep abreast of new articles being published on a particular topic. If you are interrupted while searching, do save the steps of your search so that you can come back and complete it later. Similarly, if you think you may need to tweak the strategy, save the search. By saving the search history, you can start searching exactly where you left off. You will not need to retype any of the search statements you have entered before saving the search history. Let's consider an example of why you would save a search history. As an advanced practice nurse, Joni is in charge of updating her institution's nursing standards. Her organization has recently partnered with a hospital that is inserting ventricular assist devices (VADs), and she needs to develop a nursing standard that will inform nursing practice. Joni has completed an initial in-depth search for nursing care of the VAD patient and has used relevant studies to create the recommendations for the newly developed nursing standard. She also saved search histories in the multiple databases that she searched. When it is time to review the standard, Joni is able to run the saved search, and she does not have to start from scratch. With a saved search, Joni is able to reduce the amount of time she spends searching because she already has her search strategy established and only needs to look at citations that have been added to the database since the last time she searched by limiting by publication date. She may not want to use exactly the same approach (e.g., keywords, subject headings, and combinations), but it is easy to make adjustments. Joni can introduce new keywords or look to see if a subject heading has recently been added as she considers how she needs to change her search strategy and resave her search. You can consult the user guide or help section of any database to learn more about saving your search (Competency 5A, Figure 3.1).

If you feel that you won't be revisiting the topic, then printing the search history or taking a screenshot will allow you to keep a record of the search steps you used and will help you to duplicate your search history in other databases you will be searching (Competency 5A, Figure 3.1). Most databases will allow searchers to immediately print out the search history, and this is the easiest way to obtain a print copy of how you searched. To take a screenshot, use the print screen function on your computer and insert the "screenshot" into a PowerPoint slide presentation or a Word document. By keeping a printed record or a screenshot of how the search was run, you can also share the search history with others so they know how you searched. A caveat when printing or capturing a screenshot of your search history is that you will lose the ability to automatically run the search strategy again. The search strategy will need to be manually reentered.

Here are a few more tips on taking a screenshot of your search history: To capture your search history screenshot, be sure that the search strategy is clear on your computer screen. If the history is long and does not fit completely on a single computer screen without scrolling up or down, you will need to take more than one screenshot to document the entire search strategy. The screenshot should include only the steps you took in your search, not the citations of articles in the results list. Your screenshot should resemble Figures 3.6 and 3.7. If you are unfamiliar with how to capture a screenshot, use this perfect opportunity to use keywords to search your favorite web-based database to find the steps for capturing a screenshot.

Keepers: Managing Citations of Interest

Once a search is completed, each database will provide options for managing the "keeper" citations. Most databases provide methods for printing, saving, or e-mailing citations. Databases may also provide other specialized features for dealing with selected citations. For example, PubMed has the clipboard, while CINAHL uses folders. Databases may also allow users to set up individual accounts that offer customization of certain features or the ability to save desired settings. Familiarizing yourself with these options can spare you frustration and may save you a great deal of time. To gain mastery in understanding the special features of databases, seek out "Help" documentation that can assist in learning about them (Competency 3A, Figure 3.1), or collaborate with a librarian to learn about these time-saving options (Competency 2C, Figure 3.1).

Organizing Results: Beyond the Basic Competency

Often, there is a need to organize the evidence found, because the large number of articles retrieved can be overwhelming (Stillwell et al., 2010). Practitioners need to organize evidence in some way so that they may easily find the evidence through each step of their EBP journey. Reference management software (RMS) is one solution (Competency 5B, Figure 3.1). Often referred to as citation managers/management, this software is designed to offer options that save, search, sort, share, and continuously add, delete, and organize promising citations. Some web-based examples of **reference managers** include RefWorks and Endnote. Many libraries provide this type of software for their users; therefore, readers should check with their library before purchasing any RMS software. If clinicians must select an RMS product, they need to compare purchase/subscription fees, features, ease of use, and speed. Approximate annual fees for individuals can range from $100 to $300 per year, depending on vendor/ desired features. Ovid also offers a built-in version of a reference management tool called My Projects that allows searchers to organize and share references collected from Ovid. If your library offers some type of RMS, you will want to find out more about it. In addition to subscription-based RMS, there are many open-source RMS options. Mendeley and Zotero are two free reference management tools that promote collaboration among researchers.

Practitioners can work with teams at multiple sites or their own institution using web-based RMS that is designed to import/export citations from all of the commonly searched databases as well as sort the citations by author, journal title, and keywords. Organizing the evidence in folders by clinical meaningfulness, specific PICOT concepts, or strength of evidence allows clinicians or teams to add to and keep track of the relevant information they find and use. By sharing citations with the team or organizing them for their own initiatives, clinicians can reduce the time invested in evidence retrieval and improve access to current information for the entire team.

Check out these free reference management software options:

Zotero: http://www.zotero.org

Mendeley: http://www.mendeley.com

Support and Strategy 4: Choosing the Right Database

Of the many databases that index healthcare literature, some are available through several vendors at a cost, some are free of charge, and some are available, at least in part, both free of charge and through a vendor for a fee (Competencies 2A and 2B, Figure 3.1). As noted previously, MEDLINE can be accessed free of charge through the NLM's PubMed or obtained by subscription through other providers (e.g., Ovid). Table 3.1 contains information about access to some of these databases.

This chapter focuses primarily on the following databases:

- Cochrane Databases
- MEDLINE
- Trip
- CINAHL
- Embase
- PsycINFO

MEDLINE and CINAHL are among the best-known comprehensive databases that contain much of the scientific knowledge base in healthcare. However, the amount of information in healthcare exceeds the capacity of either of these databases. In addition to MEDLINE and CINAHL, there are other types of databases that provide more readily available information in summaries and synopses (e.g., UpToDate, Nursing Reference Center). Some of these databases are highly specialized, and their numbers are growing in response to clinicians' desire for quick access to evidence.

Cochrane Databases

Classified as an international not-for-profit organization, the Cochrane Collaboration represents the efforts of a global network of dedicated volunteer researchers, healthcare professionals, and consumers who prepare, maintain, and promote access to the Cochrane Library's five current databases: (1) **CDSR**, (2) **Cochrane Central Register of Controlled Trials** (CENTRAL), (3) **Cochrane Methodology Register**, (4) **Health Technology Assessment**, and (5) **NHS Economic Evaluation Database**.

The *Cochrane handbook for systematic reviews of interventions* (Higgins & Green, 2011) is a free, authoritative, online handbook that documents the process that should be used by clinicians who are conducting a systematic review. For searchers, it provides an entire section on how to systematically search for studies to support EBP.

 The Cochrane handbook is available online at http://handbook.cochrane.org/

Cochrane Database of Systematic Reviews. The Cochrane Library's gold standard database is the CDSR. It contains Cochrane full-text systematic reviews and should be searched first to answer intervention questions. Although the CDSR is a fairly small database, in part because systematic reviews are still relatively new and few, it contains a large number of valuable, synthesized (i.e., critically appraised, compiled, and integrated) RCTs. Unlike MEDLINE (e.g., 23 million citations) and CINAHL (e.g., 3.6 million citations), the CDSR contains a few thousand citations and is limited to a single publication type—systematic reviews—including meta-analyses. A single word search in the MEDLINE or CINAHL databases can easily result in thousands of hits. Because the CDSR is a small database, the broadest search is likely to retrieve only a small, manageable number of hits. This makes the database easy to search and the results easy to review. With regard to the search results, the label "Review" refers to a completed Cochrane review, and the label "Protocol" applies to Cochrane reviews that are in the initial stages of gathering and appraising evidence. It is helpful to know that protocols are in the pipeline; however, it can be disappointing not to find a full review. If a full Cochrane review is retrieved during a search, clinicians can save time because they do not need to conduct the critical appraisal and synthesis of primary studies, because that has already been done. However, they need to critically appraise the systematic review itself. Chapter 5 contains more information on critically appraising systematic reviews.

Clinicians may access the citations (as well as abstracts of systematic reviews) free of charge. A paid subscription allows searchers to view the full text of all reviews and protocols. On February 1, 2013, authors producing a systematic review could choose, at the time of publication, one of two options for publishing their review: gold or green **open access**. Gold open access allows immediate access to the entire review if the authors agree to pay the publication charge fee. Green open access offers free access to the full review 12 months after publication. Systematic reviews published before February 1, 2013, will remain accessible by abstract only without a paid subscription. Check to see if your library has a subscription.

If it doesn't, you can use another option, namely, to access the full-text version of a review by paying for it separately (pay-per-view). This option is offered on each abstract summary page. Both MEDLINE and CINAHL index Cochrane's systematic reviews; therefore, don't miss these when searching these databases.

CENTRAL Database. The CENTRAL database serves as the most comprehensive source of reports of controlled trials. CENTRAL contains citations identified from MEDLINE, Embase, other databases and a **handsearch** (Lefebvre et al., 2011a; Lefebvre, Manheimer, & Glanville, 2011b, 2011c). Clinicians without access to Embase or other evidence sources, including **grey literature**, would be wise to search CENTRAL to identify additional trials that may be helpful in answering their PICOT question.

 The databases produced by The Cochrane Collaboration can be accessed via
http://www.cochranelibrary.com/

Guidelines International Network

Guidelines International Network (G-I-N) is a non-profit organization with a website that can be searched to find clinical practice databases. The website is designed and intended to facilitate communication among G-I-N members to foster engagement and collaboration. There is a fee for membership. G-I-N offers some information about how the guidelines were developed and tested, as well as recommendations for use. Clinical practice guidelines (CPGs) each describe a plan of care for a specific set of clinical circumstances involving a particular population. CPG developers, which include many professional associations, use various evidence sources to craft current and relevant recommendations that make up their guidelines (see Chapter 8), including PubMed, Embase, CINAHL, and PsycINFO. Links to the electronic version of the latest set of guidelines may be available. The best intervention guidelines are based on the rigorous scientific evidence obtained from systematic reviews or RCTs and other evidence. Some guidelines are a consensus of expert opinion and, although they are not the strongest evidence, can still assist in decision making.

There are several reasons why clinicians should seek out evidence-based guidelines. First, it is important to know what CPGs are available and then to compare two or more existing guidelines. This comparison allows clinicians to focus on how the recommendations within the guideline address their clinical question. It should be noted that guidelines themselves do not address PICOT questions; however, recommendations within guidelines may. The proper approach to using a guideline to answer a PICOT question is to cite the supporting evidence of the recommendation that addresses the question.

The G-I-N mission is to lead, strengthen and support the use of guidelines. They focus on development, adaptation and implementation of CPGs, as well as facilitating networking among those using the guidelines in their database. G-I-N also offers conferences, communities, and work groups to enhance collaboration around development and implementation of CPGs.

 G-I-N is online at http://www.g-i-n.net/home.

MEDLINE

MEDLINE is one of the world's largest searchable databases covering medicine, health, and the biomedical sciences. MEDLINE is a premier database produced by the NLM and is available through PubMed at no charge from any computer with Internet access. The NLM also leases the MEDLINE data to vendors (see Figure 3.3). These companies load the database into their own interface and sell subscriptions to their database. Ovid is one of several companies that do this. It is important to know that the original file of indexed citations is the same MEDLINE product in PubMed as in any of these other vendors' versions of the file. It contains citations from more than 5,600 worldwide journals in 39 languages, although its primary focus tends to be on North American journals (National Library of Medicine, 2016). Coverage spans the period 1946 to the present. MEDLINE uses MeSH to index articles and facilitate searches.

The MEDLINE database is available free of charge through PubMed at
https://www.ncbi.nlm.nih.gov/pubmed

Trip

Trip first came on the scene in 1997 and has evolved into one of the leading clinical search engines for evidence-based content. While Trip is a commercial company, the cofounders assert that the business is run more like a not-for-profit company. Access to the website continues to be free, although a low yearly subscription grants access to TRIP Premium, which enables more search functionality such as **adjacency searching** and the ability to use Boolean connectors. Trip loads the content of PubMed every 2 weeks and loads **secondary sources** of evidence such as summaries, synopses, and syntheses once a month. The process for adding these secondary sources of evidence has been developed by the founders of the database and, over the years, users have suggested sources as well. Clinicians can find research evidence as well as other content (e.g., images, videos, patient information leaflets, educational courses, and news).

The first step to optimize the Trip search experience is to register. Registering enables clinicians to take advantage of other features such as automated searches and the ability to track Continuing Professional Development/Continuing Medical Education.

Trip offers four PICO search boxes that follow the first four elements of a PICO question. This helps to focus searchers. It is not necessary to enter a term for each element, but it would be wise for searchers to use as many of the elements as possible for better results.

The limits in the Trip database are found in the Refine Results menu on the right side of the webpage. It allows searchers to limit results to the type of content that will best answer their clinical question and to further limit by publication date or clinical area.

Trip is available free of charge at http://www.tripdatabase.com

CINAHL

The CINAHL database is produced by EBSCOhost and contains citations from many subject areas, including nursing, biomedicine, 17 allied health disciplines, and alternative/complementary medicine. CINAHL includes more than 3.6 million citations from over 3,100 journals as well as more than 70 full-text journals. Available only through a library subscription, CINAHL retrieves content from journals, books, drug monographs, and dissertations and includes images that are often difficult to locate in other databases. CINAHL can be searched by keywords that retrieve the keyword in any of the indexed fields. The CINAHL database provides subject headings (CINAHL headings) that can be used instead of or in conjunction with keyword searching.

Searchers should be aware that checking the box for "suggest subject terms" will force a subject heading search. To enable keyword searching, choose your keywords at the bottom of the list of proposed subject headings. This will render a combined search of the chosen subject heading as well as your keywords.

 Video tutorials for searching (Competency 3A, Figure 3.1) are available through EBSCOhost's YouTube Channel at www.youtube.com/user/ebscopublishing/
More information about the CINAHL database is available at http://www.ebscohost.com/cinahl/

Embase

Embase provides comprehensive coverage of biomedicine, with a strong emphasis on drugs and pharmacology. It holds more than 31 million records, among which are 8,500-plus journals, including all journals indexed by MEDLINE and 2,900 unique journals. Embase is produced by the publishing company Elsevier, Inc. and is available only by subscription.

 More information about Embase is available at http://www.embase.com

PsycINFO

PsycINFO is a database produced by the American Psychological Association (APA) and includes scattered publications from 1597 to the present and comprehensive coverage from the late 1800s to the present. Available by subscription only, this database indexes literature in psychology, behavioral sciences, and mental health and contains more than 4 million citations. PsycINFO includes citations to books and book chapters, comprising approximately 11% of the database. Dissertations can also be found within this database.

 More information about PsycINFO is available at http://www.apa.org/psycinfo/

Searching the literature can be both rewarding and challenging, primarily because the volume of healthcare literature is huge. The MEDLINE database alone provides reference to more than 23 million citations; however, it cannot cover *all* worldwide healthcare journals. Searching multiple databases can increase the number of relevant articles found during the search (Competency 3H, Figure 3.1). The databases discussed here impose organization on the chaos that is the journal literature. Each database offers coverage that is broad and sometimes overlapping. Knowing which databases to search first and for what information is necessary for a successful, efficient search (Competency 2A, Figure 3.1).

Never give up, for that is just the place and time that the tide will turn.

HARRIET BEECHER STOWE

A Unique Case: PubMed

PubMed is a completely free database produced and maintained by the National Center for Biotechnology Information (NCBI) at the NLM. PubMed's primary component is MEDLINE, but it also contains citations from additional life science journals that submit full-text articles to PubMed Central as well as citations for the majority of books and book chapters available on the NCBI Bookshelf. Currently, the oldest citations date back to 1945.

NCBI has made it possible for libraries to link their electronic and print serial holdings to citations in the database, making it easy for their clientele to access full-text articles they own through the PubMed database and to identify which articles are available in print at the library. Any clinician affiliated with a library should check with that library to learn more about how to use PubMed and access their full-text and print resources (Competency 2C, Figure 3.1).

Although MEDLINE resides within the PubMed database, PubMed contains more citations than MEDLINE. Citations that are in PubMed but not in MEDLINE—approximately 8%—are *not* indexed with MeSH terms. To facilitate full use of the information in PubMed, the NLM developed automatic term mapping, which searches the keywords entered in the search box and maps them to any appropriate MeSH terms. This enables keywords to more effectively search *both* indexed and nonindexed citations in PubMed. In addition, a particular logic has been built into automatic term mapping to make it even more effective. There are three steps to this process:

1. **MeSH term:** Automatic term mapping first looks for a match between what is typed into the search box and a table of MeSH terms. If there is a match with a MeSH term, the MeSH term plus the keyword will be used to run the search.
2. **Journal title:** If there is no match with a MeSH term, what has been typed in the search box is next compared with a table of journal titles. If there is a match, the journal title is used to run the search.
3. **Author name:** If there is no match with either a MeSH term or a journal title, the words in the search box are then compared with a table of author names. If there is a match, that author name is used to run the search.

Automatic term mapping begins with the words entered into the search box as a single unit. If it cannot find a match in any of the three tables, it will drop the word that is farthest to the right in the search string, look at the remaining words, and run through the three steps of automatic term mapping, looking for a match. If a match is found, then automatic term mapping will use the match (MeSH term, journal title, or author name) plus the keyword as part of the search and return to process the term that was previously dropped.

An example of automatic term mapping is presented in Box 3.1. After thoroughly exploring her first clinical question, the nurse manager in our example then poses her second PICOT question: *In new nurses providing patient care (P) how does journaling (I) compared with focus groups (C) affect compassion fatigue rates (O) over their first year in the profession (T)?* She begins with typing compassion fatigue as one of the search terms in the search box in PubMed and runs the search. To better understand the results, she clicks on "Details," which shows how PubMed used automatic term mapping to process the search.

Once the search was run, PubMed provided the option to further refine retrieval by using filters. Some of these filters are called limits in other databases. To access these filters, the nurse manager clicks on the Show Additional Filters located on the left of the page. Limiting

BOX 3.1 *Details of PubMed Automatic Term Mapping for Compassion Fatigue*

"compassion fatigue"[MeSH Terms] OR ("compassion"[All Fields] AND "fatigue"[All Fields]) OR "compassion fatigue" [All Fields]
- The "compassion fatigue" [MeSH Terms] portion of the search will retrieve relevant information containing the MeSH term from the indexed portion of the MEDLINE database.
- The ("compassion" [All Fields] AND "fatigue" [All Fields]) OR "compassion fatigue" [All Fields] portion of the search will retrieve information from the nonindexed portion of the database.

to certain dates of publication, certain languages, human or animal studies, and types of publications (e.g., clinical trial, meta-analysis) are some of the options. Figure 3.8 shows some examples of the many filters that can be applied.

When she reviews the search results in PubMed, she remembers that it is important to note that search results appear in the order in which they were added to the database. This means that the first citation is the one that meets the search criteria and was most recently added to the database. To find the most recently published article, she uses the "Sort by Pub Date" option that can be found in the Display Settings dropdown menu (Figure 3.9).

The nurse manager is careful to design the search strategy using her second PICOT question as a guide and enters the appropriate keywords into the advanced search box in PubMed and clicks run. She applies her carefully selected filters (limits), and the results are sorted. The nurse manager considers that she can further separate the citations of interest from others that have been retrieved with the Send To option in PubMed (e.g., e-mail, clipboard; Figure 3.10).

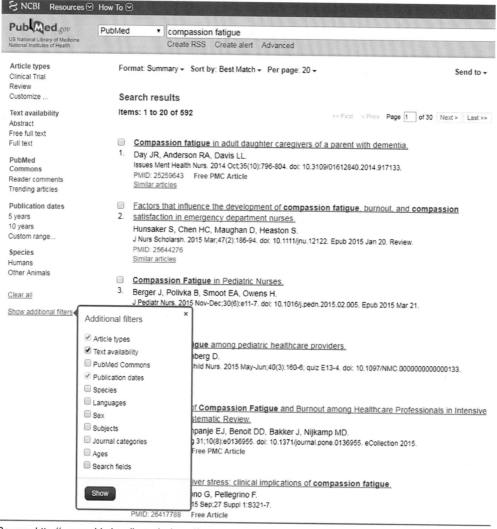

Source: *http://www.ncbi.nlm.nih.gov/pubmed/*

Figure 3.8: Filters in PubMed. (From National Library of Medicine, www.pubmed.gov.)

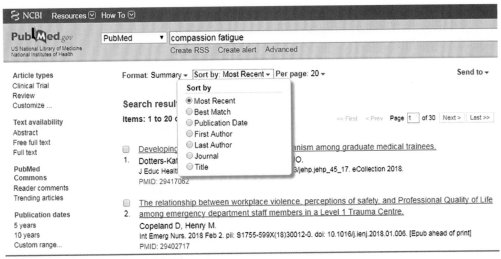

Source: *http://www.ncbi.nlm.nih.gov/pubmed/*

Figure 3.9: "Sort by" in PubMed. (From National Library of Medicine, www.pubmed.gov.)

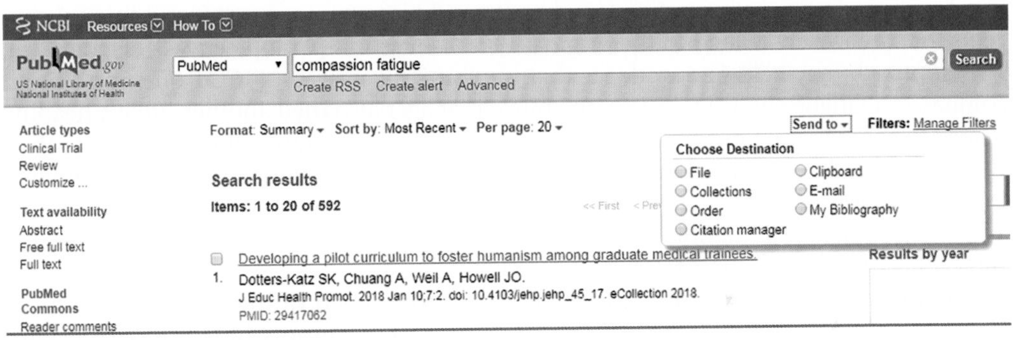

Source: *http://www.ncbi.nlm.nih.gov/pubmed/*

Figure 3.10: "Send to" options in PubMed. Note: This option saves citations but does not save the search history. (From National Library of Medicine, www.pubmed.gov.)

This has been a brief introduction to PubMed. A tutorial and quick start guide on searching PubMed can be found on the PubMed home page. And don't forget that healthcare librarians in your organization or partnering agency are always willing to help. To help with mastery of basic searching strategies, first complete your search in CINAHL and PubMed to find evidence to answer the above clinical question. Then compare your strategy with the searching examples that can be found under Suggested Answers on thePoint®.

Support and Strategy 5: Advanced Searching Competencies—Helping Find the Needle

Up until this point, basic searching competencies have primarily been highlighted. It is an expectation that all healthcare professionals who are searching for evidence will possess the basic competencies, whereas advanced searchers will need to be proficient in all the basic competencies as well as the more advanced competencies. More importantly, all searchers should continue to use these competencies to support systematic searching *throughout* their career. Support and Strategy 5 covers the majority of the additional advanced competencies highlighted in the orange sections of Figure 3.1. These advanced skills help an advanced searcher leverage technology or apply additional strategies to locate evidence as quickly and efficiently as possible.

Finding Additional Articles When There Isn't Much Out There

There are times when there are not be many articles on a specific topic. Most databases offer searchers the option to find other relevant articles like the keeper articles they have found with a single click (Competency 3I, Figure 3.1). In CINAHL, this feature is called *Find Similar Results*. In Ovid, it is referred to as the *Find Similar* feature, and in PubMed it is labeled *Similar Articles*. If you have very few relevant citations, this is definitely another method to increase the number of relevant articles being retrieved.

Scanning through the list of references (bibliography) at the end of your keeper articles may also reveal other articles that are relevant to your PICOT question that have not turned up in your search (Competency 6C, Figure 3.1). This is called the **ancestry method**.

By conducting a title search, you can identify appropriate articles and can discover the subject headings that were used. If you have not used these subject headings yet in your search, this approach will enable you to incorporate them into your search strategy and potentially increase your yield. To help with mastery of finding additional subject headings to enhance your search strategy, review Figure 3.4.

Another advanced approach to try when the yield is low is to search for additional concepts that are closely related to the original PICOT question (Competency 3J, Figure 3.1). This approach may help find evidence that can partially answer a PICOT question. In our compassion fatigue clinical scenario, the nurse manager also tried another subject heading related to compassion fatigue—*burnout, professional*. By incorporating this strategy into their systematic search, clinicians may retrieve additional evidence that is related to the original PICOT question.

Take a look at the Examples on thePoint® to see how the nurse manager utilized similar subject headings in her CINAHL and PubMed searches.

In some cases, truncation should be considered when doing keyword searching (Competency 3K, Figure 3.1). Truncation uses special symbols in combination with words or word parts to enhance the likelihood of finding relevant studies. Truncation is usually indicated by a word or part of a word followed by an asterisk (*). In PubMed, Ovid MEDLINE and CINAHL, the asterisk may be used to replace any number of letters at the end of the word. For example, in PubMed, to truncate the phrase "new graduate," one would use "new* grad*" to retrieve new grad, new grads, new graduate, new graduates, or newly graduated. Again, a librarian and the help section of individual databases can offer guidance to determine relevant search characters or symbols (Competencies 3A and 3G, Figure 3.1).

Adjacency may also be helpful in finding additional information that closely matches a PICOT concept because it enables searchers to find words that are next to each other in the specified order or within x words of each other regardless of the order (Competency 3K, Figure 3.1). Ovid uses the adjacency operator (adj), whereas CINAHL uses the **proximity searching** connectors near (N) or within (W). Consult the field guide of any database for additional information.

Another advanced competency to try when the yield is sparse is to search for British spelling variations (Competency 3L, Figure 3.1). For example, a competent searcher will remember to use both the terms "hematology" and "haematology" when broadening the search for relevant citations.

Clinicians should also perform an author search if they notice that a particular author has published extensively in their field. This will often turn up additional citations related to the PICOT question (Competency 3M, Figure 3.1).

Another tool in the advanced competency arsenal is utilizing database alert features (Competency 3N, Figure 3.1). Most databases allow searchers to save their search history and offer the option of having the database automatically run the search strategy against newly added citations to the database. Searchers are able to choose how frequently they receive a list of newly indexed citations. This feature may be of interest to clinicians who need to be aware of new publications that may affect protocols they are currently using or are in charge of updating.

RSS, also known as Rich Site Summary or Really Simple Syndication (Competency 3N, Figure 3.1), is a format for pushing out newly posted or regularly developed web content. For example, you may wish to know when the American College of Chest Physicians releases a new anticoagulation guideline. You need to have a Feed Reader or News Aggregator on your computer that allows you to read the RSS feeds from sites you have selected. Microsoft Outlook even allows you to save/store RSS feeds in a separate folder within your e-mail account. Look for this symbol on webpages and within databases to request that new content be pushed out to you.

 More information about RSS can be found in the tutorial from Common Craft at https://www.commoncraft.com/video/rss

---

When searches in indexed databases do not lead to evidence of sufficient quality, clinicians may wish to explore what other evidence is available. Google may be helpful when searching for *grey literature* (Competency 3M, Figure 3.1). Grey literature is unpublished evidence that has not been included in databases that clinicians routinely search. It may take the form of reports, unpublished drug trials, or unpublished conference proceedings. Grey literature can be elusive, so using search engines such as Google or Google Scholar can provide value; however, caution should be used, and careful evaluation of the evidence retrieved from these sources is required. Clinicians should follow an appraisal process to ensure the information is reliable. While major search engines may help clinicians get started in finding grey literature, much of this type of literature lies in the **deep web**, which is estimated to be 400 to 550 times larger than the surface web (Olson, 2013). Healthcare librarians are best able to navigate the deep web, and collaboration with the librarian is crucial when searching for grey literature. The Cochrane Collaboration attempts to seek out deep web sources of evidence and asserts that 10% of its citations come from grey literature (Lefebvre et al., 2011a). Identifying professional associations that have developed relevant guidelines or other agencies that may have published grey literature is important (Competency 7A, Figure 3.1), and clinicians should also search association websites.

Additional databases to check for grey literature include OpenGrey, http://www.opengrey.eu/ and Grey Literature Report, http://www.greylit.org/

Clinicians should try to determine whether there are **listservs** or **discussion boards** on the web where they might post a question to the readership (Competency 7B, Figure 3.1). Often, professional associations maintain listservs, so check with associations related to your profession. Listservs distribute messages to subscribers through an electronic mailing list, so the content is only sent to subscribers. Discussion boards allow anyone on the web to read and post comments. Posting to a listserv or discussion board allows clinicians to determine whether anyone else is wrestling with the same issue or PICOT question and is also a good place to try finding external evidence to benchmark against (Competency 7C, Figure 3.1).

Lastly, it is important for clinicians to identify internal evidence within their organization that might help or at least better shape their PICOT question (Competency 7C, Figure 3.1).

Specialized Database Search Functions: Another Strategy for the Advanced Searcher

Many databases have specialized search functions to help busy clinicians find evidence as quickly as possible. This section discusses the specific search functions available in PubMed, Ovid MEDLINE, and CINAHL that can assist in finding relevant evidence quickly.

PubMed Special Queries. PubMed provides several filters for busy clinicians to quickly find the needle in their haystack. Clinicians may wish to check out Clinical Queries and Topic-Specific Queries under PubMed Tools on the PubMed home page.

Clinical Queries contains two very useful search options: clinical study category and systematic reviews. The clinical study category search filter was developed by Haynes and associates and provides a quick way to limit results to a specific study category. When using this feature, search terms are entered in the query box, the type of clinical question must be selected (etiology, diagnosis, therapy, prognosis, or clinical prediction guide), and the scope of the search is selected (broad or narrow), as shown in Figure 3.11 (see also Table 3.2). Clinicians who are looking to decrease a large number of results should select the Systematic Reviews clinical query because it is a good way to identify those citations that have a higher level of evidence rating (Competency 4B, Figure 3.1).

When a search is run, PubMed applies specific search filters to limit retrieval to the desired evidence. This means that PubMed automatically adds terms to the search in order to find the type of evidence needed. A quick look at the Details box after running a search will show what terms were added. PubMed also provides a link to the filter table that shows the different search filters and the terms associated with them.

Systematic reviews are retrieved automatically when you enter your keyword in the search box on the Clinical Query page (see Figure 3.11).

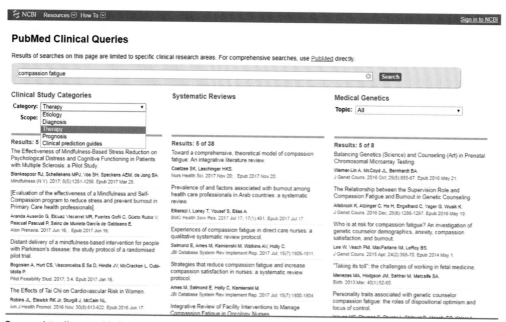

Source: *http://www.ncbi.nlm.nih.gov/pubmed/*

Figure 3.11: Clinical study categories in PubMed. (From National Library of Medicine, www.pubmed.gov.)

Clinical Queries in Ovid MEDLINE. Ovid Clinical Queries (OCQ) limits retrieval to best evidence and what Ovid refers to as clinically sound studies. To access OCQ, a searcher enters search statements in the main search box. Results are displayed on Ovid's main search page within Search History. To limit retrieved results, select Additional Limits to view Ovid's menu of limits. Find the Clinical Queries' dropdown menu and select the clinical query that best serves the purposes of your PICOT question.

The OCQ dropdown menu offers limits that retrieve clinically sound studies. Searchers select a query based on what the PICOT question is targeting (e.g., therapy, diagnosis, prognosis, reviews, clinical prediction guides, qualitative studies, etiology, costs, economics). Additionally, within each query, there are options to further refine the search. The refinement options include "Sensitive" (i.e., most relevant articles but probably some less relevant ones), "Specific" (i.e., mostly relevant articles but probably omitting a few), and "Optimized" (i.e., the combination of terms that optimizes the trade-off between sensitivity and specificity). Again, consult your healthcare librarian if you need help with using Ovid's clinical queries (Competency 3G, Figure 3.1).

Clinical Queries "Limiter" in CINAHL. Like PubMed and Ovid MEDLINE, CINAHL also offers a quick way to retrieve clinically relevant and scientifically sound results. These strategies were created in collaboration with the Health Information Research Unit (HIRU) at McMaster University and are designed for clinicians to use. There are five choices in CINAHL that can be applied to the search based on the type of PICOT question being asked: (1) Therapy, (2) Prognosis, (3) Review, (4) Qualitative, and (5) Causation (Etiology). CINAHL also provides an additional option within its Special Interest category of limits called Evidence-Based Practice. Selecting the EBP limiter allows you to narrow your results to articles from EBP journals, about EBP, research articles (including systematic reviews, clinical trials, meta-analyses, and so forth), and commentaries on research studies.

A Final Support and Strategy: Time and Money

Producing, maintaining, and making databases available is financially costly and time consuming. Although computer technology has revolutionized the print industry and made it easier to transfer documents and information around the world in seconds, the task of producing databases still relies on people to make decisions about what to include and how to index it. Databases produced by government agencies, such as MEDLINE, are produced with public money and are either very inexpensive or without cost to searchers. The MEDLINE database is available to anyone in the world who has access to the Internet through PubMed. The data in MEDLINE can be leased by vendors and placed in a variety of databases that will be accessed by healthcare providers, librarians, and others (Figure 3.3). Private organizations that produce biomedical databases, such as CINAHL or the CDSR, license their products. If there is no in-house library, it is worth the time and effort to locate libraries in the area and find out their access policies for these databases.

Clinicians must have access to databases in order to practice on the basis of evidence. Costs for supporting databases include licensing fees, hardware, software, Internet access, and library staff to facilitate users' searches and access to the evidence. Institutions must make decisions about what databases to subscribe to, and these decisions may be based on the resources available. Not all healthcare providers have libraries in their facilities. In these situations, clinicians or departments should consult with partnering librarians about securing access to databases that they consider critical to evidence-based care.

Although there is a cost associated with searching databases for relevant evidence, regular searching for answers to clinical questions has been shown to save money and improve patient outcomes. Researchers conducted an outcome-based, prospective study to measure the economic impact of MEDLINE searches on the cost both to the patient and to the participating hospitals (Klein, Ross, Adams, & Gilbert, 1994). They found that searches conducted early (i.e., in the first half) in patients' hospital stays resulted in significantly lower cost to the patients and to the hospitals, as well as shorter lengths of stay. Almost 20 years later, a multisite study found that 7% of physicians, residents, and nurses who utilized library and information sources reported a reduction in length of stay (Marshall et al., 2013).

Clinicians must remember the costs of both searching and obtaining relevant evidence, as well as the costs of not searching for and applying relevant evidence. Computerized retrieval of medical information is a fairly complex activity. It begins by considering the kind of information needed, creating an answerable PICOT question, planning and executing the search in appropriate databases, and analyzing the retrieved results.

❝

Do not go where the path may lead, go instead where there is no path and leave a trail.

RALPH WALDO EMERSON

HOW TO KNOW YOU HAVE FOUND THE NEEDLE

Successfully searching for relevant evidence is as important as asking a well-built PICOT question. For clinicians to get the answers they need to provide the best care to their patients, they must choose appropriate databases; design an appropriate search strategy using keyword, title, and subject headings; use limits; and successfully navigate the databases they are searching. In addition, clinicians must consider the cost of *not* searching for the best evidence. Commitment to finding valid, reliable evidence is the foundation for developing the skills that foster a sound search strategy, which, in turn, helps to reduce frustration and save time. Box 3.2 details the steps of an efficient search.

BOX 3.2	***Steps to an Efficient Search to Answer a Clinical Question***

- Begin with PICOT question—generates keywords.
- Establish inclusion/exclusion criteria *before* searching so that the studies that answer the question are easily identifiable. Apply these criteria after search strategy is complete.
- Use subject headings, when available.
- Expand the search using the explode option (Competency 3E, Figure 3.1), if not automatic.
- Use available mechanisms to focus the search so that the topic of interest is the main point of the article.
- Combine the searches generated from the PICOT keywords and the subject headings using Boolean connector AND.
- Limit the *final* cohort of studies with meaningful limits, such as language, human, type of study, age, and gender.
- Organize studies in a meaningful way using RMS.

The key to knowing whether the needle has been found is to further evaluate the selected studies from a successfully executed search. This evaluation method is called *critical appraisal*, the next step in the EBP process (see Chapters 4 to 7). Some journals are dedicated to the pre-appraisal of existing literature. Most of these articles are not syntheses (e.g., systematic reviews) but rather critical appraisals of current single studies. For example, the journal *Evidence-Based Nursing* reviews over 50 journals and about 25,000 articles per year. It identifies and publishes approximately 96 reviews of articles (both quantitative and qualitative) annually. The *ACP Journal Club* is another publication dedicated to preappraised literature. More than 100 journals are scanned for evidence relevant to clinicians. Specific criteria are applied to the appraised articles, and the appraisals are published bimonthly in the journal.

> Do what you can, with what you have, where you are.

THEODORE ROOSEVELT

These types of journals assist clinicians in reducing the time it takes from asking the question to applying valid evidence in clinical decision making.

NEXT STEPS

What can be done when a thorough search to answer a compelling clinical question yields either too little valid evidence to support confident practice change (i.e., inconclusive evidence) or no evidence? In most cases, clinicians are not in positions to do full-scale, multisite clinical trials to determine the answer to a clinical question, and the science may not be at the point to support such an investigation. However, determining what is effective in the clinicians' own practice by implementing the best evidence available can generate internal evidence. In addition, generating external evidence by conducting smaller scale studies, either individually or with a team of researchers, is an option. Chapters 19 and 20 address how to generate evidence to answer clinical questions. However, the starting place for addressing any clinical issue is to gather and evaluate the existing evidence using strategies and methods described in this chapter.

EBP FAST FACTS

- Good searching starts with a well-formulated clinical question.
- Systematic searching takes skills and practice (i.e., time).
- Searching all relevant databases is essential to find the body of evidence to answer a PICOT question.
- Although limiting to full text can be a useful tool to get a rapid return on a search, there may be relevant studies that are not captured in such a limited search.
- PubMed is a free database that uses automatic mapping for subject headings.
- Boolean connectors are AND (narrows search) and OR (expands search).
- There are three major search strategies that should be used in this order: (1) keywords (from PICOT question); (2) subject headings; (3) title (if necessary).
- There are basic search competencies expected of all clinicians and advanced search competencies to challenge clinicians who want to dig deeper.

> ## WANT TO KNOW MORE?
>
> A variety of resources are available to enhance your learning and understanding of this chapter.
> * Visit thePoint® to access:
>   * Suggested Answers to the case study outlined in this chapter, including searching examples on both PubMed and CINAHL
>   * Articles from the AJN EBP Step-By-Step Series
>   * Journal articles
>   * Checklists for rapid critical appraisal
> * Lippincott CoursePoint combines digital text content with video case studies and interactive modules for a fully integrated course solution that works the way you study and learn.

References

Fineout-Overholt, E. & Stillwell, S. (2015). Asking compelling clinical questions. In B. M. Melnyk & E. Fineout-Overholt (Eds.), *Evidence-based practice in nursing and healthcare: A guide to best practice* (3rd ed., pp. 25–39). Philadelphia, PA: Wolters Kluwer.

Hartzell, T. A., & Fineout-Overholt, E. (2017). The evidence-based practice competencies related to searching for best evidence. In B. M. Melnyk, L. Gallagher-Ford, & E. Fineout-Overholt (Eds.), *Implementing the evidence-based practice (EBP) competencies in healthcare: A practical guide to improving quality, safety, and outcomes.* Indianapolis, IN: Sigma Theta Tau International.

Haynes, B. (2007). Of studies, syntheses, synopses, summaries, and systems: The "5S" evolution of information services for evidence-based healthcare decisions. *Evidence-Based Nursing, 10*(1), 6–7.

Higgins, J. P. T, & Green, S. (Eds.). (2011). *Cochrane handbook for systematic reviews of interventions (version 5.1.0)* [updated March 2011]. London, England: The Cochrane Collaboration. Retrieved from www.handbook.cochrane.org.

Institute of Medicine (US) Roundtable on Evidence-Based Medicine. (2009). *Leadership commitments to improve value in healthcare: Finding common ground: Workshop summary.* Washington, DC: National Academies Press.

Klein, M. S., Ross, F. V., Adams, D. L., & Gilbert, C. M. (1994). Effect of online literature searching on length of stay and patient care costs. *Academic Medicine, 69,* 489–495.

Lefebvre, C., Manheimer, E., & Glanville, J. (2011a). Chapter 6: Searching for studies. In J. P. T. Higgins & S. Green (Eds.), *Cochrane handbook for systematic reviews of interventions (version 5.1.0).* London, England: The Cochrane Collaboration.

Lefebvre, C., Manheimer, E., & Glanville, J. (2011b). 6.2.1 Bibliographic databases. In J. P. T. Higgins & S. Green (Eds.), *Cochrane handbook for systematic reviews of interventions (version 5.1.0).* London, England: The Cochrane Collaboration.

Lefebvre, C., Manheimer, E., & Glanville, J. (2011c). 6.2.1.8 Grey literature databases. In J. P. T. Higgins & S. Green (Eds.), *Cochrane handbook for systematic reviews of interventions (version 5.1.0).* London, England: Cochrane Collaboration.

Marshall, J. G., Sollenberger, J., Easterby-Gannett, S., Morgan, L., Klem, M. L., Cavanaugh, S. K., & Hunter, S. (2013). The value of library and information services in patient care: Results of a multisite study. *Journal of the Medical Library Association, 101*(1), 38–46. doi:10.3163/1536-5050.101.1.007

National Library of Medicine. (2016). *Fact sheet: PubMed®: MEDLINE® retrieval on the world wide web.* Retrieved from http://www.nlm.nih.gov/pubs/factsheets/pubmed.html

Nourbakhsh, E., Nugent, R., Wang, H., Cevik, C., & Nugent, K. (2012). Medical literature searches: A comparison of PubMed and Google scholar. *Health Information & Libraries Journal, 29*(3), 214–222. doi:10.1111/j.1471-1842.2012.00992.x

Olson, C. A. (2013). Using the grey literature to enhance research and practice in continuing education for health professionals. *Journal of Continuing Education in the Health Professions, 33*(1), 1–3. doi:10.1002/chp.21159

Richardson, W. S., Wilson, M. C., Nishikawa, J., & Hayword, R. S. (1995). The well-built clinical question: A key to evidence-based decisions. *ACP Journal Club, 123*(3), A12–A13.

Stevens, K. R. (2001). Systematic reviews: The heart of evidence-based practice. *AACN Clinical Issues: Advanced Practice in Acute and Critical Care, 12*(4), 529–538.

Stillwell, S. B., Fineout-Overholt, E., Melnyk, B. M., & Williamson, K. M. (2010). Evidence-based practice, step by step: Searching for the evidence. *American Journal of Nursing, 110*(5), 41–47. doi:10.1097/01.NAJ.0000372071.24134.7e

Wright, A., Pang, J., Feblowitz, J. C., Maloney, F. L., Wilcox, A. R., Ramelson, H. Z., . . . Bates, D. W. (2011). A method and knowledge base for automated inference of patient problems from structured data in an electronic medical record. *Journal of the American Medical Informatics Association, 18*(6), 859–867.

| **A SUCCESS STORY**

Using an Evidence-based, Autonomous Nurse Protocol to Reduce Catheter-Associated Urinary Tract Infections in a Long-term Acute Care Facility

Tina L. Magers, PhD, MSN, RN-BC

STEP 0 The Spirit of Inquiry Ignited

Catheter-associated urinary tract infections (CAUTIs) are the most common hospital-associated infections. Approximately 25% of all hospitalized patients will experience a short-term urethral catheter (UC) (Gould et al., 2009). Long-term acute care hospitals (LTACHs) are particularly challenged with hospital-associated infections due to the population experiencing complicated healthcare conditions and an average length of stay of greater than 25 days. The most common mitigating factor in all patients with a UC is the number of days catheterized. Multiple studies have described the use of a nurse-driven protocol to evaluate the necessity of continued urethral catheterization with positive results in the reduction of catheter days (CDs) and CAUTIs. Some of the nurse-driven protocols are autonomously used by the nurse, and some require a reminder system to the provider. Clinical experts in acute care often agree that the providers may forget the patient has a UC and literature supports the observations (Saint et al., 2000). However, a reminder system may delay unnecessary catheters being removed promptly, thus increasing risk to the patient (Gokula et al., 2012). The evidence indicates that autonomous nurse-driven protocols result in continuous evaluation of the patient's necessity for a UC and result in prompt removal of UCs (Agency for Healthcare Research and Quality, 2015), thus reducing the risk of infection for the patient.

In 2011, the Mississippi Hospital for Restorative Care, a LTACH, in Jackson, Mississippi, was led by an EBP mentor in a practice change to reduce CAUTIs and CDs. Working with a multidisciplinary team, the change was designed to include a nurse-driven protocol to identify unnecessary UCs and a subsequent reminder system requesting that the UC be removed. The team proposed the nurse-driven protocol to be autonomous, but the physicians preferred the reminder system. Even so, in the first 6 months results demonstrated a reduction in CDs ($\downarrow$26%; $p \leq 0.001$) and CAUTI rates ($\downarrow$33%; $p = 0.486$) (Magers, 2013).

In 2012, Joint Commission's National Patient Safety Goals included that evidence-based strategies should be implemented to reduce unnecessary CDs in acute care hospitals. The LTACH was part of Baptist Health Systems and had shared their improvements to reduce CDs and CAUTI rates with the UC protocol using a reminder system. The following describes continued improvements experienced in the LTACH.

STEP 1 The PICOT Question Formulated

In adult patients hospitalized in an LTACH (P), how does the use of an autonomous nurse-driven protocol for evaluating the appropriateness of short-term UC continuation or removal (I), compared with the protocol with a reminder system (C), affect the number of CDs (O_1) and CAUTI rates (O_2)?

STEP 2   Search Strategy Conducted

Guided by the PICOT question, a systematic literature search was conducted in early 2013. The databases searched included the Cumulative Index to Nursing and Allied Health Literature (CINAHL), Cochrane Database of Systematic Reviews (CDSR), Cochrane Central Register of Controlled Trials, the Database of Abstracts of Reviews of Effects (DARE), Ovid Clinical Queries, and PubMed. Keyword and controlled vocabulary searches included the following terms: *catheter-related*; *urinary catheterization*; *urinary tract infection, prevention, and control*; *catheter-associated*, limited to *urinary*; *protocol*; *and nurse driven protocol*. Several articles, guidelines, and studies found in the 2011 search were reviewed again for specificity to this PICOT question, and seven new articles were selected for rapid critical appraisal. One guideline from the Institute of Healthcare Improvement (2011) was also reviewed.

STEP3   Critical Appraisal of the Evidence Performed

The purpose of rapid critical appraisal is to determine whether the literature identified in the search is "relevant, valid, reliable, and applicable to the clinical question" (Melnyk, Fineout-Overholt, Stillwell, & Williamson, 2010). In appraising the sources, the following were considered: the level of evidence, whether the studies and reviews were well conducted, and the degree to which each answered the clinical question (Fineout-Overholt, Melnyk, Stillwell, & Williamson, 2010a). Although no studies were found involving patients in LTACHs, the studies about patients in acute and critical care facilities were considered relevant to the clinical question because patients in such facilities require hospital-level care, though for shorter periods.

Five of the nine new articles were background resources that supported a nurse-driven protocol, but did not offer evidence for synthesis. Through rapid critical appraisal, the previous 14 research studies and 4 new sources were identified as keeper studies (Apisamathanark, et al., 2007; Benoist et al., 1999; Bruminhent et al., 2010; Crouzert et al., 2007; Elpern et al., 2009; Fuchs, Sexton, Thornlow, & Champagne, 2011; Gotelli et al., 2008; Hakvoort, Elberink, Vollebregt, Van der Ploeg, & Emanuel, 2004; Huang et al., 2004; Loeb et al., 2008; Meddings et al., 2010; Parry, Grant, & Sestovic, 2013; Reilly et al., 2006; Rothfeld, & Stickley, 2010; Saint et al., 2005; Topal et al., 2005; Voss, 2009; Wenger, 2010). To organize the studies, an evaluation table was created, and synthesis tables were developed to clarify similarities and differences among the findings (Fineout-Overholt, Melnyk, Stillwell, & Williamson, 2010b). Levels of evidence ranged from level I, which represents the highest quality, seen in systematic reviews, to level VI, which characterizes descriptive studies (Fineout-Overholt et al., 2010a). The studies were a broad collection published between 2004 and 2012. All 16 studies that utilized a nurse-driven protocol as an intervention reported a decrease in CDs, CAUTIs, or both. Eleven of the 16 protocols did not associate the process with a reminder system, and all but one of those reported statistically significant reductions in CAUTIs, CDs, or both (Benoist et al., 1999; Crouzet et al., 2007; Fuchs, Sexton, Thornlow, & Champagne, 2011; Hakvoort, Elberink, Vollebregt, Van der Ploeg, & Emanuel, 2004; Loeb et al., 2008; Parry, Grant, & Sestovic, 2013; Reilly et al., 2006; Topal et al., 2005; Voss, 2009; Wenger, 2010). Gotelli et al. (2008) reported a reduction in catheter prevalence from 24% to 17% without further statistical analysis.

STEP 4   Evidence Integrated With Clinical Expertise and Patient Preferences to Inform a Decision and Practice Change Implemented

The best patient outcomes result when a change in practice is based on the best evidence and combined with clinical expertise and patient preferences (Melnyk et al., 2010). Such integration involves team building, institutional approval, project planning, and implementation.

Building a team with input from a wide range of stakeholders and gaining their trust lend valuable support to EBP projects and promote a culture that is supportive of future projects (Gallagher-Ford, Fineout-Overholt, Melnyk, & Stillwell, 2011).

The project team's role was established by defining the goals and purpose. Upon review of the external and internal evidence, the stakeholders agreed that the goal was to increase the autonomy of the nurses to remove unnecessary urinary catheters on the basis of the nurse-driven protocol implemented in 2011 without the reminder system to providers. The internal evidence demonstrated reduction in CDs and CAUTIs with the protocol and reminder system, and the external evidence supported the nurses independently removing UCs when evaluated as unnecessary. During this phase of the project, it was essential to collaborate and gain support of the chair of the Infectious Disease Committee and the chair of the Medical Executive Committee. The accreditation director was a key player to ensure the proposed standing orders (protocol) met the necessary guidelines. The protocol would become active with any order for a short-term urinary catheter insertion or existing catheter. The proposal was presented to the Medical Executive Committees of the LTACH and acute care hospital with unanimous approval. An institutional review board (IRB) application was written for approval of the EBP project and data collection. It gained approval as a minimal-risk project.

Project planning included designing the process for change in practice. Education was prepared regarding the new order set, the algorithm for determining unnecessary urinary short-term catheters, appropriate documentation, and patient education. Audiences included providers, nurses, nursing assistants, and unit clerks. New content was incorporated into onboarding education in our skills lab for newly hired nurses.

STEP 5 Outcomes Evaluated

Sources of data had been established with the first protocol in 2011. Unit charge nurses record patient days and device days at midnight each day. The infection preventionists provide data on CAUTI events and rates. Microsoft Excel 2010 data analysis add-in software was used to compare baseline data of 11 quarters to 12 quarters of postintervention data with a t-test for independent means. Device days were analyzed as raw numbers and as a utilization ratio (UR). To improve reliability of results, ratios of patient days to device days are beneficial to avoid false assumptions that results in changes due to the intervention, when in reality, the changes may have occurred due to a change in the census of a unit. The UR outcomes demonstrated a statistically significant reduction ($\downarrow$27%; $p \leq 0.001$). Infections were analyzed per quarter using CAUTI rates, and outcomes were again statistically significant ($\downarrow$19%; $p = 0.027$). Results indicated that implementing an evidence-based and autonomous nurse-driven protocol to reduce CDs and CAUTIs mitigated the risk of harm to our patients. In this context, harm is defined as unnecessary catheter days and CAUTIs.

STEP 6 Project Outcomes Successfully Disseminated

The team disseminated the project and its outcomes to both internal and external audiences. Internally, reports were provided to the Nursing Quality Council, Nursing EBP and Research Council, Nursing Leadership Council, Organization Infection Control Committee, Clinical Improvement Committee, and unit staff through unit practice council meetings. Furthermore, as a result of the 2012 success in the LTACH, in 2013, the nurses at Mississippi Baptist Medical Center, the 600-bed, short-term acute care hospital in the healthcare system, collaborated with nurses from the LTACH to develop a multidisciplinary group of stakeholders to discuss whether the protocol in the LTACH could be revised with the latest evidence to include an autonomous nurse-driven protocol. The group wondered if both hospitals could implement a revision of the original LTACH protocol to further improve patient outcomes. Challenges would include obtaining physician support at the system level for a proposal of an autonomous nurse-driven protocol to remove unnecessary catheters without the associated reminder system used in the LTACH. Stakeholders included nurses, infection preventionists, accreditation, quality improvement, and medical staff. Externally, the system project was shared through a poster presentation at the 2016 National APIC Conference by one of the infection preventionists. Such projects rarely impact only one unit, and, in this case, organizations within a healthcare system. Sharing successes is a vital part of evidence-based change.

References

Agency for Healthcare Research and Quality. (2015). Toolkit for reducing catheter-associated urinary tract infections in hospital units: Implementation guide. Retrieved from https://www.ahrq.gov/sites/default/files/publications/files/implementation-guide_0.pdf

Apisarnthanarak, A., Thongphubeth, K., Sirinvaravong, S., Kitkangvan, D., Yuekyen, C., Warachan, B., . . . Fraser, V. J. (2007). Effectiveness of multifaceted hospital-wide quality improvement programs featuring an intervention to remove unnecessary urinary catheters at a tertiary care center in Thailand. *Infection Control Hospital Epidemiology, 28*(7), 791–798.

Benoist, S., Panis, Y., Denet, C., Mauvais, F., Mariani, P., & Valleur, P. (1999). Optimal duration of urinary drainage after rectal resection: A randomized controlled trial. *Surgery, 125*(2), 135–141.

Bruminhent, J., Keegan, M., Lakhani, A., Roberts, I., & Passalacqua, J. (2010). Effectiveness of a simple intervention for prevention of catheter-associated urinary tract infections in a community teaching hospital. *American Journal of Infection Control, 38,* 689–693.

Crouzet, J., Bertrand, X., Venier, A. G., Badoz, C., Hussson, C., & Talon, D. (2007). Control of the duration of urinary catheterization: Impact on catheter-associated urinary tract infection. *Journal of Hospital Infection, 67,* 253–257.

Elpern, E., Killeen, K., Ketchem, A., Wiley, A., Patel, G., & Lateef, G. (2009). Reducing use of indwelling urinary catheters and associated urinary tract infections. *American Journal of Critical Care, 18,* 535–541. doi:10.4037/ajcc2009938

Fineout-Overholt, E., Melnyk, B. M., Stillwell, S. B., & Williamson, K. M. (2010a). Evidence-based practice: Step by step: Critical appraisal of the evidence: Part I. *American Journal of Nursing, 110*(7), 47–52.

Fineout-Overholt, E., Melnyk, B. M., Stillwell, S. B., & Williamson, K. M. (2010b). Evidence-based practice: Step by step: Critical appraisal of the evidence: Part II. *American Journal of Nursing, 110*(9), 41–48.

Fuchs, M., Sexton, D., Thornlow, D., & Champagne, M. (2011). Evaluation of an evidence-based nurse-driven checklist to prevent hospital-acquired catheter-associated urinary tract infections in intensive care units. *Journal of Nursing Care Quality, 26,* 101–109. doi:10.1097/NCQ.0b013e3181fb7847

Gallagher-Ford, L., Fineout-Overholt, E., Melnyk, B., & Stillwell, S. (2011). Evidence-based practice step by step: Implementing an evidence-based practice change. *American Journal of Nursing, 111*(3), 54–60.

Gokula, M., Smolen, D., Gaspar, P., Hensley, S., Benninghoff, M., & Smith, M. (2012). Designing a protocol to reduce catheter-associated urinary tract infections among hospitalized patients. *American Journal of Infection Control, 40*(10), 1002–1004. doi:10.1016/j.ajic.2011.12.013

Gotelli, J. M., Merryman, P., Carr, C., McElveen, L., Epperson, C., & Bynum, D. (2008). A quality improvement project to reduce the complications associated with indwelling urinary catheters. *Urologic Nursing, 28*(6), 465–473.

Gould, C., Umscheid, C., Agarwal, R., Kuntz, G., Peguess, D.; Centers for Disease Control and Prevention Healthcare Infection Control Practices Advisory Committee (HICPAC). (2009). *Guideline for prevention of catheter-associated urinary tract infections 2009.* Retrieved from http://www.cdc.gov/hicpac/pdf/CAUTI/CAUTIguideline2009final.pdf

Hakvoort, R. A., Elberink, R., Vollebregt, A., Van der Ploeg, T., & Emanuel, M. H. (2004). How long should urinary bladder catheterisation be continued after vaginal prolapse surgery? A randomized controlled trial comparing short term versus long term catheterisation after vaginal prolapse surgery. *British Journal of Obstetric Gynaecology, 111,* 828–830. doi:10.111/j.1471-0528.2004.00181.x

Huang, W. C., Wann, S. R., Lin, S. L., Kunin, C. M., Kung, M. H., Lin, C. H., . . . Lin, T. W. (2004). Catheter-associated urinary tract infections in intensive care units can be reduced by prompting physicians to remove unnecessary catheters. *Infection Control and Hospital Epidemiology, 25*(11), 974–978.

Institute for Healthcare Improvement. (2011). *How-to guide: Prevent catheter-associated urinary tract infections.* Cambridge, MA: Author. Retrieved from http://www.ihi.org/resources/Pages/Tools/HowtoGuidePreventCatheterAssociatedUrinaryTractInfection.aspx

Loeb, M., Hunt, D., O'Halloran, K., Carusone, S. C., Dafoe, N., & Walter, S. D. (2008). Stop orders to reduce inappropriate urinary catheterization in hospitalized patients: A randomized controlled trial. *Journal of General Internal Medicine, 23*(6), 816–820. doi:10.1007/s11606-008-0620-2

Magers, T. (2013). Using evidence-based practice to reduce catheter-associated urinary tract infections. *American Journal of Nursing, 113*(6), 34–42. doi:10.1097/01.NAJ.0000430923.07539.a7

Meddings, J., Rogers, M. A., Macy, M., & Saint, S. (2010). Systematic review and meta-analysis: Reminder systems to reduce catheter-associated urinary tract infections and urinary catheter use in hospitalized patients. *Clinical Infectious Disease, 51*(5), 550–560. doi:10.1086/655133

Melnyk, B. M., Fineout-Overholt, E., Stillwell, S. B., & Williamson, K. M. (2010). Evidence-based practice: Step by step: The seven steps of evidence-based practice. *American Journal of Nursing, 110*(1), 51–52.

Parry, M. F., Grant, B., & Sestovic, M. (2013). Successful reduction in catheter-associated urinary tract infections: Focus on nurse-directed catheter removal. *American Journal of Infection Control, 41*(12), 1178–1181. doi:10.1016/j.ajic.2013.03.296

Reilly, L., Sullivan, P., Ninni, S., Fochesto, D., Williams, K., & Fetherman, B. (2006). Reducing catheter device days in an intensive care unit: Using the evidence to change practice. *AACN Advanced Critical Care, 17*(3), 272–283.

Rothfeld, A. F., & Stickley, A. (2010). A program to limit urinary catheter use at an acute care hospital. *American Journal of Infection Control, 38*(7), 568–571. doi:10.1016/ajic.2009.12.017

Saint, S., Kaulfman, S. R., Thompson, M., Rogers, M. A., & Chenoweth, C. E. (2005). A reminder reduces urinary catheterization in hospitalized patients. *Joint Commission Journal on Quality and Patient Safety, 31*(8), 455–462.

Saint, S., Wiese, J., Amory, J., Bernstein, M., Patel, U., Zemencuk, J., . . .Hofer, T. (2000). Are physicians aware of which of their patients have indwelling urinary catheters? *American Journal of Medicine, 109*(6), 476–480.

Topal, J., Conklin, S., Camp, K., Morris, V., Balcezak, T., & Herbert, P. (2005). Prevention of nosocomial catheter-associated urinary tract infections through computerized feedback to physicians and a nurse-directed protocol. *American Journal of Medical Quality, 20*(3), 121–126. doi:10.1177/1062860605276074

Voss, A. (2009). Incidence and duration of urinary catheters in hospitalized older adults: Before and after implementing a geriatric protocol. *Journal of Gerontological Nursing, 35*(6), 35–41. doi:10.3928/00989134-20090428-05

Wenger, J. E. (2010). Cultivating quality: Reducing rates of catheter-associated urinary tract infection. *The American Journal of Nursing, 110*(8), 40–45. doi:10.1097/01.NAJ.0000387691.47746.b5

Step Three: Critically Appraising Evidence

> If you don't synthesize knowledge, scientific journals become spare-parts catalogues for machines that are never built.
>
> —Arthur R. Marshall

EBP Terms to Learn

Case–control study
Clinical practice guidelines
Clinical significance
Clinical wisdom and
  judgment
Cohort study
Constant comparison
Context of caring
Evidentialism
Experiential learning
Fieldwork
Integrative reviews
Keeper studies
Key informants
Levels of evidence/hierarchy
  of evidence
Lived experience
Meta-analyses
Narrative reviews
Participant observation
Patient preferences
Practice-based evidence
  (PBE)
Saturation
Statistical significance
Theoretical sampling
Type I error
Type II error

UNIT OBJECTIVES

Upon completion of this unit, learners will be able to:

1 Identify the seven steps of evidence-based practice (EBP).

2 Describe the differences among EBP, research, and quality improvement.

3 Explain the components of PICOT question: Population, Issue or Intervention of interest, Comparison of interest, Outcome, and Time for intervention to achieve the outcome.

4 Discuss basic and advanced strategies to conducting a systematic search based on the PICOT question.

5 Describe a body of evidence (BOE) based on the evidence hierarchy for specific types of clinical questions.

6 Discuss key components for rapid critical appraisal of a clinical practice guideline.

MAKING CONNECTIONS: AN EBP EXEMPLAR

Betsy, the unit EBP Council representative, and Danielle, the nurse manager, crafted the following PICOT question: *In elderly patients with low risk for falls with universal precautions in place, how does hourly rounding at night compared to no hourly rounding affect preventable fall rates within 3 months of initiation?* They brought the current BOE that Scott, the hospital librarian, found in his systematic search to answer their question to the EBP Council. The members of the EBP Council were charged with appraising the evidence to see what it told them about what should be done to help address falls within their organization (*Step 3: Critically Appraising Evidence*). They acknowledged Betsy's sense of clinical inquiry and applauded Scott for his excellent systematic search. One member who particularly liked to search, Mateo, decided to do another hand search to see if there were any studies that Scott may have missed. He found four more potential studies, all of which had the same outcomes as those Scott had found. Mateo thought that they should be added to the BOE because the description of how the fall prevention intervention of hourly rounding (FPI-HR) was delivered in these studies might help with implementation. When Mateo went to retrieve one of the articles that had been in both the systematic review and the integrative review in the BOE, he discovered that it had been retracted by the editor because it was so similar to another article that had already been published. Knowing how important valid evidence is to the EBP process, Mateo brought this information to the EBP Council. Several members of the Council were surprised to see that an article in these reviews would be retracted from publication. They asked about the validity of the two reviews because of this action. DeAndre, EBP Mentor and Clinical Nurse Specialist who guided the Council, indicated that the systematic review recommendations were substantiated sufficiently with the other studies included so they would still hold. He explained that the integrative review methodology had inherent bias and could not be used with confidence, making it level VII evidence; therefore, the inclusion of the retracted study was not influential in decision making. Scott gave a report on the interlibrary loan articles he was waiting for: One he had been unable to get and the other two from the first search were still not here. One of the remaining three articles from Mateo's hand search was now available through interlibrary loan, bringing the BOE to a total of 19 articles. [Here's the math: there are currently 16 articles in hand for the EBP Council to work with: 14 of the 17 from Scott's original systematic search (2 in interlibrary loan; 1 unavailable; final count will be 16 from Scott); 2 of the 4 from Mateo's hand search (1 in interlibrary loan; 1 retracted from publication; final count will be 3 from Mateo)].

To facilitate the work of critical appraisal, the Council divided the 16 potential studies among its members and completed the appropriate rapid critical appraisal (RCA) checklists and the general appraisal overview form to determine if the studies were valid, reliable, and applicable to the population of patients at risk for falls. From the RCA of the potential studies, the Council determined that all 16 met the criteria for retention in the BOE. After some discussion, Scott and Mateo informed DeAndre and the EBP Council that the outstanding studies from interlibrary loan did not have varying results from the existing BOE; therefore, the decision was made to keep moving forward. However, because the studies in interlibrary loan had information that could help with implementation, they decided to add the outstanding studies when they arrived.

The EBP Council then divided the studies among them to efficiently create a single evaluation table containing all of the studies. They chose to use a strategy that allowed them all to access and edit a solitary document to expedite their contributions and finalize the table (e.g., online forms). DeAndre assumed the role of editor of the evaluation table to ensure that all articles had sufficient details to synthesize. He reminded his fellow EBP Council members that any information that would be used to synthesize across studies had to be in the evaluation table. The evaluation table has 10 columns to house essential information about the studies (see Table 1 on thePoint'). EBP Council members entered the data from their assigned studies into the table. Members were careful to enter the data from the studies the way DeAndre had taught them in a work-shop—succinctly and parsimoniously. They had much discussion about the requirement of no complete sentences and the importance of using appropriate abbreviations for common elements in the studies so that it was easier to compare across studies. They placed the legend with all of the agreed upon abbreviations in the footer of their table.

Within the evaluation table, DeAndre arranged the studies in the order of the level of evidence (LOE) for intervention studies to help the Council best synthesize the data. As DeAndre cleaned up the evaluation table, he began to see patterns of information in common across studies as well as differences. He prepared several synthesis tables to share with the EBP Council at their next meeting.

DeAndre presented each synthesis table and discussed the findings of the critical appraisal portion of the EBP process. The updated LOE table helped the Council to understand that there was mostly lower LOE to answer the PICOT question (see Table 2).

TABLE 2

Synthesis: Levels of Evidence

Level of Evidence for Intervention Questions	1	2	3	4	5	6	7	8	9	10	11	12	13	14	15	16
I Systematic review/meta-analysis of randomized controlled trials											X					
II Single randomized controlled trial																
III Quasi-experimental studies/nonrandomized controlled trials	X						X					X		X		
IV Cohort or case–control studies																
V Systematic review/meta-synthesis of qualitative studies																
VI Single qualitative or descriptive studies/evidence implementation and quality improvement projects		X	X	X	X		X		X	X			X		X	X
VII Expert opinion						X										

Studies in alpha order: 1, Brown; 2, Callahan; 3, Dyck; 4, Fisher; 5, Goldsack; 6, Hicks; 7, Kessler; 8, Krepper; 9, Leone; 10, Lowe; 11, Mitchell; 12, Olrich; 13, Stefancyk; 14, Tucker; 15, Waszynski; 16, Weisgram

Despite this, there was so much evidence, across all studies and projects in the BOE, showing that FPI-HR reduced the fall rate (FR) (see Table 3) that it would be unethical not to use the findings to guide practice. Furthermore, there was no report that indicated that how the FPI-HR was scheduled had an impact on further improving the reduction in FR, such as delivered every 2 hours at night as well as hourly in the day. Therefore, the Council decided to push forward with a new initiative to revamp any previous fall prevention efforts and launch a 24-hour FPI-HR with hourly day rounds and every 2-hour nightly rounds. From the evidence, there also was reason to expect that 24-hour FPI-HR would also have some impact on call light use and patient satisfaction. These were not known issues for their organization, but as they discussed the data, it seemed prudent to include them in their planning.

To help the Council determine what type of FPI-HR works best, DeAndre presented a synthesis table with the protocols used within the studies (see Table 4). DeAndre had created a Synthesis Column in Tables 3 and 4 to help with crafting a true synthesis of the evidence versus reviewing the information study-by-study. This column in Table 4 helped the Council to see that the HR protocol that was most common across studies was an assessment of fall risk (FRisk) and the 4 Ps (Pain, Potty, Position, Placement). Based on the data from the studies, DeAndre discussed the following recommendation with the Council for implementation within their organization: All clinical settings that

TABLE
3

Synthesis Table: Impact of FPI-HR

Studies/ Outcomes	1	2	3	4	5	6	7	8	9	10
FR	↓	↓	↓	↓*	↓*	↓	↓	↓	↓	↓
CLU								↓*		
PST		↑					−	↑*		
FPI duration	2 yr	30 D	5 yr	8 Q	30 D	3 wk– 6 yr	6 yr	3 mo	8 Q	3.5 mo
24 H AM/PM	NIR	NIR	NIR	NIR	−	−	−	−	NIR	−

Studies in alpha order: 1, Brown; 2, Callahan; 3, Dyck; 4, Fisher; 5, Goldsack; 6, Hicks; 7, Kessler; 8, Krepper; 9, Leone; 10, Lowe; 11, Mitchell; 12, Olrich; 13, Stefancyk; 14, Tucker; 15, Waszynski; 16, Weisgram.

*statistically significant

CLU, call light usage; D, days; FPI, fall prevention interventions; FR, fall rate(s); FRisk, fall risk; H, hour(s); MO, month(s); NIR, not in report; PST, patient satisfaction; pt, patient; Q, quarter; w/, with; wks, weeks; yr, year(s).

have patients over 24 hours should have an interprofessional 24-hour FPI-HR program (hourly in day/every 2 hours in night) in place that includes addressing FRisk and the 4 Ps. Furthermore, having an EBP Mentor lead the program is prudent.

As the Council discussed the evidence-based recommendation for implementation, they began to consider how they could intentionally integrate patient preferences into their implementation plan. They wanted to create posters to explain the implementation project and how essential their evidence and the clinicians and the patient preferences were to the success of the implementation. Lei, the Council member who would be coordinating the implementation plan, noted that crafting a plan for implementing their hourly rounding intervention across the entire organization would require quite a bit of preparation. She searched the National Guidelines Clearinghouse and the Registered Nurses Association of Ontario (RNAO) databases to see if there were guidelines that incorporated hourly rounding addressing the 4 Ps and FRisk in a fall prevention program that could help their team with implementation. Lei brought one Falls Prevention clinical practice guideline (Registered Nurses Association of Ontario [RNAO], 2017) that had the recommendation from the Council within the guideline. She proposed that they review that recommendation and any resources offered within the guideline as guidance for implementation.

Join the group at the beginning of Unit 3 as they continue their EBP journey.

11	12	13	14	15	16	Synthesis
⬇	⬇	⬇	⬇	⬇	⬇	• All studies showed a decrease in FR
⬇					⬇	• Of the 5 studies that evaluated CLU, 3 showed reduced CLU
		⬆				• Of the 4 studies that evaluated PST, 3 showed improved satisfaction
30 D–5 yr	12 mo	2 yr	3 mo w/1 yr post	NIR	30 D	• 3 of 14 primary studies or projects = 30 D • Of these 3, 2 had at least 2 of the outcomes and showed improvement and 1 had statistically significant results • 3 of the primary studies = 3 mo • Of these 3, 1 study had all 3 outcomes that showed improvement
—	—	NIR	—	NIR	—	• 9/16 studies/projects had AM/PM intervention variations; none reported differences in HR based on delivery

Studies in alpha order: 1, Brown; 2, Callahan; 3, Dyck; 4, Fisher; 5, Goldsack; 6, Hicks; 7, Kessler; 8, Krepper; 9, Leone; 10, Lowe; 11, Mitchell; 12, Olrich; 13, Stefancyk; 14, Tucker; 15, Waszynski; 16, Weisgram.

*statistically significant

CLU, call light usage; D, days; FPI, fall prevention interventions; FR, fall rate(s); FRisk, fall risk; H, hour(s); MO, month(s); NIR, not in report; PST, patient satisfaction; pt, patient; Q, quarter; w/, with; wks, weeks; yr, year(s).

TABLE
4

Synthesis Table: Protocol and Impact

Studies	Major FPI-HR	Synthesis Risk Assmt and 4 Ps	Synthesis: Additions	IMPACT
1	"4 Ps" needs met: • pain • positioning • potty • proximity of personal items	FRisk assmt—NIR 4 Ps—Y		FR—Down

2	• FRisk assmt
	• address:
	  • pain
	  • positioning/comfort
	  • toileting
	  • personal needs
	  • safety checks
		FRisk assmt—Y
		4 Ps—Y
				FR—Down
				PST—Up

3	MFFPI w/changes: • IPP • shared vision • autonomous DM for unit-level HR delivery (flexible—not "on the hour") but within 72 H of ADM • examples for observations to record • reiteration of reassurance • prominently placed FPI logo • written algorithm poster • recognition of hard work	FRisk assmt—NIR 4 Ps NIR	Culture	FR—Down
4	• 4 Ps • education on FRisk • IPP rounds • FRisk (Morse scale) • planned interventions based on assmt • bed alarms	FRisk assmt—Y 4 Ps Y		FR—Down—SS
5	• addressing the four Ps (pain, potty, position, possessions) • add IPP LSI • add EBP Mentor	FRisk assmt—NIR 4 Ps Y	IPP LSI EBP Mentor	FR—Down—SS
6	• using key words [script] • addressing the 4 Ps (pain, potty, position, possessions) • assessing the environment for safety issues • telling the pt when staff will return	FRisk assmt—NIR 4 Ps Y		FR—Down

Studies in alpha order: 1, Brown; 2, Callahan; 3, Dyck; 4, Fisher; 5, Goldsack; 6, Hicks; 7, Kessler; 8, Krepper; 9, Leone; 10, Lowe; 11, Mitchell; 12, Olrich; 13, Stefancyk; 14, Tucker; 15, Waszynski; 16, Weisgram.

ADM, admission; assmt, assessment; CLU, call light usage; COS, culture of safety; D, days; EBP, evidence-based practice; FPI, fall prevention interventions; FR, fall rate(s); FRisk, fall risk; H, hour(s); HR, hourly rounding; IPP, interprofessional; LSI, leadership involvement; MO, month(s); NIR, not in report; NM, nurse manager; PCA, patient care assistant; PST, patient satisfaction; pt, patient; q, every; SS, statistically significant; tx, treatment; w/, with; wks, weeks; X, times; Y, yes; yr, year(s).

TABLE 4	Synthesis Table: Protocol and Impact (continued)

Studies	Major FPI-HR	Synthesis Risk Assmt and 4 Ps	Synthesis: Additions	IMPACT
7	• 1-hour didactic workshops • attention to pain, position, personal needs, placement (4 Ps) • an environmental safety check and scripted response upon leaving the room	FRisk assmt—NIR 4 Ps Y	LSI	FR—Down
8	• "rounding script" • rounding logs and timeliness of the rounds for 3 months	FRisk assmt—NIR 4 Ps NIR	Rounding logs	FR, CLU—Down PST—Up
9	• Huddle • Signage • HR • COS	FRisk assmt—NIR 4 Ps Y	Phased approach	FR—Down
10	• pain: pts' pain score • potty: pts' toileting needs • position: pts' need for help with repositioning • possessions: proximity of pts' possessions Add: • C—Communicate with compassion • A—Assist with toileting, ensuring dignity • R—Relieve pain effectively • E—Encourage adequate nutrition	FRisk assmt—NIR 4 Ps—Y	CARE	FR—Down
11	• potty • positioning • pain control • proximity of personal items	FRisk assmt—NIR 4 Ps Y		FR, CLU—Down
12	8 actions: • introduction • pain assmt and tx • potty • positioning • placement • leaving script • when returning	FRisk assmt—NIR 4 Ps Y		FR—Down CLU—no change
13	PCA asked three questions during each visit: • Do you need to use the bathroom? • Are you comfortable? • Can I do anything for you?	FRisk assmt—NIR 4 Ps partial		FR—Down PST—Up

Studies in alpha order: 1, Brown; 2, Callahan; 3, Dyck; 4, Fisher; 5, Goldsack; 6, Hicks; 7, Kessler; 8, Krepper; 9, Leone; 10, Lowe; 11, Mitchell; 12, Olrich; 13, Stefancyk; 14, Tucker; 15, Waszynski; 16, Weisgram.

ADM, admission; assmt, assessment; CLU, call light usage; COS, culture of safety; D, days; EBP, evidence-based practice; FPI, fall prevention interventions; FR, fall rate(s); FRisk, fall risk; H, hour(s); HR, hourly rounding; IPP, interprofessional; LSI, leadership involvement; MO, month(s); NIR, not in report; NM, nurse manager; PCA, patient care assistant; PST, patient satisfaction; pt, patient; q, every; SS, statistically significant; tx, treatment; w/, with; wks, weeks; X, times; Y, yes; yr, year(s).

(continued)

Synthesis Table: Protocol and Impact (continued)

Studies	Major FPI-HR	Synthesis Risk Assmt and 4 Ps	Synthesis: Additions	IMPACT
14	• offering toileting assistance • assessing and addressing pt position and comfort • placing call light, bedside table, water, TV remote • Kleenex, and garbage can within pt reach • prior to leaving the room, ask "Is there anything I can do for you before I leave? I have the time" • telling the pt that a member of the nursing staff will be back in the room in an hour on rounds • emphasizing the willingness of the staff to respond rather than the pt attempting to ambulate unassisted	FRisk assmt—NIR 4 Ps Y		FR—Down

15	• introduces himself or herself to the pt and family
	• explains purpose of visit is to help reduce falls and keep the pt safe
	• confirm FRisk with hospital's fall safety screening tool
	• check fall prevention protocol is in place
	  • wearing hospital's green fall risk bracelet
	  • green triangle on door
	  • bed or chair alarm activated
	• scan room for fall hazards and correct
	• make sure pt knows how to call for assistance
	• Record bedside check
	At end of volunteer's shift, unit NM reviews
		FRisk assmt—Y
		4 Ps Y
			LSI	FR—Down

16	q1h rounding 8 AM–10 PM; q2h 10 PM–8 AM	FRisk assmt—NIR 4 Ps NIR		FR, CLU—Down

Studies in alpha order: 1, Brown; 2, Callahan; 3, Dyck; 4, Fisher; 5, Goldsack; 6, Hicks; 7, Kessler; 8, Krepper; 9, Leone; 10, Lowe; 11, Mitchell; 12, Olrich; 13, Stefancyk; 14, Tucker; 15, Waszynski; 16, Weisgram.

ADM, admission; assmt, assessment; CLU, call light usage; COS, culture of safety; D, days; EBP, evidence-based practice; FPI, fall prevention interventions; FR, fall rate(s); FRisk, fall risk; H, hour(s); HR, hourly rounding; IPP, interprofessional; LSI, leadership involvement; MO, month(s); NIR, not in report; NM, nurse manager; PCA, patient care assistant; PST, patient satisfaction; pt, patient; q, every; SS, statistically significant; tx, treatment; w/, with; wks, weeks; X, times; Y, yes; yr, year(s).

References

*Waiting for interlibrary loan

Brown, C. H. (2016). The effect of purposeful hourly rounding on the incidence of patient falls. *Nursing Theses and Capstone Projects*. http://digitalcommons.gardner-webb.edu/nursing_etd/246

Callahan, L., McDonald, S., Voit, D., McDonnell, A., Delgado-Flores, J., & Stanghellini, E. (2009). Medication review and hourly nursing rounds: an evidence-based approach reduces falls on oncology inpatient units. *Oncology Nursing Forum, 36*(3), 72.

Dyck, D., Thiele, T., Kebicz, R., Klassen, M., & Erenberg, C. (2013). Hourly rounding for falls prevention: A change initiative. *Creative Nursing, 19*(3), 153–158.

Fisher, S. K., Horn, D., & Elliot, M. (2014). Taking a stand against falls. *Nursing, 44*(10), 15–17.

Goldsack, J., Bergey, M., Mascioli, S., & Cunningham, J. (2015). Hourly rounding and patient falls: What factors boost success? *Nursing, 45*(2): 25–30.

Hicks, D. (2015). Can rounding reduce patient falls in acute care? An integrative literature review. *MEDSURG Nursing, 24*(1): 51–55.

*Jackson, K. (2016). Improving nursing home falls management program by enhancing standard of care with collaborative care multi-interventional protocol focused on fall prevention. *Journal of Nursing Education and Practice, 6*(6), 85–96.

Kessler, B., Claude-Gutekunst, M., Donchez, M., Dries, R. F., & Snyder, M. M. (2012). The merry-go-round of patient rounding: Assure your patients get the brass ring. *MEDSURG Nursing, 21*(4), 240–245.

Krepper, R., Vallejo, B., Smith, C., Lindy, C., Fullmer, C., Messimer, S., … Myers K. (2014). Evaluation of a standardized hourly rounding process (SHaRP). *Journal for Healthcare Quality, 36*(2):62–69. doi: 10.1111/j.1945-1474.2012.00222.x

Leone, R. M., & Adams, R. J. (2016). Safety standards: Implementing fall prevention interventions and sustaining lower fall rates by promoting the culture of safety on an inpatient rehabilitation unit. *Rehabilitation Nursing, 41*(1), 26–32.

Lowe, L., & Hodgson, G. (2012). Hourly rounding in a high dependency unit. *Nursing Standard, 27*(8), 35–40.

Mitchell, M. D., Lavenberg, J. G., Trotta, R. L., Umscheid, C. A. (2014). Hourly rounding to improve nursing responsiveness: a systematic review. *Journal of Nursing Administration, 44*(9):462–472.

*Meade, C., Bursell, A., & Ketelsen, L. (2006). Effect of nursing rounds on patients' call light use, satisfaction, and safety. *American Journal of Nursing, 106*(9), 58–70.

*Morgan, L., Flynn, L., Robertson, E., New, S., Forde-Johnston, C., & McCulloch, P. (2017). Intentional rounding: A staff-led quality improvement intervention in the prevention of patient falls. *Journal of Clinical Nursing, 26*(1/2), 115–124.

Olrich, T., Kalman, M., & Nigolian, C. (2012). Hourly rounding: A replication study. *MEDSURG Nursing, 21*(1): 23–36.

Registered Nurses' Association of Ontario. (2017). *Preventing falls and reducing injury from falls* (4th ed.). Toronto, ON: Author.

Stefancyk, A. L (2009). Safe and reliable care: addressing one of the four focus areas of the TCAB initiative. *American Journal of Nursing, 109*(7), 70–71.

Tucker, S. J., Bieber, P. L., Attlesey-Pries, J. M., Olson, M. E., & Dierkhising, R. A. (2012). Outcomes and challenges in implementing hourly rounds to reduce falls in orthopedic units. *Worldviews on Evidence-Based Nursing, 9*(1), 18–29.

Waszynski, C. (2012). More rounding means better fall compliance. *Healthcare Risk Management, 34*(2), 21.

Weisgram, B., & Raymond, S. (2008). Military nursing. Using evidence-based nursing rounds to improve patient outcomes. *MEDSURG Nursing, 17*(6), 429–430.

Critically Appraising Knowledge for Clinical Decision Making

Ellen Fineout-Overholt and Kathleen R. Stevens

An investment in knowledge pays the best interest.
—*Benjamin Franklin*

EBP Terms to Learn

Clinician expertise
Critical appraisal
Internal evidence
Quality improvement [QI]
  data
Narrative reviews
Meta-analyses
Patient choices
Practice-based evidence
  (PBE)
Systematic reviews

Learning Objectives

After studying this chapter, learners will be able to:

1 Describe sources of evidence for clinical decision making.

2 Describe how practice-based evidence, research, and evidence-based practice are complementary and supportive processes.

3 Discuss improvement and implementation research.

4 Discuss the importance of measurement of intended outcomes for demonstration of sustainable impact of evidence.

Evidence is a collection of facts that grounds one's belief that something is true. To discover evidence to guide which actions to take in a given clinical situation, practitioners ask carefully crafted clinical questions such as the following: (a) In adult surgical patients, how do videotaped preparation sessions compared with one-to-one counseling affect anxiety just before surgery? (b) In homebound older adults, how does a fall prevention program compared with no fall prevention program affect the number of fall-related injuries over one quarter? Now that you have mastered how to ask a searchable clinical question in PICOT format and conduct a systematic search for external evidence from indexed databases and beyond to answer it, consider how clinicians attempt to select the most effective action based on the best knowledge available. This knowledge may be derived from a variety of sources, such as research, theories, experience, tradition, trial and error, authority, or logical reasoning (Stevens, 2013; Stevens & Clutter, 2007)

In addition to the knowledge gained from their clinical experiences, healthcare providers are increasingly compelled to use evidence from research to determine effective strategies for implementing system-based change to improve care processes and patient outcomes (American Nurses Credentialing Center, 2008, 2014; Institute of Medicine [IOM], 2011). Often, this array of knowledge and evidence is so diverse that clinicians are challenged to determine which action(s) will be the most effective in improving patient outcomes.

Critical appraisal of such evidence for decision making is one of the most valuable skills that clinicians can possess in today's healthcare environment. Distinguishing the best evidence from unreliable evidence and unbiased evidence from biased evidence lies at the root of the impact that clinicians' actions will have in producing their intended outcomes.

In this unit, you learn how to critically appraise quantitative and qualitative external evidence as well as integrate this evidence with patient preferences and your expertise.

This chapter provides an overview of foundational information that helps you maximize your learning about evidence appraisal and clinical decision making.

KNOWLEDGE SOURCES

The healthcare professions have made major inroads in identifying, understanding, and developing an array of knowledge sources that inform clinical decisions and actions. We now know that systematic inquiry in the form of research produces the most reliable knowledge on which to base practice. In addition, practitioners' expertise and patients' choices and concerns must be taken into account in providing effective and efficient healthcare. Research, **clinician expertise**, and **patient choices** are all necessary evidence to integrate into decision making, but each alone is insufficient for best practice (see Chapter 1, Figure 1.2).

We discuss two processes here that offer clinicians sources of knowledge: (1) **practice-based evidence (PBE)** and (2) research. These two sources of evidence fuel evidence-based practice (EBP). Their processes and outcomes overlap somewhat and are intertwined, but they are distinct in the knowledge they produce to influence clinical decision making.

Practice-Based Evidence Through Quality Improvement

In the past, most clinical actions were based solely on logic, tradition, or conclusions drawn from keen observation (i.e., expertise). Although effective practices sometimes have evolved from these knowledge sources, the resulting practice has been successful less often than hoped for in reliably producing intended patient outcomes. Additionally, conclusions that are drawn solely from practitioner observations can be biased because such observations usually are not systematic. Similarly, non-evidence-based practices vary widely across caregivers and settings. The result is that, for a given health problem, a wide variety of clinical actions are taken without reliably producing the desired patient outcomes. That said, the process for generating PBE (e.g., **quality improvement [QI] data** or **internal evidence**) has become increasingly rigorous and must be included in sources of knowledge for clinical decision making. These data can be very helpful in demonstrating the scope of the clinical issue that underpins the PICOT question. Clinicians without PBE to establish the existence of the clinical issue (i.e., undesirable outcomes) cannot convince others of the importance of their clinical questions or the need for improved outcomes. Every EBP project begins with PBE data.

Whereas external evidence is generated from rigorous research and is typically conducted to be used across clinical settings, internal evidence is that generated by outcomes management, QI, or EBP implementation projects. Unlike external evidence, the generation of internal evidence is intended to improve clinical practice and patient outcomes within the local setting where it is conducted (see Chapter 10).

At the core of local QI and PBE is the planned effort to test a given change to determine its impact on the desired outcome. The **Plan-Do-Study-Act (PDSA)** cycle has become a widely adopted and effective approach to testing and learning about change on a small scale. In PDSA, a particular change is planned and implemented, results are observed (studied), and action is taken on what is learned. The PDSA cycle is considered a scientific method used in action-oriented learning (Institute for Healthcare Improvement, 2010; Speroff & O'Connor, 2004). The original approach is attributed to Deming and is based on repeated small trials, consideration of what has been learned, improvement, and retrial of the improvement. The PDSA cycle tests an idea by putting a planned change into effect on a temporary and small-trial basis and then learning from its impact. The approach suggests a conscious and rigorous testing of the new idea within a specific context. (See Box 4.1 for the steps of the original PDSA cycle.) Small-scale testing incrementally builds the knowledge about a change

> **BOX 4.1**   *Four Stages of the Plan-Do-Study-Act (PDSA) Cycle*
>
> The four stages of the PDSA cycle include the following:
>
> 1. **PLAN:** Plan the change and observation.
> 2. **DO:** Try out the change on a small scale.
> 3. **STUDY:** Analyze the data and determine what was learned.
> 4. **ACT:** Refine the change, based on what was learned, and repeat the testing.
>
> Finally, the action is based on the probability that the change will improve the outcome; however, without external evidence to support this improvement, the degree of certainty for any PDSA cannot be 100%.

in a structured way. By learning from multiple small trials, a new idea can be advanced and implemented with a greater chance of success on a broad scale. There have been revisions to the PDSA process over its almost four-decade use within healthcare; however, though some expect to include external evidence in PDSA, there is still no requirement to bring external evidence into decision making (Taylor et al., 2014). Also, there could be consideration that PDSA informs clinical expertise in the EBP paradigm (see Figure 1.2). Good decision making, in which PDSA is combined with external evidence and corroborates the practice change, will increase the effectiveness of the carefully evaluated outcome for sustained change.

Research

It is well recognized that systematic investigation (i.e., research) holds the promise of deepening our understanding of health phenomena, patients' responses to such phenomena, and the probable impact of clinical actions on resolving health problems. Following this realization, research evidence (i.e., **external evidence**) has become highly valued as the basis for clinical decisions.

Several definitions of research may be explored; however, all of them include systematic investigation designed to contribute to or develop generalizable knowledge (Department of Health and Human Services, 2003; RAND, 2012). Knowledge generated from research must be usable by clinicians—beyond the researchers and clinicians who generated the research. This is the definition of generalizability. Often referred to as new knowledge generation, research offers insights into how healthcare best operates. Exploration and discovery are found through different methods to examine issues, with quantitative and qualitative research as primary examples. Simply put, quantitative research involves quantifying outcomes (as the name implies). Examples include how many falls are prevented by a fall prevention intervention program or how many barriers to EBP clinicians list. Qualitative research focuses on the human experience to help clinicians understand the context of the experience and the intervention delivery. To ensure that this information is reliable, a rigorous process is required.

The first step in the research process is to ask a research question and define the purpose of study. Research questions are directional (e.g., improved outcomes). Next, researchers conduct a search for relevant literature and review it. There may or may not be a systematic approach to this search. Though not every study includes this step, there should be a conceptual framework designated to guide the study. From the framework, the research objectives, hypotheses, variables, and study design are defined. The design includes the study population, the sample, and study setting—all of which are imperative for generalizability. Hypotheses are then tested or research questions are answered by the actual study by measuring various outcomes and collecting data that is analyzed to help the researchers draw conclusions about their findings. Researchers then share their study results with others, including practice implications and study limitations (Fineout-Overholt, 2015). Careful adherence to this process enables clinicians to have increased confidence in the study findings, which explains why research and PBE are embodied within the EBP paradigm and process.

Evidence-Based Practice

Sometimes EBP is confused with research utilization (RU). Both RU and EBP movements escalated attention to the knowledge base of clinical care decisions and actions. In the mid-1970s, RU represented a rudimentary approach to using research as the prime knowledge source on which to base practice. In the early stages of developing research-based practice when electronic sources of information were not readily available, RU approaches promoted using results from a single study as the basis for practice.

Several problems arise with the RU approach, particularly when more than one study on the same topic has been reported. Multiple studies can be difficult to summarize and may produce conflicting findings, and large and small studies may hold different conclusions. To improve the process of moving research knowledge into practice, mechanisms to enhance the external evidence produced through research have improved, and more sophisticated and rigorous approaches for evaluating research have been developed. This helps researchers conduct better research and clinicians improve their competence in evaluation of research to use it to underpin their clinical decisions as well as expected outcomes.

Table 4.1 offers a comparison of the QI, research, and EBP processes and Table 2.3 shows how questions differ across these related, yet separate, healthcare improvement approaches. A graphic that may help in understanding the interface of QI/PBE, research, and EBP is the umbrella (Fineout-Overholt, 2014; Figure 4.1). The overarching practice paradigm is EBP—represented by the fabric of the umbrella (i.e., the everyday representation of EBP). The handle that supports the umbrella is research, and the stretchers that support the fabric are QI/PBE (i.e., knowing how well everyday EBP is working). If the stretchers fail (i.e., if QI/PBE data reflect poor process/outcomes), then EBP fails and the handle has increased pressure on it to keep the fabric functional within the daily stressors of clinical practice. If the handle fails (i.e., insufficient quality or quantity of research to establish best practice), the umbrella is faulty. For practice to be the best, these processes should operate well both independently and interdependently. To help understand how these three important processes work together to help clinicians care best for their patients, remember that researchers *generate* new knowledge that can be used in practice to influence what we do; clinicians use the EBP process to *translate* research into clinical practice to achieve best outcomes; and QI *monitors* how well the practice is working through generation and evaluation of PBE.

"

What I like best is the challenge of learning
something I didn't know how to do, going beyond
my comfort level.

RUTH REICHL

WEIGHING THE EVIDENCE

The EBP movement has catapulted the use of knowledge in clinical care to new heights of sophistication, rigor, and manageability. A key difference between the mandate to "apply

TABLE 4.1	Comparison of the EBP, Research, and QI processes		
EBP Process	**Research Process (Scientific Method)**	**PDSA QI Process**	
Step 0: Foster clinical inquiry	Step 1: Ask a research question and define the purpose of study.	**PLAN:** Plan the change and observe.	
Step 1: Formulate a searchable, answerable question in PICOT format.	Step 2: Search for and review relevant literature.		
Step 2: Conduct a systematic search for evidence to answer the clinical question (using the PICOT question as the driver of the search).	Step 3: Define a conceptual framework to guide the study.		
Step 3: Critically appraise the evidence: • Rapid critical appraisal for keeper studies • Evaluation of keeper studies • Synthesis of a body of evidence • Recommendations for practice from the evidence	Step 4: Develop research objectives, hypothesis, variables, and study design, including population, sample, and setting.		
Step 4: Integration of synthesis of valid and reliable evidence combined with internal evidence, clinical expertise, and patients' preferences and values into practice.	Step 5: Test your hypothesis or answer your research questions by doing a study (e.g., experiments; usually a pilot study).	**DO:** Try out the change on a small scale.	
Step 5: Evaluate to determine if expected outcome is achieved.	Step 6: Collect and analyze study data and draw conclusions.	**STUDY:** Analyze the data and determine what was learned.	
Step 6: Disseminate outcome of translation of evidence into practice to others through any/all available mechanisms.	Step 7: Communicate study results, implications, and limitations.	**ACT:** Refine the change, based on what was learned, and repeat the testing.	

EBP, evidence-based practice; QI, quality improvement. Modified from Fineout-Overholt, E. (2014). EBP, QI & research: Kindred spirits or strange bedfellows. In C. B. Hedges & B. Williams (Eds.), *Anatomy of research for nurses: A practical approach*. Indianapolis, IN: Sigma Theta Tau International.

research results in practice" and today's EBP paradigm is the acknowledgment of the relative weight and role of various knowledge sources as the basis for clinical decisions (Stevens, 2015; Stevens & Clutter, 2007).

Best Practice and EBP

"Evidence" is now viewed and scrutinized from a clinical epidemiological perspective. This means that practitioners take into account the validity and reliability of the specific evidence when clinical recommendations are made (Fineout-Overholt, Melnyk,

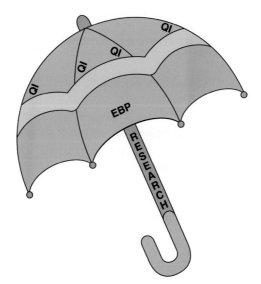

Figure 4.1: Relationship between evidence-based practice (EBP), research, and qualitative improvement (QI)/practice-based evidence (PBE) in clinical practice. (Modified from Fineout-Overholt, E. [2014]. EBP, QI & research: Kindred spirits or strange bedfellows. In C. B. Hedges & B. Williams [Eds.], *Anatomy of research for nurses: A practical approach*. Indianapolis, IN: Sigma Theta Tau International.)

Stillwell, & Williamson, 2010a, 2010b, 2010c; Stevens, Abrams, Brazier, Fitzpatrick, & Lilford, 2001). The EBP approach addresses variation in ways of managing similar health problems and the deficit between scientific evidence and clinical practice. In other words, clarifies the external evidence underlying effective practice (i.e., best practice) and specifies actions for addressing insufficient scientific evidence. In addition, EBP methods such as systematic reviews increase our ability to manage the ever-increasing volume of information produced in order to develop best practices. Indeed, systematic reviews are identified by quality care experts as the key link between research and practice (IOM, 2008, 2011; Stevens, 2013). To gain mastery in understanding the benefits of systematic reviews and other research designs as evidence, review Chapter 5.

Best practice is not new to healthcare providers. For example, mandatory continuing education for licensure in many states is regulatory testimony to the value of staying abreast of new developments in healthcare. However, emphasis on best practice has shifted from keeping current through traditional continuing education to keeping current with the latest and best available evidence that has been critically appraised for quality and impact when it is needed. Reliance on inexplicit or inferior knowledge sources (e.g., tradition or trial and error) is rapidly becoming unacceptable practice in today's quality-focused climate of healthcare. Rather, the focus is changing to replacing such practices with those based on a quality of knowledge that is said to include certainty and, therefore, predictability of outcome.

❝

We don't receive wisdom; we must discover it for ourselves after
a journey that no one can take for us or spare us.

MARCEL PROUST

CERTAINTY AND KNOWLEDGE SOURCES

The goal of EBP is to use the highest quality of knowledge in providing care to produce the greatest positive impact on patients' health status and healthcare outcomes. This entails using the following knowledge sources for care:

- Valid research evidence as the primary basis of clinical decisions (i.e., external evidence);
- Clinical expertise to best use research by filling in gaps and combining it with PBE (i.e., internal evidence) to tailor clinical actions to individual patient context;
- Patient choices and concerns for determining the acceptability of evidence-based care to the individual patient.

In clinical decisions, the key criterion for quality of underlying knowledge is certainty. Certainty is the level of sureness that the clinical action will produce the intended or desired outcome. Because clinical actions are intended to assist patients achieve a health goal, we can say with high certainty that what we do with patients is likely to move them toward that intended goal. To appraise certainty, the practitioner must first uncover the source of knowledge underlying the contemplated clinical action and then appraise the quality of that knowledge.

66

What is important is to keep learning, to enjoy challenge,
and to tolerate ambiguity. In the end there are
no certain answers.

MARTINA HORNER

RATING STRENGTH OF THE SCIENTIFIC EVIDENCE

EBP experts have developed a number of taxonomies to rate varying levels of evidence as well as strength of evidence (i.e., the level of evidence plus the quality of evidence). These assessments of the strength of scientific evidence provide a mechanism to guide practitioners in evaluating research for its applicability to healthcare decision making. Most of these taxonomies or hierarchies of evidence are organized around various research designs. For example, when asking a question about interventions, many refer to the syntheses of randomized controlled trials (RCTs) as a research design of the highest order, and most taxonomies include a full range of evidence, from systematic reviews of RCTs to expert opinions. However, simply assigning levels to evidence is not sufficient to assess quality or impact of evidence.

The Agency for Healthcare Research and Quality (AHRQ, 2002) established some time ago that grading the strength of a body of evidence should incorporate three domains: quality, quantity, and consistency. These are defined as follows:

- **Quality:** the extent to which a study's design, conduct, and analysis have minimized selection, measurement, and confounding biases (internal validity) (p. 19;)
- **Quantity:** the number of studies that have evaluated the clinical issue, overall sample size across all studies, magnitude of the treatment effect, and strength from causality assessment for interventions, such as relative risk or odds ratio (p. 25);
- **Consistency:** whether investigations with both similar and different study designs report similar findings (requires numerous studies) (p. 25).

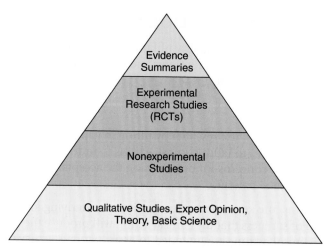

Figure 4.2: Strength-of-evidence rating pyramid. RCTs, randomized controlled trials. (© Stevens, K. R., & Clutter, P. C. [2007]. *Research and the Mandate for Evidence-based Quality, and Patient Safety. In M. Mateo & K. Kirchhoff [Eds.], Research for advanced practice nurses: From evidence to practice.* New York, NY: Springer Publishing. Used with permission.)

The challenge remains that there is no standardized approach to evaluating evidence. In 2002, AHRQ established that out of 19 systems for reviewing evidence, 7 included all 3 domains. Four of the seven indicated that systematic reviews of a body of literature represented the highest level of evidence for interventions, and five of the seven included expert opinion as evidence. The domains to evaluate to establish quality of evidence were updated to include the following (Agency for Healthcare Research and Quality, 2012):

- **Study limitations:** The likelihood of studies included in the synthesis are adequately protected against bias by the study design and how the study was conducted (p. 13).
- **Directness:** Two criteria include whether (a) evidence demonstrates association of interventions to specific outcomes; and (b) comparisons studies are head-to-head (p. 13).
- **Consistency:** Whether investigations with both similar and different study designs report similar findings (requires numerous studies; p. 14).
- **Precision:** The extent to which certainty surrounds the effect estimate and if sufficiency of sample size and number of events assumptions are met (p. 14).
- **Reporting bias:** The bias inherent in selectively publishing or reporting only research findings that are in the desired direction or magnitude of effect (p. 14).

Box 1.3 presents a sample system to determine the level of evidence for intervention questions. The level combined with the quality of the evidence that is assessed through critical appraisal reflects the strength of evidence, which determines the impact. This is a key concept for clinicians to understand when applying external evidence to practice. Figure 4.2 illustrates a basic strength-of-evidence rating hierarchy for interventions (Stevens & Clutter, 2007). The higher the evidence is placed on the pyramid, the more confident the clinician can be that the intervention will cause the targeted health effect.

APPRAISING KNOWLEDGE SOURCES

Critical appraisal of evidence is a hallmark of EBP. Although critical appraisal is not new, it has become a core skill for those who plan to use evidence to support healthcare decisions (Stevens et al., 2001). The evolution of EBP from evidence-based medicine (EBM) has heavily influenced the current emphasis on critical appraisal of evidence. At times, EBP has been criticized as having a sole focus on appraisal of RCTs. However, EBM leaders did not intend for appraisal of RCTs to be the final point of critical appraisal. The *Cochrane handbook for systematic reviews of interventions* (Higgins & Green, 2011), the most highly developed methodological source for conducting systematic reviews, states that for intervention questions RCTs are the first focus of current systematic reviews; however, other evidence is reviewed when relevant, making it explicit that the focus on RCTs is an interim situation (Box 4.2).

The Cochrane Handbook is currently being updated. Please check the url for updates http://training.cochrane.org/handbook.

EBP methodologists are actively developing and using methods for systematically summarizing the evidence generated from a broad range of research approaches, including qualitative research. Evidence from all health science disciplines and a broad array of healthcare topics, including nursing services, behavioral research, and preventive health, are available to answer clinical questions (Stevens, 2002).

The meaning of *evidence* is fully appreciated within the context of best practice, which includes the following (Stevens, 2002):

- Research evidence
- Clinical knowledge gained via the individual practitioner's experience
- Patients' and practitioners' preferences
- Basic principles from logic and theory

An important task in EBP is to identify which knowledge is to be considered as evidence for clinical decisions. The knowledge generated from quantitative and qualitative research, clinical judgment, and patient preferences forms the crucial foundation for practice. Depending on the particular source of knowledge, varying appraisal approaches can be used to determine its worth to practice. The chapters in Unit 2 describe appraisal approaches for the main types of evidence and knowledge to guide clinical practice:

- Evidence from quantitative research
- Evidence from qualitative research
- Clinical judgment
- Knowledge about patient concerns, choices, and values

The authors of the following chapters apply generic principles of evidence appraisal to the broad set of knowledge sources used in healthcare. The purpose of critically appraising these sources is to determine the certainty and applicability of knowledge, regardless of the source.

BOX 4.2	*Randomized Controlled Trials (RCTs) and Systematic Reviews*

Early on, the Cochrane Collaboration expressed through its colloquia and the Cochrane Reviewers' Handbook, an explanation of their focusing initial efforts on systematic reviews of RCTs: such study designs are more likely to provide reliable information about "what works best" in comparing alternative forms of healthcare (Kunz, Vist, & Oxman, 2003). At the same time, the Collaboration highlighted the value of systematically reviewing other types of evidence, such as that generated by cohort studies, using the same principles that guide reviews of RCTs. "Although we focus mainly on systematic reviews of RCTs, we address issues specific to reviewing other types of evidence when this is relevant. Fuller guidance on such reviews is being developed." (Alderson, Green, & Higgins, 2004, p. 14)

USING INTERNAL EVIDENCE TO TRACK OUTCOMES OF EVIDENCE-BASED PRACTICE

The EBP process comes full circle in that PBE is used to demonstrate the outcome of evidence implementation. Sustainability is the purpose of evidence implementation. Therefore, the availability of numerous scientifically sound systems of quality indicators can provide the foundational evidence for tracking quality of care over time. The value of such internal evidence is that impact of improvement in innovations can be traced, overall performance can be documented at regular intervals, and further areas for improvement can be targeted for intervention. Several quality indicator systems offer opportunities for individual healthcare agencies to survey their own organizations and compare their results with national benchmarks (see Chapter 10). Three of the quality indicator systems that compile comparative internal evidence (i.e., PBE) are described in the following sections.

Agency for Healthcare Research and Quality National Healthcare Quality Report

A notable addition to national quality indicators in the United States is the AHRQ *National Healthcare Quality Report*. The purpose of the report is to track the state of healthcare quality for the nation on an annual basis. In terms of the number of measures and number of dimensions of quality, it is the most extensive ongoing examination of quality of care ever undertaken in the United States or in any major industrialized country worldwide (Agency for Healthcare Research and Quality, 2013).

This evidence is used as a gauge of improvement across the nation. These reports measure trends in effectiveness of care, patient safety, timeliness of care, patient centeredness, and efficiency of care. Through these surveys, clinicians can locate indices on quality measures, such as the percentage of heart attack patients who received recommended care when they reached the hospital or the percentage of children who received recommended vaccinations.

The first report, in 2004, found that high-quality healthcare is not yet a universal reality and that opportunities for preventive care are often missed, particularly opportunities in the management of chronic diseases in the United States. Subsequent surveys have found that healthcare quality is improving in small increments (about 1.5% to 2.3% improvement) and that more gains than losses are being made. Core measures of patient safety improvements reflect gains of only 1% (AHRQ, 2012). These national data as well as others described in the following sections can help organizations to make clinical decisions. Best practice would be when these data are combined with external evidence supporting action to improve outcomes.

National Quality Forum

Other internal evidence useful in QI may be gleaned from a set of quality indicators that were developed by the National Quality Forum (NQF). The NQF is a not-for-profit membership organization created to develop and implement a national strategy for healthcare quality measurement and reporting. The NQF is regarded as a mechanism to bring about national change in the impact of healthcare quality on patient outcomes, workforce productivity, and healthcare costs. It seeks to promote a common approach to measuring healthcare quality and fostering system-wide capacity for QI (National Quality Forum [NQF], 2008).

The NQF endorsed a set of 15 consensus-based nursing standards for inpatient care. Known as the NQF-15, these measures represent processes and outcomes that are effected, provided, and/or influenced by nursing personnel. These factors and their structural proxies (e.g., skill mix and nurse staffing hours) are called *nursing-sensitive measures*. The NQF's endorsement of these measures marked a pivotal step in the efforts to increase the understanding of nurses' influence on inpatient hospital care and promote uniform metrics for use in internal QI and public reporting activities. The NQF-15 includes measures that examine nursing contributions to hospital care from three perspectives: patient-centered outcome measures (e.g., prevalence of pressure ulcers and inpatient falls), nursing-centered intervention measures (e.g., smoking cessation counseling), and system-centered measures (e.g., voluntary turnover and nursing care hours per patient day) (NQF, 2008).

 More can be learned about NQF-15 by accessing http://www.qualityforum.org /Projects/n-r/Nursing-sensitive_Care_Initial_Measures/Nursing_Sensitive_Care__Initial _Measures.aspx

In NQF's strategic plan, the charge to identify the most important measures to improve U.S. healthcare is key in that specific measures will help establish consistency in how to demonstrate QI and safety of the healthcare industry. Furthermore, measurement of quality is imperative to demonstrating cost-efficient care (National Quality Forum, 2016).

National Database of Nursing Quality Indicators

In 1998, the National Database of Nursing Quality Indicators (NDNQI) was established by the American Nurses Association to facilitate continued indicator development and further our understanding of factors influencing the quality of nursing care. The NDNQI provides quarterly and annual reports on structure, process, and outcome indicators to evaluate nursing care at the unit level. The structure of nursing care is reflected by the supply, skill level, and education/certification of nursing staff. Process indicators reflect nursing care aspects such as assessment, intervention, and registered nurse job satisfaction. Outcome indicators reflect patient outcomes that are nursing sensitive and improve if there is greater quantity or quality of nursing care, such as pressure ulcers, falls, and IV infiltrations. There is some overlap between NQF-15 and NDNQI because of the adoption of some of the NDNQI indicators into the NQF set. The NDNQI repository of nursing-sensitive indicators is used in further QI research.

Other Quality Improvement Initiatives

New QI initiatives have put into play new expectations for generating evidence and sources and applications of evidence. The National Strategy for Quality Improvement in Health Care (Department of Health and Human Services, 2012) was established by the Department of Health and Human Services to serve as a blueprint across all sectors of the healthcare community—patients, providers, employers, health insurance companies, academic researchers, and all government levels—to prioritize QI efforts, share lessons, and measure collective success. Success is targeted toward three aims: (1) improving the patient experience of care (including quality and satisfaction); (2) improving the health of populations; and (3) reducing the per capita cost of healthcare. With this national initiative comes the need to generate evidence about the effectiveness of improvement innovations in terms of the three aims as outcomes. National consensus on key quality measures is also evolving. Nurse scientists and their clinical partners will generate new evidence using these measures and the evidence will be suited for informing decisions about care and care delivery. In this new movement, *remaining current* will be an important challenge as the rapid-paced National Strategy achieves rapid-cycle testing of new healthcare delivery models and cost impact.

In the world of QI, PBE holds an important place. Such evidence detects the trends within a given setting so that improvement goals can be set against best practice. At the same time, a hybrid field of improvement science is emerging as a framework for research that focuses on healthcare delivery improvement. The goal of the field is to determine which improvement strategies work as we strive to assure safe and effective care (Improvement Science Research Network, 2017). In other words, the field generates evidence about EBP—how to process it and how to promote uptake and sustainment of it.

The importance of evidence on the topic of "integrating best practice into routine care" is suggested in the *Future of Nursing* report (IOM, 2010). This report recommends that, as best practices emerge, it is essential that all members of the healthcare team be actively involved in making QI changes. Together with members of other disciplines, nurses are called on to be leaders and active followers in contributing to these improvements at the individual level of care, as well as at the system level of care (IOM, 2010). According to the University of Pennsylvania Prevention Research Center (2016), implementation research offers understanding of the methods used to improve the translation of evidence into practice for sustainable change across healthcare settings. Improvement science is described as a framework for discovery of the strategies that are most effective in improving healthcare outcomes (Improvement Science Research Network, 2017). Accountable leaders of integration of EBP will rely on results of improvement and implementation research to inform their improvement initiatives. The field is growing, and nurses are leading in significant advances to produce the evidence needed for improvement (Stevens, 2009, 2012).

Another initiative affecting EBP is that of the Patient-Centered Outcomes Research Institute (PCORI). The stated mission of PCORI is to "help people make informed health care decisions, and improve health care delivery and outcomes, by producing and promoting high integrity, evidence-based information that comes from research guided by patients, caregivers and the broader health care community" (Patient-Centered Outcomes Research Institute, 2013). The work of PCORI assures that new forms of evidence enter our decision making—that of the voice of the patient, family, and caregivers. In addition, patient-centered outcomes research results are formed in such a way that it is useful to these same stakeholders as they make informed healthcare decisions in assessing the value of various healthcare options and how well these meet their preferences.

OVERVIEWS OF THE FOLLOWING FOUR CHAPTERS

In the next four chapters of this unit, you learn how to consider evidence from quantitative studies, qualitative studies, and clinical practice guidelines (CPGs) as you apply critical appraisal techniques to discern how to integrate valid and reliable external evidence with patient preferences and your expertise in good decision making with your patients. In Unit 3, the decisions made will be implemented into practice.

Critical Appraisal of Quantitative Evidence: Chapter 5

The nature of evidence produced through quantitative research varies according to the particular design utilized. Chapter 5, "Critically Appraising Quantitative Evidence for Clinical Decision Making," details the various types of quantitative research designs, including case studies, case-control studies, and cohort studies, as well as RCTs, and concludes with a discussion of systematic reviews. Distinctions among **narrative reviews**, **systematic reviews**, and **meta-analyses** are drawn. Helpful explanations about systematic reviews describe how data are combined across multiple research studies. Throughout, critical appraisal questions and hints are outlined.

Critical Appraisal of Qualitative Evidence: Chapter 6

Given the original emphasis on RCTs (experimental research design) in EBP, some have inaccurately concluded that there is no role for qualitative evidence in EBP. Chapter 6, "Critically Appraising Qualitative Evidence for Clinical Decision Making," provides a compelling discussion on the ways in which qualitative research results answer clinical questions. The rich understanding of individual patients that emerges from qualitative research connects this evidence strongly to the elements of patient preferences and values—both important in implementing EBP.

Integration of Patient Preferences and Values and Clinician Expertise into Evidence-Based Decision Making: Chapter 7

Chapter 7 focuses on the roles of two important aspects of clinical decision making: patient choices and concerns and clinical judgment or expertise. The discussion emphasizes patient preferences not only as perceptions of self and what is best, but also as what gives meaning to a person's life. The role of clinical judgment emerges as the practitioner weaves together a narrative understanding of the patient's condition, which includes social and emotional aspects and historical facts. Clinical judgment is presented as a historical clinical understanding of an individual patient—as well as of psychosocial and biological sciences—that is to be combined with the evidence from scientific inquiry. The roles of clinical judgment, clinical expertise, and patient values, choices, and concerns are essential to evidence-based care.

Critical appraisal of evidence and knowledge used in clinical care is a requirement in professional practice. These chapters provide a basis for understanding and applying the principles of evidence appraisal to improve healthcare.

Advancing Optimal Care With Robust Clinical Practice Guidelines: Chapter 8

Chapter 8 addresses the development, appraisal, and implementation of CPGs. These are sets of evidence-based recommendations that speak of safe and effective management of a clinical issue. When making decisions about what constitutes best practice, considering recommendations within CPGs and their associated supporting studies as sources of evidence offers clinicians further options for defining what needs to be implemented in practice. Clinicians use the knowledge gained within Chapters 5 and 6 to engage the tools available to appraise CPGs and their recommendations. Furthermore, knowledge gained in Chapter 7 about patient preferences and clinician expertise is incorporated when considering how these recommendations provide structure for evidence-based decision making. Understanding the value of valid and reliable CPGs and their underpinning evidence sets clinicians up for moving from evidence to action.

> **"**
> Knowledge speaks, but wisdom listens.
>
> **JIMI HENDRIX**

EBP FAST FACTS

- External evidence is scientific research.
- Internal evidence is practice-generated evidence.
- The strength of the evidence is a combination of the level of evidence in a hierarchy and how well the research was conducted and reported.
- QI process is distinct but related to EBP and research processes.
- Critical appraisal of evidence is imperative for EBP to thrive.
- EBP is about sustainability of best practices and associated outcomes.
- PBE starts and ends the EBP process.

WANT TO KNOW MORE?

A variety of resources is available to enhance your learning and understanding of this chapter.

- Visit thePoint® to access
  - Articles from the AJN EBP Step-By-Step Series
  - Journal articles
  - Checklists for rapid critical appraisal and more!
- Lippincott CoursePoint combines digital text content with video case studies and interactive modules for a fully integrated course solution that works the way you study and learn.

References

Agency for Healthcare Research and Quality. (2002). *Systems to rate the strength of scientific evidence* (AHRQ Publication No. 02-E016). Rockville, MD: Author. Retrieved from https://archive.ahrq.gov/clinic/epcsums/strenfact.pdf

Agency for Healthcare Research and Quality. (2012). *Grading the strength of a body of evidence when assessing health care interventions for the effective health care program of the Agency for Healthcare Research and Quality: An update*. Rockville, MD: Author. Retrieved from https://effectivehealthcare.ahrq.gov/sites/default/files/pdf/methods-guidance-grading-evidence_methods.pdf

Agency for Healthcare Research and Quality. (2013). *National healthcare quality report: Acknowledgments*. Rockville, MD: Author. Retrieved from https://archive.ahrq.gov/research/findings/nhqrdr/nhqr13/2013nhqr.pdf

Alderson, P., Green, S., & Higgins, J. P. T. (Eds.). (2004). Cochrane reviewers' handbook 4.2.2 [updated March 2004]. In *The Cochrane library*, Issue 1. Chichester, UK: John Wiley & Sons.

American Nurses Credentialing Center. (2008). *A new model for ANCC's MAGNET® recognition program*. Silver Spring, MD: Author.

American Nurses Credentialing Center. (2014). *2014 MAGNET® application manual*. Silver Spring, MD: Author.

Department of Health and Human Services. (2003). *OCR HIPAA privacy*. Retrieved from https://www.hhs.gov/sites/default/files/ocr/privacy/hipaa/understanding/special/research/research.pdf?language=es

Department of Health and Human Services. (2012). *2012 Annual progress report to congress*. Washington, DC: National Strategy for Quality Improvement in Health Care.

Fineout-Overholt, E. (2014). EBP, QI & research: Kindred spirits or strange bedfellows. In C. B. Hedges & B. Williams (Eds.), *Anatomy of research for nurses: A practical approach*. Indianapolis, IN: Sigma Theta Tau International.

Fineout-Overholt, E., Melnyk, B. M., Stillwell, S. B., & Williamson, K. M. (2010a). Evidence-based practice, step by step: Critical appraisal of the evidence: Part III. *American Journal of Nursing, 111*(11), 43–51.

Fineout-Overholt, E., Melnyk, B. M., Stillwell, S. B., & Williamson, K. M. (2010b). Evidence-based practice, step by step: Critical appraisal of the evidence: Part II. *American Journal of Nursing, 110*(9), 41–48.

Fineout-Overholt, E., Melnyk, B. M., Stillwell, S. B., & Williamson, K. M. (2010c). Evidence-based practice step by step: Critical appraisal of the evidence: Part I. *American Journal of Nursing, 110*(7), 47–52.

Fineout-Overholt, E. (2015). Getting best outcomes: Paradigm and process matter. *Worldviews on Evidence-Based Nursing,* 12(4): 183–186.

Higgins, J. P. T., & Green, S. (Eds.). (2011). *Cochrane handbook for systematic reviews of interventions (version 5.1.0)* [updated March 2011]. London, UK: The Cochrane Collaboration. Available from http://training.cochrane.org/handbook

Improvement Science Research Network. (2017). *What is improvement science?* Retrieved from https://isrn.net/about/improvement_science.asp

Institute for Healthcare Improvement. (2010). *Plan-Do-Study-Act (PDSA).* Retrieved from http://www.ihi.org/resources/Pages/HowtoImprove/default.aspx. Accessed June 15, 2017.

Institute of Medicine. (2008). *Knowing what works in health care: A roadmap for the nation.* Washington, DC: National Academies Press.

Institute of Medicine. (2010). *The future of nursing: Focus on scope of practice* [Committee on the Robert Wood Johnson Foundation Initiative on the Future of Nursing]. Washington, DC: National Academies Press.

Institute of Medicine. (2011). *Finding what works in health care: Standards for systematic reviews* [Committee on Standards for Systematic Reviews of Comparative Effective Research; Board on Health Care Services]. Washington, DC: National Academies Press.

Kunz, R., Vist, G., & Oxman, A. D. (2003). Randomisation to protect against selection bias in healthcare trials (Cochrane Methodology Review). In *Cochrane library,* Issue 1. Oxford, UK: Update Software.

National Quality Forum. (2008). *About us.* Retrieved from http://www.qualityforum.org/about/

National Quality Forum. (2016). *NQF's strategic direction 2016-2019: Lead, prioritize, and collaborate for better healthcare measurement.* Retrieved from http://www.qualityforum.org/NQF_Strategic_Direction_2016-2019.aspx

Patient-Centered Outcomes Research Institute. (2013). *Mission and vision.* Retrieved from http://www.pcori.org/research-results/about-our-research

RAND. (2012). *Appendix B. Government-wide and DOD definitions of R&D.* Retrieved from https://www.rand.org/content/dam/rand/pubs/monograph_reports/MR1194/MR1194.appb.pdf.

Speroff, T., & O'Connor, G. T. (2004). Study designs for PDSA quality improvement research. *Quality Management in Health Care, 13*(1), 17–32.

Stevens, A., Abrams, K., Brazier, J., Fitzpatrick, R., & Lilford, R. (Eds.). (2001). *The advanced handbook of methods in evidence based healthcare.* London, UK: Sage.

Stevens, K. R. (2002). The truth, the whole truth . . . about EBP and RCTs. *Journal of Nursing Administration, 32*(5), 232–233.

Stevens, K. R. (2009). *A research network for improvement science: The Improvement Science Research Network, 2009* ($3.1 million NIH 1 RC2 NR011946-01). Retrieved from http://era.nih.gov/commons/

Stevens, K. R. (2012). Delivering on the promise of EBP. *Nursing Management, 3*(3), 19–21.

Stevens, K. R. (2013). The impact of evidence-based practice in nursing and the next big ideas. *Online Journal of Nursing Issues, 8*(2), 4.

Stevens, K. R. (2015). Stevens Star Model of EBP: Knowledge transformation. *Academic center for evidence-based practice.* San Antonio, TX: The University of Texas Health Science Center. Retrieved from www.acestar.uthscsa.edu

Stevens, K. R., & Clutter, P. C. (2007). Research and the mandate for evidence-based quality, and patient safety. In M. Mateo & K. Kirchhoff (Eds.). *Research for advanced practice nurses: From evidence to practice.* New York, NY: Springer Publishing.

Taylor, M. J., McNicholas, C., Nicolay, C., Darzi, A., Bell, D., & Reed, J. E. (2014). Systematic review of the application of the plan-do-study-act method to improve quality in healthcare. *British Medical Journal of Quality and Safety, 23*(4), 290–298.

University of Pennsylvania Prevention Research Center. (2016). *Implementation science institute.* Retrieved on from http://www.upennprc.org/training/implementation-science-institute-march-9-11-2017/#.WUNVIuvyuUk

5

Critically Appraising Quantitative Evidence for Clinical Decision Making

Dónal P. O'Mathúna and Ellen Fineout-Overholt

> A dream doesn't become reality through magic; it takes sweat, determination and hard work.
>
> —Colin Powell

EBP Terms to Learn

Absolute risk increase (ARI)
Absolute risk reduction (ARR)
Atheoretical
Body of evidence
Case–control study
Clinical significance
Cohort study
Critical appraisal
Hierarchy of evidence
Keeper studies
Levels of evidence
Meta-analysis
Number needed to harm (NNH)
Number needed to treat (NNT)
Odds ratio (OR)
p value

Placebo
Reference population
Relative risk (RR)
Relative risk reduction (RRR)

Statistical significance
Type I error
Type II error

Learning Objectives

After studying this chapter, learners will be able to:

1. Describe how different quantitative research designs best answer different types of clinical questions.
2. Explain the four phases of critical appraisal.
3. List the three key questions to ask of all studies.
4. Explain the markers of good research for different types of quantitative research designs.
5. Discuss the role of interpreted statistics in clinical decision making.
6. Discuss how recommendations for practice come from a body of evidence.

Rigorously engaging the evidence-based practice (EBP) process is an imperative for sustainable change. After reading Chapters 2 and 3 and engaging the online resources, you will have mastered asking a clinical question in PICOT format and systematically searching for the best evidence to answer the question. This chapter focuses on understanding various quantitative research methodologies and designs that can offer reliable guidance for clinical decision making. This step (#3) of the EBP process is called critical appraisal. This step has four sequential phases. Phase one begins with determining which studies should be retained to help answer the clinical question (i.e., rapid critical appraisal [RCA] for identifying **keeper studies**); phase two focuses on extracting data from individual studies to establish agreement or disagreement among the keepers by carefully reviewing the extracted data and comparing across studies (i.e., evaluation); phase three pulls data together to paint the picture of what the body of evidence tells us (i.e., synthesis that reflects what we know about a topic); and phase four concludes this step by recommending next steps for practice that should be applied to all patients who are within the population described in the question (i.e., recommendation). To accomplish critical appraisal, there must be an appreciation of clinicians' skills in using the four sequenced phases, much like the young lumberjack who, on the first day of his first job, felled numerous trees with his handsaw. The foreman was so impressed with the young man that he provided a chain saw for the next day's work. At the end of the second day, the foreman was shocked to find out that the young lumberjack had only taken down one tree the entire day. When the foreman started up the chain saw, the lumberjack jumped back and said, "Is that thing supposed to sound that way?" All day long he had been using the chain saw as the tool he knew how to use—the handsaw. Mastering the use of research, including both quantitative and qualitative designs (Chapter 6), requires investment of time and energy and begins by understanding the available tools. Clinicians and patients alike will reap the rich rewards afforded by basing clinical decisions on the best available evidence.

For decades, clinicians have read healthcare literature to keep up-to-date with the rapid changes in care delivery or to stay current with relevant research results in their field. With the advent of EBP, clinicians increasingly use research evidence to help them make informed decisions about how best to care for and communicate with patients to achieve the highest quality outcomes. EBP is a paradigm that supports multidisciplinary decision making that is now common across dentistry, medicine, nursing, physiotherapy, respiratory therapy, and many other fields of health and social care.

The EBP decision making paradigm involves integrating clinical expertise, patient values and preferences, and the current best research evidence. However, few clinicians, if any, can keep up with all the research being published, even with various electronic tools currently available (Loher-Niederer, Maccora, & Ritz, 2013). With current competing priorities in healthcare settings, it is challenging to determine which studies are best for busy clinicians to use for clinical decision making. In addition, researchers may propose various, sometimes contradictory, conclusions when studying the same or similar issues, making it quite baffling to determine upon which studies clinicians can rely. Even the usefulness of preappraised studies, such as level one systematic reviews, is sometimes difficult to discern.

As a result, evidence-based clinicians must evaluate the appropriateness of evidence to answer clinical questions. This requires mastery of the skills necessary to critically appraise the available studies to answer the question. Establishing how well the studies were conducted and how reliable the findings are can help determine the strength of the evidence, which supports the confidence to act. In critical appraisal, the gestalt of all studies in the body of evidence (i.e., more than a simple summary of the studies) is underpinned by the evaluation of each study for its strengths, limitations, and value/worth to practice (i.e., how well it informs clinician decision making to have an impact on outcomes). Clinicians cannot focus only on the flaws of research, but must weigh the limitations with the strengths to determine the worth of the body of evidence to practice. Appraising research is similar to how a jeweler appraises gemstones, weighing the characteristics of a diamond (e.g., clarity, color, carat, and cut) before declaring its worth (Fineout-Overholt, 2008).

First, it is important to determine the best match between the kind of question being asked and the research methodology available to answer that question (see Chapter 2, Table 2.4). Different **levels of evidence** are described in Chapter 2, and those levels will be referred to in the discussion of critical appraisal of various quantitative research methodologies.

Understanding quantitative studies begins with what is called a general appraisal overview (GAO). General questions that apply to quantitative research designs are included in the GAO, such as purpose of the study, independent variables (IVs; i.e., intervention or condition), and dependent variables (DVs; i.e., outcomes). The GAO is a working form that enables clinicians to document their thinking about a particular study as they record factual information about the study. Appendix B is an example that also contains *tips* about how to use the form. Beginning with these questions is essential for every clinician to successfully use the tools of research. The GAO is followed by RCA, which includes the hierarchy of evidence for intervention questions (levels of evidence) and a detailed analysis of the specific questions that are markers of good research design. Each design within quantitative evidence has its own specific questions. By addressing these questions, study validity, reliability, and applicability can be established to determine which studies are keeper studies. Issues such as bias, confounding results, effect size, and confidence intervals (CIs) are some of the elements of research methods that are important to understanding each study's worth to practice. Applying appraisal principles to different types of research designs (such as case studies, case–control studies, cohort studies, randomized controlled trials [RCTs], and systematic reviews) allows clinicians to develop a body of evidence (i.e., what is known on the topic). These study designs are described in special sections that discuss the unique characteristics of each design type and provide specific appraisal questions for that type of design. Each section concludes with a worked example in a clinical scenario entitled "What the Literature Says: Answering a Clinical Question." Readers are encouraged to read the material about the research design first (the instruction manual) and then read the application in a clinical scenario to see a demonstration of the RCA checklist.

PRELIMINARY QUESTIONS TO ASK: GENERAL APPRAISAL OVERVIEW

Quantitative research papers generally follow a convention when presenting results. This approach can assist with critical appraisal by identifying standard criteria by which each study should be appraised. To help with mastery of the GAO, Box 5.1 provides a list of questions that should be asked of each quantitative study. These will be reviewed in the following sections.

BOX 5.1 *General Appraisal Overview (GAO) Elements and Questions for Critical Appraisal of Quantitative Studies*

PICOT Question
Overview of the study
• Why was the study done (purpose)?
• What was the study design?
• Was appropriate ethics review reported?

General Description of the Study
Research Questions or Hypothesis
Sampling
• What was the sampling technique?
• What was the sample size?
• What were the sample characteristics?

Major Variables Studied
• What are the major variables, independent and dependent?
• Are the measurements of major variables valid and reliable?
• How were the data analyzed? Were the statistics used appropriate?
• Were there any untoward events during the conduct of the study?
• How do the results fit with previous research in the area?
• What does this research mean for clinical practice?

Conclusion

Why Was the Study Done?

A clear explanation of why the study was carried out (i.e., the purpose of the study) is crucial and should be stated succinctly in the report being critically appraised. The purpose can be elaborated on in the aims of the study, which are usually more specific statements for how the purpose will be achieved. The brief background literature presented in a study should identify what we know about the topic along with the gap that this research was designed to fill. This provides readers with an understanding of how the current research fits within the context of reported knowledge on the topic.

Studies may have research questions, hypotheses, or both that provide the focus of the study—why it is being conducted. Research questions are researchers' queries that arise independently of the current evidence because it provides no guidance about what relationships can be expected. In contrast, hypotheses are reasonable statements based on current evidence that describe predictable relationships. By knowing the research questions or hypotheses of a study, users of evidence can identify the purpose and aims of studies, particularly when these are not explicitly stated.

What Is the Sample Size?

One of the keys to well-conducted, reliable quantitative evidence is that an appropriate sample size be used. Adequate sample size provides reasonable confidence that chance was minimized as a contributor to the study results and that the true effect of the intervention was demonstrated. Researchers should conduct an a priori (i.e., done before starting the study) calculation called a power analysis to assist them in determining what the sample size should be to minimize chance findings. In addition, evidence users need to be aware of two general types of errors. **Type I errors** occur when researchers conclude from an experiment that a difference exists between interventions (i.e., false positives), when in reality there is no difference. **Type II errors** occur when there truly is a difference between interventions, but researchers conclude that one does not exist (i.e., false negatives; Table 5.1). Power analyses

TABLE 5.1	*Implications of Study Results Found by Chance*

		Study Results	
		Researchers Found That the Intervention Worked (i.e., They Rejected the Null* Hypothesis)	**Researchers Found That the Intervention Did Not Work Better Than the Comparison Intervention (i.e., They Accepted the Null* Hypothesis)**
Reality options	True positive (statistically significant, $p < 0.05$)	On target finding	Oops—made a **Type II error** (false negative—said it did not work, when in reality it did)
	True negative (statistically significant, $p > 0.05$)	Oops—made a **Type I error** (false positive—said it did work when in reality it did not)	On target finding

*Null hypothesis: there is no difference between the intervention and comparison groups (the intervention did not work).

help to minimize such errors and should be reported in the methods section of the research report. If a power analysis is not reported, the adequacy or inadequacy of the sample size cannot be assumed. Sometimes ethical, economic, and other practical considerations impact the sample size of a study. How the sample size affects the validity of findings should be carefully considered when appraising a study. Sample characteristics should be noted as well. This enables clinicians to consider if there is a match between their patient population and the study participants.

Are the Measurements of Major Variables Valid and Reliable?

Identifying the major variables in studies is essential to understanding the value of evidence to clinical decision making. The IV is what has been implemented to achieve an outcome (i.e., the DV). All quantitative research designs do not have an intervention (i.e., something implemented to achieve an outcome). In those studies, the condition is the IV. Condition such as smoking or a disease can be associated with an outcome, which is the DV. The IVs must be clearly defined. There are several definitions to consider, including conceptual and operational definitions. Conceptual definitions come from the theory guiding the research, and operational definitions are how the variables are measured in the study. For example, EBP implementation conceptually may be defined as using research and other evidence in practice, and operationally may be defined by the Evidence-based Implementation Scale (Melnyk, Fineout-Overholt, & Mays, 2008).

All operational definitions should include the concepts of validity and reliability, that is, the accuracy and consistency of the measures. A valid instrument is one that measures what it is purported to measure. For example, an instrument that is expected to measure fear should indeed measure fear (and not anxiety, for example). A reliable instrument is one that is stable over time (i.e., it performs the same way each time responders answer the questions) and is composed of individual items or questions that consistently measure the same construct. Several statistical techniques can be applied to instrument results to determine their reliability (e.g., Cronbach's alpha).

Published research reports should discuss the validity and reliability of the outcome measures used in the study in the methods section. Investigators should address issues or concerns they have with the validity or reliability of their results in the discussion section of the research report. It is important for the critical appraiser to keep in mind that without valid and reliable measurement of outcomes, the study results are not clinically meaningful.

How Were the Data Analyzed?

Clear descriptions of how researchers conducted their statistical analyses assist the reader in evaluating the reliability and applicability of the study results and protect against data dredging. Clinicians do not need to be familiar with a large number of complex approaches to statistical analysis. Even experts in statistics have challenges keeping up with current statistical techniques. Although statistical methods can be challenging, clinicians need a general understanding of how to interpret some common statistical tests and the types of data that are appropriate for their use. For those new to critical appraisal, spotting common mistakes in statistics can be a great opportunity to learn the methods (Gagnier & Morgenstern, 2017; George et al., 2016). Some common statistical errors include the following:

- *Focusing only on the p value.* Choosing a statistical test because it gives the answer for which the investigator had hoped (e.g., statistical significance) is ill-advised.

A statistical test should be chosen on the basis of its appropriateness for the type of data collected. Authors should give clear justifications for using anything other than the most commonly used statistical tests.

- *Data dredging,* or conducting a large number of analyses on the same data. This can be problematic because the more analyses conducted, the more likely that a significant result will be found because of chance.
- *Confusing statistical significance with clinical importance.* A small difference between large groups may be statistically significant, but may be such a rare event that few will benefit from it. For example, if an intervention reduces blood pressure by 2 mm Hg, the finding might be statistically significant in a study with a large sample, but it would not be clinically meaningful. On the other hand, a large difference between small groups may not be statistically significant, but may make an important clinical difference.
- *Missing data.* Incomplete data are surprisingly common, and, when noted, should raise questions during critical appraisal. Researchers should indicate in their report how they addressed any incomplete data. If this issue is not addressed, the problem may be an oversight in the report, a restrictive word count from the publisher, or a poorly conducted study—all of which should be considered carefully. If the issue is an oversight in reporting or word count restriction, contacting the researcher is in order to discuss how missing data were addressed.
- *Selective reporting.* Inappropriately publishing only outcomes with statistically significant findings can lead to missing data. This can occur where only studies with positive findings are published—leading to publication bias—or where only positive outcomes within a study are published—leading to selective outcome reporting bias (Howland, 2011). Within a study, a flowchart is an efficient mechanism to account for all patients and show how the various groups progressed through the study. Figure 5.1 is an example of a flowchart that visually summarizes the study design and how participants moved through the study. The numbers in the flowchart should match those used in the statistical analyses (e.g., 396 were analyzed from the intervention group; 405 from the control group; total in the final sample 801).

Once the GAO has been completed, evidence users can begin to formulate a conclusion about whether the study is valid and other considerations should be addressed in preparation for engaging the appropriate RCA checklist. The final conclusion about keeping the study is not reached until RCA is completed.

OTHER CONSIDERATIONS FOR QUANTITATIVE RESEARCH DESIGNS

Were There Any Untoward Events During the Conduct of the Study?

During critical appraisal, it is important to understand how problems that arose during a study influenced the final results. These issues may be unpredictable and occur randomly or they may arise because of a flaw or flaws in the original study design. One such problem is loss to follow-up (i.e., study attrition), which results in missing data and introduction of bias. Research reports should provide explanations for all adverse events and withdrawals from the study and how those events affected the final results (supported by evidence regarding how those conclusions were reached).

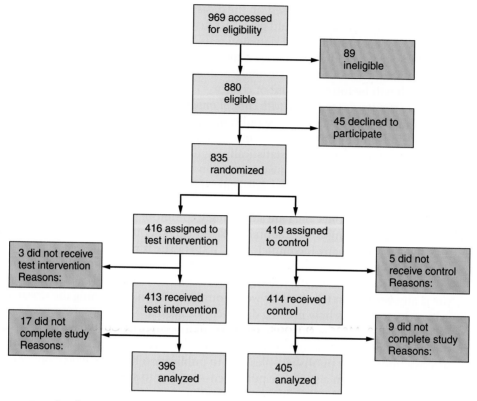

Figure 5.1: Study participant flowchart.

How Do the Results Fit With Previous Research in the Area?

Except on rare occasions when researchers investigate completely new areas of interest, studies fit into a growing body of research evidence. A study report should begin with a **systematic review** of previous literature that substantiates why this study was conducted. In a study report, the evidence review is the context in which the current research is meaningful. This review should provide confidence that the researchers took advantage of previous researchers' experiences (positive and negative) in conducting studies on this topic. In addition, the discussion section of the report should discuss the study findings in light of what is already known and how those findings complement or contradict previous work. In writing the report, the evidence review and discussion should be framed in such a way that the clinician will understand the purpose and context of the research.

What Does This Research Mean for Clinical Practice?

The point of critical appraisal of all research and subsequent evidence-based decision making in healthcare is to apply research findings to improve clinical practice outcomes. Therefore, asking what the research means for clinical practice is one of the most important questions to keep in mind during critical appraisal. Clinicians should look at the study population and ask whether the results can be extrapolated to the patients in *their*   .

Although it is imperative that these general questions are asked of every study, it is also important to ask additional, design-specific appraisal questions to determine the worth of each study to clinical decision making. The following sections provide those design-specific questions.

HIERARCHY OF EVIDENCE

A **hierarchy of evidence** is the same as levels of evidence and provides guidance about the types of research studies, if well done, that are more likely to provide reliable answers to a specific clinical question (Figure 5.2). There are various hierarchies, or levels, of evidence; which hierarchy is appropriate depends on the type of clinical question being asked. For intervention questions, the most appropriate hierarchy of evidence ranks quantitative research designs (e.g., a systematic review of RCTs) at the highest level of confidence compared with designs that give lower levels of confidence (e.g., descriptive studies). Other types of questions are best answered by other hierarchies.

The higher a methodology ranks in the hierarchy, if well done, the more likely the results accurately represent the actual situation and the more confidence clinicians can have that the intervention will produce the same health outcomes in similar patients for whom they care. An RCT is the best research design for providing information about cause-and-effect relationships. A systematic review of RCTs provides a compilation of what we know about a topic from multiple studies addressing the same research question, which ranks it higher in the hierarchy than a single RCT. A systematic review (i.e., a synthesis of these studies) of a large number of high-quality RCTs of similar design (i.e., have **homogeneity**) is the strongest and least biased method to provide confidence that the intervention will consistently bring about a particular outcome (Fineout-Overholt, O'Mathúna, & Kent, 2008; Guyatt, Rennie, Meade, & Cook, 2015; Turner, Balmer, & Coverdale, 2013). Such systematic reviews have been considered the "heart of evidence-based practice" for some time (Stevens, 2001). Despite this designation, there may be a reluctance for evidence users or faculty teaching EBP to accept that a body of evidence can contain only a systematic review and a few newer single studies; they may feel more comfortable with more single studies. However, as EBP increasingly becomes the basis for achieving healthcare

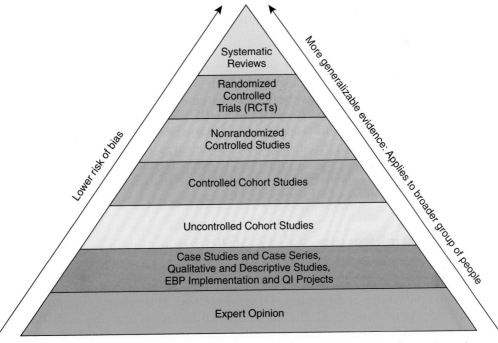

Figure 5.2: Hierarchy of evidence for intervention questions. EBP, evidence-based practice; QI, quality improvement.

outcomes, the conduct and use of systematic reviews will be essential as the mainstay of evidence for decision making.

CRITICAL APPRAISAL PRINCIPLES OF QUANTITATIVE STUDIES

Searching the literature to answer a clinical question can be exasperating if it reveals multiple studies with findings that do not agree. It can be disappointing to find a new study where a promising intervention is found to be no more effective than a **placebo**, particularly when an earlier study reported that the same intervention was beneficial. (Placebos are pharmacologically inert substances [like a sugar pill] and will be discussed later in the chapter when examining RCTs.) Given the resulting confusion and uncertainty, it is reasonable for clinicians to wonder if external evidence (i.e., research) is really that helpful.

Ideally, all studies would be designed, conducted, and reported perfectly, but that is not likely. Research inherently has flaws in how it is designed, conducted, or reported; however, study results should not be dismissed or ignored on this basis alone. Given that all research is not perfect, evidence users must learn to carefully evaluate research reports to determine their worth to practice through critical appraisal. The critical appraisal process hinges on three overarching questions that apply to any study (Fineout-Overholt, Melnyk, Stillwell, & Williamson, 2010a; Guyatt et al., 2015):

1. Are the results of the study valid? (Validity)
2. What are the results? (Reliability)
3. Will the results help me in caring for my patients? (Applicability)

This process provides clinicians with the means to interpret the quality of studies and determine the applicability of the synthesis of multiple studies' results to their particular patients (Brignardello-Petersen, Carrasco-Labra, Glick, Guyatt, & Azarpazhooh, 2015; Fineout-Overholt et al., 2010a; Fineout-Overholt, Melnyk, Stillwell, & Williamson, 2010b, 2010c; University College London, 2017).

When appraising quantitative studies, it is important to recognize the factors of validity and reliability that could influence the study findings. Study validity and reliability are determined by the quality of the study methodology. In addition, clinicians must discern how far from the true result the reported result may be (i.e., compare the study result with the outcome that can be replicated in practice [can I get what they got?]). Because all studies have some flaws or limitations, the process of critical appraisal should assist the clinician in deciding whether a study is flawed to the point that it should be discounted as a source of evidence (i.e., the results cannot reliably be used in practice). Interpretation of results requires consideration of the **clinical significance** of the study findings (i.e., the impact of the findings clinically), as well as the **statistical significance** of the results (i.e., the results were not found by chance).

Are the Study Results Valid? (Validity)

The validity of a study refers to whether the results of the study were obtained via sound scientific methods (i.e., following the research process). Bias and/or confounding variables may compromise the validity of the findings (Higgins & Green, 2011; Melnyk, Morrison-Beedy, & Cole, 2015; Polit & Beck, 2016). The less influence these factors have on a study, the more likely the results will be valid. Therefore, it is important to determine whether the study was conducted properly before being swayed by the results. Validity must be ascertained before the clinician can make an informed assessment of the size and precision of the effect(s) reported.

Bias

Bias is anything that distorts study findings in a systematic way and arises from the study methodology (Guyatt et al., 2015; Polit & Beck, 2016). Bias can be introduced at any point in a study. When critically appraising research, the clinician needs to be aware of possible sources of bias, which may vary with the study design. Every study requires careful examination regarding the different factors that influence the extent of potential bias in a study.

Selection Bias. An example of bias could be how participants are selected for inclusion into the different groups in an intervention study. This selection may occur in a way that inappropriately influences who ends up in the experimental group or comparison group. This is called selection bias and is reduced when researchers **randomly assign** participants to experimental and comparison groups. This is the "randomized" portion of the RCT, the classic experimental study. In an RCT, all other variables should be the same in each group (i.e., the groups should be homogeneous). Differences in the outcomes should be attributable to the different interventions given to each group. A controlled trial in which researchers do not properly randomize participants to the study groups will likely have a different outcome when compared with one using the best randomization methods, as there is inherently more bias in poorly randomized studies (Brignardello-Petersen et al., 2015; Polit & Beck, 2016). Other study designs (e.g., quasi-experimental, cohort, case studies) do not randomly allocate participants and risk introduction of selection bias into the research.

Figure 5.3 shows participant progression within an experimental study from the **reference population** to the intervention or control group. For example, researchers want to study the effect of 30 minutes of daily exercise in adults who are over 80 years of age. The ideal, but usually infeasible, sample to include in a study is the reference population, that is, those people in the past, present, and future to whom the study results can be generalized. In this case, the reference population would be all those over 80 years of age. Given the difficulty of obtaining the reference population, researchers typically use a study population that they assume will be representative of the reference population (e.g., a random sample of adults older than 80 years of age who live in or within a 25-mile radius of a metropolitan city in a rural state).

However, clinicians need to keep in mind that bias could be introduced at each point where a subgroup is selected. For example, the study population will include some people willing to participate and others who refuse to participate in the study. If participants are drawn from those whom the researchers can easily contact (i.e., a convenience sample), those who volunteer may differ from those who do not volunteer in some characteristic that influences the outcomes in some way. For example, in a study of the impact of exercise on the health of adults older than 80 years, those who volunteer for a study may start with a

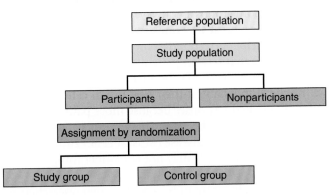

Figure 5.3: Study population.

more positive attitude toward exercise and adhere to the study protocol better. If the study involved only such people, this could affect the study outcomes and make them inapplicable to the reference population. This type of effect is particularly relevant in studies where people's attitudes or beliefs are being explored because these may be the very characteristics that influence their decision to participate or not (Polit & Beck, 2016). Evidence users must be aware that despite the best efforts of the investigators to select a sample that is representative of the reference population, there may be significant differences between the study sample and the general population.

Knowing Who Receives Which Intervention. Another type of bias in RCTs is introduced by participants, clinicians, or researchers knowing who is receiving which intervention. To minimize this bias, participants and those evaluating outcomes of the study are kept blind or "in the dark" about who receives which intervention (i.e., the experimental and the comparison groups). These studies are called double-blind studies. Increasingly, triple-blind studies are conducted to control against the potential bias coming from those administering interventions. The three groups blinded in triple-blind studies are usually the participants, those administering the interventions, and those assessing the outcomes.

Gatekeepers. Another element known to introduce bias is a well-intentioned person acting as a gatekeeper, particularly in studies involving vulnerable populations. For example, researchers conducting a study with patients receiving palliative care may have difficulty recruiting sufficient number of people into the study because the patients' caregivers may consider it too burdensome to ask patients who are quite ill to participate in research. If the gatekeepers only ask healthier patients, this introduces bias as healthier patients may respond differently to the intervention and thus lead to different outcomes than if a more representative sample of palliative care patients was enrolled in the study.

Measurement Bias. Another concern that may influence study results is measurement bias (i.e., how the data are measured). For example, *systematic error* can occur through using an incorrectly calibrated device that consistently gives higher or lower measurements than the true measurement. Data collectors may deviate from established data collection protocols or their individual personality traits may affect how patients provide information in studies involving interpersonal methods of collecting data, such as interviews or surveys. Longitudinal studies, in general, have challenges with measurement bias.

Recall Bias. One type of longitudinal, retrospective study that compares two groups is a **case–control** study, in which researchers select a group of people with an outcome of interest, the cases (e.g., cases of infection), and another group of people without that outcome, the controls (e.g., no infection). Both groups are surveyed in an attempt to find the key differences between the groups that may suggest why one group had the outcome (i.e., infection) and the other group did not. Participants respond to surveys about what they did in the past. This is referred to as *recall*. Studies that rely on patients remembering data are subject to "recall bias" (Callas & Delwiche, 2008). Recall may be affected by a number of factors. For example, asking patients with brain tumors about their past use of cellular phones might generate highly accurate or falsely inflated responses because those patients seek an explanation for their disease, compared with people who do not have tumors and whose recall of phone use may be less accurate in the absence of disease (Muscat et al., 2000). Bias can be a challenge with case–control studies in that people may not remember things correctly.

Information Bias. Another related form of bias occurs when researchers record different information from interviews or patient records. The risk of such information bias is higher when researchers know which participants are in the case group and which are controls (Callas & Delwiche, 2008). One form of longitudinal study that has to battle information bias is a **cohort study**. This type of study focuses prospectively on one group of people who have been exposed to a condition and another group that has not. For example, people living in one town might be put into one cohort and those in another town into a second cohort—the town they lived in would be the selection criterion. All of the participants would be followed over a number of years to identify differences between the two cohorts that might be associated with differences between the towns and specific outcomes (e.g., environmental factors and breast cancer).

Loss to Follow-Up. In longitudinal studies, such as cohort studies, loss of participants to follow-up may contribute to measurement bias. For example, if people stop the intervention because of an adverse event, and this is not followed up on or reported, the reported outcomes may mask important reasons for observed differences between the experimental intervention and control groups. Possible reasons for loss of participants (i.e., study attrition) could include unforeseen side effects of the intervention or burdensome data collection procedures. Although such factors are often out of the control of researchers, they can lead to noncomparable groups and biased results. Therefore, they should be noted and addressed in reports of studies.

Contamination. Contamination is another form of measurement bias. This occurs when participants originally allocated to a particular group or arm of a study are exposed to the alternative group's intervention (i.e., the comparison intervention). For example, in a study of asthmatic schoolchildren that compares retention of asthma management information given to the children in written form and by video, results may be compromised if those in the video group lend their videos to those in the written information group. Another example would be if patients in a placebo-controlled trial somehow become aware that they have been assigned to the placebo group and, believing they should be in the intervention arm of the study, find some way to access the intervention.

In critical appraisal of a research study, specific questions should be asked about the report to identify whether the study was well designed and conducted or whether risks of bias were introduced at different points. Chapter 21 contains more information on these research designs and ways of reducing bias. In Appendix B and on thePoint', readers can find GAO and RCA checklists for study designs that provide standardized criteria to be applied to each study methodology to determine if it is a valid study.

Confounded Study Results

When interpreting results presented in quantitative research papers, clinicians should always consider that there may be multiple explanations for any effect reported in a study. A study's results may be confounded when a relationship between two variables is actually due to a third, either known or unknown variable (i.e., a confounding variable). The confounding variable relates to both the intervention (i.e., the exposure) and the outcome, but is not directly a part of the causal pathway (i.e., the relationship) between the two. Confounding variables are often encountered in studies about lifestyle and health. For example, clinicians' confounding variables should be considered in a report linking caffeine intake with the incidence of headaches among hospital workers fasting for Ramadan (Awada & al Jumah, 1999). Headache sufferers consumed significantly more caffeine in beverages such as tea and coffee compared to those who did not get headaches. The reduction in caffeine consumption during fasting for Ramadan led to caffeine withdrawal, which the researchers stated was the most likely cause of the headaches. Intuitively, this may sound likely; however, if the study population includes people engaged in shift work, which is very likely because the participants were hospital staff, the irregular working hours or a combination of variables may have contributed to the headaches, not solely caffeine withdrawal. Figure 5.4 demonstrates how confounding variables

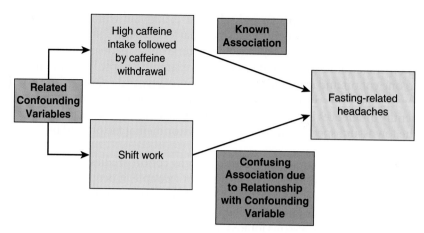

Figure 5.4: Model of possible confounding variables in a study examining the association between caffeine intake and symptoms.

can lead to confusing results. The shift work is related to both the exposure (i.e., reduced high caffeine intake and subsequent withdrawal) and the outcomes (i.e., headaches). However, it is not directly causal (i.e., irregular working hours do not cause headaches).

When critically appraising a study, clinicians must evaluate whether investigators considered the possibility of confounding variables in the original study design, as well as in the analysis and interpretation of their results. Minimizing the possible impact of confounding variables on a study's results is best addressed by a research design that utilizes a randomization process to assign participants to each study group. In this way, confounding variables, either known or unknown, are expected to equally influence the outcomes of the different groups in the study.

Confounding variables may still influence a study's results despite investigators' best efforts. Unplanned events occurring at the same time as the study may have an impact on the observed outcomes. This is often referred to as *history*. For example, a study is launched to determine the effects of an educational program regarding infant nutrition (i.e., the experimental intervention group). The control group receives the usual information on infant growth and development provided at maternal and child health visits. Unknown to the researchers, the regional health department simultaneously begins a widespread media campaign to promote child health. This confounding historical event could impact the results and thereby make it difficult to directly attribute any observed outcomes solely to the experimental intervention (i.e., information on infant nutrition). Finally, inclusion and exclusion criteria should be used to select participants and should be prespecified (i.e., a priori). Often these criteria can be controls for possible confounding variables (see Rapid Critical Appraisal checklists in Appendix B and on thePoint®.).

What Are the Results? (Reliability)

Quantitative studies use statistics to report their findings. Having evaluated the validity of a study's findings, the numerical study results need to be examined. Clinicians planning to use the results of quantitative studies need a general understanding of how to interpret the numerical results. The main concerns are the size of the intervention's effect (the effect size) and how precisely that effect was estimated (i.e., the CI). Together, these determine the reliability of the study findings. This goes beyond understanding the study's results to evaluating how likely it is that the intervention will have the same effect when clinicians use it in their practices. This part of critical appraisal examines the numerical data reported in the results section of a study and will be examined in the following sections.

> ❝
>
> Nothing in the world can take the place of Persistence . . . Persistence and determination alone are omnipotent. The slogan "Press On" has solved and always will solve the problems of the human race.
>
> CALVIN COOLIDGE

Reporting the Study Results: Do the Numbers Add Up?

In all studies, the total number of participants approached and the number consenting to participate in the study should be reported. The total number of those participating is abbreviated as N (i.e., the total sample). In addition, in RCTs, the *total number* in each group or arm of a study (e.g., intervention or comparison group) should be reported, as these values will usually be included in the statistical calculations involving the study findings. In the results section and subsequent analyses, the numbers of participants with various outcomes of interest are reported as n. When appraising a study, clinicians should check whether the sum of all n values equals the original N reported (see Table 5.2). This is particularly important, as a discrepancy represents loss of participants to follow-up (i.e., attrition). Participants may withdraw from a study for various reasons, some of which are very relevant to the validity of the study results. Regardless of the reasons, researchers should account for any difference in the final number of participants in each group compared to the number of people who commenced the study. For example, a study reporting the effectiveness of depression management that uses frequent individual appointments with a professional may report fewer participants at the end of the study than were originally enrolled. A high attrition rate may have occurred because participants found it difficult to attend the frequent appointments. Participant numbers described here are represented in Table 5.2, called a two-by-two table

TABLE 5.2	*Measures of Effect (Two-by-Two Table)*		

	Expected Outcome Occurred		
Exposure to Intervention	**Yes**	**No**	**Total**
Yes	a	b	a + b
No	c	d	c + d
Total	a + c	b + d	a + b + c + d

Notes: $a + b + c + d$ is the total number of study participants, N.

$a + b$ is the total number of study participants in the intervention arm of the study.

a is the number of participants exposed to the intervention who had the expected outcome.

b is the number of participants exposed to the intervention who did not have the expected outcome.

$c + d$ is the total number of study participants in the unexposed or comparison arm of the study.

c is the number of participants not exposed to the intervention who nevertheless had the expected outcome.

d is the number of participants not exposed to the intervention and who did not have the expected outcome.

$a + c$ is the total number of study participants, both exposed and not exposed to the intervention, who had the expected outcome occur.

$b + d$ is the total number of study participants in the control and intervention groups who did not have the expected outcome occur.

because it has two primary rows and two primary columns of data. The other rows or columns are totals. This table will be used to facilitate further understanding of concepts presented later in the chapter, so be sure to refer back to it.

A well-conducted study would attempt to discover participants' reasons for withdrawing. These factors are important to consider because sometimes even if interventions were found to be effective in a study, they may be difficult to implement in the real world.

Magnitude of the Effect

Quantitative studies are frequently conducted to find out if there is an important and identifiable difference between two groups. Some examples could be (a) why one group is diagnosed with breast cancer and not the other group, (b) the quality of life for older people living at home compared to those living in nursing homes, or (c) outcomes of taking drug A compared to taking drug B. A study will pick one or more outcomes to determine whether there are important differences between the groups. The **magnitude of effect** refers to the degree of the difference or lack of difference between the various groups (i.e., experimental and control) in the study. The effect is the **rate of occurrence** in each of the groups for the outcome of interest. It is helpful when trying to determine the magnitude of effect to use a two-by-two table—two columns and two rows of data. Table 5.3 is a two-by-two table in which one column lists those who had the outcome and the other column lists those without the outcome. Each row provides the outcomes for those exposed to the different interventions or those with or without the different conditions.

Statistical tests that researchers may conduct to determine if the effects differ significantly between groups may be included in such tables. Although it is important for clinicians to understand what these statistics mean, they do not need to carry statistical formulas around in their heads to critically appraise the literature. Some knowledge of how to interpret commonly used statistical tests and when they should be used is adequate for the appraisal process. However, keeping a health sciences statistics book nearby or using the Internet to refresh one's memory can be helpful when evaluating a study.

Table 5.3 presents data to facilitate mastery in understanding how to use a two-by-two table. The outcome chosen here is dichotomous, meaning that the outcome is either present or absent (e.g., Do you smoke? Either a "yes" or "no" answer is required). Data can also be continuous across a range of values (e.g., 1 to 10). Examples of continuous data include age, blood pressure, or pain levels. Dichotomous and continuous data are analyzed using different statistical tests. For example, the effect measured in the hypothetical study in Table 5.3 was whether smokers or nonsmokers developed a hypothetical disease, *ukillmeousus*, or not (i.e., dichotomous data, with an outcome of either "yes" or "no").

Another approach to evaluating the response of a population to a particular disease is reporting the risk of developing a disease (e.g., how likely it is that a smoker will develop the disease at some point). Other terms used to describe outcomes are *incidence* (i.e., how often

| TABLE 5.3 | Two-by-Two Table of Smokers' and NonSmokers' Incidence of Ukillmeousus |

Outcome: Incidence of *Ukillmeousus**			
Condition	Yes	No	Total
Smokers	3	97	100
Nonsmokers	2	98	100

*Ukillmeousus is a hypothetical disease.

the outcome occurs or the number of newly diagnosed cases during a specific time period) or *prevalence* (i.e., the total number of people at risk for the outcome or total number of cases of a disease in a given population in a given time frame). For the purposes of this discussion about understanding the magnitude of a treatment effect, the focus will be on risk. People are often concerned about reducing the risk of a perceived bad outcome (e.g., developing colon cancer), usually through choosing the treatment, screening, or lifestyle change that best minimizes the risk of the outcome occurrence.

Strength of Association

In the example in Table 5.3, the risk is the probability that a smoker who is currently free from *ukillmeousus* will develop the disease at some point. This risk can be expressed in a few different ways. The absolute risk (AR) of smokers developing *ukillmeousus*, often referred to as the probability (i.e., risk) of the outcome in the exposed group (Re), is 3 out of 100. This risk can also be expressed as a proportion, 1 in 33 (0.03), or a percentage, 3%. This risk is derived by dividing the number of those who had the outcome by the total number of those who could have had the outcome (i.e., 3/100). The risk for nonsmokers developing *ukillmeousus* (i.e., the probability of the outcome occurring in the unexposed group [Ru]) is 2 out of 100 (or 1 in 50 [0.02] or 2%). Table 5.4 contains the general formulas for these and other statistics. The following paragraphs will use the formulas and data in Tables 5.2 to 5.4 to show how the results of studies can be used to make clinical decisions.

When comparing groups, whether testing an intervention or examining the impact of a lifestyle factor or policy, people are often concerned about risk. Some examples of common concerns about risk include (a) colon screening to reduce the risk of colon cancer deaths; (b) high-fiber, low-fat diets to reduce the risk of cardiovascular disease; (c) high-school coping programs to reduce the risk of suicide in adolescents; and (d) lipid medications to reduce the risk of cardiovascular disease. Often, we are interested in the difference in risks of an outcome between a group that has a particular intervention and one that does not. When groups differ in their risks for an outcome, this can be expressed in a number of different ways. One is the absolute difference in risks between the groups. The **absolute risk reduction (ARR)** for an undesirable outcome is when the risk is less for the experimental/condition group than for the control/comparison group. The **absolute risk increase (ARI)** for an undesirable outcome

TABLE 5.4	*Statistics to Assist in Interpreting Findings in Healthcare Research*	
Statistic	**Formula**	***Ukillmeousus* Example**
AR	Re = a/(a + b)	3/(3 + 97) = 3/100 = 0.03
	Ru = c/(c + d)	2/(2 + 98) = 2/100 = 0.02
ARR	Ru − Re = ARR	Not appropriate
ARI	Re − Ru = ARI	0.03 − 0.02 = 0.01
		0.01 × 100 = 1%
RR	RR = Re/Ru	0.03/0.02 = 1.5
RRR	RRR = {|Re − Ru|/Ru} × 100%	{|0.03 − 0.02|/0.02} = 0.01/0.02 = 0.5 × 100 = 50%
OR	Odds of exposed = a/b	Odds of smokers 3/97 = 0.03
	Odds of unexposed = c/d	Odds of nonsmokers 2/98 = 0.02
	OR = (a/b)/(c/d)	OR = 0.03/0.02 = 1.5

AR, absolute risk; ARI, absolute risk increase; ARR, absolute risk reduction; OR, odds ratio; Re, risk in exposed; RR, relative risk; RRR, relative risk reduction; Ru, risk in unexposed.

is when the risk is more for the experimental/condition group than the control/comparison group. These values can also be referred to as the risk difference (RD).

In the previous example, the risk (or probability) for the undesirable outcome of *ukill-meousus* is higher in the smoker (i.e., condition) group than in the comparison group (i.e., nonsmokers). Therefore, the ARI is calculated as 3% (risk of *ukillmeousus* for smokers) − 2% (risk of *ukillmeousus* for nonsmokers) = 1% (or, in proportions, 0.03 − 0.02 = 0.01). To put it in a sentence, the AR for developing *ukillmeousus* is 1% higher for smokers than that for nonsmokers.

Risks between two groups can also be compared using what is called **relative risk** or risk ratio (RR). This indicates the likelihood (i.e., risk) that the outcome would occur in one group compared to the other. The group with the particular condition or intervention of interest is usually the focus of the study. In our example, the condition is smoking. Relative risk is calculated by dividing the two AR values (that of the condition of interest or intervention group divided by that of the control group). In the example, the RR is AR for smokers/AR for nonsmokers: 0.03/0.02 = 1.5. To use it in a sentence, smokers are 1.5 times more likely to develop *ukillmeousus* compared to nonsmokers. RR is frequently used in prospective studies, such as RCTs and cohort studies. If the outcome is something we want, an RR greater than 1 means the treatment (or condition) is better than control. If the outcome is something we do not want (like *ukillmeousus*), an RR greater than 1 means the treatment (or condition) is worse than control. In the example, the outcome of *ukillmeousus* is not desirable and the RR is greater than 1; therefore, the condition of a smoker is worse than the condition of a nonsmoker.

A related way to express this term is the **relative risk reduction (RRR)**. This expresses the proportion of the risk in the intervention/condition group compared to the proportion of risk in the control group. It can be calculated by taking the risk of the condition ($Re = 0.03$) minus the risk of the control ($Ru = 0.02$), dividing the result by the risk for the control (Ru), and then multiplying by 100 (to make it a percentage) ($[0.03 − 0.02]/0.02) \times 100 = 50\%$. To state this in a sentence, being a nonsmoker reduces the risk of developing *ukillmeousus* by 50% relative to being a smoker.

Notice here the importance of understanding what these terms mean. An RRR of 50% *sounds* more impressive than a 1% RD (i.e., ARI). Yet both of these terms have been derived from the same data. Other factors must be taken into account. For example, a 1% RD may not be very noteworthy if the disease is relatively mild and short-lived. However, it may be very noteworthy if the disease is frequently fatal. If the differences between the groups are due to treatment options, the nature and incidence of adverse effects will also need to be taken into account (see Example One later in this chapter).

Risk can also be understood in terms of "odds." In quantitative studies, calculating the odds of an outcome provides another way of estimating the strength of association between an intervention and an outcome. The odds of the outcome occurring in a particular group are calculated by dividing the number of those exposed to the condition or treatment who had the outcome by the number of people without the outcome. This differs from risk calculations where the same number is divided by the total number of people in the study (see Table 5.4). In the example comparing smokers and nonsmokers, the odds of a smoker getting the disease are 3/97 = 0.031. The odds of a nonsmoker getting *ukillmeousus* are 2/98 = 0.020. The **odds ratio (OR)** is the odds of the smokers (0.031) divided by the odds of the nonsmokers (0.020) = 1.5. To use it in a sentence, smokers have 1.5 greater odds of developing *ukillmeousus* than nonsmokers. As seen in this example, the OR and RR can be very similar in value. This happens when the number of events of interest (i.e., how many developed the observed outcome) is low; as the event rate increases, the values can diverge.

Interpreting results that are presented as an ARR, ARI, RR, or OR sometimes can be difficult not only for the clinician but also for the patient—whose understanding is essential in the healthcare decision making process. A more meaningful way to present the study results is through calculation of the **number needed to treat (NNT)**. NNT is a value that can permit all stakeholders in the clinical decision to better understand the likelihood of developing the outcome if a patient has a given intervention or condition. The NNT represents the number of people who would need to receive the therapy or intervention to prevent one bad outcome or cause one additional good outcome. If the NNT for a therapy was 15, this would mean 15 patients would need to receive this therapy before you could expect one additional person to benefit. Another way of putting this is that a person's chance of benefiting from the therapy is 1 in 15. The NNT is calculated by taking the inverse of the ARR (i.e., 1/ARR). For example, if smoking cessation counseling is the treatment, the outcome is smoking cessation, and the ARR for smoking cessation is 0.1, the NNT to see one additional person quit smoking using this treatment is 1/0.1 or 10. Ten people would need to receive the counseling to result in one additional person stopping smoking.

A related parameter to NNT is the **number needed to harm (NNH)**. This is the number of people who would need to receive an intervention before one additional person would be harmed (i.e., have a bad outcome). It is calculated as the inverse of the ARI (i.e., 1/ARI). In the *ukillmeousus* example, the ARI for the condition of smoking versus nonsmoking was 0.01; the NNH is 1/0.01 = 100. For every 100 persons who continue to smoke, there will be one case of *ukillmeousus*. While one case of *ukillmeousus* in 100 smokers may seem small, if we assume that this disease is fatal, clinicians may choose to put more effort and resources toward helping people stop smoking. The interpretation of a statistic must be made in the context of the severity of the outcome (e.g., *ukillmeousus*) and the cost and feasibility of the removal of the condition (e.g., smoking) or the delivery of the intervention (e.g., smoking cessation counseling).

Interpreting the Results of a Study: Example One

You are a clinician who is working with patients who want to quit smoking. They have friends who have managed to quit by using nicotine chewing gum and wonder whether this might also work for them. You find a clinical trial that measured the effectiveness of nicotine chewing gum versus a placebo (Table 5.5). Among those using nicotine chewing gum, 18.2% quit smoking (i.e., risk of the outcome in the exposed group [Re]). At the same time, some participants in the control group also gave up smoking (10.7%; i.e., risk of the outcome in the unexposed group [Ru]). The RD for the outcome between these groups (i.e., these two percentages subtracted from one another) is 7.5% (i.e., the ARR is 0.075). The NNT is the inverse of the ARR, or 13.3. In other words, 13 smokers need to use the gum for one additional person to give up smoking. Nicotine gum is a relatively inexpensive and easy-to-use treatment, with few side effects. Given the costs of smoking, treating 13 smokers to help 1 stop smoking is reasonable.

The size of the NNT influences decision making about whether or not the treatment should be used; however, it is not the sole decision making factor. Other factors will influence the

| TABLE 5.5 | The Effectiveness of Nicotine Chewing Gum |

Exposure	Quit, n (%)	Did Not Quit, n (%)	Total
		Outcome	
Nicotine gum	1,149 (18.2)	5,179 (81.8)	6,328
Placebo	893 (10.7)	7,487 (89.3)	8,380
Total	2,042	12,666	

decision making process and should be taken into account, including patient preferences. For example, some smokers who are determined to quit may not view a treatment with a 1 in 13 chance of success as good enough. They may want an intervention with a lower NNT, even if it is more expensive. In other situations, a treatment with a low NNT may also have a high risk of adverse effects (i.e., a low NNH). Clinicians may use NNT and NNH in their evaluation of the risks and benefits of an intervention; however, simply determining that an NNT is low is insufficient to justify a particular intervention (Barratt et al., 2004). Evidence-based clinical decision making requires not only ongoing consideration but also an active blending of the numerical study findings, clinicians' expertise, and patients' preferences.

> **"**
>
> Permanence, perseverance and persistence in spite of all obstacles, discouragements, and impossibilities: It is this that in all things distinguishes the strong soul from the weak.
>
> **THOMAS CARLYLE**

Measures of Clinical Significance

Clinicians involved in critical appraisal of a study should be asking themselves: Are the reported results of actual clinical significance? In everyday language, "significant" means "important," but when statistics are used to determine that a study's results are significant, this has a very specific meaning (to be discussed later). When appraising a study, clinicians (and patients) want to know the importance of these results for the clinical decision at hand. This is referred to as *clinical* significance, which may be very different from *statistical* significance (Fethney, 2010). Without understanding this, the reported significance of study findings may be misleading. For example, the ARR reported in study results is calculated in a way that considers the underlying susceptibility of a patient to an outcome and thereby can distinguish between very large and very small treatment effects. In contrast, RRR does not take into account existing baseline risk and therefore fails to discriminate between large and small treatment effects.

Interpreting the Results of a Study: Example Two

In a hypothetical example, assume that researchers conducted several RCTs evaluating the same antihypertensive drug and found that it had an RRR of 33% over 3 years (Barratt et al., 2004). A clinician is caring for two 70-year-old women: (a) Pat, who has stable, normal blood pressure, and her risk of stroke is estimated at 1% per year; and (b) Dorothy, who has had one stroke, and although her blood pressure is normal, her risk of another stroke is 10% per year. With an RRR of stroke of 33%, the antihypertensive medication seems like a good option. However, the underlying risk is not incorporated into RRR, and therefore ARR must be examined in making clinically relevant decisions.

In the first study conducted on a sample of people with low risk for stroke, the ARR for this medication was 0.01 or 1%. In the second study, conducted on a sample of individuals at high risk for stroke, the ARR was 0.20 or 20%.

Without treatment, Pat has a 1% risk per year of stroke, or 3% risk over 3 years. An ARR of 1% means that treatment with this drug will reduce her risk to 2% over 3 years. From the low-risk study (i.e., the participants looked most like Pat), 100 patients would need to be treated before one stroke would be avoided (i.e., NNT). Without treatment, Dorothy has a 10% risk of stroke each year, or 30% over 3 years. From the second study (i.e., the participants looked most like Dorothy), with an ARR of 20%, the drug would reduce her risk to 10% over 3 years, and five patients would need to be treated to reduce the incidence of stroke by one (i.e., NNT). In this case, it appears that this medication can be beneficial for both women; however, Dorothy will receive more benefit than Pat. The clinical significance of this treatment is much higher when used in people with a higher baseline risk. The ARR and NNT reveal this, but the RRR does not.

For both of these patients, the risk of adverse effects must be taken into account. In these hypothetical RCTs, researchers found that the drug increased the RR of severe gastric bleeding by 3%. Epidemiologic studies have established that women in this age group inherently have a 0.1% per year risk of severe gastric bleeding. Over 3 years, the risk of bleeding would be 0.3% without treatment (i.e., R_u) and 0.9% with the medication (i.e., R_e), giving an ARI of 0.6%. If Pat takes this drug for 3 years, she will have a relatively small benefit (ARR of 1%) and an increased risk of gastric bleeding (ARI of 0.6%). If Dorothy takes the drug for 3 years, she will have a larger benefit (ARR of 20%) and the same increased risk of gastric bleeding (ARI of 0.6%). The evidence suggests that Dorothy is more likely to benefit from treatment than Pat; however, the final decision will depend on their preferences (i.e., how they weigh these benefits and harms).

Precision in the Measurement of Effect: Reliability of Study Results

Random Error. Critical appraisal evaluates systematic error when checking for bias and confounding variables. This addresses validity and accuracy in the results. However, error can also be introduced by chance (i.e., random error). Variations as a result of chance occur in almost all situations. Here are three examples of random error: (1) A study might enroll more women than men for no particular reason other than pure chance. If the researchers were to draw some conclusion about the outcome occurring in men or women, the interpretation would have to consider that the variations in the outcome could have occurred randomly because of the disproportionate number of men to women in the sample; (2) If participants were not randomly assigned to groups, very sick people could enroll in one group purely by chance and that could have an impact on the results; (3) A hospital could be particularly busy during the time a research study is being conducted there, and that could distort the results. Random error can lead to reported effects that are smaller or greater than the true effect (i.e., the actual impact of an intervention which researchers do their best to determine, without being 100% certain they have found it). Random error influences the precision of a study's findings.

The chances of random error having an impact on the results can be reduced up to a point by study design factors such as increasing the sample size or increasing the number of times measurements are made (i.e., avoiding measurements that are a snapshot in time). When repeated measures of the same outcome are similar in a study, it is presumed that there is low random error. The extent to which random error may influence a measurement can be reported using statistical significance (p values) or by CIs.

Statistical Significance. The aim of statistical analysis of outcomes is to determine whether an outcome (i.e., observed effect) happens because of the study intervention or has occurred by chance. In comparing two groups, the research question can be phrased as a hypothesis (i.e., what we think will happen) and data collected to determine if the hypothesis is confirmed. For example, the hypothesis might be that an experimental drug relieves pain better than a placebo (i.e., the drug has effects beyond those of suggestion or the personal interactions between those involved in the study). Usually, researchers describe what they expect to happen as their study hypothesis. In contrast, the **null hypothesis** would be that there will be *no difference* in effect between the drug and placebo (i.e., the opposite position to the study hypothesis). When an intervention study is conducted and statistical analysis is performed on study data (i.e., hypothesis testing), a p value is calculated that indicates the probability that the null hypothesis is true. The smaller the p value, the less likely that the null hypothesis is true (i.e., the decreased likelihood that the study findings occurred by chance); therefore, it is more likely that the observed effect is due to the intervention. By convention, a p value of 0.05 or less is considered a statistically significant result in healthcare research. This means that it has become acceptable for the study findings to occur by chance 1 in 20 times.

While the p value is widely reported in healthcare literature, it has raised concerns since it was first introduced. In spite of being "a useful statistical measure, it is commonly misused and misinterpreted" (Wasserstein & Lazar, 2016, p. 131). Such problems have become so rampant that some journals discourage statements about results being "significant" or not based on a p value (Greenland et al., 2016). The American Statistical Association in 2016 took the unprecedented step of issuing an official policy statement on p values to help correct misunderstandings (Wasserstein & Lazar, 2016). Part of the problem is that p values can lead to an "either–or" conclusion (i.e., statistically significant or not significant) and do not assist in evaluating the strength of an association. Very small p values can arise when small differences are found in studies with large samples. These findings can be interpreted as statistically significant, but may have little clinical meaningfulness. Conversely, studies with small sample sizes can have strongly associated outcomes with large p values, which may be dismissed as statistically not significant, but could be clinically meaningful. In addition, the "cutoff" of $p \leq 0.05$ is set arbitrarily, and this can contribute to dichotomous decision making. Hence, studies reporting only p values tend to be classified as statistically significant (i.e., a positive finding) or statistically not significant (i.e., a negative study finding). The impression given is that the intervention is either useful or useless, respectively. In clinical settings, the study finding is more or less likely to be useful depending on several other factors that clinicians have to take into account when hoping to obtain similar results with their patients.

For example, patients can require mechanical ventilation because of different injuries and diseases. However, mechanical ventilation itself can cause further lung damage, especially if high tidal volumes are used. In an RCT, patients were randomly assigned to receive either low or high levels of a therapy called positive end-expiratory pressure (PEEP). The number of deaths in each group in this study is given in Table 5.6 (Brower et al., 2004). The ARI for death in the high PEEP group was 3%. When researchers investigated whether

TABLE 5.6 *Two-by-Two Table of the Incidence of Death in Comparing High PEEP to Low PEEP*

Exposure	Outcome (Death) Yes	No	Total
High PEEP	76	200	276
Low PEEP	68	205	273
Calculations			
AR	Re = a/(a + b) Ru = c/(c + d)	Re = 76/(76 + 200) = 0.28 Ru = 68/(68 + 205) = 0.25	
ARI	ARI = Re − Ru	= 0.28 − 0.25 = 0.03 0.03 × 100 = 3% increase in risk of death with high PEEP	
In Clinical Scenario for ARI	$CI = ARI \pm 1.96 \sqrt{\{Re(100 - Re) / a + b\} + \{Ru(100 - Ru) / c + d\}}$ CI = 0.03 ± 1.96 (0.44) = 0.03 ± 0.86 95% CI: −0.83 to 0.89		

AR, absolute risk; ARI, absolute risk increase; CI, confidence interval; PEEP, positive end-expiratory pressure; Re, risk in exposed; Ru, risk in unexposed.

or not there was a difference between the two groups, they found that the probability of the null hypothesis (i.e., no differences in the groups) being true was $p = 0.48$, which was corroborated by the CI (see Table 5.6). Therefore, the researchers concluded that there were no significant differences in mortality between the two levels of PEEP. However, if the study was simply classified as "statistically not significant," other important information would have been missed, as will be shown later.

Interpreting the Results of a Study: Example Three

Another potential problem with p values occurs if researchers collect a lot of data without clear objectives (i.e., hypotheses) and then analyze everything looking for some significant correlation. In these situations, it is more likely that chance alone will lead to significant results. When the level of statistical significance for the p value is set at 0.05, the probability of saying that the intervention worked when it did not (i.e., getting a false-positive result; Type I error) can be calculated as $(1 - 0.95)$ or 0.05 (i.e., 1 in 20 positive results will be found by chance). Multiple hypothesis testing is a commonly found example of poor research design (Goodacre, 2008). When two hypotheses are tested, the probability of a chance finding is increased to $(1 - [0.95 \times 0.95])$ or 0.0975 (i.e., about 1 in 10 positive results will be found by chance). With five tests, the probability moves to 0.23 (i.e., almost a one in four chance that a positive result will be found by random chance).

There are circumstances in which testing several hypotheses may be legitimate (e.g., when several factors are known to impact an outcome). In such cases, there are statistical analyses that can avoid the problems of multiple hypothesis testing (e.g., the Bonferonni correction; Bono & Tornetta, 2006). Researchers generally select one primary outcome; however, secondary outcomes may also be appropriate when they arise from the study's conceptual background and objectives. In contrast, "fishing expeditions" or "data dredging" occurs when the sole purpose of data collection is to find statistically significant results. Often a clue to data dredging is when subgroups are created without any conceptual basis and these groups differ significantly on an outcome. Subgroups should be planned prior to starting the study (i.e., a priori) and should be formed based on the conceptual framework that underpins the study. For example, a large RCT of high-dose steroids to treat spinal cord injuries has become a landmark example of the criticisms of multiple statistical tests (Bracken et al., 1997). More than 100 p values were presented in the report without specifying which one was planned as the primary analysis (Bono & Tornetta, 2006). The main results table gave 24 p values for various outcomes at different time intervals, of which one was statistically significant. With the convention for probability set at $p < 0.05$, 1 positive test in every 20 tests is likely to be found by chance; therefore, 1 positive test out of the 24 tests in the study example would very likely be due to chance. One positive finding was that patients had statistically significant better neurologic outcome scores when treated with intravenous steroids within 8 hours of a spinal cord injury. However, no significant differences in neurologic outcomes were found for the entire study population. One problem was that the 8-hour cutoff was not identified before the study was conducted, nor was there evidence from basic research as to why treatment prior to 8 hours would make a significant difference (Coleman et al., 2000). Researchers, including one involved in the original study, have expressed concerns that multiple statistical tests were run until a statistically significant difference was discovered, resulting in an artificially created subgroup (Lenzer, 2006). This has important clinical implications as this study continues to determine the standard of care even though many clinicians and researchers have questioned the reliability of its conclusion (Lenzer & Brownlee, 2008). Statistical significance cannot be the sole marker for whether or not a study finding is valuable to practice. Clinical meaningfulness (i.e., the clinician can achieve similar outcomes to the study) is another mechanism that can assist clinicians in evaluating the value of a study's results to patient care.

Confidence Intervals. A CI describes the range in which the true effect lies with a given degree of certainty. In other words, the CI provides clinicians a range of values in which they can be reasonably confident (e.g., 95%) that they will find a result when implementing the study findings. The two most important values for clinicians are the study point estimate and the CI. The point estimate, given the study sample and potentially confounding variables, is the best estimate of the magnitude and direction of the experimental intervention's effect compared with the control (Higgins & Green, 2011). Clinicians need to know the degree to which the intervention brought about the study outcome, and they need to know how confident they can be that they can achieve similar outcomes to the study. In general, researchers present a 95% CI, which means that clinicians can have 95% confidence that the value they can achieve (i.e., the true value) falls within this range of values. Studies can report 90% or 99% CI if this level of confidence is more appropriate, although 95% CI remains the most common in healthcare research (He & Fineout-Overholt, 2016).

Although a CI can be calculated easily, it is not the calculation that clinicians need to remember; rather, they need to understand what information the CI provides. A CI is appropriate to provide clinical meaningfulness for the measured effect of (a) an intervention in one group, (b) the difference the intervention made between two groups, or (c) the intervention's effect with multiple samples pooled together in a **meta-analysis**. A CI's range can be expressed numerically and graphically (Figure 5.5).

The width of the CI is the key to its interpretation. In general, narrower CIs are more favorable than wider CIs. The narrower the CI around the study point estimate, the lesser the margin of error for the clinician who is choosing to implement the study findings. In Figure 5.5, the CI is wider, leading to lesser confidence in the study findings. When the CI contains the line of no difference (also called the line of no effect), the difference between the groups (i.e., the study point estimate) is not statistically significant. The actual numerical value for this line can vary depending on the statistic used (e.g., for OR or RR, no effect = 1; for effect size, no effect = 0). The CI in Figure 5.5 crosses the center line of no effect, and therefore the results are not statistically significant.

CI width can be influenced by sample size. Larger samples tend to give more precise estimates of effects (i.e., a narrower CI) and tend to more likely yield statistically significant

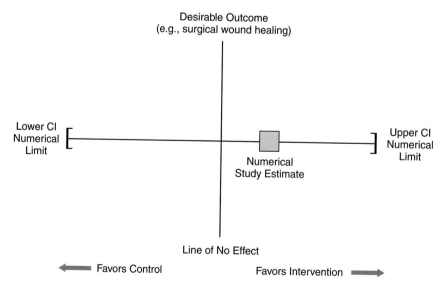

Figure 5.5: Graphic representation of a confidence interval (CI) and study estimate.

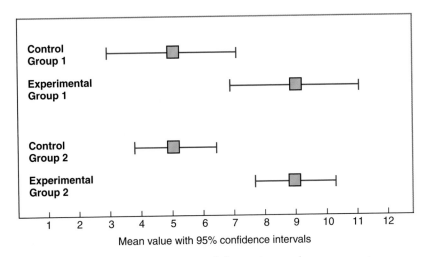

Figure 5.6: Influence of sample size on confidence intervals.

effects. In Figure 5.6, outcome estimates for the intervention and control groups and the accompanying CIs are shown for two studies. In the second study, the sample size is doubled and the same values are found. Though the mean values remain the same, the 95% CI is more narrowly defined. Clinicians can have more confidence in the findings of the second study. For continuous outcomes (e.g., blood pressure), in addition to sample size, the CI width also depends on the natural variability in the outcome measurements. Because of the limitations of p values, healthcare journals, more commonly, ask researchers to report CIs in their statistical analyses (Goodacre, 2008).

The information provided by a CI accommodates the uncertainty that is inherent in real-world clinical practice. This uncertainty is not reflected when interventions are described solely as either statistically significant or not. Although we can never be absolutely certain whether or not an intervention will help our patients, we can be reasonably confident in the outcome when we have a narrow CI and an effective intervention.

Interpreting the Results of a Study: Example Four

Look over the data in Table 5.6 from the study comparing the incidence of death with high PEEP and low PEEP in mechanical ventilation (Brower et al., 2004). The study point estimate indicates that those participants with low PEEP had lower mortality rates. Although the difference in death rate between the two groups was not statistically significant (CI crosses the line of no effect with ARI = 0.03; p = 0.48), the 95% CI provides additional information that is clinically meaningful for patient care. The 95% CI for ARI is somewhat narrow (−0.83 to 0.89), indicating that clinicians should be cautious about their confidence that they too can get a very small increase in mortality rates using high PEEP (Figure 5.7). Although the small increase in death rate is not statistically significant, it is clinically meaningful. However, it would be unwise to decide whether or not to use high PEEP based solely on results of this single study. A more definitive conclusion would require a body of evidence including further trials with more participants. In addition, because the outcome is death, it would be advisable to decrease the acceptable error to 1 in 100 or a 99% CI.

Interpreting the Results of a Study: Example Five

CIs can also be useful in examining the clinical significance of trials with statistically significant results. A blinded, multicenter trial enrolled almost 20,000 patients with vascular disease and randomized them to either aspirin or clopidogrel (CAPRIE Steering

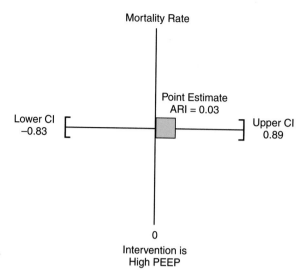

Figure 5.7: Interpretation of study findings. ARI, absolute risk increase; CI, confidence interval; PEEP, positive end-expiratory pressure.

Committee, 1996). Both drugs have been recommended to reduce the risk of serious adverse events, especially ischemic stroke, myocardial infarction, or vascular death. Researchers found an annual risk of these outcomes of 5.32% with clopidogrel (i.e., Re) and 5.83% with aspirin (i.e., Ru), giving an RRR of 8.7% in favor of clopidogrel ($p = 0.043$; 95% CI, 0.3 to 16.5).

As discussed earlier, for clinical decision making, the NNT expresses study results more meaningfully. This is calculated as the inverse of the ARR. In this case, the ARR = 0.51% (95% CI, 0.02 to 0.9) and the NNT = 1/0.51% = 100/0.51 = 196. Put into a sentence, 196 patients would need to be treated with clopidogrel instead of aspirin for one serious adverse event to be avoided each year. Sometimes, clinicians consider comparing NNT per 1,000 patients; for this example, for every 1,000 patients treated with clopidogrel instead of aspirin, about five serious adverse events would be avoided each year (i.e., adverse events avoided per 1,000 patients = 1,000/196 = 5.1).

Expressing data in terms of NNT may help clinicians discuss these results with patients. They may get a better sense of the risks involved when expressed this way. On the other hand, patients and clinicians may realize that the evidence is not available to provide clear recommendations. They may need to await the results of larger clinical trials to provide the needed evidence for more confident decision making.

Will the Results Help Me in Caring for My Patients? (Applicability)

The last couple of examples have moved into the area of applying results to an individual patient or local situation. Clinicians who are appraising evidence should always keep application to patients in mind as the ultimate goal. Each study design has specific questions that, when answered, assist clinicians in critically appraising those studies to determine their worth to practice (i.e., validity, reliability, and usefulness for clinical decision making). Several study designs will be discussed later in the chapter regarding their distinctive appraisals and how to interpret the results for application to patient care.

CRITICAL APPRAISAL OF DIFFERENT RESEARCH DESIGNS

The three rapid appraisal questions—Are the results of the study valid? What are the results? Will the results help me in caring for my patients?—are asked of all studies. These questions have design-specific issues that must be addressed before the different quantitative studies can be determined as valuable for clinicians' decision making (RCA checklists can be found in Appendix B and on thePoint®). The first phase is called rapid critical appraisal and is intended to quickly determine if a study is worthy of consideration.

Different types of quantitative study designs will be discussed in the remainder of the chapter. The first studies discussed—case, case–control, and cohort studies—fall within the nonexperimental category of study designs, meaning that there was no intervention or treatment in the study. There may be a condition that the participants have encountered or a choice the participants have made that puts them in a category that merits study. For example, a group of participants self-identifies as using cell phones at least 4 hours per day and having been diagnosed with brain cancer. This self-identification creates a cohort. They may also be the cases, and the controls would be like individuals who self-identify as using cell phones at least 4 hours per day, but reported no diagnosis of brain cancer. These groups would be compared on other variables of interest. Finally, a single person who has been diagnosed with brain cancer may report cell phone usage and other variables of interest that make the case worth reporting to the healthcare community as an example.

The next category of quantitative designs are sometimes referred to as pre-experimental designs that contain one group's outcome(s) being evaluated either before and after or just after an intervention. These studies do not offer any more confidence in their reliable impact (i.e., how they can be used by clinicians to support best practice) than the nonexperimental studies because of the bias inherent in the designs.

The next two categories of study designs have interventions that are expected to achieve outcomes. The first category is called quasi-experimental, in which there is an intervention expected to have an impact on the outcome; however, participants self-select into the groups being compared (e.g., intervention group and control or comparison group). These studies are also called nonrandomized studies because the participants are not randomly assigned to these groups. Quasi-experimental studies also include such studies as those with pre–post designs, which are studies in which the intervention is delivered to the same group with data collected preintervention and then postintervention to determine impact. The goal of these studies is to offer generalizable knowledge that can be applied more broadly than the study sample itself. This study design should not be confused with evidence implementation, which is implementing what has already been shown through research as an intervention that reliably leads to an outcome. Evidence implementation is focused only on the patients with whom the intervention is delivered. There is no expectation of generalizability for these projects. They are not studies/research and should not be considered any higher in the intervention hierarchy of evidence than level VI (see Table 2.2).

The next category of quantitative study designs is called true experimental designs as in these studies the intervention is randomly assigned to some participants and not to others. Random assignment offers the opportunity to equalize across all the groups variables that may unduly influence the relationship between the intervention and outcome (i.e., did the intervention cause the outcome?), thereby reducing bias. Often called an RCT, this type of study is the only one that offers the opportunity to establish cause-and-effect relationships. Other study designs fall short of this goal because these designs inherently have higher risks of bias. The best they can establish is an association between an intervention or condition and an outcome.

The final category of research studies that we will address is a systematic review. This is a compilation of studies that offers a synthesis of the evidence on a topic (i.e., what we know about it). Well-done systematic reviews provide the pinnacle of evidence (level 1). Within the systematic review, the types of study designs may be varied (e.g., RCTs, cohort, and predictive correlational studies and evidence implementation projects) or may be all the same (e.g., all RCTs); however, it is important to note that systematic reviews should include the body of evidence (i.e., all that we know) that best answers the clinical question. These studies offer us confidence to know what consistently works with predictable outcomes. The goal for all bodies of evidence is to include rigorous systematic reviews.

Just as with the EBP process, each study design has a rigorous method that should be followed to ensure the design is valid and the results reliable. Those markers of the rigorous process are defined in the RCA checklists used to determine which studies should be kept in the analysis and which to discard. To help gain mastery in understanding the hierarchy of a body of evidence and available quantitative research designs that should inform practice, review Table 2.4.

CRITICAL APPRAISAL OF CASE STUDIES

Case studies, also called case reports, have played an important role in identifying new issues in healthcare. Case studies were some of the first publications that led to the identification of such diverse conditions as thalidomide adverse effects, AIDS, and Zika infections (Riley et al., 2017). At the same time, case studies are historically ranked lower in the hierarchy of evidence for intervention questions because of their lack of objectivity (Chapter 1, Box 1.3). Publication bias is an important factor because most case studies found in the literature have positive outcomes. Analyses of published case studies have found that they frequently omit important items that would help clinicians interpret the relevance of the reports to their patients (Miguel, Gonzalez, Illing, & Elsner, 2018). Guidelines aimed at improving the reporting of case studies have been published (Riley et al., 2017).

Are the Results of the Study Valid? (Validity)

Case studies describe the history of a single patient (or a small group of patients), usually in the form of a story. These publications are often of great interest to clinicians because of the appealing way in which they are written and because of their strong clinical focus. However, because case studies describe one person's situation (or very few), they are not reliable for clinicians to use as the sole source of evidence. Therefore, the validity of a case study is challenging to establish. Case studies must be used with caution to inform practice, and any application requires careful evaluation of the outcomes. Case studies play important roles in alerting clinicians to new issues and rare and/or adverse events in practice and to assist in hypothesis generation. Any such hypotheses must be tested in other, less bias-prone research.

What Are the Results? (Reliability)

Case studies can be beneficial in providing information that would not necessarily be reported in the results of clinical trials or survey research. Publications reporting a clinician's experience and a discussion of early indicators and possible preventive measures can be an extremely useful addition to the clinician's knowledge base. Given that a case series would present a small number of patients with similar experiences or complications and their outcomes, statistical analyses are rarely, if ever, appropriate.

Will the Results Help Me in Caring for My Patients? (Applicability)

A major caution that impacts critical appraisal of case studies is that the purpose of such studies is to provide a patient's story about little-known health issues and not to make generalizations applicable to the general population. Therefore, case studies can inform the clinical question, but not provide much confidence in answering it.

What the Literature Says: Answering a Clinical Question

In Clinical Scenario 5.1, the clinical question, a prognosis question, you may want to ask is: In infants who have had cardiac surgery **(P)**, how often does removing pulmonary artery catheters **(I)** compared with leaving pulmonary artery catheters in place **(C)** influence cardiac tamponade **(O)** within the first week after surgery **(T)**? In your search, you find a case study that describes a similar complication to one you have just experienced: Johnston and McKinley (2000).

Clinical Scenario 5.1

You are caring for an infant 4 days after cardiac surgery in the pediatric intensive care unit. Platelets and albumin were administered the night before because of the infant's abnormal clotting profile. In consultation with the healthcare team, you remove the pulmonary artery catheter. You notice continuous ooze from the site and a marked deterioration in the patient's condition. Cardiac tamponade is diagnosed, and the patient requires a reopening of the sternotomy and removal of 200 mL of blood from the pericardial sac. At the end of your shift, you wonder how rare such a complication is in this patient population and decide to look at the literature.

The article is a case report of one patient who experienced cardiac tamponade after removal of a pulmonary artery catheter. The article focuses on describing the pathophysiology of tamponade. The report states that this complication occurs with a frequency rate of 0.22%. The authors give details of their experience with a single patient and provide some recommendations for limiting the potential for bleeding complications in this patient population. You take a copy of the paper to your unit for discussion. You realize that this one case study is not enough to make practice change, so you search for stronger studies (e.g., controlled trials) to assist in developing an addition to your unit protocol manual to create awareness of possible complications arising from removal of monitoring catheters and how to prevent such complications.

CRITICAL APPRAISAL OF CASE–CONTROL STUDIES

A **case–control study** investigates why certain people develop a specific illness, have an adverse event with a particular treatment, or behave in a particular way. An example of a clinical question (written in the PICOT format discussed in Chapter 2) for which a case–control study could be the appropriate design to provide an answer would be, In patients who have a family history of obesity (body mass index [BMI] > 30) **(P)**, how does dietary carbohydrate intake **(I)** influence healthy weight maintenance (BMI < 25) **(O)** over 6 months **(T)**? Another clinical question that could be answered by a case–control study could be, In patients who have cystic fibrosis **(P)**, how does socioeconomic status **(I)** influence their engagement with and adherence to their healthcare regimen **(O)**? Investigators conducting a case–control study try to identify factors that explain the proposed relationship between a condition and a disease or behavior. The case–control method selects individuals who have an outcome (disease, adverse event, behavior) and retrospectively looks back to identify possible conditions that may be associated with the outcome. The characteristics of these individuals (the cases) are compared with those of other individuals who do not have the outcome (the controls). The assumption underpinning this methodological approach is that differences found between the groups may be likely indicators of why the "cases" became "cases."

For example, a landmark situation where the case–control methodology played a crucial role was in identifying the connection between a rare cancer in women and diethylstilbestrol (DES; Herbst, Ulfelder, & Poskanzer, 1971). A prospective design would have been challenging because the adverse event took 20 years to develop and an RCT could not be used for ethical reasons (i.e., it would be unethical to ask pregnant women to take a drug to determine whether or not it increased the risk of birth defects). Eight women with cancer (vaginal adenocarcinoma) were enrolled in the study as cases, and 32 women without cancer were enrolled as controls in the study. Various risk factors were proposed, but found to be present in cases and controls. In contrast, mothers of seven of the women with cancer (i.e., cases) received DES when pregnant, whereas none of the control mothers did. The association between having the cancer and having a mother who took DES was highly significant ($p < 0.00001$) and was subsequently demonstrated in cohort studies (Troisi et al., 2007). The combination of (a) the huge impact vaginal adenocarcinoma had on women's lives, (b) the final outcome of death, and (c) the strong association established between the occurrence of the cancer and mothers taking DES while pregnant led to a common acceptance that DES causes this cancer (Reed & Fenton, 2013). However, causation cannot be established by a case–control study. Instead, a strong association was found between taking DES while pregnant and vaginal adenocarcinoma in the adult child. In addition, this case–control study played an important role in alerting people to the potential adverse effects of using any medications during pregnancy.

Rapid Appraisal Questions for Case–Control Studies

Are the Results of the Study Valid? (Validity)

The validity of a case–control hinges on how the cases and their controls were selected and how data were collected. The following questions help discern the validity of a case–control study.

How Were the Cases Obtained? When appraising a case–control study, the clinician first determines how the cases were identified. The investigators should provide an adequate description or definition of what constitutes a case, including the diagnostic criteria, any exclusion criteria, and an explanation of how the cases were obtained (e.g., from a specialist center, such as an oncology unit, or from the general population). In the DES study, all the cases were identified in the same hospital in Boston over a period of a few years (Herbst et al., 1971). Cases coming from one geographical area could represent another explanation for the findings. Controls would need to be from the same geographical area to control for that possible confounding variable.

The source of the cases has important implications for the appraisal of the study. For example, recruitment of patients from an outpatient chemotherapy unit could include patients with well-established and managed disease and exclude those who are newly diagnosed. Bias could be introduced when cases are recruited from a general population because the potential participants could be at various stages in their disease or have a degree of the behavior of interest. Similarly, bias may arise if some of those cases sought are not included in the study for whatever reason. Patients who choose to become involved in research studies can have characteristics that distinguish them from those who avoid research studies. Care must be taken to ensure that these characteristics are not confounding variables that could influence the relationship between the condition being investigated and the outcome.

Were Appropriate Controls Selected? Selection of controls should be done so that the controls are as similar as possible to the cases in all respects except that they do not have the disease or observed behavior under investigation. In the DES study, the control women were born within 5 days of a case in the same hospital and with the same type of delivery and were from the same geographical area (Herbst et al., 1971). In general, controls may be selected from a specialist source or from the general population. The controls in case–control studies may be recruited into the study at the same time as the cases (concurrent controls). Alternatively, they may be what are referred to as historical controls (i.e., the person's past history is examined, often through medical records). Case–control studies with historical controls are generally viewed as lower on the hierarchy of evidence than those studies with concurrent controls, because the likelihood of bias is higher.

Were Data Collection Methods the Same for the Cases and Controls? Data collection is another potential source of bias in a case–control study. Recall bias, which is inaccurately remembering what occurred, needs to be considered because of the retrospective approach to determining the possible predictive factors. For example, people who have developed a fatal disease may have already spent a considerable amount of time thinking about why they might have developed the disease and therefore be able to recall in great detail their past behaviors. They may have preconceived ideas about what they think caused their illness and report these rather than other factors they have not considered.

In contrast, the disease-free controls may not have considered their past activities in great detail and may have difficulty recalling events accurately. The time since the event can influence how accurately details are recalled. Therefore, the data should ideally be collected in the same way for both the case and control groups. Blinding of the data collector to either the case or the control status or the risk factors of interest assists in reducing the inherent bias in a case–control approach and thus provides more accurate information.

Additional Considerations. The possibility of confounding variables needs to be considered when interpreting a case–control study. Confounding variables are other extrinsic factors that unexpectedly (or unknowingly) influence the variables expected to be associated with the outcome. Coffee consumption is no longer associated with the risk of pancreatic cancer (Turati et al., 2012), but concerns about an association between the two can be traced back to a case–control study (MacMahon, Yen, Trichopoulos, Warren, & Nardi, 1981). The researchers found a strong association ($p = 0.001$) that would account for a substantial proportion of the cases of pancreatic cancer in the United States, but stated that the association would need to be supported by other research. However, other research failed to replicate these findings, which are now regarded as false-positive results (Type I error—accepting that there was an effect when in fact there was none). In the original study, individuals with a history of diseases related to cigarette smoking or alcohol consumption were excluded from the control group, but not the cases (Boffetta et al., 2008). These activities are highly correlated with coffee consumption, suggesting that coffee consumption may have been lower among the controls than among the cases because of how the cases were selected. This methodological error generated an uncontrolled confounding variable that may have been the reason for the apparent association between coffee and pancreatic cancer and gives an alert appraiser reason to question the validity of the study findings. Subsequent case–control and cohort studies have failed to support an association between coffee and pancreatic cancer (Turati et al., 2012). All findings must be carefully evaluated to determine the validity of a study's conclusions and how applicable they are to practice.

What Are the Results? (Reliability)

Results in case–control studies often are provided in terms of the risk or odds of the outcome occurring in the group exposed to the condition (i.e., the cases) compared to it occurring in the control group. Some statistics that could be used include RR and OR (see prior explanation). Bias is inherent in the results of these studies because of self-report—sometimes called information bias. Also, bias could be introduced in case–control studies because of a common variable across the cases and controls that researchers didn't consider. For example, researchers are evaluating lung cancer in smokers. They select from primary care practice their cases of patients diagnosed with lung cancer that live within a specific community. Their controls are drawn from all other persons within the community. As the study progresses, they find out that those within the case group live within a 10 block radius, which seems like a great finding—what is creating this situation. However, when they evaluate the controls, they find that only 10% of them live in the same 10 block radius, which makes their information less relevant and, therefore, potentially biases any results from the study.

Will the Results Help Me in Caring for My Patients? (Applicability)

Were the Study Patients Similar to My Own? Sample characteristics must be provided in all studies. Comparing those characteristics to those of the patients for whom clinicians care is imperative to know if study results can be applicable to them.

Will the Results Compare With Previous Studies? Case–control findings, like other less reliable study designs, must be compared to previous studies to see how they agree (or not). Strength of evidence comes with agreement across studies, demonstrating reliability of effect.

What Are My Patient's/Family's Values and Expectations for the Outcomes? Patient-centered care demands that clinicians consider any information on patient expectations and values as they are planning treatment. Regularly collecting patient preference information is a hallmark of an evidence-based clinician.

Clinical Scenario 5.2

A concerned relative follows you into the hall from the room of a family member who has just been diagnosed with a rare brain tumor. He tells you he recently saw a program on television that described research linking cellular phone use to the development of some forms of cancer. His relative has used a cellular phone for many years, and he wonders whether that may have caused the tumor. You would like to know what the research literature has to say about this issue.

What the Literature Says: Answering a Clinical Question

The clinical question for Clinical Scenario 5.2 could be: In patients admitted with brain tumors (**P**), how does cell phone usage (more cell phone usage [**I**] compared to less cell phone usage [**C**]) influence brain tumor incidence (**O**)? When conducting a quick search of the literature, you find the following study and believe it may help answer the question from the family member in your practice (Inskip et al., 2001):

Enrolled in the study were 782 case participants with histologically confirmed glioma, meningioma, or acoustic neuroma. Participants came from a number of hospitals. The control participants were 799 patients admitted to the same hospitals as the cases but with nonmalignant conditions. The predictor measured was cellular phone usage, which was quantified using a personal interview to collect information on duration and frequency of use. Once the details of the study are evaluated, the general critical appraisal questions should be answered. The RCA questions for case–control studies found in Box 5.2 can assist in critically appraising this study to determine its value in answering this relative's question.

Are the Results of the Study Valid? (Validity)

This case–control study describes in detail how cases were selected from eligible patients who had been diagnosed with various types of tumors. Tumor diagnosis was confirmed by objective tests. Validity can be compromised in case–control studies if cases are misdiagnosed. Control patients were concurrently recruited from the same healthcare centers and were matched for age, sex, and ethnicity.

A research nurse administered a computer-assisted personal interview with the patient or a proxy if the patient could not participate. Participants were asked about the frequency of cellular phone usage. Reliance on recall rather than a more objective way to measure cell phone usage is a weakness in this study. Other studies have used computer databases of actual cell phone usage to overcome this limitation (Guyatt et al., 2015). Although case patients were matched on certain demographic variables, other variables that influenced the outcome may not have been considered. In addition, recall bias would be a serious threat to the validity of this study. Although the data analysis did not support the hypothesis that cellular phone usage causes brain tumors, possible inaccuracies in patient recall or use of different types of cellular phones raises questions about the validity of the results. Overall, the study suggested that cellular phone usage does not increase or decrease the risk of brain tumors. However, subsequent research has raised conflicting results, leading to the World Health Organization accepting the 2011 declaration of the International Agency for Research on Cancer that wireless devices were a "possible human carcinogen" (Hardell, Carlberg, &

BOX **5.2**	*Rapid Critical Appraisal Questions for Case–Control Studies*

1. Are the results of the study valid?
   a. How were the cases obtained?
   b. Were appropriate controls selected?
   c. Were data collection methods the same for the cases and controls?
2. What are the results?
   a. Is an estimate of effect given (do the numbers add up)?
   b. Are there multiple comparisons of data?
   c. Is there any possibility of bias or confounding?
3. Will the results help me in caring for my patients?
   a. Were the study patients similar to my own?
   b. How do the results compare with previous studies?
   c. What are my patient's/family's values and expectations for the outcome?

Hansson Mild, 2013). This classification is used when a causal association is considered credible, but chance, bias, or confounding cannot be ruled out (World Health Organization, 2014). Given the widespread use of cellular phones, further research is being conducted on their risks, with the consensus continuing to be that cell phones do not cause brain tumors (Chapman, Azizi, Luo, & Sitas, 2016). Given the controversy surrounding their risks, clinicians will need to keep abreast of this field if they are to have confidence in the validity of any individual study's findings.

What Are the Results? (Reliability)

Returning to the Inskip et al. study, comparisons were made between those who never or very rarely used a cellular phone and those who used one for more than 100 hours. The RR for cellular phone usage was: RR = 0.9 for glioma (95% CI, 0.5 to 1.6); RR = 0.7 for meningioma (95% CI, 0.3 to 1.7); RR = 1.4 for acoustic neuroma (95% CI, 0.6 to 3.5); and the overall RR = 1.0 (95% CI, 0.6 to 1.5) for all tumor types combined. Although some studies indicated that the RR of certain types of brain tumors increased with cell phone use, the overall result from this group of studies indicated an RR of 1. This indicates that a person who has used a cell phone for more than 100 hours is just as likely (RR = 1.0) to have a tumor as someone who has not used a cell phone. The CIs reportedly give us an estimate of the precision of the measurement of effect of cell phone use in this study. Note that all the CIs in this example include the value of 1. Remember that when the CI contains what is called the line of no effect, which for RR is 1, the results are not statistically significant.

For example, from this study's findings, the RR for meningioma was 0.7 with a CI of 0.3 to 1.7, which includes 1 and therefore is not statistically significant. Because in this study the sample size is moderate to large, we would expect the CIs to be narrow. The narrower the CI, the more precise the finding is for the clinician (i.e., the more likely clinicians can get close to the study finding). A 95% CI enables clinicians to be 95% confident that their findings, if they do the same thing (e.g., use the cell phone for so many hours), will be within the range of the CI. In studies with a high-risk outcome (e.g., death), having 95% confidence in knowing the outcome they will achieve may not be sufficient. In studies of these types, clinicians will want to know more specifically what they can expect and would be likely to choose a 99% CI.

Will the Results Help Me in Caring for My Patients? (Applicability)

When evaluating the results of this study and the associated limitations, it is difficult to find helpful information for clinical decision making. When critically appraising all studies, a basic aspect of applicability is to evaluate the study patients in comparison with the patients to whom the evidence would be applied (i.e., the clinician's own patients). Because this study has known limitations, it is more challenging to determine if the results would lead directly to selecting or avoiding cell phone use. However, the results of the study assist researchers in understanding the need for more research about cell phone usage and the possible sequelae of brain tumors. For the patient's family members, the information from this one study would not be definitive. To provide appropriate counsel to healthcare consumers, it would be important to find other studies that could help answer the clinical question (e.g., Hardell et al., 2013).

CRITICAL APPRAISAL OF COHORT STUDIES

The **cohort study** design is especially suitable for investigating the course of a disease or the unintended consequences of a treatment (Guyatt et al., 2015). A *cohort* refers to a study population sharing a characteristic or group of characteristics. Cohort studies can be conducted with and without a control group. Without a control group, researchers identify a cohort exposed to the characteristic of interest and monitor them over time to describe various outcomes. For example, a cohort could be adolescents experiencing their first episode of psychosis. The study could follow the cohort over time and report on what was observed and measured. Alternatively, a control group could be included by selecting another cohort of adolescents that is similar in every way, yet who have not experienced psychosis. As with case–control studies, exposed and unexposed cohorts should have a similar risk of the target outcome.

The largest long-term cohort study of women's health is the Nurses' Health Study. More than 121,000 nurses were enrolled in the study in 1976 and were mailed questionnaires every 2 years. In 1989, Nurses' Health Study 2 enrolled almost 117,000, and Nurses' Health Study 3 began enrolling 100,000 more nurses and nursing students in 2010. Several correlations have been identified through these cohorts. For example, women under 60 years (but not older) who sleep 5 or fewer hours per night are more likely to have high blood pressure compared to those sleeping 7 hours per night (Gangwisch, Feskanich, Malaspina, Shen, & Forman, 2013). The results were statistically significant (OR = 1.19 and 95% CI, 1.14 to 1.25). The cohorts were selected from within Nurses' Health Study 1 and 2 based on answers to a question about sleep duration.

Because cohort studies generally follow people over a period of time to determine their outcomes, they are longitudinal. In prospective studies, a cohort exposed to a drug, surgery, or particular diagnosis may be followed for years while collecting data on outcomes. For example, in studying DES and cancer, cohort studies have been running since the initial case studies reported in the 1970s and now involve three generations of people who have been impacted by this association (Troisi et al., 2007). Because such prospective studies can take many years to complete, cohort studies are often retrospective. In retrospective studies, the outcome under investigation (e.g., occurrence of a disease or condition) has already occurred and researchers go even further into the past to select those characteristics they believe might be associated with the given outcome. The cohort is followed from that point forward to determine what influenced the development of the outcome and when those influences occurred. Because participants are not randomly assigned to a cohort, cohort studies do not have an experimental research design. These studies therefore have the limitations of all observational studies.

A landmark example of the limitations that may accompany a cohort study can be seen in the data supporting or refuting the benefits of hormone replacement therapy for heart health. A meta-analysis of 16 cohort studies of women taking postmenopausal estrogen therapy concluded that the medication gave women a lower risk of coronary heart disease (CHD), with an RR of 0.5 and 95% CI of 0.44 to 0.57 (Stampfer & Colditz, 1991). Practice was based on these studies for quite a long time; however, standards of care were challenged when the highly publicized Women's Health Initiative RCT showed that hormone replacement therapy actually increased the risk of CHD in postmenopausal women (Rossouw et al., 2002). The quandary for clinicians is deciding which studies provide the most valid and reliable evidence for making decisions with their patients. RCTs are the strongest evidence for making decisions about interventions; however, without the existence of this type of evidence, cohort studies may be the only evidence available to guide practice.

Rapid Appraisal Questions for a Cohort Study

The design-specific RCA questions for cohort studies that can assist the clinician in quickly determining the value of a cohort study can be found in Box 5.3.

BOX
5.3

Rapid Critical Appraisal Questions for Cohort Studies

1. Are the results of the study valid?
   a. Was there a representative and well-defined sample of patients at a similar point in the course of the disease?
   b. Was follow-up sufficiently long and complete?
   c. Were objective and unbiased outcome criteria used?
   d. Did the analysis adjust for important prognostic risk factors and confounding variables?
2. What are the results?
   a. What is the magnitude of the relationship between predictors (i.e., prognostic indicators) and targeted outcome?
   b. How likely is the outcome event(s) in a specified period of time?
   c. How precise are the study estimates?
3. Will the results help me in caring for my patients?
   a. Were the study patients similar to my own?
   b. Will the results lead directly to selecting or avoiding therapy?
   c. Would the results be used to counsel patients?

Are the Results of the Study Valid? (Validity)

Was There a Representative and Well-Defined Sample of Patients at a Similar Point in the Course of the Disease? When appraising a cohort study, establishing the characteristics of the patients or clients under study is important. These characteristics, such as the severity of symptoms or stage in the illness trajectory, will strongly influence the impact an intervention may have on the patient's condition or the resulting outcomes. A suitably detailed description of the population and how the cohorts were defined (i.e., how the exposure [and nonexposure, if appropriate] cohorts were established) is necessary for the clinician to draw any conclusions about the validity of the results and whether they are generalizable to other populations.

Was Follow-Up Sufficiently Long and Complete? The length of follow-up for a cohort study will depend on the outcomes of interest. For example, wound breakdown as a consequence of an early discharge program after surgery would require a shorter follow-up period than a study examining hospital admissions for management of acute asthma subsequent to an in-school education strategy. Insufficient time for outcomes to be demonstrated will bias the study findings.

Clinicians appraising a cohort study would need to evaluate if people withdrew from the study and, if so, why (i.e., to determine if there was something unique about those participants). Patients enrolled in a cohort study, particularly over a long time, may be lost to follow-up. Furthermore, the condition of interest in a cohort study may predispose patients to incomplete or nonadherent participation in a study. Cohort studies involving patients with a terminal or end-stage illness commonly must deal with patients dying during the study before follow-up data are completely collected. Although unavoidable, the extent of loss to follow-up may bias the study results.

Were Objective and Unbiased Outcome Criteria Used? When evaluating outcomes in the cohort, researchers can use both subjective and objective measurements. Subjective measures introduce bias (e.g., recall) into the study, whereas ideally, objective measures have less bias and provide more reliable data. Patient self-reporting and clinician diagnosis are outcome measures that are subject to some bias. Objective measures will be based on a reference standard, such as a biochemical test or clinical interview conducted by a psychologist. Research reports should contain the validity and reliability of the measures that were used. The clinician should also integrate clinical expertise with appraisal skills when thinking about the measurement of the outcomes of interest.

Did the Analysis Adjust for Important Prognostic Risk Factors and Confounding Variables? Clinicians need to consider what, if any, other prognostic (i.e., predictive) factors could have been included in the study, but were not. If there are other factors identified, clinicians must determine how those would affect the validity of the current findings. In addition, other factors must be considered that could muddy the relationships among the existing identified factors and the outcomes. For example, a cohort study may be designed to study the risk of gastric bleeding in nonsteroidal anti-inflammatory drug (NSAID) users compared to nonusers. Incidence of gastric bleeding (i.e., the event rate) is so low that an enormous number of participants would be needed for an RCT, making a cohort study more feasible. However, a cohort of NSAID users may inherently be older than a cohort of NSAID nonusers and bring with them increased risk for gastric bleeding. In this case, age could be a confounding variable if it is not controlled for when selecting the cohorts.

What Are the Results? (Reliability)

What Is the Magnitude of the Relationship Between Predictors (i.e., Prognostic Indicators) and Targeted Outcome? For cohort studies, clinicians must evaluate the final results. Often studies may report an incident rate or a proportion for the outcome occurring within the exposed and unexposed cohorts as well as the differences in those rates or proportions. Evaluating the strength of association between exposure and outcome is imperative (e.g., RR, ARR, or NNT).

How Likely Is the Outcome Event(s) in a Specified Period of Time? Often the strength of association is provided for a given time period. For example, researchers may state that the NNT is 15 with an antihypertensive medication to prevent one more stroke within 3 years.

How Precise Are the Study Estimates? CIs must be provided, along with p values, to determine precision of the findings (i.e., whether a clinician can replicate the results).

Will the Results Help Me in Caring for My Patients? (Applicability)

Were the Study Patients Similar to My Own? As with all studies, it is important to note how similar or dissimilar the sample is to the clinicians' patients.

Will the Results Lead Directly to Selecting or Avoiding Therapy? and Would the Results Be Used to Counsel Patients? After clinicians evaluate the findings to see if they are reliable and applicable to their patients, they must determine how they can be used to assist those patients in their healthcare management. Caution must be used here, as cohort studies are not RCTs and inherently have bias in their design; therefore, confidence in replicating their findings should always be lower. Nevertheless, providing information to patients regarding the study findings is important to having evidence-based consumers who use the best evidence to make their healthcare decisions.

Clinical Scenario 5.3

You have been working in a community mental health program for a number of years. Young people who have experienced their first episode of schizophrenia make up a large proportion of your client base. Your colleagues have suggested that differences in the disease and social course of schizophrenia may arise depending on clients' age at onset. You volunteer to find a paper for the next journal club that investigates the influence of age at onset on the symptom-related course of the disease.

What the Literature Says: Answering a Clinical Question

The clinical question for Clinical Scenario 5.3 could be: In adolescent patients who have schizophrenia (P), how does age of onset (early onset [I] compared to later onset [C]) influence the social course of the disease (O)? The following study may help answer the question about adolescents and schizophrenia: Häfner, Hambrecht, Löffler, Munk-Jørgensen, and Riecher-Rössler (1998). Using the RCA questions, this study will be evaluated to determine whether it provides valid, relevant evidence to address this clinical question.

The participants in the study were 1,109 patients first admitted to a mental health institution with a broad diagnosis of schizophrenia at ages 12 to 20, 21 to 35, or 36 to 59 years. Symptoms were assessed at 6 months and at 1, 2, 3, and 5 years after first admission. The outcome measured was symptom severity as determined by scores on the symptom-based Present State Examination (PSE), using a computer program to arrive at diagnostic classifications (PSE-CATEGO). The higher the score on the PSE-CATEGO, the more severe the illness.

Are the Results of the Study Valid? (Validity)

There are several questions that help determine if a cohort study is valid. The first is: Was there a representative and well-defined sample of patients at a similar point in the course of the disease? Because the participants in this study were admitted into the study at their first admission and their onset and course before the first admission were assessed retrospectively with a standardized instrument, the study sample seems representative for patients at similar points for schizophrenia. The second question is: Was follow-up sufficiently long and complete? In this study, ensuing symptoms and social consequences were prospectively followed over 5 years. Although there was no explanation for why a 5-year follow-up period was chosen, nor was any information given on losses to follow-up, 5 years is probably sufficiently long enough for follow-up. The third question is: Were objective and unbiased outcome criteria used? Symptomatology, functional impairment, and social disability were assessed by clinically experienced, trained psychiatrists and psychologists using previously validated instruments. The fourth and final question to assess study validity is: Did the analysis adjust for important prognostic risk factors? In the study, symptoms of schizophrenia as well as onset of formal treatment were considered for their impact on functional impairment and social disability. Given these methods, the study findings are valid and can help in determining practice.

What Are the Results? (Reliability)

In this study, participants with early-onset schizophrenia, especially men, presented with higher PSE-CATEGO scores than did study participants with late-onset disease. In men, symptom severity decreased with increasing age of onset. In women, symptom severity remained stable, although there was an increase in negative symptoms with late onset. Disorganization decreased with age, but delusions increased markedly across the whole age of onset range. The main determinant of social course was level of social development at onset. Inferential statistics were used to determine any differences between groups, and p values were reported; however, there were no CIs provided, and precision of the effect is difficult to determine.

Will the Results Help Me in Caring for My Patients? (Applicability)

Some of the study participants are similar in age and social development to those in your clinic population. Although much of the data show trends rather than statistically significant differences, the authors of the study developed some suggestions about why any differences exist that are clinically meaningful. You and your colleagues could use this information, along with other studies, to plan early intervention programs with the goal of limiting the negative consequences of schizophrenia in young people. This study is applicable to your practice and should assist in making decisions. Always keep in mind, however, that any time you use evidence to make clinical decisions, subsequent evaluation of the difference the evidence makes in your own practice is essential.

Perfection is not attainable, but if we chase perfection
we can catch excellence.

VINCE LOMBARDI

CRITICAL APPRAISAL OF RCTS

RCTs are the most appropriate research design to answer questions of efficacy and effectiveness of interventions because their methodology provides confidence in establishing cause and effect (i.e., increased confidence that a given intervention leads to a particular outcome). As individual studies, RCTs rank as Level II evidence in this hierarchy of evidence because a well-conducted study should have a low risk of bias. A synthesis of RCTs is considered Level I evidence for answering questions about interventions for the same reason (see Chapter 1, Box 1.3). An RCT compares the effectiveness of different interventions. This can involve one group that gets the intervention under investigation (intervention group) and another group that gets one of four comparative options (comparison group) to determine whether the intervention or comparison is better at producing the outcome. The four options for the comparison group include (1) no intervention (i.e., a true control group), (2) a placebo, (3) another treatment (i.e., comparison intervention), or (4) the current standard of care. RCTs are experimental studies in which participants are *randomly* assigned to the intervention or comparison group in what are often referred to as the "arms" of a study. An RCT often has two arms, but may have more than two, such as when an intervention (arm 1) is being compared with no intervention (arm 2) and a placebo (arm 3). RCTs are also prospective and longitudinal in that participants are studied over a period of time to assess the effects of an intervention or treatment on selected outcomes.

In crossover trials, participants are given the experimental intervention and then the comparison or placebo-controlled intervention in consecutive periods and thus serve as their own controls. For example, a crossover design was used to study the effectiveness of two combinations of dental hygiene products on bad mouth odor (Farrell, Barker, Walanski, & Gerlach, 2008). The study used four periods in which participants were randomly assigned to either combination A (antibacterial toothpaste, antibacterial mouth rinse, and an oscillating-rotating toothbrush) or combination B (regular toothpaste and manual toothbrush). The participants were allowed 2 days between each intervention to permit the effects of the previous intervention to subside or washout, hence the name "washout period." Combination A led to a 35% reduction in bad breath as determined by an instrument widely used to measure breath volatiles ($p < 0.001$). Crossover trials allow comparisons of the same participants' responses to the two interventions, thus minimizing variability caused by having different people in each intervention group. The crossover design works well for short-lasting interventions, such as the dental hygiene products used in this study. The major concern with crossover trials is carryover, in which the effects of the first intervention linger into the period of testing of the second intervention (Higgins & Green, 2011). It is important to consider this introduction of bias when critically appraising a crossover trial.

RCTs, in general, are sometimes considered to be overly artificial because of the control investigators exert over most aspects of the study. Predetermined inclusion and exclusion criteria are used to select participants and provide a homogeneous study population (i.e., all the participants in the sample are alike). The investigators must carefully consider how to recruit participants for the intervention, the control, and the comparison groups before starting the study. The outcomes of interest are also predetermined. Since some suggest that the results of an RCT are really only generalizable to the particular population studied in the trial because of this artificiality, two approaches to conducting RCTs have been developed.

The two approaches to conducting RCTs are called the efficacy study and the effectiveness study (Singal, Higgins, & Waljee, 2014). The efficacy has to be established first (i.e., how well the intervention works in ideal settings) before an effectiveness trial is done (i.e., how well the intervention works in the real world). The distinction rests with the sort of research question that each study attempts to answer. In an efficacy study (sometimes also called an explanatory study), everything is controlled as tightly as possible to ensure the two groups differ only in regard to how they respond to the intervention. Such studies give the best information on whether and how well the intervention works, but may not be as readily applicable to clinical practice. Effectiveness studies (also called pragmatic studies) address the value of an intervention in clinical practice. In an effectiveness study, controls are kept to a minimum to ensure the research setting is as similar to routine practice as possible. Although the degree to which RCT findings are generalizable must be kept in mind when applying the results to individual patients, RCTs remain the most valid and rigorous study design for assessing the benefits or harms of an intervention and supporting cause-and-effect relationships.

Rapid Appraisal Questions for Randomized Controlled Trials

Although all the issues and standard appraisal questions discussed earlier in this chapter apply to RCTs, there are additional questions that are specific to this methodology. Rapid appraisal questions for RCTs can assist the clinician in quickly determining a particular study's value for practice (Box 5.4).

BOX 5.4	*Rapid Critical Appraisal Questions for Randomized Controlled Trials*

1. Are the results of the study valid?
   a. Were the participants randomly assigned to the experimental and control groups?
   b. Was random assignment concealed from the individuals who were first enrolling participants into the study?
   c. Were the participants and providers kept blind to the study group?
   d. Were reasons given to explain why participants did not complete the study?
   e. Were the follow-up assessments conducted long enough to fully study the effects of the intervention?
   f. Were the participants analyzed in the group to which they were randomly assigned?
   g. Was the control group appropriate?
   h. Were the instruments used to measure the outcomes valid and reliable?
   i. Were the participants in each of the groups similar on demographic and baseline clinical variables?
2. What are the results?
   a. How large is the intervention or treatment effect (NNT, NNH, effect size, level of significance)?
   b. How precise is the intervention or treatment effect (CI)?
3. Will the results help me in caring for my patients?
   a. Were all clinically important outcomes measured?
   b. What are the risks and benefits of the treatment?
   c. Is the treatment feasible in my clinical setting?
   d. What are my patient's/family's values and expectations for the outcome being pursued and the treatment itself?

CI, confidence interval; NNH, number needed to harm; NNT, number needed to treat.

Are the Results of the Study Valid? (Validity)

Were the Participants Randomly Assigned to the Experimental and Control Groups? Because the purpose of an RCT is to determine the efficacy or effectiveness of an intervention in producing an outcome, beyond that due to chance, the groups assigned to either the experimental treatment or the comparison need to be equivalent in all relevant characteristics (e.g., age, disease severity, socioeconomic status, gender) at the beginning of the study, before the intervention is delivered. The best method to ensure baseline equivalency between study groups is to randomly assign participants to the experimental treatment or intervention and to the comparison or placebo-controlled group. This became more obvious when awareness of bias in observational studies arose in the 1980s. Several studies were published that showed how observational studies tended to have more favorable outcomes than an RCT on the same research question (Kunz & Oxman, 1998). In one early review, the researchers found significant differences between the outcomes of 145 trials investigating different treatments for acute myocardial infarction (Chalmers, Celano, Sacks, & Smith, 1983). Within this body of evidence, the frequency of significant outcomes for observational trials for a given treatment was 25%, for nonconcealed RCTs was 11%, and for concealed RCTs was 5%. The average RRR for a myocardial infarction per study type was 34%, 7%, and 3%, respectively. More recent comparisons of study designs have found that observational studies can produce similar results to RCTs with certain types of interventions, which suggests that the general quality of observational studies has improved (Benson & Hartz, 2000; Concato, Shah, & Horwitz, 2000). However, this is not always the case. A review of studies comparing oral and depot antipsychotics for schizophrenia found no significant difference between the two formulations in RCTs, whereas observational trials showed a significant benefit for depot injections (Kirson et al., 2013). This shows the importance of examining the impact of research design on study outcomes.

In a large review of treatments for 45 conditions, researchers found that although randomized and nonrandomized trials of the same treatment tend to agree on whether the treatment works, they often disagree on the size of the effect (Ioannidis et al., 2001). Observational studies may often be preferred in evaluating the harms of medical treatments; however, RCTs of the same treatments usually found larger risks of harm than observational trials, though not always (Papanikolaou, Christidi, & Ioannidis, 2006). In general, it appears that if the clinician chooses which patients receive which treatment or if patients self-select the treatment they will receive, important demographic and clinical variables are introduced that impact the outcomes. Where possible, random assignment should be used to minimize such bias.

The method of randomization should be reported in the methods section of the published research report. To avoid selection bias, the random sequence for assigning patients should be unpredictable (e.g., a random number table, a computer random number generator, or tossing a coin). Researchers sometimes assign participants to groups on an alternate basis or by such criteria as the participants' date of birth or the day of the week, but these methods are not adequate because the sequence can introduce bias. For example, significantly higher death rates after elective surgery have been demonstrated if the surgery is carried out on Friday or at the weekend compared to other days of the week (Aylin, Alexandrescu, Jen, Mayer, & Bottle, 2013). If participants in a study were assigned to a surgical intervention according to the day of the week, the day would be a confounding variable. Such kinds of assignment methods are called *pseudo-* or *quasi-randomization* and have been shown to introduce assignment bias (Schulz & Grimes, 2002b). Often such approaches are used because they are more convenient; however, the higher risk of bias makes them less desirable.

Variations on the simple randomization method described previously do exist. *Cluster randomization* is a method whereby groups of participants are randomized to the same treatment together (Torgerson, 2001). The unit of measurement (e.g., individual clinician, patient unit, hospital, clinic, or school) in such a study is the experimental unit rather than individual participants. When critically appraising a cluster randomized trial, attention must be paid to whether the results were analyzed properly. Analysis of a standard RCT is based on individuals being randomized between groups, but this does not happen with cluster randomization and the analysis needs to take this into account. A review of such trials in primary care found that 41% did not take account of the clustering in their analyses (Eldridge, Ashby, Feder, Rudnicka, & Ukoumunne, 2004). *Block randomization* is where participants from groups with characteristics that cannot be manipulated (e.g., age, gender) are randomly assigned to the intervention and control groups in equal numbers (i.e., 40 men out of a group of 100 men and 40 women out of a group of 100 women). **Stratified randomization** ensures an equal distribution of certain patient characteristics (e.g., gestational age or severity of illness) across the groups.

Was Random Assignment Concealed From Those Enrolling Participants Into the Study? Bias can be introduced when recruiting participants into a study. If those recruiting know to which group the participants will be assigned, they may consciously or subconsciously recruit those going into the intervention group differently than those going into the comparison or control group. Therefore, random assignment should be concealed until after the participants are recruited into the study. This can be accomplished with a method as simple as having designated recruiters who are not investigators or by placing the assignment in an envelope and revealing the assignment once recruitment is complete, to something as elaborate as using an assignment service independent of the study investigators. Using a sealed, opaque envelope to conceal the randomly generated treatment allocation can be susceptible to bias if recruiters are determined to ensure a specific allocation for a particular participant (Schulz & Grimes, 2002a). This susceptibility was illustrated in a study in which researchers anonymously admitted they had held semiopaque envelopes up to a bright light to reveal the allocation sequence or searched a principal investigator's files to discover the allocation list (Schulz, 1995). Although such investigators may have rationalized that their actions were well intended, they probably introduced bias into their studies, which could have undermined the conclusions. To avoid such issues, a central research facility could be used where someone other than the study researchers e-mails or texts the enrollment of a new participant. The central facility determines the treatment allocation and informs the researcher. Such *distance randomization* removes the possibility of researchers introducing bias by attempting to ensure that a patient receives the treatment they believe would be most beneficial; however, the increased cost of this option may prohibit using it.

Were the Participants and Providers Kept Blind to Study Group? Blinding, sometimes referred to as "masking," is undertaken to reduce the bias that could arise when those observing the outcome know what intervention was received by the study participants. Clinicians may be familiar with the term *double blind*, in which neither the person delivering the intervention nor the participant receiving it knows whether it is the treatment or comparison intervention; however, they may not be as familiar with other degrees of blinding, such as *single blind* and *triple blind* (Devereaux et al., 2001). All research reports should describe precisely which groups of people were blinded to treatment allocation and how this was done. Double blinding is very important because it mitigates the placebo effect (i.e., participants respond to an intervention simply because they received something from the researchers rather than because the intervention itself was effective). Studies have demonstrated that the size of a treatment effect can be inflated when patients, clinicians, data collectors, data analyzers, or report authors know which patients received which interventions (Devereaux et al., 2001). When everyone involved is blinded, the expectations of those involved in the study are less likely to influence the results observed.

The degree of blinding utilized in a study partly depends on the intervention being studied and the outcome of interest. For example, death as an outcome is objective and unlikely to be influenced by knowledge of the intervention. However, quality-of-life or pain scores are relatively subjective measures and may be influenced by the participants' knowledge, if outcomes are self-reporting, or by the health professionals' knowledge, if they are collecting the data.

The **placebo** intervention is another method used for blinding. When investigators report on using a placebo, it should appear like the treatment in all aspects. For example, a placebo medication should look, smell, and taste just like the experimental drug and should be given via the same mode of delivery. A placebo can be developed for many types of interventions. Surgical procedures have been tested in patient-blinded trials using "sham surgery" in which patients receive only an incision. Although ethically controversial, they are viewed by some as necessary to adequately evaluate surgical procedures (Swift, 2012).

When the intervention cannot be blinded, usually due to ethical considerations, researchers can ensure that outcome assessment is blinded to reduce bias. For example, patients with burns could be allocated to either the currently used dressing type or an experimental bioengineered dressing. The patients and their caregivers would be aware of the dressing that they were receiving; however, through taking photographs of the wounds and having assessors score the degree of healing without knowing which patients received which dressing, healing could be measured in a blinded fashion.

Were Reasons Given to Explain Why Participants Did Not Complete the Study? Researchers conducting RCTs prospectively follow people over a period of time, sometimes for years. Evidence users critically appraising such studies should examine the number of participants originally enrolled in the study and compare that number with the final numbers in the analyzed outcome data. Ideally, the status of every patient enrolled in the study will be known at the study's completion and reported. When large numbers of participants leave a study and therefore have unknown outcomes, the validity of the study is potentially compromised or bias may be introduced. This is especially important if the study arms differ in how many people did not complete the study. Participants may leave a study for many reasons, including adverse outcomes, death, a burdensome protocol, or because their symptoms resolved and they did not return for assessment. When critically appraising a study, consider whether those who were lost to follow-up differed from those who finished the trial. Although a commonly accepted dropout rate is 20% or less (i.e., 80% retention), this arbitrary rate is inadvisable as a sole marker of study validity.

Consider an example where researchers conducting a well-done study with severely ill participants plan to enroll more participants than they know is necessary according to a **power analysis**. These are done to reduce making a Type II error (i.e., accepting that the intervention really did not work, the null hypothesis, when it did). They enroll additional participants because they anticipate a high dropout rate. For example, if the power calculation determines they need 100 participants to avoid a Type II error, and they anticipate a 50% dropout rate, they may enroll 200 participants to ensure that at least 100 participants complete the study. This is why it is important to note not only the number of participants who completed the study but also other factors that influence such studies (e.g., conducted over very long periods or involving severely ill participants) that may lead to unavoidably high incompletion rates. Often researchers will compare the demographic variables of those who did not complete the study to those who remained in the study. They may also assess the impact of loss to follow-up by assuming the worst outcome for those who withdrew and by repeating the analysis. If researchers find that this worst-case scenario has the same treatment effect, clinicians can consider that the validity of the study has not been compromised.

Were the Follow-Up Assessments Conducted Long Enough to Fully Study the Effects of the Intervention? In critically appraising an intervention study, clinicians consider how long it takes for the intervention to produce the outcome. For example, if an intervention was given in hospital, and a study measured the outcome at discharge, insufficient time may have passed to adequately evaluate the outcome. Follow-up assessment might need to be weeks or months later. In critically appraising a study, clinicians should use their experience with patient populations to guide them in determining the appropriate time frame for a study.

Were the Participants Analyzed in the Group to Which They Were Randomly Assigned? Another way to ask this question is: Was an intention-to-treat analysis conducted? Despite the best efforts of investigators, some patients assigned to a particular group may not receive the allocated treatment throughout the entire study period. For example, some people allocated an experimental drug might not take it. In the Chocolate Happiness Undergoing More Pleasantness (CHUMP) study (Chan, 2007), participants in one treatment group traded treatments with another treatment arm of the study, muddying the analysis for both arms of the study.

One approach to addressing these cross-contamination issues could be to exclude from the analysis the data of everyone who did not adhere to their assigned intervention. However, this approach could potentially introduce bias as patients who change treatment or drop out of a study may be systematically different from those who do not. The intention-to-treat principle states that data should be analyzed according to the group to which the patient was originally allocated. Researchers follow this principle to preserve the value of random assignment (Higgins & Green, 2011). If the comparability of groups is to be maintained through the study, patients should not be excluded from the analysis or switched.

The intention-to-treat principle tends to minimize Type I errors but is more susceptible to Type II errors (Table 5.1). The alternative approach would be to analyze patient data according to the intervention they actually obtained in the study (i.e., per-protocol analysis), but this method is vulnerable to bias. Any study that deviates substantially from its protocol may have methodological problems or a higher risk of bias and should be evaluated carefully before being applied to practice (Ruiz-Canela, Martínez-González, & de Irala-Estévez, 2000).

Another alternative would be for researchers to exclude patients from final data analysis. It is commonly accepted that patients who were actually ineligible to be enrolled in the trial and who were mistakenly randomized may be excluded, as well as patients who were prematurely enrolled in a trial but who never received the intervention. Excluding such patients from analysis may not introduce bias; however, clinicians should consider the implications these reductions would have on sample size and the study's ability to detect important differences (Fergusson, Horwood, & Ridder, 2005).

Was the Control Group Appropriate? The only difference between the experimental and control groups should be the study intervention. What the researchers choose for the comparison or control intervention can assist in understanding whether or not the study results are valid. If an intervention involves personal attention, time spent with participants, or other activities, the participants in the treatment group must be provided the same attention, time, or activities as the comparison group. This is because the attention, time, or other activity could impact the outcomes. For example, an RCT was conducted to evaluate the effect of a complementary therapy, Therapeutic Touch (TT), on women's mood (Lafreniere et al., 1999). Participants in the experimental group removed their shoes, laid on a hospital bed, and listened to soft music while receiving TT. They rested for 5 to 10 minutes and were taken to a testing room where they completed study questionnaires. Those in the control group went directly to the testing room to complete the questionnaires, without any of the attention or time that the experimental group received. The indicators of mood differed significantly between the groups, but the choice of control made it inappropriate to attribute the differences to TT alone. The soft music, relaxing environment, 10 minutes of rest, or any combination of those confounding variables could have contributed to the observed outcomes, making the study findings unreliable for clinicians to use in practice. Another study found that when irritable bowel syndrome patients were informed that they would be given a placebo, their outcomes were significantly better than those assigned to a no treatment control (Kaptchuk et al., 2010). In this case, the professional interaction between patients and researchers impacted the outcomes, even though the patients knew their treatment was an inert placebo.

If treatments used in a research study are to be used in clinical practice, a clear description of the intervention and control is essential. If the description is unclear, clinicians' delivery of the interventions may differ, thereby resulting in a different outcome. For example, drug dosages, details of written information given to participants, or number of clinic visits, if relevant, should be described adequately. The description of the interventions in the methods section also should report any other interventions that differed between the two groups, such as additional visits from clinicians or telephone calls, because these may affect the reported outcomes.

Were the Instruments Used to Measure the Outcomes Valid and Reliable? The instruments researchers use to measure study outcomes are important in determining how useful the results are to clinicians. If the measures are valid (i.e., they measure what they are intended to) and are reliable (i.e., the items within the instrument are consistent in their measurement, time after time), then clinicians can have more confidence in the study findings. Chapter 21 has more information on validity and reliability of outcome measurement.

Were the Participants in Each of the Groups Similar on Demographic and Baseline Clinical Variables? Sufficient information about how the participants were selected should be provided in the research paper, usually in the methods section. The study population should be appropriate for the question the study is addressing. Clinicians can decide whether the results reported are relevant to the patients in their care. The choice of participants may affect the size of the observed treatment effect. For example, an intervention delivered to people with advanced disease and cared for in a specialist center may not be as effective for or relevant to those with early-stage disease managed in the community.

The characteristics of all intervention groups should be similar at baseline if randomization did what it is expected to do. These data are often the first data reported in the results section of a research paper. This can include demographic variables of the groups, such as age and gender, stage of disease, or illness severity scores. Investigators generally indicate if the groups differed significantly on any variables. If the groups are different at baseline, clinicians must decide whether these reported differences invalidate the findings, rendering them clinically unusable.

As an example, let's say that researchers attempted to determine the effectiveness of oral sucrose in alleviating procedural pain in infants. The participating infants were randomized to treatment (sucrose) or control (water) groups. Statistical tests found that the two groups did not differ significantly in gestational age, birth weight, and the like. However, by chance and despite the appropriate randomization, a statistically significant difference in the severity of illness scores existed between the two groups and in the number of infants in each group who used a pacifier as a comfort measure. As clinicians evaluate these results, they must decide about the usefulness of the study findings. If the outcome of interest was incidence of infection, these differences may be irrelevant. However, in the hypothetical study described here, the outcome (i.e., pain scores associated with a procedure) could very well be influenced by the infants' use of a pacifier for comfort. In this case, the baseline differences should be taken into account when reporting the observed effects. If the groups are reported as being significantly different on certain baseline variables, clinicians should look for how investigators controlled for those baseline differences in their statistical analyses (e.g., analysis of covariance tests).

What Are the Results? (Reliability)

How Large Is the Intervention or Treatment Effect? and How Precise Is the Intervention or Treatment Effect? How the size and precision of the effect are reported is extremely important. As discussed earlier in this chapter, trials should report the total number of study participants assigned to the groups, the numbers available for measurement of outcomes, and the occurrence or event rates in the groups. If these data are not reported, the measures of effect, such as RR and OR, cannot be calculated. CI and/or p values (or the information required to calculate these) should also be included in the results presented to identify the precision of the effect estimates.

Clinicians have to decide on the usefulness or clinical significance of any statistical differences observed. As discussed earlier, statistically significant differences and clinically meaningful differences are not always equivalent. If the CI is wide and includes the point estimate of no effect, such as an RR of 1 or a reported p value of greater than 0.05, the precision of the measurement is likely to be inadequate and the results unreliable. Clinicians cannot have confidence that they can implement the treatment and get similar results. Clinicians must also ask, because the results are not significant and the CI is wide, if it is possible that the sample size was not large enough. A larger sample would likely produce a shorter CI. In addition, trials are increasingly conducted across a large number of healthcare sites. If the findings are consistent across different settings, clinicians could be more confident that the findings were reliable.

Will the Results Assist Me in Caring for My Patients? (Applicability)

Are the Outcomes Measured Clinically Relevant? EBP requires integration of clinical expertise with the best available research evidence and patient values, concerns, and choices. Clinicians need to utilize their own expertise at this point in the critical appraisal process to decide whether the outcomes measured in a study were clinically important. They also need to assess whether the timing of outcome measurement in relation to the delivery of the intervention was appropriate. For example, it may be important to measure the effectiveness of an intervention, such as corticosteroid administration in the management of traumatic brain injury, by measuring survival to discharge from the intensive care unit. However, in determining the effectiveness of a cancer therapy, survival up to 5 years may be more relevant. Outcome measures such as mortality would appear appropriate in these examples but would not likely be relevant in trials with patients with dementia or chronic back pain. Quality-of-life scores or days lost from work would be more useful measures in the studies of these types of conditions.

Investigators may be interested in more than one outcome when designing a study, such as less pain and an improved quality of life. Researchers should designate the primary outcome of interest in their research report and should clarify what outcome formed the basis of their a priori power calculation (assuming one was carried out). This should minimize problems with multiple measures or data dredging in attempts to ensure that a significant result is found.

Clinical Scenario 5.4

At a recent meeting of the surgical division managers of your hospital, the budget was discussed. An idea was proposed that a legitimate cost-cutting measure may be found by discharging women earlier after surgery for breast cancer. Debate about the advantages and disadvantages of such a change to health service provision continued until it was decided to investigate the available evidence.

What the Literature Says: Answering a Clinical Question

The following study may begin to help answer the question that arises from Clinical Scenario 5.4. In women who have had surgery for breast cancer **(P)**, how does early discharge **(I)** compared to current length of stay **(C)** affect coping with the challenges of recovery **(O)** (physical and psychosocial) within the first 3 months after discharge **(T)**? (Bundred et al., 1998). Using the general critical appraisal questions, clinicians can critically appraise this study to determine whether it provides valid, reliable, and relevant evidence.

The participants in the study were 100 women who had early breast cancer and who were undergoing (a) mastectomy with axillary node clearance ($n = 20$) or (b) breast conservation surgery ($n = 80$). The intervention and comparison were early discharge program versus routine length of stay. The outcomes measured were physical illness (i.e., infection, seroma formation, shoulder movement) and psychological illness (i.e., depression and anxiety scores). The timing of follow-up was first preoperatively, then 1 and 3 months postoperatively.

Are the Results of the Study Valid? (Validity)

After patients were recruited into the study, they were randomized in clusters for each week of admissions by a research nurse who opened a sealed envelope containing the randomization code. A flowchart was provided in the report to identify the recruitment, participation, and follow-up of participants. Before the study began (i.e., a priori), a power calculation was undertaken to determine how large the sample needed to be to lessen the chance of accepting that there was no effect when there was one (i.e., Type II error). Participants were analyzed using an intention-to-treat analysis. Participants were not blinded to the intervention and no mention was made of whether the investigators assessing the outcomes were blinded. A detailed description of the intervention and the control management was given. The groups were reported as similar at baseline. Based on these methods, the study results should be considered valid.

What Are the Results? (Reliability)

Results are expressed as OR with 95% CI, and p values are provided where there was statistical significance. Women discharged early had greater shoulder movement (OR = 0.28; 95% CI, 0.08 to 0.95) and less wound pain (OR = 0.28; 95% CI, 0.10 to 0.79) at 3 months compared with the standard length of stay group. Symptom questionnaire scores were significantly lower in the early discharge group at 1 month. It is difficult to determine whether there were clinically meaningful differences in the psychological measures because a total of six tools were used to measure psychological illness. Multiple measurements in themselves are more likely to lead to significant results.

Will the Results Help Me in Caring for My Patients? (Applicability)

The results presented in this research report are those of a planned interim analysis (i.e., the analysis was done to confirm that there were no adverse consequences of early discharge). This approach is reasonable to protect the participants. The results of the full study, when and if completed, would be important to evaluate. From this interim analysis, it would appear that early discharge might be appropriate if women are given sufficient support and resources. However, an outcome that may affect the usefulness of the findings is cost. A cost analysis was not undertaken, so further research that addresses this point may need to be found and appraised before making any final decisions about changing an entire health service model. Based on these issues, this evidence will assist clinicians to consider early discharge but will not answer the clinical question of whether it is the best option for most women who have had surgery for breast cancer.

CRITICAL APPRAISAL OF SYSTEMATIC REVIEWS

A systematic review is a compilation of similar studies that address a specific clinical question (Table 5.7). To conduct a systematic review, a detailed search strategy is employed to find the relevant evidence to answer a clinical question. The researchers determine beforehand what inclusion and exclusion criteria will be used to select identified studies. Systematic reviews of RCTs, considered Level I evidence, are found at the top of the hierarchy of evidence for intervention studies (see Chapter 1, Box 1.3). Systematic review methodology is the most rigorous approach to minimization of bias in reviewing studies.

A systematic review is not the same as a literature review or narrative review (O'Mathúna, 2010a). The methods used in a systematic review are specific and rigorous, whereas a narrative review usually compiles published papers that support an author's particular point of view or serve as general background discussion for a particular issue. In contrast to systematic review,

TABLE 5.7	Definitions of Different Types of Research Evidence Reviews
Review	**Definition**
Systematic review	A compilation of like studies to address a specific clinical question using a detailed, comprehensive search strategy and rigorous appraisal methods for the purpose of summarizing, appraising, and communicating the results and implications of all the research available on a clinical question. A systematic review is the most rigorous approach to minimization of bias in summarizing research
Meta-analysis	A statistical approach to synthesizing the results of a number of studies that produce a larger sample size and thus greater power to determine the true magnitude of an effect. Used to obtain a single-effect measure (i.e., a summary statistic) of the results of all studies included in a systematic review
Integrative review	A systematic review that does not have a summary statistic because of limitations in the studies found (usually because of heterogeneous studies or samples)
Narrative review	A research review that includes published papers that support an author's particular point of view and usually serves as a general background discussion of a particular issue. An explicit and systematic approach to searching for and evaluating papers is usually not used

these types of reviews would be considered level VII evidence for intervention questions. A systematic review is a methodology to summarize, appraise, and communicate the results and implications of several studies that may have contradictory results.

Research trials rarely, if ever, have flawless methodology and a large enough sample size to provide a conclusive answer to questions about clinical effectiveness. Archie Cochrane, an epidemiologist after whom the Cochrane Collaboration is named, recognized that the increasingly large number of RCTs of variable quality and differing results were seldom made available to clinicians in useful formats to improve practice. "It is surely a great criticism of our profession that we have not organised a critical summary, by specialty or subspecialty, adapted periodically, of all relevant randomised controlled trials" (Cochrane, 1979, p. 9). For this reason, the systematic review methodology has been gradually adopted and adapted to assist healthcare professionals take advantage of the overwhelming amount of information available in an effort to improve patient care and outcomes. According to the Cochrane Collaboration, which facilitates the production of healthcare systematic reviews and provides much helpful information on the Internet, the key characteristics of a systematic review are (Higgins & Green, 2011):

- A clearly stated set of objectives with predefined eligibility criteria for studies
- An explicit, reproducible methodology
- A systematic search that attempts to identify all studies that would meet the eligibility criteria
- A standardized assessment of the validity of the findings of the included studies, for example, through the assessment of risk of bias
- A systematic presentation of the synthesis of studies, including the characteristics and findings of the studies included in the review

A systematic review is a form of *secondary research* because it uses previously conducted studies. The study types discussed previously in this chapter would be *primary research* studies.

Because it is such an obviously different research approach, it requires unique critical appraisal questions to address the quality of a review.

> ❝
>
> Excellence is an art won by training and habituation. We do not act rightly because we have virtue or excellence, but we rather have those because we have acted rightly. We are what we repeatedly do. Excellence, then, is not an act but a habit.
>
> ARISTOTLE

Rapid Appraisal Questions for Systematic Reviews

Systematic reviews have multiple phases of development, with each one designed to reduce bias. This entire process requires attention to detail that can make it time-consuming and costly (O'Mathúna, Fineout-Overholt, & Kent, 2008). Clinicians have specific questions that they must ask in appraising a systematic review (Box 5.5), just as they should do with other study designs to determine their value for practice (O'Mathúna, 2010b). (Please note that the discussion of critical appraisal of systematic reviews follows a slightly different format than prior research design sections.)

BOX 5.5

Rapid Critical Appraisal Questions for Systematic Reviews

1. Are the results of the review valid?
   a. Are the studies contained in the review RCTs?
   b. Does the review include a detailed description of the search strategy to find all relevant studies?
   c. Does the review describe how validity of the individual studies was assessed (e.g., methodological quality, including the use of random assignment to study groups and complete follow-up of the participants)?
   d. Were the results consistent across studies?
   e. Were individual patient data or aggregate data used in the analysis?
2. What were the results?
   a. How large is the intervention or treatment effect (odd ratio, relative risk, effect size, level of significance)?
   b. How precise is the intervention or treatment effect (CI)?
3. Will the results assist me in caring for my patients?
   a. Are my patients similar to the ones included in the review?
   b. Is it feasible to implement the findings in my practice setting?
   c. Were all clinically important outcomes considered, including risks and benefits of the treatment?
   d. What is my clinical assessment of the patient and are there any contraindications or circumstances that would inhibit me from implementing the treatment?
   e. What are my patient's and his or her family's preferences and values about the treatment under consideration?

CI, confidence interval; RCTs, randomized controlled trials.

Are the Results of the Study Valid? (Validity)

Phase 1 of a systematic review identifies the clinical practice question to be addressed and the most suitable type of research design to answer it. The next step, Phase 2, develops inclusion criteria for the studies to be included and exclusion criteria for those studies that will not be included in the analysis. These steps are completed prior to gathering any evidence.

Once Phase 2 of planning is completed, Phase 3 begins the process of searching for and retrieving published and unpublished literature related to the study question. Rigorous search strategies are developed to ensure that research findings from all relevant disciplines and in all languages are found. Multiple computer databases (e.g., MEDLINE, CINAHL, Embase) are searched, and some researchers conducting systematic reviews will also search for conference proceedings, dissertations, and other "grey literature." Grey literature is unpublished studies or studies published by governmental agencies or other organizations that are not peer-reviewed (Higgins & Green, 2011). The section of the research report that discusses Phase 3 will answer the critical appraisal questions: Are the studies contained in the review RCTs? Does the review include a detailed description of the search strategy to find all relevant studies?

Are the Studies Contained in the Review RCTs? and Does the Review Include a Detailed Description of the Search Strategy to Find All Relevant Studies? Systematic reviews minimize bias by the way in which the literature pertaining to the research question is identified and obtained. The research literature comprises the raw data for a review. When appraising a systematic review, the clinician looks for a detailed description of the databases accessed, the search strategies used, and the search terms. Researchers conducting systematic reviews make many decisions about which databases to search, for which years, whether to include grey literature and non-English language studies. Each of these decisions has the potential to introduce bias, and should be carefully evaluated during critical appraisal of the resulting systematic review. To assist with this, reports of systematic reviews should be very detailed. The databases searched should be specified, as should the years searched. MEDLINE and CINAHL are probably the best-known healthcare publication databases used in such studies. Although these databases index thousands of journals, not all journals are indexed by any one database. Reviewers should indicate whether they limited the retrieved information to English language studies only. If they include only English language sources, they risk omitting studies that addressed their particular research question. For example, EMBASE is a European database of healthcare research that includes many studies in non-English languages. Some languages, such as Spanish, German, and Chinese, have their own journal databases. However, the cost of accessing these databases and translating non-English language papers may create challenges.

Search terms used should be clearly described so the reader of the systematic review can make an informed decision about whether all relevant publications were likely to be found. For example, a review of antibiotic therapy for otitis media might use the search terms *otitis media* and *glue ear*. However, *red ear* is also used commonly for this disorder, and omission of the term from the search strategy may lead to the review missing some studies. Most electronic databases provide an index or thesaurus of the best terms to use in searching, such as MeSH terms in MEDLINE (O'Mathúna et al., 2008).

Clinicians should be able to clearly see from the systematic review which studies were included and which were excluded. The studies are usually presented in a table format and provide clinicians with information about the study populations, settings, and outcomes measured. Ideally, included studies should be relatively homogeneous (i.e., the same) with respect to these aspects. Reasons for exclusion, such as study design or quality issues, also should be included in a table. The information presented in these tables assists clinicians to decide whether it was appropriate to combine the results of the studies.

Both published and unpublished research should be identified and retrieved where possible because of publication bias. This term applies to the finding that studies reporting positive or highly significant results have a greater chance of being published compared to those with nonsignificant results (*PLoS Medicine*, 2011). Publication bias arises for several reasons and means that the results of systematic reviews or meta-analyses that include only published results could be misleading. Including grey literature in the search strategy is one way to overcome publication bias. Reviewers will sometimes search relevant journals by hand, called hand searching, and examine the reference lists of previously retrieved papers for possible studies. In addition, reviewers might contact researchers in the field of interest to identify other studies, or to ask questions about a researcher's own publication if details were missing from the published report. This process of exhaustive literature retrieval can be time-consuming and costly, and clinicians need to consider whether the absence of such complete searching affects the conclusions drawn in the review.

Given publication bias, the failure to include unpublished studies is likely to exaggerate the size of any effect. One way researchers may indicate that they evaluated the presence of selection bias is through the use of a statistical test called the "funnel plot." This method is a scatterplot in which each study's sample size is plotted on the horizontal axis and each study's effect size is plotted on the vertical axis of the graph. When the risk of publication bias is low, a symmetrical inverted funnel is expected. An asymmetrical plot may indicate selection bias through the absence of some studies.

Does the Review Describe How Validity of the Individual Studies Was Assessed (e.g., Methodological Quality, Including the Use of Random Assignment to Study Groups and Complete Follow-Up of the Participants)? This question can be answered in the section addressing Phases 4 and 5 of a systematic review. These phases involve assessing the quality and validity of the included studies. The systematic review should report precisely how this was conducted and against what criteria evaluations were made. A clear report of how the review was conducted can assist clinicians in determining the worth of the gathered studies for practice.

The critical appraisal process itself shows that primary research is of varying quality. A rigorous, high-quality systematic review should base its primary conclusions only on high-quality studies. A clear description of the basis for quality assessment should be included in the review. Although a review with a rigorous methodology that includes only RCTs is considered the highest level of evidence for intervention questions, other clinical questions (e.g., questions of prognosis) that are not appropriate for an RCT design should also include the types of study designs that are most appropriate to answer those questions (e.g., cohort studies).

The systematic review report should inform clinicians about how data were extracted from the individual studies (Phase 6) and provide an overview of the evaluation of the included studies (Phase 7). Data should be extracted and the quality of included studies assessed independently by at least two members of the review team. The independent assessment further reduces the possibility of bias regarding evaluation of the studies. This process should be discussed in a systematic review as well as how the researchers resolved any disagreement they may have had regarding study findings.

Were the Results Consistent Across Studies? and Were Individual Patient Data or Aggregate Data Used in the Analysis? The studies included in a systematic review often have varying designs and inconsistent results, which may allow for only a descriptive evaluation of the studies. When studies are similar enough to be combined in a quantitative synthesis (e.g., comparing effect size, ORs), this can be very helpful to clinicians. The statistical approach to synthesizing the results of two or more studies is called a meta-analysis. A **meta-analysis**

is a quantitative systematic review, but not all systematic reviews are meta-analyses (Higgins & Green, 2011). When critically appraising these studies, clinicians must keep in mind that overviews or integrative reviews do not apply statistical analyses to the results across studies, generally because the studies are not amenable to that kind of analysis. Instead, these reviews or evidence syntheses often culminate in recommendations based on descriptive evaluations of the findings or they indicate to clinicians that the included studies on a given topic cannot be synthesized, for a myriad of reasons.

This section of the systematic review report is helpful in answering the critical appraisal questions about consistent results across studies and whether individual patient data or aggregate data are used in the analysis. The latter question reflects whether pooling the data was suitable or not from across the included studies. If it is possible (i.e., the researchers studied the same variables, defined them the same way, measured them the same way), given what you know about the sample size from your prior reading, consider how researchers could have more reliable findings with a larger pooled sample (e.g., 1,000) than 10 smaller samples (e.g., 100).

Chance alone would suggest that some variation will arise in the results of individual studies examining the same question. The differences in studies and the reported findings (i.e., heterogeneity) can be due to study design. Formal statistical methods can be used to test whether there is significant heterogeneity among the studies that precludes them being combined. Generally, reviewers will report using such a test. However, as with all statistical tests, statistical significance is not the same as clinical meaningfulness.

What Are the Results? (Reliability)

How Large Is the Intervention or Treatment Effect (e.g., NNT, NNH, Effect Size, Level of Significance)? and How Precise Is the Intervention or Treatment? Common statistics seen in systematic reviews are ORs and effect sizes. If the study is a meta-analysis, these values will assist the clinician in determining the magnitude of effect. The CI is the indicator of the preciseness of the study findings (i.e., can clinicians get what the researcher got, if they repeat the intervention?). A major advantage of a systematic review is the combining of results from many studies. In meta-analyses, combining the results of several studies produces a larger sample size and thus greater power to accurately determine the magnitude of the effect. Because of the strength of this type of evidence, this relatively new methodology has become a hallmark of EBP (Stevens, 2001).

Meta-analysis is the statistical method used to obtain a single-effect measure of the summarized results of all studies included in a review. Although the technique may sound complicated, clinicians do not require even moderate understanding of the mathematics involved in such methods. A solid understanding of how to interpret the results is what is needed. The meta-analysis of a number of trials recognizes how sample size of the studies may influence findings and, thereby, provides a more precise estimate of treatment effect than individual studies. A "forest plot" (Figure 5.8) is a diagrammatic representation of the results of trials included in a meta-analysis, along with their CIs. You can now apply what you learned from the explanation of OR and CI given earlier in this chapter. In the forest plot, each square is the measure of effect of an individual study, and the horizontal line shows its CI. The larger the square, the more important the contribution of that particular study is to the meta-analysis (Lewis & Clarke, 2001). The diamond at the bottom of the forest plot is the summary treatment effect of all studies, with the vertical points of the diamond being the result and the horizontal points of the diamond being the CI for that overall result.

To interpret these data, clinicians must consider the outcome first. If there is no difference in outcomes between the treatment and control groups, the resulting OR is 1.0. If the CI crosses the line of no treatment effect (OR = 1.0), the study is not statistically significant. If the outcome is something you do not want (e.g., death, pain, or infection), a square to

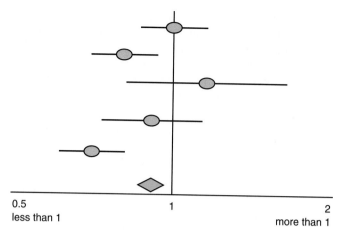

Figure 5.8: Example of a forest plot.

the right of the line means that the treatment was worse than the control in the trial (i.e., there were more deaths in the treated group compared to the comparison or control group). Usually, this is not the desired result. For a negative outcome, the desired result is to see the treatment decrease the outcome, and this would be reflected in a square to the left of the line of no effect. A square to the left of the line means that the treatment was better, which is what would be desired for outcomes you want (e.g., stopping smoking or continuation of breast-feeding).

The forest plot gives a way to make an informed estimate of study homogeneity. A forest plot with study estimates that are scattered all over and have wide CIs suggests excessive heterogeneity in the measurement and precision of effect. Bringing together all of the studies to answer a particular clinical question provides important information; however, studies are often too dissimilar to combine their results. If possible, reviewers can quantify the effectiveness of the intervention in a summary statistic that can be compared across these studies. Alternatively, the studies may not be of sufficient quality to combine or compare, which provides information to researchers regarding the need for additional high-quality research.

Clinicians must also watch for reports in which reviewers have analyzed by subgroups when no overall effect was found. Study subsets may be analyzed on the basis of particular patient demographics or methodological quality of the included studies. However, in such an analysis, the purpose of the initial randomization to treatment and control groups in the underlying studies is essentially lost because the balance afforded by randomization does not extend to subgroupings generated after the fact. However, some subgroup analyses may be legitimate. For example, if an overall effect is found, but individual studies varied widely in quality, subgroup analysis based on study quality may be warranted and important. For example, researchers conducting a meta-analysis of chromium supplements for diabetes found some beneficial outcomes, but when subgroup analyses were conducted based on study quality, those studies with the lowest quality had significantly more favorable outcomes than the high-quality studies (Balk, Tatsioni, Lichtenstein, Lau, & Pittas, 2007). This suggests that the overall beneficial results of the meta-analysis were unduly influenced by low-quality studies, and therefore the overall results of the meta-analysis should be applied with caution in clinical practice.

Another tool for clinicians is a sensitivity analysis, which is done to help determine how the main findings may change as a result of pooling the data. It involves first combining the results of all the included studies. The studies considered of lowest quality or unpublished studies are then excluded, and the data are reanalyzed. This process is repeated sequentially, excluding studies until only the studies of highest quality are included in the analysis. An alteration in the overall results at any point in study exclusion indicates how sensitive the conclusions are to the quality of the studies included.

The final issue for clinicians in critically appraising this portion of a systematic review is to determine if the reviewers justified their conclusions. EBP requires integrating the best evidence with clinical expertise and patient values, choices, and concerns. Poor-quality systematic reviews exist, just as there are poor-quality primary studies. Clinicians need to ask whether the interpretations of the reviewers are justified and valid based on the strength of the evidence presented in the review.

Will the Results Help Me in Caring for My Patients? (Applicability)

The final questions in critically appraising systematic reviews are: (a) Are my patients similar to the ones included in the review? (b) Is it feasible to implement the findings in my practice setting? (c) Were all clinically important outcomes considered, including risks and benefits of the treatment? (d) What is my clinical assessment of the patient and are there any contra-indications or circumstances that would inhibit me from implementing the treatment? and (e) What are my patient's and his or her family's preferences and values about the treatment under consideration? Common sense may appear to answer some of the questions, but without careful attention to the details, important application issues can be missed.

Interpreting the Results of a Study: Example Six

You are thinking of establishing an early discharge program for first-time mothers, but are concerned that such a program may be associated with unplanned readmissions for breast-feeding-related problems. You find three RCTs with different sample sizes. The smallest study ($n = 50$) reports that there is no difference in readmissions between the early discharge and routine length of stay groups. A study with a larger sample size ($n = 100$) reports an increase in readmissions in the experimental group. The study with the largest sample size ($n = 1,000$) reports an increase in readmissions in the control group. All three studies are rigorously conducted trials with very similar patient demographics. How can these three studies be synthesized for clinical decision making?

While the study with the larger sample size is more likely to capture the variation in the reference population and thus represent a more accurate estimation of the effect of such a program, the other studies need to be considered as well, as they may have small samples, but clinically meaningful results. Ideally, you would like to have a meta-analysis that combines the results of all three studies and pools the study samples. This would provide a sample size of 1,150 and important evidence to guide decision making.

Clinical Scenario 5.5

Nursing staff on your unit in a residential elder care facility have just completed an audit of falls in the previous 12 months. A total of 45 falls were documented during the period, but the actual number could have been higher. Interested and concerned clinicians meet to discuss the results and consider options for reducing this incidence. A few people bring copies of trials with them that discuss the efficacy of fall prevention programs that incorporated various interventions. All the trials look like high-quality studies, but they all show different results. Which one to believe? It would be nice to have one study that summarizes all the available evidence for you and presents the implications for clinical practice.

What the Literature Says: Answering a Clinical Question

The following study may help answer the clinical question for Clinical Scenario 5.5. In older adults living in residential care facilities **(P)**, how do fall prevention programs **(I)** compared to no fall prevention **(C)** affect fall rates **(O)** within the first quarter after program completion **(T)**? Cameron et al. (2012) conducted a systematic review in which the objective was to assess the effects of interventions designed to reduce the incidence of falls in older people in care facilities and hospitals. The literature search was conducted on the Cochrane Bone, Joint and Muscle Trauma Group Specialised Register (March 2012), the Cochrane Library (2012, Issue 3), MEDLINE (1966 to March 2012), EMBASE (1988 to March 2012), CINAHL (1982 to March 2012), and ongoing trial registers (to August 2012). A hand search of reference lists of articles was conducted, and field researchers were contacted. The selection criterion was that studies had to be randomized trials of interventions designed to reduce falls in older people in residential or nursing care facilities or in hospitals. The primary outcomes of interest were the rates or numbers of falls or numbers of fallers. Trials reporting only intermediate outcomes (like improved balance) were excluded. The data collection and analysis methods involved two reviewers independently assessing the trial quality and extracting data. Data were pooled using the **fixed effect model** where appropriate. In the fixed effect model, it is assumed that the event rates are fixed in both control and treatment groups. Therefore, if the event rates have any variation, this can be attributed to chance.

> If the trials being combined are truly clinically homogeneous and have been designed properly (for example, with balanced arms), which is the situation that will commonly pertain, then in this (and only in this) case it is appropriate to pool raw data.
>
> (Moore, Gavaghan, Edwards, Wiffen, & McQuay, 2002, p. 3)

The systematic review included 60 trials, 43 in care facilities and 17 in hospitals. Thirteen trials tested exercise interventions, but the results were inconsistent, and overall meta-analysis showed no significant differences between intervention and control groups in either rate of falls or risk of falls. However, post hoc subgroup analysis by level of care showed reduced falls in intermediate-level facilities and increased falls in high-level facilities. Vitamin D supplementation reduced the rate of falls but not the risk of falling. Multifactorial interventions showed some benefit in reducing falls in hospitals, but their impact on risk of falling was inconclusive. Many different interventions were tested in different trials, making it difficult to determine the effectiveness of any individual component.

The reviewers' conclusions were that interventions to prevent falls that are likely to be effective are now available. Costs per fall prevented have been established for four of the interventions. Some potential interventions are of unknown effectiveness, and further research is indicated.

Are the Results of the Study Valid? (Validity)

Only RCTs that met quality inclusion criteria were included in the review. A large number of databases were searched, and both English and non-English language sources were searched. Two reviewers independently assessed the quality of trials and extracted the data. Tables of included and excluded studies were provided. These methods produced valid results.

What Are the Results? (Reliability)

A rate ratio (RaR) with 95% CI was used to compare rates of falls and an RR with 95% CI for the risk of falling. For the trials testing exercise interventions, no significant differences were found for the rate of falls (RaR = 1.03; 95% CI, 0.81 to 1.31) or risk of falling (RR = 1.07; 95% CI, 0.94 to 1.23). In both cases, the 95% CI crosses the line of no effect at 1. Similar statistics were reported for the other intervention groupings and subgroup analyses. However, because the subgroup analysis by level of care was conducted post hoc (and not a priori), the results should be interpreted somewhat cautiously. The overall protocol was published prior to completion of the review (standard practice for Cochrane reviews), and the pooled study results were tested for heterogeneity. The results of the review can be viewed as reliable.

Will the Results Help Me in Caring for My Patients? (Applicability)

Although there was variation in the study settings, types of patients, and interventions included in this review, the authors provided a description of the circumstances in which a particular intervention may be beneficial. Economic outcomes were not reported, and there were no trials of reducing the serious consequences of falls. Given the clinical question of reducing falls in an elder care facility, the evidence is applicable.

❝

Be a yardstick of quality. Some people aren't used to an environment where excellence is expected.

STEVE JOBS

EVALUATION AND SYNTHESIS: FINAL STEPS IN CRITICAL APPRAISAL

Once each study that was retrieved from the systematic search has been rapidly critically appraised and the keeper studies have been determined, the next phase of critical appraisal begins—evaluation. Evaluation is digging deeper into each of the studies in the body of evidence to determine how well they agree. The agreement across studies is then melded together into a synthesis upon which to base practice and standards of care. Clinical decisions at the point of care may use already synthesized or synopsized resources, as described in Chapter 3; however, when sustainable practice changes are required, careful evaluation and synthesis of evidence are necessary. To provide best care, we must act on what we currently know and understand from what we synthesize as the best available evidence (Fineout-Overholt, 2008). The PICOT question is the driver for the evaluation table and synthesis tables. The goal is to find the answer to the question.

Evaluation

All studies should be evaluated using a single evaluation table that contains several columns with the essential elements of evaluation listed as headings (see evaluation table template in Appendix C). Each of these elements is discussed below. In rare occurrences, there may be other elements that clinicians feel are important to their studies that can be added. The purposes of evaluation include capturing the data from each study to (1) ensure there is no need to search the volume of articles in the body of evidence more than one time and (2) establish patterns across studies.

Citation

In the first column of the evaluation table, enter each study's first author, date of publication, and title of the article. To put all of the citation information in the column will clutter it with too much detail. Parsimony is required for evaluation data. Too much information, or information in complete sentences, clogs the table and slows the comparison across studies process.

Purpose of the Study

The purpose of the study is entered into the second column. Evidence users need to know why the study was conducted. Sometimes, the study purpose is not clearly stated. In those cases, consider the research question, hypotheses, or specific aims of the study to help identify the purpose of the study. The purpose is the general reason why the study was conducted; the study aims are more specific about what is to be accomplished within the study and the research question/hypotheses are reflective of the relationships expected within the study. Consider how to abbreviate the elements of the purpose, aims, and research questions/hypotheses to allow a rapid comparison across studies. Finding those studies that have similar purposes, aims, and research questions/hypotheses is the first commonality for synthesis.

Conceptual Framework

The third column in the evaluation table is the conceptual (or theoretical) framework that underpins the research. A brief explanation of how the framework guides the research is helpful for clinicians because that same framework would guide translation of the research into practice. However, often the research is **atheoretical**, that is, without a guiding framework. Without a guiding framework, the conduct of the study is guided by a hunch. Whether guided by a conceptual framework or not, the primary focus for researchers has to be on sound methodology.

It is important to note that there may be some varied perspectives on the importance of conceptual or theoretical guidance for conducting research that is reflected in bodies of evidence. Some disciplines hold conceptual basis for how research is conducted as an essential, such as nursing, and other disciplines do not consider this as a foundational research principle, such as medicine. Whether or not a given discipline values a conceptual basis for research, if one is provided, it is important to consider it in critical appraisal. If a common framework has underpinned studies within the table, it provides guidance as clinicians consider how to apply a body of evidence.

Study Design and Method

Users of evidence must identify the study research design. Sometimes this is clearly defined in the report and sometimes it is not. If it is not, consider the GAO elements first to determine the study design (see resources available on thePoint®). To help gain mastery in understanding markers for identifying specific research methods, review the critical appraisal checklists in Appendix B.

A brief description of research methods (i.e., what they did in the study) helps in evaluation and synthesis. This description focuses primarily on the protocol for the intervention or identification so that these can be compared as well as used for making the recommendation in the last phase of appraisal.

Sample and Setting

Describing the sample is imperative for critical appraisal. The sample size that was defined in the GAO, along with the sample characteristics, needs to be extracted onto the evaluation table. Succinctly placed information allows for quickly comparing samples across studies.

Where a study is conducted (i.e., the setting) is of utmost importance. Comparing the study settings will enable users to understand how broadly the issue has been investigated as well as identify the populations to which the study findings can be applied. As with all information within the evaluation table, using succinct abbreviations to convey the information will allow for easy comparison.

Major Variables Studied and Definitions

The major variables in the studies are either the IV, the intervention or the issue of interest, or the DV or outcome. In this column, the abbreviation of IV and DV is used to identify these variables. In addition, they are numbered if more than one exists, for example, IV1 and IV2, DV1 and DV2.

The second piece of information in this column should be all the conceptual definitions of these variables. These are important because without them it may be unclear whether or not different studies included exactly the same IV or DV. Unfortunately, sometimes, conceptual definitions are not provided by researchers.

Measurement of Major Variables

How the DVs are measured is called the operational definition for the variable. The operational definitions of the outcome variables are critical. If they are different, then, in essence, the DVs are different. Furthermore, the IVs often have certain operational definitions that are important to understand, such as blood pressure as a predictor variable of heart disease. Without a description of how the variables were measured, the studies cannot be adequately compared.

Data Analysis

Although many statistics may be reported in a study, the data analysis column requires only those statistics that assist you in answering the PICOT question. List only the statistic, such as "*t*-test," that would be used to compare differences between groups. Remember to keep information within the table succinct. Another caveat is that it is not appropriate to place the statistical software used to conduct that analyses in this column.

Study Findings

As with data analysis, only the findings that are relevant to the clinical question should be placed in the table. For each statistic listed in the Data Analysis column, there should be a corresponding numerical result. It is appropriate to provide the variable and then the result. For example, DV1: $t = 1.83$, $p < 0.063$. This column should never contain a conclusion. Another example would be, if the statistic was an OR for DV2, the finding would be the value of the OR, along with the p value or CI, DV2: $OR = 0.54$; 95% CI, 0.33 to 0.67.

Worth to Practice

This is the column where evidence users enter the information that reflects the appraisal information demonstrating the study's worth to practice, beginning with the level of evidence. The strength of the evidence (i.e., level of evidence + quality [study methods, strengths, and limitations]) is key to understanding its benefit to practice. The risk, or harm, if the study interventions or findings are implemented should be carefully described. Clinical expertise is required to best convey this information. Next, indicate the feasibility of using the findings of this study in practice. Consider sustainability of the study findings, as well as simple implementation issues that could stymie the worth to practice. For example, consider that political issues, cultural issues, or financial issues could prevent the findings from being feasible or sustainable.

Once all of these pieces are entered into the worth to practice column, it is important to consider using standardized methodology to compare across studies using standardized criteria (e.g., United States

Preventive Services Task Force [USPSTF] GRADE criteria) or whether to evaluate the studies without such criteria.

 There is grading criteria posed by the USPSTF grading schema:
https://www.uspreventiveservicestaskforce.org/Page/Name/grade-definitions

As evidence users consider the value of the studies to practice, they also should consider if there are any gems or caveats in the studies that would help in comparing across them or help with implementation of the body of evidence, for example, a protocol list or barriers to implementation list. The final two pieces in the worth to practice column include (1) the evidence user's conclusions regarding the message from the study findings (i.e., not the researchers' conclusion) and (2) the recommendation the evidence user must make based on the data across the columns about the use of the study to practice. If the evidence user is PhD prepared or studying in a PhD program, recommendations for further research can be made. However, clinicians using this recommendation indicate that there was insufficient evidence to guide practice. The options for next steps include making a recommendation for one of the following, 1) clinicians with PhD-prepared scientists to study the clinical issue, 2) quality monitoring using evidence-based quality improvement strategies, or 3) benchmarking with what is known from research and other like clinical agencies.

 To gain mastery in understanding evaluation of a body of evidence, review the online completed evaluation table: http://download.lww.com/wolterskluwer_vitalstream_com /PermaLink/AJN/A/AJN_110_11_2010_10_12_AJN_0_SDC1.pdf

Keep the order of information placed in the table clear and simple so that comparisons across studies are easily synthesized. Process the information from the left side of the table to the right. As information is entered into the table, consider the information in studies below and above. Some suggestions to make the table user-friendly are to (a) use abbreviations (e.g., RCT) with a legend for interpretation, (b) keep the order of the information the same in each study (e.g., a variable is abbreviated MS consistently across studies and when entered into the variable column would appear at the top of the variables section for each study), and (c) place similar statistics in the same order in each study for easy comparison (Fineout-Overholt, 2008). Appendix C contains a template for an evaluation table.

Synthesis

Synthesis starts as clinicians enter the study data into the evaluation table (Fineout-Overholt, 2008). Each study is compared to the others for how it agrees or disagrees with the others in the table. Fineout-Overholt (2008) outlines some principles of synthesis that can assist clinicians in making determinations about how to use the data extracted from across the studies. One of the principles of synthesis is making decisions about which study details and findings need to be synthesized. The clinical question drives this decision making. Often, clinicians can cluster studies around different aspects of methods or findings (e.g., study design, interventions, outcome measurement, or findings). Synthesis requires thoughtful consideration of inconsistencies as well as consistencies across studies. These can give great insights into what is not known, what is known, and what researchers need to focus on to improve the body of evidence to address a particular clinical question. Pulling together the conclusions or major findings from a study can be of great help in clinical decision making. In addition, carefully discussing how studies' strengths, limitations, and level of evidence match or do not match can assist in the final conclusion regarding what should be done in practice. Synthesis tables are the best way to formulate and communicate the information that is essential for comparison across studies. To gain mastery in understanding how to construct a synthesis table, review Table 5.8. A caveat about synthesis is in order here: Synthesis is not reporting the findings of consecutive studies (sometimes referred to as reporting study-by-study); rather, it is combining, contrasting, and interpreting a body of evidence (i.e., the gestalt) to reach a conclusion about what is known and what should be done with that knowledge to improve healthcare outcomes, which adds confidence to the final step of critical appraisal, making recommendations for practice.

Evaluation and synthesis tables differ in that evaluation tables contain information about each individual study, whereas synthesis tables contain only those aspects of the individual studies that are common or unique across studies (e.g., level of evidence, study design, outcomes). Such tables should have the advantages of clarity and simplicity. Synthesis tables enable clinicians to confidently make clinical decisions about the care that is provided to their patients by making evidence from studies readily useable for clinical decision making (Fineout-Overholt, 2008). Chapter 9 speaks to implementation of evidence, which is the next step after critical appraisal (i.e., RCA, evaluation, synthesis, and recommendations).

Recommendations

The final phase of critical appraisal is formulating recommendations for practice based on the body of evidence. These recommendations are not tentative; they are clear, definitive

---

TABLE 5.8   *Example of a Synthesis Table*

Sample Clinical Question: In adolescents at risk for depression (P), how does relaxation and visual imagery (I1) and/or music (I2) compared to yoga (C) affect depression (O) over 5 months (T)?*

Study Author	Year	Number of Participants	Mean Age (or Other Sample Characteristic That Is Pertinent to Your Question)	Study Design	Intervention	Major Finding That Addresses Your Question and Direction of Outcome
Carrigan	2018	15	15	R	Yoga	↓ D
Johnson	2015	280	17	Q	Relaxation/ visual imagery	— D
Meade	2016	51	19	Q	Music	↓ D
Smith	2012	1,400	14	R	Relaxation/ visual imagery + music	↑ D

*Example is hypothetical.

D, depression; Q, quasi-experimental study; R, randomized controlled trial (all studies measured depression using the Beck Depression Scale); ↓, decreased; ↑, increased; —, no effect.

evidence-based statements of best practice that are expected of all clinicians. Recommendations guide implementation, so the statements should include what should be done, any information about how it should be done, and what outcome(s) should be expected. Also, recommendations apply to all patients in the population. In evidence implementation, there is no sample, informed consent, or comparison group; therefore, these should not be part of a recommendation. The recommendation should be implemented because the evidence indicates with confidence that when the intervention is delivered or issue is addressed as it is in the studies, the outcomes are predictable. For example, in the American Journal of Nursing EBP Step-by-Step Series, the recommendation could be that all acute care organizations should implement rapid response teams on all shifts and monitor code rates and code-associated mortality rates prior to implementation and on a monthly basis for the expected reduction in these outcomes. Organizations with limited budgetary resources should train and expect code teams also to serve as rapid response teams (Fineout-Overholt et al., 2010a, 2010b, 2010c). In this example, the body of evidence supported these clear recommendations; however, this is not always the case. Recommendations must match the support the body of evidence provides. If the evidence cannot support a definitive recommendation, then the recommendation could be to continue current practice and monitor practice outcomes as well as the literature for further studies. Furthermore, if the evidence user is a PhD-prepared scientist or PhD student, the recommendation may be to conduct research to strengthen a weak body of evidence; however, this is not an acceptable recommendation for clinicians. Providing a recommendation is the fourth and final phase of critical appraisal and without this phase, critical appraisal is not complete.

CONCLUSIONS

Evidence-based healthcare decision making requires the integration of clinical expertise with the best available research evidence and the patients' values, concerns, and choices. To do this, clinicians must develop skills in critically appraising available research studies and applying the findings to practice. This begins by matching the appropriate research design to the clinical question asked. Assessing the validity and reliability of study findings by evaluating how well researchers used study design principles in their studies enables clinicians to understand how studies agree or disagree within a body of evidence. Accessing and regularly using one of the many available critical appraisal guides will build mastery skills in critical appraisal. Strong evidence results in strong recommendations that facilitate appropriate use of research in practice; however, not all bodies of evidence are strong. Nonetheless, recommendations must follow evaluation and synthesis of the evidence. Completing the four phases of critical appraisal will boost clinicians' confidence to act on existing evidence to improve healthcare outcomes, thereby helping clinicians learn more about the scientific basis for health management and lead to best practice decision making.

❝

Thinking is the hardest work there is, which is probably the reason why so few [choose to] engage in it . . . If you think you can do a thing or think you can't do a thing, you're right.

HENRY FORD

EBP FAST FACTS

- There are four phases of critical appraisal that are focused on finding the worth of research to practice (1) RCA, in which studies that should be retained, called keeper studies, are identified; (2) evaluation, in which data are extracted from individual studies to establish agreement across studies; (3) synthesis, in which data are pulled together to paint the picture of what the body of evidence tells us; and (4) recommendation, in which next steps for practice are clearly articulated for all patients who are within the population described in the question.
- EBP requires critical appraisal of all studies before they are used to influence clinical decision making, even if they are published in high-impact, peer-reviewed journals.
- The three key questions to ask of all studies: (1) Are the results valid? (2) What are the results? and (3) Are the results helpful in caring for my patients?
- Additional questions should be asked of each study; these questions are study design specific and reflect the research methodology that defines a good study.
- Some knowledge of how to interpret statistics is required to appraise research studies, especially distinguishing between statistical significance and clinical significance.
- Having critically appraised relevant studies, the final step in critical appraisal is to make a recommendation from the synthesized study findings that guides using them to influence practice and standards of care.

WANT TO KNOW MORE?

A variety of resources are available to enhance your learning and understanding of this chapter.

- Visit thePoint® to access:
  - Articles from the AJN EBP Step-By-Step Series
  - Journal articles
  - Checklists for rapid critical appraisal and more!
- Lippincott CoursePoint combines digital text content with video case studies and interactive modules for a fully integrated course solution that works the way you study and learn.

References

Awada, A., & al Jumah, M. (1999). The first-of-Ramadan headache. *Headache, 39*(7), 490–493.

Aylin, P., Alexandrescu, R., Jen, M. H., Mayer, E. K., & Bottle, A. (2013). Day of week of procedure and 30 day mortality for elective surgery: Retrospective analysis of hospital episode statistics. *British Medical Journal, 346,* f2424.

Balk, E. M., Tatsioni, A., Lichtenstein, A. H., Lau, J., & Pittas, A. G. (2007). Effect of chromium supplementation on glucose metabolism and lipids: A systematic review of randomized controlled trials. *Diabetes Care, 30*(8), 2154–2163.

Barratt, A., Wyer, P. C., Hatala, R., McGinn, T., Dans, A. L., Keitz, S., . . . For, G. G.; Evidence-Based Medicine Teaching Tips Working Group. (2004). Tips for learners of evidence-based medicine: 1. Relative risk reduction, absolute risk reduction and number needed to treat. *Canadian Medical Association Journal, 171*(4), 353–358.

Benson, K., & Hartz, A. J. (2000). A comparison of observational studies and randomized, controlled trials. *New England Journal of Medicine, 342*(25), 1878–1886.

Boffetta, P., McLaughlin, J. K., La Vecchia, C., Tarone, R. E., Lipworth, L., & Blot, W. J. (2008). False-positive results in cancer epidemiology: A plea for epistemological modesty. *Journal of the National Cancer Institute, 100*(14), 988–995.

Bono, C. M., & Tornetta III, P. (2006). Common errors in the design of orthopaedic studies. *Injury, 37*(4), 355–360.

Bracken, M. B., Shepard, M. J., Holford, T. R., Leo-Summers, L., Aldrich, E. F., Fazl, M., . . . Young, W. (1997). Administration of methylprednisolone for 24 or 48 h or tirilazad mesylate for 48 h in the treatment of acute spinal cord injury. Results of the Third National Acute Spinal Cord Injury Randomized Controlled Trial. National Acute Spinal Cord Injury Study. *Journal of the American Medical Association, 277*(20), 1597–1604.

Brignardello-Petersen, R., Carrasco-Labra, A., Glick, M., Guyatt, G. H., & Azarpazhooh, A. (2015). A practical approach to evidence-based dentistry: III: How to appraise and use an article about therapy. *Journal of the American Dental Association, 146*(1), 42–49.

Brower, R. G., Lanken, P. N., MacIntyre, N., Matthay, M. A., Morris, A., Ancukiewicz, M., . . . Thompson, B. T.; National Heart, Lung, and Blood Institute ARDS Clinical Trials Network. (2004). Higher versus lower positive end-expiratory pressures in patients with the acute respiratory distress syndrome. *New England Journal of Medicine, 351*(4), 327–336.

Bundred, N., Maguire, P., Reynolds, J., Grimshaw, J., Morris, J., Thomson, L., . . . Baildam, A. (1998). Randomised controlled trial of effects of early discharge after surgery for breast cancer. *British Medical Journal, 317*(7168), 1275–1279.

Callas, P. W., & Delwiche, F. A. (2008). Searching the biomedical literature: Research study designs and critical appraisal. *Clinical Laboratory Science, 21*(1), 42–48.

Cameron, I. D., Gillespie, L. D., Robertson, M. C., Murray, G. R., Hill, K. D., Cumming, R. G., & Kerse, N. (2012). Interventions for preventing falls in older people in care facilities and hospitals. *Cochrane Database of Systematic Reviews, 12*, CD005465.

CAPRIE Steering Committee. (1996). A randomised, blinded, trial of clopidogrel versus aspirin in patients at risk of ischaemic events (CAPRIE). *Lancet, 348*(9038), 1329–1339.

Chalmers, T. C., Celano, P., Sacks, H. S., & Smith, H., Jr. (1983). Bias in treatment assignment in controlled clinical trials. *New England Journal of Medicine, 309*(22), 1358–1361.

Chan, K. (2007). A clinical trial gone awry: The Chocolate Happiness Undergoing More Pleasantness (CHUMP) study. *Canadian Medical Association Journal, 177*(12), 1539–1541.

Chapman, S., Azizi, L., Luo, Q., & Sitas, F. (2016). Has the incidence of brain cancer risen in Australia since the introduction of mobile phones 29 years ago? *Cancer Epidemiology, 42*, 199–205.

Cochrane, A. L. (1979). 1931–1971: A critical review, with particular reference to the medical profession. In G. Teeling-Smith & N. Wells (Eds.), Medicines for the year 2000 (pp. 1–11). London, UK: Office of Health Economics.

Coleman, W. P., Benzel, E., Cahill, D., Ducker, T., Geisler, F., Green, B., . . . Zeidman, S. (2000). A critical appraisal of the reporting of the National Acute Spinal Cord Injury Studies (II and III) of methylprednisolone in acute spinal cord injury. *Journal of Spinal Disorders, 13*(3), 185–199.

Concato, J., Shah, N., & Horwitz, R. I. (2000). Randomized, controlled trials, observational studies, and the hierarchy of research designs. *New England Journal of Medicine, 342*(25), 1887–1892.

Devereaux, P. J., Manns, B. J. H., Ghali, W. A., Quan, H., Lacchetti, C., Montori, V. M., . . . Guyatt, G. H. (2001). Physician interpretations and textbook definitions of blinding terminology in randomized controlled trials. *Journal of the American Medical Association, 285*(15), 2000–2003.

Eldridge, S. M., Ashby, D., Feder, G. S., Rudnicka, A. R., & Ukoumunne, O. C. (2004). Lessons for cluster randomized trials in the twenty-first century: A systematic review of trials in primary care. *Clinical Trials, 1*(1), 80–90.

Farrell, S., Barker, M. L., Walanski, A., & Gerlach, R. W. (2008). Short-term effects of a combination product night-time therapeutic regimen on breath malodor. *Journal of Contemporary Dental Practice, 9*(6), 1–8.

Fergusson, D. M., Horwood, L. J., & Ridder, E. M. (2005). Tests of causal linkages between cannabis use and psychotic symptoms. *Addiction, 100*(3), 354–366.

Fethney, J. (2010). Statistical and clinical significance, and how to use confidence intervals to help interpret both. *Australian Critical Care, 23*(2), 93–97.

Fineout-Overholt, E. (2008). Synthesizing the evidence: How far can your confidence meter take you? *AACN Advanced Critical Care, 19*(3), 335–339.

Fineout-Overholt, E., Melnyk, B. M., Stillwell, S. B., & Williamson, K. M. (2010a). Evidence-based practice, step by step: Critical appraisal of the evidence: Part I. *The American Journal of Nursing, 110*(7), 47–52.

Fineout-Overholt, E., Melnyk, B. M., Stillwell, S. B., & Williamson, K. M. (2010b). Evidence-based practice, step by step: Critical appraisal of the evidence: Part II: Digging deeper—Examining the "keeper" studies. *The American Journal of Nursing, 110*(9), 41–48.

Fineout-Overholt, E., Melnyk, B. M., Stillwell, S. B., & Williamson, K. M. (2010c). Evidence-based practice, step by step: Critical appraisal of the evidence: Part III. *The American Journal of Nursing, 110*(11), 43–51.

Fineout-Overholt, E., O'Mathúna, D. P., & Kent, B. (2008). Teaching EBP: How systematic reviews can foster evidence-based clinical decisions: Part I. *Worldviews on Evidence-Based Nursing, 5*(1), 45–48.

Gagnier, J. J., & Morgenstern, H. (2017). Misconceptions, misuses, and misinterpretations of P values and significance testing. *Journal of Bone and Joint Surgery, 99*(18), 1598–1603.

Gangwisch, J. E., Feskanich, D., Malaspina, D., Shen, S., & Forman, J. P. (2013). Sleep duration and risk for hypertension in women: Results from the nurses' health study. *American Journal of Hypertension, 26*(7), 903–911.

George, B. J., Beasley, T. M., Brown, A. W., Dawson, J., Dimova, R., Divers, J., . . . Allison, D. B. (2016). Common scientific and statistical errors in obesity research. *Obesity, 24*(4), 781–790.

Goodacre, S. (2008). Critical appraisal for emergency medicine 2: Statistics. *Emergency Medicine Journal, 25*(6), 362–364.

Greenland, S., Senn, S. J., Rothman, K. J., Carlin, J. B., Poole, C., Goodman, S. N., & Altman, D. G. (2016). Statistical tests, P values, confidence intervals, and power: A guide to misinterpretations. *European Journal of Epidemiology, 31*(4), 337–350.

Guyatt, G., Rennie, D., Meade, M. O., & Cook, D. J. (2015). *Users' guide to the medical literature: A manual for evidence-based clinical practice* (3rd ed.). New York, NY: McGraw Hill.

Häfner, H., Hambrecht, M., Löffler, W., Munk-Jøgensen, P., & Riecher-Rössler, A. (1998). Is schizophrenia a disorder of all ages? A comparison of first episodes and early course across the life-cycle. *Psychological Medicine, 28*(2), 351–365.

Hardell, L., Carlberg, M., & Hansson Mild, K. (2013). Use of mobile phones and cordless phones is associated with increased risk for glioma and acoustic neuroma. *Pathophysiology, 20*(2), 85–110.

He, Z., & Fineout-Overholt, E. (2016). Understanding confidence intervals helps you make better clinical decisions. *American Nurse Today, 11*(3), 39–58.

Herbst, A. L., Ulfelder, H., & Poskanzer, D. C. (1971). Adenocarcinoma of the vagina: Association of maternal stilbestrol therapy with tumor appearance in young women. *New England Journal of Medicine, 284*(15), 878–881.

Higgins, J. P. T., & Green, S. (Eds.). (2011). *Cochrane handbook for systematic reviews of interventions, Version 5.1.* Retrieved from http://training.cochrane.org/handbook

Howland, R. H. (2011). Publication bias and outcome reporting bias: Agomelatine as a case example. *Journal of Psychosocial Nursing and Mental Health Services, 49*(9), 11–14.

Inskip, P., Tarone, R., Hatch, E., Wilcosky, T., Shapiro, W., Selker, R., . . . Linet, M. S. (2001). Cellular-telephone use and brain tumors. *New England Journal of Medicine, 344*(2), 79–86.

Ioannidis, J. P. A., Haidich, A. B., Pappa, M., Pantazis, N., Kokori, S. I., Tektonidou, M. G., . . . Lau, J. (2001). Comparison of evidence of treatment effects in randomized and nonrandomized studies. *Journal of the American Medical Association, 286*(7), 821–830.

Johnston, L. J., & McKinley, D. F. (2000). Cardiac tamponade after removal of atrial intracardiac monitoring catheters in a pediatric patient: Case report. *Heart and Lung, 29*(4), 256–261.

Kaptchuk, T. J., Friedlander, E., Kelley, J. M., Sanchez, M. N., Kokkotou, E., Singer, J. P., . . . Lembo, A. J. (2010). Placebos without deception: A randomized controlled trial in irritable bowel syndrome. *PLoS ONE, 5*(12), e15591.

Kirson, N. Y., Weiden, P. J., Yermakov, S., Huang, W., Samuelson, T., Offord, S. J., . . . Wong, B. J. (2013). Efficacy and effectiveness of depot versus oral antipsychotics in schizophrenia: Synthesizing results across different research designs. *Journal of Clinical Psychiatry, 74*(6), 568–575.

Kunz, R., & Oxman, A. D. (1998). The unpredictability paradox: Review of empirical comparisons of randomised and nonrandomised clinical trials. *British Medical Journal, 317*(7167), 1185–1190.

Lafreniere, K. D., Mutus, B., Cameron, S., Tannous, M., Giannotti, M., Abu-Zahra, H., & Laukkanen, E. (1999). Effects of therapeutic touch on biochemical and mood indicators in women. *Journal of Alternative and Complementary Medicine, 5*(4), 367–370.

Lenzer, J. (2006). Study break: NIH secrets. *The New Republic.* Retrieved from https://newrepublic.com /article/65022/national-institutes-health-fred-geisler-spinal-cord

Lenzer, J., & Brownlee, S. (2008). An untold story? *British Medical Journal, 336*(7643), 532–534.

Lewis, S., & Clarke, M. (2001). Forest plots: Trying to see the wood and the trees. *British Medical Journal, 322*(7300), 1479–1480.

Loher-Niederer, A., Maccora, J., & Ritz, N. (2013). Positive linking: A survival guide on how to keep up-to-date with pediatric infectious diseases literature using internet technology. *Pediatric Infectious Disease Journal, 32*(7), 786–787.

MacMahon, B., Yen, S., Trichopoulos, D., Warren, K., & Nardi, G. (1981). Coffee and cancer of the pancreas. *New England Journal of Medicine, 304*(11), 630–633.

Melnyk, B. M., Fineout-Overholt, E., & Mays, M. (2008). The evidence-based practice beliefs and implementation scales: Psychometric properties of two new instruments. *Worldviews on Evidence-Based Nursing, 5*(4), 208–216.

Melnyk, B. M., Morrison-Beedy, D., & Cole, R. (2015). Generating evidence through quantitative research. In B. Melnyk & E. Fineout-Overholt (Eds.), *Evidence-based practice in nursing & healthcare: A guide to best practice* (pp. 439–475). Philadelphia, PA: Wolters Kluwer.

Miguel, D., Gonzalez, N., Illing T., & Elsner, P. (2018). Reporting quality of case reports in international dermatology journals. *British Journal of Dermatology, 178*(1), e3–e4. doi:10.1111/bjd.15696

Moore, R., Gavaghan, D., Edwards, J., Wiffen, P., & McQuay, H. (2002). Pooling data for number needed to treat: No problems for apples. *BMC Medical Research Methodology, 2*, 2.

Muscat, J., Malkin, M., Thompson, S., Shore, R., Stellman, S., McRee, D., . . . Wynder, E. L. (2000). Handheld cellular telephone use and risk of brain cancer. *Journal of the American Medical Association, 284*(23), 3001–3007.

O'Mathúna, D. P. (2010a). The role of systematic reviews. *International Journal of Nursing Practice, 16*(2), 205–207.

O'Mathúna, D. P. (2010b). Critical appraisal of systematic reviews. *International Journal of Nursing Practice, 16*(4), 414–418.

O'Mathúna, D. P., Fineout-Overholt, E., & Kent, B. (2008). Teaching EBP: How systematic reviews can foster evidence-based clinical decisions: Part II. *Worldviews on Evidence-Based Nursing, 5*(2), 102–107.

Papanikolaou, P. N., Christidi, G. D., & Ioannidis, J. P. A. (2006). Comparison of evidence on harms of medical interventions in randomized and nonrandomized studies. *Canadian Medical Association Journal, 174*(5), 635–641.

PLoS Medicine (Ed.). (2011). Best practice in systematic reviews: The importance of protocols and registration. *PLoS Medicine, 8*(2), e1001009.

Polit, D., & Beck, C. (2016). *Nursing research: Generating and assessing evidence for nursing practice* (10th ed.). Philadelphia, PA: Lippincott Williams & Wilkins.

Reed, C. E., & Fenton, S. E. (2013). Exposure to diethylstilbestrol during sensitive life stages: A legacy of heritable health effects. *Birth Defects Research. Part C, Embryo Today, 99*(2), 134–146.

Riley, D. S., Barber, M. S., Kienle, G. S., Aronson, J. K., von Schoen-Angerer, T., Tugwell, P., . . . Gagnier, J. J. (2017). CARE guidelines for case reports: Explanation and elaboration document. *Journal of Clinical Epidemiology, 89*, 218–235.

Rossouw, J. E., Anderson, G. L., Prentice, R. L., LaCroix, A. Z., Kooperberg, C., Stefanick, M. L., . . . Ockene, J.; Writing Group for the Women's Health Initiative Investigators. (2002). Risks and benefits of estrogen plus progestin in healthy postmenopausal women: Principal results from the Women's Health Initiative randomized controlled trial. *Journal of the American Medical Association, 288*(3), 321–333.

Ruiz-Canela, M., Martínez-González, M. A., & de Irala-Estévez, J. (2000). Intention to treat analysis is related to methodological quality [letter]. *British Medical Journal, 320*(7240), 1007–1008.

Schulz, K. F. (1995). Subverting randomization in controlled trials. *Journal of the American Medical Association, 274*(18), 1456–1458.

Schulz, K. F., & Grimes, D. A. (2002a). Allocation concealment in randomised trials: Defending against deciphering. *Lancet, 359*(9306), 614–618.

Schulz, K. F., & Grimes, D. A. (2002b). Generation of allocation sequences in randomised trials: Chance, not choice. *Lancet, 359*(9305), 515–519.

Singal, A. G., Higgins, P. D., & Waljee, A. K. (2014). A primer on effectiveness and efficacy trials. *Clinical and Translational Gastroenterology, 5*, e45.

Stampfer, M. J., & Colditz, G. A. (1991). Estrogen replacement therapy and coronary heart disease: A quantitative assessment of the epidemiologic evidence. *Preventive Medicine, 20*(1), 47–63.

Stevens, K. R. (2001). Systematic reviews: The heart of evidence-based practice. *AACN Clinical Issues, 12*(4), 529–538.

Swift, T. L. (2012). Sham surgery trial controls: Perspectives of patients and their relatives. *Journal of Empirical Research on Human Research Ethics, 7*(3), 15–28.

Torgerson, D. J. (2001). Contamination in trials: Is cluster randomisation the answer? *British Medical Journal, 322*(7282), 355–357.

Troisi, R., Hatch, E. E., Titus-Ernstoff, L., Hyer, M., Palmer, J. R., Robboy, S. J., . . . Hoover, R. N. (2007). Cancer risk in women prenatally exposed to diethylstilbestrol. *International Journal of Cancer, 121*(2), 356–360.

Turati, F., Galeone, C., Edefonti, V., Ferraroni, M., Lagiou, P., La Vecchia, C., & Tavani, A. (2012). A meta-analysis of coffee consumption and pancreatic cancer. *Annals of Oncology, 23*(2), 311–318.

Turner, T. L., Balmer, D. F., & Coverdale, J. H. (2013). Methodologies and study designs relevant to medical education research. *International Review of Psychiatry, 25*(3), 301–310.

University College London. (2011). *Critical appraisal of a journal article*. Retrieved from https://www.ucl.ac.uk/ich/support-services/library/training-material/critical-appraisal

Wasserstein, R. L., & Lazar, N. A. (2016). The ASA's Statement on *p*-values: Context, process, and purpose. *American Statistician, 70*(2), 129–133.

World Health Organization. (2014). *Electromagnetic fields and public health: Mobile phones*. Retrieved from http://www.who.int/mediacentre/factsheets/fs193/en

6 Critically Appraising Qualitative Evidence for Clinical Decision Making

Mikki Meadows-Oliver

> What is important is to keep learning, to enjoy challenge, and to tolerate ambiguity. In the end, there are no certain answers.
>
> —*Martina Horner*

EBP Terms to Learn

Basic social process (BSP)
Constant comparison
Culture
Emic
Essences
Etic
Fieldwork
Key informants
Lived experience
Participant observation
Pragmatism
Saturation
Symbolic interaction
Theoretical sampling

Learning Objectives

After studying this chapter, learners will be able to:

1. Discuss the impact qualitative evidence has on clinical decisionmaking.

2. Describe the role qualitative studies have in helping answer clinical questions that address the *how* of healthcare interventions.

3. Discuss the unique language and concepts that are encountered in the qualitative literature.

4. Discuss appropriate critical appraisal criteria for qualitative evidence that are required to accurately translate these studies into practice.

All scientific evidence is important to clinical decision making, and all evidence must be critically appraised to determine its contribution to that decision making. Part of critical appraisal is applying clinicians' understanding of a field of science to the content of a research report, that is, how well the research answers the clinical question (for more on clinical questions, see Chapter 2). Qualitative evidence may not be as familiar to clinicians as quantitative evidence—methods, language, and especially how it can be useful in guiding practice. Qualitative evidence is defined as information that is narrative, reflective, or anecdotal, and requires judgment to interpret the data. Qualitative evidence answers clinical questions about the human experience, such as how mothers with physical disabilities perceive their mothering experiences during their children's infancy. Answering these types of questions can provide clinicians with the *why* for practice, whereas answering questions that require quantitative evidence tends to provide the *how*. Therefore, this chapter offers information to help clinicians with principles and queries for appraising of qualitative evidence for clinical decision making, including the following:

- Language and concepts that will be encountered in the qualitative literature;
- Aspects of qualitative research known to have raised concerns for readers less familiar with different qualitative methods;
- Issues surrounding the use of evaluative criteria that, if not understood, could lead to their misuse in the appraisal of studies and subsequent erroneous conclusions.

With adequate knowledge, clinicians can extract what is good and useful to clinical decision making by applying appropriate method-specific and general appraisal criteria to qualitative research reports. Glossary boxes are provided throughout the chapter to assist the reader understand common terms and concepts that support and structure the chapter discussion.

It is important for clinicians to gain the knowledge and ability required to appreciate qualitative studies as sources of evidence for clinical decision making. As with all knowledge, application is the best way to gain proficiency. Readers are invited to review a demonstration of how to use the rapid critical appraisal checklist in Box 6.1 with a variety of sample articles found in Appendix D (available on thePoint'). Reading these articles is the best way to fully appreciate how to apply the checklist. Firsthand appraisal of qualitative studies requires active engagement with the evidence. This chapter prepares clinicians to engage with and move beyond the material presented to apply it when appraising the research in their particular fields of practice.

"

Learning is not attained by chance; it must be sought for with ardor and attended to with diligence.

ABIGAIL ADAMS

BOX
6.1 *Rapid Critical Appraisal of Qualitative Evidence*

Are the results valid/trustworthy and credible?

1. How were study participants chosen?
2. How were accuracy and completeness of data assured?
3. How plausible/believable are the results?

Are implications of the research stated?

1. May new insights increase sensitivity to others' needs?
2. May understandings enhance situational competence?

What is the effect on the reader?

1. Are the results plausible and believable?
2. Is the reader imaginatively drawn into the experience?

What were tµhe results of the study?

1. Does the research approach fit the purpose of the study?

How does the researcher identify the study approach?

1. Are language and concepts consistent with the approach?
2. Are data collection and analysis techniques appropriate?

Is the significance/importance of the study explicit?

1. Does review of the literature support a need for the study?
2. What is the study's potential contribution?

Is the sampling strategy clear and guided by study needs?

1. Does the researcher control selection of the sample?
2. Do sample composition and size reflect study needs?
3. Is the phenomenon (human experience) clearly identified?

Are data collection procedures clear?

1. Are sources and means of verifying data explicit?
2. Are researcher roles and activities explained?

Are data analysis procedures described?

1. Does analysis guide direction of sampling and when it ends?
2. Are data management processes described?
3. What are the reported results (description or interpretation)?

How are specific findings presented?

1. Is presentation logical, consistent, and easy to follow?
2. Do quotes fit the findings they are intended to illustrate?

How are the overall results presented?

1. Are meanings derived from data described in context?
2. Does the writing effectively promote understanding?

Will the results help me in caring for my patients?

1. Are the results relevant to persons in similar situations?
2. Are the results relevant to patient values and/or circumstances?
3. How may the results be applied in clinical practice?

THE CONTRIBUTION OF QUALITATIVE RESEARCH TO DECISION MAKING

In the past, critical appraisal seems to have been the portion of the evidence-based practice (EBP) process that has received the most attention, with efforts focusing on helping clinicians develop their skills in retrieving, critically appraising, and synthesizing largely quantitative studies. There is growing awareness, however, that qualitative research provides clinicians with guidance in deciding how findings from quantitative studies can be applied to patients. Qualitative research can also help clinicians understand clinical phenomena with emphasis on understanding the experiences and values of patients (Straus, Richardson, Glasziou, & Haynes, 2010). Clinical practice questions that focus on interventions, risk, and etiology require different hierarchies of evidence that do not designate qualitative evidence as "best evidence" (for more on hierarchies [Levels] of evidence and associated clinical questions, see Chapter 2). Multiple types of qualitative research are present in cross-disciplinary literature. When addressing a meaning question (i.e., about the human experience), synthesis of qualitative research is considered Level 1 evidence—the top of the hierarchy. Knowledge derived from syntheses of qualitative and quantitative research evidence to answer respective clinical questions enables the integration of all elements of EBP in a manner that optimizes clinical outcomes. Therefore, both a challenge and an opportunity are present for clinicians—to utilize the appropriate evidence to answer their questions about quality patient care.

Expanding the Concept of Evidence

Given that healthcare is an intervention-driven industry, from its inception as a clinical learning strategy used at Canada's McMaster Medical School in the 1980s, clinical trials and other types of intervention research have been a primary focus of EBP. Also, the international availability of systematic reviews (for more information on systematic reviews, see Chapter 5) provided by the Cochrane Collaboration and the incorporation of intervention studies as evidence in clinical decision support systems have made this type of evidence readily available to point-of-care clinicians. Previously, when compared with quasi-experimental and nonexperimental (i.e., comparative, correlational, and descriptive) designs, randomized controlled trials (RCTs) easily emerged as the designated gold standard for determining the effectiveness of a treatment. The one-size-fits-all "rules of evidence" (determination of weakest to strongest evidence with a focus on the effectiveness of interventions) often used to dominate discussions within the EBP movement. That has been minimized with new hierarchies of evidence that help identify the best evidence for different kinds of questions. Now, evidence hierarchies that focus on quantitative research provide the guidance for selection of studies evaluated in EBP reviews to answer **intervention** questions. In turn, evidence hierarchies focused on qualitative research guide selection of studies to answer meaning questions.

Nevertheless, the use of qualitative studies remains less clear than is desirable for clinical decision making. Often clinicians and researchers consider that intervention strength-of-evidence pyramids (i.e., a rating system for the hierarchy of evidence) are universal for all types of clinical questions. In this hierarchy, qualitative studies continue to be ranked as weaker forms of evidence at or near the base of the pyramids, along with descriptive, evaluative, and case studies, with the strongest research design being RCTs at or near the apex. When this hierarchy of evidence is used to address meaning questions, qualitative research genres are misrepresented because applying the linear approach used to evaluate intervention studies does not fit the divergent purposes and nonlinear nature of qualitative research traditions and designs.

We know that systematic reviews of RCTs provide best evidence for intervention questions. Best evidence for diagnosis and prognosis questions are systematic reviews of descriptive prospective cohort studies. Grace and Powers (2009) proposed some time ago that recognition of two additional question domains is important to delivery of patient-centered care: human response and meaning. The strongest evidence to answer these questions arises from qualitative research traditions. This supports the use of different evidence hierarchies for different types of questions (see Chapter 2 for more information on levels of evidence that are appropriate for different types of questions).

Furthermore, a need to balance scientific knowledge gained through empirical research with practice-generated evidence and theories in clinical decision making is part of the work of expanding the concept of evidence. For several years, nurse leaders have been calling for evidence to include theoretical sources, such as ethical standards and philosophies, personal experiences, and creative, aesthetic arts (Fawcett, Watson, Neuman, Hinton-Walker, & Fitzpatrick, 2001).

Efforts to expand the concept of evidence are consistent with fundamental tenets of the EBP movement. A clear example is the conceptual framework put forward in this chapter, in which the goal of EBP is the successful integration of the following elements of clinical care (see Figure 1.2):

- Best research (e.g., valid, reliable, and clinically relevant) evidence;
- Clinical expertise (e.g., clinical skills, past experience, interpretation of practice-based evidence [PEB]);
- Patient values (e.g., unique preferences, concerns, and expectations);
- Patient circumstances (e.g., individual clinical state, practice setting, and organizational culture).

Recognizing Research Relevant to Practice

Science and art come together in the design and execution of qualitative studies. For clinicians to critically appraise qualitative research, they must have an appreciation for and basic knowledge of its many methodologies and practices, which are rooted in the social and human sciences. Questions asked by qualitative researchers are influenced by the focus of qualitative traditions on in-depth understanding of human experiences and the contexts in which the experiences occur.

In the health sciences, knowledge generated by qualitative studies may contain theoretical bases for explicit (specific) interventions. However, more often, qualitative studies promote better understanding of what health and illness situations are like for people, how they manage, what they wish for and expect, and how they are affected by what goes on around them. These valuable insights must influence how clinicians practice. For example, heightened sensitivity or awareness of healthcare experiences from patients' vantage points may lead to changes in how clinicians deliver their care for those persons. Furthermore, understanding these vantage points may prompt reflection on and discussions about practical actions that would be important not only on an individual basis, but also on a larger scale.

Significant growth in qualitative health science literature over recent decades has occurred at least in part because these approaches were capable of addressing many kinds of questions that could not be answered by other research methods. Because of the expansion and evolution of qualitative methods, clinicians across disciplines will encounter a more varied mix of articles on different clinical topics. Therefore, to keep up to date on the latest developments in their fields, clinicians need to be able to recognize and judge the validity of relevant qualitative as well as quantitative research studies.

> **"**
>
> The heights by great men reached and kept were not obtained by sudden flight. But they, while their companions slept, were toiling upward in the night.
>
> HENRY WADSWORTH LONGFELLOW

SEPARATING WHEAT FROM CHAFF

When we critically appraise a study, we are separating the wheat from the chaff (imperfections) so that only the good and useful remains. There are no perfect studies, so the task becomes one of sifting through and deciding whether good and useful elements outweigh a study's shortcomings. To critically appraise qualitative research reports, readers need a sense of the diversity that exists within this field (i.e., a flavor of the language and mindset of qualitative research) to appreciate what is involved in using any set of criteria to evaluate a study's validity (or trustworthiness) and usefulness. This decreases the possibility of misconstruing such criteria because of preconceived notions about what they signify and how they should be used. The sections that follow provide brief overviews of how qualitative approaches differ and a synthesis of basic principles for evaluating qualitative studies.

Managing Diversity

Qualitative research designs and reporting styles are very diverse. In addition, there are many ways to classify qualitative approaches. Therefore, it is necessary to be able to manage this diversity through an awareness of different scientific traditions and associated research methods and techniques used in qualitative studies.

External Diversity Across Qualitative Research Traditions

Qualitative research traditions have origins within academic disciplines (e.g., the social sciences, arts, and humanities) that influence the language, theoretical assumptions, methods, and styles of reporting used to obtain and convey understanding about human experiences.

Therefore, despite similarities in techniques for data gathering and management, experiences are viewed through different lenses, studied for different purposes, and reported in language and writing styles consistent with the research tradition's origins. Among qualitative traditions commonly used in health sciences research (i.e., research about healthcare) are ethnography, grounded theory, phenomenology, and hermeneutics.

Ethnography. Ethnography involves the study of a social group's **culture** through time spent combining **participant observation** (Box 6.2), in-depth interviews, and the collection of artifacts (i.e., material evidence of culture) in the informants' natural setting. This appreciation of culture—drawing on anthropologic (i.e., human development) theory and practice—provides the context for a better understanding of answers to specific research questions. For example, cultural understanding may help answer questions about the following:

- The provision of psychosocial care to children with cancer (Brage & Vindrola-Padros, 2017); parental experiences of caring for a child with attention deficit hyperactivity disorder (ADHD) (Laugesen, Lauritsen, & Jorgensen, 2017);
- Communication between physicians and nurses (Michel, 2017); communication between nurses during patient hand-offs (Bunkenborg, Hansen, & Holge-Hazelton, 2017);
- Patterns of behavior in families of critically ill patients in the emergency room (Barreto, Marcon, & Garcia-Vivar, 2017); the use of health information technology in the ICU (Leslie, Paradis, & Gropper, 2017).

Fieldwork is the term that describes all research activities taking place in or in connection with work in the study setting (i.e., field). These activities include the many social and personal skills required when gaining entry to the field, maintaining field relationships, collecting and analyzing data, resolving political and ethical issues, and leaving the field. Researchers may have **key informants** (in addition to other informants) who help them establish rapport and learn about cultural norms. Research reports are descriptions and interpretations that attempt to capture study informants' **emic** points of view balanced against the researcher's **etic** analytic perspectives (De Chesnay, 2015).

Grounded Theory. The purpose of grounded theory, developed by sociologists Glaser and Strauss (1967), is to generate a theory about how people deal with life situations grounded in empirical data and that describes the processes by which they move through experiences

---

BOX
6.2   *Ethnography Research Terms*

Culture: Shared knowledge and behavior of people who interact within distinct social settings and subsystems.

Participant observation: The active engagement (i.e., observation and participation) of the researcher in settings and activities of people being studied (i.e., everyday activities in study of informants' natural settings).

Fieldwork: All research activities carried out in and in relation to the field (informants' natural settings).

Key informant: A select informant/assistant with extensive or specialized knowledge of his/her own culture.

Emic and etic: Contrasting "insider" (emic) views of informants and the researcher's "outsider" (etic) views.

Grounded Theory Research Terms

Symbolic interaction: Theoretical perspective on how social reality is created by human interaction through ongoing, taken-for-granted processes of symbolic communication.

Pragmatism: Theoretical perspective that problems of truth and meaning need to be arrived at inductively; understood in terms of their utility and consequences; and modified to fit the circumstances of time, place, and the advent of new knowledge.

Constant comparison: A systematic approach to analysis that is a search for patterns in data as they are coded, sorted into categories, and examined in different contexts.

Theoretical sampling: Decision making, while concurrently collecting and analyzing data, about the data and data sources that are needed further to develop the emerging theory.

Saturation: The point at which categories of data are full and data collection ceases to provide new information.

Core variable: A theoretical summarization of a process or pattern that people go through in specified life experiences.

over time. Movement is often expressed in terms of stages or phases (e.g., stages/phases of living with a chronic illness, adjusting to a new situation, or coping with challenging circumstances). For example, Lawler, Begley, and Lalor (2015) studied the transition process to motherhood for women with a disability using grounded theory. In another example, Babler and Strickland (2015) used grounded theory to describe the experiences of adolescents transitioning to successful diabetes self-management. Philosophical underpinnings of this tradition are **symbolic interaction** and **pragmatism** (Wuest, 2012; see Box 6.3). Data collection and analysis procedures are similar to those of ethnographic research, but the focus is on symbolic meanings conveyed by people's actions in certain circumstances, resultant patterns of interaction, and their consequences.

The goal is to discover a core variable through procedures of constant comparison and theoretical sampling. **Constant comparison** is coding, categorizing, and analyzing incoming data while consistently seeking linkages by comparing informational categories with one another and with new data. **Theoretical sampling** directs data gathering toward **saturation** of categories (i.e., completeness).

The *core variable*, or **basic social process (BSP)**, is the basis for theory generation. It recurs frequently, links all the data together, and describes the pattern followed, regardless of the various conditions under which the experience occurs and different ways in which persons go through it. In the literature, the reader may encounter terms that are used to further describe the types of BSP (e.g., a basic social psychological process [BSPP] and a basic social structural process [BSSP]). Researchers will typically describe the meaning of these terms within the context of the study. For example, Quinn (2016) described the BSP of *becoming someone different* in early through late stages of their pregnancies to help explain how nurses in the United States navigated the various transitions they experienced as they integrated pregnancy and 12-hour shift work.

Phenomenology. Phenomenology is the study of **essences** (i.e., meaning structures, Box 6.4) intuited or grasped through descriptions of **lived experience**. Husserl's philosophy described lived experience (i.e., the lifeworld) as understandings about life's meanings that lie outside a person's conscious awareness. Thus, in studying the meaning, or essence, of an experience

Phenomenology/Hermeneutics Research Terms

Essences: Internal meaning structures of a phenomenon grasped through the study of human lived experience.

Lived experience: Everyday experience, not as it is conceptualized, but as it is lived (i.e., how it feels or what it is like).

Introspection: A process of recognizing and examining one's own inner state or feelings.

Bracketing: Identifying and suspending previously acquired knowledge, beliefs, and opinions about a phenomenon.

Phenomenological reduction: An intellectual process involving reflection, imagination, and intuition.

Hermeneutics: Philosophy, theories, and practices of interpretation.

(phenomenon), researchers need to recognize their own personal feelings (**introspection**) and suspend their beliefs about what the experience is like (**bracketing**), particularly if they are using the Husserlian approach to phenomenology. Interpretive insights are derived by collecting experiential descriptions from interviews and other sources and engaging in intellectual analytic processes of reflection, imagination, and intuition (**phenomenological reduction**). Use of certain philosophers' perspectives to direct the analysis (e.g., Husserl, Heidegger, Merleau-Ponty) can affect methodological processes.

Phenomenology, represented as a school of thought within philosophy, offers perspectives shaped through ongoing intellectual dialogs rather than explicit procedures. Descriptions of research processes have come from outside the parent discipline of philosophy. Processes often cited are as follows:

- The philosophically, language-oriented, descriptive-interpretive phenomenology of educator Max van Manen (the German Dilthey-Nohl and the Dutch Utrecht schools of phenomenological pedagogy). An example of this type of phenomenology would be a study of the experience of young adults who grew up infected with perinatally acquired human immunodeficiency virus (Williams et al., 2017).
- The empirical descriptive approaches of the Duquesne school of phenomenological psychology (i.e., Giorgi, Colaizzi, Fischer, and van Kaam). An example of this type of phenomenology would be a study of nurses' experiences of caring for people with intellectual disability and dementia (Cleary & Doody, 2016).

In writing about the usefulness of phenomenology in nursing research, Matua (2015) states that phenomenology is commonly used to expand the understanding of human phenomena relevant to nursing practice. Examples of phenomena of interest to clinical researchers include what various illness experiences are like for persons or how a sense of hope, trust, or being understood is realized in their lives. Insights offered through research reports range in style from lists of themes and straightforward descriptions (i.e., empiric descriptions) to philosophical theorizing and poetizing (i.e., interpretations).

Hermeneutics. Hermeneutics has a distinct philosophical history as a theory and method of interpretation (originally associated with the interpretation of Biblical texts). However, various philosophers (e.g., Dilthey, Heidegger, Gadamer, Hirsch, and Ricoeur) have contributed to its development beyond a focus on literal texts to viewing human lived experience as a text that is to be understood through the interpreter's dialogical engagement (i.e., thinking that is like a thoughtful dialog or conversation) with life.

There is not a single way to practice hermeneutics. A variety of theories and debates exists within the field. However, although separated by tradition, it may also be associated with phenomenology and certain schools of phenomenological thought. Thus, *hermeneutic phenomenology* sometimes is the terminology used to denote orientations that are interpretive, in contrast to, or in addition to, being descriptive (van Manen, 1990/1997). For instance, Feeley and Thomson (2016) draw on the hermeneutic traditions of Heidegger and Gadamer in their study exploring factors that influence women to give birth without a trained professional present. The complex realities of women's decisionmaking experiences regarding childbirth are presented. Clinicians can obtain a fuller appreciation of how hermeneutic research contributes to understanding clinical practice through firsthand reading of these types of reports, engaging reflectively with the actual words of the written text, and experiencing the total effect of the narrative.

Internal Diversity Within Qualitative Research Traditions

Qualitative research traditions vary internally as well as externally. For example, there are several reasons why ethnographic, grounded theory or phenomenological accounts may assume a variety of forms, including

- when a tradition acts as a vehicle for different representational styles and theoretical or ideological conceptualizations;
- when historical evolution of a tradition results in differing procedural approaches;
- when studies differ individually in terms of their focus on description, interpretation, or theory generation.

Representation and Conceptualization. **Representation** of research findings (i.e., writing style, including authorial voice and use of literary forms and rhetorical devices) should not be a matter of dictate or personal whim. Rather, it is part of the analytic process that, in qualitative research, gives rise to a great variety of representational styles. Both classic and more recent journal articles and books have been devoted to the topic of representation (Denzin, 2014; Morse, 2007; Richardson, 1990; Sandelowski, 1998b, 2004, 2007; Van Maanen, 1988; van Manen, 1990/1997, 2002; Wolcott, 2009). Qualitative research reports may be conversational dialogs. They may contain researchers' personal reflections and accounts of their experiences; poetry, artistic, and literary references; hypothetical cases; or fictional narratives and stories based on actual data, using study informants' own words in efforts to increase sensitivity and enhance understanding of a phenomenon.

Although researchers should not abuse artistic license, readers should also not see a research report as unconventional if that report is enriched by using an alternative literary form as a faithful representation that best serves a legitimate analytic purpose. If the representation is meaningful to the reader, it meets a criterion of analytic significance in keeping with the scholarly norms of these traditions. For example, qualitative researchers have used photovoice (i.e., combines photography with community-based participatory research) to make research findings more accessible and relevant to select audiences (Colon-Ramos, Monge-Rojas, & Cremm, 2017; Gilbert, 2017; Wahab, Mordiffi, Ang, & Lopez, 2017). An additional example of different representational strategies in qualitative health research is the use of *autoethnography* (i.e., personal/autobiographical experience). Haugh (2016) conducted an autoethnography that represented her journey into motherhood and her first experiences with breastfeeding her newborn infant.

Some standard forms of representation also are used with ethnographic, phenomenological, and grounded theory designs to bring out important dimensions of the data. For example, Creswell (2013) discussed how case studies and biography could serve as adjuncts to these types of studies as well as traditions in their own right.

Major qualitative traditions may also be vehicles for distinctive theoretical or ideological concepts. For example, a critical ethnography combines ethnographic methods with methods of **critical inquiry** or cultural critique. The reader should expect to find an integration of empirical analysis and theory related to a goal of emancipation from oppressive circumstances or false ideas. Ross, Rogers, and Duff (2016) note that critical ethnography is suitable for studies involving vulnerable populations and workplace culture. For example, Batch and Windsor (2015) conducted a critical ethnography of the culture of communication for nurses in a healthcare facility.

Similarly, feminist research, traditionally, has focused critique on issues of gender and gender inequity/inequality (Flick, 2014). However, a feminist perspective may be brought to bear on research interest in any area of social life that would benefit from the establishment of collaborative and nonexploitative relationships and sensitive, ethical approaches. For those conducting research from a feminist perspective, Im (2013) provided 10 categories that can be used as guidelines for designing the research project. Among these are guidelines regarding gender and ethnic diversity in a research team, getting participant feedback, and the contextual interpretation of study findings. Regarding gender and ethnic diversity, the author stated, "contemporary feminist researchers trust that researchers from both genders could understand women's experience through multiple methods (e.g., self-reflection)" (p. 141). Im (2013) stressed the importance of getting participant feedback because "the findings of feminist research should be viewed by the research participants as their own experience, opinions, values, and attitudes" (p. 142). Additionally, she implored feminist researchers to consider the contextual interpretation of study findings. She stated that when interpreting study findings, "feminist researchers need to consider what are the sociopolitical and cultural contexts of the study findings rather than simply interpreting study findings from an objective stance" (p. 143). Similarly, **feminist epistemologies** emphasize these tenets from a ways of knowing or theory of knowledge point of view (Box 6.5).

BOX **6.5**	*General Qualitative Research Terms*

Representation: Part of the analytic process that raises the issue of providing a truthful portrayal of what the data represent (e.g., essence of an experience; cultural portrait) that will be meaningful to its intended audience.

Case study: An intensive investigation of a case involving a person or small group of people, an issue, or an event.

Biography: An approach that produces an in-depth report of a person's life. Life histories and oral histories also involve gathering of biographical information and recording of personal recollections of one or more individuals.

Critical inquiry: Cultural critique guided by theories/approaches to the study of power interests between individuals and social groups, often involving hegemony (domination or control over others) associated with ideologies that operate to create oppression and constrain multiple competing interests in order to maintain the status quo.

Feminist epistemologies: A variety of views and practices inviting critical dialog about issues arising in areas of social life that involve such concerns as inequality, neglect of diversity, exploitation, insensitivity, and ethical behavior.

BOX
6.6

General Qualitative Research Terms

Interpretive ethnography: Loosely characterized as a movement within anthropology that generates many hybrid forms of ethnographic work because of crossing a variety of theoretical boundaries within social science.

Axial coding: A process used to relate categories of information by using a coding paradigm with predetermined subcategories in one approach to grounded theory (Corbin & Strauss, 2014; Strauss & Corbin, 1990).

Emergence: Glaser's (1992) term for conceptually driven ("discovery") versus procedurally driven ("forcing") theory development in his critique of Strauss and Corbin (1990).

Theoretical sensitivity: A conceptual process to accompany techniques for generating grounded theory (Glaser, 1978).

Discourse analysis: Study of how meaning is created through the use of language (derived from linguistic studies, literary criticism, and semiotics).

Semiotics: The theory and study of signs and symbols applied to the analysis of systems of patterned communication.

Sociolinguistics: The study of the use of speech in social life.

Critical theory: A blend of ideology (based on a critical theory of society) and a form of social analysis and critique that aims to liberate people from unrecognized myths and oppression in order to bring about enlightenment and radical social change.

Historical Evolution. Use over time may refine, extend, or alter and produce variations in the practice of a research tradition. One example of this within anthropology is the developing interest in **interpretive ethnography** (Box 6.6). This occurred as researchers crossed disciplinary boundaries to combine theoretical perspectives from practices outside the discipline to inform their work (e.g., the humanistic approaches of phenomenology and hermeneutics; **discourse analysis**, evolving from **semiotics** and **sociolinguistics**; and **critical theory**). Of course, said influencing practices may also be qualitative approaches in their own right. For example, Mosman, Poggenpoel, and Myburgh (2015) use interpretive phenomenology and ethnography to describe the life stories of women who perceived rejection from the mothers. Findings revealed that these women had difficulty forming and sustaining relationships with others because of that perceived rejection.

Another example of historical evolution within a tradition began with controversy between Glaser and Strauss, the originators of grounded theory over Strauss's interpretation of the method (Corbin & Strauss, 2014; Strauss & Corbin, 1990, 1998), which included *axial coding*, a procedure not featured in earlier texts (Chenitz & Swanson, 1986; Glaser, 1978; Glaser & Strauss, 1967). When appraising qualitative evidence, clinicians may see axial coding, which involves the use of a prescribed coding paradigm with predetermined subcategories (e.g., causal conditions, strategies, context, intervening conditions, and consequences) intended to help researchers pose questions about how categories of their data relate to one another. All qualitative researchers did not embrace this new technique. Glaser (1978, 1992) indicated that coding should be driven by conceptualizations about data. These and other concerns (e.g., inattention to earlier developed ideas about BSPs and saturation of categories) led Glaser to assert that Strauss and Corbin's model is a new method no longer oriented to the discovery, or **emergence**, of the grounded theory method as originally conceived by Strauss and himself (Melia, 1996).

These and subsequent developments in grounded theory offer clear choices not only between Straussian and Glaserian methods of analysis, but also between both Glaser's and

Strauss and Corbin's versions and other approaches that expand its interpretive possibilities, because a growing number of scholars apply grounded theory's basic guidelines to research agendas that involve a wider variety of philosophical perspectives and theoretical assumptions (Charmaz, 2014). For clinicians, it is important to note which approach was used in conducting the research to fully understand the interpretation of the data.

Description, Interpretation, and Theory Generation. Qualitative researchers amass many forms of data: recorded observations (fieldnotes), interview tapes and transcripts, documents, photographs, and collected or received artifacts from the field. There are numerous ways to approach these materials.

All researchers write descriptively about their data (i.e., the empirical evidence). The act of describing necessarily involves interpretation of the facts of an experience through choices made about what to report and how to represent it. Researchers also refer to Geertz's (1973) notion of **thick description** (as opposed to thin description; Box 6.7) as what is needed for interpretations. Thick description not only details reports of what people say and do, but also incorporates the textures and feelings of the physical and social worlds in which people move and—always with reference to that context—an interpretation of what their words and actions mean. Although Sandelowski (2004) wrote that "thick description" is a phrase that "ought not to appear in write-ups of qualitative research at all" (p. 215), researchers continue to apply the phrase to qualitative research descriptions. Hengst, Devanga, and Mosier (2015) discussed the use of thick versus thin descriptions when analyzing the translatability into practice of research about the lifeworlds of people with acquired communication disorders. These researchers found that there were more published communication sciences and disorder studies using thin description than thick, making evidence translation potentially challenging for clinicians.

Describing meaning in context is important because it is a way to try to understand what informants already know about their world. Informants do not talk about what they take for granted (i.e., tacit, personal knowledge) because their attention is not focused on it. And sometimes what they do is different from what they say because everyday actions in familiar settings also draw on tacit understanding of what is usual and expected. Thick descriptions attempt to take this into account. They are the researcher's interpretations of what it means to experience life from certain vantage points through written expression that is "artful and evocative" as well as "factual and truthful" (Van Maanen, 1988, p. 34).

It is the researcher's choice to report research findings in more factual, descriptive terms (allowing the empirical data to speak for itself) or more interpretive terms (drawing out the evidence that illuminates circumstances, meanings, emotions, intentions, strategies, and motivations). However, this mostly is a matter of degree for researchers whose work in a designated tradition tends to push them toward more in-depth interpretation. Additionally, the venue and intended audiences influence decisions about how to represent research findings.

Theory generation also is a proper goal in ethnography and an essential outcome in grounded theory. In these traditions, theories are empirical, evidence-based explanations of how cultural, social, and personal circumstances account for individuals' actions and interactions with others. Analyzed data supply the evidence on which the theories are grounded.

BOX
6.7   *General Qualitative Research Terms*

Thick description: Description that does more than describe human experiences by beginning to interpret what they mean.

General Qualitative Research Terms

Qualitative description: Description that "entails a kind of interpretation that is low-inference (close to the 'facts') or likely to result in easier consensus (about the 'facts') among researchers" (Sandelowski, 2000b, p. 335).

Naturalistic research: Commitment to the study of phenomena in their naturally occurring settings (contexts).

Field studies: Studies involving direct, firsthand observation and interviews in informants' natural settings.

Theory generation is not expected in phenomenological or hermeneutic approaches. The purpose of these studies is to understand and interpret human experience (i.e., to provide a mental picture or image of its meaning and significance), not to explain it (e.g., to describe or theorize about its structure and operation in terms of causes, circumstances, or consequences).

Qualitative Descriptive Studies. Descriptive studies may be used in quantitative research as a prelude to experiments and other types of inquiry. However, qualitative descriptive studies (Box 6.8) serve to summarize factual information about human experiences with more attention to the feel of the data's subjective content than usually found in quantitative description. Sandelowski (2000b) suggested that researchers "name their method as qualitative description [and] if . . . designed with overtones from other methods, they can describe what these overtones were, instead of inappropriately naming or implementing these other methods" (p. 339). Shorey et al. (2017) used qualitative description to research the experiences of 15 first-time fathers. They found that the first-time fathers felt unsupported and unprepared for the reality of fatherhood.

Generic Qualitative Studies. Researchers may identify their work in accordance with the technique that was used (e.g., observation study or interview study). Other generic terms are **naturalistic research** (Lincoln & Guba, 1985), which largely signifies the intellectual commitment to studying phenomena in the natural settings or contexts in which they occur, or **field study**, implying research activities that involve direct, firsthand observations and interviews in the informants' natural settings. Whiteside-Mansell, Nabaweesi, and Caballero (2017) used a naturalistic approach to compare parent reports of infant sleep environments to observed assessments of the same environments.

Qualitative Evaluation and Action Research Studies. Some studies that use qualitative research techniques need to retain their unique identities. For example, evaluation of educational and organizational programs, projects, and policies may use qualitative research techniques of interviewing, observation, and document review to generate and analyze data. Also, various forms of **action research**, including **participatory action research** (PAR; see Box 6.9), may use field techniques of observation and interviewing as approaches to data collection and analysis. Munns, Toye, and Hegney (2017) used PAR to explore the feasibility and effectiveness of a parent support home visiting program.

Favored Research Techniques

Favored techniques used in qualitative research reflect the needs of particular study designs. It is appropriate for them to appear last in a discussion of methods because techniques do not

Qualitative Research Terms

BOX 6.9

Qualitative evaluation: A general term covering a variety of approaches to evaluating programs, projects, policies, and so forth using qualitative research techniques.

Action research: A general term for a variety of approaches that aim to resolve social problems by improving existing conditions for oppressed groups or communities.

Participatory action research (PAR): A form of action research that is participatory in nature (i.e., researchers and participants collaborate in problem definition, choice of methods, data analysis, and use of findings); democratic in principle; and reformatory in impulse (i.e., has as its objective the empowerment of persons through the process of constructing and using their own knowledge as a form of consciousness raising with the potential for promoting social action).

drive research questions and designs. They are the servants, not the masters, and they are not what make a study qualitative. Nevertheless, a secure knowledge of techniques and their uses has important consequences for successful execution, evaluation, and translation of studies.

Observation and Fieldnotes. In fieldwork, observation, combined with other activities, takes on different dimensions, sometimes described as complete observer, observer as participant, participant as observer, and complete participant (Flick, 2014). **Participant observation** (i.e., active engagement of the researcher in settings and activities of people being studied; Box 6.10) encompasses all of these social roles with less time spent at the extremes. Most time is spent in the middle where distinctions between observer as participant and participant as observer are blurred. This is similar to everyday life in which the emphasis shifts back and forth as people take more or less active roles in interactions (e.g., speaking and listening, acting and watching, taking the initiative and standing by), depending on the situation.

Fieldnotes are self-designed observational protocols for recording notes about field observation. Most are not actually recorded in the field, where researchers may only be able to do "jottings" (e.g., phrases and key words as memory aids) until it is possible to compose an expanded account. Fieldnotes are highly detailed records of all that can be remembered of observations, as well as researcher actions and interactions. They may include maps and drawings of the environment, as well as conversations and records of events. **Analytic notes** (also called *reflective notes* or *memos*) are notes researchers write to themselves about ideas for analysis, issues to pursue, people to contact, questions, personal

Qualitative Research Terms

BOX 6.10

Observation continuum: A range of social roles encompassed by participant observation and ranging from complete observer to complete participant at the extremes.

Fieldnotes: Self-designed observational protocols for recording notes about field observations.

Analytic notes (memos): Notes that researchers write to themselves to record their thoughts, questions, and ideas as a process of simultaneous data collection and data analysis unfolds.

Qualitative Research Terms

Unstructured, open-ended interviews: Informal conversations that allow informants the fullest range of possibilities to describe their experiences, thoughts, and feelings.

Semistructured interviews: Formal interviews that provide more interviewer control and question format structure but retain a conversational tone and allow informants to answer in their own ways.

Structured, open-ended interviews: Formal interviews with little flexibility in the way the questions are asked but with question formats that allow informants to respond on their own terms (e.g., "What does . . . mean to you?" "How do you feel/think about . . .?").

Focus groups: This type of group interview generates data on designated topics through discussion and interaction. Focus group research is a distinct type of study when used as the sole research strategy.

emotions, understandings, and confusions brought into focus by writing and thinking about the field experience. This process illustrates how data collection and analysis occur simultaneously throughout the study.

Interviews and Focus Groups. Although a variety of interview forms and question formats are used in qualitative research, their common purpose is to provide ways for informants to express and expand on their own thoughts and remembrances, reflections, and ideas. Informal conversational interviews that occur in the natural course of participant observation are the **unstructured, open-ended** type (Box 6.11). Formal interviews, however, often involve the use of interview guides that list or outline in advance the topics and questions to be covered. Interviews remain conversational, and the interviewer has the flexibility to decide sequence and wording of questions based on how the conversation is flowing, but the **semistructured interview** approach makes data collection more comprehensive and systematic from one informant to another.

Some studies also use **structured, open-ended** question formats, where informants answer the same exactly worded question(s) but are free to describe their experiences in their own words and on their own terms. Although this discussion covers several interview methods, it does not exhaust possible interview approaches.

Group interviews may be used in addition to individual interviews in field research. **Focus groups** may be used as a sole research strategy or in combination with other forms of data collection. When used as the sole research strategy, the focus group interview represents a distinct type of study with a history in marketing research. Thus, researchers should limit their naming of the method to "focus group" and refer to primary sources for information on specific focus group strategies when planning to use this as the central data collection technique (e.g., Krueger & Casey, 2014). Focus groups may also be used in combination with other forms of data collection in both qualitative and quantitative research studies to generate data on designated topics through discussion and interaction. Group moderators direct interaction in structured or semistructured ways, depending on the purpose of the interview. Lora, Cheney, and Branscum (2017) used focus groups as the sole research strategy to explore Hispanic mothers' views of the fathers' role in promoting healthy behaviors at home. El-Banna, Whitlow, and McNelis (2017) used a focus group as part of a mixed methods study researching nursing students' experiences and satisfaction with the flipped classroom environment.

Narrative and Content Analysis. Analysis in qualitative research involves extracting themes, patterns, processes, essences, and meanings from textual data (i.e., written materials such as fieldnotes, interview transcripts, and various kinds of documents). However, there is no single way to go about this. For instance, narrative, discourse, and content analysis are examples of broad areas (paradigms) within which researchers work; each comprises many different approaches.

Narrative analysis examines how people make sense of their life events. The focus of this type of research is the participant's complete story. This type of inquiry is distinguished from other qualitative research methods by its focus on the wide boundaries of the narrative (Polit & Beck, 2017). Stories analyzed as part of a narrative approach are not broken into sections. A classic and well-known example of a narrative analysis is Kleinman's (1988) *The illness narratives: Suffering, healing & the human condition.* A more recent example is Shorten and Ruppel's (2017) narrative analysis of the experiences of nursing students who participated in a maternal-newborn simulation. Although qualitative researchers commonly deal with stories of individuals' experiences, narrative analysis is a particular way of dealing with stories. Therefore, the term should not be used casually to refer to any form of analysis that involves narrative data.

Discourse analysis is a term covering widely diverse approaches to the analysis of recorded talk. This type of analysis strives to understand the structure of conversations and texts. The general purpose is to draw attention to how language/communication shapes human interactions. Data are typically from transcripts of naturally occurring conversations, which are situated within a social, cultural, political, and historical context (Polit & Beck, 2017).

> *Discourse analysis uses "conventional" data collection techniques to generate texts . . . [which] could be interview transcripts, newspaper articles, observations, documents, or visual images . . . Although the methods of generating texts and the principles of analysis may differ . . . the premises on which the research being reported has drawn need to be clearly articulated.*
>
> (Cheek, 2004, pp. 1145–1146)

An example is Arousell, Carlbom, and Johnsdotter's (2017) discourse analysis on the how healthcare providers incorporated gender equality ideals into multicultural contraceptive counseling.

Qualitative **content analysis** is most commonly mentioned in research reports in connection with procedures that involve breaking down data (e.g., coding, comparing, contrasting, and categorizing bits of information), then reconstituting them in some new form, such as description, interpretation, or theory. Ethnographers refer to this as *working data* to tease out themes and patterns. Grounded theorists describe *procedural sequences* involving different levels of coding and conceptualization of data. Phenomenologists may also use **thematic analysis** as one of many analytic strategies. Hsieh and Shannon (2005) discussed three approaches to qualitative content analysis: conventional content analysis, direct content analysis, and summative content analysis. With conventional content analysis, the coding categories originate directly from the text data. With a directed approach, analysis starts with relevant research findings or a particular theory as guidance for initial codes. A summative content analysis usually involves counting and comparisons of keywords or content, followed by an interpretation of the underlying context. Graneheim, Lindgren, and Lundman (2017), in discussing the challenges associated with conducting a qualitative content analysis, cautioned researchers to "avoid surface descriptions and general summaries" (p. 30) and "to keep abstraction levels and interpretation degrees logical and congruent throughout the analysis" (p. 31). An example of a content analysis is Dispenza, Harper, and Harrigan's (2016) study in which subjective health among lesbian, gay, bisexual, and transsexual persons living with disabilities was explored. Participants stressed two themes: (1) the importance of their physical well-being and (2) their emotional strength.

Sampling Strategies. *Sampling* decisions involve choices about study sites or settings and people who will be able to provide information and insights about the study topic. A single setting may be chosen for in-depth study, or multiple sites may be selected to enlarge and diversify samples or for purposes of comparison. Some studies of human experiences are not specific to a particular setting. Within and across sites, researchers must choose activities and events that, through observation and interview, will yield the best information. For example, if in a study of older adults' adjustment to congregate living, data gathering is limited to interviews in individuals' private quarters, there will be a loss of other individuals' perspectives (e.g., family members, service providers) and the ability to observe how participants interact with others in different facets of community life.

The choice of participants (i.e., informants or study subjects in qualitative studies) is based on a combination of criteria, including the nature and quality of information they may contribute (i.e., **theoretic interest**), their willingness to participate, their accessibility, and their availability. A prominent qualitative sampling strategy is purposeful.

Purposeful/purposive sampling (Box 6.12) enables researchers to select informants who will be able to provide particular perspectives that relate to the research question(s). In grounded theory, this is called **theoretical sampling** (i.e., sampling used in specific ways to build theory). **Nominated** or **snowball sampling** may also be used, in which informants assist in recruiting other people they know to participate. This can be helpful when informants are in a position to recommend people who are well informed on a topic and can provide a good interview. **Volunteer/convenience samples** are also used when researchers do not know potential informants and solicit for participants with the desired experience who meet study inclusion criteria. With all types of sampling, researcher judgment and control are essential to ensure that study needs are met.

Researchers' judgments, based on ongoing evaluation of quality and quantity of different types of information in the research database, determine the number and variety of informants needed (Creswell, 2013; Marshall & Rossman, 2016). Minimum numbers of informants needed for a particular kind of study may be estimated, based on historical experience. If a study involves multiple interviews of the same people, fewer informants may be needed. If the quality of information that informants supply is not good or sufficient to answer questions or saturate data categories (the same information keeps coming up), more informants will be needed. When discussing the issue of sample size in qualitative research, Cleary, Horsfall, and Hayter (2014) stated that it is "important that qualitative researchers justify their sample size on the grounds of quality data" (p. 473). They further stated that it is also important that "the majority of participants are represented in the presentation of data" (p. 473). Decisions to stop collecting data depend on the nature and scope of the

---

BOX
6.12   *Qualitative Research Terms*

Purposeful/purposive sampling: Intentional selection of people or events in accordance with the needs of the study.
Nominated/snowball sampling: Recruitment of participants with the help of informants already enrolled in the study.
Volunteer/convenience sampling: A sample obtained by solicitation or advertising for participants who meet study criteria.
Theoretical sampling: In grounded theory, purposeful sampling used in specific ways to build theory.

study design; the amount, richness, and quality of useable data; the speed with which types of data move analysis along; and the completeness or saturation (Morse, 2000).

> *An adequate sample size . . . is one that permits—by virtue of not being too large—the deep, case-oriented analysis that is a hallmark of all qualitative inquiry, and that results in—by virtue of not being too small—a new and richly textured understanding of experience.*

> (Sandelowski, 1995, p. 183)

Quality markers of quantitative methods should not be applied to qualitative studies. For example, **random sampling**, often used in quantitative studies to achieve statistically representative samples, does not logically fit with purposes of qualitative designs. Rather, purposive sampling in which researchers seek out people who will be the best sources of information about an experience or phenomenon is more appropriate.

Data Management and Analysis. In appraising qualitative studies, it is important to understand how data are managed and analyzed. Qualitative studies generate large amounts of narrative data that need to be managed and manipulated. Personal computers and word processing software facilitate data management (Box 6.13), including the following:

- Data entry (e.g., typing fieldnotes and analytic memos, transcribing recorded interviews);
- "Cleaning" or editing;
- Storage and retrieval (e.g., organizing data into meaningful, easily located units or files).

Data manipulation involves coding, sorting, and arranging words, phrases, or data segments in ways that advance ongoing analysis. Various types of specialized software have been developed to support management and manipulation of textual data. There is no inherent virtue in using or not using qualitative data analysis software (QDAS). It is wise to consider the advantages and disadvantages (Creswell, 2013). Most important to remember is that QDAS packages, unlike statistical software, may support but do not perform data analyses. Users need to be certain that the analyses they must perform do not suffer because of inappropriate fit with the limits and demands of a particular program or the learning curve that may be involved.

Data analysis occurs throughout data collection to ensure that sampling decisions produce an appropriate, accurate, and sufficiently complete and richly detailed data set to meet the needs of the study. Also, to manage the volume of data involved, ongoing analysis is needed to sort and arrange data while developing ideas about how to reassemble and represent them as descriptions, theories, or interpretations.

Sorting may involve making frequency counts, coding, developing categories, formulating working hypotheses, accounting for negative cases (instances that contradict other data or do

---

BOX 6.13 *Qualitative Research Terms*

Qualitative data management: The act of designing systems to organize, catalog, code, store, and retrieve data. (System design influences, in turn, how the researcher approaches the task of analysis.)

Computer-assisted qualitative data analysis: An area of technological innovation that in qualitative research has resulted in use of word processing and software packages to support data management.

Qualitative data analysis: A variety of techniques that are used to move back and forth between data and ideas throughout the course of the research.

not fit hypotheses), or identifying concepts that explain patterns and relationships among data. Research design and specific aims determine one of the many analytic techniques that will be used (e.g., phenomenological reduction, constant comparison, narrative analysis, content analysis).

Similarly, the results of data analysis may take many forms. A common example is thematic analysis that systematically describes recurring ideas or topics (i.e., themes) that represent different yet related aspects of a phenomenon. Data may be organized into tables, charts, or graphs or presented as narratives using actual quotes from informants or reconstructed life stories (i.e., data-based hypothetical examples). Data may also be presented as metaphors where the authors use figurative language to evoke a visual analogy (Polit & Beck, 2017). Beck and Watson (2016) used the metaphor of an "earthquake" in their study on posttraumatic growth after the experience of childbirth trauma. As noted previously in discussing issues of representation, researchers may also use drama, self-stories, and poetry to immerse the reader in the informants' world, decrease the distance between the author and the reader, and more vividly portray the emotional content of an experience. These kinds of evaluation are important to critical appraisal of qualitative studies.

Mixing Methods. It is unhelpful to view qualitative research as a singular entity that can be divorced from the assumptions of the traditions associated with different methods or reduced to a group of data collection and analysis techniques. Because there are so many choices that necessarily involve multilevel (e.g., paradigm, method, and technique; Box 6.14) commitments (Sandelowski, 2000a), seasoned researchers have cautioned against nonreflective, uncritical mixing of qualitative perspectives, language, and analytic strategies (i.e., hybridized qualitative studies) to produce results that do not meet rigorous scholarly standards, which clinicians should be aware of when appraising qualitative evidence. This is coupled with a concern about researchers who rely on textbooks or survey courses for direction rather than expert mentorship. For novice researchers, the concern is that their ability to recognize within-method and across-method subtleties and nuances, identify decision points, and anticipate consequences involved in the research choices they make may be compromised because of the insufficient depth of understanding offered by these limited knowledge bases (Morse, 1997a). Clinicians who are novice readers of qualitative research (and beginning researchers) are advised first to learn about pure methods so that they will be able to proceed with greater knowledge and confidence, should they later encounter a hybrid (combined qualitative) or mixed-method (combined qualitative and quantitative) approach.

BOX 6.14	*Qualitative Research Terms*

Paradigm: A worldview or set of beliefs, assumptions, and values that guide all types of research by identifying where the researcher stands on issues related to the nature of reality (ontology), relationship of the researcher to the researched (epistemology), role of values (axiology), use of language (rhetoric), and process (methodology; Creswell, 2013).

Method: The theory of how a certain type of research should be carried out (i.e., strategy, approach, process/overall design, and logic of design). Researchers often subsume description of techniques under a discussion of method.

Techniques: Tools or procedures used to generate or analyze data (e.g., interviewing, observation, standardized tests and measures, constant comparison, document analysis, content analysis, statistical analysis). Techniques are method-neutral and may be used, as appropriate, in any research design—either qualitative or quantitative.

APPRAISING INDIVIDUAL QUALITATIVE STUDIES

A variety of method-specific and general criteria has been proposed for evaluating qualitative studies. In fact, there is a large variety of rules related to quality standards, but there is no agreed-upon terminology or preset format that bridges the diversity of methods enough to dictate how researchers communicate about the rules they followed. Only part of the judgment involves what researchers say they did. The other part is how well they represent research results, the effect of the presentation on readers, and readers' judgments about whether study findings seem credible and useful.

Method-Specific Criteria for Evaluating Qualitative Studies

Some criteria for evaluating scientific rigor specifically relate to central purposes and characteristics of traditional methods. Classic evaluation criteria remain relevant for qualitative researchers today. For example, ethnography's historic emphasis on understanding human experience in cultural context is reflected by six classic variables proposed by Homans (1955) to evaluate the adequacy of field studies: *time, place, social circumstance, language, intimacy,* and *consensus.*

Elaboration on these variables relates to values placed on prolonged close engagement of the researcher with study participants, active participation in daily social events, communication, and confirmation of individual informant reports by consulting multiple informants. Appraisals of an ethnographic/field study's accuracy (credibility) may be linked to how well values such as these appear to have been upheld.

Similarly, the ultimate goal of grounded theory-influenced evaluative criteria was summarized by Glaser and Strauss (1967) as *fit, grab, work,* and *modifiability* (Box 6.15).

The pedagogic, semiotic/language-oriented approach to phenomenology of van Manen (1990/1997) is reflected in his four conditions or evaluative criteria of any human science text. The text must be *oriented, strong, rich,* and *deep* (Box 6.16).

These are just a few examples of how active researchers working within specific traditions have conceptualized their craft. Because there is such diversity in qualitative inquiry, no single set of criteria can serve all qualitative approaches equally well. However, there have been efforts to articulate criteria that may more generally apply to diverse qualitative research approaches (Creswell, 2013; Flick, 2014; Marshall & Rossman, 2016). The method-specific criteria to some extent drive these general criteria. However, the primary driver for the variety of attempts to develop general criteria has been perceived as communication gaps between qualitative and quantitative researchers whose use of language and worldviews often differ. Despite these attempts, there is no agreement among qualitative researchers about how or whether it is appropriate to use the general appraisal criteria.

BOX
6.15

Glaser and Strauss's Evaluative Criteria for a Grounded Theory Study

- **Fit:** Categories must be indicated by the data.
- **Grab:** The theory must be relevant to the social/practical world.
- **Work:** The theory must be useful in explaining, interpreting, or predicting the study phenomenon.
- **Modifiability:** The theory must be adaptable over time to changing social conditions.

Van Manen's Evaluative Criteria for a Phenomenological Study

BOX 6.16

- **Oriented:** Answers a question of how one stands in relation to life and how one needs to think, observe, listen, and relate
- **Strong:** Clear and powerful
- **Rich:** Thick description/valid, convincing interpretations of concrete experiences
- **Deep:** Reflective/instructive and meaningful

General Criteria for Evaluating Qualitative Studies

Examples of general evaluative criteria are those proposed by Lincoln and Guba (1985) that offer qualitative equivalents to quantitative concepts of validity and reliability. These help explain the scientific rigor of qualitative methods to quantitatively oriented persons. However, it has been argued that by framing discussion on the basis of the belief structures of quantitative researchers and drawing attention away from other criteria of equal importance, the criteria fail to address paradigmatic differences. The differences reflected by qualitative researchers' world views are in the ways they perceive reality as subjective and multiple, ontological differences; the way they view the relationship between the researcher and the researched as close and collaborative, epistemologic differences; the belief that all research is value laden, and biases that are naturally present need to be dealt with openly, axiologic differences; the conviction that effective use of personal and literary writing styles are key to meaningful representation of research results, rhetorical differences; and the ways in which inductive logic is used to draw out and encourage development of emerging understanding of what the data mean, methodological differences (Creswell, 2013).

Trustworthiness Criteria

When appraising qualitative research, applying the classic and often cited work of Lincoln and Guba's (1985) trustworthiness criteria can be helpful. These criteria include *credibility*, *transferability*, *dependability*, and *confirmability* (Box 6.17). These four criteria parallel the quantitative criteria for good research, namely internal validity, external validity, reliability, and objectivity.

Lincoln and Gubas's Evaluative Criteria: Trustworthiness Criteria

BOX 6.17

- **Credibility:** Accuracy and validity assured through documentation of researcher actions, opinions, and biases; negative case analysis; appropriateness of data; adequacy of the database; verification/corroboration by multiple data sources; validation of data and findings by informants and colleague consultation.
- **Dependability:** Ensuring study findings are consistent and repeatable by verifying the consistency between researchers' findings and raw data collected from study participants.
- **Transferability:** Providing information sufficient for clinicians to determine whether the study findings are meaningful to other people in similar situations, often using thick description.
- **Confirmability:** Confidence that study findings reflect participants' perspectives versus researcher perceptions.

Credibility. Credibility is demonstrated by accuracy and validity that are assured through documentation of researcher actions, opinions, and biases; negative case analysis (e.g., accounting for outliers/exceptions); appropriateness of data (e.g., purposeful sampling); adequacy of the database (e.g., saturation); and verification/corroboration by use of multiple data sources (e.g., triangulation), validation of data and findings by informants (e.g., member checks, respondent validation, participant validation), and consultation with colleagues (e.g., peer debriefing).

Much like internal validity in quantitative methods (the extent to which you can infer causality), there are some caveats about the above indicators of credibility that merit mentioning. Member checks can be problematic when researchers' findings uncover implicit patterns or meanings of which informants are unaware. Thus, they may not be able to corroborate findings and may need to reexamine the situation and "check out results for themselves" (Morse, 1994, p. 230).

When reading a qualitative report, member checks may or may not be present. Also, they are seldom useful for corroborating reports that are a synthesis of multiple perspectives, because individuals are not positioned well to account for perspectives beyond their own. Therefore, member checks should be seen as an ongoing process for assuring that informants' recorded accounts accurately and fairly reflect their perceptions and experiences. However, as an ultimate check on the final interpretation of data, they are not required; it is up to the researcher to decide when and how they may be useful (Morse, 1998; Sandelowski, 1993, 1998a).

Birt, Scott, Cavers, Campbell, and Walter (2016) discussed potential methodological and ethical issues related to member checks. Methodologically, the authors stated that the process of member checking should be consistent with the study's epistemological stance. Examples of member checking documents and responses from participants to such documents should be provided. Steps taken to handle additional data or disconfirming cases should be noted. An ethical issue that may arise during member checks is that participants may become embarrassed or distressed while reading their narratives.

Birt et al. (2016) also reported on their in-depth method of member checking called Synthesized Member Checking (SMC). Within this process, synthesized data from the final stages of analysis were returned to participants alongside illustrative quotes. Participants were then asked to comment on whether the results resonated with their experiences. During this process, the participants were also provided with the opportunity for further comments.

Varpio, Ajjawi, Monrouxe, O'Brien, and Rees (2017) discussed the epistemological and ontological origins of the term "member checks." They concluded by cautioning researchers to avoid using qualitative terms uncritically and nonreflexively.

Peer debriefing involves seeking input (substantive or methodological) from knowledgeable colleagues as consultants, soliciting their reactions as listeners, and using them as sounding boards for the researcher's ideas. It is up to the researcher to decide when and whether peer debriefing will be useful. It is important to distinguish peer debriefing from quantitative researchers' use of multiple raters and expert panels. In qualitative research, it is not appropriate to use individuals outside of the research to validate the researcher's analyses and interpretations, because these are arrived at inductively through closer contact and understanding of the data than an outside expert could possibly have (McConnell-Henry, Chapman, & Francis, 2011; Morse, 1994, 1997b, 1998; Sandelowski, 1998a). Because peer debriefing may not always be useful, the reader should not expect to encounter this credibility criterion in every qualitative report.

Transferability. Transferability is demonstrated by information that is sufficient for a research consumer to determine whether the findings are meaningful to other people in similar situations (analytic or theoretical vs. statistical generalizability). Statistical generalization and analytic or theoretic generalization are ***not*** the same thing. In quantitative traditions, external validity is concerned with *statistical generalization*, which involves extending or transferring implications of study findings to a larger population by using mathematically based probabilities. *Analytic or theoretic generalization*, on the other hand, involves extending or *transferring* implications of study findings to a larger population by logically and pragmatically based possibilities, which is appropriate for qualitative research.

The practical usefulness of a qualitative study is judged by its

- ability to represent how informants feel about and make sense of their experiences;
- effectiveness in communicating what that information means and the lessons it teaches.

Dependability. Dependability is demonstrated by a research process that is carefully documented to provide evidence of how conclusions were reached and whether, under similar conditions, a researcher might expect to obtain similar findings (i.e., the concept of the audit trail). In quantitative traditions, reliability refers to consistency in findings across time. This is another example of what is called parallelism—parallel concepts within the qualitative and quantitative traditions; however, these concepts are entirely different in meaning and application.

Confirmability. Confirmability is demonstrated by providing substantiation that findings and interpretations are grounded in the data (i.e., links between researcher assertions and the data are clear and credible). The parallel concept of objectivity in quantitative traditions speaks to reduction of bias through data-driven results.

Other general criteria are linked to concepts of credibility and transferability but relate more to the effects that various portrayals of the research may have. For example, a second set of criteria developed by Guba and Lincoln (1989) has overtones of a critical theory view that when the goal of research is to provide deeper understanding and more informed insights into human experiences, it may also prove to be empowering (Guba & Lincoln, 1994).

Authenticity Criteria

Box 6.18 lists Guba and Lincoln's (1989) evaluative *authenticity criteria*. Ontological and educative authenticity, in particular, is at the heart of concerns about how to represent research results. That is, to transfer a deeper understanding of a phenomenon to the reader, researchers may strive for literary styles of writing that make a situation seem more "real" or "alive." This is also called making use of *verisimilitude*, an important criterion of traditional validity (Creswell, 2013; Denzin, 2014), and describes when the readers are drawn *vicariously into the multiple realities of the world that the research reveals* from perspectives of both the informant and researcher.

BOX **6.18**	*Guba and Lincoln's Evaluative Criteria: Authenticity Criteria*

- **Fairness:** Degree to which informants' different ways of making sense of experiences (i.e., their "constructions") are evenly represented by the researcher
- **Ontological authenticity:** Scope to which personal insights are enhanced or enlarged
- **Catalytic authenticity:** How effectively the research stimulates action
- **Tactical authenticity:** Degree to which people are empowered to act
- **Educative authenticity:** Extent to which there is increased understanding of and appreciation for others' constructions

Evaluation Standards

Authenticity criteria (Guba & Lincoln, 1989) are not as well recognized or cited as regularly by quantitative researchers and clinicians as Lincoln and Guba's (1985) trustworthiness criteria. Trustworthiness criteria seem to be more universally understandable and serve to impose a sense of order and uniformity on a field that is diverse and sometimes difficult to understand. Thus, some readers have greater confidence in qualitative reports that use the classic trustworthiness criteria terminology to explain what researchers did to assure *credibility, transferability, dependability,* and/or *confirmability.*

However, it does not mean that reports that do not do so are necessarily deficient. Many qualitative researchers and clinicians resist using words that mirror the concepts and values of quantitative research (e.g., our example of the parallel concepts of internal validity and credibility), because they think that it may detract from better method-specific explanations of their research (a matter of training and individual preference). Some also think, as a matter of principle, that it could undermine the integrity of qualitative methods themselves. Furthermore, they know that methods to ensure quality and rigor are different for different kinds of qualitative studies and, therefore, attempts to talk about the general properties of qualitative designs and findings pose many constraints. As a result, there is a threat to integrity if general criteria come to be viewed as rigid rules that must apply to every qualitative study. Therefore, it is incumbent upon clinicians to assimilate more active knowledge about the differences, similarities, and nuances of qualitative research to conduct a fair and accurate appraisal of qualitative evidence.

WALKING THE WALK AND TALKING THE TALK: CRITICAL APPRAISAL OF QUALITATIVE RESEARCH

We began by comparing critical appraisal of individual research reports with separation of the wheat from the chaff. Separating out the chaff involves applying readers' understanding of the diversity within qualitative research to the content of the report. Next, extracting what is good and useful involves applying the appropriate method-specific and general evaluative criteria to the research report. A degree of familiarity with the diversity of characteristics, language, concepts, and issues associated with qualitative research is necessary before using the guide in Box 6.1 to appraise qualitative research studies.

The guide adopts the EBP format of basic quick appraisal questions followed by more specific questions, but there are caveats. One is that no individual study contains the most complete information possible about everything in the appraisal guide. Sometimes, as in quantitative reports, the information is available and built into the design itself, but depends on the reader's knowledge of the method. At other times, because the volume of data and findings may require a series of reports that focus on different aspects of the research, authors sometimes direct readers to introductory articles more focused on the methods and broad overviews of the study. The final caveat is that space limitations and a journal's priorities determine the amount of detail that an author may provide in any given section of the report.

"

That inner voice has both gentleness and clarity. So, to get to authenticity, you really keep going down to the bone, to the honesty, and the inevitability of something.

MEREDITH MONK

Putting Feet to Knowledge: Walking the Walk

It is time to put feet to the knowledge the reader has gained through this chapter. The reader is encouraged to use Appendix D (available on thePoint®) that demonstrates a rapid critical appraisal application of the appraisal guide for qualitative evidence. The appendix contains exemplars of qualitative research reports. The range of topics appearing in the literature confirms that clinical researchers across professions and specialty areas are "walking the walk and talking the talk" and using a variety of qualitative approaches with attendant methodologies, terms, and concepts as described earlier.

The choice of exemplars presented here was guided by the following criteria:

- A mix of articles representing a variety of concerns across different areas of clinical interest;
- A range of qualitative research designs that illustrate the achievement of valid results;
- A range of research purposes that illustrate a variety of ways in which results may help readers care for their patients.

The following factors may affect reader response to the appraisal of articles using the rapid critical appraisal format:

1. Individual preference: In the real world, people choose topics that interest them.
2. The ease with which the report submits to appraisal: Appreciation and understanding of qualitative reports depend on individual reading of and engagement with the report in its entirety. Therefore, the articles lose some of their communicative and evocative qualities when parsed apart and retold.

The results of the appraisal process combined with individual preference may affect the studies' initial appeal. Because in every case evaluations of an article's plausibility and generalizability (transferability) require the use of independent reader judgments, firsthand reading is recommended.

> ❝
> Changes may not happen right away, but with effort even the difficult may become easy.
>
> **BILL BLACKMAN**

KEEPING IT TOGETHER: SYNTHESIZING QUALITATIVE EVIDENCE

Synthesizing qualitative evidence is not a new endeavor, given the history of the *meta-study* in the social sciences. A meta-study is not the same as a critical literature review or a secondary analysis of an existing data set. Instead, meta-studies involve distinct approaches to the analysis of previously published research findings in order to produce new knowledge (a synthesis of what is already known).

In quantitative research, *meta-analysis* is the research strategy designed to ask a new question on multiple studies that address similar research hypotheses using comparable methodologies, reanalyzing, and combining their results to conclude on what is known about the issue of interest. In qualitative research, various strategies for performing *metasynthesis* have been proposed.

Several methodological approaches to synthesizing qualitative data have been used in the nursing and healthcare literature. Many studies use the "meta-ethnography" approach of Noblit and Hare (1988). This approach involves seven steps in which the included studies are compared and translated into each other. Thorne, Jensen, Kearney, Noblit, and Sandelowski (2004) presented their distinct perspectives on metasynthesis methodology in order to underscore what it is not (i.e., it is not an integrative critical literature review) and to explore the various methodological conventions they used and/or recommended. Other methodological approaches include *Meta-study of qualitative health research: A practical guide to meta-analysis and meta-synthesis* (Paterson, Thorne, Canam, & Jillings, 2001) and *Handbook for synthesizing qualitative research* (Sandelowski & Barroso, 2007).

Despite the lack of a single set of agreed-upon techniques for synthesizing qualitative studies, there is an appreciation for the basic definition and underlying purposes of meta-synthesis and the general procedural issues that any approach to it will need to address. Basically, metasynthesis is a holistic translation, based on comparative analysis of individual qualitative interpretations, which seeks to retain the essence of their unique contributions. Although individual studies can provide useful information and insights, they cannot give the most comprehensive answers to clinical questions. A benefit of metasynthesis methods is that they provide a way for researchers to build up bodies of qualitative research evidence that are relevant to clinical practice. The result of various approaches to qualitative metasyn-thesis can be a formal theory or a new refined interpretive explanation of the phenomenon.

Specific approaches to metasynthesis need to address the following issues:

- How to characterize the phenomenon of interest when comparing conceptualizations and interpretations across studies;
- How to establish inclusion criteria and sample from among a population of studies;
- How to compare studies that have used the same or different qualitative strategies;
- How to reach new understandings about a phenomenon by seeking consensus in a body of data where it is acknowledged that there is no single "correct" interpretation (Jensen & Allen, 1996).

Appraisal of metasynthesis research reports requires an appreciation for the different perspectives that may be guiding the analysis. Mechanisms described by Sandelowski and Barroso (2007) for promoting valid study procedures and outcomes include the following:

- Using all search channels of communication and maintaining an audit trail (Rodgers & Cowles, 1993) tracking search outcomes as well as procedural and interpretive decisions;
- Contacting primary study investigators;
- Consulting with reference librarians;
- Independent search by at least two reviewers;
- Independent appraisal of each report by at least two reviewers;
- Ensuring ongoing negotiation of consensual validity (Belgrave & Smith, 1995; Eis-ner, 1991) facilitated by collaborative efforts by team members to establish areas of consensus and negotiate consensus in the presence of differing points of view;
- Securing expert peer review (Sandelowski, 1998a) by consultation with experts in research synthesis and with clinical experts.

Written reports will vary in their use or mention of these approaches and in their detailing of research procedures. Readers will have to be alerted about references to a named methodology; explanation of the search strategy that was used; clarity in the manner in which findings (data that comprise the study sample) are presented; and the originality, plausibility, and perceived usefulness of the synthesis of those findings.

Examples of metasynthesis and meta-ethnography in the literature include Nolte, Downing, Temane, and Hastings-Tolsma's (2017) metasynthesis on compassion fatigue in nursing and

Keedle, Schmied, Burns, and Dahlen's (2017) meta-ethnography on women's experiences of vaginal birth after a cesarean section. Nolte et al. (2017) included nine articles in their metasynthesis, generating four central themes: (1) physical symptoms; (2) emotional symptoms; (3) factors contributing to compassion fatigue; and (4) measures to prevent or overcome compassion fatigue. Keedle et al. (2017) included 20 articles in their meta-ethnography, which yielded one overarching theme "the journey from pain to power." Four subthemes also emerged: (1) "the hurt me" subtheme described the previous cesarean experience and resultant feelings; (2) the subtheme of "peaks and troughs" described women's moving from their previous experience of a cesarean to their experience of vaginal birth after a cesarean; (3) "powerful me" described the sense of achieving a vaginal birth after a cesarean; and (4) the resultant benefits described in the subtheme "the ongoing journey." These studies are powerful for assisting clinicians make decisions about how they will care for moms attempting vaginal births after a cesarean section while considering their compassion fatigue as they engage in the care.

❝

You will come to know that what appears today to be a sacrifice [learning to appraise qualitative evidence is hard work!] will prove instead to be the greatest investment that you will ever make.

GORDEN B. HINKLEY

EBP FAST FACTS

- Qualitative evidence has an impact on clinical decision making, providing relevant, influential information for patients, families, and systems.
- Qualitative studies help answer clinical questions that address the how of healthcare interventions.
- Unique language and concepts are encountered in the qualitative literature, including such terms as purposive sampling, saturation, and participant observation.
- Qualitative evidence requires a different approach to appraisal than quantitative evidence.
- Intentional understanding of the appropriate evaluative criteria for qualitative evidence is required to avoid misuse of appraisal of studies and subsequent erroneous conclusions.

WANT TO KNOW MORE?

A variety of resources is available to enhance your learning and understanding of this chapter.

- Visit thePoint® to access:
  - Appendix D: Walking the Walk and Talking the Talk: An Appraisal Guide for Qualitative Evidence
  - Articles from the AJN EBP Step-By-Step Series
  - Journal articles
  - Checklists for rapid critical appraisal and more!

- Lippincott CoursePoint combines digital text content with video case studies and interactive modules for a fully integrated course solution that works the way you study and learn.

References

Arousell, J., Carlbom, A., & Johnsdotter, S. (2017). Unintended consequences of gender equality promotion in Swedish multicultural contraceptive counseling: A discourse analysis. *Qualitative Health Research, 27*, 1518–1528.

Babler, E., & Strickland, C. (2015). Moving the journey towards independence: Adolescents transitioning to successful diabetes self-management. *Journal of Pediatric Nursing, 30*, 648–660.

Barreto, M., Marcon, S., & Garcia-Vivar, C. (2017). Patterns of behaviour in families of critically ill patients in the emergency room: A focused ethnography. *Journal of Advanced Nursing, 73*, 633–642.

Batch, M., & Windsor, C. (2015). Nursing casualization and communication: A critical ethnography. *Journal of Advanced Nursing, 71*, 870–880.

Beck, C., & Watson, S. (2016). Posttraumatic growth after birth trauma: "I Was Broken, Now I Am Unbreakable". *MCN: The American Journal of Maternal-Child Nursing, 41*, 264–271.

Belgrave, L. L., & Smith, K. J. (1995). Negotiated validity in collaborative ethnography. *Qualitative Inquiry, 1*, 69–86.

Birt, L., Scott, S., Cavers, D., Campbell, C., & Walter, F. (2016). Member checking: A tool to enhance trustworthiness or merely a nod to validation? *Qualitative Health Research, 26*, 1802–1811.

Brage, E., & Vindrola-Padros, C. (2017). An ethnographic exploration of the delivery of psychosocial care to children with cancer in Argentina. *European Journal of Oncology Nursing: The Official Journal of European Oncology Nursing Society, 29*, 91–97.

Bunkenborg, G., Hansen, T., & Holge-Hazelton, B. (2017). Handing over patients from the ICU to the general ward—a focused ethnographical study of nurses' communication practice. *Journal of Advanced Nursing, 73*, 3090–3101.

Charmaz, K. (2014). *Constructing grounded theory* (2nd ed.). London, UK: Sage Publications.

Cheek, J. (2004). At the margins? Discourse analysis and qualitative research. *Qualitative Health Research, 14*, 1140–1150.

Chenitz, W. C., & Swanson, J. M. (1986). *From practice to grounded theory.* Menlo Park, CA: Addison-Wesley.

Cleary, J., & Doody, O. (2016). Nurses' experience of caring for people with intellectual disability and dementia. *Journal of Clinical Nursing, 26*, 620–631.

Cleary, M., Horsfall, J., & Hayter, M. (2014). Data collection and sampling in qualitative research: Does size matter? *Journal of Advanced Nursing, 70*, 473–475.

Colon-Ramos, U., Monge-Rojas, R., & Cremm, E. (2017). How Latina mothers navigate a "food swamp" to feed their children: A photovoice approach. *Public Health Nutrition, 20*, 1–12.

Corbin, J., & Strauss, A. (2014). *Basics of qualitative research: Techniques and procedures for developing grounded theory* (4th ed.). Thousand Oaks, CA: Sage Publications.

Creswell, J. (2013). *Research design: Qualitative, quantitative and mixed methods approaches* (4th ed.). Thousand Oaks, CA: Sage Publications.

De Chesnay, M. (2015). Ethnographic methods. In M. de Chesnay (Eds.). *Nursing research using ethnography.* New York, NY: Springer Publishing.

Denzin, N. K. (2014). *Interpretive ethnography: Ethnographic practices for the 21st century* (2nd ed.). Thousand Oaks, CA: Sage Publications.

Dispenza, F., Harper, L., & Harrigan, M. (2016). Subjective health among LGBT persons living with disabilities: A qualitative content analysis. *Rehabilitation Psychology, 61*, 251–259.

Eisner, E. W. (1991). *The enlightened eye: Qualitative inquiry and the enhancement of educational practice.* New York, NY: Macmillan.

El-Banna, M., Whitlow, M., & McNelis, A. (2017). Flipping around the classroom: Accelerated Bachelor of Science in Nursing students' satisfaction and achievement. *Nurse Education Today, 56*, 41–46.

Fawcett, J., Watson, J., Neuman, B., Hinton-Walker, P., & Fitzpatrick, J. J. (2001). On theories and evidence. *Journal of Nursing Scholarship, 33*, 115–119.

Feeley, C., & Thomson, G. (2016). Why do some women choose to freebirth in the UK? An interpretative phenomenological study. *BMC Pregnancy and Childbirth, 16*(59), 1–12.

Flick, U. (2014). *An introduction to qualitative research* (5th ed.). London, UK: Sage Publications.

Geertz, C. (1973). *The interpretation of cultures.* New York, NY: Basic Books.

Gilbert, L. (2017). Photovoice: A link between research and practice for prostate cancer advocacy in Black communities. *Journal of Racial and Ethnic Health Disparities, 4*, 364–375.

Glaser, B. G. (1978). *Theoretical sensitivity.* Mill Valley, CA: Sociology Press.

Glaser, B. G. (1992). *Emergence vs. forcing: Basics of grounded theory analysis.* Mill Valley, CA: Sociology Press.

Glaser, B. G., & Strauss, A. L. (1967). *The discovery of grounded theory: Strategies for qualitative research.* New York, NY: Aldine.

Grace, J. T., & Powers, B. A. (2009). Claiming our core: Appraising qualitative evidence for nursing questions about human response and meaning. *Nursing Outlook, 57*, 27–34.

Graneheim, U., Lindgren, B., & Lundman, B. (2017). Methodological challenges in qualitative content analysis: A discussion paper. *Nurse Education Today, 56,* 29–34.

Guba, E. G., & Lincoln, Y. S. (1989). *Fourth generation evaluation.* Newbury Park, CA: Sage.

Guba, E. G., & Lincoln, Y. S. (1994). Competing paradigms in qualitative research. In N. K. Denzin & Y. S. Lincoln (Eds.), *Handbook of qualitative research* (pp. 105–117). Thousand Oaks, CA: Sage.

Haugh, B. (2016). Becoming a mother and learning to breastfeed: An emergent autoethnography. *Journal of Perinatal Education, 25,* 56–68.

Hengst, J., Devanga, S., & Mosier, H. (2015). Thin versus thick description: Analyzing representations of people and their life worlds in the literature of communication sciences and disorders. *American Journal of Speech-Language Pathology, 24,* S838–S853.

Homans, G. C. (1955). *The human group.* New York, NY: Harcourt Brace.

Hsieh, H. F., & Shannon, S. E. (2005). Three approaches to qualitative content analysis. *Qualitative Health Research, 15,* 1277–1288.

Im, E. O. (2013). Practical guidelines for feminist research in nursing. *ANS. Advances in Nursing Science, 36,* 133–145.

Jensen, L. A., & Allen, M. N. (1996). Meta-synthesis of qualitative findings. *Qualitative Health Research, 6,* 553–560.

Keedle, H., Schmied, V., Burns, E., & Dahlen, H. (2017). The journey from pain to power: A meta-ethnography on women's experiences of vaginal birth after caesarean. *Women and Birth: Journal of the Australian College of Midwives, 31*(1), 69–79.

Kleinman, A. (1988). *The illness narratives: Suffering, healing & the human condition.* New York, NY: Basic Books.

Krueger, R., & Casey, M. (2014). *Focus groups: A practical guide for applied research* (5th ed.). Thousand Oaks, CA: Sage Publications.

Laugesen, B., Lauritsen, M., & Jorgensen, R. (2017). ADHD and everyday life: Healthcare as a significant lifeline. *Journal of Pediatric Nursing, 35,* 105–112.

Lawler, D., Begley, C., & Lalor, J. (2015). (Re)constructing myself: The process of transition to motherhood for women with a disability. *Journal of Advanced Nursing, 7,* 1672–1683.

Leslie, M., Paradis, E., & Gropper, M. (2017). An ethnographic study of health information technology use in three intensive care units. *Health Services Research, 52,* 1330–1348.

Lincoln, Y. S., & Guba, E. G. (1985). *Naturalistic inquiry.* Beverly Hills, CA: Sage.

Lora, K., Cheney, M., & Branscum, P. (2017). Hispanic mothers' views of the fathers' role in promoting healthy behaviors at home: Focus group findings. *Journal of the Academy of Nutrition and Dietetics, 117,* 914–922.

Marshall, C., & Rossman, G. B. (2016). *Designing qualitative research* (6th ed.). Thousand Oaks, CA: Sage Publications.

Matua, G. (2015). Choosing phenomenology as a guiding philosophy for nursing research. *Nurse Researcher, 22,* 30–34.

McConnell-Henry, T., Chapman, Y., & Francis, K. (2011). Member checking and Heideggerian phenomenology: A redundant component. *Nurse Researcher, 18,* 28–37.

Melia, K. M. (1996). Rediscovering Glaser. *Qualitative Health Research, 6,* 368–378.

Michel, L. (2017). A failure to communicate? Doctors and nurses in American hospitals. *Journal of Health Politics, Policy and Law, 42,* 709–717.

Morse, J. M. (1994). Designing funded qualitative research. In N. K. Denzin & Y. S. Lincoln (Eds.), *Handbook of qualitative research* (pp. 220–235). Thousand Oaks, CA: Sage.

Morse, J. M. (1997a). Learning to drive from a manual? *Qualitative Health Research, 7,* 181–183.

Morse, J. M. (1997b). "Perfectly healthy, but dead": The myth of inter-rater reliability. *Qualitative Health Research, 7,* 445–447.

Morse, J. M. (1998). Validity by committee. *Qualitative Health Research, 8,* 443–445.

Morse, J. M. (2000). Determining sample size. *Qualitative Health Research, 10,* 3–5.

Morse, J. M. (2007). Quantitative influences on the presentation of qualitative articles. *Qualitative Health Research, 17,* 147–148.

Mosman, S., Poggenpoel, M., & Myburgh, C. (2015). Life stories of young women who experience rejection from their mothers. *Curationis, 38*(1), 1–8.

Munns, A., Toye, C., & Hegney, D. (2017). Peer-led Aboriginal parent support: Program development for vulnerable populations with participatory action research. *Contemporary Nurse, 53,* 1–18.

Noblit, G. W., & Hare, R. D. (1988). *Meta-ethnography. Synthesizing qualitative studies.* Newbury Park, CA: Sage.

Nolte, A., Downing, C., Temane, A., & Hastings-Tolsma, M. (2017). Compassion fatigue in nurses: A metasynthesis. *Journal of Clinical Nursing, 26,* 1–17.

Paterson, B. L., Thorne, S. E., Canam, C., & Jillings, C. (2001). *Meta-study of qualitative health research: A practical guide to meta-analysis and meta-synthesis.* Thousand Oaks, CA: Sage.

Polit, D, & Beck, C. (2017). Qualitative research design and approaches. In D. Polit & C. Beck *Nursing research: Generating and assessing evidence for nursing practice* (10th ed.). Philadelphia, PA: Wolters Kluwer.

Quinn, P. (2016). A grounded theory study of how nurses integrate pregnancy and full-time employment. *Nursing Research, 65*(3), 170–178.

Richardson, L. (1990). *Writing strategies: Reaching diverse audiences.* Newbury Park, CA: Sage.

Rodgers, B. L., & Cowles, K. V. (1993). The qualitative research audit trail: A complex collection of documentation. *Research in Nursing and Health, 16,* 219–226.

Ross, C., Rogers, C., & Duff, D. (2016). Critical ethnography: An under-used research methodology in neuroscience nursing. *Canadian Journal of Neuroscience Nursing, 38,* 4–7.

Sandelowski, M. (1993). Rigor or rigor mortis: The problem of rigor in qualitative research revisited. *Research in Nursing and Health, 16,* 1–8.

Sandelowski, M. (1995). Sample size in qualitative research. *Research in Nursing and Health, 18,* 179–183.

Sandelowski, M. (1998a). The call to experts in qualitative research. *Research in Nursing and Health, 21,* 467–471.

Sandelowski, M. (1998b). Writing a good read: Strategies for re-presenting qualitative data. *Research in Nursing and Health, 21,* 375–382.

Sandelowski, M. (2000a). Combining qualitative and quantitative sampling, data collection, and analysis techniques in mixed methods studies. *Research in Nursing and Health, 23,* 246–255.

Sandelowski, M. (2000b). Whatever happened to qualitative description? *Research in Nursing and Health, 23,* 334–340.

Sandelowski, M. (2004). Counting cats in Zanzibar. *Research in Nursing and Health, 27,* 215–216.

Sandelowski, M. (2007). Words that should be seen but not written. *Research in Nursing and Health, 30,* 129–130.

Sandelowski, M., & Barroso, J. (2007). *Handbook for synthesizing qualitative research.* New York, NY: Springer.

Shorey, S., Dennis, C., Bridge, S., Chong, Y., Holroyd, E., & He, H. (2017). First-time fathers' postnatal experiences and support needs: A descriptive qualitative study. *Journal of Advanced Nursing, 73,* 1–10.

Shorten, A., & Ruppel, H. (2017). Looking for zebras and finding horses: A qualitative narrative study of pre-RN licensure nursing students' experience of a "normal" postnatal simulation. *Nurse Education Today, 48,* 185–189.

Straus, S. E., Richardson, W. S., Glasziou, P., & Haynes, R. B. (2010). *Evidence-based medicine: How to practice and teach it* (4th ed.). Edinburgh, Scotland: Churchill Livingstone/Elsevier.

Strauss, A. L., & Corbin, J. (1990). *Basics of qualitative research: Grounded theory procedures and techniques.* Newbury Park, CA: Sage.

Strauss, A. L., & Corbin, J. (1998). *Basics of qualitative research: Techniques and procedures for developing grounded theory* (2nd ed.). Thousand Oaks, CA: Sage.

Thorne, S., Jensen, L., Kearney, M. H., Noblit, G., & Sandelowski, M. (2004). Qualitative metasynthesis: Reflections on methodological orientation and ideological agenda. *Qualitative Health Research, 14,* 1342–1365.

Van Maanen, J. (1988). *Tales of the field.* Chicago, IL: University of Chicago Press.

van Manen, M. (1990/1997). *Researching lived experience.* London: University of Western Ontario & State University of New York Press.

van Manen, M. (2002). *Writing in the dark: Phenomenological studies in interpretive inquiry.* London: University of Western Ontario.

Varpio, L., Ajjawi, R., Monrouxe, L., O'Brien, B., & Rees, C. (2017). Shedding the cobra effect: Problematising thematic emergence, triangulation, saturation and member checking. *Medical Education, 51,* 40–50.

Wahab, S., Mordiffi, S., Ang, E., & Lopez, V. (2017). Light at the end of the tunnel: New graduate nurses' accounts of resilience: A qualitative study using photovoice. *Nurse Education Today, 52,* 43–49.

Whiteside-Mansell, L., Nabaweesi, R., & Caballero, A. (2017). Assessment of safe sleep: Validation of the parent newborn sleep safety survey. *Journal of Pediatric Nursing, 35,* 30–35.

Williams, E., Ferrer, K., Lee, M., Bright, K., Williams, K., & Rakhmanina, N. (2017). Growing up with perinatal human immunodeficiency virus—A life not expected. *Journal of Clinical Nursing, 26,* 1–17.

Wolcott, H. (2009). *Writing up qualitative research* (3rd ed.). Thousand Oaks, CA: Sage Publications.

Wuest, J. (2012). Grounded theory: The method. In P. L. Munhall (Ed.), *Nursing research: A qualitative perspective* (5th ed., pp. 225–257). Sudbury, MA: Jones & Bartlett Learning.

7

Integration of Patient Preferences and Values and Clinician Expertise into Evidence-Based Decision Making

Ellen Fineout-Overholt, Lisa English Long, and Lynn Gallagher-Ford

One of the most sincere forms of respect is actually listening to what another has to say.

—*Bryant H. McGill*

EBP Terms to Learn
Clinical wisdom and judgment
Clinical expertise
Context of caring
Epistemic justification
Evidentialism
Experiential learning
Patient preferences

Learning Objectives

After studying this chapter, learners will be able to:

1. Explain the importance of clinician expertise and patient preferences and values to evidence-based decision making.

2. Discuss the impact of how clinicians think about their practice on clinical decisions.

3. Explain how evidence alone cannot substantiate a clinical decision or a practice change.

Evidence-based practice (EBP) is the integration of **patient preferences** and values, **clinical expertise**, and rigorous research to make decisions that lead to improved outcomes for patients and families (Figure 7.1). To improve these outcomes, transdisciplinary clinicians collaborate with patients and families in the decision making processes. Although this may seem a logical approach to clinical care, it may not be the most used. Therefore, it is imperative for clinicians practicing from the EBP paradigm to combine **external evidence** with patient preferences and clinical expertise. The focus of the health industry on gathering, appraising, and synthesizing evidence to make recommendations for practice change does not necessarily guarantee that patient preferences and clinician expertise are included as essentials in decision making that affects patients and families. It is also prudent to consider that these decisions are best achieved within a **context of caring**. For clinicians and students alike, reflection on how these are integrated into their learning, decision making, and care practices is critical. This chapter discusses the importance of engaging patients and families in the decision making process as well as helping clinicians realize their unique contributions to jointly achieving best outcomes.

In Clinical Scenario 7.1 and many others like it across multiple contexts, clinicians actualize on a daily basis what the American Nurses Association's (ANA, 2014) official position statement on professional role competence states—that the public has a right to expect clinicians to be accountable for and demonstrate their professional competence. This is accomplished in association

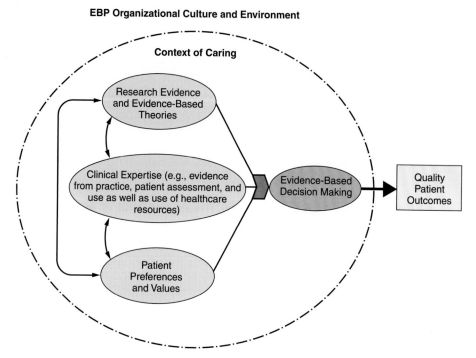

Figure 7.1: Integration of external evidence, clinical expertise (wisdom and judgment), and patient preferences and values into evidence-based decision making. (© 2003 Melnyk & Fineout-Overholt, used with permission.)

Clinical Scenario 7.1

Gillian has just started her shift at 7 AM. She receives report that the new mom, Mrs. Blum, in room 26B has a moderately distended bladder, cannot void, and will need to be catheterized; however, the patient has not been out of bed yet after her vaginal delivery at 5 AM. Gillian pops into 26B and tells the patient she will be in shortly to do her catheterization. She gathers her supplies to do a straight catheterization, and goes over it in her mind several times because she has not done a lot of these procedures. She walks into Mrs. Blum's room and notes that she is crying. Gillian realizes that her assessment has not been complete. She puts down her materials and lets Mrs. Blum know she is here to help. Mrs. Blum informs Gillian that all night the nurse caring for her and the resident who came in the morning were all focused on her emptying her bladder. No one asked about her baby, and she is concerned because the night nursery nurses did not bring back the baby for her early morning feeding. Gillian further assesses Mrs. Blum's bladder and asks her if she thinks she can void if she goes into the bathroom and sits on the toilet. She informs Mrs. Blum that after she voids, they will go to the nursery to see her daughter. Mrs. Blum agrees; after assessing Mrs. Blum's balance, together they walk to the bathroom. Mrs. Blum expresses appreciation for being able to sit on the toilet as the bedpan "is just unbearable." She promptly voids 450 mL of amber urine. Gillian then helps her to clean up and gets a wheelchair to conserve her energy so that she can focus on her daughter. On arrival at the nursery, Mrs. Blum is visibly relieved and pleased to see and hold her daughter. She indicates to Gillian that she cannot thank her enough for taking the time to treat her "like a person versus a procedure."

Clinical Scenario 7.2

Marc Siegel describes a determined 93-year-old female tap dancer. A former teacher of dance at Julliard, she has, for the past 50 years since her retirement, been an avid tap dancer at amateur shows and recitals, until it was discovered that she had a "bulging disc in her neck, tissue so inflamed that it encroached on the space intended for the spinal cord, the crucial super-highway of the nervous system." All scientific evidence on prognosis for someone of her age undergoing spinal surgery unanimously showed that the risks outweighed the benefits, even though this particular patient's heart was in excellent health and she was also in excellent physical condition. When Siegel enumerated the risks of having the surgery, and the almost certain continued pain and incapacitation without the surgery, she asked, "Can the surgery make me dance again?" To which he replied, "It's possible." "Then," she responded, "I'll take my chances." Dr. Siegel was able to find a neurosurgeon willing to do the surgery, and when the patient returned to Dr. Siegel's office, she appeared a vigorous woman whose vitality was returning. Her walking had already progressed beyond her presurgical capacities. And several weeks later, Dr. Siegel received an invitation to her first postsurgical tap dancing recital. She explained to Dr. Siegel: "You see," she said, "we patients are not just statistics. We don't always behave the way studies predict we will."

with the respective health profession, which is also responsible to the public to shape and guide any process that guarantees clinician competence. The competent clinician is expected to deliver the best care possible, which, as demonstrated by patient outcomes, is care that is supported by evidence. However, the fact that evidence from research and clinician assessment is not the only influence on clinical decision making should be considered. Patients and their families are increasingly savvy about what they want from a healthcare experience. Clinicians must use this regularly gathered data to care for patients holistically.

Integration of the concepts of patient preferences and values as well as clinical expertise with evidence from well-conducted studies become part of everyday decision making within a context of caring—whether inserting a urinary catheter or simply holding a hand during a painful procedure. This principle is wonderfully illustrated in Clinical Scenario 7.2 from a *New York Times* article entitled "When doctors say don't and the patient says do" (Siegel, 2002).

In this story, multiple processes were occurring simultaneously that reflected integration of research evidence, patient preferences and values, and clinical expertise. These occurred throughout the patient and clinicians' relationship. Evidence-based decision makers do not have a magic formula that guides them; rather, their care is delivered with careful discernment about how to integrate their best knowledge and expertise with what researchers have found to be best practice and what patients have identified as their preferences in a particular healthcare encounter. To successfully engage in evidence-based decision making, clinicians must first understand the meaning of evidence, from both practical and theoretical perspectives (also see Chapters 4 to 6), as well as actively participate in decision making with patients and families.

EVIDENCE-BASED DECISION MAKING

When learning about EBP, clinicians and student often have challenges with the language. For example, patient preference, internal evidence external evidence, randomized controlled trials, synthesis, and expertise are all critical concepts in EBP—and there are more. If the barrier of language is not mitigated, then the EBP paradigm and process are hard to embrace. Therefore, gaining proficiency with EBP language is incumbent upon everyone to learn, understand, and implement evidence-based decision making. Readers have the opportunity to review and learn the glossary of terms for this book. This list of critical terms is compiled from the book chapters and is a great resource for laying the foundation for learning how to make evidence-based decisions. The words we use to discuss a clinical topic matter, as does how clinicians consider how best to guide patients through a healthcare decision.

> ❝
> An expert is someone who knows some of the worst mistakes that can be made in his subject and how to avoid them.
>
> **WERNER HEISENBERG**

Evidence: What It Is and How Good It Is

Evidence is generally defined in the dictionary as "(1) that which tends to prove or disprove [support or not support] something: ground for belief; proof [and] (2) something that makes plain or clear; an indication or sign" (Dictionary.com, 2017). In some disciplines, the term evidence refers solely to information derived from experimental research designs. Randomized controlled trials (RCTs) are the most rigorous of these designs, and therefore, it is expected that RCTs offer what is considered in these disciplines to be the most valued information for clinical decision making. However, in healthcare, the term evidence is a more complex concept in that clinicians are seeking to find what works best for human beings, which could be a wide range of interventions that would make research designs such as RCTs unrealistic or unethical to perform. Other research designs may be more appropriate.

Furthermore, evidence in healthcare encompasses more than research. Clinicians gather evidence about clinical issues on a daily basis. They cannot function in their roles without assessment data. In the same way, research (i.e., external evidence) is a central source of evidence in clinical decision making and cannot be missed. Researchers (evidence generators) in any particular situation select a particular research design that matches the healthcare concern they are investigating. This establishes that there are numerous research designs that can be useful to clinicians; each one must be matched to the proper clinical issue (see Chapter 2). Depending on the type of clinical question, the range of available research designs includes RCT (the most rigorous design for intervention questions) to descriptive or qualitative designs (the best for addressing meaning questions; see Chapter 2 for more on forming clinical questions). To provide best care for all types of clinical issues encountered in healthcare on a daily basis, clinicians (i.e., evidence users) must be knowledgeable and skilled in *reading and interpreting* a wide range of research studies (external evidence). External evidence is combined with internal evidence in decision making, making it an imperative that clinicians are proficient at gathering and using internal evidence (quality improvement data, outcomes data).

It is important to note that both internal and external evidence are introduced and brokered within the decision making process through the clinician. Clinical expertise cannot be considered apart from clinicians' use of the range of internal and external evidence available to them, including knowledge of (a) the psychosocial and basic sciences (e.g., psychology, physiology, anatomy, biochemistry, pharmacology, genetics); (b) appraised research from a range of methodologies; (c) clinical reasoning across time based on experiences with patients; and (d) individual patient's concerns and preferences. Clinicians must understand and interpret evidence in light of the patient's concerns, history, family, and cultural context. Furthermore, clinical reasoning enables clinicians to integrate their understanding of disease trajectory with what they know about the way the evidence was produced (how well researchers conducted the study) and what it offers clinical practice (how sure clinicians can be that they can get the same outcomes as the study if they implement the study intervention, for example); these are also called the validity and reliability of external evidence. All evidence must be carefully evaluated for its relevance for a particular patient (see Chapter 5). This process of evaluation, called critical appraisal, applies to single studies; syntheses, summaries, and synopses of comparative evidence; and guidelines.

Part of critical appraisal is considering all possible flaws in a research study before applying study findings. For example, clinicians must evaluate whether there were biased commercial influences in the design, presentation, or dissemination of the research; or, if the study is credible, whether the study can be directly applied to particular patients. Sometimes research is robust and convincing; at other times, it is weaker and more conflicted. Yet other times, the clinical trial that would address the issue for a particular patient has not been done. As part of the evaluation process, clinicians have an obligation to patients to constantly clarify practice patterns, skills, and clinical insights (i.e., thoughtful questioning and reflection about particular patient outcomes and a careful review of the basic science supporting associated interventions and their effectiveness) as they make joint decisions.

> **"**
>
> Reason obeys itself: ignorance submits to what is dictated to it.
>
> THOMAS PAINE

How You Think About Evidence Matters

Clinicians daily evaluate multiple data points and weigh their reliability, validity, and usefulness for making decisions. Validity of the data is determined by the correct data gathered for the correct issue (e.g., 124/68 is reported as a blood pressure, not pulse). Reliability is determined by data gathering methods resulting in data consistency (i.e., always measures the same way). Validity and reliability comprise data's credibility. The usefulness of these data is determined by what clinicians have deemed as credible pieces of information. It is important for clinicians to understand how credibility of information used in making clinical decisions is established.

Conee and Feldman (2004) articulated a theory called **evidentialism** that explains what is required for clinicians to have credible information as the basis of clinical decisions (e.g., justified belief about something; the evidence). One of the most important underpinnings for evidence-based decision making is the degree to which clinicians consider evidence as foundational to their decisions about the care they provide. In EBP, the evidence is categorized in two ways: (1) the sources of information, ranging from highly reliable sources to opinions of experts (i.e., levels of evidence) and (2) the quality of the information produced by these sources.

Conee and Feldman (2004) call the justified belief **"epistemic justification."** For clinicians, this means that the information available at a particular time justifies the decisions at that time—that is, the credibility of the available evidence establishes the credibility of the decision. Therefore, it is important to establish the validity, reliability, and applicability of evidence before it is applied to a clinical situation. In addition, epistemic justification reinforces the importance of continually learning throughout one's career (i.e., lifelong learning). For clinicians to have their best decisions justified, they must have evidence that supports it at that particular time. Clearly, should the evidence or circumstances change, the same decision may not be justified.

To better understand clinical decision making, three central themes of evidentialism are provided:

1. Evidence is mental information, which means that clinicians must be aware of or know about the information needed to make decisions (i.e., assessment; systematic searching).
2. Beliefs are based on current evidence, which means clinicians' beliefs are based on what they know at that moment.
3. Clinicians' experiences count as evidence.

Every theory has assumptions—what we believe to be true without proof. The assumptions underpinning the role of **clinical wisdom and judgment** in evidence-based decision making include the following:

- Only decisions that result from *thoughtfully responsible behavior* are justified.
- External evidence that supports a conclusion about patient care cannot be considered the sole source of information that makes a conclusion clinically meaningful.
- As available evidence changes, decision makers' responses should change too.
- Decisions made from a body of external evidence depend on the validity, reliability, and applicability (i.e., credibility) of the evidence and clinicians' understanding of the evidence (clinical wisdom).
- Having a belief without supportive external evidence is unjustified. An unjustified belief will affect all decisions connected to that unjustified belief.

These assumptions reinforce why clinical wisdom and judgment are critical to evidence-based decision making and how integration of clinical wisdom and judgment along with external evidence is imperative. Patients rely on clinicians to be clinically wise and make sound judgments as experts in their profession. When clinicians do not meet this expectation, they fail patients and communities.

Clinical wisdom and judgment may help fulfill the professional role responsibility to modify or override external evidence as appropriate. Aikin (2006) argues that making decisions based solely on external evidence could cause harm. He argues that evidence must be intentionally included in decision making, and that there will be times when the prudent, pragmatic, and/or moral decision may not align with the external evidence. Decisions should be evaluated by wise, experienced clinicians as to their credibility, including the nature and quality of the supporting evidence, whether patients' preferences and values were fully considered, and whether the context is supportive of a caring relationship. Evidentialism provides clear and ethical support for clinicians to shift from tradition-based practice to EBP, and thereby fulfill their professional obligation to make the best decisions with their patients.

CLINICAL EXPERTISE

To continuously improve practice, different clinical interventions and consequent outcomes must be compared. The goal is for practice to be self-improving through application of external evidence and experiential clinical learning (i.e., use of internal evidence and clinical expertise) that leads to correction and improvement, rather than practice that is stagnant and based on tradition with the potential to repeat errors. **Experiential learning** and clinical inquiry are equally important to individual clinicians and organizations.

Organizations cannot be self-improving without every clinician actualizing self-improvement in the everyday course of his or her practice.

In the classic work by Gadamer (1976), experience is never a mere passage of time or exposure to an event. To qualify as experience, a turning around of preconceptions, expectations, sets, and routines or adding some new insights to a particular practical situation needs to occur. Experiential learning is at the heart of improving clinical judgment and directly contributes to clinical expertise, which is a core aspect of the EBP process. Learning can be from past or present experiences that involve the examination of evidence when considering a practice change.

> **"**
>
> ## Everything that occurs to us in life is a resource, an experience that we can learn from and grow from.
>
> **KILROY J. OLDSTER**

Although there is a considerable amount of literature that refers to and discusses clinical expertise, there is a paucity of literature that clearly describes the nature and purpose of such expertise. In general, expertise is defined as including "the possession of a specialized body of knowledge or skill, extensive experience in that field of practice, and highly developed levels of pattern recognition . . ." (Jasper, 1994). More specifically, McCracken and Corrigan (2004), defined clinician expertise as "a set of cognitive tools that aid in the interpretation and application of evidence. This set of tools for thinking develops over a period of extended practice such that the individual with experience in a decision area is likely to respond very differently from the novice" (p. 302). These authors suggested that clinicians' expertise includes three overlapping knowledge and skill sets: clinical, technical, and organizational. The clinical set includes knowledge, skills, and experience related to direct practice with clients and includes diagnosis, assessment, engagement, relationships, communication related to warmth and genuineness as well as knowledge of theory, and mastery of skills related to specific care models and interventions (Barlow, 2004; Lambert & Barley, 2001). The technical set includes knowledge, skills, and experience related to formulating questions, conducting a systematic electronic search, and evaluating validity and reliability of findings for use in evidence-based decision making (Gibbs, 2003). The organizational set includes knowledge, skills, and experience related to teamwork, organizational design and development, and leadership (McCracken & Corrigan, 2004).

The application of clinical expertise to evidence-based decision making highlights the fluid interaction that must occur for the best decisions to be made, particularly with a patient/family who is in unique moments and spaces. In everyday clinical practice, individual perceptions, decisions, and actions are influenced by the current situation as well as clinicians' experience. To deliver best care, there must be a continuous flow of external evidence into practice and out to the patients. What evidence supports as best practice is what counts as good practice in any particular discipline. Clinicians, then, have an obligation to develop mastery of this flow of external evidence so that they become clinical experts. In their expert roles, they can effectively use their clinical wisdom and judgment to integrate patient preferences in a decision making relationship with the patient.

Clinical expertise, while inclusive of skills, knowledge, and experience of clinicians, also incorporates experiences of applying external evidence to contextualized (i.e., different clinical settings), situated, clinical experiences. Clinical expertise is on a continuum of experiential learning and can be described as clinicians becoming more expert through decision making within such contextualized experiences (e.g., clinical rotations for exposure to various circumstances and decisions). At any point in the experiential learning continuum, clinicians are able to perform at their best and progress in expertise as they engage in additional clinical decision making experiences. This is supported by Benner's (1984/2001) novice to expert framework.

Much of the literature on clinical expertise is implicitly based on the assumption that expertise is based on tacit (inferred) knowledge and intuition that cannot be described. Kinchin, Cabot, and Hay (2008) suggested that although the development of expertise is highly regarded, its indicators have often been described as an "opaque phenomenon" (Benner, 1984/2001; Dreyfus & Dreyfus, 1986) and labeled as intuition or implicit (i.e., not readily describable or hidden). These descriptions, according to Kinchin et al., have clouded what is actually happening and that indeed expertise is not implicit or indescribable, it has simply not been described adequately with the tools and vocabulary that we have applied to other aspects of decision making. New tools, such as concept maps and other advanced technology applications, are available to explicate the multidimensionality of clinical expertise-related concepts and how they interact. Individuals can use these concepts and their interactions to describe their decision making and growth in experiential learning.

Beginning evidence-based decision makers start their experiential learning journey through perceived assessment and evaluation of simple indicators of competence (i.e., tasks), with a linear progression of assimilation of activities (e.g., how many tasks have I done on my checklist) that do not necessarily reflect clinicians' capacities to perform or excel in the inevitable uncertainties of real-world clinical practice, in which evidence-based decision making with patients is imperative. Clinical expertise is cultivated in teaching and precepted experiences in clinical settings in which the interaction of external evidence, clinical expertise, and patient preference is demonstrated, learned, assessed, scrutinized, valued, and ultimately actualized. All clinicians can engage in evidence-based decision making; however, the ability to embrace the ambiguity in healthcare and anticipate the complexity in a patient situation is key to demonstrating clinical expertise.

How You Think About Care Matters

As potential clinicians enter their basic preparation, it is interesting to ask why they made their choice. Health professions' educators often hear many indicate that they were encouraged by their parents, mentor, or teacher to pursue their career in the health professions because they "would be so good at helping people." However, nursing and other healthcare professions include far more than "helping people." Developing good thinking, as Dr. John Maxwell (2009) calls it, is imperative. Good thinking requires embracing big-picture thinking, which in this discussion means to embrace the research, clinical expertise, and patient preference/values in each decision. However, focused thinking is also required, in which the perspective gained by big-picture thinking is used to bring the decision to fruition. For example, in the story of the 93-year-old tap dancer, the complexity of thinking required for the neurosurgeon to make the decision with her to pursue surgery is revealed in the links between ethical and clinical decision making. These challenges are magnified in the dancer's comment about the problematic implications of instinctively applying population-based research findings to individual patients. Both clinician and patient had to choose to see the big picture first (e.g., in the current context, what does the patient want and can it be obtained) and then use focused thinking to make the best decision to achieve the patient's desired outcome (e.g., how do we make this happen).

How you think matters more than what you think.

PHILIP E. TETLOCK

Within this framework, good clinical judgment requires the clinician to discern what is good in a particular situation. Good judgment comes with purposeful reflection on how learners consider their learning to become a clinician and then how clinicians approach their profession. It is important to note that decisions based on scientific facts are wonderful *if* those facts are interwoven with clinical wisdom and sound judgment that lead to careful consideration of the influence of patient preferences on a decision.

As much as clinicians like certainty, uncertainty is part of healthcare decision making (Kamhi, 2011). Patients do not represent an average statistical life to a possible medical intervention; rather, each patient is concerned with his or her particular chances and has only the particular life they have. Every clinical judgment has ethical aspects about the potential benefits and harms in a particular situation. The clinician must act in the patient's best interests and do as little harm and as much good as possible, demonstrating a relationship grounded in clinical stewardship and patient trust. In our example, the patient presented evidence that she experienced an exceptional health and fitness level, far different from projections based on the "average" 93-year-old person. For this woman, the social aspects weighed in heavily in this decision, as they do in many other clinical decisions. The patient explained that tap dancing was her life, and she literally could not imagine a life without tap dancing. She also had robust confidence in her physical and emotional ability to withstand the surgery successfully. It is her life and her choice, and in the end, her outcomes demonstrated that she was right. This is a great example of evidence-based decision making in which science is weighed and considered and indicates one path for treatment, but the patient's values and preferences were what really drove the decision making toward a different intervention (i.e., the evidence was "outplayed"). Furthermore, evidence-based decision making includes clinicians using their judgment to help patients make decisions that are best for them. In this example, this clinical wisdom extended to subsequently finding a surgeon to bring the patient's decision to fruition (use of focused thinking). This example has helped many people who have heard this story to understand the imperative of including patient information, preferences, values, and concerns in evidence-based decision making.

PATIENT PREFERENCES AND VALUES

Patient-centeredness is required for the integration of patient preferences and values in evidence-based decision making. Patient-centeredness is not a new concept in the delivery of healthcare. Early work in the areas of skills, attitudes, and knowledge of physicians relationships and interactions with patients focused specifically on training, components, and drivers of patient satisfaction; dysfunction and improvement strategies in doctor–patient communication; and deeper understanding of what patients want to know and how to help them discover what they want to know (Hibbard, 2007; Korsch, 1999; Roter & Hall, 2006; Ware, Snyder, Wright, & Davies, 1983). System-wide patient-centeredness leads to patient-centered care, which is imperative for evidence-based decision making.

Patient-centered care has been defined as "Providing care that is respectful of and responsive to individual patient preferences, needs and values, and ensuring that patient values *guide* all clinical decisions" (Institute of Medicine, 1999). Nonconsumer-focused stakeholders are sometimes not aware of what is truly important to patients and, therefore, do not engage them in the decision making process. The Institute for Healthcare Improvement (IHI, 2013) describes "patient-centered" as placing an intentional focus on patients' cultural traditions, values and personal preferences, family issues, social circumstances, and lifestyles. Including patient preferences and values in decision making leads to higher level of patient engagement, and engaged patients seem to have better perceived health outcomes (Gill, 2013a, 2013b).

Of note, not only individual clinicians provide patient-centered care but systems also must focus on patient-centered healthcare (International Alliance of Patients' Organizations, 2006). An additional resource designed to catapult the incorporation of patient preferences and values into healthcare decision making processes is the Patient-Centered Outcomes

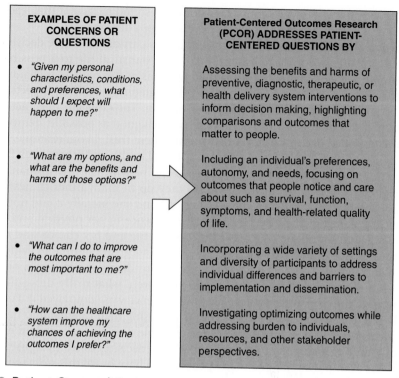

EXAMPLES OF PATIENT CONCERNS OR QUESTIONS	Patient-Centered Outcomes Research (PCOR) ADDRESSES PATIENT-CENTERED QUESTIONS BY
• *"Given my personal characteristics, conditions, and preferences, what should I expect will happen to me?"*	Assessing the benefits and harms of preventive, diagnostic, therapeutic, or health delivery system interventions to inform decision making, highlighting comparisons and outcomes that matter to people.
• *"What are my options, and what are the benefits and harms of those options?"*	Including an individual's preferences, autonomy, and needs, focusing on outcomes that people notice and care about such as survival, function, symptoms, and health-related quality of life.
• *"What can I do to improve the outcomes that are most important to me?"*	Incorporating a wide variety of settings and diversity of participants to address individual differences and barriers to implementation and dissemination.
• *"How can the healthcare system improve my chances of achieving the outcomes I prefer?"*	Investigating optimizing outcomes while addressing burden to individuals, resources, and other stakeholder perspectives.

Figure 7.2: Patient-Centered Outcomes Research Institute responses to patient concerns. (From Patient Centered Outcomes Research Institute [PCORI]. [2013]. *Patient-centered outcomes research.* Retrieved from http://pcori.org/research-we-support/pcor/on September 8, 2013.)

Research Institute (PCORI). The PCORI conducts research to provide information about the best available evidence to help patients and their healthcare providers make more informed decisions. Proposals for comparative effectiveness research studies must include patient preferences in their research design to be considered by PCORI. The vision of PCORI is for patients and the public to have the information they need to make decisions that reflect their desired outcomes. The work of PCORI answers clinical questions for both the clinician and the consumer and shares that information with the broader healthcare community (Figure 7.2).

In other work on an individual patient approach, Montori (2012) and the Mayo clinic focused on the development of decision aids. Decision aids provide specific options for patients to make decisions in collaboration with their physician. Intervention studies focused on providing support for patients and families making care decisions using decision aids have been conducted for some time in both inpatient and outpatient settings (Brinkman et al., 2013; Degner & Sloan, 1992; Gillies, Skea, Politi, & Brehaut, 2012; Kremer & Ironson, 2008). Decision aids help patients clearly elucidate the decision at hand by providing potential interventions, pathways, and outcomes that are clarified by applying personal values to the decision making process. Decision aids offer a valuable tool to clinicians as they counsel patients (Patient Decision Aids, 2017).

Studies conducted to address patient-centeredness and shared decision making (SDM) provide insight into the importance of patient engagement in their care. Decisions need to be realized through the interactions of patients and transdisciplinary healthcare providers. In addition, the evidence produced through studies that address patient-centeredness and transdisciplinary collaborative care may guide future actions and outcomes for healthcare staff, patients, and families. Légaré et al. (2011) conducted their first mixed methods study to determine the validity of an interprofessional (IP) approach to an SDM model with stakeholders, which typically includes patients. The data were analyzed using thematic analysis of transcripts and descriptive analysis of questionnaires. Results showed that most stakeholders believed that the concepts for interprofessional shared decision making (IPSDM) and relationships between those concepts were clear. With all IP healthcare providers valuing patient preferences in their decision making, the focus can easily turn to improving patient outcomes.

> ❝
> It is much more important to know what sort of a patient has a disease than what sort of a disease a patient has.
>
> **WILLIAM OSLER**

Légaré et al. (2013) later evaluated health professionals' intentions to engage the same IPSDM in home care and explore factors associated with the intent for SDM. Researchers of the mixed methods study reported factors associated with this intention vary depending on the healthcare provider, even within the same setting. In addition, researchers described barriers and facilitators to engaging in IPSDM. The greatest barrier reported was a lack of time to engage in the process, in addition to lack of resources and high staff turnover. A third finding that could influence decision making was that perceived behavioral control ("respondent's perception of barriers and facilitators to his/her performing the behavior," Légaré et al., 2013, p. 215) was most closely associated with the intention to engage in IPSDM.

Hesselink et al. (2012) explored barriers and facilitators to patient-centered care in the hospital discharge process in a qualitative study. Researchers identified four themes as barriers:

1. Time constraints and competing care obligations interfere with healthcare providers' prioritization in discharge consultations with patients and families.
2. Discharge communication ranged from instruction to SDM.
3. Patients did not feel prepared for discharge and post discharge care was not individualized.
4. Discharge process was affected by pressure for use of available beds. Researchers suggested increased communication between providers, patients and families, the hospital, and community care providers as a future intervention. These findings support the need for change in the process of SDM and the incorporation of patient preferences and values within the agreed upon IPSDM framework.

Berwick (2009) discusses the need for a radical change in care delivery and disruptive shift in control and power. The shift involves moving control and power out of the hands of those who give care and into the hands of those who receive care. He has proposed a new definition of patient-centered care: "the experience (to the extent the informed, individual patient desires it) of transparency, individualization, recognition, respect, dignity, and choice in all matters, without exception, related to one's person, circumstances, and relationships in health care" (p. w560). In exploring the concept of patient-centeredness, three slogans were developed: "(1) The needs of the patient come first; (2) Nothing about me without me; and (3) Every patient is the only patient" (p. w560). Based on the patient as a member of the healthcare system, Berwick proposed the following radical changes to patient care:

- Hospitals would have no restrictions on visiting: restrictions would be decided upon by the individual and/or family.
- Patients would determine what food they eat and what clothes they wear in hospitals based on patient condition.

- Rounding would include the patient and family member(s).
- Medical records would belong to the patient: healthcare providers would need permission to access patient healthcare information.
- Operating room schedules would change with the aim of minimizing wait time for patients as opposed to schedules based on clinician choice.
- Patients physically capable of self-care would have the option to do it (Berwick, p. 561).

Berwick (2009), knowing the need for quality in healthcare design and systems to support patient-centeredness, suggests the following statement become a part of a healthcare providers ending interaction with each person: "Is there anything at all that could have gone better today from your point of view in the care you experienced?" (p. w563).

How You Think About Shared Decision Making Matters

A clinician's approach to SDM in any healthcare setting can affect the effectiveness of outcomes to patients, families, staff, and the overall organization. Just as the language of EBP is essential for the EBP paradigm and process, the language we use in SDM can affect the understanding of those making the decision and the difference SDM can make in the overall success of the EBP process. Healthcare literacy includes use of a common language that fosters engagement in SDM aimed at achieving the best outcomes for patients, families, and staff regardless of the healthcare setting (Long, 2018).

Montori's (2012) interactions with patients in SDM revealed that addressing communication and perception issues were imperative when engaging patients in mutual decision making. Clinicians are cautioned to refrain from making judgments about what patients may or may not expect or desire related to their physical and psychological care needs. To learn more, review examples of discussions with patients that focus on potential treatments and the overall care the patients preferred (Montori, 2012; https://www.youtube.com/watch?v=NECp7TtEzM4).

Long (2018) interviewed nurses about their perspectives on SDM with parents of hospitalized children. Two main themes emerged: communication and team approach. The two-way communication between nurses and parents in making decisions is essential, which is often opposed to the more traditional unilateral approach to healthcare decision making. In addition, nurses discussed the importance of team approach when providing care to children and their parents. Within the team approach, nurses reported that discussions with parents revolved around an essential component of understanding the desired involvement of parents/guardians in SDM. Nurses indicated that clear communication and clarity in understanding parent involvement was essential for the patient preferences and values component of EBP to be integrated into everyday patient care.

Understanding how clinicians think about SDM and its effect on practice can help them shift from considering discussions with the patient or family as "just another thing to do" to removing the potential for suffering by involving them in daily decision making. Integrating patients into care teams' decision making processes offers clarity in plans of care and desired outcomes, which can result in patient and family empowerment.

CONCLUSIONS: EVIDENCE-BASED DECISION MAKING LEADS TO OUTCOMES

Evidence-based decision making must be contextualized by the clinician in any particular clinical setting through actualizing particular patient–provider relationships, concerns, and goals. EBP can provide guidance and intelligent dialogue that brings best practice options to particular situations; however, clinicians need to intentionally seek out EBP knowledge for this to occur successfully. It cannot be assumed that all clinicians have current scientific knowledge or that knowledge flows only from science to practice. Knowledge also results from direct experiential learning in practice. Patient/family and healthcare values and concerns, practice-based knowledge, understanding change processes, and impact on patients and families all must be central to the dialogue between patient and clinician that incorporates the patients' values, concerns, and choices. In patient care, evidence-based decision making incorporates developing expertise and use of clinical judgment in conjunction with understanding patient preferences and applying valid external evidence to provide the best possible care.

EBP FAST FACTS

- Patient preferences and clinician expertise are essential to making clinical decisions that affect the health and well-being of patients and families.
- Clinical expertise includes clinicians' use of the range of internal and external evidence available to them, their clinical reasoning across time based on experiences with patients, and assessment of individual patient's concerns and preferences.
- Good thinking—evidence-based thinking—requires embracing big picture thinking (i.e., the research, clinical expertise, and patient preference/values in each decision).
- Patient/family and healthcare values and concerns, practice-based knowledge, understanding change processes, and impact on patients and families are integral to evidence-based initiatives.
- How clinicians think greatly influences how they practice.
- Evidence-based decision making is the precursor to implementing evidence in practice.
- Patients expect clinicians to communicate and work together to ensure they get the best care possible.

WANT TO KNOW MORE?

A variety of resources is available to enhance your learning and understanding of this chapter.

- Visit thePoint° to access:
  - Articles from the AJN EBP Step-By-Step Series
  - Journal articles
  - Checklists for rapid critical appraisal and more!

- Lippincott CoursePoint combines digital text content with video case studies and interactive modules for a fully integrated course solution that works the way you study and learn.

References

Aikin, S. (2006). Modest evidentialism. *International Philosophical Quarterly, 46*(3), 327–343.

American Nurses Association. (2014). *Professional role competence.* Retrieved from https://www.nursingworld.org/practice-policy/nursing-excellence/official-position-statements/

Barlow, D. H. (2004). Psychological treatments. *American Psychologist, 59,* 869–878.

Benner, P. (1984/2001). *From novice to expert: Excellence and power in clinical nursing practice.* Menlo Park, CA: Addison-Wesley.

Berwick, D. (2009). What "patient-centered" should mean: Confessions of an extremist. *Health Affairs, 28*(4), w555–w565.

Brinkman, W. B., Majcher, J. H., Poling, L. M., Shi, G., Zender, M., Sucharew, H., Britto, M. T., & Epstein, J. (2013). Shared decision-making to improve attention-deficit hyperactivity disorder care. *Patient Education & Counseling, 93*(1), 95–101. doi: 10.1016/j.pec.2013.04.009.

Conee, E., & Feldman, R. (2004). *Evidentialism: Essays in epistemology.* Oxford, UK: Clarendon Press.

Degner, L., Sloan, J. (1992). Decision making during serious illness: What role do patients really want to play? *Journal of Clinical Epidemiology, 45,* 941-950. http://dx.doi.org/10.1016/0895-4356(92)90110-9.

Dictionary.com. (2017). *Evidence.* Retrieved from http://dictionary.reference.com/browse/evidence?s=t

Dreyfus, H. L., & Dreyfus, S. E. (1986). *Mind over machine: The power of human intuition and expertise in the era of the computer.* New York, NY: Free Press.

Gadamer, H. G. (1976). *Truth and method.* (G. Barden & J. Cummings, Eds. and Trans.). New York, NY: Seabury.

Gibbs, L. E. (2003). *Evidence-based practice for the helping professions.* Pacific Grove, CA: Brooks/Cole.

Gill, P. S. (2013a). Improving health outcomes: Applying dimensions of employee engagement to patients. *The International Journal of Health, Wellness and Society, 3*(1), 1–9.

Gill, P. S. (2013b). Patient engagement: An investigation at a primary care clinic. *International Journal of General Medicine, 6,* 85–98. doi:10.2147/IJGM.S42226

Gillies, K., Skea, Z., Politi, M. C., Brehaut, J. C. (2012). Decision support interventions for people making decisions about participation in clinical trials (Protocol). *Cochrane Database of Systematic Reviews,* Issue 3. doi: 10.1002/14651858.CD009736.

Hesselink, G., Flink, M., Olosson, M., Barach, P., Dudzik-Urbaniak, E., Orrego, C., . . . Wollersheim, H. (2012). Are patients discharged with care? A qualitative study of perceptions and experiences of patients, family members and care providers. *BMJ Quality and Safety, 21,* i39–i49.

Hibbard, J. (2007). Consumer competencies and the use of comparative quality information: It isn't just about literacy. *Medical Care Research and Review, 64*(4), 379–394.

Institute for Healthcare Improvement. (2013). *Across the chasm aim #3: Health care must be patient-centered.* Retrieved from http://www.ihi.org/knowledge/Pages/ImprovementStories/AcrosstheChasmAim3Health-CareMustBePatientCentered.aspx

Institute of Medicine. (1999). *Crossing the quality chasm: A new health system for the 21st century.* Retrieved from https://www.ncbi.nlm.nih.gov/pubmed/25057539

International Alliance of Patients' Organizations. (2006). *Declaration on patient-centred healthcare.* Retrieved from http://www.patientsorganizations.org/showarticle.pl?id=712&n=312

Jasper, M. A. (1994). Expert: A discussion of the implications of the concept as used in nursing. *Journal of Advanced Nursing, 20*(4), 769–776.

Kamhi, A. (2011). Balancing certainty and uncertainty in clinical practice. *Language, Speech and Hearing Services, 42,* 88–93.

Kinchin, I. M., Cabot, L. B., & Hay, D. B. (2008). Using concept mapping to locate the tacit dimension of clinical expertise: Towards a theoretical framework to support critical reflection on teaching. *Learning in Health and Social Care, 7*(2), 93–104.

Korsch, B. M. (1999). Current issues in communication research. *Health Communication, 1*(1), 5–9.

Kremer, H., Ironson, G. (2008). Spirituality and HIV. In T. G. Plante & C. E. Thoresen (Eds.), *Spirit, Science, and Health: How the Spiritual Mind Fuels Physical Wellness.* Westport, CT: Greenwood Publishing Group.

Lambert, M. J., & Barley, D. E. (2001). Research summary on the therapeutic relationship and psychotherapy outcome. *Psychotherapy, 38,* 357–361.

Légaré, F., Stacey, D., Brière, N., Fraser, K., Desroches, S., Dumont, S., . . . Aubé, D. (2013). Healthcare providers' intentions to engage in an interprofessional approach to shared decision-making in home care programs: A mixed methods study. *Journal of Interprofessional Care, 27,* 214–222.

Légaré, F., Stacey, D., Gagnon, S., Dunn, S., Pluye, P., Frosh, D., . . . Graham, I. D. (2011). Validating a conceptual model for an inter-professional approach to shared decision making: A mixed methods study. *Journal of Evaluation in Clinical Practice, 17,* 554–564.

Long, L. (2018). *Perceptions of nurses and parents of hospitalized pediatric patients' engagement in shared decision-making* (Unpublished doctoral dissertation). University of Louisville, Louisville, KY.

Maxwell, J. (2009). *How successful people think.* New York, NY: Center Street Press.

McCracken, S. G., & Corrigan, P. W. (2004). Staff development in mental health. In H. E. Briggs & T. L. Rzepnicki (Eds.), *Using evidence in social work practice: Behavioral perspectives* (pp. 232–256). Chicago, IL: Lyceum.

Montori, V. (2012). *Shared decision making: An interview.* Retrieved from https://www.youtube.com/watch?v=NECp7TtEzM4

Patient Decision Aids. (2014, April 17). Retrieved from https://decisionaid.ohri.ca/

Roter, D. L., & Hall, J. A. (2006). *Doctors talking with patients/patients talking with doctors: Improving communication in medical visits.* Westport, CT: Prager.

Siegel, M. (2002, October 29). When doctors say don't and the patient says do. *New York Times, (Science),* p. D7.

Ware, J. E., Jr., Snyder, M. K., Wright, W. R., & Davies, A. R. (1983). Defining and measuring patient satisfaction with medical care. *Evaluation and Program Planning, 6*(3/4), 247–263.

8

Advancing Optimal Care With Robust Clinical Practice Guidelines

Doris Grinspun, Bernadette Mazurek Melnyk, and Ellen Fineout-Overholt

> **Whatever you can do or dream you can, begin it. Boldness has genius, power, and magic in it.**
> —*Johann Wolfgang von Goethe*

EBP Terms to Learn
Clinical practice guidelines
Integrative reviews
Systematic review
Internal evidence
Level of evidence
Meta-analysis
Randomized controlled trials

Learning Objectives
After studying this chapter, learners will be able to:

1. Discuss how clinical practice guidelines can reduce variation in care and optimize population health outcomes.

2. Describe attributes of good guideline development.

3. Identify reliable sources of clinical practice guidelines.

4. Discuss key components for rapid critical appraisal of a clinical practice guideline.

INTRODUCTION

Governments around the world are aiming to improve healthcare and optimize outcomes through initiatives that accelerate the systematic integration of clinical care based on the best evidence. Therefore, it is not surprising to see entire programs dedicated to this endeavor (Bajnok, Grinspun, Lloyd, & McConnell, 2015; Grinspun, 2011, 2015, 2016a). However, the problem is that clinical practice variations continue to persist (Melnyk, Grossman, & Chou, 2012; Runnacles, Roueche, & Lachman, 2018). More than 40 years have passed since Wennberg and Gittelsohn (1973, 1982) first described the variation in treatment patterns in New England and other parts of the United States. Since then, researchers have continued to document large variations in service use and healthcare spending across geographic regions (Institute of Medicine, 2013). These remarkable practice differences in the diagnosis, treatment, and management of patients continue to permeate healthcare everywhere and lead to problematic results.

The Dartmouth Atlas of Health Care (Wennberg, McAndrew, & the Dartmouth Medical School Center for Evaluative Clinical Sciences Staff, 1999) has long offered many queries that can assist in graphically demonstrating the variability of healthcare services in the United States. Features allow comparisons of states and resource utilization (Table 8.1). In Canada, similar reports are available through the Institute for Clinical Evaluative Sciences. These regional variations in care and resource utilization are reflections of the many factors that influence outcomes of healthcare delivery.

One critical factor that may hold the key to reducing variation in outcomes is the availability, uptake, and consistent utilization of clinical evidence at the point of care in the form of **clinical practice guidelines** and rigorously developed evidence-based

TABLE 8.1	Example of Data That Can Be Accessed From Dartmouth Health Atlas		
State Name	State No.	No. of Deaths*	Registered Nurses Required Under Proposed Federal Standards per 1,000 Decedents During the Last 2 Years of Life
Arizona	3	15,568	38.73
Nevada	29	6,020	48.18
New Mexico	32	6,344	35.82

* No. of deaths are from 20% sample.

Source: http://www.dartmouthatlas.org/index.shtm

recommendations by groups such as the U.S. Preventive Services Task Force (USPSTF), Guidelines International Network (G-I-N), the Community Preventive Services Task Force, and the Registered Nurses' Association of Ontario (RNAO). Clinical practice guidelines are statements that include recommendations for practice based on a systematic review of evidence along with the benefits and harms of interventions intended to optimize patient care and outcomes.

Practice based on evidence includes the integration of individual clinical expertise, including **internal evidence** (i.e., practice-generated data; see Chapter 4) and patient preferences and values with the best available evidence from systematic research (Melnyk & Fineout-Overholt, 2015). Robust practice guidelines also include a cost-benefit analysis. A good example of these comprehensive criteria is present in the best practice guidelines of RNAO. It incorporates a synthesis of the best evidence about recommendations for care in clinical and workplace issues that respond to specific questions. They are developed by panels of experts and based on systematic reviews, along with all aspects to be considered for determining a clinical decision. This includes risk, prognosis, age, costs, patient values, and institutional resources, maintaining a balance between the benefits and the risk of a recommendation (Grinspun, 2016b).

Evidence-based practice (EBP) requires clinicians to determine the clinical options that are supported by high-quality scientific evidence and corroborated with the internal evidence. Gaining access to up-to-date scientific clinical information can be very challenging, particularly where access to healthcare journals is limited. Synthesizing the information can be even more challenging. PubMed contains more than 27 million citations to articles from thousands of journals published worldwide making it impossible for the individual clinician to fully master a body of emerging evidence in a particular area. The reality of information overload is especially difficult for busy point-of-care providers who find themselves already overwhelmed by competing clinical priorities.

During a landmark workshop on clinical practice guidelines organized by the American Thoracic Society and the European Respiratory Society that drew experts from more than 40 international organizations, a vision statement was created that highlighted 10 key visions for guideline development and use (Schünemann et al., 2009). These included the following:

1. Globalize the evidence (i.e., make the evidence applicable on a worldwide basis).
2. Focus on questions that are important to patients and clinicians and include relevant stakeholders in guideline panels.
3. Undertake collaborative evidence reviews relevant to healthcare questions and recommendations.

4. Use a common metric to assess the quality of evidence and strength of recommendations.
5. Consider comorbidities in guideline development.
6. Identify ways that help guideline consumers (clinicians, patients, and others) understand and implement guidelines using the best available tools.
7. Deal with conflicts of interest and guideline sponsoring transparently.
8. Support development of decision aids to assist implementation of value- and preference-sensitive guideline recommendations.
9. Maintain a collaboration of international organizations.
10. Examine collaborative models for funding guideline development and implementation.

GUIDELINES AS TOOLS

Overwhelming evidence, competing clinical priorities, and ever-increasing accountability highlight the importance of synthesis studies and clinical practice guidelines. **Meta-analyses** (the highest form of systematic review) and **integrative reviews** (a narrative evidence review that synthesizes research on a given topic) facilitate practitioners' ability to base their interventions on the strongest, most up-to-date, and relevant evidence, rather than engaging with the challenging task of individually appraising and synthesizing large volumes of scientific studies. Evidence-based practice guidelines (EBPGs), which are systematically developed statements based on the best available evidence, including syntheses, make recommendations in order to assist practitioners with decisions regarding the most effective interventions for specific clinical conditions across a broad array of clinical diagnoses and situations (Tricoci, Allen, Kramer, Califf, & Smith, 2009). They also are designed to allow some flexibility in their application to individual patients who fall outside the scope of the guideline or who have significant comorbidities not adequately addressed in a particular guideline. These tools are increasingly being used to reduce unnecessary variations in clinical practice.

Rigorously and explicitly developed EBPGs can help bridge the gap between published scientific evidence and clinical decision making (Davies, Edwards, Ploeg, & Virani, 2008; Grinspun, Virani, & Bajnok, 2002; Miller & Kearney, 2004). As expected, the dramatic growth in guideline development is not without unintended consequences. The rigor of guidelines varies significantly as does the reporting on how a particular guideline is formulated. In a review of 53 guidelines on 22 topics by the American College of Cardiology (ACC) and the American Heart Association (AHA), Tricoci et al. (2009) found that the recommendations issued in these guidelines were largely developed from lower levels of evidence (e.g., nonrandomized trials, case studies) or expert opinion. As another example, Belamarich, Gandica, Stein, and Racine (2006) found that none of the 162 verbal health advice directives from 57 policy statements by the American Academy of Pediatrics, on which pediatric healthcare providers should counsel patients and parents, included evidence to support the efficacy of the advice (empirical data to support the advice produce positive outcomes). The findings from the Tricoci and Belamarich reviews indicate that the process of developing guidelines and recommendations needs to continuously improve, and the research base from which guidelines are derived needs to be tighter. The varied quality of guidelines produced points to the importance of clinicians having the knowledge and skills to critically appraise clinical practice guidelines and recommendation statements to ensure selection and implementation of high-quality guidelines.

At times, one can find guidelines with conflicting recommendations, posing dilemmas for users and potentially hindering, rather than advancing, quality patient care and outcomes. For example, some professional organizations continue to recommend routine lipid screening in children with cardiovascular risk factors when there is insufficient and less than high-quality evidence to support this recommendation (Grossman, Moyer, Melnyk, Chou, & DeWitt, 2011). Guidelines also are often developed and written in ways that clinicians and organizations may find difficult to implement, which limits their effectiveness and impact on clinical practice and improving patient outcomes. Despite these limitations or "growing pains," the increased emphasis over the past two decades on evidence-based guideline development, implementation, and evaluation is a welcome direction toward evidence-based decision making at the point of care. This chapter offers clinicians a brief overview of EBPGs and ways to access, critically appraise, and use these tools to improve the care and health outcomes of their patients.

HOW TO ACCESS GUIDELINES

In the past, finding EBPGs was a formidable challenge. The large number of guideline developers and topics, coupled with the various forms of guideline publication and distribution, made identification of guidelines difficult and unpredictable. Fortunately today, a two-step Google search brings forward the most commonly used EBPG sites. If the term *practice guideline* is used, you will immediately access the Centre for Health Evidence (CHE), the Canadian Medical Association (CMA), the Registered Nurses' Association of Ontario (RNAO), and other such reliable sources of EBPG. In addition, in order to make finding EBPGs easier, the term *practice guideline* can be used as a limit to define a publication type when searching the National Library of Medicine's (NLM) PubMed database:

 Access CCHE at http://www.cche.net/

Access CMA at http://www.cma.ca/

Access PubMed at http://www.ncbi.nlm.nih.gov/pubmed

Access RNAO at http://www.RNAO.ca/

Using the Google search term *practice guideline* alone, without any qualifiers, yields 23,100,000 results (0.47 seconds). Most of these citations are not actual guidelines but studies of guideline implementation, commentaries, editorials, or letters to the editor about guidelines. Thus, once a specific site (e.g., PubMed, G-I-N, RNAO, USPSTF) is accessed, it is important to refine the search by adding the clinical areas or interventions of interest. Searching citation databases for EBPGs can present challenges, because not all guidelines are published in indexed journals or books, making it difficult to locate them in traditional healthcare databases.

In the last decade, individual collections that distribute international, regional, organizational, or specialty-specific guidelines have matured (Box 8.1). The list of individual guideline developers is long, and the distribution venues for guidelines can be as plentiful as the number of developers.

In Canada, the RNAO disseminates its production of over 50 rigorously developed best practice guidelines (those supported by evidence from robust research) on its website; 44 of these guidelines are clinical and 11 focus on a healthy work environment or system. All are freely downloadable and widely used across Canada and internationally, having been translated into multiple languages, including French, Spanish, Chinese, and Italian. The RNAO clinical guidelines are kept up to date by being reviewed every 5 years. They have been adopted by individual clinicians, by entire healthcare organizations that join as Best Practice Spotlight Organizations (BPSOs), and by governments such as Investen in Spain and the Ministry of Health (MINSAL) in Chile.

BOX 8.1 *Selected Guideline Databases*

General

- U.S. Preventive Services Task Force: http://www.uspreventiveservicestaskforce.org/
- The Community Guide: https://www.thecommunityguide.org/
- Primary Care Clinical Practice Guidelines: http://medicine.ucsf.edu/education/resed/ebm/practice_guidelines.html
- Registered Nurses' Association of Ontario: http://rnao.ca/bpg/guidelines
- Canadian Medical Association Infobase, Clinical Practice Guidelines: https://www.cma.ca/En/Pages/clinical-practice-guidelines.aspx
- Health Services/Health Technology Assessment Text: https://www.nlm.nih.gov/hsrph.html
- Guidelines Advisory Committee: http://www.gacguidelines.ca
- Scottish Intercollegiate Guidelines Network: http://www.sign.ac.uk/guidelines/index.html
- National Institute for Health and Clinical Excellence: http://www.nice.org.uk
- New Zealand Guidelines Group: http://www.nzgg.org.nz
- Guidelines International Network: https://www.g-i-n.net/home

Specific

- American College of Physicians: http://www.acponline.org/clinical_information/guidelines
- American Cancer Society: http://www.cancer.org/
- American College of Cardiology: http://www.acc.org/guidelines
- American Association of Clinical Endocrinologists: https://www.aace.com/publications/guidelines
- American Association of Respiratory Care: http://www.aarc.org/resources/
- American Academy of Pediatrics: http://pediatrics.aappublications.org/content/114/3/874.full
- American Psychiatric Association: https://psychiatryonline.org/guidelines
- Ministry of Health Services, British Columbia, Canada: http://www.gov.bc.ca/health/
- New York Academy of Medicine: http://www.ebmny.org/resources-for-evidence-based.html
- Veterans Administration: http://www.va.gov/health/index.asp, https://www.healthquality.va.gov/
- National Kidney Foundation: https://www.kidney.org/professionals/guidelines
- American Medical Directors Association: https://paltc.org/product-type/cpgs-clinical-practice-guidelines
- Association of Women's Health, Obstetric, and Neonatal Nurses: http://awhonn.org
- National Association of Neonatal Nurses: http://www.nann.org
- Oncology Nursing Society: http://www.ons.org
- University of Iowa Gerontological Nursing Interventions Research Center: https://nursing.uiowa.edu/csomay/evidence-based-practice-guidelines

The CMA, also in Canada, maintains its InfoBase of clinical practice guidelines for physicians. Guidelines are included in the CMA InfoBase only if they are produced or endorsed in Canada by a national, provincial/territorial, or regional medical or health organization, professional society, government agency, or expert panel.

 Access CMA InfoBase at http://www.cma.ca/clinicalresources/practiceguidelines

---

In the United Kingdom, another country-specific guideline collection is the Scottish Intercollegiate Guidelines Network (SIGN) sponsored by the Royal College of Physicians. Also, the National Institute for Health and Clinical Excellence (NICE) in England maintains a collection of guidelines to advise the National Health Service. In New Zealand, the New Zealand Guidelines Group (NZGG) maintains a collection of guidelines developed under its sponsorship.

 Access SIGN at http://www.sign.ac.uk/our-guidelines.html
Access NICE at http://www.nice.org.uk
Access NZGG at https://www.health.govt.nz/publications?f%5B0%5D=im_field_publication_type%3A26

In the United States, the USPSTF produces rigorously developed evidence-based recommendations about clinical preventive services, such as screenings, counseling services, or preventive medications, that are released in an annual updated pocket guide for clinicians entitled Guide to Clinical Preventive Services (http://www.ahrq.gov/professionals/clinicians-providers/guidelines-recommendations/guide/index.html), which is an authoritative source for making decisions about preventive services. The USPSTF is composed of 16 national experts in prevention and EBP who work to improve the health of all Americans through their evidence-based recommendations, which are based on a rigorous review of the literature and an analysis of benefits and harms of the recommended clinical practice. Similar to the Guide to Clinical Preventive Services, the Guide to Community Preventive Services is a free resource rigorously developed by a panel of national experts to help clinicians choose programs and policies to improve health and prevent disease in their communities.

 Access USPSTF at http://www.ahrq.gov/professionals/clinicians-providers/guidelines-recommendations/guide/index.html
Access the Guide to Community Preventive Services at http://www.thecommunityguide.org/index.html

---

Several individual professional societies and national groups in the United States also maintain collections of guidelines specific to a particular practice, professional specialty, disease screening, prevention, or management. The ACC and the AHA have joint guideline panels and publish their guidelines in a variety of formats. The American Cancer Society (ACS) also convenes multidisciplinary panels to develop cancer-related guidelines and to make the guidelines available on the Internet.

Access the ACC at http://www.acc.org/guidelines
Access the ACS at http://www.cancer.org/

In addition, there is an international collaboration of researchers, guideline developers, and guideline implementers called the ADAPTE Collaboration that promotes the development and use of clinical practice guidelines through adaptation of existing guidelines. This collaboration develops and validates a generic adaptation process that fosters valid and high-quality adapted guidelines.

 Access ADAPTE Collaboration at http://www.g-i-n.net/library/international-guidelines-library/

Although it is useful to have collections of guidelines that are specific to a disease or specialty, this can make it difficult to find guidelines in more than one clinical area. In 1998, the U.S. Agency for Health Care Policy and Research, now the Agency for Healthcare Research and Quality (AHRQ), released the National Guideline Clearinghouse (NGC).

The NGC was developed in partnership with the American Medical Association and the American Association of Health Plans. In developing the NGC, AHRQ intended to create a comprehensive database of up-to-date English language EBPGs (Box 8.2). NGC supported AHRQ's mission to produce evidence to make healthcare safer, higher quality, more accessible, equitable, and affordable by providing objective, detailed information on clinical practice guidelines, and to further their dissemination, implementation, and use in order to inform healthcare decisions. On July 16th, 2018, the NGC was no longer publicly available due to a lack of federal funding to AHRQ to continue it. However, since other stakeholders have expressed interest in continuing this type of guideline repository, it is hoped that sometime in the near future a similar type of guideline repository will be publicly available. At the time of its closure, the NGC contained well over 10,000 clinical guidelines from developers all over the world.

Organizations or developers who submitted guidelines to NGC had to meet the strict criteria for trustworthiness of clinical practice guidelines recommended by the Institute of Medicine's (IOM) landmark publication entitled *Clinical Guidelines We Can Trust*, published in 2011. In this publication, the IOM recommended that trustworthy clinical practice guidelines should

- be based on a systematic review of the existing evidence;
- be developed by a knowledgeable, multidisciplinary panel of experts and representatives from key affected groups;
- consider important patient subgroups and patient preferences, as appropriate;
- be based on an explicit and transparent process that minimizes distortions, biases, and conflicts of interest;
- provide a clear explanation of the logical relationships between alternative care options and health outcomes, and provide ratings of both the quality of evidence and the strength of recommendations;
- be reconsidered and revised as appropriate when important new evidence warrants modification of recommendations.

BOX	
8.2	*Elements of a Comprehensive Database of Up-to-Date Evidence-Based Practice Guidelines (EBPGs)*

Sample database features

- Structured abstracts (summaries) about the guideline and its development, fully downloadable
- Links to full-text guidelines, where available, and/or ordering information for print copies
- A guideline comparison utility that gives users the ability to generate side-by-side comparisons for any combination of two or more guidelines
- Unique guideline comparisons that allow for comparing guidelines covering similar topics, highlighting areas of similarity and difference
- A mechanism for exchanging information on clinical practice guidelines and their development, implementation, and use
- Annotated bibliographies on guideline development, methodology, structure, evaluation, and implementation
- Expert commentaries
- Guideline archive

Sample EBPG inclusion criteria

- Contains systematically developed statements including recommendations intended to optimize patient care and assist health care practitioners and patients to make decisions about appropriate health care for specific clinical circumstances.
- Produced under the auspices of a healthcare specialty, organization or plan, professional society, private or public organization, or government agency, not by an individual(s) without support of such agencies.
- Based on a systematic review of evidence.
- Contains an assessment of the benefits and harms of recommended care and alternative care options.
- Available to the public upon request (for free or for a fee).
- Developed, reviewed, or revised within the past 5 years, as evidenced by appropriate documentation (e.g., the systematic review or detailed description of methodology).

The NCG database was updated at least weekly with new content and provided guideline comparison features so that users could explore differences among guidelines, facilitating critical appraisal. An important feature of the NGC was the guideline synthesis, which enabled users to access comprehensive information with the best available evidence to support recommendations. Expert commentaries were also available at the NCG website.

Of the various guideline collections and databases, the NGC contained the most descriptive information about guidelines. It was also the most selective about the guidelines included in its database. Inclusion criteria were applied to each guideline to determine whether or not they would be incorporated in the database. Furthermore, guidelines in the NGC database reflected the most current version. In nursing, almost all of RNAO clinical guidelines were posted on the NGC.

A very helpful website is the NLM Gateway. The Gateway allows users to enter a search term that is then sent out to eight different NLM databases. One of these, Health Services/ Health Technology Assessment Text (HSTAT), is especially practical. HSTAT is unique because it takes large guidelines, systematic reviews, and technology assessments and enables their texts to be searchable on the Internet, making them much easier to navigate electronically.

 Access the NLM Gateway at http://gateway.nlm.nih.gov/gw/Cmd

There is no shortage of guideline-related sites on the Internet. The challenge is finding the source of guidelines that is easiest to use and provides the best mechanisms for making sure the contents are up to date. Because so many guideline resources are now on the Internet, it is wise to consider the quality of the website when choosing a source. Extremely useful databases of evidence-based guidelines exist. Many of these resources provide users with the guidelines, and some also provide additional information on how guidelines are developed and used. Evaluation of guideline databases is necessary to ensure that the information is reliable and current.

FINDING THE RIGHT GUIDELINE

Locating and reviewing current guidelines on a particular subject are often overwhelming. Even after a guideline has been identified, it can be difficult to determine critical information of the guideline, such as who developed and funded it, who was on the panel, how the guideline was developed, and what dates the literature review covered. Guidelines should provide this background and be explicit in their discussion of the evidence supporting their recommendations as well as in identifying the benefits and harms of interventions (DiCenso, Ciliska, Dobbins, & Guyatt, 2005; Rey, Grinspun, Costantini, & Lloyd, 2018; Grinspun & Bajnok, 2018). Guidelines developed using evidence of established benefit and harms of treatments or interventions have the potential to improve healthcare and health outcomes as well as decrease morbidity and mortality (Grimshaw, Thomas, & MacLennan, 2004; Melnyk et al., 2012). However, low-quality guidelines may harm patients and should be carefully appraised for validity and reliability of their information and supporting evidence.

Users of guidelines need to keep in mind that "one size *does not* fit all." In a landmark work, Hayward, Wilson, Tunis, Bass, and Guyatt (1995) from the Evidence-Based Medicine Working Group identified three main questions to consider when using EBPGs: (a) What are the guideline recommendations? (b) Are the guideline recommendations valid? (c) How useful are the recommendations? Lastly, experts remind us that evidence alone is never sufficient to make clinical decisions. One must weigh the evidence in context, always accounting for the values and preferences of patients with the goal of achieving optimal shared decision making; risk; prognosis; age; costs; and institutional resources, always maintaining a balance between the benefits and the risk of a recommendation (Grinspun, 2016b; Rey, Grinspun, Costantini, & Lloyd, 2018; Straus & Hayenes, 2009). These authors add that key to supporting clinicians is ensuring that information resources are reliable, relevant, and readable.

How to Read and Critically Appraise Recommendations

The strength of a guideline is based on the validity and reliability of its recommendations. In addition, guideline usefulness depends highly on the meaningfulness and practicality of the recommendations. Practicality relates to the ease with which a recommendation can be implemented. The recommendations should be as unambiguous as possible. They should address how often screening and other interventions should occur to achieve optimal outcomes. In addition, the recommendations should be explicit about areas where informing the patient of choices can lead to varying decisions. Furthermore, recommendations should address clinically relevant actions. The developers' assessment of the benefits against the harms of implementing the recommendation should be part of the supporting documentation for the recommendation.

It is important to know whether the developers focused on outcomes that are meaningful to patients and whether they were inclusive in considering all reasonable treatment options for a given condition or disease. The user should consider whether the developers assigned different values to the outcomes they evaluated, taking patient preferences into consideration. Developers need to fully describe the process used to systematically search and review the evidence on which the guideline recommendations are based. When combining the evidence, it is important to note whether the developer used a rating scheme or similar method to determine the quality and strength of the studies included, both primary studies and syntheses. Developers often use letter grades or words such as *strongly recommend* to rate their assessment of the strength of the evidence for a given recommendation. In 2002, the Research Training Institute at the University of North Carolina at Chapel Hill (RTI-UNC) Evidence-Based Practice Center completed a **systematic review** of schemes used to rate the quality of a body of evidence. While there is no universal consensus on grading evidence or determining the strength of a body of evidence supporting a recommendation, there are well-established norms. The most notable process for grading recommendations is the one used by the USPSTF (Harris et al., 2001; U.S. Preventive Services Task Force, 2008; Box 8.3).

BOX
8.3

The USPSTF System for Evaluating Evidence to Support Recommendations

A: The USPSTF recommends the service. There is high certainty that the net benefit is substantial. Offer or provide this service.

B: The USPSTF recommends the service. There is high certainty that the net benefit is moderate or there is moderate certainty that the net benefit is moderate to substantial. Offer or provide the service.

C: The USPSTF recommends selectively offering or providing this service to individual patients based on professional judgment and patient preferences. There is at least moderate certainty that the net benefit is small. Offer or provide this service for selected patients depending on individual circumstances.

D: The USPSTF recommends against the service. There is moderate or high certainty that the service has no net benefit or that the harms outweigh the benefits. Discourage the use of this service.

I: The USPSTF concludes that the current evidence is insufficient to assess the balance of benefits and harms of the service. Evidence is lacking, of poor quality, or conflicting, and the balance of benefits and harms cannot be determined. Read the clinical considerations section of the USPSTF Recommendation Statement. If the service is offered, patients should understand the uncertainty about the balance of benefits and harms.

USPSTF, U.S. Preventive Services Task Force.
Source: https://www.uspreventiveservicestaskforce.org/Page/Name/methods-and-processes

As another example of grading recommendations in clinical practice guidelines, the ACC and the AHA use a system based on level of evidence and class or recommendation (see http://www.acc.org and http://www.aha.org). The **level of evidence** integrates an objective description of the existence and type of studies supporting the recommendation and expert consensus according to one of three categories:

- Level of evidence A (i.e., the recommendation is based on evidence from multiple **randomized controlled trials** or **meta-analyses**);
- Level of evidence B (i.e., the recommendation is based on evidence from a single randomized trial or nonrandomized studies);
- Level of evidence C (i.e., the recommendation is based on expert opinion, case studies, or standards of care).

The class of recommendation indicates the strengths and weaknesses of the evidence as well as the relative importance of the risks and benefits identified by the evidence. The following are definitions of classes used by the ACC and AHA:

- Class I: conditions for which there is evidence and/or general agreement that a given procedure or treatment is useful and effective;
- Class II: conditions for which there is conflicting evidence and/or a divergence of opinion about the usefulness/efficacy of a procedure or treatment;
- Class IIa: weight of evidence/opinion is in favor of usefulness/efficacy;
- Class IIb: usefulness/efficacy is less well established by evidence/opinion;
- Class III: conditions for which there is evidence or general agreement that the procedure/treatment is not useful/effective and in some cases may be harmful (Tricoci et al., 2009).

Because guidelines reflect snapshots of the evidence at a given point in time, they require consistent updating to incorporate new evidence. Thus, it is critical that developers commit to a cyclical systematic review of their guidelines. In addition, developers can alert guideline users to ongoing research studies that may have an impact on the recommendations in the future. It is advisable that guidelines undergo peer review and pilot testing in actual practice before being released. Stakeholders' review allows a reality check to identify last-minute inconsistencies or relevant evidence that might have been overlooked. Pilot testing allows organizational or functional problems with implementing the guideline to be identified, including the cost of implementing the guideline. These can then be corrected or accommodated to enhance the chances of the guideline being implemented.

Widely used today is the *Grading of Recommendations Assessment, Development, and Evaluation* (GRADE), which provides a common and transparent approach to grading quality (or certainty) of evidence and strength of the recommendations provided in clinical practice guidelines. This is important because, as was previously discussed, systematic reviews of the effects of a given intervention—even when based on strong evidence—are essential but not sufficient information for making well-informed decisions. GRADE provides a systematic and explicit approach to making judgments that can help prevent errors, facilitate critical appraisal of these judgments, and help improve communication of this information (GRADE Working Group, 2017.

GRADE provides a framework for specifying healthcare questions, choosing outcomes of interest and rating their importance, evaluating the available evidence, and bringing together the evidence with considerations of values and preferences of patients and society to arrive at recommendations. Using GRADE enables us to be transparent in our judgment as to the quality of the evidence and the strength of the recommendations related to each of the outcomes and their importance. The system specifies three categories of outcomes according to their importance for decision making: (1) critical; (2) important but not critical; and (3) of limited importance. It enables one to categorize the strength of recommendations, ranging from a strong recommendation to a weak recommendation. A *strong recommendation* is one where the guideline panel is confident that the desirable effects of an intervention outweigh its undesirable effects. Using GRADE, a strong recommendation implies that most or all individuals will be best served by the recommended course of action. However, strong recommendations are not necessarily high priority recommendations because that will depend on the importance of the outcome. A *weak recommendation* is one in which the undesirable effects probably outweigh the desirable effects, but appreciable uncertainty exists. A weak recommendation implies that not all individuals will be best served by the recommended course of action. There is a need to consider more carefully than usual the individual patient's circumstances, preferences, and values. GRADE recommends that, when there are weak recommendations, caregivers need to allocate more time to shared decision making, making sure that they clearly and comprehensively explain the potential benefits and harms to a patient (Schünemann, Brożek, Guyatt, & Oxman, 2013).

Will the Recommendations Help Patient Care?

Applying a guideline on management of heart failure in the ambulatory setting is not the same as using a guideline on management of heart failure in the hospital. Similarly, a guideline on management of heart failure in children is not comparable with a guideline on management of heart failure in adults. The guideline should (a) fit the setting of care and the age and gender of the patients; (b) be usable by the type of clinicians providing the care; and (c) take into consideration the presence of any comorbidities. Ultimately, both the guideline user and developer must keep in mind the role evidence plays in developing recommendations. For example, unique characteristics of individuals, including comorbidities and clinical settings, are often not taken into consideration in experimental studies. Although EBPGs do not always take into account multiple conditions and patients generally do not present with only one disease or condition, guidelines can help point clinicians in the right direction when looking for the right care for their patients. Practitioners have the responsibility to individualize guideline implementation for their patients' circumstances.

Tools for Critically Appraising Guidelines

Finding the right guideline to use is contingent on being able to critically appraise the validity and reliability of a guideline. There is ample evidence that guideline developers do not always adhere to best practices in guideline development. Two landmark studies of guidelines developed by medical specialty societies found that a significant percentage did not adhere to accepted methodological practices in their development (Grilli, Magrini, Penna, Mura, & Liberati, 2000; Shaneyfelt, Mayo-Smith, & Rothwangl, 1999). In another landmark work, the IOM identified the following eight attributes of good guideline development:

1. Validity
2. Reliability and reproducibility
3. Clinical applicability
4. Clinical flexibility
5. Clarity
6. Documentation
7. Development by a multidisciplinary process
8. Plans for review

BOX 8.4	*Rapid Critical Appraisal Questions to Ask of Evidence-Based Guidelines*

- Who were the guideline developers?
- Were the developers representative of key stakeholders in this specialty (interdisciplinary)?
- Who funded the guideline development?
- Were any of the guideline developers funded researchers of the reviewed studies?
- Did the team have a valid development strategy?
- Was an explicit (how decisions were made), sensible, and impartial process used to identify, select, and combine evidence?
- Did its developers carry out a comprehensive, reproducible literature review within the past 12 months of its publication/revision?
- Were all important options and outcomes considered?
- Is each recommendation in the guideline tagged by the level/strength of evidence on which it is based and linked with the scientific evidence?
- Do the guidelines make explicit recommendations (reflecting value judgments about outcomes)?
- Has the guideline been subjected to peer review and testing?
- Is the intent of use provided (e.g., national, regional, local)?
- Are the recommendations clinically relevant?
- Will the recommendations help me in caring for my patients?
- Are the recommendations practical/feasible? Are resources (people and equipment) available?
- Are the recommendations a major variation from current practice? Can the outcomes be measured through standard care?

Guidelines are complex and heterogeneous documents with many different components; therefore, evaluating them is often difficult. However, with a good guide, critical appraisal of guidelines can be accomplished (see Appendix B for a rapid critical appraisal [RCA] checklist for clinical practice guidelines).

Rapid Critical Appraisal Checklist

The RCA of a guideline can be accomplished by applying standardized criteria when evaluating the attributes of the guideline (Box 8.4). The answer to each question in the RCA checklist supplies the end user with information that, when weighed together, enables the clinician to decide whether the given guideline is the best match for his or her setting, patient, and desired outcomes.

AGREE Instrument for Assessing Guidelines

In 1992, the U.K. National Health Services Management Executive set in motion the development of an appraisal instrument for the National Health Services (Cluzeau, Littlejohns, Grimshaw, Feder, & Moran, 1999). This was the first attempt to formally evaluate the usefulness of a guideline appraisal instrument. Subsequently, the European Union provided funding for the development of the Appraisal of Guidelines for Research and Evaluation (AGREE) instrument.

 The AGREE instrument can be found at http://www.agreetrust.org

The AGREE instrument (Box 8.5) was developed and evaluated by an international group of guideline developers and researchers. Since its original release in 2003, the AGREE instrument has been translated into many languages and has gained significant acceptance as the standard guideline appraisal tool. It is important to note that some studies raised serious

---

BOX 8.5 **AGREE II Instrument**

Scope and Purpose

Item 1: The overall objective(s) of the guideline is (are) specifically described.
Item 2: The health question(s) covered by the guideline is (are) specifically described.
Item 3: The population (e.g., patients, public) to whom the guideline(s) is (are) meant to apply are specifically described.

Stakeholder Involvement

Item 4: The guideline development group includes individuals from all relevant professional groups.
Item 5: The views and preferences of the target population (e.g., patients, population) have been sought.
Item 6: The target users of the guideline are clearly defined.

Rigor of Development

Item 7: Systematic methods were used to search for evidence.
Item 8: The criteria for selecting the evidence are clearly described.
Item 9: The strengths and limitations of the body of evidence are clearly described.
Item 10: The methods for formulating the recommendations are clearly described.
Item 11: The health benefits, side effects, and risks have been considered in formulating the recommendations.
Item 12: There is an explicit link between the recommendations and the supporting evidence.
Item 13: The guideline has been externally reviewed by experts prior to its publication.
Item 14: A procedure for updating the guideline is provided.

Clarity and Presentation

Item 15: The recommendations are specific and unambiguous.
Item 16: The different options for management of the condition or health issue are clearly presented.
Item 17: The key recommendations are easily identifiable.

Applicability

Item 18: The guideline describes facilitators and barriers to implementation.
Item 19: The guideline provides advice and/or tools on how it can be put into practice.
Item 20: The potential resource implications of applying the recommendations have been considered.
Item 21: The guideline presents monitoring and/or auditing criteria.

Editorial Independence

Item 22: The views of the funding body have not influenced the content of the guideline.
Item 23: Competing interests of the guideline development group members have been recorded and discussed.

Adapted from Brouwers, M., Kho, M. E., Browman, G. P., Cluzeau, F., Feder, G., Fervers, B., ... Makarski, J; AGREE Next Steps Consotrium. (2010). Agree II: Advancing guideline development, reporting and evaluation in healthcare. *Canadian Medical Association Journal, 182*, E839–E842, Table 1, p. E841.

questions regarding the interrater reliability of the AGREE instrument and suggested that the tool could benefit from further detailed appraisal (Wimpenny & van Zelm, 2007). The tool was further refined, and the AGREE II version was released in 2010.

The instrument contains 6 quality domains (areas or spheres of information) and 23 items. The domain scores remain the same as in the original one and are not meant to be aggregated into one overall score for the guideline. Thus, using the instrument to evaluate the robustness (strength) of clinical practice guidelines will produce individual domain scores and not an overall rating for a guideline. The revised instrument uses a 7-point Likert scale (up from the 4-point Likert scale) from 1 being "strongly disagree" to 7 being "strongly agree" depending on completeness and quality of reporting. The instrument allows the appraiser to give a subjective assessment of the guideline based on review of the individual domain scores. The AGREE instrument recommends there be more than one appraiser for each guideline—preferably four—to increase confidence in the reliability of the instrument.

Alternative appraisal instruments are being developed that address more than the guidelines along other sources of evidence. A promising example is the GRADE instrument (Atkins et al., 2004).

Conference on Guideline Standardization

The Conference on Guideline Standardization (COGS) Statement recommends standardizing the development and reporting of a guideline; hence, developers can ensure the quality of their guidelines and make their implementation easier (Shiffman et al., 2003).

 More can be learned about the COGS appraisal guides at http://gem.med.yale.edu/cogs/welcome.do

---

HOW GUIDELINES ARE DEVELOPED

Determining when to develop guidelines should be systematically approached owing to the amount of resources, skill, and time needed to accomplish these activities. In 1995, the IOM issued guidance on setting priorities for clinical practice guidelines (Field, 1995). The report emphasized the importance of considering whether the guideline had the potential to change health outcomes or costs and the availability of scientific evidence on which to develop the recommendations (Field, 1995). Other criteria used by organizations include the following:

- The topic is clinically important, affecting large numbers of people with substantial morbidity or mortality (the burden of illness).
- The topic is complex and requires clinical practice clarity.
- There is evidence of substantive variation between actual and optimal care.
- There are no existing valid or relevant guidelines available to use.
- There is evidence available to support evidence-based guideline development.
- The topic is central to healthy public policy and serves to introduce innovation.

When it is determined that there is uncertainty about how to treat or when gaps between optimal practice and actual practice have been identified, an organization may decide to develop a clinical practice guideline. Because it is difficult and expensive to develop guidelines, many organizations would be better served by adopting or adapting existing guidelines. Critically appraising already developed guidelines will allow an organization to screen for the best developed and suited guidelines for their organization.

Processes and Panels

When the decision is made that a guideline will be developed, several important steps must take place. Guidelines can be developed at a central level with a good scientific basis and broad validity, or they can follow a local approach in the form of care protocols agreed upon by a department or institution. The emphasis of the latter is on practical feasibility and support of care processes. These local guidelines can be developed using informal consensus, formal consensus, evidence-based methodologies, and explicit methodologies, either alone or in any combination. However, it is highly recommended that development focus on more formal and explicit processes so that another developer using similar techniques would likely come to the same conclusions.

Next, the guideline panel must be identified. The process for development of the panel should include multidisciplinary major stakeholders for the guideline, including users and patients (Scottish Intercollegiate Guideline Network, 2008). Guideline panels should be composed of members who can adequately address the relevant interventions and meaningful outcomes and can weigh benefits and harms. To increase the feasibility of implementation, it is advisable that panels be composed of subject experts who bring the different perspectives of research, clinical practice, administration, education, and policy (Grinspun et al., 2002; McQueen, Montgomery, Lappan-Gracon, Evans, & Hunter, 2008). Variations in the composition of the guideline development panel, the developing organization, and the interpretation of the evidence are often the source of differing recommendations on the same clinical topic across guidelines (DiCenso & Guyatt, 2005).

Review Questions

The next step in guideline development is the formal assessment of the clinical questions to be reviewed. This can be aided by the development of an analytic framework or causal pathway (Harris et al., 2001). These diagrams provide a roadmap for the precise description of the target population, setting of care, interventions, and intermediate as well as final health outcomes. They also help focus the most meaningful questions that will guide the literature review and subsequent recommendations. Figure 8.1 shows an analytic framework for prevention screening used by the USPSTF (Harris et al., 2001).

The numbers in the diagram relate to the key questions that will be considered. For example, (1) relates to whether the screening test actually reduces morbidity and/or mortality; and (5) asks the important question of whether treatment of clinically diagnosed patients results in reduced morbidity and/or mortality.

Literature Search and Review

After the key questions have been identified, a formal search and review of the literature take place. It is easiest if a systematic review has already been identified by searching databases such as the Cochrane Library, MEDLINE, Cumulative Index of Nursing and Allied Health Literature (CINAHL), and Embase. If an already completed systematic review is not found, it is necessary to develop one. The first step is to determine what types of evidence will be considered, including study design, dates of publication, and language. A search strategy of relevant citation database should be developed, preferably with the assistance of a medical librarian familiar with electronic searches. Once the search is completed, a process for screening titles and abstracts for relevance is conducted. The remaining titles are retrieved for evaluation. These articles are then screened and data are extracted from the studies. The individual articles are reviewed for internal and external biases, and their quality is often rated

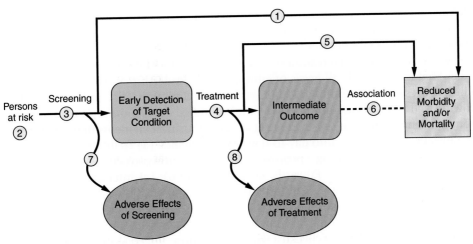

Figure 8.1: Example of an analytic framework with key questions for prevention screening evidence-based recommendations used by the U.S. Preventive Services Task Force. (Reprinted from Harris, R. P., Helfand, M., Woolf, S. H., Lohr, K. N., Mulrow, C. D., Teutsch, S. M., Atkins, D.; Methods Work Group; Third US Preventive Services Task Force. [2001]. Current methods of the U.S. Preventive Services Task Force: A review of the process. *American Journal of Preventive Medicine, 20*[3 Suppl.], 21–35. With permission from Elsevier.)

based on standardized criteria. Once data are extracted from the individual studies, the results are summarized, sometimes using meta-analysis to combine results from similar studies.

Evidence-Based Recommendations

The formal search, review, and appraisal of the literature lead to developing recommendations based on the strength of the evidence for each of the questions that were identified in the analytic framework. Some guideline panels choose to make recommendations based solely on evidence, whereas others use expert opinion when the evidence is poor or lacking. When expert opinion is used, it should be identified as such and be gathered using formal, explicit methods (Grinspun et al., 2002).

Peer Review and Dissemination

After the guideline recommendations are formulated, the guideline should be subjected to peer review to uncover any omissions or misinterpretations. In some cases, pilot testing will uncover that it is not feasible to implement a certain guideline or will offer tips to facilitate contextual modifications that ease adoption. Following the peer review and pilot testing, if necessary, the guideline is revised. Then, it is published and broadly disseminated.

IMPLEMENTING EVIDENCE-BASED GUIDELINES

It is important to understand that evidence and the quality of a guideline are vital, but are only two of many factors influencing guideline utilization. Implementing evidence-based guidelines into daily clinical practice requires a multifaceted and sustained approach with individual and systemic interventions. Indeed, despite the increasing availability of high-quality guidelines, their utilization remains low (Melnyk et al., 2012; Melnyk, 2015). Thus, the process for implementation is as important as that for selecting a robust guideline; it must be purposeful and well thought out.

Assessing organizational readiness for best practice guidelines implementation is a critical step that must include all levels of administrative leadership and clinical practice staff. Studies report successful results and improvements in clinical practice and patient outcomes following well-thought-out multilevel and multibundled interventions (O'Connor, Creager, Mooney, Laizner, & Ritchie, 2006; Ploeg et al., 2010). Critical elements that assist in uptake and translation of evidence into day-to-day practice include (a) facilitating staff to use best practice guidelines; (b) creating a positive milieu and securing structures and processes that inspire EBP (Gifford, Davies, Edwards, & Graham, 2006); (c) interactive education with skills building practice sessions and attention to patient education (Davies et al., 2008; Straus et al., 2011); (d) use of reminders (Cheung et al., 2012); (e) electronic gathering and dissemination systems offering real-time feedback and access to guidelines (Davies et al., 2008; Doran et al., 2009); (f) a checklist with interventions linked to times (Runnacles et al., 2018); (g) changing organizational policies and procedures to reflect best clinical practices and making staff aware of these changes (St-Pierre, Davies, Edwards, & Griffin, 2007); (h) prioritizing interventions when care bundles are used (Runnacles et al., 2018); (i) integrating evidence-based guidelines into care pathways when comorbid conditions exist; and (j) organizational and unit-based champions or EBP mentors, teamwork and collaboration, professional association's support, interorganizational collaboration, networks, and administrative leadership (Melnyk & Fineout-Overholt, 2015). Sandström, Borglin, Nilsson, and Willman (2011) discuss in detail the pivotal role that managerial leadership plays in securing uptake of research evidence by point-of-care clinical staff.

Several strategies are available to facilitate knowledge transfer. An effective example is the use of best practice champions (Ploeg et al., 2010). Best practice champions are nurses who promote, support, and influence the utilization of nursing best practice guidelines (RNAO, 2008). Similar to best practice champions, EBP mentors as first proposed in the Advancing Research and Clinical practice through close Collaboration (ARCC) Model (Melnyk & Fineout-Overholt, 2002) also are an effective strategy for implementation and sustainability of evidence-based guidelines and care with demonstrated outcomes of improving quality of care and patient outcomes (Melnyk & Fineout-Overholt, 2015; Melnyk, Fineout-Overholt, Giggleman, & Choy, 2017). EBP mentors, typically advanced practice nurses who have in-depth knowledge and skills in EBP as well as individual and organizational change strategies, work with direct care staff to use high-quality clinical practice guidelines and promote evidence-based care.

A review of guidelines conducted by Gagliardi, Brouwers, Palda, Lemieux-Charles, and Grimshaw (2011) shows that guideline producers do not, generally, include content about guideline implementation. However, there are excellent toolkits to facilitate the implementation process (RNAO, 2012). Implementation in nursing and other health sciences educational programs also is of critical importance in preparing future nurses and healthcare providers to "take a consistent evidence-based approach to care." Workshops with clinical instructors have been shown to be an effective way to assist faculty in initiating integration of practice guidelines in undergraduate nursing education (Higuchi, Cragg, Diem, Molnar, & O'Donohue, 2006). Quality measurement and feedback mechanisms can help determine whether the guideline is actually being used in practice. Lastly, implementing guidelines at the system level is a major undertaking that requires a whole systems approach. Edwards and Grinspun (2011) explain that to produce whole systems change requires the engagement of institutional, political, and educational stakeholders at the micro, meso, and macro levels of the system. In Canada, such a whole system change approach for cross-country clinical practice guidelines implementation is being spearheaded since 2011 by the Council of the Federation (2012).

Once best practice guidelines are successfully implemented, it is vital to ensure that utilization is sustained over time. This is critical to ensure long-lasting practice changes, improved clinical outcomes for patients, and organizational and system effectiveness. On-going administrative support and staff engagement are critical elements, as is embedding the evidence in policies, procedures, and plans of clinical care. Organizational learning theory provides a complementary perspective to understand the sustainability of practice changes. A critical aspect of this approach is that of "organizational memory," which refers to the various ways knowledge is stored within organizations for current and future use (Virani, Lemieux-Charles, Davis, & Berta, 2008).

Do Context and Culture Matter?

The ability of practitioners to implement evidence-based care and a guideline's recommendations highly depends on the **context** (i.e., the milieu or environment) and culture of an organization (Melnyk, 2016). A teaching hospital that has multiple clinical supports in the United States or urban Canada may differ greatly from a hospital with fewer supports in rural and remote areas in the same countries, let alone in developing nations. The level of staffing and skill mix impact guideline implementation as well as the organizational model of care delivery.

A critical success factor is the continuity of the care provider within the model of care delivery.

Practice guidelines can serve to build capacity and improve clinical practice across all sectors of care. However, strategies to promote uptake may be different in public health, hospital care, nursing homes, or home healthcare agencies.

Despite the need to account for practice context and culture, most practice guidelines focus only on clinical recommendations and overlook the critical role that work environments play, leaving it to individuals to determine the appropriate method for implementation. However, there are some guidelines that are improving on this development process. For example, RNAO's best practice guidelines contain clinical, work environment, and educational recommendations making them easier to implement in practice (Bajnok et al., 2015; Grinspun et al., 2002; RNAO, 2012). Gagnon et al. (2014) conducted a systematic review of instruments to assess organizational readiness for knowledge translation. They found that only 18 of 26 instruments were valid and reliable. One of these is the tool of Melnyk, Fineout-Overholt, and Mays (2008). Furthermore, Squires et al. (2014, 2015) conducted a comprehensive concept analysis of clinical practice contexts to better understand what facilitates and what mitigates against the uptake of research evidence by clinicians. These implementation science scholars aim to identify the domains of context that are important for the uptake of evidence into day-to-day clinical practice and to develop a pragmatic framework to facilitate knowledge translation. Similarly, Craig et al. (2017) tested a structured decision support procedure, using a survey, to identify and prioritize barriers to successful implementation of complex healthcare interventions. Edwards and Grinspun (2011) and Grinspun (2016a) discuss the leverages and blockages that enable whole system change to happen at the macro health system level. These authors give us a sober perspective of how evidence, as important as it is, is but one element to advance healthy public policy. Advocacy, in its various facets, is a key ingredient to overcome challenges at the health system level (Grinspun & Bajnok, 2018; Grinspun, Botros, Mulrooney, Mo, Sibbald & Penney, 2018).

IMPLICATIONS FOR PATIENT CARE

Evidence-based clinical practice guidelines have the potential to dramatically improve patient care, health outcomes, and organizational/system performance. When developed rigorously and implemented consistently, they can achieve their purpose of improving healthcare quality and patient outcomes. Guidelines can be an important vehicle for translating complex research findings into recommendations that can be acted upon. Because organizations still struggle with the best mechanisms to implement research into practice, guideline developers need to continue to strive toward collaboration and avoidance of duplication. Increasing collaboration between developers and implementers will result in practice recommendations that are readily usable by point-of-care practitioners as well as more easily utilized in electronic health records and clinical decision support tools. An encouraging sign is that developers also are condensing guidelines for download onto today's technology devices (e.g., NGC, RNAO). Collaboration among healthcare providers and joint clinical decision making also are central to improving patients' clinical outcomes (Grinspun, 2007; Grinspun & Bajnok, 2018). Moreover, transdisciplinary EBPGs can serve as a catalyst for positive team work.

In 2002, a new international organization, the Guidelines International Network (G-I-N) was formed. This not-for-profit organization is made up of 93 guideline developers from throughout the world. Its mission is to improve the quality of healthcare by promoting systematic development of EBPGs and their application into practice by supporting international collaboration. The presence of G-I-N is indicative of the move toward globalizing evidence while still promoting localized decision making. Given the complexity and expense of developing EBPGs, this type of initiative is essential. Moreover, this collaboration signifies a universal awareness that clinical decisions can no longer be made without being informed by the best available evidence.

 Find G-I-N online at http://www.G-I-N.net

NEXT FRONTIERS: CLINICAL DECISION TOOLS AND EVALUATION

The next 10 years will bring new developments to the area of EBPGs. Most notable are clinical decision tools derived from EBPGs and available application into electronic medical records to support decision making and documentation at the point of care and outcome evaluation of EBPGs. The RNAO is a leading organization in these two fields. RNAO's Nursing Order Sets are designed to be embedded within clinical information and decision support systems. These Nursing Order Sets are derived from RNAO's clinical-based practice guidelines and are coded using standardized terminology language based on the International Classification for Nursing Practice (ICNP; Wilson, Bajnok, & Costa, 2015).

RNAO also is heavily engaged in outcomes evaluation. The launching in 2012 of Nursing Quality Indicators for Reporting and Evaluation (NQuIRE) indicates the maturity of RNAO's EBPG program. NQuIRE collects, analyzes, and reports comparative data on nursing-sensitive indicators reflecting the structure, process, and outcomes of care arising from EBPG implementation. For now, NQuIRE focuses only on BPSOs. These are organizations with a formal agreement with RNAO to systematically implement, sustain, and evaluate RNAO's guideline—over 500 health service organizations such as public health units, primary care organizations, hospital, home care agencies and long-term care facilities, as well as academic entities—in Australia, Belgium, Canada, Chile, China, Colombia, Italy, Spain, and South Africa, are part of the BPSO movement. These healthcare organizations use NQuIRE data to inform where and how nursing is providing valuable benefits to patient, organization, and system outcomes by using evidence-based decision making to optimize safe, quality healthcare; (Grinspun, 2015, 2016b; Grdisa, Grinspun, Toor, Owusu, Naik & Smith, 2018; Van De Velde-Coke et al., 2012).

The RNAO's NQuIRE database can be viewed at https://nquire.rnao.ca/

Early results are promising both in the reception and adherence to the RNO BPSO program, as well as its clinical outcomes. For example, hospitals have reported improvements in falls risk assessment and reassessments, a reduction in the use of side rails (which is one of the key and most complex recommendation of RNAO's best practice guidelines on falls prevention) alongside the improved outcome of decreased injuries after a fall. Similarly, substantive improvements have been achieved by many BPSOs in the nursing care and interventions to prevent pressure injuries, alongside a decrease in their overall prevalence and the complete elimination of levels III and IV pressure injuries (Cortés et al., 2016; Esparza-Bohórquez, Granados-Oliveros, & Joya-Guevara, 2016). An important result across the board is a growing organizational culture of evidence-based care, a point seen in the eight BPSO hospitals in Spain (Albornos-Muñoz, González-María, & Moreno-Casbas, 2015; Moreno-Casbas, González-María & Albornos-Muñoz, 2018).

"

To think is easy. To act is hard. But the hardest thing in the world is to act in accordance with your thinking.

JOHANN WOLFGANG VON GOETHE

EBP FAST FACTS

- Clinical practice guidelines are statements that include recommendations for practice based on a systematic review of evidence along with the benefits and harm of interventions intended to optimize patient care and outcomes.
- Clinical practice guidelines that are rigorously developed reduce variations in care and enhance healthcare quality and patient outcomes.
- Not all clinical practice guidelines that are published follow rigorous methods in their development, which is why critical appraisal of guidelines before adopting them for implementation in clinical practice settings is necessary.
  - An excellent exemplar of the process used to develop rigorous evidence-based clinical recommendations can be found in the procedure manual used by the U.S. Preventive Services Task Force (see https://www.uspreventiveservicestask-force.org/Page/Name/procedure-manual).
- Implementing evidence-based guidelines in daily clinical practice requires a multifaceted and sustained approach with individual and systemic interventions, including individual skills building, along with factors such as developing a culture and context that support EBP, providing EBP champions and mentors, and administrative support that includes the provision of tools that support implementation of evidence-based guidelines and recommendations.

WANT TO KNOW MORE?

A variety of resources is available to enhance your learning and understanding of this chapter.

- Visit thePoint® to access:
  - Articles from the AJN EBP Step-By-Step Series
  - Journal articles
  - Checklists for rapid critical appraisal and more!

- Lippincott CoursePoint combines digital text content with video case studies and interactive modules for a fully integrated course solution that works the way you study and learn.

References

Albornoz-Muñoz, L., González-María, E., & Moreno-Casbas, T. (2015). Implantación de guías de buenas prácticas en España. Programa de centros comprometidos con la excelencia de cuidados [Implementation of good practice guides in Spain. Program of centers committed to the excellence of care]. *MedUNAB, 17*(3), 163–169.

Atkins, D., Eccles, M., Flottorp, S., Guyatt, G. H., Henry, D., Hill, S., . . . Williams, J. W. Jr.; The GRADE Working Group. (2004). Systems for grading the quality of evidence and the strength of recommendations I: Critical appraisal of existing approaches The GRADE Working Group. *BMH Health Services Research, 4,* 38.

Bajnok, I., Grinspun, D., Lloyd, M., & McConnell, H. (2015). Leading quality improvement though best practice guideline development, implementation and measurement science. *MedUNAB, 17*(3), 155–162.

Belamarich, P. F., Gandica, R., Stein, R. E. K., & Racine, A. D. (2006). Drowning in a sea of advice: Pediatricians and American Academic of Pediatrics Policy Statements. *Pediatrics, 118*(4), e964–e978.

Cheung, A., Weir, M., Mayhew, A., Kozloff, N., Brown, K., & Grimshaw, J. (2012). Overview of systematic reviews of the effectiveness of reminders in improving healthcare professional behavior. *Systematic Review, 1,* 36.

Cluzeau, F. A., Littlejohns, P., Grimshaw, J. M., Feder, G., & Moran, S. E. (1999). Development and application of a generic methodology to assess the quality of clinical guidelines. *International Journal of Quality Health Care, 11*(1), 21–28.

Cortés, O. L., Serna-Restrepo, A., Salazar-Beltrán, L., Rojas-Castañeda, J. A., Cabrera-González, S., & Arévalo-Sandoval, I. (2016). Implementation of clinical practice guidelines of the Registered Nurses' Association of Ontario-RNAO: A nursing experience in a Colombian Hospital. *MedUNAB, 19*(2), 103–114.

Council of the Federation. (2012). *From innovation to action: The first report of the health care innovation working group.* Ottawa, ON: Author. Retrieved from http://www.canadaspremiers.ca/council-of-the-federation-to-meet-in-victoria-on-january-16-17-2012/

Craig, L. E., Churilov, L., Olenko, L., Cadilhac, D. A., Grimley, R., Dale, S., . . . Middleton, S. (2017). Testing a systematic approach to identify and prioritize barriers to successful implementation of a complex healthcare intervention. *BMC Medical Research Methodology, 17*(1), 24.

Davies, B., Edwards, N., Ploeg, J., & Virani, T. (2008). Insights about the process and impact of implementing nursing guidelines on delivery of care in hospitals and community settings. *BMC Health Services Research, 8*(29), 1–44.

DiCenso, A., Ciliska, D., Dobbins, M., & Guyatt, G. (2005). Moving from evidence to actions using clinical practice guidelines. In A. DiCenso, G. Guyatt, & D. Ciliska (Eds.), *Evidence-based nursing: A guide to clinical practice* (pp. 154–169). Philadelphia, PA: Elsevier Mosby.

DiCenso, A., & Guyatt, G. (2005). Interpreting levels of evidence and grades of health care recommendation. In A. DiCenso, G. Guyatt, & D. Ciliska (Eds.), *Evidence-based nursing: A guide to clinical practice* (pp. 508–525). Philadelphia, PA: Elsevier Mosby.

Doran, D., Carryer, J., Paterson, J., Goering, P., Nagle, L., Kushniruk, A., . . . Srivastava, R. (2009). Integrating evidence-based interventions into client care plans. *Nursing Leadership, 143,* 9–13.

Edwards, N., & Grinspun, D. (2011). *Understanding whole systems change in healthcare: The case of emerging evidence-informed nursing service delivery models.* Ottawa, ON: Canadian Health Services Research Foundation.

Esparza-Bohórquez, M., Granados-Oliveros, L. M., & Joya-Guevara, K. (2016). Implementation of the good practices guide: Risk assessment and prevention of pressure ulcers, an experience at "Fundacion Oftalmológica of Santander" (FOSCAL). *MedUNAB, 19*(2), 115–123.

Field, M. J. (Ed.). (1995). *Setting priorities for clinical practice guidelines.* Washington, DC: National Academy Press.

Gagliardi, A. R., Brouwers, M. C., Palda, V. A., Lemieux-Charles, L., & Grimshaw, J. M. (2011). How can we improve guideline use? A conceptual framework of implementability. *Implementation Science, 6,* 26.

Gagnon, M. P., Attieh, R., Ghandour, E. K., Legare, F., Ouimet, M., Estabrooks, C. A. & Grinshaw, J. (2014). A systematic review of instruments to assess organizational readiness for knowledge translation in health care. *PLoS One, 9*(12), e114338.

Gifford, W. A., Davies, B., Edwards, N., & Graham, I. (2006). Leadership strategies to influence the use of clinical practice guidelines. *Nursing Research, 19*(4), 72–88.

GRADE Working Group. Downloaded on April 16, 2017. http://www.gradeworkinggroup.org/

Grdisa, V., Grinspun, D., Toor, G., Owusu, Y., Naik, S., & Smith, K. (2018). Evaluating BPG impact: Development and refinement of NQuIRE. In D. Grinspun & I. Bajnok (Eds.), *Transforming nursing through knowledge: Best practices for guideline development, implementation science, and evaluation.* Indianapolis, IN, USA: Sigma Theta Tau International Honor Society of Nursing.

Grilli, R., Magrini, N., Penna, A., Mura, G., & Liberati, A. (2000). Practice guidelines developed by specialty societies: The need for a critical appraisal. *Lancet, 355,* 103–105.

Grimshaw, J. M., Thomas, R. E., & MacLennan, G. (2004). Effectiveness and efficiency of guidelines dissemination and implementation strategies. *Health Technology Assessment, 8*(6), 1–84.

Grinspun, D. (2007). Healthy workplaces: The case for shared clinical decision making and increased full-time employment. *Healthcare Papers, 7,* 69–75.

Grinspun, D. (2011). Guías de práctica clínica y entorno laboral basados en la evidencia elaboradas por la Registered Nurses' Association of Ontario (RNAO). *EnfermClin, 21*(1), 1–2.

Grinspun, D. (2015). Transforming nursing practice through evidence [Editorial]. *MedUNAB, 17*(3), 133–134.

Grinspun, D. (2016a). Health policy in changing environments. In E. Staples, S. Ray, & R. Hannon (Eds.), *Canadian perspectives on advanced nursing practice: Clinical practice, research, leadership, consultation and collaboration* (pp. 285–299). Toronto, ON: Canadian Scholar's Press.

Grinspun, D. (2016b). Leading evidence-based nursing care through systematized processes [Editorial]. *MedUNAB, 19*(2), 83–84.

Grinspun, D., & Bajnok, I. (2018). *Transforming nursing through knowledge: Best practices for guideline development, implementation science, and evaluation.* Indianapolis, IN, USA: Sigma Theta Tau International Honor Society of Nursing.

Grinspun, D., Botros, M., Mulrooney, L.A., Mo, J., Sibbald, R.G., & Penney, T. (2018). Scaling deep to improve people's health: From evidence-based practice to evidence-based policy. In D. Grinspun & I. Bajnok (Eds.), *Transforming nursing through knowledge: Best practices for guideline development, implementation science, and evaluation.* Indianapolis, IN, USA: Sigma Theta Tau International Honor Society of Nursing.

Grinspun, D., Virani, T., & Bajnok, I. (2002). Nursing best practice guidelines: The RNAO project. *Hospital Quarterly, Winter, 4,* 54–58.

Grossman, D. C., Moyer, V. A., Melnyk, B. M., Chou, R., & DeWitt, T. G. (2011). The anatomy of a US Preventive Services Task Force recommendation: Lipid screening for children and adolescents. *Archives of Pediatrics and Adolescent Medicine, 165*(3), 205–210.

Harris, R. P., Helfand, M., Woolf, S. H., Lohr, K. N., Mulrow, C. D., Teutsch, S. M., Atkins, D.; Methods Work Group; Third US Preventive Services Task Force. (2001). Current methods of the U.S. Preventive Services Task Force: A review of the process. *American Journal of Preventive Medicine, 20*(3 Suppl.), 21–35.

Hayward, R. S., Wilson, M. C., Tunis, S. R., Bass, E. B., & Guyatt, G. (1995). Users' guides to the medical literature. VIII. How to use clinical practice guidelines. A. Are the recommendations valid? *JAMA, 274,* 570–574.

Higuchi, K. A., Cragg, C. E., Diem, E., Molnar, J., & O'Donohue, M. S. (2006). Integrating clinical guidelines into nursing education. *International Journal of Nursing Education Scholarship, 3*(1), article 12.

Institute of Medicine. (2013). *Variation in health care spending: Target decision-making, not geography.* Washington, DC: The National Academies Press.

Lohr, K. N., & Field, M. J. (1992). A provisional instrument for assessing clinical practice guidelines. In M. J. Field, & K. N. Lohr (Eds.), *Guidelines for clinical practice: From development to use* (pp. 346–410). Washington, DC: National Academy Press.

McQueen, K., Montgomery, P., Lappan-Gracon, S., Evans, M., & Hunter, J. (2008). Evidence-based recommendations for depressive symptoms in postpartum women. *Journal of Obstetric, Gynecologic, and Neonatal Nursing, 37*(2), 127–135.

Melnyk, B. M. (2015). Important information about clinical practice guidelines Key tools for improving quality of care and patient outcomes. [Editorial] *Worldviews on Evidence-based Nursing, 12*(1), 1–2.

Melnyk, B. M. (2016). Culture eats strategy every time: What works in building and sustaining an evidence-based practice culture in healthcare systems. *Worldviews on Evidence-Based Nursing, 13*(2), 99–101.

Melnyk, B. M., & Fineout-Overholt, E. (2002). Putting research into practice. *Reflections on Nursing Leadership, 28*(2), 22–25.

Melnyk, B. M., & Fineout-Overholt, E. (2015). *Evidence-based practice in nursing & healthcare. A guide to best practice* (3rd ed.). Philadelphia, PA: Wolters Kluwer/Lippincott Williams & Wilkins.

Melnyk, B. M., Fineout-Overholt, E., Giggleman, M., & Choy, K. (2017). A test of the ARCC® model improves implementation of evidence-based practice, healthcare culture, and patient outcomes. *Worldviews on Evidence-Based Nursing, 14*(1), 5–9.

Melnyk, B. M., Fineout-Overholt, E., & Mays, M. Z. (2008). The evidence-based practice beliefs and implementation scales: Psychometric properties of two new instruments. *Worldviews on Evidence-Based Nursing, 5,* 208–216.

Melnyk, B. M., Grossman, D., & Chou, R. (2012). USPSTF perspective on evidence-based preventive recommendations for children. *Pediatrics, 130*(2), e399–e407.

Miller, M., & Kearney, N. (2004). Guidelines for clinical practice: Development, dissemination and implementation. *International Journal of Nursing Studies, 41*(1), 813–821.

O'Connor, P., Creager, J., Mooney, S., Laizner, A. M., & Ritchie, J. (2006). Taking aim at falls injury adverse events: Best practices and organizational change. *Healthcare Quarterly, 9*(Special Issue), 43–49.

Ploeg, J., Skelly, J., Rowan, M., Edwards, N., Davies, B., Grinspun, D., . . . Downey, A. (2010). The role of nursing best practice champions in diffusing practice guidelines: A mixed methods study. *Worldviews on Evidence-Based Nursing, 7*(4), 238–251.

Rey, M., Grinspun, D., Costantini, L., & Lloyd, M. (2018). The anatomy of a rigorous best practice guideline development process. In D. Grinspun & I. Bajnok (Eds.), *Transforming nursing through knowledge: Best practices for guideline development, implementation science, and evaluation.* Indianapolis, IN, USA: Sigma Theta Tau International Honor Society of Nursing.

Registered Nurses' Association of Ontario. (2008). *Who are best practice champions.* Retrieved from http://www.rnao.org/

Registered Nurses' Association of Ontario. (2012). *Toolkit: Implementation of clinical practice guidelines* (2nd ed.). Toronto, ON: Author.

Research Training Institute. (2002). *RTI-UNC evidence-based practice center.* Retrieved from http://www.rti.org

Runnacles, J., Roueche, A., & Lachman, P. (2018). The right care, every time: Improving adherence to evidence-based guidelines. *Archives of Disease in Childhood. Education and Practice Edition, 103*(1), 27–33.

Sandström, B., Borglin, G., Nilsson, R., & Willman, A. (2011). Promoting the implementation of evidence-based practice: A literature review focusing on the role of nursing leadership. *Worldviews on Evidence-Based Nursing, 8*(4), 212–223.

Schünemann, H., Brożek, J., Guyatt, G., Oxman, A. (2013). *GRADE handbook.* Retrieved from http://gdt.guide-linedevelopment.org/app/handbook/handbook.html#ftnt_ref1

Schünemann, H. J., Woodhead, M., Anzueto, A., Buist, S., MacNee, W., Rabe, K. F., & Heffner, J. (2009). A vision statement on guideline development for respiratory disease: The example of COPD. *Lancet, 373,* 774–779.

Scottish Intercollegiate Guideline Network. (2008). *SIGN 50: A guideline developers' handbook. An introduction to SIGN methodology for the development of evidence-based clinical guidelines.* Edinburgh, Scotland: Author.

Shaneyfelt, T. M., Mayo-Smith, M. F., & Rothwangl, J. (1999). Are guidelines following guidelines? The methodological quality of clinical practice guidelines in the peer-reviewed medical literature. *JAMA, 281,* 1900–1905.

Shiffman, R. N., Shekelle, P., Overhage, J. M., Slutsky, J., Grimshaw, J., & Deshpande, A. M. (2003). Standardized reporting of clinical practice guidelines: A proposal from the Conference on Guideline Standardization. *Annals of Internal Medicine, 139*(6), 493–498.

Squires, J. E., Graham, I. D., Hutchinson, A. M., Linklater, S., Brehaut, J. C., Curran, J., . . . Grimshaw, J. M. (2014). Understanding context in knowledge translation: A concept analysis study protocol. *Journal of Advanced Nursing, 71*(5), 1146–1155.

Squires, J. E., Graham, I. D., Hutchinson, A. M., Michie, S., Francis, J. J, Sales, A., . . . Grimshaw, J. M. (2015). Identifying the domains of context important to implementation science: A study protocol. *Implementation Science, 10,* 135.

St-Pierre, I., Davies, B., Edwards, N., & Griffin, P. (2007). Policies and procedures: A tool to support the implementation of clinical guidelines. *Nursing Research, 20*(4), 63–78.

Straus, S. E., Brouwers, M., Johnson, D., Lavis, J. N., Légaré, F., Majumdar, S. R., . . . Grimshaw, J.; KT Canada Strategic Training Initiative in Health Research (STIHR). (2011). Core competencies in the science and practice of knowledge translation: Description of a Canadian strategic training initiative. *Implementation Science, 6,* 127.

Straus, S., & Haynes, B. (2009). Managing evidence-based knowledge: The need for reliable, relevant and readable resources. *Canadian Medical Association Journal, 180*(9), 942–945.

Tricoci, P., Allen, J. M., Kramer, J. M., Califf, R. M., & Smith, S. C. (2009). Scientific evidence underlying the ACC/AHA Clinical Practice Guidelines. *JAMA, 301*(8), 831–841.

U.S. Preventive Services Task Force. (2008). *The guide to clinical preventive services.* Rockville, MD: The Agency for Healthcare Research and Quality.

Van De Velde-Coke, S., Doran, D., Grinspun, D., Hayes, L., Sutherland-Boal, A., Velji, K., & White, P. (2012). Measuring outcomes of nursing care, improving the health of Canadians: NNQR(C), C-HOBIC, and NQuIRE. *Canadian Journal of Nursing Leadership, 25*(2), 26–37.

Virani, T., Lemieux-Charles, L., Davis, D., & Berta, W. (2008). Sustaining change: Once evidence-based practices are transferred, what then? *Hospital Quarterly, 12*(1), 89–96.

Wennberg, J. E., McAndrew, C., & the Dartmouth Medical School Center for Evaluative Clinical Sciences Staff. (1999). *The Dartmouth atlas of health care.* Washington, DC: The American Hospital Association.

Wennberg, J., & Gittelsohn, A. (1973). Small area variations in health care delivery. *Science, 182*(117), 1102–1108.

Wennberg, J., & Gittelsohn, A. (1982). Variations in medical care among small areas. *Scientific American, 246*(4), 120–134.

Wilson, R., Bajnok, I., & Costa, T. (2015). Promoting evidence-based care through nursing order sets. *MedUNAB, 17*(3), 176–181.

Wimpenny, P., & van Zelm, R. (2007). Appraising and comparing pressure ulcer guidelines. *Worldviews on Evidence-Based Nursing, 4*(1), 40–50.

Intradermal Lidocaine Intervention on the Ambulatory Unit: An Evidence-Based Implementation Project

Amanda Thier, RN, FNP, MSN

STEP 0 | The Spirit of Inquiry Ignited

Healthcare organizations are nationally measured and reimbursed based on patient satisfaction scores and individualized patient experiences. The Press Ganey (2017) patient experience survey includes scientifically developed patient-centered questions to provide a more comprehensive view of the overall patient experience. Scores from the survey revealed how well the intravenous (IV) service was provided by a nurse and led to an immediate evidence-based practice (EBP) change at a Heart and Vascular Hospital (HVH) in central south United States.

After discharge, a Press Ganey survey is sent to each ambulatory patient at HVH. This follow-up survey asks multiple questions regarding the patient's care, including a specific question about "The skill of the nurse starting the IV." Survey results indicated that the ambulatory unit at HVH was in the 41st percentile for the months of November and December of 2014. Along with the mailed Press Ganey survey, each patient receives a follow-up phone call within 1 day of discharge from a registered nurse within the facility. Data from these phone calls revealed at least one compliant made each day related to the pain or discomfort of a peripherally inserted IV catheter. Specific comments made by patients included "My IV really hurt" or "The nurse stuck me multiple times." Taken together, the low patient satisfaction rate and patient complaints revealed a critical opportunity for improvement in patient satisfaction related to the quality and experience of the IV start.

STEP 1 | Asking the Clinical Question in PICOT Format

Therefore the question arises: In ambulatory surgery patients requiring a peripheral IV (P), how does intradermal lidocaine use (I) compared to no pain reduction intervention (C) affect patient's satisfaction (O) during the start of an IV (T)?

STEP 2 | Searching for Evidence

In order to provide the strongest evidence for confident clinical decision making, an exhaustive systematic search was conducted. The three electronic databases used for the systematic search were PubMed, the Cumulative Index of Nursing and Allied Health Literature (CINAHL), and the Cochrane Database of Systematic Reviews. Keyword and controlled vocabulary searches included the following terms: *lidocaine, IV insertion, venipuncture, pain, patient satisfaction, vascular access device, venipuncture,* and *intradermal lidocaine.* The systematic search strategy was completed using the same search terms across all databases. In order to make the search inclusive, if the database had its own indexing language or subject headings, the search was conducted using those terms.

The identified PICOT question asks about an intervention, comparing the use of a pain reduction intervention to no intervention. The best study design to answer this specific question is a systematic review or meta-analysis of randomized controlled trials (RCT), or a single RCT. Therefore, these limits were considered for the search. Furthermore, inclusion criteria for the search were that studies had to: (1) be published in English between 1998 and 2014, (2) report findings of empirical research in the form of a RCT or meta-analysis study, and (3) examine the effect of patient satisfaction related to intradermal lidocaine prior to the IV insertion. The single exclusion criterion was that studies could not involve participants under the age of 18.

The CINAHL search yielded 31 articles that likely would answer the clinical question. After review of the abstracts, eight articles were relevant to the purpose of the evidence synthesis. A hand search of the eight articles' reference lists yielded two additional studies. The PubMed search yielded 20 studies, with 5 studies retained for review. The Cochrane Database of Systematic Review yielded two studies, but only one abstract was relevant to the PICOT question. The retained 16 studies were then moved into critical appraisal.

STEP 3 Critical Appraisal of the Evidence

Rapid critical appraisal (RCA) of the retrieved studies was done to determine which studies were keeper studies, i.e., were they relevant, valid, and applicable to the PICOT question. The RCA involved choosing a proper RCA checklist for each study on the basis of the study's research design. An RCA checklist and a general appraisal overview (GAO) form were completed on all studies. Six studies were discarded and 10 moved forward to evaluation (see sample RCA and GAO on thePoint˚).

In the evaluation phase of critical appraisal, one single evaluation table was used to organize data from the studies (see Table 1 on thePoint˚). This phase was critical because it identified what the literature indicated was best practice regarding the pain perception after implementing a pain reduction intervention. Completing one evaluation table organized data so comparisons and relationships could be easily identified and used to make the appropriate recommendations for a practice change. From the evaluation table, three synthesis tables were developed to provide an overall understanding of the entire body of evidence (BOE), craft a recommendation, and formulate the basis for the project implementation plan.

In the first synthesis table, the level of evidence was presented and the specific variables throughout the 10 studies were identified. The final BOE included one systemic review study, one meta-analysis, and eight RCTs (see Table 2). In review of the sample for the identified RCTs, samples ranged from 50 to 376 participants within the sample and settings column of the evaluation table. All 10 trials were completed within the last 20 years and all 8 RCT studies were conducted in the United States. Each RCT used similar design methods, such as comparable IV needle sizes, subcutaneous needle sizes, and amount of local anesthetic injected. The independent variables across the studies included a control of no local anesthesia, 4% lidocaine cream, bacteriostatic normal saline, 1% buffered lidocaine, 1% lidocaine, and ethyl chloride spray within multiple practice settings (see Table 2). In each study, the participants were identified as adults older than 18 years of age; however, one study used medical students to make up the participant group, which may be perceived as different from the patient population.

Another comparison made across studies was how intradermal lidocaine prior to IV insertion effected patient satisfaction. Although none of the studies exclusively addressed patient satisfaction, the studies measuring the perception of pain were considered relevant to the clinical question because pain perception is directly related to patient satisfaction. Scales used to measure perception of pain included valid and reliable scales. Studies showed that patient perception of pain decreased with the use of intradermal lidocaine before IV insertion (see Table 3). Local anesthetics used to decrease pain during venipuncture have been studied with equivocal results; however, researchers from level I studies determined that lidocaine was most effective in reducing pain in adults (see Table 3). Additionally, across all ten studies, those that used lidocaine showed pain reduction, regardless of needle gauge of the catheter or the intradermal needle or the amount of lidocaine injected (see Table 2).

TABLE 2

Level of Evidence and Intervention Description Synthesis Table

Study	Halm	Gater-Ristz	Deguzman	Brown	Winfield	Kahre	McNaughton	Burke	Oman	Hattula
Level of Evidence	SR	RCT	RCT	RCT	RCT	RCT	RCT	RCT	MA	RCT
Size (N)	N = 180	N = 252	N = 376	N = 100	N = 94	N = 56	N = 68	N = 145	Combined N = 1,559	N = 24
IV	Control 1% Lido	1% Lido BLD BNS	BL BNS	Control 1% Lido	1% Lido BNS Pain Ease Spray	BL BNS	Control 4% LC 1% BL	BL BNS	Control BLD 1% Lido BNS NS	Control BL BNS
IV Gauge	18, 20	20	18, 20, 22	18, 20	16	20	20	16–22	16–22	18, 20
Lido Dose ML (ID)	0.3 mL (25–29)	0.8 ± 1 (27)	0.1–0.2 (27)	0.1	0.1–0.3 (27)	1 ± 1.3 (30)	0.1–0.2 (30)	0.2 (30)	0.01–1.3 (25–30)	1.32 ± 1.0 (25)
BNS Dose ML (ID)	NA	0.1 (27)	0.2 (27)	NA	0.1–0.3 (27)	0.2 (30)	NA	0.2 (30)	0.1–0.5 (25–30)	0.2 (25)

BL, buffered lidocaine; BNS, bacteriostatic normal saline; ID, intradermal lidocaine needle size; IV, independent variables; LA, local anesthetic; Lido, lidocaine; M ± SD, mean (standard deviation); MA, meta-analysis; MES, mean effect size; NA, not applicable; PS, pain score; RCT, randomized controlled trial; SR, systematic review; VPS, verbal pain scale.

(continued)

TABLE 2 · *Level of Evidence and Intervention Description Synthesis Table (continued)*

Study	Halm	Gater-Ristz	Deguzman	Brown	Winfield	Kahre	McNaughton	Burke	Oman	Hattula
Pain scale used	VPS (0–10)	VPS (0–10)	VPS (0–10)	VPS (0–10)	Verbal rating	Visual (FACES)	VPS (0–10)	VPS (0–10)	VPS FACES	VPS (0–10)
Lido PS: M ± SD	Males 1.6 ± 1.74 Females 2.4 ± 2.1	Lido 0.8 ± 1.0 BLD 0.8 ± 1.1	1.19 ±1.59	1.4 ± 1.96	1% Lido had least pain (p < 0.001)	0.093 ± 1.3	1 ± 3	1.56 ± 1.99	Decreased PS in 10 studies	1.32 ± 1.0
BNS PS M ± SD	NA	1.4 ± 2.1	1.72 ± 1.58	NA	ID BNS: Pain "same as"	2.36 ± 1.45	NA	2.58 ± 2.50	Decreased PS in 2 studies	2.68 ± 1.42
Control PS M ± SD	Males 3.24 ± 2.7 Fe 3.2 ± 2.75	NA	NA	2.8 ± 2.49	NA	NA	7 ± 3	NA	NA	3.11 ± 1.85
Mean reduction reported pain (raw score)	Males (−1.64) Fe (−0.8)	Lido (−0.5) BL (-0.1)	−0.18	−1.4	Poor study design No M ± SD	−2.267	−6	−1.02	−0.46 (MES calculated using z score)	−1.36

BL, buffered lidocaine; BNS, bacteriostatic normal saline; ID, intradermal lidocaine needle size; IV, independent variables; LA, local anesthetic; Lido, lidocaine; M ± SD, mean (standard deviation); MA, meta-analysis; MES, mean effect size; NA, not applicable; PS, pain score; RCT, randomized controlled trial; SR, systematic review; VPS, verbal pain scale.

260

TABLE 3

Intervention and Patient Perception of Pain (Outcome) Synthesis Table

Study	Halm	Gater-Ristz	Deguzman	Brown	Winfield	Kahre	McNaughton	Burke	Oman	Hattula
Level of Evidence	SR	RCT	RCT	RCT	RCT	RCT	RCT	RCT	MA	RCT
1% Lido	↓*	↓*		↓*	↓†				↓*	
BL		↓*	↓*			↓*	↓†	↓*	↓*	↓*
BNS		↑	↑		↓†	↑		↑	↓	↑
No Intervention (control)	↑			↑			↑↑		↑	↑
LA Spray Or LA Cream					↑↑		↑↑			

↑, pain increased with intervention agent; ↓, pain decreased with intervention agent.

*Statistically significant.

†Some statistically significant data.

BL, buffered lidocaine; BNS, bacteriostatic normal saline; LA, local anesthetic; Lido, lidocaine; MA, meta-analysis; RCT, randomized controlled trial; SR, systematic review.

Although there are multiple factors that influence patients' perceptions of pain, offering a pain-reducing agent prior to venipuncture could positively impact the patient perception of pain. The BOE demonstrates that an adult's pain perception can be decreased by the use of intradermal lidocaine prior to IV insertion, regardless of the buffered or unbuffered solution (see Table 2). Both lidocaine agents produced similar results; it was clear from the synthesis tables that patient satisfaction and the perception of pain could be positively affected by the use of intradermal lidocaine prior to venipuncture. This evidence-based project was feasible and important to clinical practice decisions. Therefore, the recommendation from the BOE is to implement intradermal lidocaine before peripheral IV catheter insertion on all patients requiring such access.

STEP 4   Implementation - Linking Evidence to Action

The plan for this project based on the evidence found included the implementation of intradermal lidocaine before IV insertion, assess its feasibility, and the outcomes related to patient satisfaction with ambulatory surgery patients treated at HVH. When patients were admitted to the ambulatory surgery unit at HVH, the placement of an IV catheter was required prior to the procedure for the administration of fluids, blood products, sedation, and medications. The existing standard of practice at the facility for all ambulatory surgery patients involved no pain-reducing intervention prior to the IV catheter insertion. The pain of the needle insertion is not a life-threatening discomfort, and the current practice of insertion of an IV catheter was effectively completed without an anesthetizing agent. However, literature strongly supported the injection of intradermal lidocaine as the most effective anesthetizing agent to reduce the perception of pain and provide optimal patient comfort during the catheter insertion process. In terms of patient preference and satisfaction, most patients want to experience minimal to no pain during the IV catheter insertion and throughout their entire day-surgery experience. The 10 experienced ambulatory surgery nurses, with their expertise and skills in IV catheter insertion, helped apply the evidence from current literature in the EBP project using intradermal lidocaine before the insertion of an IV catheter.

In order to facilitate safe and effective nursing practice change on the ambulatory surgery unit, the Stetler model (Dang et al, 2015) was used to guide implementation, combined with the collaboration of active and passive stakeholders. The EBP model outlined a series of five progressive phases: (1) preparation; (2) validation; (3) comparative evaluation/decision making; (4) translation/application; and (5) evaluation. During phase I, preparation for evidence-based change project was completed. Phase II included validation of the evidence, that is, critical appraisal. Stetler's Model was introduced in phase III with a detailed EBP implementation plan for how to execute the intradermal lidocaine intervention on the ambulatory unit, including how to collect baseline data to effectively evaluate the impact of intradermal lidocaine on patient satisfaction. In phase IV, the Advancing Research and Clinical Practice Through Close Collaboration (ARCC) model (Dang et al., 2015) was used to translate the evidence into practice.

The translation/application phase of the Stetler model incorporated moving evidence into action with a well-planned and executed implementation of the evidence-based change—beginning with identifying key stakeholders and acquiring necessary approval for the project. EBP mentors were identified to support sustainable change. All interprofessional team member were sought out and approvals obtained for the project.

Each checkpoint in the ARCC model timeline was completed. Baseline data collection process showed patient satisfaction scores of 41% on the Press Ganey survey question, "The degree pain was controlled during the IV insertion procedure." Furthermore, the ambulatory unit received on average about 20 to 30 patient complaints a week related to excessive pain with IV insertion. The Standards and Measures hospital-wide council and the electronic health record (EHR) were sources of baseline data. The goal for outcomes for the project included increased Press Ganey scores and decreased patient complaints after the evidence-based intervention. A data collection tool was implemented to complete at the end of each shift to track project outcomes across the three-month implementation period.

As per phase VI of the Stetler model, a data collection protocol and project protocol were used to facilitate smooth project processes. An IV education course was implemented to help clinical staff use Mosby's education resources as foundational sources of information for all ambulatory nurses to help substantiate the appropriate process for intradermal lidocaine injection. As the project was starting and planning was completed, all team members, including the mentors and stakeholders, participated in a poster presentation to gear up for final plan implementation. Multiple hurdles were encountered and processes were put into place to overcome the challenges. A major struggle throughout the implementation period was nurse buy-in. The charge nurse indicated that nurses were consistently implementing the evidence-based intervention, but staff was frustrated because it was taking additional time to insert the IV catheter. Key personnel engaged the nurses in the third week of implementation to help with ease of the lidocaine process. The additional education allowed the nurses to improve their skills and confidence with the lidocaine process. Evidence-based practice projects must be owned by all stakeholders, not just the project director. Shared ownership by various individuals, providing enthusiasm and help toward one common goal of improved patient satisfaction, moved the project forward. The role of project leader is not to own the project, but to keep the project on track, keep stakeholders informed, remain organized, and, most importantly, ensure that the intervention has fidelity as well as the outcomes are evaluated to with validity and accuracy.

The evidence-based intervention of intradermal lidocaine prior to IV insertion was implemented from September 7th until October 2nd. Throughout the implementation timeframe, there was an effort to foster effective communication among project team members, including mid-project meetings of all key stakeholders.

STEP 5   Outcomes Evaluation

Finally, the last stage of Stetlers Model merged with the ARCC Model timeline, and the final data collection for the project evaluation was conducted with a review of the project processes—particularly were project goals and milestones achieved. A total of 247 ambulatory patients received 1% lidocaine prior to IV insertion. Each week total pain scores on the ambulatory unit were manually gathered from the electronic health record, averaged, and organized in tables. The mean, median, and standard deviation results were calculated using Excel. After the 4-week implementation timeframe, the entire mean pain score was generated. The mean pain score of 1.8 strongly correlates with the expected outcomes in the literature, indicating that lidocaine was an effective pain reduction agent in the ambulatory population. Process indicators suggested that premedication with 1% lidocaine can be effectively executed. Furthermore, there was improvement in the Press Ganey survey results about the extent to which pain was controlled with IV insertion (baseline 1.57 [standard deviation (SD) 0.37]; postimplementation 1.82 [SD 0.33]) and an increase in perception of nurse skill with IV insertion (score at baseline 91.9; post implementation 93.4), all of which indicates successful implementation of the evidence-based intervention.

STEP 6   Dissemination

The success of the project prompted conversations with the nursing director and project mentor around how such a simple intervention impacted patients' perceptions of their care. Involvement of medical and nursing leadership, ambulatory staff, the Standards and Measures Council, and other staff in the ambulatory setting within the organization made the implementation of the project a success. Because of the success of this project and how it fostered interprofessional collaboration, the organization chose to pursue taking the evidence-based intervention system-wide. The focus of the initiative was achieving patient-centered care goals, promoting safety, and accelerating change within the Magnet environment, further realizing that a nursing-initiated EBP change within the organization demonstrates the requirements to remain a Magnet-recognized organization.

References

Dang, D., Melnyk, B. M., Fineout-Overholt, E., Ciliska, D., DiCenso, A., Cullen, L., Cvach, M., Larrabee, J., Rycroft-Malone, J., Schulz, A., Stetler, S., & Stevens, K. (2015). Models to Guide Implementation and Sustainability of Evidence-Based Practice. In B.M. Melnyk & E. Fineout-Overholt, *Evidence-based Practice in Nursing and Healthcare: A Guide to Best Practice*. (3rd ed.). Philadelphia, PA: Wolters Kluwer. (pp. 274–315).
Press Ganey. (2017). *Patient Satisfaction Surveys*. Retrieved from http://www.pressganey.com/resources/patient-satisfaction-surveys

3

Steps Four and Five: Moving From Evidence to Sustainable Practice Change

> A good plan executed now is better than a perfect plan tomorrow.
>
> — *George Patton*

EBP Terms to Learn

Clinician judgment
Competency
Delphi study
EBP barriers
EBP integration
EBP mentors
EBP process
Effect size
Evidence-based leadership
Evidence-based practice guideline
Evidence-based quality improvement project
Innovation leadership
Integrative review
Internal evidence
Interval data
Level of evidence
Meta-analysis
Outcome measures
Outcomes evaluation
Outcomes research
Patient preferences and values
Process measures
Systematic review
Transformational leadership

UNIT OBJECTIVES

Upon completion of this unit, learners will be able to:

1. Describe how best to integrate patient concerns, choices, and clinical judgment in evidence-based practice (EBP).

2. Discuss qualities of well-developed best practice clinical guidelines.

3. Create a plan for how best to implement an EBP change project.

4. Identify EBP competencies for practicing nurses and advanced practice nurses.

5. Describe important elements of an evidence-based quality improvement project, including evaluation of outcomes.

6. Discuss leadership qualities that are essential for sustaining an EBP culture.

MAKING CONNECTIONS: AN EBP EXEMPLAR

Based on the systematic search to answer their PICOT question (*In elderly patients with low risk for falls with universal precautions in place, how does hourly rounding at night compared to no hourly rounding affect preventable fall rates within 3 months of initiation?*) and critical appraisal (rapid critical appraisal, evaluation, synthesis, and recommendation) of the body of evidence (BOE) found, a decision was made by the EBP Council to implement an interprofessional 24-hour fall prevention intervention with hourly rounding program (every hour during the day and every 2 hours during the night) that includes assessing FRisk (fall risk) and the four Ps (pain, potty, positioning, placement) (*Step 4: Integrate the Evidence with Clinical Expertise and Patient/Family Preferences to Make the Best Clinical Decision*). Lei, the Council member coordinating the implementation plan, pointed out that their plan actually agreed with three of the recommendations from the Registered Nurses Association of Ontario (RNAO, 2017) evidence-based guideline, Preventing Falls and Reducing Injury from Falls: "1.2a: Complete comprehensive FRisk assessment, including multifactorial assessment (p. 11); 5.1 Ensure a safe environment through universal precautions and altering physical environment for safety (p. 14); and 5.3: Implement rounding as a strategy to proactively meet the person's needs and prevent falls (p. 14)." The Council also recommended that patient/family preferences be taken into consideration with implementation of the four Ps as well.

Lei and the other EBP Council members met to develop a strategic plan for widespread dissemination and implementation of the evidence-based recommendations that would result in success. The group knew, from reading prior studies on system-wide implementation of an EBP change, that education of staff on the importance of the practice change would not be enough in itself to ensure its ongoing success. They discussed several other key factors that would be necessary to accomplish the system-wide practice change, including top leadership/managerial buy-in and support, staff beliefs about the value of changing their current practice, buy-in from interprofessional team members, clear communication, and ongoing mentorship of the staff as the practice change is made (Li, Jeffs, Barwick, & Stevens, 2018; RNAO, 2017). Council members discussed current barriers that might impede implementation success in their system, including the fact that some clinicians do not like to change and are comfortable with the status quo (i.e., doing things the way that they always have done them). Given their knowledge of Rogers' Diffusion of Innovation Theory (2003), Council members believed the first step would be to identify innovators and early adopters on each of the targeted units (those individuals with "a twinkle in their eye and a fire in their belly" to improve practice for best population health outcomes) and begin working with them first on the practice change. The Council members also realized that individuals who resist change often have fears; having direct conversations with those individuals who were reluctant to engage in the change effort would be critical. The group also discussed how important it would be to create a team vision on each unit and raise people's emotions to help strengthen their beliefs about the value of this practice change and assist them in adopting it. Therefore, they planned to make a video of Sam, the patient who experienced a fall while hospitalized and whose story began this search for best practices in fall prevention, to highlight the adverse physical health, mental health, and cost outcomes of a fall and the negative impact the fall had on Sam and his family.

Lei reminded the Council members that it was critical to monitor the change as it was being implemented and to have a solid evaluation plan (*Step 5: Evaluate the Outcomes of the Practice Change Based on Evidence*). The group decided that the plan should include ongoing monitoring of the number of falls, call light use, and patient satisfaction, along with a cost analysis that included calculation of the dollars saved by the institution with the expected fall rate (FR) decline. The outcomes evaluation data that they gathered would be shared on a quarterly basis with the hospital's C-Suite executives (e.g., the Chief Executive Officer, the Chief Financial Officer, the Chief Nurse Executive) and staff. If hospital dollars were saved by a decrease in FR, they would make a request to the C-Suite executive team to designate a portion of those funds to the EBP Council to further fuel other important evidence-based change initiatives.

The EBP Council decided to appoint a team who would be responsible for the project's implementation and outcomes evaluation. A decision was made for the team to include the following members: Lei (lead for the project as she was an EBP expert and seasoned mentor), DeAndre, Mateo, Scott, a respected high-level nurse leader, a physician from the hospital's leadership team, the hospital's chief quality officer, and a clinical nurse specialist from each unit who would also function as an EBP mentor to the staff. Lei, as the Council member coordinating the implementation plan, would be responsible for reaching out to the other identified members and inviting them to participate on the team.

The EBP Council outlined the major phases of the implementation plan as follows:

i. Develop the video that captures the emotional story of Sam's fall to be shared in information sessions with leaders and educational sessions with staff.

ii. Present to the C-Suite executive team, including the rationale for the EBP change, to obtain their support for the project and the resources necessary for implementation.

iii. Invite all individuals who will be part of the implementation team to an initial meeting where a shared exciting vision would be created that explained why this EBP change is key to reducing FR and improving outcomes throughout the hospital. At this meeting, the implementation plan would be shared and input gathered. Goals would be set and their time frames and persons responsible specified.

iv. Meet with the clinical nurse specialists on the units who will serve as EBP mentors to review the EBP change and strategies for implementation as well as to obtain their input on the practice change, including the best means of working with staff who are resistant to behavior change and strategies to overcome other barriers they might encounter.

v. Engage staff by creating a team vision for the practice change while conducting interprofessional educational sessions on implementation of the new evidence-based fall prevention practice.

vi. Create posters for each unit that highlight the evidence-based recommendations as a visual reminder of the steps in the practice change.

vii. Conduct bimonthly sessions with the EBP mentors to discuss challenges with implementation and strategies to overcome them.

viii. Ask the chief quality officer to appoint individuals whose job will be to review patient care plans and charts on a monthly basis to ensure adherence to the steps in implementing the EBP change.

ix. If it is found on review that implementation is not occurring with full fidelity, conduct review sessions with EBP mentors and staff on a regular ongoing basis that include recognition and appreciation for their efforts.

x. Collect outcome data on a quarterly basis to determine whether implementation of the fall prevention EBP is resulting in improved outcomes.

Join the group at the beginning of Unit 4 as they continue their EBP journey.

References

Li, S. A., Jeffs, L., Barwick, M., & Stevens, B. (2018). Organizational contextual features that influence the implementation of evidence-based practices across healthcare settings: A systematic integrative review. *Systematic Reviews, 7*(1): 72.

Registered Nurses' Association of Ontario. (2017). *Preventing Falls and Reducing Injury from Falls* (4th ed.). Toronto, ON: Author.

Rogers, E. M. (2003). *Diffusion of innovations* (5th ed.). New York, NY: Free Press.

9

Implementing Evidence in Clinical Settings

Cheryl C. Rodgers, Terri L. Brown, and Marilyn J. Hockenberry

> **I never worry about action, only inaction.**
> —*Winston Churchill*

EBP Terms to Learn
Barriers to EBP
EBP integration
EBP mentors
EBP process
EBP vision
External evidence
Internal evidence
Outcome measures
Patient-centered quality care measures
Quality care improvement measures
Shared mental framework

Learning Objectives
After studying this chapter, learners will be able to:

1. Identify strategies to develop a vision for change.
2. Discuss activities to promote engagement in evidence-based practice (EBP).
3. Describe steps to integrate EBP into the clinical environment.
4. Evaluate EBP activities with clinical outcomes.

It is not enough to have knowledge of the best evidence to guide clinical practice; knowledge must be translated into clinical practice to improve patient care and outcomes. Because evidence-based practice (EBP) is known to improve the quality of healthcare and patient outcomes as well as decrease healthcare costs, there is currently an increased emphasis in clinical settings on promoting EBP. However, delivery of care based on evidence requires support and commitment throughout the organization (Melnyk, 2016). This chapter describes essential concepts for developing an environment that fosters a culture of EBP and key strategies for successful implementation of EBP in clinical settings. Essential mechanisms for creating an evidence-based clinical environment, which include vision, engagement, integration, and evaluation, will be highlighted (Figure 9.1; Hockenberry, Walden, Brown, & Barrera, 2007).

An EBP environment promotes excellence in clinical care resulting in improvement of patient outcomes. Transforming a healthcare institution into a setting where an EBP culture exists requires persistence, patience, and perseverance (Hockenberry et al., 2007). Persistence—to maintain steadiness on a course of action—allows time to realize how EBP can improve clinical outcomes and is a partner with wisdom when change may create significant stress for staff. Patience—showing the capacity for endurance—provides the strength to wait for change to occur. Perseverance—adhering to a purpose—allows the team to survive the change process by resolve and dedication during a time when it is essential to stay the course and believe that EBP can transform a clinical environment (Hockenberry et al., 2007).

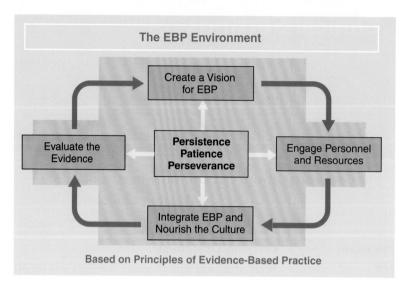

Figure 9.1: Evidence-based practice (EBP) environment model. (With permission from Hockenberry, M., Walden, M., Brown, T., & Barrera, P. [2007]. Creating an evidence-based environment: One hospital's journey. *Journal of Nursing Care Quality, 22*[3], 223.)

A VISION FOR EVIDENCE-BASED PRACTICE

Healthcare institutions with successful EBP programs begin with a vision and an understanding of the goals to be accomplished. A clear vision gives substance to the actions needed to transform a healthcare setting into an EBP environment. The **EBP vision** provides a compelling and motivating image of desired changes that result in excellence in clinical practice throughout the healthcare organization. An image of the future, defined as a **shared mental framework**, is created to begin the transformation process (Box 9.1).

Reasons for transforming a clinical culture into an EBP environment are numerous, depending on the type of clinical setting and its mission. For many institutions, the vision for EBP is based on regulatory initiatives and insurance-mandated outcomes. One such regulation is the Centers for Medicare and Medicaid Services' (CMS's) decision to move from a volume-based payment model to a value-based model by stopping reimbursement for "preventable complications" in hospitalized patients. Numerous hospital-acquired conditions with current evidence-based guidelines for prevention were among the list that CMS ruled as nonreimbursable in late 2008. These complications and hospital readmissions that

BOX
9.1   *A Shared Mental Framework*

A **shared mental framework** exemplifies an institution's most closely held values and ideals that inspire and motivate administrators, researchers, and clinicians to participate in practice changes.

It serves as the catalyst for change within the organization. With increasing emphasis on quality patient care and outcome metrics, a new image is emerging at hospitals that place tremendous value in providing excellent care throughout the organization. A new, shared mental framework is established by administration's willingness to increase resources for quality initiatives and evidence-based practice programs.

result from medical errors or improper care could have reasonably been avoided through the application of evidence-based guidelines (Sung-Heui, 2017).

In 2011, to provide further perspective on the importance of creating a vision for transforming healthcare, the U.S. Department of Health & Human Services (DHHS) released the inaugural report to Congress on the National Strategy for Quality Improvement in HealthCare (2012). The National Quality Strategy has three aims:

1. *Better Care:* Improve the overall quality of care by making healthcare more patient-centered, reliable, accessible, and safe.
2. *Healthy People/Healthy Communities:* Improve the health of the U.S. population by supporting proven interventions to address behavioral, social, and environmental determinants of health in addition to delivering higher quality care.
3. *Affordable Care:* Reduce the cost of quality healthcare for individuals, families, employers, and government.

This strategy calls clinical institutions into action to develop and share methods for data collection, measurement, and reporting that support measurement and improvement efforts of both public and private sector stakeholders at the national and community level (National Strategy for Quality Improvement in Health Care, 2012).

The Magnet Recognition Program also provides specific expectations for transforming a nursing culture into an environment that promotes superior performance through EBP (American Nurses Credentialing Center [ANCC], 2014). This program recognizes hospitals that demonstrate quality patient care, nursing excellence, and innovations in practice. Magnet hospitals must promote quality and disseminate best practices throughout nursing, attainable only through the pursuit of an EBP environment. Magnet recognition requirements include specific demonstration of expected outcomes for 2 years prior to submission of the Magnet application (ANCC, 2014). To acquire this type of evidence over time for nursing practice, an environment must promote staff use of an EBP approach to everyday care.

Understanding the importance of cultural change within a clinical environment frequently begins with a few passionate individuals who have a shared mental framework for the kind of quality care they want to provide their patients and families. The vision of a dedicated EBP team is critical to the success of project implementation (Melnyk, 2016). Chapter 12 elaborates on creating a vision and motivating a change to EBP.

Early involvement of clinical experts and **EBP mentors** (i.e., clinicians who have advanced knowledge and skills in EBP as well as individual and organizational change strategies [Kowalski, 2017]) shapes the future vision for EBP at any institution. While increased knowledge and understanding are important to any EBP initiative, a key to changing actual behaviors is ownership of change. An effective method to obtain clinical support is to include experts or mentors at the beginning of an EBP project, preferably when the vision for change is first established. Administrative support for the vision is obtained as soon as those involved have organized their shared vision or mental framework. When possible, the project should be designated as an organizational priority before the first formal meeting. (See Box 9.2 for how the vision for a successful EBP change project at Texas Children's Hospital was created.)

Keys to accomplishing a successful vision include preparation and planning. The old saying "begin with the end in mind" serves vision planners well at this stage of an EBP initiative. Selecting strategies that promote small changes over time is known to be more effective than conducting large-scale initiatives. Effective programs capture the momentum by acting quickly to disseminate the vision and by emphasizing small goals that are easily attainable (Table 9.1). Small goals with measurable outcomes provide concrete examples of motivating the vision for change.

BOX
9.2

An Example of Creating a Vision for Change: Pain Prevention for Hospitalized Children at Texas Children's Hospital

The first formal EBP initiative at the Texas Children's Hospital involved developing an EBP pain prevention protocol for use throughout the hospital. A procedural pain leadership group consisting of clinical nurse specialists from Acute Care, the Pediatric Intensive Care Unit, the Neonatal Intensive Care Unit, the Cancer Center, the chair of the Clinical Practice Council, a nurse researcher, and research assistant was established.

- **Small steps toward change**
  - The pain prevention initiative began with small steps toward change. Leaders of this initiative recognized that the vision for change needed to start within nursing.
  - Specific nursing interventions that commonly cause pain for children were selected, and an intensive evidence review provided strategies for improving pain management.
  - Changes in practice began as a purposeful, selected focus rather than an attempt to transform pain management across all disciplines at once.
- **Focusing awareness**
  - The evidence-based pain prevention initiative began by increasing awareness that pain remains a major problem for hospitalized children.
  - Many clinicians believed that pain intervention was not necessary for common nursing procedures, and routinely performed painful procedures without intervention for a number of reasons because the painful period of time was limited for the child, or the clinician felt like such an expert at performing the procedure that the pain experienced was minimal.
  - Because the procedural pain leadership group had completed an extensive review of the evidence and found that pain experiences of hospitalized children are significant and long lasting, regardless of the length of procedure or expertise of the provider, a new awareness of pain practices throughout the hospital was an essential first step for the EBP pain prevention program's vision.

EBP, evidence-based practice.

Sharing the vision for excellence in practice is perhaps the most essential catalyst for promoting EBP. Initiatives that are most effective in changing the environment engage strategies that share the vision for change as early as possible. Expert clinicians may be less aware of the need for change than their inexperienced colleagues. Emphasizing the need for change must be direct and to the point. Recognizing that one's own patient care is less than excellent is often painful for clinicians. Box 9.3 highlights the strategies for sharing the vision for the EBP change project at Texas Children's Hospital. Establishing the direction for EBP in a clinical environment sets the stage for an organized approach for all future initiatives. Although change takes time, establishing a clear direction for change provides focus toward a common goal—improved patient outcomes.

TABLE
9.1

EBP Vision: Transforming a Clinical Environment

Objective	Strategies
Develop a mental framework	• Develop a written summary of what you want to accomplish. • Brainstorm with colleagues regarding the environment you want to create.
Establish a motivating image for change	• Use creativity to capture attention of the clinical staff. • Take advantage of real clinical scenarios to stress the need for changes in practice.
Create specific goals	• Focus on short-term, attainable goals. • Establish only two to three goals at a time.
Gain administrative support	• Contact administrators responsible for clinical practice. • Create a presentation that reflects the need for transforming the culture into an EBP environment. • Seek administration support for the project to be identified as an organizational priority.
Establish a leadership team	• Identify key personnel with a passion for EBP. • Conduct small focus group meetings.
Involve experts and EBP mentors in clinical practice	• Identify clinical experts and EBP mentors focused on the area. • Engage clinical expert support.

EBP, evidence-based practice.

BOX
9.3

Sharing the Vision for Change

To develop a vision for needed changes in pain management, the project at the Texas Children's Hospital began by increasing awareness that hospitalized infants and children commonly experience pain.

- A video was used to create a dramatic image and raise nurses' emotions regarding the need for change.
- The video demonstrated two infants undergoing a heel stick; one infant was given a sucrose/pacifier intervention and the other infant underwent the heel stick without pain intervention.
- The video showed dramatic differences in infant behavior during the heel stick procedure. The infant who received standard care without pain intervention cried, moved, and thrashed his arms and legs throughout the entire procedure. The infant who received the pain intervention quietly sucked on the pacifier without movement during the entire heel stick.
- Although a written summary of the evidence supporting sucrose as a pain intervention for young infants was given to all staff, the video was much more powerful in creating a needed change in the mental framework for managing pain.
- After viewing the video, numerous staff began using the sucrose/pacifier intervention prior to heel sticks as well as for other painful procedures.

PROMOTE ENGAGEMENT

Recent studies stress the importance of healthcare systems' commitment to carrying out activities that promote quality clinical care (Friesen, Brady, Milligan, & Christensen, 2017; Nilsen, Reg, Ellstrom, & Gardner, 2017). As healthcare systems continue to evolve, it is evident that high quality clinical practice depends on its connection with ongoing, systematic learning. EBP mentors along with staff engagement are essential for successful implementation of evidence to improve patient care (Nilsen et al., 2017; Friesen et al., 2017). This requires that staff at all levels must be engaged in high-priority clinical issues to develop a successful, supportive environment (Table 9.2). Clinical staff are best positioned to identify variations in practice and ineffective processes, because they often have a vested interest in streamlining inefficiencies. Administrators responsible for the clinical areas where changes will occur and who engage early in the planning process are likely to share ownership. A key strategy for success is involvement of staff and leaders of all disciplines who are directly affected by the potential change, including likely early adopters as well as those who may have difficulty accepting the change.

Assess and Eliminate Barriers

Barrier assessment is an integral component throughout the engagement and integration phases of EBP implementation (Powell et al., 2017). Change, even when welcome, is stressful

TABLE 9.2	*Promoting Engagement in EBP*
Objective	**Strategies**
Engage staff and stakeholders in assessing and eliminating barriers	• Engage stakeholders to identify educational content and strategies to learn about the practice change. • Seek information about attitudes toward the affected practice directly from staff. • Involve influential staff and leaders in conducting discussions with colleagues.
Prioritize clinical issues	• Select clinical issues of direct interest and responsibility of clinician stakeholders. • Choose issues with solid empiric evidence to begin an organizational area's EBP endeavors.
Evaluate the infrastructure	• Determine the individuals and committees with decision making authority. • Gain administrative support for adequate time and personnel for the initiative. • Enlist experts to lead EBP initiatives. • Ensure access to databases, search engines, and full-text articles.
Develop experts in the evidence-based process	• Utilize leaders within the organization or form an academic partnership to provide expertise in research, EBP design, and evaluation. • Provide formal classes and/or small-group sessions on finding and evaluating evidence. • Mentor staff in critically appraising research studies and formulating practice recommendations.

EBP, evidence-based practice.

| BOX 9.4 | *Staff and Stakeholders to Engage at All Levels* |

- Staff clinicians
- Leadership team members (e.g., executives, administrators)
- Advanced practice registered nurses
- Stakeholders of all disciplines directly affected
- Physicians
- Family advisory board
- Allied health professionals
- Doctorally prepared nurse researchers
- Evidence-based practice mentors

to everyone. Chapter 12 provides additional information on organizational change concepts that support processes for moving a culture toward EBP. Stakeholder resistance to change must be explored early, because it frequently results from numerous factors including hesitation to break traditional practice, unfamiliarity with how evidence will improve patient outcomes, or misconceptions regarding time and effort needed to implement practice change. See Box 9.4 for stakeholders who are important to engage when planning an EBP change project.

Common **barriers to EBP** implementation include inadequate knowledge and skills, weak beliefs about the value of EBP, lack of EBP mentors, social and organizational influences, and economic restrictions (Brennan, Greenhalgh, & Pawson, 2017; Liddy et al., 2017; Melnyk, 2016).

Lack of knowledge and skills can create barriers to daily evidence-based care owing to inadequate understanding of EBP principles, unawareness of how evidence will improve patient outcomes, and unfamiliarity with how to implement change. The best evidence-based policies are of no value to the patients when the staff lack knowledge of how to implement them in practice; the right information must be in the right place at the right time and presented in a meaningful way (Aasekjaer, Waehle, Ciliska, Nordtvedt, & Hjalmhult, 2016).

Weak beliefs about the value of EBP and attitudinal barriers can be more difficult to overcome than knowledge barriers. Negative attitudes about research and EBP can make it difficult for staff to engage in EBP (Sharma, Pandit, & Tabassum, 2017; Spiva et al., 2017). Focus group discussions and anonymous electronic surveys can be valuable in identifying beliefs and attitudes about current and proposed practice changes. Traditional educational techniques (e.g., lectures and web-based training), when used alone, are usually ineffective in changing attitudes. Interactive discussions with influential colleagues, seeing the positive impact of change, and removal of perceived barriers can be powerful in overcoming resistance. Box 9.5 provides an example of barrier assessment and strategies used for elimination during an EBP procedural pain initiative.

Findings from research have indicated that a lack of EBP mentors in the environment can also be a barrier to implementing EBP by point-of-care staff (Spiva et al., 2017). Mentors who have in-depth knowledge and skills in both EBP and individual and organizational change strategies are also a key strategy for sustaining change once it is realized. Chapter 15 expands on the role of the EBP mentor in advancing best practice in clinical settings.

Social and organizational barriers to change include lack of support by leaders, disagreement among clinicians, and limited resources to support change (Best et al., 2016). Effective barrier assessment includes discerning knowledge, attitudes, and beliefs of mid-level and upper-level administrators surrounding practice change and their perceived roles in

---

| BOX **9.5** | *Assessing and Eliminating Barriers* |

In the procedural pain initiative at the Texas Children's Hospital, staff members identified several barriers to prevent pain prior to performing venipunctures. The project team members implemented multiple solutions to eliminate the barriers at the organizational level.

Assessing Barriers

- Prolonged time to obtain orders and medications and implement interventions
- Lack of knowledge about what is in the hospital formulary
- Attitude: "Even if pain medication is used, children are already stressed out/crying"; perception that medications cause vasoconstriction leading to multiple sticks; "I'm good so it only hurts for a moment."
- Unit culture: Unaccustomed to medicating prior to needlesticks

Eliminating Barriers

- Time demands were reduced through the development of a procedural pain protocol that bundled multiple medications with varying onset times: immediate (oral sucrose, vapocoolant spray), 12 minutes (buffered lidocaine injection), 10 minutes (lidocaine iontophoresis), and 30 minutes (lidocaine cream). Nurses could select floor stock medications within the protocol that were appropriate for the child's age, procedural urgency, and developmental considerations. A pharmacist reviewed and entered the protocol into the patient's medication profile on admission to the hospital.
- Additional medications were brought into the formulary to accommodate urgent needs. Bundling the medications into a protocol increased the knowledge about what was available to prevent venipuncture pain. Educational modules and skills sessions were conducted to familiarize staff nurses with new and unfamiliar medications and administration techniques.
- A multifaceted approach was used to change individual attitudes and unit cultures. Videos of infants receiving heel sticks with and without sucrose and of older children talking about their venipuncture experiences with and without lidocaine premedication were shown. Results of published research studies on the intermediate and long-term effects of unrelieved pain during procedures were disseminated through online modules. A commitment to evaluate the medication in several children was obtained from several unit IV experts. Unit administrators communicated support for the practice in staff meetings and with individual nurses. Champions for change routinely asked colleagues what medications were used when starting IVs.

IV, intravenous.

---

communicating support for this change. Peer group discussions can be very influential, and informal leaders may weigh in even stronger than formal leaders on whether practice change will actually occur. Overlooked process details can impede a well-accepted practice change, including anticipated economic and workload implications. Exploring the economic and workload impact of a practice change early in a project and securing administrative support when there may be potential increase in cost or workload can prevent these barriers from impeding progress. Economic considerations must include the fact that an increase in one type of cost may be readily offset with savings in time (i.e., workload), satisfaction, or the additional expense of patient complications when best practices are not implemented.

Prioritize Clinical Issues

In order to spark EBP, it is best to start with a clinical issue of direct interest to clinicians, because changing one's own practice can be much easier than changing the practice of another discipline or specialty. Box 9.6 provides an example of prioritizing clinical issues for EBP initiatives. Initial efforts should focus on maximizing the likelihood of success. EBP changes are most likely to be successful when they are based on solid **external** as well as **internal evidence**, provide clear steps for change, and fit within the parameters of the clinician's routine practice and patient population (Brennan et al., 2017). When an organization's readiness for change is assessed, regardless of whether the change will have a large or small impact, an easy win is more likely to occur. A practice issue that aligns with the organization/administrators' key priorities or is a focus of quality initiatives mandated by regulatory agencies, such as the Joint Commission or the Institute for Healthcare Improvement, is likely to gain administrative support more readily than an isolated initiative.

Evaluate the Infrastructure

Organizational leaders must dedicate resources, including time, to provide support for staff and their EBP mentors to ask clinical questions; search for and critically appraise evidence; analyze internal evidence; develop practice recommendations; plan changes; and develop, implement, and evaluate the EBP project. Although administrative support is crucial, it is

BOX
9.6

Prioritize Clinical Issues

Procedures that nurses most often perform were selected as the first phase of the procedural pain initiative at the Texas Children's Hospital. Peripheral intravenous access, venipuncture for specimens, port access, and injections were identified as the highest priority procedures for pain prevention. Nasogastric tube and urinary catheter insertions were also considered but dropped early in the initiative. These two procedures were performed less frequently than needlesticks, and there was scant and conflicting evidence on pain prevention techniques. Although important, they would have delayed protocol implementation and have a weaker evidence foundation than the other procedures.

Narrow Focus Through PICO Questions

- In children, how does EMLA compared with LMX affect join pain during PIV access, venipuncture, and injections?
- In children, how does lidocaine iontophoresis compared with usual care affect pain during PIV access?
- In infants 16 months old, how does 24% sucrose compared with 50% or 75% sucrose affect crying time during and after PIV insertion?
- In children, how does buffered lidocaine compared with usual care affect pain during PIV insertion?
- In children, how does ethyl chloride compared with usual care affect pain during PIV access and venipuncture?
- In children, how does ethyl chloride compared with usual care affect pain during port access?

PIV, peripheral intravenous.

only one of the starting points and will not lead to success on its own. Administrators should seek guidance from expert clinicians, EBP mentors, and researchers within the organization while providing authoritative as well as financial support for the EBP initiative.

Resources that support the ability to locate and critically appraise relevant literature are essential for EBP implementation (Miglus & Froman, 2016). Access to an academic medical library, databases, search engines, and full-text articles should be available for the EBP team to be successful in securing evidence to support practice change. Although PubMed and the Cochrane Library are free to search and view abstracts, access to electronic full-text articles requires a subscription to electronic journals, some of which can be accessed only through specific databases. Chapter 3 provides sources and strategies for finding relevant evidence.

Working within already established committees and councils can effectively gain momentum for an EBP environment. Team members should be engaged in identifying how an EBP project fits within the committee's responsibilities, priorities, and agenda. Involving multiple approval bodies within the organizational hierarchy in the engagement phase can increase the number of individuals and teams eager to ensure an EBP project's success. To allow extended time for topic exploration, focus groups may need to be formed within existing committees.

Gaining consensus for a shared vision to improve patient outcomes can help break down process silos (processes separated by departments or other divisions within a healthcare institution with different departments fixing just their part) and communication barriers. Agreement that practice changes are based on evidence, rather than individual preferences or tradition, is a critical component that EBP teams may need to revisit several times during group discussions and workshops (Melnyk et al., 2016).

Develop Experts in the Evidence-Based Practice Process

Expertise available to lead an EBP team may exist within an organization or may require a partner from an academic or other healthcare setting. Expertise in critically appraising and synthesizing the research literature is crucial. Education related to all steps of the **EBP process** through formal classes and/or small-group skill-building sessions can expand the pool of EBP experts and mentors. Staff and clinical experts may be inexperienced at critically appraising research studies and evaluating evidence. With education and mentorship, clinicians who are novices in the EBP process can learn to analyze evidence and formulate practice recommendations within a structured environment (Benner, 1984). Gaining understanding of the concepts of EBP prior to the actual practice change is essential. Mentoring clinical staff eager to learn the steps of the EBP process is an important strategy that eventually develops EBP clinical experts throughout the institution (Spiva et al., 2017).

EVIDENCE-BASED PRACTICE INTEGRATION

Integrating EBP into clinical practice is one of the most challenging tasks faced by clinicians and leaders in healthcare settings (Best et al., 2016; Brennan et al., 2017). Evidence-based education and mentoring initiated during the engagement phase should continue during the integration phase, which is now directed toward overcoming knowledge and skill deficits along with stakeholder skepticism to enhance the likelihood of a positive EBP change (Spiva et al., 2017). Bridging the gap between evidence and practice is essential to bring about cultural change within a clinical environment. Education alone will not change behavior. Interventions need to be tailored to target groups and settings and include individual, team, and organizational approaches (Melnyk & Gallagher-Ford, 2015). Professional development systems, such as clinical ladders, can serve as incentives to increase nurses' engagement and proficiency with

> **"**
> Ideas without action are worthless.
>
> **HELEN KELLER**

EBP (Melnyk & Gallagher-Ford, 2015). Successful integration occurs when evidence is robust (i.e., being strong enough to withstand intellectual challenge), the physical environment is receptive to change, and the change process is appropriately facilitated (Table 9.3).

| TABLE 9.3 | *Build Excitement While Integrating EBP into the Clinical Environment* |

Objective	Strategies
Build excitement for EBP	• Demonstrate the link between proposed EBP changes and desired patient outcomes. • Build a "burning platform" (i.e., a passionate, compelling case) to drive change. • Create a level of discomfort with status quo by sharing evidence of better outcomes at other healthcare settings.
Establish formal implementation teams	• Integrate experts in change theory at the systems level, such as advanced practice registered nurses. • Include expert staff members to ensure clinical applicability, feasibility, and adoption into practice. • Exhibit passion for the practice change. • Enlist local opinion leaders who can attest to the need for practice change. • Bring in outside speakers who have the potential to connect and inspire key stakeholders. • Create discomfort with status quo.
Disseminate evidence	• Utilize multifaceted strategies to overcome knowledge deficits, skill deficits, and skepticism. • Promote experience sharing to emphasize the need for change and positive outcomes of change. • Provide time to assimilate new practices.
Develop clinical tools	• Anticipate tools and processes that the staff will need to transform practice. • Revise patient care documentation records. • Ensure easy access to clinical resources. • Integrate alerts and reminders into workflow processes at the point of care. • Repeatedly expose the staff to evidence-based information.
Pilot the evidence-based change	• Choose pilot sites with consideration to unit leadership strength, patient population diversity, acuity, and geographic location. • Address the root causes of problems. • Decide to adopt, adapt, or abandon at the end of the pilot.
Preserve energy sources	• Engage support personnel. • Implement smaller, more manageable projects. • Anticipate setbacks and be patient and persistent.
Allow enough time to demonstrate the project's success	• Develop incremental project steps. • Establish a timeline.
Celebrate success	• Acknowledge the staff instrumental in the process. • Ensure recognition by supervisors and administration. • Recognize the staff in presentations.

EBP, evidence-based practice.

Establish Formal Implementation Teams

Establishing a formal EBP project implementation team early in the process is essential to success. This team guides EBP changes, and engages informal and formal coordinators at the unit and organizational levels to champion EBP (Aarons et al., 2014; Gardner et al., 2016). Advanced practice registered nurses are change agents adept at systems-level project design and often have the advantage of clinical experience with practice variations and outcome evaluation (Harbman et al., 2017). An implementation team that includes masters and/or doctorally prepared nurses and expert staff nurses is essential to determine the clinical applicability and feasibility of practice change recommendations and the likelihood of integrating evidence into practice and evaluating patient outcomes.

Build Excitement While Implementing EBP

One of the key factors to success of any EBP change is building excitement during implementation. Team members who exhibit passion can ignite a fire in their colleagues. Recognized national experts lend stature and credibility to the idea of implementing a practice change, whereas experts within the organization can attest to the relevance of the practice in local settings and add synergy for change. Younger nurses with less clinical experience often have more knowledge and enthusiasm for EBP then seasoned nurses; however, all nurses need guidance to implement EBP (Bovino et al., 2017; Warren et al., 2016). It is essential to engage nurses by demonstrating the link between proposed EBP changes and desired patient outcomes. Building a "burning platform" (i.e., a passionate, compelling case to drive change) to drive change can be strengthened with baseline practice-based data (e.g., quality and performance improvement data). Creating a level of discomfort with status quo by sharing evidence of better outcomes at other healthcare settings can create a readiness for change. Fostering enthusiasm by unit/service-based staff and leaders can lead to a shared ownership in the success of an EBP initiative.

Disseminate Evidence

Passive educational approaches such as dissemination of clinical practice guidelines and didactic educational sessions are usually ineffective and unlikely to result in practice change (Gardner et al., 2016). Education should be planned to overcome knowledge and skill deficits and skepticism. Eliminating knowledge deficits includes not only communicating what should be done (how to change) but also why a change will be beneficial (i.e., the outcome) and the evidence to support the change. It is important to share positive outcomes of the change including external evidence, internal evidence (e.g., quality improvement data), actual patient experiences, and stories from authentic voices (i.e., practitioners using the recommended practice). Raising the level of emotion through sharing experiences is a powerful way to increase motivation toward the practice change. Stories provide not only powerful images of the need for change but also a mechanism to communicate the outcomes associated with change. The impetus for change is different for each individual; therefore, multifaceted interventions for disseminating evidence are more likely to produce change than a singularly focused endeavor, such as education alone (Higuchi, Edwards, Carr, March, & Abdullah, 2015).

Strengthening beliefs about the value of EBP, an important strategy for increasing EBP implementation, and changing attitudes can be more challenging than imparting knowledge. A shared understanding of the problem and identified gaps in outcomes can be a foundation to valuing the change in practice. Evidence summaries should be shared with practitioners, along with persons involved in consensus building. Perceived barriers need to be removed, and processes may need to be streamlined to create time and support for the new practice.

Develop Clinical Tools

To enact change, the EBP implementation team must anticipate new processes and tools that the staff will need to transform practice. Development of resources that match interventions and overall strategies can greatly facilitate changes in clinical practices (Melnyk, Gallagher-Ford, Long, & Fineout-Overholt, 2014). Clinical tools to enhance appropriateness and consistency of care may include guidelines, EBP summaries, order sets, decision support embedded within the electronic medical record, clinical pathways, and algorithms (Box 9.7). Availability and ease of use are key to the successful adoption of any of these resources.

Alerts and reminders can help if well integrated into workflow processes. Whether electronic or paper, optimal timing and placement of reminders in relation to decision making about the care practices are essential. Guideline prompts at the point of care can be programmed into an electronic medical record, medication administration record, or even "smart" infusion pumps. Clinical decision support systems that provide electronic links to EBP information within an electronic health record or organizational website can positively influence an evidence-based practitioner's use of recommended practice changes.

Pilot Test the Evidence-Based Practice Change

Implementing a new EBP change requires restructuring of the flow of daily work so that routine processes make it natural for the clinician to give care in a new way. Even educated and motivated providers can have difficulty practicing in the desired manner without daily environmental supports. Piloting small tests of change with a commitment to modify and improve the practice change with staff feedback can promote positive attitudes along with engagement in the new practice. Plan to quickly respond to questions and concerns and address the root causes of problems during the pilot phase. Early evaluation results should be shared with staff at the end of each pilot cycle, and a decision should be made to adopt, adapt, or abandon the proposed practice.

BOX
9.7

Example of an Evidence-Based Practice Critical Appraisal Template

Ask the question   **Question**
                                 Background summary
Search for the evidence   **Search strategies**
                                 Dates/search limits
                                 Key words/terms/controlled vocabulary

Rapidly critically appraise, evaluate, and synthesize the evidence
Summary of findings
Integrate the evidence
Recommendation for practice, research, or education
References
Cite all references

Pilot testing in a select number of patient care areas, or target areas, before moving to widespread implementation can help identify issues of clinical applicability and feasibility that will have an impact on future efforts at successful EBP implementation (Curtis, Fry, Shaban, & Considine, 2017).

Leadership capacity, populations served, patient acuity, and geographic location are some of the initial considerations for choosing a pilot site. In addition, sites that are known to have early adopters as well as those known to be difficult or resistant implementation sites are important to consider in choosing the site to conduct a pilot project. Early adopters can serve as training sites for later adopters. Well-managed programs with a long history of successful implementation of initiatives are likely to establish practice change early in the pilot phase. However, establishing an EBP change on a struggling unit can communicate to others that change can occur even in difficult clinical settings.

Preserve Energy Sources

Change in a dynamic healthcare environment adds stress on clinicians in the care setting. When implementing EBP changes, it is important to develop strategies to maintain excitement and preserve energy resources. Implementing smaller, more manageable projects in phases rather than introducing a single large EBP project may reduce fatigue and build confidence that the recommended change is achievable and sustainable given adequate time and resources (Box 9.8). Informal and formal leaders, referred to as "champions," can help with sustainability by bringing new energy and ownership during specific phases of a project (Fleiszer, Semenic,

---

BOX 9.8   *Small Steps of Change*

During the engagement phase of the procedural pain initiative at the Texas Children's Hospital, many nurses became uncomfortable with status quo and were eager to have broader access to pain prevention medications. The protocol was anticipated to take several months to allow for critically appraising evidence, building algorithms, gaining consensus, and piloting.

Sucrose had been used for years in the hospital's Neonatal Intensive Care Unit (NICU), but young infants admitted to other areas were not given sucrose.

- The first step of change was to establish an upper age limit for sucrose and permit its use anywhere in the organization.
- The second step was to remove a time barrier by adding sucrose and LMX (4% lidocaine cream) to floor stock in many areas. Additional medications were added to the formulary and available for use by individual order as the third step of the initiative.
- The final step was to implement the procedural pain protocol, a group of medications for multiple procedures, and expand floor stock availability.

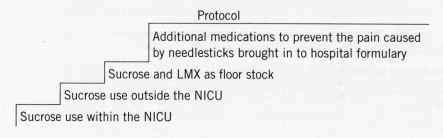

Protocol

Additional medications to prevent the pain caused by needlesticks brought in to hospital formulary

Sucrose and LMX as floor stock

Sucrose use outside the NICU

Sucrose use within the NICU

Ritchie, Richer, & Denis, 2016). Project leaders and teams should anticipate setbacks with patience and persistence. Periodically sharing small successes along the way can foster continued excitement for the project and reduce fatigue often associated with lagging outcomes.

Allow Enough Time for Success

Planning practice changes for an EBP project includes evaluating current practice, identifying gaps in "what is" and "what is desired," establishing incremental steps of the project, and setting timelines. Competing priorities within an area or organization can influence the timing needed to embark on a successful EBP project. When conducting a large change, often it is easier to accomplish it when customarily busy periods are over or when leaders are as free as possible from competing responsibilities. Project timelines for EBP changes vary extremely and can be influenced by many environmental issues, such as the size of the project, staff time commitment, EBP expertise, expediency of decision making, and the urgency of the need for practice change (Box 9.9).

BOX 9.9 | *Sample EBP Implementation Project Plan*

Project timelines for EBP changes are highly variable. Several project components may overlap or occur simultaneously.

Project component	Timeframe
Develop a vision for change	Variable
Identify and narrow practice topic	1–3 weeks
Evaluate current practice and analyze recent quality data	4–6 weeks
Engage staff and stakeholders	4 weeks
Evaluate the infrastructure and establish formal teams	4 weeks
Develop and refine PICO questions	2–4 weeks
Develop search strategy and conduct search	4–6 weeks
Critically appraise, evaluate, and synthesize the evidence	4–8 weeks
Formulate practice recommendations	2 weeks
Celebrate success of progress to date!	Ongoing
Gain stakeholder support	2–4 weeks
Assess and eliminate barriers	Variable
Develop clinical tools	Variable
Conduct rapid cycle pilot	Variable
Celebrate success of progress to date!	Ongoing
Gain approval for change	Variable
Disseminate evidence and educate staff	4 weeks
Implement practice change	1 week
Celebrate success of progress to date!	Ongoing
Measure clinical outcomes	Ongoing
Analyze measurement data and refine practice and processes	Ongoing
Celebrate success!	Ongoing

Celebrate Success

Celebrate success early in the development phases of practice change recommendations. It is important to acknowledge members of the project team who are instrumental in the planning and implementation process in meetings where the practice is discussed, in hospital newsletters, or in any venue in which materials related to the project are presented. Recognize individuals and teams who adopt and implement the new practice. Positive outcomes from preliminary measurements of success should be shared with all point-of-care providers as well as other key stakeholders. Clinicians and administrators who see the positive results of an EBP project will be more likely to engage in and support future EBP initiatives. Leaders and point-of-care providers responsible for promoting EBP change should be encouraged to share their findings through presentations and publications so that other professionals and institutions may benefit from their EBP endeavors.

EVALUATION: LINKING EVIDENCE-BASED PRACTICE TO CLINICAL OUTCOMES

One of the most difficult aspects of EBP is ensuring that change has occurred and, even more importantly, has resulted in positive, sustained outcomes. All too frequently, patient care outcomes in clinical settings indicate a need for changes that demand immediate action by administrators and leaders, which may place clinicians in a practice environment shaped by practice standards and initiatives that are not well thought out or evaluated for successful outcomes. This crisis orientation to clinical practice change results in less than impressive results. Well-intentioned administrators often demand changes without considering the time taken to change a culture. Policy changes that make it difficult for the clinician to provide quality care in a timely manner will never succeed. For example, EBP that requires supplies and resources that are not readily available to the clinicians will not produce positive clinical outcomes because the clinicians will not integrate changes in their practice that are difficult or impossible to perform. Redesign and standardization of workflows are commonly needed to integrate EBP at the point of care. For sustainable change to occur, time must be taken to evaluate influence of EBP on patient care processes.

Evaluating outcomes produced by clinical practice changes is important at the patient, clinician, and unit, departmental, organizational, or system level. Outcomes reflect the impact of the process changes or structural changes. Outcomes may vary when translation of an effective intervention from research to real-world clinical practice does not control for confounding variables or involve similar patient populations. Evaluating outcomes of an EBP change is important to determine whether the findings from research are similar when translated into the real-world clinical practice setting. It is important to measure outcomes before (i.e., baseline), shortly after (i.e., short-term follow-up), and for a reasonable length of time after (i.e., long-term follow-up) the practice change. Each of these points in time provides data on the sustainable impact of the EBP change.

The complexity of health-related outcomes associated with clinical practice presents an opportunity to evaluate the impact of EBP in the environment from multiple perspectives. Table 9.4 highlights six key indicators of evidence that are important for evaluation.

These indicators reflect evidence in the environment that demonstrates effective changes in clinical practice. Health outcome measures must be a part of the EBP environment to determine whether healthcare interventions actually make a difference.

TABLE 9.4	EBP Evaluation in the Clinical Environment
Objective	**Measurement Description**
Outcome measures	Outcome measures quantify medical outcomes such as health status, death, disability, iatrogenic effects of treatment, health behaviors, and the economic impact of therapy and illness management.
Quality care improvement	Examples of health-related quality of life measures include symptom burden such as pain, fatigue, nausea, sleep disturbances, and depression caused by many acute and chronic diseases and improving self-perception, sense of well-being, and social participation.
Patient-centered quality care	Measures include effective communication with healthcare personnel; open, unrushed interactions; presentation of all options for care; open discussion of the illness or disease; sensitivity to pain and emotional distress; consideration of the cultural and religious beliefs of the patient and family; being respectful and considerate; nonavoidance of specific issues; empathy; patience; equitable access and treatment; and a caring attitude and environment.
Efficiency of processes	Optimal timing of interventions, effective discharge planning, elimination of waste such as duplication of tests, and efficient utilization of hospital beds are exemplars of efficiency of processes indicators.
Environmental changes	Evaluation of policy and procedure adherence, unit resource availability, and healthcare professional access to supplies and materials essential to implement best practices.
Professional expertise	Knowledge and expertise of clinical staff

EBP, evidence-based practice.

Outcome Measures

Outcome measures are defined as those healthcare results that can be quantified, such as health status, death, disability, iatrogenic (undesirable or unwanted) effects of treatment, health behaviors, and the economic impact of therapy and illness management (Institute of Medicine [IOM], 2000). Health outcome measures are used to evaluate changes in clinical practice, support healthcare decision making, and establish new policies or practice guidelines. Two well-recognized frameworks for large-scale population health outcome measures have been established by the Institute for Healthcare Improvement Whole Systems Measures (Martin, Nelson, Rakover, & Chase, 2016) and the Institutes of Medicine Core Metrics (IOM, 2015). Over the last two decades, there has been an explosion of outcomes measures developed or endorsed by various professional societies, quality improvement associations, and governmental agencies. Public clearinghouses for healthcare measures exist such as the National Quality Forum and the Agency for Healthcare Research and Quality.

 The National Quality Forum (http://www.qualityforum.org) is a nonprofit, nonpartisan organization that improves health and healthcare quality through national collaboration and measurement. The website contains information on public and private efforts of six priority areas: health and well-being, prevention and treatment of leading causes of mortality, person- and family-centered care, effective communication, patient safety, and affordable care.

Agency for Healthcare Research & Quality (http://www.ahrq.gov) is an agency of the U.S. DHHS that focuses on producing evidence to make healthcare safer, better, more accessible, equitable, and affordable. Their website contains information about funding and grants, clinical and educational programs, research findings and reports, clinical tools, and links to data sources.

Important questions to ask regarding measurement of outcomes from an EBP implementation project include the following:

- Are the outcomes of high importance to the current healthcare system?
- Are the outcomes of interest sensitive to change over time?
- How will the outcome(s) of interest be measured (e.g., subjectively through self-report and/or objectively by observation)?
- Are there existing valid and reliable instruments to measure the outcomes of interest?
- Who will measure the outcomes, and will training be necessary?
- What is the cost of measuring the outcomes?

Identifying these aspects of measurement of outcomes will assist in the quality of outcomes obtained.

Quality Care Improvement

Quality care improvement measures complement established health outcome measures by further quantifying how interventions affect the quality of life of patients and families. Effectively managing common symptoms caused by many acute and chronic diseases can provide specific data to demonstrate quality care improvement in clinical practice. Often, quality indicators demonstrate the existence of a clinical issue as well as provide information about successful evidence of implementation and change. The Healthy People 2020 (2017) campaign provides examples of validated measurement tools for health-related quality of life in multiple domains.

Patient-Centered Quality Care

Increasing emphasis has been placed on **patient-centered quality care measures**. These measures are defined as the value patients and families place on the healthcare received. Patient-centered quality care requires a philosophy of care that views the patient as an equal partner rather than a passive recipient of care, much like the EBP paradigm, in which patient preferences must be part of the decision making (Box 9.10). Commonly, patient-centered

 BOX **9.10**   *Patient-Centered Quality Care*

Crucial to promoting patient-centered quality care is open, honest discussion of the illness or disease.
- Consideration of the cultural and religious beliefs of the patient and family, being respectful and considerate, nonavoidance of specific issues, empathy, patience, and a caring attitude and environment are all important.
- Use of measures that critically evaluate key aspects of patient-centered quality care within a healthcare organization can provide crucial evidence that differentiates a good healthcare setting from an outstanding one.
- Busy hospital environments often prevent family coping strategies from effectively being utilized even though evidence supports the importance of family presence.
- Time constraints often prevent patient-centered quality care.

One family at the Texas Children's Hospital felt strongly that they needed to place a prayer rug under their child and say a prayer over the child immediately before anesthesia. Although this activity added a few more minutes to the preanesthesia preparation, it resulted in the child being relaxed and fully cooperating with the anesthesiologist once the prayer was completed. The child went to sleep without a struggle lying on the prayer rug. Parents left the anesthesia induction room feeling that their needs were met and patient/family-centered care was provided.

quality care measures have been described as "soft" indicators and historically received limited attention. Policy makers, healthcare organizations, and healthcare professionals now recognize the importance of organizing and managing health systems to ensure patient-centered quality care. Today, patient and family ratings of hospitals and providers can affect reimbursement. To spotlight excellence in healthcare quality, some payer agencies, such as the CMSs, make key measures and scores easily accessible on the internet.

 Hospital Consumer Assessment of Healthcare Providers and Systems (HACHPS) is available at http://www.medicare.gov/hospitalcompare

Efficiency of Processes

As healthcare organizations become more sophisticated in evaluation strategies, it becomes essential to evaluate the efficiency of healthcare delivery processes. Information technology provides numerous EBP strategies to improve care delivery methods at every level in the organization. Efficiency in providing EBP care and evaluating the best possible process for implementing these practices lead to excellence in care and cost containment. Appropriate timing of interventions, effective discharge planning, and efficient utilization of hospital beds are examples of efficiency of process indicators. These indicators are directly associated with outcomes (Box 9.11).

Barriers That Influence Efficiency of Process Changes

Barriers to EBP implementation often impede measurable clinical outcomes.
- Implementation of an evidence-based guideline for managing bronchiolitis demonstrated a resistance to change that significantly influenced the efficiency of the EBP implementation process.
- An EBP review revealed that earlier discharge could occur when discharge planning was initiated earlier during hospitalization.
- During the implementation phase of this guideline, two different healthcare disciplines refused to compromise over who would notify the physician about early discharge orders, stating it was not their role to obtain the order.
- Rather than evaluate what was best for the patient and family, these professionals refused to change their practice and the administrators had to intervene to persuade a compromise.

EBP, evidence-based practice.

Environmental Changes

Environmental change evaluation reflects the creation of a culture that promotes the use of EBP throughout the organization. Environmental outcome measures are uniquely different in comparison with efficiency of processes in that a process can change or patient outcomes change, yet there is no impact on the environment. This difference is often observed with policy and procedure changes that are carefully updated and filed into procedure manuals, yet no practice changes actually occur in the clinical setting. Examples of indicators of environmental changes include evaluation of policy and procedure adherence, unit resource availability, and healthcare professional use of supplies and materials essential to implement best practices.

Professional Expertise

Excellence in providing the best possible healthcare cannot occur without expert providers. Increasing sophistication in healthcare technology places significant demands on institutions to employ healthcare professionals with appropriate expertise. Professional expertise promotes excellence by establishing expectations for adherence to accepted standards of care essential for best practice. Without the expertise of healthcare providers, institutions are often unable to determine why specific outcomes are not being met (Box 9.12).

BOX
9.12   *Linking Clinical Outcomes to Professional Expertise*

Placement of NG tubes in infants and children is a common and often difficult nursing procedure.

- Using the gold standard (radiographic documentation), Ellett, Croffie, Cohen, and Perkins (2005) found that more than 20% of NG tubes were incorrectly placed in 72 acutely ill children.
- Other studies quote misplacement as high as 43.5% in children (Ellett & Beckstrand, 1999; Ellett, Maahs, & Forsee, 1998). Displaced NG tubes can create significant morbidity and mortality.
- Throughout numerous children's hospitals across the country, changes in assessing NG tube placement are being implemented because there is substantial evidence that the traditional method of auscultation is not effective in determining proper placement (Westhus, 2004).
- A combination of measures to ensure NG tube placement, including pH, tube length, and physical symptoms, has been shown to be more effective in the assessment of NG tube placement in children (Ellett, 2004, 2006; Ellett et al., 2005; Gilbertson, Rogers, & Ukoumunne, 2011; Metheny et al., 2005; Metheny & Stewart, 2002; Stock, Gilbertson, & Babl, 2008).

    However, there is significant discussion throughout the country that it is difficult to change traditional nursing practice even when there is evidence to indicate that auscultation for proper NG tube placement is not safe practice. Policy changes without education and reinforcement of this new evidence-based practice approach to NG tube placement will never be effective in producing measurable change in clinical outcomes.

NG, nasogastric.

IMPLEMENTING EVIDENCE IN CLINICAL SETTINGS: EXAMPLE FROM THE FIELD

The following example from the field of successful EBP implementation projects started with identification of a clinical problem because of a spirit of inquiry (Melnyk, 2015).

McCommons, Wheeler, and Houston (2016) describe the practice change from air to carbon dioxide insufflation during colonoscopies using the EBP process. Nurses had concerns about patient experiences of discomfort, bloating, flatus, and satisfaction during colonoscopy procedures and were interested in using carbon dioxide as an alternative to air insufflation during the procedure (Step 0 in the EBP process). It was identified that evidence was needed to evaluate the outcomes of carbon dioxide versus air insufflation. Therefore, the following patient population, intervention or *issue* of interest, comparison intervention or group, outcome, and time frame) PICOT question (Step 1 in the EBP process) was developed:

> *In the general adult population undergoing colonoscopy (P), how does carbon dioxide insufflation (I) compared with air insufflation (C) affect postoperative pain (O)?*

A search for the evidence to answer the PICOT question (Step 2 in the EBP process) revealed 12 relevant publications, of which 10 were research and 2 were editorials. Critical appraisal, evaluation, and synthesis of these studies (Step 3 of the EBP process) led to the following conclusions: A statistically significant decrease in postprocedural pain and discomfort along with less residual gas was noted in carbon dioxide groups after the procedure. Therefore, a recommendation was made to change insufflation from air to carbon dioxide during a colonoscopy procedure.

Based on the evidence, an interprofessional team with team champions was formed to develop the practice change (Step 4 in the EBP process) that included educating staff, obtaining and piloting the equipment, and developing a data collection tool. At staff meetings, healthcare professionals were educated on the evidence and process of carbon dioxide insufflation. The project was implemented and evaluated (Step 5 in the EBP process). Patient discomfort decreased from 11% to 1.6% immediately after the procedure and 14% to 3% 15 minutes after the procedure. These results were shared with organizational leaders and healthcare professionals, and the policy remains in place (Step 6 in the EBP process).

EBP FAST FACTS

- Essential components for successful EBP implementation in clinical settings include creating a vision (a shared mental framework), developing specific goals, identifying a dedicated EBP team, involving EBP experts, and promoting engagement by eliminating barriers, prioritizing clinical issues, and evaluating the infrastructure.
- Key factors for a successful EBP change implementation include the following:
  1. **Establish a formal implementation team:** Integrate staff nurses and masters/doctorally prepared nurses.
  2. **Build excitement:** Engage staff, raise awareness of the need for change, foster enthusiasm, encourage ownership of EBP initiative.
  3. **Disseminate evidence:** Communicate the process and rationale for the change and share experiences to increase motivation to change.
  4. **Develop clinical tools:** Written guidelines, preprinted orders, or algorithms will encourage adoption of new practices; alerts and reminders can help influence change.

5. **Pilot the evidence-based change:** Evaluating changes on a small scale before moving to widespread implementation can promote positive attitudes to engage in new practices, but early evaluation results should be shared with staff promptly along with time to address questions and concerns.
6. **Preserve energy sources:** Implementing smaller, more manageable projects in phases may reduce fatigue and build confidence; integrating new "champions for change" for each phase can bring new energy and enthusiasm.
7. **Develop a timeline for success:** Competing priorities or environmental issues should be considered with project timelines for EBP change.
8. **Celebrate success:** Acknowledge project team members, early adopters, and positive outcomes of the change.

- Evaluating clinical practice outcomes is an important but commonly overlooked step in the EBP process. It is important to measure outcomes before, shortly after, and at a reasonable length of time after the practice change implementation.

WANT TO KNOW MORE?

A variety of resources is available to enhance your learning and understanding of this chapter.

- Visit thePoint® to access:
  - Articles from the AJN EBP Step-By-Step Series
  - Journal articles
  - Checklists for rapid critical appraisal and more!

- Lippincott CoursePoint combines digital text content with video case studies and interactive modules for a fully integrated course solution that works the way you study and learn.

References

Aarons, G. A., Fettes, D. L., Hurlburt, M. S., Palinkas, L. A., Gunderson, L., Willging, C. E., & Chaffin, M. J. (2014). Collaboration, negotiation, and coalescence for interagency-collaborative teams to scale-up evidence-based practice. *Journal of Clinical Child and Adolescent Psychology, 43*(6), 915–928.

Aasekjaer, K., Waehle, H. V., Ciliska, D., Nordtvedt, M. W., & Hjalmhult, E. (2016). Management involvement—a decisive condition when implementing evidence-based practice. *Worldviews on Evidence-Based Nursing, 13*(1), 32–41.

American Nurses Credentialing Center. (2014). *Magnet recognition program: Application manual.* Silver Spring, MD: Author.

Benner, P. (1984). *From novice to expert: Excellence and power in clinical nursing practice.* Menlo Park, CA: Addison-Wesley.

Best, A., Berland, A., Herbert, C., Bitz, J., van Dijk, M. W., Krause, C., . . . Millar, J. (2016). Using systems thinking to support clinical system transformation. *Journal of Health Organization and Management, 30*(3), 302–323.

Bovino, R., Aquila, A. M., Bartos, S., McCurry, T., Cunningham, C. E., Lane, T., . . . Quiles, J. (2017). A cross-sectional study on evidence-based nursing practice in the contemporary hospital setting: Implications for nurses in professional development. *Journal for Nurses in Professional Development, 33*(2), 64–69.

Brennan, C., Greenhalgh, J., & Pawson, R. (2017). Guidance on guidelines: Understanding the evidence on the uptake of health care guidelines. *Journal of Evaluation in Clinical Practice.* doi: 10.1111/jep.12734

Curtis, K., Fry, M., Shaban, R. Z., & Considine, J. (2017). Translating research findings to clinical nursing practice. *Journal of Clinical Nursing, 26*(5–6), 862–872.

Ellett, M. L. (2004). What is known about methods of correctly placing gastric tubes in adults and children. *Gastroenterology Nursing, 27*(6), 253–259.

Ellett, M. L. (2006). Important facts about intestinal feeding tube placement. *Gastroenterology Nursing, 29*(2), 112–124.

Ellett, M. L., & Beckstrand, J. (1999). Examination of gavage tube placement in children. *Journal of the Society of Pediatric Nurses, 4*(2), 51–60.

Ellett, M. L., Croffie, J. M., Cohen, M. D., & Perkins, S. M. (2005). Gastric tube placement in young children. *Clinical Nursing Research, 14*(3), 238–252.

Ellett, M. L., Maahs, J., & Forsee, S. (1998). Prevalence of feeding tube placement errors & associated risk factors in children. *MCN. The American Journal of Maternal Child Nursing, 23*(5), 234–239.

Fleiszer, A. R., Semenic, S. E., Ritchie, J. A., Richer, M., & Denis, J. (2016). Nursing unit leaders' influence on the long-term sustainability of evidence-based practice improvements. *Journal of Nursing Management, 24,* 309–318.

Friesen, M. A., Brady, J. M., Milligan, R., & Christensen, P. (2017). Findings from a pilot study: Bringing evidence-based practice to the bedside. *Worldviews on Evidence-Based Nursing, 14*(1), 22–34.

Gardner, K., Kanaskie, M. L., Knehans, A. C., Salisbury, S., Doheny, K. K., & Schirm, V. (2016). Implementing and sustaining evidence based practice through a nursing journal club. *Applied Nursing Research, 31,* 139–145.

Gilbertson, H. R., Rogers, E. J., & Ukoumunne, O. C. (2011). Determination of a practical pH cutoff level for reliable confirmation of nasogastric tube placement. *JPEN. Journal of Parenteral and Enteral Nutrition, 35*(4), 540–544.

Harbman, P., Bryant-Lukosius, D., Martin-Misener, R., Carter, N., Covell, C. L., Donald, F., . . . Valaitis, R. (2017). Partners in research: Building academic-practice partnerships to educate and mentor advanced practice nurses. *Journal of Evaluation in Clinical Practice, 23*(92), 382–390.

Healthy People 2020 [Internet]. (2017). *Health-related quality of life and well-being.* Washington, DC: U.S. Department of Health & Human Services, Office of Disease Prevention and Health Promotion. Retrieved from www.healthypeople.gov/2020/about/foundation-health-measures/Health-Related-Quality-of-Life-and-Well-Being

Higuchi, K. S., Edwards, N., Carr, T., March, P., & Abdullah, G. (2015). Development and evaluation of a workshop to support evidence-based practice change in long-term care. *Journal for Nurses in Professional Development, 31*(1), 28–34.

Hockenberry, M., Walden, M., Brown, T., & Barrera, P. (2007). Creating an evidence-based practice environment: One hospital's journey. *Journal of Nursing Care Quality, 22*(3), 221–231.

Institute of Medicine. (2000). *To err is human: Building a safer health system.* Washington, DC: The National Academies Press.

Institute of Medicine. (2015). *Vital signs: Core metrics for health and health care progress.* Washington, DC: The National Academies Press.

Kowalski, M. O. (2017). Strategies to heighten EBP engagement. *Nursing Management, 48*(2), 13–15.

Liddy, C., Rowan, M., Valiquette-Tessier, S., Drosinis, P., Crowe, L., & Hogg, W. (2017). Improved delivery of cardiovascular care (IDOCC): Findings from narrative reports by practice facilitators. *Preventive Medicine Reports, 5,* 214–219.

Martin, L., Nelson, E., Rakover, J., & Chase, A. (2016). *Whole system measures 2.0: A compass for health system leaders.* Cambridge, MA: Institute for Healthcare Improvement. Retrieved from www.ihi.org

Melnyk, B. M. (2015). Transforming quality improvement into evidence-based quality improvement: A key solution to improve healthcare outcomes. *Worldviews on Evidence-Based Nursing, 12*(5), 251–252.

Melnyk, B. M. (2016). Culture east strategy every time: What works in building and sustaining an evidence-based practice culture in healthcare systems. *Worldviews on Evidence-Based Nursing, 13*(2), 99–101.

Melnyk, B. M., & Gallagher-Ford, L. (2015). Implementing the new essential evidence-based practice competencies in real-world clinical and academic settings: Moving from evidence to action in improving healthcare quality and patient outcomes. *Worldviews on Evidence-Based Nursing, 12*(2), 67–69.

Melnyk, B. M., Gallagher-Ford, L., Long, L. E., & Fineout-Overholt, E. (2014). The establishment of evidence-based practice competencies for practicing registered nurses and advanced practice nurses in real-world clinical settings: Proficiencies to improve healthcare quality, reliability, patient outcomes, and costs. *Worldviews on Evidence-Based Nursing, 11*(1), 5–15.

Melnyk, B. M., Gallagher-Ford, L., Thomas, B. K., Troseth, M., Wyngarden, K., & Szalacha, L. (2016). A study of chief nurse executives indicates low prioritization of evidence-based practice and shortcomings in hospital performance metrics across the United States. *Worldviews on Evidence-Based Nursing, 13*(1), 6–14.

Metheny, N. A., Schnelker, R., McGinnis, J., Zimmerman, G., Duke, C., Merritt, B., . . . Oliver, D. A. (2005). Indicators of tubesite during feedings. *Journal of Neuroscience Nursing, 37*(6), 320–325.

Metheny, N. A., & Stewart, B. J. (2002). Testing feeding tube placement during continuous tube feedings. *Applied Nursing Research: ANR, 15*(4), 254–258.

McCommons, R., Wheeler, M., & Houston, S. (2016). Colonoscopy comfort: An evidence-based practice project. *Gastroenterology Nursing, 39*(3), 212–215.

Miglus, J. D., & Froman, R. D. (2016). Evaluation of an evidence-based practice tutorial for nurses: A useful tool and some lessons learned. *Journal of Continuing Education in Nursing, 47*(6), 266–271.

National Strategy for Quality Improvement in Health Care. (2012). *Annual progress report to congress.* Washington, DC: U.S. Department of Health & Human Services.

Nilsen, P., Reg, M. N., Ellstrom, P., & Gardner, B. (2017). Implementation of a evidence-based practice from a learning perspective. *Worldviews on Evidence-Based Nursing, 14,* 192–199.

Powell, B. J., Beidas, R. S., Lewis, C. C., Aarons, G. A., McMillen, J. C., Proctor, E. K., & Mandell, D. S. (2017). Methods to improve the selection and tailoring of implementation strategies. *Journal of Behavioral Health Services and Research, 44*(2), 177–194.

Sharma, S., Pandit, A., & Tabassum, F. (2017). Potential facilitators and barriers to adopting standard treatment guidelines in clinical practice. *International Journal of Health Care Quality Assurance, 30*(3), 285–298.

Spiva, L., Hart, P. L., Patrick, S., Waggoner, J., Jackson, C., & Threatt, J. L. (2017). Effectiveness of an evidence-based practice nurse mentor training program. *Worldviews on Evidence-Based Nursing, 14*(3), 183–191.

Stock, A., Gilbertson, H., & Babl, F. E. (2008). Confirming nasogastric tube position in the emergency department. *Pediatric Emergency Care, 24*(12), 805–809.

Sung-Heui, B. (2017). CMS nonpayment policy, quality improvement, and hospital-acquired conditions: An integrative review. *Journal of Nursing Care Quality, 32*(1), 55–61.

Warren, J. I., McLaughlin, M., Bardsley, J., Eich, J., Esche, C. A., Kropkowski, L., & Risch, S. (2016). The strengths and challenges of implementing EBP in healthcare systems. *Worldviews of Evidence-Based Nursing, 13*(1), 15–24.

Westhus, N. (2004). Methods to test feeding tube placement in children. *MCN. The American Journal of Maternal Child Nursing, 29*(5), 282–287.

10 The Role of Outcomes and Evidence-Based Quality Improvement in Enhancing and Evaluating Practice Changes

Anne W. Alexandrov, Tracy L. Brewer, and Barbara B. Brewer

> **Quality in a service or product is not what you put into it. It is what the client or customer gets out of it.**
>
> —*Peter Drucker*

EBP Terms to Learn

Aim statement
Balancing measures
Categorical variables
Demographics
Effect size
Electronic health records (EHRs)
Evidence-based practice improvement (EBPI)
Evidence-based quality improvement
Frequencies
Health insurance portability and accountability act (HIPAA) regulations
Histogram
Hospital consumer assessment of healthcare providers and systems (HCAHPS)
Institutional review board (IRB)

Internal evidence
Interval data
Key driver diagram
Key stakeholders
Model for improvement
Outcomes
Outcome measures
Outcomes management
Outcomes research
Pareto chart

Process measures
Provider skill mix
Quality improvement
Readmission rates
Run charts
Science of improvement
Structure measures
Systematic review
Taxonomy
Value-based purchasing (VBP)

Learning Objectives

After studying this chapter, learners will be able to:

1. Discuss the importance of outcomes in healthcare.

2. Describe sources of data.

3. Discuss how quality models can improve clinical outcomes.

3. Discuss various methods to display outcomes for making clinical decisions.

Monitoring outcomes is essential to delivery of best practices because our knowledge of the "results of our care" determines the quality of our services by making known their impact on the patient, health service systems, and cost (Melnyk, Morrison-Beedy, & Moore, 2012). It makes perfect sense that practitioners discovering new evidence, for example, a new **systematic review** supporting use of a specific type of fall prevention program for use in older adult long-term care residents, would ultimately want to measure whether implementation does indeed produce better results as the systematic review indicates, in this case, fewer falls (the outcome). Donabedian (1980) first described outcomes in his quality framework, along with structure and process components. Yet healthcare providers were slow to embrace outcomes measurement; instead, providers recognized the importance of structure and rapidly adopted process measurement activities alone in an attempt to determine healthcare quality. In fact, it was not until almost two decades later that a focus on outcomes measurement and management began to take hold in the late 1990s (Wojner, 2001).

This chapter focuses on understanding the role of outcomes within **evidence-based quality improvement (EBQI)**, enabling a comparison of traditional practice with new evidence-based interventions. Measurement and evaluation of the results or outcomes of EBQI are fundamental to the provision of excellent healthcare and therefore essential for all healthcare providers to integrate into their practice.

BLENDING TRADITIONAL QUALITY IMPROVEMENT WITH EVIDENCE-BASED PRACTICE

Quality improvement (QI) is broadly defined as "a data-driven approach by which individuals work together to improve specific internal systems, processes, costs, productivity, and quality outcomes within an organization" (Haughom, 2016; Shirey et al., 2011, p. 61). QI methods were originally aimed at reducing the variation found in the quality and efficiency of industrial work and were not adopted by healthcare as an improvement framework until the 1980s (Haughom, 2016; Parry, 2014). Despite differences, both evidence-based practice (EBP) and QI employ a systematic approach for problem solving within the context of a system, with the aim of improving results (Fitzpatrick, 2016; Glasziou, Ogrinc, & Goodman, 2011; Institute for Healthcare Improvement [IHI], 2017a; Shirey et al., 2011).

Both Glasziou et al. (2011) and Levin et al. (2010) were early proponents of "blending" the quality and EBP paradigms as a logical step toward addressing the research–practice gap. However, Levin (2008) suggested that the "jargon" or terminology within each model increased confusion and could impede understanding of how "processes" for each could support knowledge and practice change. Overall, EBP and QI have similar objectives for focusing on clinical or system problems, with data serving as a means of decision making to support improvement. However, EBP and QI focus on different aspects of a problem. For example, the EBP process concentrates on "doing the right thing" through the appraisal and synthesis of the "best" available evidence for informing clinicians and patients of practice recommendations (Glasziou et al., 2011, p. i13; Parry, 2014), whereas the QI process is more focused on "doing things right" (Glasziou et al., 2011, p. i13) or evaluating "how we are doing" with less of a focus on identifying best practice evidence. The marriage of EBP and QI to create EBQI produces a system whereby internal evidence of patient-based results or outcomes is used to systematically and continuously improve health services and, ultimately, the health status or health outcomes of targeted patient groups (U.S. Department of Health & Human Services, 2011a). The **evidence-based practice improvement (EBPI)** model showcases the merger of EBP with QI using the well-known Plan (P), Do (D), Study (S), and Act (A) approach (Levin et al., 2010). However, what seems like a simple, linear approach to EBPI often fails full implementation because of misunderstandings of what constitute health outcomes and how to measure them.

In healthcare, **outcomes** are *"health status results"* experienced by patients (e.g., blood pressure, anxiety, disease severity, functional status, the cost of health services, recidivism, etc.), that surface between two or more time points and are *caused by the care that is provided, in combination with discrete modifiable or nonmodifiable patient or environmental factors.* **Outcomes research** uses a rigorous scientific process that generates new knowledge (external evidence) about the outcomes of certain healthcare practices (e.g., a randomized controlled trial that tests for differences in patient outcomes [such as weight loss] using a currently accepted method [such as standardized patient discharge teaching on diet and activity level], compared to a new method [such as the addition of a health coaching smartphone app]). Unlike outcomes research, an EBPI approach utilizes data collected through QI processes and routine documentation, termed "**internal evidence**," to guide continuous assessment and improvement of healthcare services (Glasziou et al., 2011, p. i16).

" "

In planning anything, the best place to begin is at the end.
What outcome do you want?
How do you want the story to end?

MICHAEL HYATT

UNDERSTANDING OUTCOMES: THE "END-RESULT IDEA"

In 1917, Ernest Codman had the audacity to propose that hospitals and physicians should be promoted on the basis of outcomes that they produce, something considered outrageous within the capitalistic health economic framework of the United States. Simply named the "end-result idea," Codman boldly suggested that hospitals and physicians should measure the results of their healthcare processes and make them available to the general public. Those agencies with optimal outcomes would then command a leadership position within the healthcare market, whereas those with suboptimal performance would be challenged to improve, resign, or go out of business. Sadly for Codman (1934), his suggestion was deemed nothing short of dangerous in the context of a paternalistic medical philosophy, which held that patients were uneducated and cognitively ill equipped to participate in both health decision making and determination of medical provider excellence. Until the emergence of Donabedian's (1980) quality framework, the healthcare community remained silent on outcomes measurement.

In 1988, Paul Ellwood took up the charge for outcomes measurement, proposing a framework for **outcomes management** (OM). Ellwood described OM as "a technology of patient experience designed to help patients, payers, and providers make rational medical care-related choices based on better insight into the effect of these choices on patient life" (p. 1549). The principles supporting OM ascribed by Ellwood included the following:

- Emphasizing practice standards that providers can use to select interventions;
- Measuring patient functional status, well-being, and disease-specific clinical outcomes;
- Pooling outcome data on a massive scale;
- Analyzing and disseminating outcomes, in relation to the interventions used, to appropriate decision makers and stakeholders.

Ellwood's framework for OM was published in response to a new emphasis in the mid-1980s on healthcare costs in relation to service quality and was the first to provide context for use of what were then called "best practices" (Wojner, 2001). Nursing case management also emerged in the late 1980s in response to a focus on healthcare efficiency as key to controlling healthcare costs and improving quality. Case management used methods that first surfaced in psychiatric social work (Wojner, 1997b). Although these methods sharpened the focus on process efficiency, which continues to be significant today, they did little to promote the use of evidence-based interventions and failed to detail measurement of health outcomes.

In 1997, the Health Outcomes Institute's OM model (Figure 10.1) was the first to take the Ellwood framework and build in actual steps to guide measurement of the impact of new interventions on improving healthcare outcomes (Wojner, 1997a). The model includes four phases:

- *Phase 1:* Definition of outcome measures, along with contributing structure (e.g., infrastructure of the organization, technology) and **process measures** (what is done and how it is done), and construction of a database to capture targeted variables. Measurement of baseline performance allows improvement to be clearly identified in relation to a shift in practice.

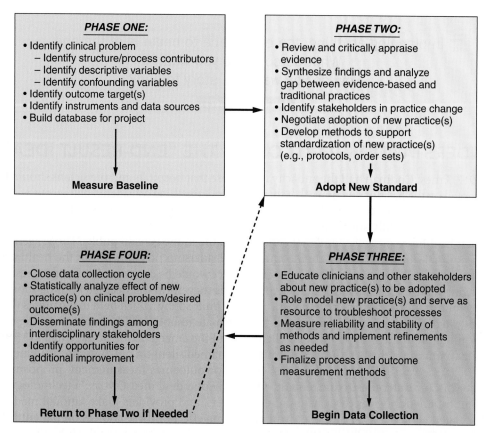

Figure 10.1: Outcomes management model. (© Health Outcomes Institute, Inc.)

- *Phase 2:* Contrasting and comparing traditional practice methods with those identified in the literature as best practices, interdisciplinary negotiation, adoption of new evidence-based initiatives, and construction of structured care methods (e.g., order sets, protocols) to ensure practice standardization for the purpose of improved outcomes. Emphasis is placed on interdisciplinary team engagement to encourage acceptance of new practice methods.
- *Phase 3:* Implementation of new evidence-based initiatives. This step involves role modeling and teaching new practices, making clear interdisciplinary expectations for use of newly adopted practices, determining the stability and reliability of new practices to ensure uniform use, and measuring outcome targets.
- *Phase 4:* Analysis of process and outcome targets in relation to newly adopted evidence-based initiatives. The focus is on interdisciplinary evaluation and dialogue about the findings achieved, including the ability to generate new research questions or hypotheses for testing, ultimately driving refinement of standardized processes (Wojner, 1997a).

The Health Outcomes Institute's OM model provided a road map for transdisciplinary evaluation of care, causing practitioners to define outcome targets, establish measurement methods, identify practices supported by evidence, educate and train healthcare providers in the use of these methods, and subsequently measure the impact associated with implementation of new interventions on healthcare quality (Wojner, 2001).

QUANTIFYING THE IMPACT OF INTERVENTIONS: OUTCOMES MEASUREMENT FOR OUTCOME MANAGEMENT

The process of measuring and managing health outcomes is inherent to both OM and EBPI, promoting clinical decision making by understanding the success or failure of the implementation of an evidence-based initiative. When substandard results are achieved, new EBPs should be tested in an attempt to improve outcome targets (Ellwood, 1988; Wojner, 2001).

Attitudes and beliefs that clinicians attach to traditional practices often make changing practice difficult. However, practice outcomes are a powerful change promoter. For example, by using internal evidence to make substandard results from traditional practice widely known within the healthcare setting, providers are well positioned to negotiate changes that aim to standardize use of new evidence-based best practices. Without making clear the results/outcomes of their care, providers are unlikely to successfully promote change and continuously improve performance.

In the current healthcare system, significant pressure has been placed on healthcare providers to implement practices associated with the highest quality outcomes, especially with the advent of the **value-based purchasing (VBP)** program for U.S. hospitals (U.S. Department of Health & Human Services, 2011b). VBP evaluates hospital performance measures annually and ties performance to financial incentives (Brooks, 2016). VBP scores are calculated in different domains; the number of domains and associated quality measures, as well as how each domain is weighted, varies from year to year based on emerging priorities in healthcare (Brooks, 2016). At the time of this writing, four domains exist—*clinical care process and outcomes; safety; patient experience of care; and efficiency*. Reimbursement is based on performance results, and a total performance score is calculated by a mathematical formula (Brooks, 2016). Additionally, numerous measures exist today, with more under development each year. The measure development journey often begins with the testing and refinement of proposed process or outcome metrics by a sponsoring professional or scientific organization, such as the American Heart Association or the American Association of Neurology. Measures must be supported by evidence demonstrating that proposed measures meet the following criteria:

- The measure is important (the measure is impactful, and an opportunity exists for improvement);
- The measure is scientifically acceptable (the measure is **valid** and **reliable**);
- The measure is feasible (the required data for the measure are available, preferably in an electronic format with consistent **taxonomy**);
- The measure is usable (the intended audience [payers, patients, providers, policymakers] can understand the data and use them to make healthcare decisions; National Quality Forum, 2017).

Measures ready for submission are brought forward for review and ultimately endorsement by the National Quality Forum (NQF), and endorsed measures are then adopted into the Centers for Medicare and Medicaid Services (CMS) core measure dataset for VBP that now spans hospital to outpatient care.

Measures are often categorized into Donabedian (1980) groupings. As mentioned previously, **outcome measures** are those that capture "results." Although the intention of an outcome measure is to understand how healthcare processes affect patient results (IHI, 2017b), the contribution of inherent patient and environmental factors must be considered (Wojner, 2001). Examples of outcome measures include disease severity, functional status, mortality, quality of life, complication incidence, readmissions, and personal healthcare costs. Process measures allow us to quantify the methods used to provide care and to determine fidelity in use of standardized care. Most measures in use today, including those in the VBP program, are classified as process measures, with the aim of determining the degree of standardization/uniformity of care. Examples of process measures include the following: time for delivery of reperfusion treatment in patients with vascular emergencies such as acute ischemic stroke and acute myocardial infarction; administration of anticoagulation to prevent venous thromboembolism; providing smoking cessation counseling; completing focused patient/family teaching; measurement and documentation of ejection fraction in patients with heart failure; and bundled measures such as for sepsis (within 3 hours, measure lactate, collect blood cultures before administration of antibiotics, administer broad-spectrum antibiotic, and administer 30 mL/kg of crystalloid for hypotension or lactate greater than 4 mmol/L). **Structure measures** refer to those that capture components such as manpower, use of a specific specialty unit for patient management, and the availability of technology or highly specialized services. Lastly, the IHI (2017b) classified "unanticipated findings" that arise during new practice testing as **balancing measures** that are useful to account for so that approaches to implementation can be tweaked and improved upon.

Healthcare organizations possess a virtual "treasure trove" of internal data generated by multiple disciplines, often housed in numerous disparate and disconnected systems. For example, data are generated during the course of caring for patients, as a result of tests or treatments, and by billing and financial systems. However, healthcare providers may have limited knowledge of how to access or how to interpret the data to improve their services. As transparency and VBP pressures have grown, knowledge of how to access and use data has become paramount. The following are examples of available data:

- Use of specific medications
- Timing of antibiotics
- Specific patient education
- Targeted discharge instructions

In addition, data on the following outcomes are also collected:

- Fall rates
- Catheter-related infections
- Urinary tract infections
- Pressure ulcer rates and stage progression

Collection of individual process and outcome data is time consuming and expensive. Therefore, use of internal evidence from existing data sources is essential.

> "
> Uncontrolled variation is the enemy of quality.
>
> **EDWARD DEMING**

Sources of Internal Evidence

Internal evidence sources include data from the quality management, finance, and human resource departments; clinical systems; administration; and **electronic health records (EHRs)**. Selected sources and examples of internal evidence discussed in the following sections are not intended to be exhaustive, because there may be data sources in other departments and systems within an organization.

Quality Management

In most organizations, quality management departments house data generated from incident reports, which may include falls, sentinel events (i.e., an unexpected event that culminates in death or serious injury), medication errors, and near misses (i.e., an event that could have resulted in harm but was corrected prior to it occurring). These types of data may be examined for trends related to types, locations, or other factors associated with care process errors, or they may be correlated with structural indicators such as staffing patterns (e.g., number of nurses scheduled to work). Other types of data that may be housed in quality management are patient satisfaction results and data collected through chart reviews submitted to regulatory or accreditation bodies.

Finance

Data housed in finance departments are frequently the most robust within an organization. Many of the data elements found within financial systems are generated by billing and registration systems and are used for billing purposes. Examples of these types of data are charges for tests, medications, equipment or supplies, patient days, **readmission rates**, and patient **demographics** such as name, age, ethnicity, gender, and nursing unit. Other data frequently housed in finance departments are codes for patient diagnosis, including Medicare-Severity Diagnosis Related Groups (MS-DRG) and International Statistical Classification of Diseases and Related Health Problems Version 10 (ICD-10) codes. These types of data are routinely used to measure patient volume, to understand care processes (types of medications used or tests done), or to risk-adjust for patient outcomes. They may also be used to evaluate the incidence of errors within certain patient populations. For example, patients who have certain comorbid conditions, such as cancer or diabetes, may have a higher incidence of hospital-acquired infections. Evaluation of these data would assist in determining the severity of this association.

Human Resources

Data housed in human resource departments generally include those generated from employee and payroll systems. Data generated by employee systems include turnover and staff education levels. Frequently, if available, staff education levels reflect those at the time of hire and therefore may not reflect the current position. Data available from payroll systems include hours by pay category or labor category and contract labor use. In some organizations, contract labor use and expense may be housed in financial systems used for expense reporting. Hours by labor category may be used to calculate **provider skill mix**. Hours by pay category may be used to calculate staffing.

Clinical Systems

Clinical systems are data collection and management mechanisms that can store many kinds of data. For example, these systems may house test results such as laboratory tests or point-of-care tests. They may also house pharmacy data such as numbers of doses of a medication or types of medications, which may be used to evaluate care process compliance or evaluate relationships among different medications and patient outcomes. In some organizations, the clinical system is the source of data for reporting outcomes in integrated reviews, such as dashboards, which are discussed in detail later in this chapter.

Administration

Administrative departments, such as hospital administration, may provide data related to patient complaints about care and services. Such data may be in the form of a call log or table containing information about the source, type, location, and resolution of complaints. Administrative outcomes may include data on patients' perspectives on hospital care collected through mandated surveys such as the **Hospital Consumer Assessment of Healthcare Providers and Systems (HCAHPS)**.

Electronic Health Records

Since 2014, what is called meaningful use of EHRs has been required for all providers of healthcare—both public and private. Meaningful use refers to using data from the EHRs to improve healthcare quality and outcomes. Within EHRs, the numbers and types of internal data available for use in evaluating impact are vast. Data may include patient-level information, such as vital signs and weights, non–charge-generating clinical interventions (e.g., indwelling urinary catheter use) or essentially any data element captured through documentation of clinical care.

One caveat related to collection of data from EHRs is that data aggregation requires standardization of language in order to collect the entire group of incidences of a particular intervention, care process, or event. Many data abstracting queries (i.e., requesting information from the EHR) use a process similar to searching for articles through an electronic database. Some searches return articles based on the precise term or terms used for the search, resulting in missing articles filed in the database under synonyms of the search term. Searching an EHR in some systems may work the same way. Events or care processes documented using a synonym for the search term may not be included in the query results.

BRINGING EBPI AND OUTCOMES MEASUREMENT TO LIFE: THE SCIENCE OF IMPROVEMENT

Several approaches to QI such as *Six Sigma* and *Lean* have been used in a variety of industrial settings and have their foundation in Deming's theory of "profound knowledge," which emerged in the 1950s (Bisognano, Cherouny, & Gullo, 2014; Haughom, 2016). Associates in Process Improvement (API), in collaboration with the Institute for Healthcare Improvement (IHI), used Deming's theory to develop an approach to improve healthcare that incorporates systems thinking, human psychology, knowledge formation, and understanding variation, known as the **science of improvement** (see Box 10.1 for detailed definition) (Associates in Process Improvement, 2017; IHI, 2017c).

The **Model for Improvement** emerged from this work, providing a systematic approach to accelerate the pace of improvement within the healthcare system (IHI, 2017d), with the intent to develop, test, implement, and spread changes that result in improved outcomes. Using rapid-cycle tests of change, a QI team is positioned to plan a practice change on a small scale, try the change, observe the results/outcomes in real time, and act upon what is learned so that when further change is needed, they are armed with the knowledge of where, how, and when to implement a new EBP (Bisognano et al., 2014, p. 811; IHI, 2017a; Parry, 2014). Fundamental to the use of the Model for Improvement is the need for OM to determine the results of EBPI initiatives (Haughom, 2016).

Using the Model for Improvement

Box 10.2 provides an exemplar of the Model for Improvement in action. Selection of a strong team of individuals is crucial for the success of any type of change project. The team must consist of individuals from varying roles and disciplines with the knowledge, skills, and commitment to facilitate organizational change (IHI, 2017d). Chapter 14 details team formation.

BOX 10.1 *The Science of Improvement*

"The **science of improvement** is an applied science that emphasizes innovation, rapid-cycle testing in the field, and spread in order to generate learning about what changes, in which contexts, produce improvements. It is characterized by the combination of expert subject knowledge with improvement methods and tools. It is multidisciplinary—drawing on clinical science, systems theory, psychology, statistics, and other fields" (IHI, 2017a).

| BOX 10.2 | *An Exemplar of a Model for Improvement* |

The following exemplar demonstrates how an interdisciplinary team improved patient outcomes on an acute pediatric care unit, guided by the Model for Improvement (Tucker, Brewer, Baker, Demeritt, & Vossmeyer, 2009).

What Are We Trying to Accomplish?

A team of nurses, physicians, and interdisciplinary staff on an acute pediatric medical unit concerned about the frequency of codes occurring outside the PICU came together to form a CSI team. Baseline data from the QI department revealed that a code occurred on average every 88 days on their unit. The pediatric medical center had recently implemented a MRT, but this did not reduce the number of codes on the unit during the corresponding year. Causative factors considered by the CSI team included whether

- bedside nurses knew how to recognize early clinical deterioration so that they could call the MRT in a timely manner or
- bedside nurses knew to communicate important clinical changes to the healthcare team.

The medical director presented a study using an objective tool called the PEWS and suggested, as an intervention, teaching the bedside nurses how to use the tool on the unit.

How Will We Know That a Change Is an Improvement?

The CSI team developed an operational definition of a "preventable code" as "patients who had shown signs of deterioration prior to the initiation of chest compressions and bag valve mask ventilation outside the PICU." The outcomes targeted for the project were the number of preventable codes and the number of calendar days since the previous MRT preventable code. The CSI team decided to test the project initially on one 24-bed acute pediatric medical unit.

Establishing a Data Collection Plan

The CSI team determined that the data on preventable codes and MRT performance were already routinely collected by the QI department; however, to ensure the data accurately reflected the performance of the intervention on the intended population of patients, the CSI team would review cases to determine they were indeed preventable once data collection commenced. Once the PEWS had been fully implemented, data would be collected over a 36-month period in 12-month intervals.

What Change Can We Make That Will Result in Improvement?

The suggested intervention was the use of the PEWS tool as an objective method to determine clinical deterioration. The CSI team debated whether to "just do it" and test the PEWS or whether to formulate a PICOT (patient population, intervention or *issue* of interest, comparison intervention or group, outcome, and time frame) question and then search/critically appraise the literature to determine the best method to reduce preventable codes in pediatric patients outside the PICU. Given the emerging evidence regarding early Pediatric warning mechanisms, a decision was made to try the PDSA process using the PEWS, thus establishing the best process for implementing this intervention in their organization. The Plan (P) was to teach and implement the PEWS tool by the bedside nurses as a means for objective assessment of deterioration in patients' conditions. Three nurses were chosen to roll out the use

(continued)

BOX
10.2 — *An Exemplar of a Model for Improvement* **(continued)**

of the PEWS tool for their patients in the Do (D) phase. These nurses documented the score in the EHR and each nurse also placed a colored dot that corresponded with the patient's room number on a dry erase board located on the unit. The nurses then used a decision making algorithm to support the determination of the next steps in each patient's plan of care. At the end of the shift, the three nurses huddled (Study [S] phase) with the CSI team members to discuss the process, what they have learned, and what action had been taken based on the PEWS findings. Initial huddles showed that there was a need to involve pediatric medical residents in the use of the PEWS tools. So the team included physicians-in-training in their next round of education and engaged a resident to join the CSI team. Over the next several months, the PEWS intervention was fully implemented with more and more staff fully integrated into the process. Additional refinements included adding an MRT trigger into the decision algorithm and regular reporting of "days between codes" to unit staff, patients, and families.

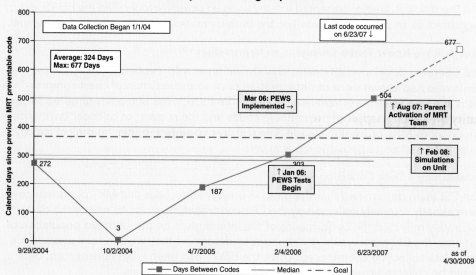

Figure 10.2: Example run chart from PEWS project.

Spreading the Change

After using the PEWS tool on the unit for 15 months, the CSI team decided to share their findings at a hospital grand rounds presentation and was proud to report that the average number of days between codes had increased to 259 days from the original 88 days. This led to hospital leadership spreading use of the PEWS to other units throughout the organization.

CSI, clinical systems improvement; EHR, electronic health record; MRT, medical response team; PEWS, pediatric early warning score; PICU, pediatric intensive care unit; QI, quality improvement.

To implement the Model for Improvement, team members must answer three guiding questions:

1. What are we trying to accomplish?
2. How will we know that a change is an improvement?
3. What change can we make that will result in improvement? (IHI, 2017b)

To guide their work, the team should develop an **aim statement** to ensure clarity of direction (Crowl, Sharma, Sorge, & Sorensen, 2015; IHI, 2017e). A well-written aim statement should be *time specific, measurable,* and define the *specific* population of patients affected. For example, the following aim statement was used to guide the work showcased in Box 10.2: *"To reduce codes outside the Pediatric Intensive Care Unit (PICU) to 0 within 12 months."* Teams may also want to develop a **key driver diagram** to assist with initial planning by illustrating the pathway from development of the aim statement to achievement of the outcome. The diagram links goals (aim) with factors (primary drivers) and interventions (secondary drivers), providing a method to ensure inclusion of key steps and stakeholders in the process (Bennett & Provost, 2015).

> ❝
>
> Quality is never an accident; it is always the result of high intention, sincere effort, intelligent direction and skillful execution; it represents the wise choice of many alternatives.
>
> WILLIAM A. FOSTER

Internal evidence plays a pivotal role in answering these questions, yet clinicians often struggle to obtain access to these data within their organizations. Barriers to accessing needed data are common and may be driven by differences in how clinicians describe what they need and why the data are important, or often concerns about personal health information security and even inappropriate sharing of findings with competitors. Additionally, the ability to make sense of these internal data requires an a priori understanding of the level of different variables and the anticipated analysis that needs to be executed. For example, if the team's intent were to improve glucose control in an effort to improve neurologic outcomes after stroke, patient-specific data based on a primary admitting ICD-10 code for stroke would be needed, such as medical record numbers, names, nursing units, both point-of-care and laboratory glucose results collected at specific dates/times, admitting physician, secondary diagnosis of diabetes, and a measure of stroke severity such as the NIH Stroke Scale. These data elements may be generated and housed in financial, clinical, and EHR systems in an organization. Getting these data in an integrated report may require someone with specialized skills to write a query that draws data from different databases, *if* an organization has a query system to achieve this kind of integration, and once received a skilled statistician would help understand baseline performance.

Note how this process of obtaining and using internal evidence ties not only to the Model for Improvement, but also to the OM model and PDSA, ensuring that a *measurable starting point* is set from which to launch improvement initiatives. Being clear about what data are needed from the outset will help avoid repeated requests for additional data elements needed to complete the analysis and will facilitate the timely acquisition of data, often a challenging process. Generally, those individuals within an organization with report writing skills and access to the necessary databases are few in number and in high demand. As with any person in high demand, limited time is available to meet requests that are beyond normal workload requirements. Finding someone within the organization willing to mentor staff members who are novices at using internal evidence will minimize "forgotten" or unrecognized data needs, avoid repeated requests, foster relationships with database owners, and may speed up the turnaround time for data requests.

Asking for data in a usable format is also important. When asking for a report, always inquire whether the data are available in an electronic format. Many systems can run queries that will download data in a text file or in a format that can be opened and manipulated in spreadsheet software, such as Excel. Doing so can eliminate hours of data entry, which is necessary to convert a paper report of results into an analyzable format. Electronic formatted data also avoid potential data entry errors that can occur when entering data from a paper report to data analysis software (e.g., Excel or SPSS). Before requesting data analysis, carefully consider the data format that will require the least amount of manipulation (e.g., entry from paper) and cleaning (e.g., addressing missing information) to prepare for analysis. Once data have been prepared for analysis, statistical tests may be run using spreadsheet software, or the data file can be easily transferred to statistics software for further analysis.

Incremental Testing to Determine Impact and Next Improvement Steps

Once the team's mission is clear and a baseline performance point has been established, the testing phase can begin. Using either the OM model or the PDSA approach, tests of change can be undertaken in repetitive cycles, with each new test building on what was learned in the previous test. When limited external evidence exists to support a practice change, the cycle can focus on small, incremental changes using a "let's see what happens" approach. However, when a solid evidence base exists to support immediate adoption and testing of an intervention, repeated cycles may shift their focus to examining a graduated approach to implementation, whereby select pieces of a new process are added slowly over time so as not to overwhelm clinicians. In both cases, when measurable improvement occurs, testing spreads to the larger system until the practice is embedded throughout the entire service or organization (IHI, 2017f).

Data required to measure the impact of evidence-based interventions on specified outcomes may not be found in preexisting sources. Therefore, it is important to discuss collection and measurement of data. By recognizing data that you may never have access to, you are also able to acknowledge the limitations of your findings, which is key to your preparation and presentation of results. If data cannot be extracted from a preexisting data source, the method of data collection may be the most important strategy to consider. Gathering meaningful data in an efficient manner takes forethought, ingenuity, and familiarity with how data are best collected and the importance of measurement. Consideration of which patient characteristics and contextual elements might affect the outcome target can increase the likelihood of collecting valid (i.e., unbiased) data. For example, if an evidence-based oral care program were initiated to reduce the incidence of ventilator-associated pneumonia (VAP), it would not be adequate to collect data solely on the frequency of oral care delivery and the VAP rate. Other factors, such as patient severity, preexisting pulmonary disease, or mode of suctioning (data that may not exist in the EHR), need to be measured because they may influence patients' risk for development of VAP. Additionally, collection of data by those involved in the delivery of care can be tricky because it may introduce an element of bias. As described in Phase 3 of the Health Outcomes Institute's OM model, using methods that capture the stability of processes, such as control charts, can assist in ensuring that data are collected uniformly, resulting in accurate data (Wojner, 2001).

> **"**
> One accurate measurement is worth a thousand expert opinions.
> **GRACE HOPPER**

Measurement Accuracy: Establishing Validity and Reliability

Measurement instruments, whether developed in practice or through research, should be valid and reliable so that users will be confident about the accuracy of data when collected.

Validity

Validity indicates that the measure or instrument actually measures what it is supposed to measure. For example, if you choose a valid instrument designed to measure fear, it should truly measure fear and not anxiety. There are several types of validity. For our purposes, we focus on content validity, which is often reflected through an expert review of the instrument. Experts indicate whether or not they view the questions or items on the instrument as measuring the construct. For example, if a practice-developed instrument was said to measure satisfaction with the Situation-Background-Assessment-Recommendation (SBAR) communication technique, a group of experts in verbal handoffs between patients would review the instrument to indicate whether the items or questions on the measure did reflect satisfaction with SBAR.

Reliability

Reliability means that an instrument will measure the construct consistently every time it is used. Often, this is indicated through a statistic called Cronbach's alpha. A Cronbach's alpha of 0.80 or greater indicates an instrument that should perform reliably each time it is used. There are many other elements of both validity and reliability of measures that go beyond the scope of this chapter. Clinicians may be tempted to develop their own instrument; however, that is ill-advised unless they have established that valid and reliable measures do not exist. If practice-developed instruments are used, it is important to take the time to establish content validity and assess reliability. Given that whole books are dedicated to understanding measurement, including establishing validity and reliability, it would be wise for clinicians who are developing measures to use experts in the field to facilitate accurate measurement.

Understanding Results: Making Sense of the Data

How data are analyzed is driven by the level of data available. In larger organizations, there may be a department or portions of a department that take on this role. However, not all organizations have such resources, so we will briefly discuss data analysis. Further information on data analysis may be found in other resources that focus on this topic.

There are two basic types of data, categorical and numeric. **Categorical variables** are those that are grouped due to a defined characteristic, such as gender, presence or absence of a disease, or possession of particular risk factors. Numbers are commonly used to label categorical data, but these numbers have no meaning and only facilitate grouping of cases into like data bundles. Likert scales, which allow ranking of data (e.g., not at all, somewhat, moderately so, very much so), are also categorical in nature in that they group data by ranks. However, data analysts often consider these types of scales numerical. Generally, the statistical methods used to analyze categorical data are **frequencies** (Kellar & Kelvin, 2013).

Numeric data potentially have an infinite number of possible values, such as measures for height, weight, mean arterial pressure, and heart rate. Unlike categorical data, the mathematical intervals that separate numeric data are equal. For example, the interval between the numbers 20 and 21 is equal to the interval between 21 and 22, namely 1.

Levels of Data

Categorical and numeric data fall within four possible levels of measurement: nominal, ordinal, interval, and ratio. When defining the outcomes to be measured, clinicians must carefully consider the instruments to measure them so that they are most accurately reflected. For example, if a project were conducted to evaluate an evidence-based weight loss strategy, the outcome of weight loss could be measured at the categorical–nominal level (e.g., "body mass index [BMI] < 25," "BMI 25–29," "BMI 30–34," "BMI 35–39," and "BMI ≥ 40") or at the ratio level by using actual weight loss (e.g., in pounds or kilograms). Using pounds or kilograms (i.e., ratio level) would enable those evaluating the outcome to use more powerful statistical analyses. Measurement of the impact of a practice change on outcomes denotes the need to use statistical analyses that detect a difference in the outcome target that can be attributed to the evidence-based intervention. Although it is beyond the scope of this chapter to provide detailed instruction on selection and use of different forms of statistical analyses, the information presented here is meant to provide some considerations for the context of outcome measurement and analysis. Collaborating with a biostatistician is a wise decision for clinicians who are analyzing more than outcome frequencies or means. The purpose of the project and the level of the data drive the selection of the statistical methods that will be used to measure the impact of the practice change. The clinical issues that would fit within each level of measurement are discussed in the following sections.

Nominal Level Data

Data measured at the nominal level are the least sophisticated and lowest form of measurement. Nominal measurement scales assign numbers to unique categories of data, but these numbers have no meaning other than to label a group. Scales that describe the quality of a symptom by some descriptive format are nominal. For example, a nominal measure of the quality of pain may include categories such as "throbbing," "stabbing," "continuous," "intermittent," "burning," "dull," "sharp," "aching," "stinging," or "burning" (McHugh, 2003).

Ordinal-Level Data

Ordinal measures use categorical data as well. Numbers assigned to categories in ordinal measures enable ranking from lowest to highest so that the magnitude of the variable can be captured. However, it is important to note that although numbers are assigned to enable sorting of findings by rank, the absolute difference in each level on an ordinal scale does not possess an equal or "true" mathematical difference in the values. Likert scales provide clinicians with ordinal-level data using selections such as "very dissatisfied," "dissatisfied," "neither dissatisfied nor satisfied," "satisfied," and "very satisfied." Clearly, each level of progression from very dissatisfied to very satisfied describes higher satisfaction, but "very satisfied" could not be described as four times more satisfied than "very dissatisfied." When developing instruments, researchers typically use four or five categories from which to rank the variable of interest on a Likert scale.

Interval and Ratio-Level Data

Interval measures are the next highest level of measurement and are purely derived from numeric data with equal and consistent mathematical values separating each discrete measurement point. Although ratio-level data possess this same characteristic, the difference between these two levels of measurement is that **interval data** do not possess an absolute zero point. The best examples of interval-level data are temperature measures derived from the Fahrenheit scale that assigns 32° instead of zero as the point where water freezes.

Measures derived from a ruler and temperatures measured on the Centigrade scale are both examples of ratio-level data. Data measured at the interval and ratio levels allow virtually all types of algebraic transformations, and therefore, the greatest number of statistical options can be applied (Kellar & Kelvin, 2013). Given the significant amount of numeric variables used routinely in healthcare settings, many outcome targets—for example, those associated with objective, quantitative physiologic data—are defined at the interval or ratio level (e.g., weight, mean arterial pressure, hemoglobin A_{1c}).

Reporting Outcomes to Key Stakeholders

Undertaking the implementation of new interventions and, ultimately, the measurement of their impact requires significant work on the part of the interdisciplinary healthcare team. It is paramount that all parties involved with this process (i.e., both active and passive **key stakeholders**) be afforded an opportunity to understand the results achieved, whether positive or negative. Project coordinators need to consider which reporting methods will make results easily understood by all stakeholders to enhance dissemination and further knowledge development. Once internal data have been analyzed, reports should be generated to display results using whatever means best makes clear what has occurred, what contributed to it, and what needs to happen next, thereby stimulating ownership among all stakeholders to continue the improvement journey. Below we present scorecards and dashboards along with **run charts** and bar graphs as methods to present data in an easily interpretable manner. A survey of 586 hospital leaders found that 81% used scorecards or dashboards for tracking outcome indicators of performance and quality (Gordon & Richardson, 2012).

Scorecards

Balanced scorecards are used to show how indicators from different areas may relate to each other. For example, relationships among financial performance indicators (e.g., hours per patient day) can be examined against clinical and safety indicators, such as patient falls or infection rates. Systematically evaluating performance from a balanced perspective allows clinicians and leaders to evaluate both intended and unintended consequences of practice change. For example, if an interdisciplinary team in the emergency department (ED) implemented an evidence-based care management program that resulted in patients who normally were admitted to the hospital for observation being discharged to home with home care, it would be prudent to ensure that the new program did not lead to higher hospital readmission rates for those patients (collection of balancing measures), while at the same time evaluating whether length of stay within the ED was reduced and patient satisfaction maintained or improved. Figure 10.3 provides an example of indicators that may be used in a balanced scorecard.

Scorecard

Operational	Quality	Satisfaction
• Turnover • Vacancy rate • Readmission rate • Total average length of stay • Case mix index • Hours per patient day • Contract labor use • Mean wait time in ED	• Patient falls • Pressure ulcer rate • Infection rate • Compliance with evidence-based care • Mean glucose value	• Patient satisfaction • Staff satisfaction score • Medical staff satisfaction • Patient complaint rate

Figure 10.3: Balanced scorecard indicators. ED, emergency department.

Scorecard indicators can include (a) identifiers of high-level strategic initiatives; (b) objectives linked to the organizational strategic plan, making the outcomes relevant across the organization; (c) the measures or metrics for each outcome; and (d) indicators of how things are going, usually in relation to given expectations or standards, often using colors. Including these components in the scorecard integrates the performance demonstrated by internal evidence with the organization's strategic plan and mission.

Using color to enhance interpretation of indicators is extremely helpful for viewing at a glance the impact of practice on outcomes. Many organizations use a red/yellow/green color scheme, where red generally indicates performance below and green indicates performance at or above goal or target. Yellow indicates performance within a certain percentage or standard deviation of a target, but not significantly below or above the identified markers. Using font or background color to distinguish particular outcomes sets them apart from surrounding values. Making the scorecard easy to read and interesting to look at aids in quick overall communication of current performance. Typically, scorecards are used to indicate performance over a single year. Months or quarters may be used as reporting intervals. The decision regarding which to use is often based on frequency of data collection and preference (see Figure 10.3).

Dashboards

Dashboards are graphic displays of information that are often used at the unit level to compare performance indicators for the population being cared for on that unit. As with scorecards, color-coding enables clear displays of performance indicators of excellence and deficiencies. The same red/yellow/green color scheme can be used for dashboards to achieve the same at-a-glance overview of performance (Modern Healthcare, 2006).

Dashboards can help healthcare providers see the direct impact on performance from the care they provided. Dematteis and Werstler (2006) indicated that the use of a unit dashboard encourages active participation of staff nurses in the continued improvement of quality because they could see the results of their contributions to patient care. Performance dashboards can help build in point-of-care providers the confidence that they are indeed making a difference in the outcomes of the patients for whom they care as they implement EBP.

Run Charts

Since improvement occurs over time, tracking data in real time can be a powerful aspect of QI monitoring. Run charts are line charts that display data change over time (Evergreen, 2017; Wexler, Shaffer, & Cotgreave, 2017). To develop a run chart, first determine the time to be displayed along the x-axis (horizontal line). Along the y-axis (vertical line), the values for the measure of interest are plotted at the selected time intervals. A goal line can also be added to show how close to attainment the initiative is over time. Box 10.2 contains an example of a run chart (see Figure 10.2).

Bar Graphs

Histograms and Pareto charts are examples of bar graphs that are easily interpreted by personnel of all backgrounds. A **histogram** is a bar chart that is used to display the distribution of continuous data (Evergreen, 2017; Wexler et al., 2017). **Pareto charts** are bar graphs that show the distribution of categorical data arranged in descending order to show the effect of each contributing factor (50 minutes.com, 2017; Wexler et al., 2017). The left y-axis (vertical) presents the frequency of occurrences or a chosen unit of measure. The right y-axis (vertical) shows the cumulative percentage of occurrences. The Pareto principle, simply stated, suggests that 80% of outcomes or results can be attributed to 20% of the inputs; however, it is important to point out that the numbers 80/20 are not written in stone. Instead, Pareto really means that a large part of the results is likely caused by a small part of the input—not all contributing factors. When used in QI, the Pareto principle would suggest that those intent on improving a targeted outcome will get the most "bang for their bucks" by focusing on a small number of factors that are producing the worst defects in care (50 minutes.com, 2017).

Research Designs for Comparing Traditional Practice With New Interventions

Sometimes, practitioners choose to use more formal, rigorous methods to compare differences between traditional and new practices, by conducting outcomes research with the use of either a quasi-experimental or an experimental approach (see Chapter 21 on generating evidence). There are both strengths and limitations associated with these methods, but each starts with ensuring that the study is adequately powered to find a difference when a true difference does exist.

An **effect size** (i.e., the extent of an intervention's impact on an outcome), calculated by subtracting the mean outcome score of one group from the mean outcome score of the other group and dividing by the average standard deviation, is often calculated when comparing a new intervention with traditional practice. It is typically used with the anticipated power (usually 0.80) and the probability (i.e., alpha) (usually $p = 0.05$) to determine exactly how many subjects are required in each study arm to find a difference in the outcome that is caused by the intervention. Although it may be tempting to simply conduct a small quality study that describes the performance of an existing practice in relation to a new intervention, these studies may be less than persuasive for slow adopters to embrace new practices. Additionally, the **Health Insurance Portability and Accountability Act (HIPAA) regulations** call for ethics review boards' approval (i.e., human subject or **institutional review board [IRB]** approval of all studies involving personal health information [PHI]), and in many cases initiation of informed consent. It is also important to share the knowledge learned from studies of this nature, and dissemination of findings requires IRB approval prior to the beginning of the study. Because of these factors, there can be confusion about whether implementation of evidence is considered research. Chapter 4 contains more information on differences between EBQI and research. Either approach requires IRB review to assure participant safety and to enable the demonstration of how effective a given intervention is on outcomes within a particular setting. See Chapter 21 for information about the various types of experimental research designs capable of generating external evidence.

Conclusion

Demonstrating that practice change has indeed brought about improved outcomes is imperative in this era of healthcare when many evidence-based initiatives have been endorsed by powerful professional healthcare organizations, as well as payers, as acceptable methods to use in the treatment of specific health conditions. With steadily emerging trends, such as VBP supported by use of standardized evidence-based initiatives, it is important that evaluation of outcomes be conducted in a valid and reliable manner. Outcomes must be accessible to healthcare leadership as well as to the point-of-care providers to increase ownership and encourage engagement in the continuous improvement of patient, provider, system, and community services. Using the principles of OM and EBPI described in this chapter will enable healthcare providers to improve healthcare practice for years to come.

EBP FAST FACTS

- Measurement of outcomes is essential to determine the impact on healthcare quality, costs, and patient outcomes as a result of EBP changes.
- VBP is a program in which hospitals are paid based on quality, rather than quantity, of care.
- Acceptance of new evidence-based initiatives can be fostered among clinicians through measurement of failed outcomes achieved with traditional practices. Measuring outcomes of practice should be viewed as a powerful change promoter to adopt best practices.
- Internal evidence sources include quality management, finance, and human resource departments; clinical systems; administration; and EHRs.
- Data for evaluation of outcomes are available from multiple sources within healthcare organizations, including finance (billing and coding information), quality management (errors, patient satisfaction), human resources (numbers of staff), clinical systems (laboratory values, medications), administration, and EHR.
- Before requesting data for evaluation of outcomes, it is helpful to consider thoroughly and be clear about what is needed and how it will be analyzed to ensure that all necessary data are requested in the correct format.
- The level of available data (nominal, ordinal, interval, ratio) determines the type of analyses that can be performed.
- Quantifying baseline performance is essential to an understanding of how changes in processes and systems perform comparatively over time.
- Dashboards, scorecards, run charts, and bar graphs are commonly used as methods of sharing performance results with interdisciplinary providers in an easily understandable manner.

WANT TO KNOW MORE?

A variety of resources are available to enhance your learning and understanding of this chapter.

- Visit thePoint® to access:
  - Articles from the AJN EBP Step-By-Step Series
  - Journal articles
  - Checklists for rapid critical appraisal and more!
- Lippincott CoursePoint combines digital text content with video case studies and interactive modules for a fully integrated course solution that works the way you study and learn.

References

50 minutes.com. (2017). *Pareto's principles: Expand your business with the 80/20 rule.* Retrieved from https://www.amazon.com/Paretos-Principle-Expand-your-business/dp/2806269350

Associates in Process Improvement. (2017). *W. Edwards Deming.* Retrieved from http://www.apiweb.org/

Bennett, B., & Provost, L. (2015). What's your theory? Driver diagram serves as tool for building and testing theories for improvement. *Quality Progress, 48,* 36–43.

Bisognano, M., Cherouny, P. H., & Gullo, S. (2014). Applying a science-based method to improve perinatal care. *Obstetrics and Gynecology, 124*(4), 810–814. doi:10.1097/AOG.0000000000000474

Brooks, J. A. (2016). Understanding hospital value-based purchasing. *The American Journal of Nursing, 116*(5), 63–66.

Codman, E. A. (1917). The value of case records in hospitals. *Modern Hospitals, 9,* 426–428.

Codman, E. A. (1934). *The shoulder: Rupture of the supraspinatus tendon and other lesions in or about the subacromial bursa.* Brooklyn, NY: G. Miller.

Crowl, A., Sharma, A., Sorge, L., & Sorensen, T. (2015). Accelerating quality improvement within your organization: Applying the model for improvement. *Journal of the American Pharmacists Association, 55*(4), e364–e376. doi:10.1331/JAPhA.2015.15533

Dematteis, J., & Werstler, J. (2006). Placing ownership for quality in the hands of the staff. *Critical Care Nurse, 26*(2), S38.

Donabedian, A. (1980). *The definition of quality and approaches to its management.* Ann Arbor, MI: Health Administration.

Ellwood, P. M. (1988). Outcomes management: A technology of patient experience. *The New England Journal of Medicine, 318,* 1549–1556.

Evergreen, S. D. H. (2017). *Effective data visualization: The right chart for the right data.* Thousand Oaks, CA: Sage.

Fitzpatrick, J. J. (2016). Distinctions between research, evidence based practice, and quality improvement. *Applied Nursing Research, 29,* 261.

Glasziou, P., Ogrinc, G., & Goodman, S. (2011). Can evidence-based medicine and clinical quality improvement learn from each other? *BMJ Quality and Safety, 20*(1), i13–i17. doi:10.1136/bmjqs.2010.046524

Gordon, J., & Richardson, E. (2012). Continuous improvement using balanced scorecard in healthcare. *American Journal of Health Sciences, 3,* 185–188.

Haughom, J. (2016). *Five Deming principles that help healthcare process improvement.* Health Catalyst. Retrieved from https://www.healthcatalyst.com/wp-content/uploads/2014/11/Five-Deming-Principles-That-Help-Healthcare-Process-Improvement.pdf

Institute for Healthcare Improvement. (2017a). *Science of improvement: How to improve.* Retrieved from http://www.ihi.org/resources/Pages/HowtoImprove/ScienceofImprovementHowtoImprove.aspx

Institute for Healthcare Improvement. (2017b). *Science of improvement: Establishing measures.* Retrieved from http://www.ihi.org/resources/Pages/HowtoImprove/ScienceofImprovementEstablishingMeasures.aspx

Institute for Healthcare Improvement. (2017c). *Science of improvement.* Retrieved from http://www.ihi.org/about/Pages/ScienceofImprovement.aspx

Institute for Healthcare Improvement. (2017d). *Science of improvement: Forming the team.* Retrieved from http://www.ihi.org/resources/Pages/HowtoImprove/ScienceofImprovementFormingtheTeam.aspx

Institute for Healthcare Improvement. (2017e). *Science of improvement: Setting aims.* Retrieved from http://www.ihi.org/resources/Pages/HowtoImprove/ScienceofImprovementSettingAims.aspx

Institute for Healthcare Improvement. (2017f). *How to improve.* Retrieved from http://www.ihi.org/resources/Pages/HowtoImprove/default.aspx

Kellar, S. P., & Kelvin, E. A. (2013). *Munro's statistical methods for health care research* (6th ed.). Philadelphia, PA: Wolters Kluwer Health Lippincott Williams & Wilkins.

Levin, R. F. (2008). EBP by any other name is still a rose. *Research and Theory for Nursing Practice: An International Journal, 22*(1), 7–9. doi:10.1891/0889-7182.22.1.7

Levin, R. F., Keefer, J. M., Marren, J., Vetter, M. J., Lauder, B. & Sobolewski, S. (2010). Evidence-based practice improvement: Merging 2 paradigms. *Journal of Nursing Care Quality, 25*(2), 117–126.

McHugh, M. L. (2003). Descriptive statistics, Part I: Level of measurement. *Journal for Specialists in Pediatric Nursing, 8*(1), 35–37.

Melnyk, B. M., Morrison-Beedy, D., & Moore, S. (2012). Nuts and bolts of designing intervention studies. In B. M. Melnyk & D. Morrison-Beedy (Eds.), *Designing, conducting, analyzing and funding intervention research. A practical guide for success.* New York, NY: Springer Publishing Company.

Modern Healthcare. (2006). Ten best practices for measuring the effectiveness of nonprofit healthcare boards. *Bulletin of the National Center for Healthcare Leadership, 36,* 9–20.

National Quality Forum. (2017). Retrieved from http://www.qualityforum.org/Measuring_Performance/Measuring_Performance.aspx

Parry, G. J. (2014). A brief history of quality improvement. *Journal of Oncology Practice, 10*(3), 196–199.

Shirey, M. R., Hauck, S. L., Embree, J. L., Kinner, T. J., Schaar, G. L., Phillips, L. A., & McCool, I. A. (2011). Showcasing differences between quality improvement, evidence-based practice, and research. *The Journal of Continuing Education in Nursing, 42*(2), 57–68.

Tucker, K. M., Brewer, T. L., Baker, R. B., Demeritt, B., & Vossmeyer M. T. (2009). Prospective evaluation of a pediatric inpatient early warning scoring system. *Journal for Specialists in Pediatric Nursing, 14*(2), 79–85.

U.S. Department of Health & Human Services. (2011a, April). *Quality improvement.* Washington, DC: U.S. Department of Health and Human Services Health Resources and Services Administration.

U.S. Department of Health & Human Services. (2011b, November). *Hospital value-based purchasing program.* Retrieved from http://www.cms.gov/Outreach-and-Education/Medicare-Learning-Network-MLN/MLNProducts/downloads/Hospital_VBPurchasing_Fact_Sheet_ICN907664.pdf

Wexler, S., Shaffer, J., & Cotgreave, A. (2017). *Visualizing your data using real-world business scenarios*. Hoboken, NJ: Wiley.

Wojner, A. W. (1997a). Outcomes management, from theory to practice. *Critical Care Nurse Quarterly, 19*(4), 1–15.

Wojner, A. W. (1997b). Widening the scope: From case management to outcomes management. *Case Manager, 8*(2), 77–82.

Wojner, A. W. (2001). *Outcomes management: Application to clinical practice*. St. Louis, MO: Mosby.

Implementing the Evidence-Based Practice Competencies in Clinical and Academic Settings to Ensure Healthcare Quality and Improved Patient Outcomes

Bernadette Mazurek Melnyk, Lynn Gallagher-Ford, and Cindy Zellefrow

It always seems impossible until it's done.
—Nelson Mandela

EBP Terms to Learn
Competency
Delphi study
Institutional review board

Learning Objectives

After studying this chapter, learners will be able to:

1. Discuss why achievement of the evidence-based practice (EBP) competencies is key to improving healthcare quality and population health outcomes.

2. Describe how leaders can use the EBP competencies in their healthcare organizations.

3. Discuss how the EBP competencies can be integrated into academic programs.

Evidence-based practice (EBP) is instrumental in meeting the quadruple aim in healthcare because it improves healthcare quality and patient outcomes, empowers clinicians, and reduces costs. Yet adoption of EBP among healthcare professionals, including nurses, physical therapists, dentists, social workers, and physicians, remains low throughout the world, with estimates of only one quarter to one third of clinicians consistently taking an EBP approach to care (Bellamy et al., 2013; Galbraith, Ward, & Heneghan, 2017; Melnyk, Fineout-Overholt, Gallagher-Ford, & Kaplan, 2012; Scurlock-Evans, Upton, & Upton, 2014; Skela-Savic, Hvalic-Touzery, & Pesjak, 2017; Straub-Morarend et al., 2016). Clinicians often lack the knowledge and skills they need to implement EBP, especially in the areas of searching for and critically appraising research evidence (Galbraith et al., 2017). However, even when clinicians and academics are skilled in the seven steps of EBP, the cultures of healthcare systems and academic institutions that are steeped in "that's the way we do it here" combined with a lack of infrastructure, resources, and leadership to support EBP often prevent practitioners and faculty from practicing and educating based on the best evidence.

COMPETENCY DEFINED

Competence is defined as "the ability to do something well" (Merriam Webster Dictionary, n.d.). The American Nurses Association (ANA, 2010) defines **competency** as "an expected and measurable level of nursing performance that integrates knowledge, skills, abilities, and judgement, based on established scientific knowledge and expectations for nursing practice" (p. 64). Dunn et al. (2000) contend that competency is "not a skill or task to be done, but characteristics required in order to act effectively in the nursing setting" (p. 341). Competencies are necessary in order to deliver high-quality safe care, especially in an era where the "true number of premature deaths associated with preventable harm to patients is estimated at more than 400,000 per year" (James, 2013) and medical errors are the third leading cause of death in the United States (ANA, 2010; Makary & Daniel, 2016; Melnyk, Gallagher-Ford, Long, & Fineout-Overholt, 2014). Use of competencies also can enhance clinical effectiveness, decrease variability across healthcare systems, and improve education of clinicians by serving as a guide for professional development (Mallidou et al., 2017). A number of health professions have adopted competencies to help ensure quality and safety of care. Currently, there is an increased emphasis on the use and assessment of health professionals' competencies regarding multiple patient care activities in healthcare systems throughout the United States and the world.

The Quality and Safety Education for Nurses (QSEN, 2013) project has established competencies for nursing prelicensure and graduate education to prepare nurses to achieve the knowledge, skills, and attitudes to deliver safe high-quality care. Based on the Institute of Medicine's competency recommendations for healthcare professionals, the QSEN competencies focus on the following practice areas:

- Patient-centered care
- Teamwork and collaboration
- **EBP**
- Quality improvement
- Safety
- Informatics

QSEN defines competency for EBP as the integration of best current evidence with clinical expertise, family preferences, and values for delivery of optimal care (American Association of Colleges of Nursing QSEN Education Consortium, 2012). Stevens (2005) developed EBP competencies for nursing education through a consensus process to support faculty in preparing their students for EBP and to "provide a basis for professional competencies in clinical practice" (p. 8). However, a set of EBP research-based competencies was lacking for practicing registered nurses (RNs) and advanced practice nurses (APNs). Therefore, Melnyk et al. (2014) embarked on a journey to rigorously develop a set of EBP competencies for practicing RNs and APNs with a two-step process, so that healthcare systems could ensure that RNs and APNs deliver the highest quality of evidence-based care.

DEVELOPMENT AND VALIDATION OF THE EBP COMPETENCIES FOR RNs AND APNs

Drs. Bernadette Melnyk and Ellen Fineout-Overholt, who had decades of experience advancing EBP in healthcare systems and academic institutions as well as conducting research in the field of EBP nationally and globally, drafted the first set of EBP competencies for practicing RNs and APNs. A panel of seven national EBP experts from academia and practice then convened to review the drafted competencies. Through a consensus building validation process that consisted of both e-mail exchanges and multiple telephone sessions, the national panel came to a consensus on 13 essential EBP competencies for practicing RNs and 11 additional EBP competencies for APNs (Melnyk, 2017).

Next, after **Institutional Review Board (IRB)** approval was obtained, a national Delphi study was conducted to create the final set of EBP competencies (Melnyk et al., 2014). A **Delphi study** is a method of research that uses experts to arrive at a consensus through two or more structured rounds of a survey. Delphi studies use an iterative multistage process where experts are given feedback from the first round of the survey to consider in the next round of the survey. Most Delphi studies take two to three rounds to achieve a consensus by the experts (Hasson, Keeney, & McKenna, 2000).

Eighty EBP mentors from across the United States who had previously attended an intensive 5-day EBP immersion workshop served as the experts in the Delphi EBP survey. These mentors responded to two questions: (1) whether each competency was necessary for practicing registered professional nurses (or APNs) depending on the item; and (2) whether the competency statement was clearly written (Melnyk et al., 2014).

In round one of the survey, each of the practicing RN and APN competencies reached a consensus in response to the first question about whether the competency was essential. However, four of the competencies for RNs were recommended for rewording. Therefore, those four competencies were rewritten based on the EBP mentors' feedback. In addition, it was recommended that one of those four RN competencies be split into two competencies, which meant that consensus needed to be obtained on these five newly worded RN competencies. A second round of the survey was e-mailed to the 80 EBP mentors who completed the first round; 59 of the original 80 EBP mentors responded to the round two survey, and rated the five reworded competencies for RNs. Total consensus was reached by the EBP mentors on the second round of the survey, which resulted in the final set of 13 EBP competencies for RNs and 11 additional competencies for APNs (Melnyk et al., 2014) (Table 11.1). The EBP competencies were published in 2014.

TABLE 11.1	*EBP Competencies for Practicing Registered Nurses and Advanced Practice Nurses*

EBP Competencies for Practicing Registered Professional Nurses

1. Questions clinical practices to improve the quality of care.
2. Describes clinical problems using internal evidence.*
3. Participates in the formulation of clinical questions using PICOT* format.
4. Searches for external evidence[†] to answer focused clinical questions.
5. Participates in critical appraisal of preappraised evidence (such as clinical practice guidelines, evidence-based policies and procedures, and evidence syntheses).
6. Participates in the critical appraisal of published research studies to determine their strength and applicability to clinical practice.
7. Participates in the evaluation and synthesis of a gathered body of evidence to determine its strength and applicability to clinical practice.
8. Collects practice data (e.g., individual patient data, quality improvement data) systematically as internal evidence for clinical decision making in the care of individuals, groups, and populations.
9. Integrates evidence gathered from external and internal sources to plan EBP changes.
10. Implements practice changes based on evidence, clinical expertise, and patient preferences to improve care processes and patient outcomes.
11. Evaluates outcomes of evidence-based decisions and practice changes for individuals, groups, and populations to determine best practices.
12. Disseminates best practices supported by evidence to improve quality of care and patient outcomes.
13. Participates in strategies to sustain an EBP culture.

(continued)

| TABLE 11.1 | *EBP Competencies for Practicing Registered Nurses and Advanced Practice Nurses* (continued) |

Evidence-Based Practice Competencies for Practicing Advanced Practice Nurses

All competencies of registered professional nurses AND

14. Systematically conducts an exhaustive search for external evidence[‡] to answer clinical questions.
15. Critically appraises relevant preappraised evidence (i.e., clinical guidelines, summaries, synopses, syntheses of relevant external evidence) and primary studies, including evaluation and synthesis.
16. Integrates a body of external evidence from nursing and related fields with internal evidence** in making decisions about patient care.
17. Leads transdisciplinary teams in applying synthesized evidence to initiate clinical decisions and practice changes to improve the health of individuals, groups, and populations.
18. Generates internal evidence through outcomes management and EBP implementation projects for the purpose of integrating best practices.
19. Measures processes and outcomes of evidence-based clinical decisions.
20. Formulates evidence-based policies and procedures.
21. Participates in the generation of external evidence with other healthcare professionals.
22. Mentors others in evidence-based decision making and the EBP process.
23. Implements strategies to sustain an EBP culture.
24. Communicates best evidence to individuals, groups, colleagues, and policy makers.

*Evidence generated internally within a clinical setting, such as patient assessment data, outcomes management, and quality improvement data.

[†]Evidence generated from research.

[‡]Evidence generated from research.

**Evidence generated internally within a clinical setting, such as patient assessment data, outcomes management, and quality improvement data.

*PICOT, Patient population, Intervention or area of interest, Comparison intervention or group, Outcome, Time.

Source: © Melnyk, B. M., Gallagher-Ford, L., Long, L. E., & Fineout-Overholt, E. (2014). The establishment of evidence-based practice competencies for practicing registered nurses and advanced practice nurses in real-world clinical settings: Proficiencies to improve healthcare quality, reliability, patient outcomes, and costs. *Worldviews on Evidence-Based Nursing, 11*(1), 5–15.

IMPLEMENTING THE EBP COMPETENCIES IN CLINICAL SETTINGS

Leaders in healthcare organizations should integrate the EBP competencies into their programs and processes to facilitate high-quality care, improved patient outcomes, and reduced costs. Organizations should clearly state EBP and patient-centered care as part of their vision and their mission. Very importantly, the EBP competencies should be

- presented as an expectation of all clinicians, managers, and leaders in their orientation/onboarding;
- imbedded in clinical job descriptions and performance reviews to support the expectation that meeting the EBP competencies is not an option; it is a requirement of practice (Gallagher-Ford, 2017);
- an expectation for clinicians responsible for development and/or review of clinical policies and procedures, the underpinnings of practice;
- integrated into the role expectations of clinical preceptors to reinforce expectations delineated during onboarding/orientation;

- Included in clinical ladder programs to reflect progressive expectations for clinicians pursuing practice advancement opportunities; it also can be used as an incentive to encourage clinicians to become more skilled in EBP (Melnyk & Gallagher-Ford, 2015).

In the near future, there will continue to be a wide disparity in EBP competency because there is still much variation in how academic programs across the country prepare their students, with many still teaching the rigorous process of *how to conduct research* at the bachelor's and master's levels instead of *how to be proficient in the seven-step EBP process.* Findings from a recent national study with over 2,300 nurses across the United States indicated that although master's prepared nurses reported themselves a bit higher on each of the competencies, nurses with associate, baccalaureate, and master's degrees stated that they were not meeting most of the EBP competencies (see Figure 11.1). Therefore, there is a tremendous need for healthcare systems to provide EBP educational and skills-building sessions to assist clinicians in achieving competency in evidence-based care. Investing in nurses' continuing professional development increases their knowledge, enhances competency, facilitates career development, and improves quality of care, which will help retention (Covell, 2009;

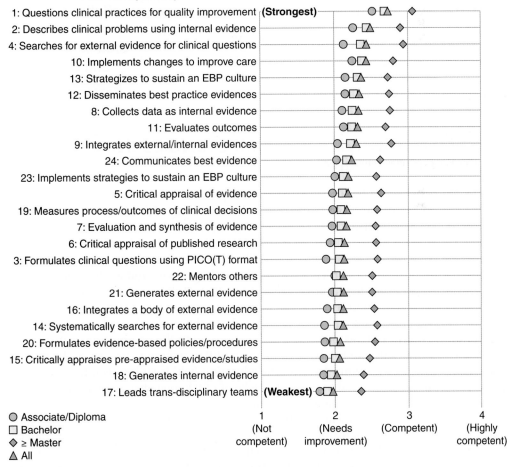

Figure 11.1: Self-reported evidence-based practice (EBP) competency in over 2,300 nurses across the United States in 2017. (From Melnyk, B. M. et al. (2017). The first U.S. study on nurses' evidence-based practice competencies indicates major deficits that threaten healthcare quality, safety, and patient outcomes. *Worldviews on Evidence-Based Nursing, 15:1, 16–25.)*

Wilcock, Janes, & Cambers, 2009). Nurses can rate themselves on each of the EBP competencies using a self-assessment format (see Appendix K). For those who have not yet reached competency, the self-assessment tool allows for the development of an efficient, effective, and targeted plan for strengthening EBP knowledge and skills. Development of a critical mass of EBP mentors, as first described in the Advancing Research and Clinical practice with close Collaboration (ARCC) model, has been demonstrated to be a very effective strategy for working with and engaging point-of-care clinicians in EBP to improve the delivery of care (Melnyk et al., 2018) (see Chapter 14). Because it is well known that appreciation and recognition are key in helping motivate and engage people, an ongoing recognition program should be launched to highlight and recognize those clinicians who achieve all of the EBP competencies (Melnyk, 2016a).

Healthcare leaders, directors, and managers should also be held to meeting the EBP competencies. Unless leaders role model EBP in their own practice decision making, as well as publicly navigate barriers to EBP and provide necessary tools and resources for EBP, including access to electronic databases for searching and a critical mass of EBP mentors, evidence-based care is not likely to thrive. See Chapter 12 for additional leadership strategies to accelerate and sustain EBP. An EBP culture that upholds evidence-based care as the norm is absolutely necessary for EBP to sustain (Melnyk, 2016a). Leaders must also facilitate the development of business plans and calculation of return on investment for EBP practice changes that result in improved outcomes within their system. Demonstrating the cost effectiveness of EBP activities and projects provides critical data (evidence) to obtain resources/support for additional EBP activities and projects in the future.

> **"**
> Culture eats strategy for breakfast, lunch, and dinner!
>
> **PETER DRUCKER**

IMPLEMENTING THE EBP COMPETENCIES IN ACADEMIC SETTINGS

One of the goals of higher education in healthcare is to produce clinicians who are evidence-based practitioners on graduation. To do so, EBP must become a way of thinking rather than a task or a project to be accomplished. This means EBP is applied to decision making surrounding not only patient care issues, but also staff, administrative, and health policy issues in both didactic and clinical courses at all levels. The EBP competencies provide structure to guide EBP integration throughout curricula at both the undergraduate and graduate levels. They should also be used in academic programs to ensure that all clinicians are competent in EBP when they enter practice settings on graduation.

EBP must be integrated and built on throughout the student's academic program; it should not be taught only as one stand-alone course with the assumption that students have mastered knowledge and skills to implement EBP in their practice settings by the end of the course. The body of knowledge in the education field is still in its infancy in terms of what teaching strategies lead to the best uptake of EBP knowledge and skills in students. Therefore, more research in this area is needed.

Many educators, especially doctorally prepared academicians, have outstanding expertise in research, but have not learned EBP. As a result, they often continue to teach students the rigorous process of how to conduct research instead of teaching them how to best find, critically appraise, and synthesize a body of literature as well as how to make and evaluate practice changes based on the best evidence. Educators cannot teach what they themselves have not mastered; therefore, it is important to first ensure that they have the needed knowledge, attitudes, and skills (i.e., they themselves should meet the EBP competencies) to teach EBP to their students. Although many educators think they are teaching EBP, research has shown that is often not the case (Melnyk, Fineout-Overholt, Feinstein, Sadler, & Green-Hernandez,

2008; Orta et al., 2016). Therefore, a large number of students are graduating from academic programs without the knowledge and skills needed to consistently engage in EBP to make decisions about best practice in all realms of healthcare.

For academics to be effective in teaching EBP, they must first have a common definition of EBP. For example, EBP is a problem-solving approach to clinical practice that integrates the conscientious use of best evidence in combination with a clinician's expertise as well as patient preferences and values to make decisions about healthcare issues. Establishing a common definition provides a foundation for EBP competency integration. Next, educators should model what it looks like to be evidence-based practitioners, integrating the language, skills, positive beliefs and attitudes around EBP into interactions with students. This supports the idea that being evidence-based practitioners is vital.

A common understanding of whether students should be users or generators of evidence is critical, yet there remains confusion in many Doctor of Nursing Practice (DNP) programs across the United States that have students conducting research for their capstone projects instead of conducting evidence-based quality improvement projects (Melnyk, 2013). PhD programs should prepare students to generate the best evidence for practice; DNP programs should prepare students to be the best rapid translators of research evidence into clinical practice to improve outcomes in real-world settings (Melnyk, 2016b). DNP students should also meet all of the EBP competencies.

EBP Competency Integration in Undergraduate Programs

As faculty focus on integrating EBP competencies 1 through 13 in both didactic and clinical courses throughout undergraduate programs, the following should be the goals for the teaching and learning of EBP:

1. Increase knowledge of EBP.
2. Build the language of EBP (e.g., "evidence-based practice," not "evidence-based research"), critically appraising the literature (EBP) versus analyzing studies (research).
3. Develop EBP skills.
4. Create positive beliefs and attitudes about EBP.
5. Generate early consistent engagement in EBP.

EBP should be introduced early in undergraduate programs and woven throughout the entire curriculum. Content to address the first 13 competencies for practicing nurses should be incorporated into both didactic and clinical courses, ensuring that students can put the knowledge and skills they are learning in the classroom into practice in real-world settings. Table 11.2 provides some examples of how EBP can be integrated throughout undergraduate curricula.

EBP Integration in Graduate Programs

The level of expectations for EBP competency rises when students enter graduate-level programming. Not only are clinicians and academicians who hold graduate degrees expected to be competent in the first 13 EBP competencies, but they should also be mentoring, teaching, and leading EBP at all levels, from unit or department-level work (more likely master's-prepared with some individuals doctorally prepared) to population/systems level and beyond (more likely doctorally prepared individuals but some master's-prepared clinicians and academicians). At this level, descriptors in EBP competencies 14 to 24 change from lower-level verbs that include "searches," "participates in critical appraisal," and "collects practice data" to higher-level action words including "systematically searches," "critically appraises," "measures," "leads," and "mentors." This means faculty must use methods to assess foundational

TABLE 11.2 *Example of Progression of EBP Integration in Undergraduate Programs*

Year	Course	Learning Activity	EBP Competency Addressed
Initial year in nursing curriculum*	Foundations/ fundamentals course	Introduce basic concepts of EBP in a lecture or two, early in the first course. Differentiate between research and EBP.	Competency 1
	EBP language and skills building integrated throughout all courses	<ul><li>Faculty integrate language of EBP and model clinical inquiry.</li><li>Create searchable questions (e.g., PICO[T] questions).</li><li>Students build awareness of databases.</li><li>Expose students to searching in databases at basic level.</li><li>Incorporate different types of literature (research articles, different types of reviews, expert opinions, clinical practice guidelines into reading materials in courses).</li></ul>	Competencies 1–4
	NOTE: Align stand-alone EBP course with semester of first clinical experiences to establish full overview of EBP process and exposure to skills.	<ul><li>Emphasize rapid critical appraisal and synthesis of various types of studies.</li><li>Introduce organizational culture's impact on EBP integration and sustainability.</li><li>Students explore where EBP is present in professional organizations, accrediting bodies, reimbursement, government agencies like CDC, AHRQ.</li><li>Templated group EBP project</li></ul>	Competencies 1–7, 13
Second year of nursing curriculum or as students progress through specialty area or clinical rotations	EBP language and skills integrated throughout all courses	<ul><li>Students explore where EBP is present in the clinical site where they are working (e.g., shared governance committees, policies, procedures)</li><li>Students engage in a group project around an issue that is of importance to the clinical site where they are working in collaboration with unit/department staff or leadership. Stop at making recommendation based on evidence.</li><li>Disseminate to clinical site staff/leadership.</li><li>Students create a hypothetical implementation plan to implement their recommended practice change in the EBP project executed in collaboration with unit/department-level staff and leadership, identifying measurable outcomes (at least one of which has a "so what" factor), key stakeholders, and proposed rollout plan.</li></ul>	Competencies 1–7, 12, 13 Competency 10

TABLE 11.2	*Example of Progression of EBP Integration in Undergraduate Programs* (continued)		

Year	Course	Learning Activity	EBP Competency Addressed
Final year of nursing curriculum or as students progress into the last of their specialty-track clinical courses and leadership and transition into professional practice courses	EBP language and skills integrated throughout all courses PLUS explore the results of EBP in the clinical setting. Explore anticipated outcomes from evidence-based decisions and projects, data collection practices, and data ownership. Understand change theory and impact on implementation and sustainability. Understand importance of stakeholder engagement across the organization. Application is at the organization level.	• Students choose a patient care issue that is benchmarked by NDNQI (National Database of Nursing Quality Indicators) or CMS, identifies unit-level data on that indicator and compares unit-level data against national-level benchmarks • Students explore organizational procedures on policy and procedure creation and maintenance. Address such questions as, "How are new policies created?" "How often are current policies reviewed?" "Is evidence provided to support policies and procedures? If so, how many articles are in the body of evidence?" "What is the date range of the body of evidence?" "Are synthesis tables provided? How does that align with what you've learned about evidence-based decision making?" "Make recommendations to strengthen policy and procedure development and review.	Competencies 2, 8, 11 Competencies 9, 13

* This is an exemplar of EBP integration across three-years of a nursing program as many programs do not direct-admit students into nursing program in their initial year in college.

AHRQ, Agency for Healthcare Research and Quality; CDC, Centers for Disease Control and Prevention; EBP, evidence-based practice.

levels of knowledge, attitudes, and skills in EBP and remediate where necessary while moving graduate students to the higher level of EBP competency. Coursework should include a strong focus on the science behind mentoring, leading change, and building cultures that support and sustain EBP as well as planning, implementing, and evaluating practice changes. Other topics that should be included in graduate programs as they relate to EBP include discovering internal data, benchmarking, national safety goals, evidence-based quality improvement processes, informatics, leadership styles and theory, bringing about organizational change, and dissemination of evidence. Again, it is necessary to ensure that students are applying concepts learned in didactic courses in their clinical practicum experiences. See Table 11.3.

Many DNP programs across the United States have students conducting research for their DNP scholarly projects instead of evidence-based quality improvement, health policy or program evaluation projects (American Association of Colleges of Nursing [AACN], 2016; Loversidge, 2016; Melnyk, 2013). PhD programs should prepare students to generate

TABLE
11.3

Progression of EBP Integration in Graduate-Level Programs

Progression of EBP Integration in Graduate-Level Programs	NOTE 1: Graduate-level students should be competent in all 24 EBP competencies by the time of graduation. Faculty should identify gaps in meeting the first 13 competencies for practicing clinicians and remediate where needed while moving students through the 11 competencies for advanced practitioners (competencies 14–24).	Note 2: Graduate-prepared practitioners may serve in a number of different practice and middle- to upper-level leadership roles, depending on many factors, including educational preparation, job description, practice setting, professional experience, size of the organization, and organizational priorities.
EBP Competency	**Master's Level Activity or Assignment**	**Doctoral Level Activity or Assignment**
14. Systematically conducts an exhaustive search for external evidence* to answer clinical questions	*FOCUS: Personal Skill Development* Identify a topic or issue of interest, create a well-designed, searchable question (in PICO[T] or similar format) and conduct a comprehensive search using multiple databases and advanced searching techniques with Medical Subject Headings (MeSH) terms.	*FOCUS: Personal Skill Development* Identify a topic or issue of interest, create a well-designed searchable question (in PICO[T]) or similar format) and conduct an exhaustive search using multiple databases and advanced searching techniques with MeSH terms.
15. Critically appraises relevant preappraised evidence (i.e., clinical guidelines, summaries, synopses, syntheses of relevant external evidence) and primary studies, including evaluation and synthesis 22. Mentors others in evidence-based decision making and the EBP process	*FOCUS: Personal Skill Development and Mentoring* Practice rapid critical appraisal of various types of literature using rapid critical appraisal tools. Lead a group of clinicians, students, or peers through rapid critical appraisal of an article in a journal club format.	*FOCUS: Personal Skill Development and Mentoring* Same as master's level AND Conduct rapid critical appraisal of a comprehensive body of evidence around a topic of interest discovered through an exhaustive search of the databases. Identify which studies are "keeper" studies that will be included in the final body of evidence.

322

(continued)

	FOCUS: *Personal Skill Development*	FOCUS: *Personal Skill Development and Leading EBP*
16. Integrates a body of external evidence from nursing and related fields with internal evidence[†] in making decisions about patient care	Explore types of data that organizations collect internally (i.e., patient assessment data, outcomes management data, benchmark and national patient safety goal data, and quality improvement data). Identify who owns that data, how to access it, and how it affects EBP.	Explore types of data that organizations collect internally, including who owns that data, how to access it, and how it affects EBP. Identify gaps in data collected and data needed to drive EBP decision making (including patient data, outcomes management data, benchmarks and national patient safety goal data, and quality improvement data). Explore how leaders can facilitate collection of relevant data and making data more accessible to front-line clinicians for use in EBP.
	FOCUS: *Personal Skill Development and Mentoring*	FOCUS: *Personal Skill Development and Mentoring*
17. Leads transdisciplinary teams in applying synthesized evidence to initiate clinical decisions and practice changes to improve the health of individuals, groups, and populations 22. Mentors others in evidence-based decision making and the EBP process	Lead group of clinicians, students, or peers who have each identified and appraised one article on a chosen topic as they collectively create a synthesis table from the body of evidence the group discovered.	Same as master's level, AND Address all aspects of a complex clinical issue and create a synthesis table from a body of evidence around each aspect of that issue. For example, in taking on an EBP approach to addressing non–ventilator-acquired pneumonia, synthesize the body of literature around all components of a care bundle (i.e., early ambulation, incentive spirometry, and oral care, as well as a synthesis table on the effect of bundling care).
	FOCUS: *Personal Skill Development*	FOCUS: *Personal Skill Development and Leading Change*
18. Generates internal evidence through outcomes management and EBP implementation projects for the purpose of integrating best practices 19. Measures processes and outcomes of evidence-based clinical decisions	Explore various change theories and processes of implementing an EBP change. Create a plan to implement a hypothetical EBP change in an organization. Identify measurable outcomes and create a plan to measure those outcomes. Explore quality improvement processes, such as PDSA/PDCA, Six Sigma, and Donabedian's Structure/Process/Outcomes cycle, recognizing the difference between quality improvement and evidence-based quality improvement.	Using either a real-life scenario or an unfolding case study, identify a change theory and apply it to leading an EBP change. Create a plan to implement a hypothetical EBP change, including what types of resources would be needed to support the EBP practice change implementation. Choose an evidence-based quality improvement process and apply it to monitoring, measuring, and trending the effectiveness of a real or hypothetical EBP practice change.

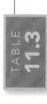

TABLE 11.3 Progression of EBP Integration in Graduate-Level Programs (continued)

23. Implements strategies to sustain an EBP culture	FOCUS: *Personal Skill Development and Mentoring* Conduct an organizational assessment to assess organizational readiness for EBP and barriers and facilitators to EBP within the organization. Identify organizational strengths and how they can be leveraged to move the culture toward being an evidence-based organization. Identify solutions to overcome barriers to EBP in the organization.	FOCUS: *Personal Skill Development and Leading EBP* Same as master's level AND Identify key players within the organization and opportunities to influence integration of EBP. Discuss how barriers and resistance to EBP would be publicly navigated. Formulate a plan to sustain an organization's EBP culture.
20. Formulates evidence-based policies and procedures 21. Participates in the generation of external evidence with other healthcare professionals 24. Communicates best evidence to individuals, groups, colleagues, and policy makers	FOCUS: *Personal Skill Development, Mentoring, and Leading* Identify what type of resources would need to be allocated to support dissemination of information at conferences and professional meetings. Engage in a team working on the generation of external evidence. Present best evidence to a group during a presentation. Prepare a health policy brief based on the best evidence.	Focus: *Personal Skill Development, Mentoring, and Leading* Same as master's level AND Present best evidence at a regional or national conference. Engage in writing and submitting a manuscript in a quality peer-reviewed journal from an EBP or evidence-based quality improvement project.

*Evidence generated from research.

†Evidence generated internally within a clinical setting, such as patient assessment data, outcomes management, and quality improvement data.

EBP, evidence-based practice; PICOT, Patient population; Intervention or area of interest; Comparison intervention or group; Outcome; Time.

the best evidence for practice, whereas DNP programs should prepare students to be the best rapid translators of evidence into practice to improve outcomes in real-world settings (AACN, 2016; Melnyk, 2016b). Establishing and celebrating the expertise each degree brings to the profession creates an environment where PhDs and DNPs can work collaboratively to address clinically meaningful and important issues in real-world settings.

The EBP competencies serve as a guide for EBP integration into curricula as well as a standard to measure the competency of clinicians and academicians alike. Appropriately preparing clinicians and academicians of the future to be evidence based is imperative to improving the current state of healthcare. To accomplish this goal, three things must happen. First, faculty must commit to acquiring expertise in EBP where they may have gaps in knowledge and skills. That expertise must then not only be integrated across curricula at all levels, but also be infused into organizational cultures in a meaningful and intentional way to sustain EBP. Second, students must embrace EBP as they actively apply the knowledge, attitudes, and skills in EBP while leveraging their position as students, serving as brokers of new ideas to practice settings (Cronje & Moch, 2010; Moch, Cronje, & Branson, 2010). When students do so throughout their education, the greatest opportunity exists to make the EBP process the way in which they think rather than a task they accomplish. Third, as students graduate, they must integrate the EBP competencies into their daily practice and encourage colleagues to join them in doing so. It is only then that a brighter future for improving the quality of healthcare and enhancing population health outcomes will be built.

EBP FAST FACTS

- Thirteen EBP research-based competencies for practicing RNs and another 11 EBP competencies for APNs have been developed to enhance healthcare quality, safety, and population health outcomes as well as decrease costs.
- EBP competencies should be integrated into healthcare systems in various forms, including job descriptions; orientations for new nurses, APNs, managers, and leaders in order to set expectations for practice, clinical ladders, and performance evaluations.
- EBP competencies should be incorporated into academic programming across undergraduate and graduate levels so that students achieve competency in EBP on graduation.

WANT TO KNOW MORE?

A variety of resources are available to enhance your learning and understanding of this chapter.

- Visit thePoint® to access:
  - Articles from the AJN EBP Step-By-Step Series
  - Journal articles
  - Checklists for rapid critical appraisal and more!
- Lippincott CoursePoint combines digital text content with video case studies and interactive modules for a fully integrated course solution that works the way you study and learn.

References

American Association of Colleges of Nursing. (2015). *The Doctor of Nursing Practice: Current issues and clarifying recommendations.* Retrieved from http://www.aacnnursing.org/Portals/42/News/White-Papers/DNP-Implementation-TF-Report-8-15.pdf

American Association of Colleges of Nursing QSEN Education Consortium. (2012). *Graduate level QSEN competencies.* Washington, DC: Author.

American Nurses Association. (2010). *Nursing. Scope and standards of practice* (2nd ed.). Washington, DC: Author.

Bellamy, J. L., Mullen, E. J., Satterfield, J. M., Newhouse, R. P., Ferguson, M., Brownson, R. C., & Spring, B. (2013). Implementing evidence-based practice education in social work: A transdisciplinary approach. *Research on Social Work Practice, 23*(4), 426–436. doi:10.1177/1049731513480528

Covell, C. (2009). Outcomes achieved from organizational investment in nursing continuing professional development. *Journal of Nursing Administration, 39*(10), 438–443.

Cronje, R. J., & Moch, S. D. (2010). Part III. Reenvisioning undergraduate nursing students as opinion leaders to diffuse evidence-based practice in clinical settings. *Journal of Professional Nursing, 26*(1), 23–28. doi:10.1016/j.profnurs.2009.03.002

Dunn, S. V., Lawson, D., Robertson, S., Underwood, M., Clark, R., Valentine, T., & Herewane, D. (2000). The development of competency standards for specialist critical care nurses. *Journal of Advanced Nursing, 31*(2), 339–346.

Gallagher-Ford, L. (2017). Integrating the evidence-based practice competencies in healthcare settings. In B. M. Melnyk, L. Gallagher-Ford, & E. Fineout-Overholt (Eds.), *Implementing the evidence-based practice competencies in healthcare. A practical guide for improving quality, safety and outcomes* (pp. 185–204). Indianapolis, IN: Sigma Theta Tau International.

Galbraith, K., Ward, A., & Heneghan, C. (2017). A real-world approach to evidence-based medicine in general practice: A competency framework derived from a systematic review and Delphi process. *BMC Medical Education, 17*(78). doi:10.1186/s12909-017-0916-1

Hasson, F., Keeney, S., & McKenna, H. (2000). Research guidelines for the Delphi survey technique. *Journal of Advanced Nursing, 32*(4), 1008–1015.

James, J. T. (2013). A new, evidence-based estimate of patient harms associated with hospital care. *Journal of Patient Safety, 9*(3), 122–128.

Loversidge, J. M. (2016). A call for extending the utility of evidence-based practice: Adapting EBP for health policy impact. *Worldviews on Evidence-Based Nursing, 13*(6), 399–401. doi:10.1111/wvn.12183

Makary, M. A., & Daniel, M. (2016). Medical error-the third leading cause of death in the US. *BMJ: British Medical Journal, 353*, i2139.

Mallidou, A. A., Atherton, P., Chan, L., Frisch, N., Glegg, S., & Scarrow, G. (2017). Protocol of a scoping review on knowledge translation competencies. *Systematic Reviews, 6*(1), 93. doi:10.1186/s13643-017-0481-z

Melnyk, B. M. (2013). Distinguishing the preparation and roles of the PhD and DNP graduate: National implications for academic curricula and healthcare systems. *Journal of Nursing Education, 52*(8), 442–448.

Melnyk, B. M. (2016a). Culture eats strategy every time: What works in building and sustaining an evidence-based practice culture in healthcare systems. *Worldviews on Evidence-Based Nursing, 13*(2), 99–101.

Melnyk, B. M. (2016b). The Doctor of Nursing Practice degree = Evidence-based practice expert. *Worldviews on Evidence-Based Nursing, 13*(3), 183–184.

Melnyk, B. M. (2017). Development of and evidence to support the evidence-based practice competencies. In B. M. Melnyk, L. Gallagher-Ford, & E. Fineout-Overholt, *Implementing the evidence-based practice competencies in healthcare. A practical guide for improving quality, safety and outcomes* (pp. 20–30). Indianapolis, IN: Sigma Theta Tau International.

Melnyk, B.M., Buck, J., & Gallagher-Ford, L. (2015). Transforming quality improvement into evidence-based quality improvement: A key solution to improve healthcare outcomes [Editorial]. *Worldviews on Evidence-based Nursing, 12*(5), 251–252. doi: 10.1111/wvn.12112

Melnyk, B. M., Fineout-Overholt, E., Feinstein, N. F., Sadler, L. S., & Green-Hernandez, C. (2008). Nurse practitioner educators' perceived knowledge, beliefs, and teaching strategies regarding evidence-based practice: Implications for accelerating the integration of evidence-based practice into graduate programs. *Journal of Professional Nursing, 24*(1), 7–13.

Melnyk, B. M., Fineout-Overholt, E., Gallagher-Ford, L., & Kaplan, L. (2012). The state of evidence-based practice in US nurses: Critical implications for nurse leaders and educators. *Journal of Nursing Administration, 42*(9), 410–417.

Melnyk, B. M., Gallagher-Ford, L., Long, L. E., & Fineout-Overholt, E. (2014). The establishment of evidence-based practice competencies for practicing registered nurses and advanced practice nurses in real-world clinical settings: Proficiencies to improve healthcare quality, reliability, patient outcomes, and costs. *Worldviews on Evidence-Based Nursing, 11*(1), 5–15.

Melnyk, B. M., Gallagher-Ford, L., & Tan, A. (2017). Self-reported evidence-based practice (EBP) competency in nurses across the United States in 2017. Columbus, OH: The Ohio State University.

Melnyk, B. M., Gallagher-Ford, L., Zellefrow, C., Tucker, S., Thomas, B., Sinnott, L. T., & Tan, A. (2018). The first U.S. study on nurses' evidence-based practice competencies indicates major deficits that threaten healthcare quality, safety, and patient outcomes. *Worldviews on Evidence-Based Nursing, 15*(1), 16–25.

Merriam Webster Dictionary. (n.d.). *Competence.* Retrieved from http://www.learnersdictionary.com/definition/competence.

Moch, S. D., Cronje, R. J., & Branson, J. (2010). Part 1. Undergraduate nursing evidence-based practice education: Envisioning the role of students. *Journal of Professional Nursing, 26*(1), 5–13. doi:10.1016/j.profnurs.2009.01.015

Orta, R., Messmer, P. R., Valdes, G. R., Turkel, M., Fields, S. D., & Wei, C. C. (2016). Knowledge and competency of nursing faculty regarding evidence-based practice. *Journal of Continuing Education in Nursing, 47*(9), 409–419. doi:10.3928/00220124-20160817-08

Quality and Safety Education for Nurses/QSEN. (2013). *Project overview: The evolution of the Quality and Safety Education for Nurses (QSEN) initiative.* Retrieved from http://qsen.org/about-qsen/project-overview/

Scurlock-Evans, L., Upton, P., & Upton, D. (2014). Evidence-based practice in physiotherapy: A systematic review of barriers, enablers and interventions. *Physiotherapy, 100*(3), 208–219. doi:10.1016/j.physio.2014.03.001

Skela-Savic, B., Hvalic-Touzery, S., & Pesjak, K. (2017). Professional values and competencies as explanatory factors for the use of evidence-based practice in nursing. *Journal of Advanced Nursing, 73*(8), 1910–1923.

Stevens, K. R. (2005). *Essential competencies for evidence-based practice in nursing* (1st ed.). Academic Center for Evidence-Based Practice, University of Texas Health Science Center at San Antonio.

Straub-Morarend, C., Wankiiri-Hale, C., Blanchette, D. R., Lanning, S. K., Bekhuis, T., Smith, B. M., . . . Spallek, H. (2016). Evidence-based practice knowledge, perceptions, and behavior: A multi-institutional, cross-sectional study of a population of U.S. dental students. *Journal of Dental Education, 80*(4), 430–438.

Wilcock, P., Janes, G., & Chambers, A. (2009). Health care improvement and continuing interprofessional education: Continuing interprofessional development to improve patient outcomes. *Journal of Continuing Education in the Health Professions, 29*(2), 84–90.

12 Leadership Strategies for Creating and Sustaining Evidence-Based Practice Organizations

Lynn Gallagher-Ford, Jacalyn S. Buck, and Bernadette Mazurek Melnyk

> **A leader is one who knows the way, goes the way, and shows the way.**
>
> —*John C. Maxwell*

EBP Terms to Learn
Authentic leaders
Evidence-based leadership
Innovative leaders
Servant leadership
Transformational
  leadership

Learning Objectives
After studying this chapter, learners will be able to:

1. Describe leadership strategies for creating and sustaining a culture of evidence-based practice in healthcare organizations.
2. Discuss common leadership styles and theories.

Today's healthcare environment is vastly complex and ever changing. Scientific knowledge continues to increase and grow at an exponential pace, yet it is well known that the time lag for translation of new knowledge into clinical practice ranges from 8 to 30 years (Sandström, Borglin, Nilsson, & Willman, 2011). There is increasing evidence that patient outcomes are linked to nurses' performance and that nurses' decision making affects quality (Melnyk, Fineout-Overholt, Giggleman, & Choy, 2017). Therefore, nurse leaders must build and promote work environments where nursing performance is maximized. In this rapidly changing healthcare environment, leaders need to be innovative and able to motivate and inspire nurses through vision and actions. In addition, leaders must implement strategies that help nurses provide safe, quality nursing care that is also caring, empathetic, and respectful. Leaders must invest in each nurse's potential, professional development, and well-being and assure they are aware of their individual responsibilities and contributions to the organization's mission, vision, and goals.

Both the Institute of Medicine (IOM), now called the National Academy of Medicine, and The Joint Commission (TJC) have identified the value of using nursing science (evidence-based practice or EBP) to improve patient outcomes, and the American Nurses Credentialing Center (ANCC) emphasizes the utilization of research and EBP as critical mechanisms to achieve best outcomes. These external influences reinforce the necessity for leaders to create work environments and cultures where EBP can arrive, survive, and thrive. An EBP environment and culture is present when clinicians have access to EBP resources (computers, databases, librarians), space for reading and reflective thinking, opportunities to collaborate with colleagues, structures and processes in place to provide education and skills building, access to EBP mentors, time to read and appraise the literature, and autonomy/capacity to change practice when indicated (Melnyk et al., 2016; Pryse, McDaniel, & Schafer, 2014; Spiva et al., 2017). An EBP environment and culture is actualized when **evidence-based decision making** is the standard approach (i.e., the norm) to all decision making.

An organization's environmental context is critical to creating a culture of EBP. The context of healthcare organizations where practice occurs is hierarchical, complex, fluid, and interactive. The structure of key factors such as hierarchy, communication patterns, teamwork, and collaboration all influence the culture where clinicians function. When these organizational factors are combined with the unique characteristics and competencies (knowledge, skills, and attitudes) of each individual practitioner, a dynamic social system is formed where decision making and practice decisions occur. This organizational environment is directly influenced by leadership in positive or negative ways to create an EBP-friendly environment, or otherwise. Leadership activities can enhance, influence, and stimulate motivation of nurses to use research in practice. Support, encouragement, giving "voice" to the clinicians, negotiating work conditions, supporting needed education and skills building, role modeling, raising a call to a common vision/purpose, continuous commitment, and keeping momentum going are all critical responsibilities that organizational and unit-based leaders must embrace and ensure to make EBP a reality.

Consistent implementation of evidence-based care in practice, whether at the individual or organizational level, requires behavior change. Behavior change of any kind requires more than the provision of didactic information and/or simply providing resources, such as computers and librarians. In order for clinicians to change their behavior and consistently implement EBP, a multitude of interventions are necessary, including

- targeted interventions to enhance cognitive beliefs about the value of EBP;
- EBP education combined with active repetitive skills building;
- EBP mentorship or facilitation and support;
- a culture and an environment that supports and sustains EBP;
- leaders and managers (who are knowledgeable in EBP and "walk the talk") who build the capacity and infrastructure, publically navigate barriers, and role model EBP in their leadership practice;
- mutual commitment to EBP among organizational leaders (e.g., chief nursing officers [CNOs]/chief nursing executives [CNEs], directors/managers/clinical leaders, advanced practice nurses [APNs], nursing professional development specialists [NPDs], clinical nurse specialists [CNSs], and clinical ladder participants); and
- resilience and perseverance to keep momentum going (Beckette et al., 2011; Bennett et al., 2016; Gerrish & Clayton, 2004; Melnyk et al., 2004; Melnyk, Fineout-Overholt, Gallagher-Ford, & Kaplan, 2011; Rycroft-Malone, Harvey et al., 2004).

In a descriptive survey by Melnyk, Fineout-Overholt et al, (2012) with a random sample of over 1,000 nurses from across the United States who were members of the American Nurses Association (ANA), barriers to EBP were identified. Although several of the barriers named by nurses were the same barriers that had been reported in previous decades, there were new developments. The long-time barriers named by survey participants included lack of time, EBP education, and resources as well as lack of availability of EBP mentors. Of particular note, the previously identified barrier of nurses not valuing EBP (Pravikoff, Tanner, & Pierce, 2005) was largely gone in the 2011 survey. This finding reflected that clinicians are more accepting of EBP as important and beneficial for patient care. The survey identified a barrier that had not been previously identified in the literature, which was resistance to EBP from managers and leaders. Traditional organizational cultures that upheld the philosophy of "that is the way we do it here" also named as a top barrier. Respondents to the survey expressed a need for support from their organizations, managers/leaders, and interdisciplinary colleagues to be able to implement EBP. In addition, clinicians identified relief from overwhelming workloads as an essential requirement for implementing EBP as well as education and access to EBP information and mentors (Melnyk et al., 2011).

The survey findings reinforced that implementation of EBP was still influenced by a multitude of factors, including

- cognitive beliefs and attitudes about EBP (Melnyk, Fineout-Overholt, & Mays, 2008; Rycroft-Malone, 2008),
- knowledge about EBP (Melnyk et al., 2004),
- organizational commitment to EBP (Dopson, FitzGerald, Ferlie, Gabbay, & Locock, 2002),
- organizational support for EBP (Hutchinson & Johnston, 2004; Rycroft-Malone, Harvey et al., 2004),
- a culture that is responsive to change (Gerrish & Clayton, 2004), and
- support for EBP ideas/initiatives.

A subsequent study was conducted by Melnyk, Gallagher-Ford, Long, and Fineout-Overholt (2014) to further explore the 2011 finding related to leader and manager resistance to EBP. The following findings were reported:

- More than one third of hospitals were not meeting benchmarks for National Database of Nursing Quality Indicators (NDNQI) performance metrics;
- Almost one third of hospitals were above national benchmarks for core measures (e.g., falls, pressure ulcers);
- CNOs believed that EBP resulted in higher quality of care, safety, and improved patient outcomes, yet very little of their budgets were allocated to EBP;
- CNOs reported their top priorities were quality and safety, yet EBP was rated as a very low priority;
- CNOs beliefs in the value of EBP were strong but their own implementation of EBP was relatively low;
- More than 50% of CNOs believed that EBP was practiced in their organization from "not at all" to "somewhat"; and
- CNOs reported that there were inadequate numbers of EBP mentors in their healthcare systems to work on EBP with direct care staff and create EBP cultures/ environments.

Shortly following this study, a forum with 150 nursing executives was held at an American Organization of Nurse Executives (AONE) annual conference to discuss the findings and strategize potential solutions. The nurse executives who attended the forum expressed their lack of understanding of how EBP was a direct "driver" leading to quality and safety outcomes; instead they perceived EBP as a competing priority that would become a higher priority once quality and safety were achieved. This disconnect was discussed in detail at the forum, and when asked what they, as CNOs, needed to help move EBP forward in their organizations, they expressed the need for tools (i.e., an EBP toolkit) to help them "make the case for EBP" at the C-suite level in their organizations. Specifically, they were interested in educational programs to facilitate building a critical mass of EBP mentors; research studies demonstrating the effectiveness of EBP programs and mentors as well as the return on investment (ROI); job description exemplars that clearly articulated the role and expected deliverables of EBP mentors; and specific expectations (competencies) for all nurses whether in staff level or in advanced practice roles.

Since then, several studies have been conducted and tools have been developed to assist leaders in making a case for building an EBP program. In 2014, Melnyk et al. published the results of their Delphi study that was conducted to develop a set of clear EBP competencies for both practicing registered nurses and APNs in clinical settings to be used by healthcare institutions to build high-performing systems that consistently implement and sustain EBP.

The interest in these competencies as an accessible and easy-to-use tool to promote EBP in healthcare organizations led to the publication of a handbook titled *Implementing the EBP competencies in healthcare: A practical guide for improving quality, safety, and outcomes* (Melnyk, Gallagher-Ford, & Fineout-Overholt, 2017), which has been widely used in a variety of organizations. The textbook includes strategies for integrating the EBP competencies into healthcare system expectations, orientations, job descriptions, performance appraisals, and clinical ladder promotion processes. Two chapters are dedicated to describing the experiences of healthcare systems that have integrated the competencies into the CNS role across a large health system and an interprofessional policy and procedure committee across a large pediatric health system. These examples highlight how integration of the EBP competencies in real-world healthcare settings has helped organizations to achieve higher quality and reliability as well as reduce healthcare costs.

In 2017, Melnyk, Fineout-Overholt et al., published another study examining the impact of preparing a critical mass of EBP mentors on patient outcomes in a health system through use of the Advancing Research and Clinical practice through close Collaboration (ARCC) Model. Healthcare professionals' EBP beliefs, EBP implementation, and organizational culture were measured with valid and reliable instruments. Patient outcomes were collected in aggregate from the hospital's medical records. Findings from the study revealed that, after developing a cadre of EBP mentors, there were significant increases in clinicians' EBP beliefs and EBP implementation along with positive movement toward an organizational EBP culture. In addition, there were substantial improvements in several patient outcomes, including significant reductions in ventilator days in the ICU with no ventilator-associated pneumonia, significant reductions in pressure ulcer rates, substantial improvements in patient satisfaction ratings, and a 15% reduction in readmissions for congestive heart failure patients.

These studies are examples of ongoing work to inform the development of tools for leaders to utilize to make the case for EBP in the C-suite of an organization. As research continues to support the development of EBP implementation tools, it is imperative that leaders use them effectively and take action to bring EBP into their organizations to improve outcomes.

The literature substantiates that leaders influence whether EBP is actualized in organizations or not. Leaders who support colleagues and create a vision for EBP in their organizations as well as influence policy to facilitate EBP and incorporate evidence into their own leadership practices are key in having an impact on EBP implementation (Rycroft-Malone, 2004; Rycroft-Malone, Harvey et al., 2004).

With all of the barriers and facilitators of EBP that have been described over the past decades, it becomes clear that a multifocal, multilayered strategy that addresses individuals as well as the overall organization must be developed. Strategies must be designed to facilitate change, shift practice from tradition-based/provider-centric care to evidence-based/patient-centered care and to create structures to sustain the new paradigm. Approaching these complex challenges to deliver best healthcare practices and outcomes will require innovative thinking and courageous acts. The solutions themselves should be derived from an evidence-based approach, and the timelines for integration of the solutions into clinical practice arenas should be immediate.

Despite the urgency to implement and adopt this new practice paradigm, the integration of evidence into practice continues to be perceived as challenging and burdensome and, as such, is often delegated, avoided, or ignored. Much of the distress related to implementing and sustaining EBP in organizations stems from a lack of EBP knowledge, skills, and/or attitudes across the system, from executive suites to the bedside. Healthcare leaders are well poised to be held accountable to address these challenges and be at the forefront of the paradigm shift to evidence-based instead of traditional care to drive better outcomes for patients, families, and clinicians.

RESPONSIBILITIES AND STANDARDS OF EVIDENCE-BASED LEADERSHIP

In a time when the nation is calling for EBP as standard of care, leaders must guide and support their organizations and clinicians through this challenge and opportunity. The basic definition of a leader is "one who guides or directs a group" (Leader, n.d.). Leadership, on the other hand, is a process through which an individual influences a group to achieve a common goal. The definition of **evidence-based leadership** is a problem-solving approach to leading and influencing organizations or groups to achieve a common goal that integrates the conscientious use of best evidence with leadership expertise and stakeholders' preferences and values. Evidence-based leadership requires two levels of commitment: (1) self-actualization of EBP and public demonstration of EBP as the foundation of daily practice and decision making and (2) facilitation of the enculturation of EBP throughout the organization(s) (Rycroft-Malone, Harvey et.al., 2004).

Evidence-based leaders must be grounded in and embrace the EBP process for decision making in their practice and across the organization as well. This requires knowledge and application of key aspects of the EBP process to leadership decisions, including

- clinical inquiry and formulating PICOT questions,
- effective searching for best evidence,
- critical appraisal of evidence,
- evaluation and synthesis of evidence/integration of evidence into decision making/implementing evidence-based changes,
- measuring and sustaining outcomes, and
- disseminating findings.

Self-actualization and demonstration of EBP by leaders includes embracing EBP in one's own practice by attaining EBP knowledge/skills, developing a pro-EBP attitude, role modeling EBP by making evidence-based leadership decisions, publicly navigating EBP barriers, building an infrastructure and culture to support EBP, and recognizing EBP achievements. Beyond leaders' individual responsibilities to embrace EBP, they are, by virtue of their position, power, and authority, accountable to facilitate the enculturation of EBP throughout their organizations. By embracing and role modeling EBP as well as creating a culture and environment that adopts, values, and implements EBP, evidence-based leaders build work environments and context where EBP can not only arrive but also survive and thrive. Yet culture change is not easy; it is character building in that only 19% of organizational change efforts tend to succeed (Gibbons, 2015). It takes a team vision, belief in the vision, and persistence through the character builders until the vision comes to fruition. Chapter 15 covers essential elements in creating a vision and leading culture change in individuals, teams, and organizations.

The EBP imperative is supported by professional leadership organizations in their scope and standards of practice statements. The American Nurses Association (ANA) *Scope and Standards of Practice for the Nurse Administrator* (2016) maintains that the nurse administrator will attain knowledge and competency reflective of contemporary current practice and integrate research findings into practice; enhance the quality and effectiveness of nursing practice, nursing services administration, and the delivery of services; evaluate nursing practice against the exiting evidence; and incorporate new knowledge to improve the quality of care. The American Organization of Nurse Executives (AONE, 2015) sets forth competencies similar to ANA for healthcare leaders in executive roles. With its vision of "shaping the future of healthcare through innovative nursing leadership," the organization recognizes that nursing leaders must be proficient and competent in leadership practice to ensure excellence in patient care (AONE). In addition, AONE emphasizes that leaders must be innovative and competent in five domains of practice: (1) communication and relationship management, (2) knowledge of the healthcare environment, (3) leadership, (4) professionalism, and (5) business skills and principles. Competencies in all of these domains are essential for the leader to influence and cultivate a culture of innovation and EBP.

The ANCC Magnet Recognition Program, considered the highest recognition for nursing excellence, acknowledges healthcare organizations for achieving quality outcomes in patient care, innovative nursing practice, and care excellence. Evidence-based practice is evident and supported throughout the Magnet model, including the requirement that organizations describe components and sources of evidence that promote superior performance and excellent outcomes in their enterprise (American Nurses Credentialing Center, 2011). healthcare organizations that have achieved Magnet status ensure that their clinicians are educated about EBP and research so they are able to search the literature and explore new and best practices for patient care. Leaders in Magnet organizations must establish infrastructures to create and sustain strong EBP and research programs. These individuals must guarantee that financial resources are secured to support and encourage scholarly inquiry, EBP, and research initiatives in the organization.

It is apparent that professional nursing organizations understand the critical function that all nursing leaders play in creating a culture of EBP. Literature from these organizations consistently conveys the expectation that leaders must demonstrate competence and enact EBP on a consistent basis to lead the transformational work needed in healthcare today and into the future.

Organizational Structure for EBP

In the majority of healthcare organizations in the United States, there are traditional leadership hierarchies that are responsible for the delivery of services. Although titles may vary, these leadership hierarchies generally include a chief nursing officer/executive, nursing directors, and unit-based nurse managers. Currently, organizations function within these inevitable structures and, for better or worse, they are the structures through which the EBP paradigm shift must be driven. For now, as EBP transformations are occurring in traditional structures, both strong leadership and strong management are necessary for optimal effectiveness. As opportunities to reinvent organizational structures arise in the future, leadership will need to take place at each and every level of the hierarchy for peak performance to be actualized, and day-to-day management functions will be merged in the leadership role. A shared EBP leadership model encourages joint accountability, partnership, and ownership of EBP and subsequent outcomes (Bennett et al., 2016).

Contributions of Managers and Leaders

Managers and leaders have always made valuable contributions to organizations; however, contributions from each has been described as unique and different (Lunenburg, 2011). Kotter (2013) defines management as a set of processes, including budgeting and planning, organizing and staffing, controlling, and problem solving. According to landmark work by Bennis (1991), managerial qualities and functions include administering, maintaining, focusing on systems and structure, relying on control, holding a short range view, asking how and when, and having their eye on the bottom line and doing "things right." When managers exercise their authority to ensure things are completed, advocating for consistency and maintaining the status quo, they reduce uncertainty and maintain stability of the organization on a day-to-day basis (Lunenburg, 2011). In contrast, leaders challenge the status quo and advocate for change and innovation. Leadership involves developing a vision and aligning people with that vision. The leader focuses on people; they motivate and inspire others to act by empowering them, thus building trust and commitment. They use their influence to create change in the organization in order to take it into the future (Kotter, 2013; Lunenburg, 2011).

This traditional model, however, is insufficient to meet today's challenges in our complex and dynamic healthcare environments. An innovative and transformational approach to creating new leadership models is an imperative. The traditional role of the nurse manager whose responsibilities are often limited to stabilizing the organization and producing efficiency and reliability must be reenvisioned to encompass the expectation of a leader who promotes change and innovation to guide the organization into the future (Kotter, 2013). Fleizer, Semenic, Ritchie, Richer, and Denis (2016) found that unit-based managers had a considerable impact on nursing practice improvements and sustainability of those practice changes. Once thought most pertinent to the more senior leaders in the organization, the findings from the Fleizer et al. study suggest that the unit-based leader had a larger role in influencing and sustaining best practices through alignment with the organizational vision and strategies. Regardless of the title held, all clinicians within the leadership structure are responsible to be evidence-based leaders. They must embrace the EBP paradigm in their own personal practice, integrate EBP into their decision making processes, and promote a culture of EBP in their sphere(s) of influence on a day-to-day basis.

LEADERSHIP STYLES AND THEORIES

Although many leadership theories exist, there are several that are particularly relevant to contemporary healthcare leadership. These models of leadership focus on the relationship between the leader and the follower to achieve a common goal. In these relationship-based theories, the leader creates an environment where individuals are supported and recognized for their work and achievements. They feel inspired and empowered to innovate and change, resulting in positive outcomes for the organization. These attributes are critical components of an EBP culture. The theoretical models of relationship-based leadership include but are not limited to innovation leadership, transformational leadership, servant leadership, and authentic leadership. Although any of these leadership theories is appropriate for the healthcare leader of today, the concept of evidence-based leadership must be synergistically incorporated in tandem with the style adopted by the leader.

As an evidence-based leader, role modeling, empowering others, and optimizing others to reach their full potential creates the infrastructure for best practice and positive outcomes.

Innovation Leadership

Innovative leaders are those individuals who create an infrastructure that weaves innovation into the DNA of their organization. Within a culture of innovation, employees are both empowered and encouraged to challenge the status quo and integrate new processes and technologies into the organization so that systems operate more effectively and efficiently.

Traditionally, healthcare organizations have tended to avoid risk and maintain comfort where costs and outcomes were controlled and well known. Innovation and risk-taking were not traditionally viewed as positive attributes of a healthcare leader. More emphasis was placed on continuing routine practices that were predictable and worked yesterday, or reworking ineffective processes, rather than taking initiative to advance innovation and move the organization to the desired future. Many contemporary leaders challenge this traditional view of leadership in light of the looming need to transform healthcare organizations into cost-effective, efficient systems where quality and patient safety are the norm. Whereas all leaders must maintain the necessary skills of planning, organizing, and evaluating, innovative leaders have the ability to support innovation and manage change (Porter-O'Grady & Malloch, 2010).

The innovative leader is an individual who can create the "context for innovation to occur; and create and implement the roles, decision making structures, physical space, partnerships, networks and equipment that supports innovative thinking and testing" (Malloch & Porter-O'Grady, 2009). The innovative leader is ideally suited to create the systems and structures that support implementation and sustainability of EBP, including fostering creativity and innovation to build systems and structures that support EBP; facilitating organizational changes needed to promote EBP as the foundation of all decision making; and development of partnerships and networks to hard-wire and embed EBPs and processes that will persist over time. To sustain an innovative culture, innovative leaders must be present and leading the organization. Malloch (2010) reveals several competencies for innovative leaders:

- Assessment for innovation: personal knowledge of one's propensity, ability, and skill with innovation work
- Future focused: actively plans for a better future and understands the value of change
- Value-driven: believes new ideas will advance performance and value

Transformational Leadership

Transformational leadership is defined as a state in which leaders and followers "find meaning and purpose in their work, and grow and develop as a result of their relationship" (Barker, Sullivan, & Emery, 2006, p. 16). Because of this relationship, leaders and followers become partners in pursuit of a common goal. Transformational leaders are energetic, compassionate, and enthusiastic. They have the ability to provide a vision, motivate, and inspire others. As a result, followers gain trust in, admiration of, and respect for their leader. The environment created by transformational leaders is change oriented, supportive of new ideas, innovative, and open (Klainberg & Dirschel, 2010). These leaders have the ability to direct change in the organization via their ability to create a supportive infrastructure and empower staff to incorporate evidence into practice (Ryan, Harris, Mattox, Camp, & Shirey, 2015). Ultimately, they create a culture where staff can be creative, innovative, and open to change (Guerrero, Padwa, Fenwick, Harris, & Aarons, 2016). The transformational leader is uniquely able to create and sustain environments where EBP can thrive by leveraging the deep trust-based relationships they have cultivated at multiple levels across the organization.

Four dimensions comprise transformational leadership, including idealized influence, inspirational motivation, intellectual stimulation, and individualized consideration (Bass & Avolio, 1993). These four dimensions of transformational leadership create a synergy within a workplace where EBP can flourish and patient care quality and satisfaction excel.

1. **Idealized influence**—serves as role model for followers and builds respect and trust. The focus is on doing things right rather than ensuring that their followers do the right things (Modassir & Singh, 2008).
2. **Inspirational motivation**—articulates a clear vision for followers and is charismatic. She or he infuses enthusiasm and optimism, and inspires and motivates others to accomplish great achievements (Bass & Riggio, 2006; Modassir & Singh, 2008).
3. **Intellectual stimulation**—encourages innovation and creativity; empowers followers to explore new ways of doing things and approach problems using EBP (Doody & Doody, 2012).
4. **Individualized consideration**—provides support and encouragement for followers; offers rewards and recognition to individuals for their unique contributions (Bass & Riggio, 2006; Modassir & Singh, 2008).

Servant Leadership

Servant leadership is both a leadership philosophy and a set of leadership behaviors. First coined by Robert K. Greenleaf in 1970, servant leadership is based on the essential elements of trust, empathy, caring, and focus on others (Greenleaf Center for Servant Leadership, 2013). Greenleaf asserted that great leadership grows out of service and great leaders are servants first (Gersh, 2006). A servant leader shares power and focuses on the growth and well-being of their followers, allowing them to reach their full potential and perform to their highest level. In that, leadership is measured not by the accumulation of exercise of power by one individual at the top of a hierarchy but rather by whether those being served develop as individuals to become more autonomous, independent, wiser, healthier, and likely to become servant leaders themselves. The servant leader can develop an EBP culture and environment by leveraging their rich relationships with individuals in the organization to build teams with strong beliefs in the value and importance of EBP. Because the servant leader is devoted to developing individuals on their teams, servant leaders are uniquely poised to cultivate committed EBP champions who perform at their highest level and encourage others to follow in their pursuit of excellence. Those who are led by servant leaders are proposed to reach their full potential and perform optimally (Greenleaf Center for Servant Leadership, 2013), thus making this theory a good fit for facilitating a culture of EBP. Spears (2010) describes 10 foundational characteristics that are central to servant leadership:

1. **Listening**—consistently listens intently and carefully to others
2. **Empathy**—values individuals for their unique characteristics and contributions; seeks to understand and empathize with their followers
3. **Healing**—helps others to solve problems and conflicts in relationships, which supports and promotes the personal growth of their followers
4. **Awareness**—views situations from a holistic standpoint, which allows awareness and better understanding of issues surrounding ethics, power, and values
5. **Persuasion**—effectively builds consensus among followers and relies on persuasion, rather than power by authority, to influence others and achieve organizational goals
6. **Conceptualization**—sees beyond the limits of the operating business and focuses on long-term goals
7. **Foresight**—learns from the past to understand the present and identify consequences of decisions for the future
8. **Stewardship**—serves the needs of others; stresses the use of openness and persuasion, rather than control
9. **Commitment to the growth of people**—is dedicated to the personal, professional, and spiritual growth and development of each individual
10. **Building community**—develops a true community among businesses

Authentic Leadership

Authentic leaders are described as individuals who are confident, hopeful, optimistic, resilient, transparent, and possess high moral character. These leaders demonstrate self-awareness; they are aware of how they think and behave. They have a keen sense of who they are and where they stand on issues, values, and beliefs (Wong & Cummings, 2009).

Authentic leaders are role models and focus on the ethical and right thing to do. The development of others is a priority, and they work to ensure that their communication is transparent and comprehended as intended (Wong & Cummings, 2009). Followers perceive them as having an intense awareness of their own and others values, moral perspectives, knowledge, and strengths (Avolio, Gardner, Walumbwa, Luthans, & May, 2004). Authentic leaders are able to create and sustain high-quality relationships with their followers via personal identification, which results in enhanced engagement, increased motivation, commitment, and job satisfaction (Avolio et al., 2004; Wong & Laschinger, 2013). The authentic leader is uniquely poised to lead the transition to an EBP culture through role modeling of EBP, engaging and motivating their teams to adopt best practices, and enthusiastically celebrating delivery of the best and most ethical care possible for patients.

Authentic leaders are able to build trust and healthier work environments through four types of behaviors, including balanced processing, internalized moral perspective, relational transparency, and self-awareness (Avolio et al., 2004; Walumbwa, Peterson, Avolio, & Hartnell, 2010; Wong & Cummings, 2009). These core behaviors resonate with competencies to promote, build, and sustain a culture of EBP.

- **Balanced processing**—objectively analyzes data to formulate decisions; solicits views that may challenge traditional ideas to come to a conclusion; possesses the capability for accurate self-assessment; and can act on these assessments without being diverted by self-protective intentions (Bamford, Wong, & Laschinger, 2013; Wong & Laschinger, 2013)
- **Internalized moral perspective**—role models high standards for moral and ethical conduct (Wong & Laschinger, 2013)
- **Relational transparency**—presents their genuine self to their followers; shares values, emotions, and goals in a transparent manner that encourages followers to be forthcoming with their ideas and opinions (Bamford et al., 2013; Wong & Laschinger, 2013); strives to achieve trust by listening to and accepting others' opinions and views and acting on recommendations (Wong & Cummings, 2009)
- **Self-awareness**—understands their own unique talents, beliefs, and desires (Wong & Cummings, 2009); uses knowledge of self to enhance leadership effectiveness (Walumbwa et al., 2010)

UNIQUE ROLE OF LEADERS IN CHANGING THE EBP PARADIGM

Healthcare leaders must leverage their power and positions within organizational hierarchies to create organizations that are ready to integrate and sustain EBP. They must have a clear understanding of EBP and implementation strategies (Guerrero et al., 2016). In addition, leaders must be knowledgeable about the current barriers and facilitators of EBP that clinicians articulate/face (Melnyk et al., 2012) and acknowledge that they have control over multiple aspects of them. Healthcare leaders must find ways to eliminate persistent barriers and advocate for clinicians to have the time, resources, and support to implement EBP. Leaders must remain tenacious and steadfast in EBP implementation despite the challenges posed (Guerrero et al., 2016). They must create and sustain work environments where the resources that clinicians need to implement EBP and provide best patient care are a reality of daily practice. Today's leaders must never forget how important it is to create a team vision for EBP and to help all members of the team stay focused on and excited about the vision; doing so will help prevent change fatigue. Some of the EBP barriers that healthcare leaders can address easily within their scope of authority and responsibility include the following:

- Arranging EBP education/skill-building opportunities so that clinicians meet the EBP competencies
- Prioritizing operational budgets to include EBP resources

- Revamping job descriptions and performance evaluation tools to reflect EBP expectations
- Integrating EBP deliverables into clinical ladder requirements
- Rewriting the organizational vision and mission statement with clear EBP language included
- Reorganizing traditional reporting structures to better align the organization with the EBP paradigm
- Creating dedicated EBP mentor positions into which individuals are hired who have robust EBP knowledge and skills in the steps of EBP as well as individual behavior and organizational change theory

There are other barriers to EBP that are more challenging for healthcare leaders to address. However, it is imperative that they be faced and addressed. Some of these barriers include allotting more time for clinicians to implement EBP and assuring that managers and leaders support EBP activities. Examples of strategies to address barriers to implementing and sustaining a culture of EBP are shown in Table 12.1.

TABLE 12.1	*Leadership Strategies to Overcome Barriers to EBP*	
Strategy	**Activities**	**Measures**
EBP education and skills building	• Develop EBP content and skill-building programs targeted to clinicians at various levels of practice including staff, managers, and directors • Include EBP content and the EBP competencies in onboarding/orientation and residency programs designed for new hires	• Number of education programs developed with outcomes • Number of education programs delivered • Number of new hires oriented to EBP content • EBP knowledge, beliefs, and implementation scores (pre/post) for all groups
Operational budgets for EBP resources	• Purchase computers dedicated for EBP work • Allot/budget time for EBP project work	• Number of dedicated EBP workstations • Number of hours allotted per EBP project reported with EBP project outcomes
Library services support	• Access to library with adequate clinical databases and journals available • Support from librarians knowledgeable in EBP steps and processes	• Number of databases available • Number of journals available • Number of librarian referrals • Number of librarian searches provided to staff
Job descriptions and performance evaluation tools	• Write or revise job descriptions with EBP competencies/expectations articulated • Write or revise performance appraisal tools with EBP outcomes/deliverables articulated	• Revised staff job descriptions • Revised staff performance appraisal tools
Clinical ladder requirements	• Write or rewrite clinical ladder application with progressive EBP requirements at each level	• New clinical ladder with EBP requirements for each level

TABLE 12.1	Leadership Strategies to Overcome Barriers to EBP (continued)	
Strategy	**Activities**	**Measures**
Organizational vision, mission, and values statements	• Write or rewrite organizational and departmental vision, mission, and values statements with EBP language integrated • Engage the team in the vision and mission and keep them focused on and excited about it	• Organizational mission, vision, and values statements written with EBP language integrated • Number of departmental mission, vision, and values statements written with EBP language integrated
EBP mentors aligned within the organization	• Develop a cadre of EBP mentors centrally within the organization to work with point-of-care clinicians to implement EBP and to promote, support, and sustain a unified message and vision of EBP • Designate a dedicated, knowledgeable EBP leader to oversee EBP mentors and activities and to help create and inspire the EBP culture	• EBP mentors reporting to a centralized leader • Organizational chart reflecting centralized EBP structure • Knowledgeable EBP leader designated
EBP mentor positions	• Create designated EBP mentor positions with specific job descriptions • Align EBP mentors centrally in the organization • Hire individuals with robust knowledge and skills in the steps of EBP as well as in individual behavior and organizational change theory to fill EBP mentor positions	• EBP mentor job description created • % of EBP mentor positions filled
Manager and leader accountability	• Write or rewrite leadership job descriptions with EBP expectations articulated • Write or revise performance appraisal tools with EBP outcomes/deliverables required	• Revised leadership job descriptions • Revised leadership performance appraisal tools

EBP, evidence-based practice.

In addition, healthcare leaders need to design spaces and systems that promote EBP at the bedside, justify positions that support EBP in their personnel budgets, and provide a professional practice work environment where clinicians have autonomy and control over their practices. Regardless of how difficult these challenges may be, it is the ethical and professional responsibility of healthcare leaders to enact bold actions to promote the EBP shift in healthcare to assure best practices and, ultimately, best care for patients. Finally, healthcare leaders must use best evidence in making their own leadership decisions, thereby modeling EBP behaviors, making the best decisions possible, and providing the best practice environment and culture for their staff and patients.

Adams and Erickson (2011) have explored the definition and scope of influence related to nursing leadership. In their work, influence is framed as "critical to chief nursing executives" and posited as a nurse leader competency (p. 186). In addition, the AONE (2015) has included influence as an essential component of nurse executive competency and the ANA identifies influence in its nurse administrator *Scope and Standards for Nursing Administration* (ANA, 2015). Adams and Erickson also state that, although healthcare leaders recognize the importance of influence related to affecting change in their organizations, they are not "familiar with how influence is acquired, enhanced, and strategically applied" (p. 186). The *Adams Influence Model* (AIM) is a framework designed to promote understanding of the factors, attributes, and process of influence and it is intended for use by healthcare leaders "as a guide to maximizing their individual influence and that of the profession" (Adams & Erickson, 2011, p. 186). The AIM recognizes that the healthcare leader's influence in a given situation is a combination of their individual influence characteristics such as authority, communication style, and knowledge as well as the particular situation being addressed. The model posits that, beyond the personal influence attributes of the leader, interpersonal and social system characteristics are interrelated and affect the leader's level of influence. The AIM model was conceptualized to provide a systematic tool for nurse executives to "consider when developing an influence strategy" (Adams & Erickson, 2011, p. 187) and, as such, is an excellent tool for healthcare leaders. The application of this or similar frameworks can help healthcare leaders build, assess, and enhance their personal influence capacity to positively influence their staff and their organizations, both in a general sense and as it relates to the shift toward an EBP paradigm. Having a better understanding of their influence and power will enable nurse executives to more effectively promote and sustain EBP. Leaders in healthcare are uniquely poised and directly responsible to implement evidence-based leadership and influence their organizations to promote best care and deliver best outcomes. By embracing and supporting EBP, leaders make a conscientious and active choice to achieve these goals.

EVIDENCE-BASED PRACTICE COMPETENCIES AS A KEY STRATEGY FOR SUSTAINING EVIDENCE-BASED CARE

Competencies are used across a variety of health professions as a mechanism for clinicians to provide high-quality safe care. The measurement of competencies related to various patient care activities is a standard ongoing activity in a multitude of healthcare organizations across the nation. For example, general competencies for nursing have been developed by the Quality and Safety Education for Nurses (QSEN) Project, which is a global nursing initiative whose purpose was to develop competencies that would "prepare future nurses who would have the knowledge, skills and attitudes necessary to continuously improve the quality and safety of the healthcare systems within which they work" (Quality and Safety Education for Nurses, 2013). This project has developed six QSEN competencies that address the following practice issues, including

1. patient-centered care,
2. teamwork and collaboration,
3. EBP,
4. quality improvement,
5. safety, and
6. informatics.

Leaders must foster these competencies and encourage interprofessional teamwork because research has supported its positive impact on care and patient outcomes.

Through a consensus-building process by a panel of seven national experts who developed an initial set of EBP competencies for practicing registered nurses (RNs) and APNs followed by two rounds of a Delphi survey with 80 EBP mentors across the United States to establish consensus, a final set of 24 competencies for practicing RNs and APNs in real-world healthcare settings now exists (Melnyk et al., 2014). See Chapter 11 for a full description of how the competencies were developed and for the list of the final competencies. Leaders should incorporate these EBP competencies into healthcare system expectations, orientation programs for new clinicians, performance appraisals, and job descriptions. These competencies also can be used for clinical ladder promotions processes in order to drive higher quality, reliability, and consistency of healthcare as well as to reduce costs.

In summary, healthcare leaders must take an evidence-based approach to decision making in their organizations and provide resources that will support EBP in their clinicians. In addition, they must create cultures and environments in which clinicians can implement and sustain EBP for the ultimate purpose of improving healthcare quality and patient outcomes as well as reducing costs. Creating a vision, mission, and goals for the organization that include EBP along with adopting the EBP competencies and incorporating them into role expectations and job performance requirements will communicate high prioritization of EBP within the institution and result in positive outcomes for both the organization and the patients who are served.

EBP FAST FACTS

- In order for clinicians to change their behavior and consistently implement EBP, a multitude of interventions are necessary, including EBP education combined with active repetitive skills building; EBP mentorship or facilitation and support; a culture and an environment that supports EBP; leaders and managers who support and role model EBP; and evidence-based strategies to overcome system barriers.
- Leaders in healthcare systems must engage in evidence-based leadership, which is a problem-solving approach to leading and influencing organizations or groups to achieve a common goal that integrates the conscientious use of best evidence with leadership expertise and stakeholders' preferences and values.
- Leaders in healthcare organizations must role model evidence-based decision making if they expect their staff to consistently deliver evidence-based care.
- Leaders must create and sustain work cultures and environments where the resources clinicians need to implement EBP and provide best patient care are a reality of daily practice.
- Incorporation of the EBP competencies into role performance expectations, evaluations, and clinical ladder systems is essential in creating and sustaining an evidence-based organization.

WANT TO KNOW MORE?

A variety of resources are available to enhance your learning and understanding of this chapter.

- Visit thePoint° to access:
  - Articles from the AJN EBP Step-By-Step Series
  - Journal articles
  - Checklists for rapid critical appraisal and more!

- Lippincott CoursePoint combines digital text content with video case studies and interactive modules for a fully integrated course solution that works the way you study and learn.

References

Adams, J. M., & Erickson, J. I. (2011). Applying the Adams influence model in nurse executive practice. *The Journal of Nursing Administration, 41*, 186–192.

American Nurses Association. (2015). *Code of ethics for nurses with interpretive statements.* Silver Spring, MD: nursesbooks.org

American Nurses Association. (2016). *Nursing: Scope and standards of practice* (2nd ed.). Silver Springs, MD: Author.

American Nurses Credentialing Center. (2011). *The magnet model components and sources of evidence: Magnet recognition program.* Silver Springs, MD: Author.

American Organization of Nurse Executives. (2015). *AONE Nurse Executive Competencies.* Chicago, IL: Author. Retrieved from http://www.aone.org/resources/nurse-leader-competencies.shtml

Avolio, B., Gardner, W., Walumbwa, F., Luthans, F., & May, D. (2004). Unlocking the mask: A look at the process by which authentic leaders impact follower attitudes and behaviors. *The Leadership Quarterly, 15*, 801–823.

Bamford, M., Wong, C. A., & Laschinger, H. (2013). The influence of authentic leadership and areas of worklife on work engagement of registered nurses. *Journal of Nursing Management, 21*, 529–540.

Barker, A. M., Sullivan, D. T., & Emery, M. J. (2006). *Leadership competencies for clinical managers: The renaissance of transformational leadership.* Sudbury, MA: Jones and Bartlett Learning.

Bass, B., & Avolio, B. (1993). Transformational leadership and organizational culture. *Public Administration Quarterly, 17*(1), 112–121.

Bass, B. M., & Riggio, R. E. (2006). *Transformational leadership* (2nd ed.). New York, NY: Psychology Press.

Beckette, M., Quiter, E., Ryan, G., Berrebi, C., Taylor, S., Cho, M., … Kahn, K. (2011). Bridging the gap between basic science and clinical practice: The role of organizations in addressing clinician barriers. *Implementation Science, 6*(1), 35. doi:10.1186/1748-5908-6-35

Bennett, S., Allen, S., Caldwell, E., Whitehead, M., Turpin, M., Flemming, J., & Cox, R. (2016). *Australian Occupational Therapy Journal, 63*, 9–18.

Bennis, W. (1991). Managing the dream: Leadership in the 21st century. *The Antioch Review, 49*(1), 22.

Doody, O., & Doody, C. M. (2012). Transformational leadership in nursing practice. *British Journal of Nursing, 21*(20), 1212–1218.

Dopson, S., FitzGerald, L., Ferlie, E., Gabbay, J., & Locock, L. (2002). No magic targets! Changing clinical practice to become more evidence based. *Healthcare Management Review, 27*(3), 35–47.

Fleizer, A., Semenic, S. Ritchie, J., Richer, M.-C., & Denis, J.-L. (2016). Nursing unit leaders' influence on the long-term sustainability of evidence-based practice improvements. *Journal of Nursing Management, 24*, 309–318.

Gerrish, K., & Clayton, J. (2004). Promoting evidence based practice: An organizational approach. *Journal of Nursing Management, 12*, 114–123.

Gersh, M. R. (2006). Servant-leadership: A philosophical foundation for professionalism in physical therapy. *Journal of Physical Therapy Education, 20*(2), 12.

Gibbons, P. (2015). *The science of successful organizational change. How leaders set strategy, change behavior, and create an agile culture.* New York, NY: Pearson Education.

Greenleaf Center for Servant Leadership. (2013). Retrieved from http://www.greenleaf.org

Guerrero, E., Padwa, H., Fenwick, K., Harris, L., & Aarons, G. (2016). Identifying and ranking implicit leadership strategies to promote evidence-based practice implementation in addiction health services. *Implementation Science, 11*(69), 1–13.

Hutchinson, A., & Johnston, L. (2004). Bridging the divide: A survey of nurses' opinions regarding barriers to, and facilitators of, research utilization in the practice setting. *Journal of Clinical Nursing, 13*, 304–315.

Klainberg, M., & Dirschel, K. (Eds.). (2010). *Today's nursing leader: Managing, succeeding, excelling.* Sudbury, MA: Jones and Bartlett Learning.

Kotter, J. (2013). *Management is (still) not leadership.* Retrieved from http://blogs.hbr.org/kotter/2013/01/management-is-still-not-leadership.html

Leader. (n.d.). In *dictionary.reference.com online dictionary.* http://www.dictionary.com/browse/leader?s=t

Lunenburg, F. C. (2011). Leadership versus management: A key distinction—at least in theory. *International Journal of Management, Business, and Administration, 14*(1), 1–4.

Malloch, K. (2010). Innovation Leadership: New perspectives for new work. *Nursing Clinics of North America, 45*, 1–9.

Malloch, K., & Porter-O'Grady, T. (2009). *Introduction to evidence-based practice in nursing and healthcare.* Sudbury, MA: Jones and Bartlett.

Melnyk, B. M. (2016). Culture eats strategy every time: What works in building and sustaining an evidence-based practice culture in healthcare systems. *Worldviews on Evidence-Based Nursing, 13*(2), 99–101.

Melnyk, B. M., Fineout-Overholt, E., Fischbeck Feinstein, N., Li, H., Small, L., Wilcox, L., & Kraus, R. (2004). Nurses perceived knowledge, beliefs, skills, and needs regarding evidence based practice: Implications for accelerating the paradigm shift. *Worldviews on Evidence-Based Nursing, 1*, 185–193.

Melnyk, B. M., Fineout-Overholt, E., Gallagher-Ford, L., & Kaplan, L. (2011). The state of evidence-based practice in U.S. nurses: Critical implications for nurse leaders and educators. *Journal of Nursing Administration, 42*(9), 410–417.

Melnyk, B. M., Fineout-Overholt, E., Gallagher-Ford, L., & Kaplan, L. (2012). The state of evidence-based practice in US nurses: critical implications for nurse leaders and educators. *Journal of Nursing Administration, 42*(9), 410–417.

Melnyk, B. M., Fineout-Overholt, E., Giggleman, M., & Choy, K. (2017). A test of the ARCC© model improves implementation of evidence-based practice, healthcare culture, and patient outcomes. *Worldviews on Evidence-Based Nursing, 14*(1), 5–9.

Melnyk, B. M., Fineout-Overholt, E., & Mays, M. Z. (2008). The evidence-based practice beliefs and implementation scales: Psychometric properties of two new scales. *Worldviews on Evidence-Based Nursing, 5*, 208–216. doi:10.1111/j.1741-6787.2008.00126.x

Melnyk, B. M., Gallagher-Ford, & Fineout-Overholt, E. (2017). *Implementing the EBP competencies in healthcare; a practical guide for improving quality, safety and outcomes.* Indianapolis, IN: Sigma Theta Tau International.

Melnyk, B. M., Gallagher-Ford, L., Long, L. A., & Fineout-Overholt, E. (2014). The establishment of evidence-based practice competencies for practicing registered nurses and advanced practice nurses in real world clinical settings: Proficiencies to improve healthcare quality, reliability, patient outcomes and costs. *Worldviews on Evidence-Based Nursing, 11*(1), 5–15. doi:10.1111/wvn.12021

Melnyk, B. M., Grossman, D. C., Chou, R., Mabry-Hernandez, I., Nicholson, W., Dewitt, T. G., ... US Preventive Services Task Force. (2012). USPSTF perspective on evidence-based preventive recommendations for children. *Pediatrics, 130*(2), e399–e407.

Modassir, A., & Singh, T. (2008). Relationship of emotional intelligence with transformational leadership and organizational citizenship behavior. *International Journal of Leadership Studies, 4*(1), 3–21.

Porter-O'Grady, T., & Malloch, K. (2010). *Quantum leadership; Advancing innovation, transforming healthcare.* Sudbury, MA: Jones and Bartlett.

Pravikoff, D. S., Tanner, A. B., & Pierce, S. T. (2005). Readiness of U.S. nurses for evidence-based practice. *American Journal of Nursing, 105*(9), 40–51.

Pryse, Y., McDaniel, A., & Schafer, J. (2014). Psychometric analysis of two new scales: the evidence-based practice nursing leadership and work environment scales. *Worldviews on Evidence-Based Nursing, 11*(4), 240–247.

Quality and Safety Education for Nurses. (2013). Retrieved from http://qsen.org/about-qsen/project-overview/

Ryan, R., Harris, K., Mattox, L., Camp, M., & Shirey, M. (2015). Nursing leader collaboration to drive quality improvement and implementation science. *Nursing Administration Quarterly, 39*(3), 229–238.

Rycroft-Malone, J. (2004). The PARIHS framework: A framework for guiding the implementation of evidence-based practice. *Journal of Nursing Care Quality, 19*(4), 297–304.

Rycroft-Malone, J. (2008). Evidence-informed practice: From individual to context. *Journal of Nursing Management, 16*, 404–408.

Rycroft-Malone, J., Harvey, G., Seers, K., Kitson, A., McCormack, B., & Titchen, A. (2004). An exploration of the factors that influence the implementation of evidence into practice. *Journal of Clinical Nursing, 13*, 913–924.

Sandström, B., Borglin, G., Nilsson, R., & Willman, A. (2011). Promoting the implementation of evidence-based practice: A literature review focusing on the role of nursing leadership. *Worldviews on Evidence-Based Nursing, 8*(4), 212–223. doi:10.1111/j.1741-6787.2011.00216.x

Spears, L. (2010). Character and servant leadership: Ten characteristics of effective, caring leaders. *The Journal of Virtues and Leadership, 1*(1), 25–30.

Spiva, L., Hart, P. L., Patrick, S., Waggoner, J., Jackson, C., & Threatt, J. L. (2017). Effectiveness of an evidence-based practice nurse mentor training program. *Worldviews on Evidence-Based Nursing, 14*(3), 183–191.

Walumbwa, F. O., Peterson, S. J., Avolio, B. J., & Hartnell, C. A. (2010). An investigation of the relationships among leader and follower psychological capital, service climate, and job performance. *Personnel Psychology, 63*(4), 937–963.

Wong, C., & Cummings, G. (2009). Authentic leadership: A new theory for nursing or back to basics? *Journal of Health Organization and Management, 23*(5), 522–538.

Wong, C., & Laschinger, H. (2013). Authentic leadership, performance, and job satisfaction: The mediating role of empowerment. *Journal of Advanced Nursing, 69*(4), 947–959. doi:10.1111/j.1365-2648.2012.06089

A SUCCESS STORY

Improving Outcomes for Depressed Adolescents With the Brief Cognitive Behavioral COPE Intervention Delivered in 30-Minute Outpatient Visits

Pamela Lusk, DNP, RN, PMHNP-BC

STEP 0 — The Spirit of Inquiry Ignited

Major depressive disorder is a treatable medical illness. Despite a prevalence of 12.8% of the U.S. population aged 12 to 17 years (SAMHSA, 2016) with major depressive disorder or depressive symptoms that impair their functioning, less than 25% of depressed adolescents receive the evidence-based treatment they need. In outpatient mental health settings, advanced practice psychiatric nurses conduct comprehensive psychiatric evaluations with adolescents; spend time learning about their strengths, symptoms, and struggles; and establish and implement treatment plans. For teens with symptoms of depression, their day-to-day life can be a painful struggle. Typically, parents come to the practice feeling helpless and wanting the best most active treatment to help their child feel less depressed and function better. We, as psychiatric advanced practice registered nurses (APRNs), know that the most robust treatment for depression in adolescents involves psychotherapy (which historically has been in 50-minute "hours") and medication (if indicated). Many psychiatric APRNs now practice in settings where there has been a shift to brief 20- to 30-minute medication visits with patients, because of agency requirements to see an increasing number of patients each work day. APRNs are expected to adhere to the clinic schedule while providing the best evidence-based care to our young patients. Often we do not know how to bridge the gap between what the research indicates is best practice for treatment of depression in teens and what is happening in practice. This led me to wonder about whether it would be possible to deliver evidence-based cognitive behavioral therapy (CBT) and improve treatment outcomes for depressed adolescents within the limitation of 30-minute medication evaluation appointments. I needed to use the evidence-based practice (EBP) process to find out.

STEP 1 — The PICOT Question Formulated

In depressed adolescents (P), how does CBT (I) compared to other psychotherapy interventions (C) improve depressive symptoms (O) over a 3-month period (T)?

STEP 2 — Search Strategy Conducted

The Cochrane Database of Systematic Reviews (CDSR) was searched first with the keywords adolescent, depression, treatment effectiveness evaluation, and psychotherapy. A systematic review by Watanabe, Hunot, Omori, Churchill, and Farukawa (2007) was found that reviewed studies of psychotherapy effectiveness for children and adolescents with depression. Next, MEDLINE, PsycINFO, and Cumulative Index to Nursing and Allied Health Literature (CINAHL) were searched using the same keywords. The search also included the National Guidelines Clearinghouse for practice guidelines to treat depression in adolescents (Cheung et al., 2007). Both level I and level II evidence studies (Melnyk & Fineout-Overholt, 2014) were found in the search process.

STEP 3 Critical Appraisal of the Evidence Performed

Rapid critical appraisal checklists were used to evaluate the validity, reliability, and applicability to practice (Melnyk & Fineout-Overholt, 2015) for each of the studies found from the search. The systematic review by Watanabe et al. (2007) supported CBT and interpersonal psychotherapy as effective treatments for adolescents with depression. In the search of PsycINFO and other databases, several meta-analyses of randomized controlled trials (RCTs), including one conducted by McCarty and Weisz (2007), supported CBT as an effective treatment for depressed adolescents. One of the RCTs, The Treatment of Adolescent Depression Study (TADS) by March, Hilgenberg, Silva, and TADS Team (2007), was a landmark 13-site RCT that compared (1) CBT, (2) placebo, (3) antidepressant medication (fluoxetine), and (4) a combination of fluoxetine and CBT. The study determined the superior effectiveness of the combination of CBT and fluoxetine in the acute and continuation treatment of adolescent major depression.

The **level I evidence**, the strongest level of evidence to guide practice, found a systematic review and a meta-analysis of RCTs that tested the efficacy of CBT for adolescent depression. Level II evidence was also found in the TADS RCT, which is the strongest study design for controlling extraneous or confounding variables (Melnyk & Fineout-Overholt, 2011) and supported that CBT is a very efficacious treatment for adolescent depression. In the studies included in the meta-analysis, individual CBT sessions were 60 minutes long. Group CBT programs for adolescents were also included in the meta-analysis.

Cited CBT treatment manuals for depressed adolescents in the studies were reviewed for their applicability to brief sessions. In these treatment manuals, the authors recommended individual CBT sessions of 60 minutes duration. For this project, a CBT-based intervention entitled Creating Opportunities for Personal Empowerment (COPE; Melnyk, 2003) was selected because it included all of the components identified in the literature that comprise effective CBT interventions for depressed adolescents. The manual for each of the seven COPE sessions is concise, and the COPE intervention is usable in 30-minute sessions. The seven CBT-based skill-building sessions in COPE had been previously embedded into a 15-session healthy lifestyle intervention for adolescents that was delivered in required high school health courses, but it had not yet been evaluated in a community health setting (Melnyk et al., 2007, 2009). Therefore, the purpose of this EBP change project was to implement and evaluate the outcomes of delivering COPE to teens in a community mental health clinic.

STEP 4 Evidence Integrated With Clinical Expertise and Patient Preferences to Inform a Decision and Practice Change Implemented

The plan for this project based on the evidence found was to translate evidence-based CBT into brief 30-minute sessions and assess its feasibility and outcomes with 12- to 17-year-old clinically depressed adolescents treated at a community mental health center in a small, rural town in the southwestern United States.

When adolescents are seen in community mental health practices and diagnosed with moderate to severe depression, the usual treatment is antidepressant medication. Antidepressants are an effective treatment to relieve symptoms of depression, but the evidence strongly supports the combination of antidepressant medication and CBT as the most effective treatment plan. In terms of patient preferences and values, many parents who bring their adolescents for treatment do not want medication as part of the treatment plan. However, some families feel that pharmacologic treatment will provide the most rapid relief for their child's depressive symptoms. The advanced practice psychiatric nurse, with education and skills in both psychotherapy and pharmacology, can provide evidence from current literature and her own practice and encourage parents and teens to share experiences, concerns, and questions related to the acceptability of various treatment options. It is helpful to provide the families with written handouts to take home, such as the American Academy of Pediatrics' (AAP) "Evidence-based Child and Adolescent Psychosocial Interventions" (2011, revised 2012, 2017-2018) PDF handout. Together, the advanced practice nurse and the family can establish a mutually agreed upon treatment plan. With the implementation of this project, informed consents by parents and teen assents were signed. None of the families seen for initial psychiatric evaluation of their adolescent declined the COPE cognitive behavioral skills building intervention when it was explained, reviewed, and offered as an option.

A pre- and postintervention outcomes evaluation was used. Fifteen adolescents aged 12 to 17 years, who came for intake to the community mental health center and presented with significant depression, were enrolled in the project. All of the adolescents, along with their parents, agreed to receive COPE, which was presented in seven 30-minute sessions scheduled at weekly intervals. They also agreed to fill out project-related outcome measures both before and after the COPE seven-session intervention. The measures included the Beck Youth Inventory, which has five subscales (anxiety, anger, depression, self-concept, and destructive behavior), a personal beliefs scale, a COPE content quiz, and a form that asked for demographic data about the teen and family. The parents and teens were both given post-COPE evaluation forms to fill out anonymously to provide feedback regarding their experiences with the COPE intervention.

STEP 5 — Outcomes Evaluated

All 15 teens enrolled completed all seven sessions of COPE. Adolescents reported significant decreases in depression, anxiety, anger, and destructive behavior as well as increases in self-concept and personal beliefs about managing negative emotions (Lusk & Melnyk, 2011a). Evaluations indicated that COPE was a positive experience for teens and parents (Lusk & Melnyk, 2011b). It was concluded that COPE is a promising brief CBT-based intervention that can be delivered within 30-minute individual outpatient visits. With this intervention, advanced practice nurses can work within busy outpatient practice time constraints and still provide evidence-based treatment for the depressed teens they manage.

STEP 6 — Project Outcomes Successfully Disseminated

This project was presented at national conferences and was published. The COPE intervention is now standard practice for treating depressed and anxious teens. Other psychiatric and pediatric advanced practice nurses in community mental health and pediatric primary care settings as well as schools across the country are now being trained in using COPE to prevent and treat depressed and anxious adolescents. Further studies and evaluation projects have continued to show positive outcomes with the cognitive behavioral skills building COPE intervention, including decreases in depression, suicidal ideation, and anxiety; improvements in self-esteem; and increases in healthy lifestyle behaviors (Hart, Lusk, Hovermale, & Melnyk, 2018; Hickman, Jacobson, & Melnyk, 2014; Kozlowski, Lusk, & Melnyk, 2015; Melnyk et al., 2013, 2015; Melnyk, Kelly, Jacobson, Arcoleo, & Shaibi, 2013; Melnyk, Kelly, & Lusk, 2014; Ritchie, 2011). A recent study published in the AAP journal *Pediatrics* (Dickerson et al., 2018) showed that a CBT delivered in a primary care setting is a cost-effective way to treat adolescents with depression declining antidepressants and the CBT intervention can be brief and still deliver long-term benefits in terms of cost and clinical outcomes. The COPE intervention is increasingly being used in schools and colleges as well as primary care clinics to assist *all* youth who are coping with current life stressors.

References

American Academy of Pediatrics. (Revised 2012, 2017-2018). *Addressing Mental Health Concerns in Primary Care: A Clinicians Toolkit.*

American Academy of Pediatrics. (2018). *Evidence-based child and adolescent psychosocial interventions.* Retrieved from https://www.aap.org/en-us/Documents/CRPsychosocialInterventions.pdf

Cheung, A., Zuckerbrot, R., Jensen, P., Ghalib, K., Laraque, D., & Stein, R. (2007). Guidelines for adolescent depression in primary care (GLAD-PC): II. Treatment and ongoing management. *Pediatrics, 120*(5), 131.

Dickerson, J., Lynch, F., Leo, M., Debar, L., Pearson, J., & Clarke, G. (2018). Cost-effectiveness of cognitive behavioral therapy for depressed youth declining antidepressants. *Pediatrics, 141*(2), 42. doi:10.1542/peds.2017-1969

Hart, B., Lusk, P., Hovermale, R., & Melnyk, B. M. (2018). Decreasing depression and anxiety in college youth using the Creating Opportunities for Personal Empowerment Program (COPE). *Journal of the American Psychiatric Nurses Association.* doi:10.1177/1078390318779205

Hickman, C., Jacobson, D., & Melnyk, B. M. (2014). Randomized controlled trial of the acceptability, feasibility, and preliminary effects of a cognitive behavioral skills building intervention in adolescents with chronic daily headaches: A pilot study. *Journal of Pediatric Health Care, 29*(1), 5–16.

Kozlowski, J., Lusk, P., & Melnyk, B. M. (2015). Pediatric nurse practitioner management of child anxiety in the rural primary care clinic with the evidence-based COPE. *Journal of Pediatric Health Care, 29*(3), 274–282.

Lusk, P., & Melnyk, B. M. (2011a). The brief cognitive-behavioral COPE intervention for depressed adolescents: Outcomes and feasibility of delivery in 30-minute outpatient visits. *Journal of the American Psychiatric Nurses Association, 17*(3), 226–236.

Lusk, P., & Melnyk, B. M. (2011b). COPE for the treatment of depressed adolescents: Lessons learned from implementing an evidence-based practice change. *Journal of the American Psychiatric Nurses Association, 17*(4), 297–309.

Majid, S., Foo, S., Luyt, B., Zhang, X., Theng, Y. L., Chang, Y. K., & Mokhtar, I. A. (2011). Adopting evidence-based practice in clinical decision making: Nurses' perceptions, knowledge, and barriers. *Journal of the Medical Library Association, 99*(3), 229–236.

March, J., Hilgenberg, D., Silva, S., & TADS Team. (2007). The treatment of adolescents with depression study (TADS): Long term effectiveness and safety outcomes. *Archives of General Psychiatry, 64*(10), 1132–1143.

McCarty, C., & Weisz, J. (2007). Effects of psychotherapy for depression in children and adolescents: What we can (and can't) learn from meta-analysis and component profiling. *Journal of the Academy of Child and Adolescent Psychiatry, 46*(7), 879–886.

Melnyk, B. M. (2003). *COPE (Creating Opportunities for Personal Empowerment) for teens (revised): A 7-session cognitive behavioral skills building program.* Columbus, OH: COPE2Thrive.

Melnyk, B. M., & Fineout-Overholt, E. (2011). *Evidence-based practice in nursing and healthcare: A guide to best practice* (2nd ed.). Philadelphia, PA: Wolters Kluwer/Lippincott Williams & Wilkins.

Melnyk, B. M., & Fineout-Overholt, E. (2014). *Evidence-based practice in nursing and healthcare: A guide to best practice* (3rd ed.). Philadelphia, PA: Wolters Kluwer/Lippincott Williams & Wilkins.

Melnyk, B. M., Jacobson, D., Kelly, S., Belyea, M., Shaibi, G., Small, L., ... Marsiglia, F. F. (2013). Promoting healthy lifestyles in high school adolescents: A randomized controlled trial. *American Journal of Preventive Medicine, 45*(4), 407–415. doi:10.1016/j.amepre.2013.05.013

Melnyk, B. M., Jacobson, D., Kelly, S. A., Belyea, M. J., Shaibi, G. Q., Small, L., ... Marsiglia, F. F. (2015). Twelve-month effects of the COPE healthy lifestyles TEEN program on overweight and depression in high school adolescents. *Journal of School Health, 85*, 861–870.

Melnyk, B. M., Jacobson, D., Kelly, S., O'Haver, J., Small, L., & Mays, M. Z. (2009). Improving the mental health, healthy lifestyle choices and physical health of Hispanic adolescents: A randomized controlled pilot study. *Journal of School Health, 79*(12), 575–584.

Melnyk, B. M., Kelly, S., Jacobson, D., Arcoleo, K., & Shaibi, G. (2013). Improving physical activity, mental health outcomes and academic retention of college students with freshman 5 to thrive: COPE/healthy lifestyles. *Journal of the American Academy of Nurse Practitioner, 26*(6), 314–322.

Melnyk, B. M., Kelly, S., & Lusk, P. (2014). Outcomes and feasibility of a manualized cognitive-behavioral skills building intervention: Group COPE for depressed and anxious adolescents in school settings. *Journal of Child and Adolescent Psychiatric Nursing, 27*(1), 3–13. doi:10.1111/jcap.12058

Melnyk, B. M., Small, L., Morrison-Beedy, D., Strasser, A., Spath, L., Kreipe, R., ... O'Haver, J. (2007). The COPE healthy lifestyles TEEN program: Feasibility, preliminary, efficacy, & lessons learned from an after-school group intervention with overweight adolescents. *Journal of Pediatric Health Care, 21*(5), 315–322.

Ritchie, T. (2011). *Evaluation of the impact of the Creating Opportunity For Personal Empowerment (COPE) healthy lifestyles Thinking, Emotions, Exercise, and Nutrition (TEEN) program in a rural high school health class* (DNP Capstone Project). Morgantown, WV: West Virginia University.

SAMHSA. (2016). *Major depression.* Retrieved from https://www.nimh.nih.gov/health/statistics/major-depression.shtml#part_155033

Watanabe, N., Hunot, V., Omori, I., Churchill, R., & Farukawa, T. (2007). Psychotherapy for depression among children and adolescents: A systematic review. *Acta Psychiatrica Scandinavica, 116*, 84–95.

Creating and Sustaining a Culture and Environment for Evidence-Based Practice

Learning and innovation go hand in hand. The arrogance of success is to think that what you did yesterday will be sufficient for tomorrow.

—William Pollard

EBP Terms to Learn
Complexity science
Context
Critical Thinking
Cybernetic evidence–Innovation
Dynamic
Data driven
EBP mentor
Evidence-based decision making
Facilitators
Fidelity of the evidence-based intervention
Implementation science
Innovation
Organizational culture of EBP
Point-of-care clinicians
Research utilization
SCOT (Strengths, Challenges, Opportunities, and Threats) analysis
Senior (C-Suite) leadership
SMART (Specific, Measurable, Achievable, Relevant, and Time bound) goals
Strategic plan
Triggers

UNIT OBJECTIVES

Upon completion of this unit, learners will be able to:

1. Describe innovation and its relationship to evidence-based practice (EBP).

2. Discuss how EBP models can improve healthcare quality and population health outcomes.

3. Identify barriers to organizational change and strategies to overcome them.

4. Explain a conceptual framework for teaching EBP.

5. Explain the importance of teaching EBP in clinical settings.

6. Discuss the importance of the EBP mentor role to sustainability of an EBP culture.

MAKING CONNECTIONS: AN EBP EXEMPLAR

As the EBP Council considered how to make the evidence implementation successfully sustainable, they reviewed the articles that Scott, the hospital librarian, and Mateo, the staff registered nurse (RN), obtained through interlibrary loan. They also had a couple of articles that DeAndre, the EBP mentor, had discovered. These articles offered insights into both barriers to and facilitators of implementing fall prevention interventions, but were not added to the evaluation table or synthesis tables because the recommendation for best practice had already been put forward. Three recommendations from the Registered Nurses, Association of Ontario (RNAO, 2017) evidence-based guideline, *Preventing Falls and Reducing Injury from Falls*, were implemented as planned on the targeted units to which older adults who were assumed to have low fall risk were admitted: *1.2a: Complete comprehensive fall risk (FRisk) assessment, including multifactorial assessment (p. 11); 5.1: Ensure a safe environment through universal precautions and altering physical environment for safety (p. 14); and 5.3: Implement rounding as a strategy to proactively meet the person's needs and prevent falls (p.14).* The Council also planned to implement the Morse Fall Scale (1989) as the fall risk (FRisk) assessment, because it was the most commonly used FRisk assessment in the synthesized studies, as well as universal precautions (see Box 1). Both were evaluated for ease of use.

The EBP Council discussed how the EBP models that their organization had chosen the previous year would influence the implementation of their initiative. DeAndre reminded them that their decision to adopt two models was key here. The organizational EBP model had already put into place structures and supports to enhance the successful implementation of this initiative. The process model was well familiar to the staff now, so when the initiative was rolled out, they would recognize the steps to evidence implementation.

As the group discussed their implementation plan, they considered the issues surrounding implementation of hourly rounding, as identified by Toole, Meluskey, and Hall (2016), which included the following:

- the burdensomeness of keeping rounding logs
- obtaining and keeping staff buy-in for both project progression and project outcomes
- how to make hourly rounding work with other competing workload priorities
- how to adequately educate and prepare staff for hourly rounding implementation
- issues with how to use or if to use the scripting process for patient engagement in hourly rounding
- issues with certain patient populations and securing leadership support for the impact and sustainment of hourly rounding within the organization.

Although less often cited by researchers, the EBP Council noted that staff did report a lack of value and recognition for their efforts to conduct hourly rounding. As the Council discussed their implementation plan, they addressed each of these issues because they wanted to ensure the success of this important initiative for their patients and families (Goldsack, Cunningham, & Mascioli, 2014; Jackson, 2016).

As the EBP Council discussed resources for educating the interprofessional team who would be implementing the project, they considered their academic partnership with the local nursing and physical therapy programs. They contacted faculty within each of these programs and requested current curricula taught about fall prevention as well as any teaching aids, practice exercises, and knowledge evaluation tools, such

BOX
1

Universal Fall Precautions

- Familiarize the patient with the environment.
- Have the patient demonstrate call light use (CLU).
- Maintain call light within reach.
- Keep the patient's personal possessions within safe reach of the patient.
- Have sturdy handrails in patient bathrooms, room, and hallway.
- Place the hospital bed in low position when a patient is resting in bed; raise bed to a comfortable height when the patient is transferring out of bed.
- Keep hospital bed brakes locked.
- Keep wheelchair's wheel locks in "locked" position when stationary.
- Keep nonslip, comfortable, well-fitting footwear on the patient.
- Use night lights or supplemental lighting.
- Keep floor surfaces clean and dry. Clean up all spills promptly.
- Keep patient care areas uncluttered.
- Follow safe patient handling practices.

Source: Agency for Healthcare Research and Quality (AHRQ). Retrieved from https://www.ahrq.gov/professionals/systems/hospital/fallpxtoolkit/fallpxtk3.html#3-2

as quizzes. They incorporated these resources into their educational plan for the staff. Faculty also provided a conceptual framework for consideration that had learner assimilation of EBP as a primary goal, which fitted the Council's goals as well. They were thankful for the faculty guidance and the framework as it helped them to consider the completeness of their educational approach and evaluate its effectiveness.

The Council formed a subcommittee of educators and staff who focused solely on planning and preparing education about hourly rounding at the hospital for leadership, physicians, nurse practitioners, allied health providers, nursing staff, families, and patients—from initiation to evaluation to dissemination (*Steps 4, 5, and 6 of the EBP process*).

When the Council members were tasked with finding resources for introducing hourly rounding to the organization, they came back with several versions of the *intentional hourly rounding guide* (IHRG) (Meade, Bursell, & Ketelsen, 2006; Morgan et al., 2016; Patterson, 2014). The Council reviewed these resources and compiled their own guide, which included the four Ps, the Morse Fall Scale FRisk assessment, the role of the EBP mentor with contact information, the implementation protocol based on the chosen EBP models for their organization, evaluation markers for outcomes (i.e., project impact), and process indicators to help determine if the project was progressing as expected. One outcome that the EBP Council wanted to evaluate that was not found across the studies, but seemed helpful to their organization, was call light use (CLU). Lei, the project coordinator, and her team put together a plan for evaluating this outcome, with checklists for staff, patients, and families to complete. Because they did not know whether or not this would be a good indicator of fall prevention outcome, they did not make this part of the electronic health record.

DeAndre consulted with Dr. Ayita, the DNP-prepared clinical expert who was the chief quality officer for the organization and the EBP Council's leadership resource, about steps for educating across the board about the background, the plan, the evaluation metrics and process, the recognition plan, and the dissemination plan for the hourly rounding initiative. After the discussion with DeAndre, Dr. Ayita worked with the Council and led the educational plan preparation and delivery, focusing on multiple opportunities for all involved in the project to learn about the IHRG and other resources and mechanisms that were available to reduce barriers to the success of the project.

Lei and the Council members discussed how to ensure that all those involved in the project were recognized for their contributions to its success. They chose to use a bucket as their mechanism for ongoing recognition because it could include patients, families, and all those involved in the care of the patient. Paper buckets were placed on the doors of the unit—one for families, one for patients, and one for personnel. Paper cutouts of water droplets were placed in the waiting room, in the patient rooms, and in the staff break rooms so that everyone could have easy access to them. Housekeeping was tasked with keeping the droplets stocked. As part of the guide, everyone associated with the patient was informed of the recognition plan mechanism and purpose. Staff were asked to initiate the first drop by recognizing families and patients engaging in hourly rounding for their role, such as making needs known.

Dr. Ayita was eager to discuss the recognition initiative with Dr. Reyansh, the nurse scientist for the organization, as Dr. Ayita could not find any evidence that this kind of plan had been part of an hourly rounding implementation. She wanted to explore the idea of conducting a pilot study of this initiative with Dr. Reyansh. In their discussion, they both agreed this was a good idea and began the process of planning the pilot study of the recognition initiative in tandem with the hourly rounding project implementation.

DeAndre helped the Council negotiate with the information technology support team and the finance department to get quarterly reports of the evaluation metrics (i.e., fall rate, CLU, patient satisfaction, and staff satisfaction) and their associated dollars saved so that ongoing evaluation of impact could be discussed. DeAndre asked Dr. Ayita, as a C-suite executive, to come to their Council meeting when the outcomes would be discussed so she could provide administrative perspective on project progress and success, as well as keep communication fluid between staff and leadership. DeAndre and Lei were committed to preserving the return on investment of the Council and worked with Dr. Ayita to secure a portion of the dollars saved by the project to seed future Council evidence-based change initiatives.

Once the plan was put together and the video created that told Sam's story (to share at hospital orientation and with families and patients at risk for falls), the Council, led by DeAndre and Lei, presented the final plan and video to Dr. Ayita for C-Suite executive approval.

Key clinical nurse specialist (CNS) personnel were tagged on each of the target units to be EBP mentors to facilitate the project implementation. They helped staff create posters that highlighted the evidence synthesis and steps of the implementation plan, along with dissemination and discussion of copies of the IHRG. These were placed in the break rooms on each unit. The group of EBP mentors had a timeline and meeting schedule to touch base with DeAndre, Lei, and each other to mark progress indicators and discuss lessons learned and strategies aimed at mitigating challenges encountered with implementation.

The CNS EBP mentors had mapped out their data collection strategy, which was similar to that of the studies, as well as a plan to present these data to the EBP Council and Dr. Ayita on a quarterly basis. As the project progressed, the CNS EBP mentors discovered that the IHRGs were extremely helpful for standardizing the implementation of the initiative. The video of Sam's story was helpful to patients and families as well as staff and ancillary personnel.

During the first quarter of the project, fall rates dropped by a third. During the second and third quarters of project implementation, fall rates dropped to single digits, saving hundreds of thousands of dollars per quarter. In addition, patient satisfaction scores were now at benchmark with national expectations. The CLU outcome was not as informative. Staff, patients, and families forgot to complete the checklists, so the evaluation data were not sufficient. Nonetheless, the project was deemed a success. As Danielle (the nurse who initiated the clinical issue) considered how well Sam's story was received, she decided to write him a note to thank him for the impact he had made on the safety and satisfaction of their patients. The entire EBP Council and Dr. Ayita signed Sam's note, thankful for the opportunity to tell his story and improve care for their patients.

The next step for the EBP Council is to tell others about their project. Join the group at the beginning of Unit 5 as they wind down their EBP journey.

References

Goldsack, J., Cunningham, J., & Mascioli, S. (2014). Patient falls: Searching for the elusive "silver bullet." *Nursing, 7,* 61–62.

Jackson, K. (2016). Improving nursing home falls management program by enhancing standard of care with collaborative care multi-interventional protocol focused on fall prevention. *Journal of Nursing Education and Practice, 6*(6), 85–96.

Meade, C. M., Bursell, A. L., & Ketelsen, L. (2006). Effects of nursing rounds: On patients' call light use, satisfaction, and safety. *American Journal of Nursing, 106*(9), 58–70.

Morgan, L., Flynn, L., Robertson, E., New, S., Forde-Johnston, C., & McCulloch, P. (2017). Intentional rounding: A staff-led quality improvement intervention in the prevention of patient falls. *Journal of Clinical Nursing, 26*(1/2), 115–124.

Morse Fall Scale. (1989). Available from https://www.ahrq.gov/professionals/systems/hospital/fallpxtoolkit/fall-pxtk-tool3h.html

Patterson, L. M. (2014). Preparing staff for intentional rounding: A process yielding success on a general surgical unit. *Journal for Nurses in Professional Development, 30*(1), 16–20.

Registered Nurses' Association of Ontario. (2017). *Preventing falls and reducing injury from falls* (4th ed.). Toronto, ON: Author.

Toole, N., Meluskey, T., & Hall, N. (2016). A systematic review: barriers to hourly rounding. *Journal of Nursing Management, 24,* 283–290.

Innovation and Evidence: A Partnership in Advancing Best Practice and High Quality Care

Kathy Malloch and Timothy Porter-O'Grady

Innovation distinguishes between a leader and a follower.

—Steve Jobs

EBP Terms to Learn
Complexity science
Cybernetic evidence–
 Innovation dynamic
Innovation

Learning Objectives
After studying this chapter, learners will be able to:

1. Describe innovation and its relationship to evidence-based practice (EBP).
2. Understand the dynamics of EBP and innovation.
3. Discuss how leaders affect innovation.
4. Describe factors necessary to facilitate a flourishing culture of innovation.

RELATIONSHIP BETWEEN INNOVATION AND EVIDENCE-BASED PRACTICE

It is often difficult to understand the relationship between evidence and **innovation**. At first glance, it appears as though these concepts are on the opposite end of the continuum. Perhaps this is because good evidence is grounded in "hard" knowledge and research skews our notions of its relationship to innovation, which is considered much more "emergent" and "fluid." However, the truth is that there is a symbiotic relationship between evidence and innovation, one that is dynamic and, at the same time, rigorous and structured. Both innovation (the introduction of something new that promises to challenge existing concepts, practices, or products) and evidence (data obtained from multiple sources from rigorous research to anecdotal information) are essentially related, because innovation frees evidence to alter the trajectory of our practice and evidence disciplines innovation to affirm the validity of practice (Malloch & Porter-O'Grady, 2009).

A fundamental requirement for understanding evidence-based practice (EBP) is that it be seen not so much as a process, but more as a dynamic (Hovmand & Gillespie, 2010). Evidence as a dynamic suggests a high level of fluidity, mobility, and portability. In fact, EBP could simply not exist in a nondigital milieu because the power and capacity of digitalization is an essential requisite to the fluidity and flow that characterizes effective EBP (Malloch & Porter-O'Grady, 2010). The massive aggregation of data and the detailed requirements of analysis and synthesis that provide the foundation for effective choice, decisions, and action is not so much a corollary, but instead, a characteristic of the essential dynamics associated with the complexities of EBP (Schultz, 2009). This sort of evidentiary dynamic represents a mosaic of interacting and interfacing elements and relationships that lead to definitive and replicable patterns of behavior that reflect measures of effectiveness, efficiency, and efficacy (E3) (Porter-O'Grady & Malloch, 2010). At the same time, this evidentiary dynamic lays the floor for good practice, creating the foundations for creativity and innovation. From here, clinicians can stretch to new levels of practice and clinical behavior through use of innovative practices that help them conceive and reach for the "ceiling" of practice excellence.

The challenge in the current healthcare environment is related to continuum-based delivery models, interprofessional collaboration, patient-guided care, supportive cultures for new work, and all the associated chaos and energy provide models to illustrate these complexities. Consider the current efforts to create a continuum-based model of care delivery in response to the mandates of value-based clinical care delivery. Key stakeholders in healthcare systems have recognized the need for increased collaboration, fully integrated system communication, and improved patient engagement in the delivery of healthcare. Working to address the redesign of the healthcare infrastructure is one of the more complex challenges faced by leaders and requires an approach that considers current evidence for effective system performance and then acknowledgment of gaps in knowledge that can be logically and systematically addressed with innovative approaches (Chan & Schaffrath, 2017).

A Cybernetic Dynamic

In order to comprehend the full range of interacting characteristics in this dynamic of evidence (evidentiary dynamics), one must understand the fluid, interacting, and cybernetic (involved with cyclical communication and control) nature of its stages/phases of movement. The concept of continuous and unending movement is critical to the complete comprehension of this evidentiary dynamic informing EBP (Tait & Richardson, 2010). The foundations of good practice are simply not established only to remain constant and changeless. The clinical history of healthcare certainly validates—to its detriment—the health system's addiction to a fixed approach to standards and practices with a procedural and policy approach (Starr, 2011). This model for defining the foundations of practice assumed that such foundations were firm and fixed in time, quite rigid, and, most often, permanent. Good practice, in this format, meant a slavish addiction to the rules and consistently and routinely repeating procedural applications. Certainly, basic rules of good process such as safety checklists, functional protocols, and procedural routines do have significant value in providing safe and effective foundations for clinical routines that require little or no variation and are not subject to the notions of human relationships, culture, and communication. Indeed, more of these would prove a significant value in reducing both risk and resource use (Lorenz, Beyea, & Slattery, 2009). Yet, even these basic and routine mechanics, if informed by insight and innovation, can be altered and radically improved or advanced in ways that could not be anticipated with the same tools and processes that created them. In spite of the often overwhelming challenges of complex changes, it is the reality of the evidence–innovation interface that provide clarity for healthcare leaders. As Sharts-Hopko (2013) noted, tackling complex ("wicked") problems is indeed the nature of much of our work.

The Cybernetic Dynamic and Wicked Problems

Such problems or challenges, described as "any complex issue which defies complete definition and for which there can be no final solution; such problems are diabolical in that they resist the usual attempts to resolve them" (Brown, Harris, & Russell, 2010, p. 302), give life to current realities and guidance as to what can or should be done to address these challenges. To be sure, the complexities of continuum of care planning and integration involve multiple individuals, multiple levels and types of knowledge, varied resources, and the ever-present reality that there is no road map to the future. Although the diabolical label (wicked) seems unusually harsh in the world of caring, it is within the realm of informed professionals not only to overcome such stubborn complexity, but also to thrive in creating systems that are more dynamic, thrive in massive amounts of data in a sophisticated digital world, and skillfully move in new ways to facilitate rather than control health processes.

Complexity Science

An important consideration for reflection is the application drawn from **complexity science**, which suggests for leaders, both clinical and administrative, that understanding the characteristics and nature of the trajectory of action is critical to understanding the connection between evidence and innovation. The trajectory of action is constantly influenced by the ability to observe, analyze, predict, and accommodate the vagaries of the relationship between the external environment and individual and collective action. The wise leader attempts to understand the converging forces between these two environments (external dynamic context and internal responsive behaviors), and create a "goodness of fit" between them that more accurately leads to a viable and sustainable response (Nalipay, Bernardo, & Mordeno, 2016).

Sharts-Hopko (2013) stated that building evidence for practice is as important as creating new healthcare policies, new delivery models, and processes to assure safe and cost-effective care. Multiple initiatives from the Institute of Medicine (IOM, 2001, 2011) drive the need for both evidence and creative approaches to improve the healthcare system specific to the infrastructure, providers, organizational cultures, and management of financial resources.

Translation to the Innovator Role

The evidence-based innovator is both grounded in and respects the discipline of the scientific process. The innovator understands the components of good science and is schooled in both the scientific process and the translational skills that help make its products amenable to guiding practice and behavior (Erickson, Ditomassi, & Adams, 2012). Science is indeed the link between evidence and innovation: the discovery and use of the laws of nature to answer questions about the world in which we live and to invent new solutions to problems (Heilbron, 2003).

At the same time, this innovator recognizes that the products of scientific process simply form the ground on which the innovator stands. The foundations established by good evidence serve as the beginning database of the subsequent creative work of translating, applying, questioning, testing, changing, and adapting. The evidence-based innovator is aware of the constancy and fluidity of the movement and interface between each element of the evidentiary journey. The innovator recognizes that within this dynamic lies the opportunity for new insight, connections, configurations, and collaborations. These, in turn, lead to new ways of seeing, defining, and doing—which can inexorably raise the bar of practice and performance (McCarthy, 2011). Moreover, the innovator is aware that this can be done at any point (gap) or at any phase or stage of the evidence-based process. New insights, information, collaboration, and wisdom can inform the data at any particular point in a way that alters the cascade of subsequent decisions or actions further down the evidence-based levels. The change at any one place along the evidence-based continuum ultimately alters the entire process.

Practice leaders need to be fluid, flexible, portable, and mobile in their own leadership capacity, being role models to these patterns of behavior as their major contribution to creating a culture of innovation. It is difficult to expect that staff can become open, responsive, dynamic, and adaptive in their practice if their leaders are rigid and procedural in the expression of their role (Marshall, 2011). Leaders must first develop a deeper and richer understanding of professional practice, the requisites of collaboration, shared decision making, science-based systems, and the characteristics of a culture of innovation (Cristofoli, Markovic, & Meneguzzo, 2014).

Models of shared governance and leadership have provided structures, processes, and outcomes that support and reinforce professional autonomy. Councils provide forums for nurse engagement and participation in advancing evidence and innovation. Bylaws, policies, and principles in the shared governance model provide direction on how decisions are made. Most importantly, the emphasis is on metrics specific to patient outcomes, nurse satisfaction, and organizational excellence. There are numerous reports and evidence supporting a shared governance model from both qualitative and quantitative perspectives (Rundquist & Givens, 2013).

When examining current shared governance models through an evidence–innovation lens, new opportunities are uncovered. Current shared governance models were never intended to be rigid and procedural; rather, they were intended to be fluid, evidence-driven, and empowering. In light of the changing healthcare environment, traditional approaches to shared governance can now be seen as incomplete for the future. Innovation is needed to advance shared governance models from models focusing on nursing autonomy and ownership to models focusing on interdisciplinary decision making, collaboration, and measurement. The need exists for an infrastructure that meaningfully supports the discussion and debate about full scope of practice not just for one discipline, but for all of the disciplines involved in the clarification, extension, and valuing of changes to role performance (Clavelle, Porter-O'Grady, Weston, & Verran, 2016). Creating divisional level shared governance structures as well as organizational and cross-setting structures can provide more robust frameworks for a system focused on continuum of care services. As multidisciplinary, continuum shared governance structures are created, new evidence and outcome measures will emerge that reflect their value.

A MODEL OF THE CYBERNETIC INNOVATION AND EVIDENCE DYNAMIC

A systematic understanding about the dynamics of EBP and innovation is critical to a scholarly and practical understanding of how evidence changes practice. A rich and detailed description of the characteristics and processes associated with EBP is presented in detail elsewhere in this book. In this chapter, we create an interface between the stages of EBP and the opportunities for innovation embedded in them.

The existence of wide gaps between clinical knowledge and practice is well known and acknowledged (Melnyk & Fineout-Overholt, 2012). In the emerging value-driven healthcare system, it will become increasingly imperative to narrow that gap and provide a relevant intersection among knowledge creation, related research activity, and practice decision making. A systematic and organized approach to knowledge translation application is an essential foundation to build evidentiary processes. In addition, establishing a systematic and cyclical understanding of the cybernetic elements that underpin evidence-based processes is a critical first step to utilizing these processes to establish good decision making and to advance practice (Brown, 2009). Valuable to both scholars and clinicians is the use of a model that links the evidence-based processes within a dynamic and cybernetic context that recognizes and accommodates the environmental, contextual, and complexity issues continuously interfacing and affecting evidence-based processes (evidentiary dynamics) (Curlee & Gordon, 2011). This model must reflect the realities of a fluid interaction between environment, organization, and people in ways that influence priorities, resources, and decisions.

The combined influence of sociopolitical and economic environmental drivers has a constant and continuous influence on strategic direction, priorities, and choices made in health systems, which ultimately influence the character and kind of decisions made in the clinical setting (Kinney, 2011). Such resource allocation priorities help determine what clinical

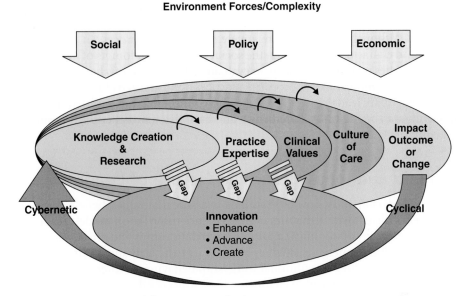

Figure 13.1: Environmental forces: complexity.

conditions or situations will ascend and the order of priority in which subsequent research and translational work will unfold. For example, the priority of the Centers for Medicare and Medicaid Services (CMS) related to hospital-acquired pressure ulcers, for which there will be no payment in the new regulations, increases the likelihood that a more intensive focus on generating data regarding approaches to adequate skin care will result in more effective approaches to care. In this scenario and others like it, a highly structured and disciplined approach to applying evidentiary processes will be used to increase the veracity and utility of the data in clinical practice decision making. This model should exemplify knowledge creation and research; the application of practice expertise; inclusion of patient, family, and clinical care values; the cultural diversity of patients and populations; and the aggregate of each of these on patient care outcomes and changes in clinical performance. Within each of the critical stages of the evidentiary process, there are opportunities (gaps) for variance assessment and solution seeking that will be useful to calibrate the process so that each stage of the process can positively inform and guide subsequent stages with an alignment of these processes that can positively affect outcomes (Kolbasovsky, Zeitlin, & Gillespie, 2012).

These outcomes essentially become the new foundation for advancing evidence, driving the cybernetic trajectory of this dynamic in a cyclical fashion back to knowledge creation and research. At each of the stages with potential gaps in the evidence-based process, opportunities for innovation abound in ways that influence conceptualizing, planning, and approaching appropriate change everywhere in the evidentiary process. This disciplines the process and frees it to be open and available for creative conceptualizing, staging, deciding, and acting (Figure 13.1).

TRANSLATIONAL INNOVATION: KNOWLEDGE CREATION AND RESEARCH

Organizations and systems attempt to "morph" knowledge and research in ways that inform practice behaviors, but face significant challenges in the interaction between innovation and evidence (Ridenour, 2010). Here, some of the foundations laid out by Everett Rogers related to diffusion of innovation, or the spread of new ideas from an individual adoption perspective, have significant applications with regard to knowledge and research adoption (Burns, 2012). Although Rogers's is a relatively simple linear process, it does identify the relationship and characteristics between the social system and adopters of innovation. More complex approaches require the capacity to evaluate data, develop mechanisms for adoption, and, finally, support diffusion of appropriate practices by all affected clinicians (Topol, 2012). The role of evidentiary leadership at this stage is to confirm that the foundations of evidence are sufficiently narrow, definitive, predictive, and establish a broad enough foundation for rational clinical action.

Leadership and Innovation: The Nature of Leadership

The nature of leadership must now be examined to assure that values, beliefs, behaviors, and outcomes are consistent with dynamics of the evidence–innovation model. Leadership that supports the complexity of nonlinear, multiple interrelationships and directions, uncertainty, and self-organizing and emergent activities is necessary to actively support the dynamic work of the future (Weberg, 2017). Traditional leadership behaviors of directing and controlling with clearly defined communication channels will obstruct the dynamic in several ways. Most notable will be the tendency to stay located in the knowledge and research stage—locking on to work that is based on high levels of evidence.

> "
> Courage to continually challenge existing evidence and practices is supported by leadership principles and values steeped in the nature of complexity.
>
> **KATHY MALLOCH & TIM PORTER-O'GRADY**

To embrace complexity leadership, leaders must engage in personal reflection and ego management, adopt a style of appreciative inquiry, develop high levels of emotional competence, use creativity and open dialogue to make decisions as a team, continually be mindful of the bigger picture in which decisions are being made, and demonstrate willingness to stretch performance (Malloch, 2010). Evidence for complexity leadership in healthcare is emerging slowly and will need ongoing examination and documentation of its ability to produce the desired outcomes.

Creativity in this scenario exists in several different frames. First, designing an infrastructure that makes knowledge translation a part of practice is essential. Creating a consistent and systematic framework for knowledge management that includes knowledge generation, translation, and application is critical to successfully using evidence-based processes. Second, embedding this infrastructure in the clinical organization's "way of doing business" requires a consistent and systematic indoctrination of the established framework so that all clinical practitioners operate using the same evidentiary set of guidelines. Third, a level of transparency around questions of translation related to the relevance, veracity, and applicability of the data within particular clinical processes is important. Clarity is essential to the comparability of the data at the outset of translation and decision making and at the point of outcome measurement. The evidence-grounded practitioner is always looking through the lens of efficiency, effectiveness, and efficacy (Straus, Tetroe, & Graham, 2013).

Using the evidence–innovation dynamic framework, there is much evidence for selected segments of the care continuum and a lack of data supporting the integration of system segments. The design of patient care delivery models that now require integrated services across the continuum of care settings, collaboration across disciplines, value-based care, and economic sustainability is a reflection of this stage of the model. First, evidence exists for many of the unit-based or discipline-based delivery models (Baggs, Ryan, Phelps, Richeson, & Johnson, 1992; Institute of Medicine, Committee on Quality Health Care in America, 2000; Salas, Sims, & Burke, 2005). The current infrastructure for healthcare delivery models focuses on the acute care experience, a physician-dominated delivery system, discipline-focused services, and control of knowledge in policy sources created by the organization. Second, the use of evidence is based on individual discipline resources and not on an integrated use of evidence from multiple disciplines focusing on the individual patient. A multidisciplinary approach to planning and coordinating patient care as a team is emerging. New evidence specific to team rounding supports the values and principles of an integrated team approach (Henneman, Kleppel, & Hinchey, 2013). Third, there is a lack of transparent and interdisciplinary evaluation of each patient's care on a routine basis related to relevance, veracity, and appropriateness. The shortcomings of these processes create gaps in existing evidence for patient care delivery models and thus opportunities for innovation (Chen, 2016).

From the current status, the gaps in the practice framework to meet the expectations and goals of IOM (2001, 2011) and other organizations focused on patient engagement and satisfaction now illuminate the need not only for a new delivery model, but also for a framework that will support meaningful change (Hast, DiGioia, Thompson, & Wolf, 2013). Innovation is needed in our complex digital system that recognizes changing patterns of interactions among individuals, environmental changes, and the introduction of new products. Creating a delivery model driven by the gaps in patient and family-centered care now becomes an innovation imperative. Redefining roles, values, accountabilities, and resources is necessary for transformation to improve the quality of the healthcare system and achieve optimal patient and family engagement.

Innovation is largely evidenced by systematic flexibility and individual adaptability such that when evidence indicates the need for a shift or change in practice, the structures of the system and the behaviors of the practitioners are responsive to that demand (Ho, 2012). Here also, the goal of innovation is to enhance effectiveness, advance practice, and create new platforms of practice excellence (MacGregor & Carleton, 2012). Innovation tools that are especially useful at this stage relate to small focused testing of evidence-based approaches with specific patient populations to determine effectiveness and the ability to replicate; technique and methodological comparisons of approach at local units of service (or against a control or standard); and, finally, comparative analysis of comprehensive EBPs with other systems and agencies serving populations with like characteristics (comparative effectiveness) (Figure 13.2).

Of course, all adaptation of research and knowledge translation assumes the veracity of the science and the rigor of methodology in the research process and data retrieval (Barton-Burke, 2016). Innovation also has implications for study design and approach and provides opportunities for the creation and generation of knowledge in ways that make best use of emerging technologies that also facilitate its translation into practice. Like the evidence-based process itself, innovation is a reflection of the good use of emergent tools that are also the product of sound innovation processes. Rather than seeing innovation as a separate or nonaligned process, it is better seen as an embedded dynamic present in each stage of the evidence-based process and essential to its success (Endsley, 2010). Clearly, it would be inappropriate to determine that each element of the process and the gaps emerging out of them is unaligned with subsequent stages, or that such stages are iterative (building on past successful processes) or linear. Often, gaps in one stage can reach back to earlier evidence-based actions and inform changes or adjustments in them in ways imperceptible during an earlier stage in the process. Sensitivity to the "re-evidencing" process cannot be

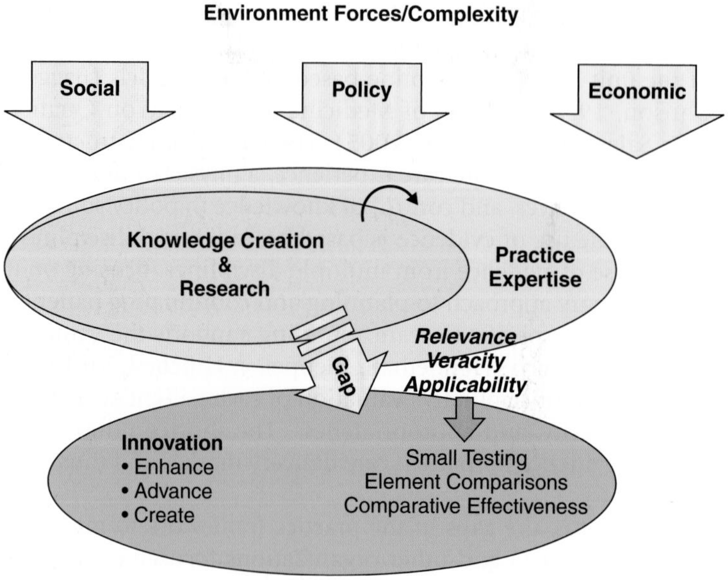

Figure 13.2: Environmental forces: innovation tools.

understated (Li et al., 2015). A strong willingness to continually challenge assumptions of current work provides incredible opportunities to advance practice excellence.

The use of Bar Code Medication Administration (BCMA) technology is an example of good rationale to reexamine the use of this evidence-driven process. In the knowledge and research stage, significant research supported the use of BCMA to decrease medication errors with the expectation of improving medication safety by automating processes of medication checking (Hook, Pearlstein, Samarth, & Cusack, 2008). As BCMA became the standard in medication administration, Koppel, Wetterneck, Telles, and Karsh (2008) noted variations from BCMA protocols, resulting in deviations, violations, or work-arounds to the designed processes. Recently, a typology was developed that identified 15 types of BCMA-related work-arounds with 31 types of causes (Koppel et al., 2008). These deviations from the intended practice can be now considered gaps in the evidence–innovation model. It is interesting to note that Lalley (2013) acknowledges that work-arounds (work efforts that accommodate impeding structures or processes) were not all necessarily negative and could, in fact, be innovations to existing processes. A careful examination of the evidence gap leads to the need for innovation—new ways to conduct medication administration.

Another source of an evidence gap can be identified when caregivers question current evidence. The notion that we have always done it this way is becoming less sacred in many healthcare organizations. In one organization, nurses queried why the Trendelenburg position was used and discovered that the 45-degree head down position was not a recommended position for many reasons (Makic, Rauen, & VonRueden, 2013). Multiple sources of evidence were examined, including the original use by Friedrich Adolph Trendelenburg in the late 1880s. Trendelenburg, a surgeon, used the position to visualize abdominal organs for surgical procedures. Today, some clinicians use the position to treat hypotensive events to shift blood volumes and to increase brain blood flow. Interestingly, in the 1960s, researchers found that in the Trendelenburg position, patient blood pressure decreased because head and neck veins became engorged, oxygen flow decreased, and the risk for retinal detachment increased. Researchers concluded that the Trendelenburg position had little positive impact on cardiac output or blood pressure (Makic et al., 2013). This new evidence created by challenging a long-held assumption is an example of the evidence–innovation dynamic in action. New evidence now requires new thinking or innovations to quickly address hypotensive events.

Experience and Application: Practice Expertise

Evidence is an aggregating dynamic that makes it always a work in progress. The science and data process grow in veracity (inherent truth) and applicability as the information regarding episodes of care or population needs increases in volume and accuracy (precision). Multiple practice variations and provider experiences contribute to the complexity of understanding practice. In the meantime, contributing to the data generation is the sum of experience and practice patterns of colleagues with specific cases, episodes, or populations (Soriano & Weberg, 2017). Mechanisms for conversations, conferences, collaboration, or care planning provide the frame for the construction of practices with no sufficient database on which practices can rely (Stanhope & Lancaster, 2010).

Collaborative sessions intended to converge around planning and constructing models, algorithms, or approaches to care create a foundation for practice for which there is yet no aggregated evidence sufficient to establish an evidentiary foundation for such practices.

Evidence for practice expertise emanates from several sources: past practices, experience, collective wisdom, and standards. Traditionally, caregivers and healthcare providers have relied on past practices and experiences to deliver care based on an institutional model with distinctly separate caregiver- and provider-role behaviors. The emphasis on the caregiver role has marginalized the role of the patient or the user of healthcare services. The challenges of limited communications among caregivers and providers, duplication of diagnostic tests, and delayed decision making have been identified as deficiencies in the existing evidence: the lack of effectiveness of current collaboration models becomes a gap and opportunity for innovation and new evidence (Davidson, 2017).

To address the gap is *care collaboration*, which is believed to have potential to bring stakeholders together to lower the cost and improve the quality of patient care (Tocknell, 2013). While shifting to a continuum-driven, population health model in which collaborative care is the cornerstone and expected to address current patient satisfaction challenges and the risk of readmissions, new quality measures will emerge and begin the dynamic to again identify the gap and create innovative processes. Working together to understand and facilitate each patient care episode by an informed team becomes the desired process to address the current gap. Working together in ways that create synergistic outcomes for patients rather than individual, segmented provider interventions is now the task in hand.

Another scenario within care collaboration is the nurse–physician relationship. Continuing work on nurse–physician relationships also is supported by evidence, because failure to achieve effective collaboration reflects the need for innovation and more evidence to address the poor relationships that still exist. This is not necessarily a failure of nurses and physicians to get along, but results from the lack of compelling evidence and rationale to change the current negative behaviors. Failure to support respectful and collaborative dialogue between these professionals will continue to obstruct progress in achieving higher levels of collaborative care. Overall, teamwork is the fundamental competency needed by all members of the team and becomes a gap when care is interrupted and delayed because of poor communication. Evidence clearly links collaborative practices to positive patient outcomes and staff satisfaction (Raup & Spegman, 2013).

Although this seems straightforward—let us all work together for the patient—it is far from easy to achieve this complex collaboration. Increasing our understanding of care collaboration processes can be examined innovatively using social network analysis (SNA). SNA is relatively new and more available in a digital environment and provides a process to gain information about the number and strength of connections among caregiver, providers, patients, and families (Merrill, Yoon, Larson, Honig, & Reame, 2013). This type of data provides information on who is involved in the care, how many times they are involved, and at what different points in time. In addition, the level and length of interactions can be identified. Progress on the desired types of communication can be tracked and evaluated with interval SNA. The patterns of SNA can then be considered in light of clinical outcomes providing best practices for collaborative care processes.

Another approach to creating effective collaborative care is through patient preferences. Finding the best evidence between nursing practice and patient-centered care has been facilitated using patient preferences (Burman, Robinson, & Hart, 2013). Patient preferences serve as the focal point in linking evidence and practitioner expertise in assuring that care is respectful and responsive to patient needs, values, and engagement. Recommendations to advance collaborative care involve more than one stage of the model—much like the interconnectedness of reality! The available knowledge and research are closely linked to practitioner expertise to enact the knowledge and research in practice. To have an impact on and advance collaborative care, recommendations address healthcare redesign, decision support, an empowered organizational culture, and informed and empowered nurses (Burman et al., 2013), further reflecting the dynamic interconnectedness of the evidence–innovation model.

Similarly, new evidence that can enhance collaborative care is emerging related to nurse staffing. Having the appropriate numbers and competencies of providers is another facet of caregiver expertise. Numerous studies link registered nurse staffing to patient outcomes, which include nurse–patient engagement (Aiken, Clarke, Sloane, Lake, & Cheney, 2008; Blegen, Goode, Spetz, Vaughn, & Park, 2011; Needleman et al., 2011). True, effective collaboration requires identifiable levels of education and certifications. Addressing gaps in staffing competencies and numbers also requires innovations to facilitate ideal staffing models (Malloch & Porter-O'Grady, 2017).

These shared opportunities for addressing the gaps in evidence in practice provide a range of opportunities for innovation in both design and execution, facilitating the journey to a stronger evidentiary foundation for these practices. The latitude in creativity is related to methods of conception and designs of practice approaches, agreements of colleagues around roles and contributions, anecdotes about experiences and evaluation of impact, and understood knowledge of practice–impact relationships (Payne, 2011). Supplementing these opportunities with preliminary data and sources of experiences in broader categories of practice referenced from other settings or environments helps strengthen the evidence of effectiveness (Gray, Coates, & Hetherington, 2013).

In the absence of collective and historical agreement on practices, the clinician is driven to construct approaches that best validate personal experiences where replication of practices shows valuable, relevant, consistent results. In these scenarios, the evidence-driven practitioner develops a level of uncertainty and discomfort, viewing the evidence as too informal and insufficiently structured to validate the tradition of practice associated with the practitioner's work. Good evidence for practice requires the clinician to connect individual practices with others' experiences to develop a collective database on which to ultimately construct an evidence-grounded approach to validate practice (Mauk, 2010). Here, the discipline of innovation requires the individual practitioner to make such practices intentional and deliberate using best approaches or best practices as seen in others' practices or in the anecdotal literature. In addition, there is nothing to stop the individual clinician from designing her or his own study of practice and establishing some foundations in practice evidence that can help move the practice closer to a standard of measure. This standard can be built upon and used as a part of the complex of individualized approaches to care that, when aggregated, begins to provide evidence of best practices or at least normative processes that lead in that direction (Figure 13.3).

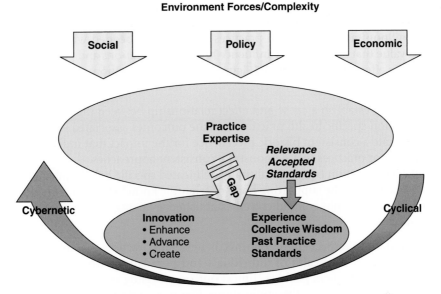

Figure 13.3: Environmental forces: aggregating evidence.

The key to transformation in practice and the innovations associated with it lies in creating a culture where exploration and "next steps" are permissible and encouraged. Healthcare providers need to be clear around expectations that (1) it is safe to take the initiative in examining individual and collective practices and (2) those practices are validated by the disciplines of research and evidence (Brynteson, 2013). Establishing the basis for particular practices that represent an approach, standard, or protocol becomes the first step in ascertaining their validity and forms the foundation for a more disciplined and structured review of the efficacies of particular practices and approaches. This culture of innovation helps support the urge for improvement, the desire to advance practice, and the goal of confirming the validity and veracity of particular approaches to patient care.

Clinical/Patient Personal and Cultural Values

In all clinical dynamics, patients bring with them a set of personal and cultural beliefs that represents grounding or traditions in faith, culture, family, and a related range of health practices (Andrews & Boyle, 2012). These beliefs can both positively and negatively affect the practice of healthy behaviors. All of these serve to bring out the patient's personal "tools" that help energize and motivate the patient toward healing and health. Some of these patient beliefs and historic and cultural norms may have some validity or evidence of value and applicability; some may not. Yet all, when integrated, may serve as a frame of reference for the patient and caring community in ways that help enable the patient to cope, confront, and address challenges and issues associated with healing and health.

Other than obviously dangerous or endangering practices, the provider may need to accommodate and incorporate particular personal and cultural characteristics and processes of healing into the complex of choices necessary to offer best service to particular patients and populations. The caring and insightful provider recognizes the value of incorporating culture and care, personality and practices, faith and healing, and history and experience into a mosaic that creates a positive and renewing interface between them to meet the needs of the person with the science of evidenced-based services (Giger, 2012). In the interests of evidence-driven innovation, it is important for practitioners to note that ample opportunity for linking culturally influenced and personal health practices to the evidentiary dynamic is a creative but important component of building evidentiary foundations for practices. Indeed, many nontraditional health practices may have embedded within them seeds of insight and value that can positively influence broader populations and provide for a strong foundation for effective health service (Figure 13.4). The innovation requisites would need to do the following:

1. Attempt to establish a cause-and-effect relationship between the cultural notions or population-specific health practices and the outcomes associated with them.
2. Enumerate a consistent historic precedence for the impact that indicates a norm of behavior or practices that demonstrate consistent approaches.
3. Make a connection between culturally delineated specific beliefs, practices, or approaches and the supporting body of scientific knowledge that correlates to it or, at least, does not contradict well-established, evidence-grounded sources of knowledge.

It is important to respect cultural norms, beliefs, and practices that demonstrate a tangible contribution to the health of individuals and populations when building evidence that supports and influences positive clinical outcomes. Using evidence-based approaches and connecting them to innovative applications does not preclude the potential for broader generalizations of culturally specific health foundations; instead, it may lead to innovations that potentially advance health and improve outcomes (Dayer-Berenson, 2011).

Creating the Culture of Care Within the Culture of Innovation

In order to both generate and sustain creative and innovative behaviors, the organizational infrastructure or culture must make it possible for those behaviors to thrive (Dodgson, Gann, & Salter, 2005). Innovation does least well in organizations that are rigidly controlled, policy dominated, with a narrow locus of control and an overpowering/overwhelming management authority structure. Although structure is certainly a requisite for all organized

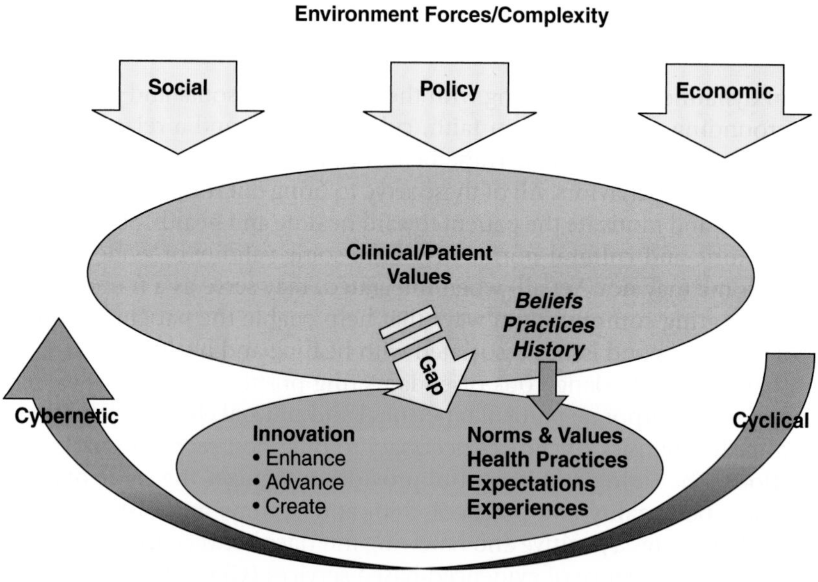

Figure 13.4: Environmental forces: embedding evidence.

human behavior, the kind of structure that advances innovation capacities and behaviors requires a considerably different design. Innovation is not successfully driven from the top of any system. Instead, it is generated from the center of the system and enabled by the institutional infrastructures to move in a way that allows the innovation to grow, adapt, and succeed (Grebel, 2011). The authoritarian, hierarchal structures with rigidly defined roles, relationships, and communication pathways are no longer effective for organizations seeking to support a dynamic evidence–innovation model. It is the point of care or intersection of the healthcare user and provider that must now be the focal and driving point of action (Weberg & Davidson, 2017).

The cultural context for innovation is created by organizational leadership from the boardroom to the first-line manager. This culture represents an availability or openness in the organization to ideas, stimulation, questioning, and drilling deeper into issues and processes that can advance the interests of the organization (Braithwaite, Hyde, & Pope, 2010). Leadership recognizes that innovation is located everywhere in the system, and that opportunities for it to arise and generate value and outcomes depend on the ability of those leaders to embrace and engage individuals and opportunities in a way that brings life and energy to the enterprise. The culture of innovation suggests that the structures and systems in place enable rather than constrain, give deference to relationships, good ideas, and processes—rather than rules and discipline—with the rigors associated with their systematic exploration and management in a way that will lead to value and impact (Anderson, 2012).

Although innovation is a dynamic as is EBP, it also is a discipline with elements and components, processes and stages, metrics and measures, and outcomes and impact (Leonard-Barton, 2011). Building a culture that supports the challenge to create and innovate while maintaining the rigors of good structure and process is no easy task for leadership. These challenges emphasize the need for innovation in the organizational structure to support both rigor and creative change. The trimodal organizational model offers an approach to integrate seemingly paradoxical work processes (Malloch, 2010), and is comprised of three major categories of work:

1. Operations, or the work of providing evidence-based patient care within a defined structure with supportive staff and resources.
2. Innovation planning is high-intensity work with the continual introduction and evaluation of new ideas. Develop new approaches to healthcare that are safer, less invasive, and more cost effective.
3. Transformation or transition work is about facilitating and assuring an effective transition between innovation and operations. The work of changing a culture requires much more than a single education session.

With specific attention to these three work processes, operations, innovation planning, and transformation are equally represented and resourced in the organization. The organization can be more nimble and responsive and increasingly able to take advantage of digital resources. The trimodal model creates a context whereby creative thinking is valued, improvement is rewarded, and individuals feel safe in recommending or initiating innovative ways of working and producing outcomes. The fully effective organization is expected to support quality, creativity, new thinking, and willingness to challenge long-held assumptions and have the means to transition between the current state and the desired future state.

Structure and leadership ability operate as a work in progress, constantly adjusting to environmental shifts, organizational responses to its market (for health systems; policy, society, users), and the vitality and viability of the organization itself (Howie, 2011). In order to thrive, the organization must remain relevant, expressing through its various functions and capacities the ability to maintain purpose, role, function, and impact in the broader landscape in which it lives (Ouden, 2012).

Innovation and Evidence

The core of both innovation and evidence is represented in what is often referred to as *associational thinking*. This represents an ability to find relationships and intersections between seemingly unrelated and unconnected components and processes. Indeed, the innovation embedded in evidence is represented by the clinician's capacity to look at precedence, past practices, metrics, and data and to draw insights from the data that challenge, inform, and advance new insights, connections, and responses that lead to improvement and enhancements in service and care (Mattimore, 2012).

Seeking out uncommon partners who further encourage us to challenge current assumptions, discard non–value-added work, and see the world in different ways provides new knowledge for consideration. The integration of clinical disciplines with architects has served to improve the environment of care and enhance the space for healing. Partnerships with engineers and "informaticists" provide invaluable insights into the documentation, categorization, analysis, and communication of complex health data. These uncommon partnerships enrich the evidence–innovation dynamic with the addition of knowledge from different perspectives.

The traditional notion that associates EBP with rule-defined parameters that eliminate judgment, initiative, creativity, and new insights is simply untrue. Evidence suggests an attachment to solid foundations, good science, research, validated practice precedence, and aggregated data. However, each of these simply provides the "floor" of practice, a foundation from which to discern, create, design, and construct next-step clinical approaches. These more effective approaches represent better, higher-level choices and actions. When taken together, these simple rules or practices can lead to improvements, enhancements, or entirely new approaches that result in better service, higher levels of quality, and new standards of clinical performance. In fact, without these dynamics at work, EBPs become no more than rote mechanisms that standardize and stabilize human action in a way to eliminate the vitality and initiative necessary to improve and advance. Building a culture of innovation that makes creativity, change, and improvement the "way of doing business" for the organization and its people is the essential context necessary to build a viable and sustainable culture of care (Kuratko, Hornsby, & Goldsby, 2012).

❝

If you always do what you always did, you will always get
what you always got.

ALBERT EINSTEIN

Creating the Culture of Care

The culture of care creates the infrastructure necessary for the dynamics and processes of EBP to make a lasting impact and lead to higher levels of quality service and care. This culture of care represents a fundamental commitment on the part of the organization and its people to focus in every arena, decisions, and activities in a way that advances service and care (Smith & Institute of Medicine, Committee on the Learning Health Care System in America, 2012). The norms and values of the organization represent a fundamental pledge to care and exemplify that commitment in the practices and behaviors of all those who represent its interests. The culture of care falls within the context of the overriding culture of innovation. This makes it possible within the care setting to design and adapt approaches to care delivery that reflect not only grounding in good science, but also gives opportunity to build approaches reflecting insights from past data, information about clinical and technological advances, the recalibration of policy and protocol, and insights from patient-related practices and experiences.

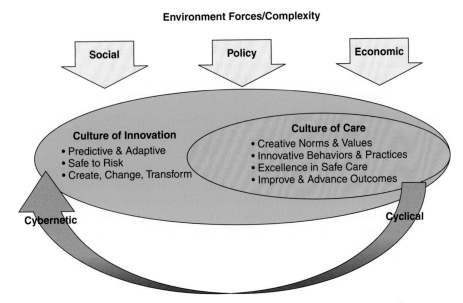

Figure 13.5: Environmental forces: coalescing of energies.

The culture of care assumes that practice unfolds within a constantly moving dynamic, ever informed by shifts in the environment, science-based evidentiary dynamics, and the dialogue and relationship between caregivers and patients. The interface of these forces represents the culture that makes possible creativity and adaptation, refinement and improvement, and advancement and enhancement of practices and processes, all of which lead to increasing intensity of relevance and value of quality care and service (Cross, 2013). The interface between the culture of innovation and care creates a sort of coalescing of energies that act as the stimuli for associational work that leads to the improvements suggested by good EBPs and processes (Figure 13.5).

The behaviors of providers and patients are the best indicators of whether an intertwined culture of innovation and care exists in the organization. There are five behavioral indicators that suggest the context of innovation and care are successfully operating within the system:

1. The ability to openly and frankly probe and question in an effort to challenge for clarity and creativity in a way that leads to a deeper look into existing decisions, processes, and actions subject to the potential for improvement and positive change;
2. The capacity to network collaterally within and across the system with a wide variety of people with diverse capacities and skills, which helps provide access to dynamic thinking and stimulates openness and availability (equity) between providers, resulting in increased value from their relationships and interactions;
3. Availability and awareness of the changing external environment and the ability of leaders and clinicians to predict and adapt internal dynamics and practices to reflect these changes and to assure that clinical and care responses are relevant, contemporary, and demonstrate the best in care;
4. Sustaining and advancing experimental awareness that no practice is permanent and that evidence-based design and practice demands a level of mobility, portability, and personal behavior that embraces the journey rather than the event. This demonstrates the role of the provider to appropriately change practice as soon as the evidence demands. This more fluid and flexible characterization of the

professional's role is essential for adaptation to ensure that clinical practice is current, relevant, and continuously effective.

5. There must be a willingness to act on evidence. Identifying areas of concern and opportunities to improve is often simpler than the courage to do something about those identified issues. Leaders must be willing to take rational risks and challenge long-held assumptions for the good of the healthcare system.

Building a culture of innovation in healthcare often seems paradoxical. We focus on reliability and consistency, yet there is an ever-present need to continue to assure that our practices are complementary to current evidence, changing environmental circumstances, and innovations. Nonetheless, the importance of being skilled in dynamic competence rather than an either–or (operations or innovation) cannot be overstated—it is a requirement.

Advancing organizational culture requires time and knowledge. Oftentimes, leaders may believe that creating initiatives and billboards and buttons will drive new behaviors. Nothing could be further from the truth. Advancing or changing a culture requires knowledge of the critical elements and the impact of cultural attributes (Schein, 2004). Numerous descriptions of organizational culture have been studied for many years. The combination of Schein and Hatch's work provides a fairly clear framework to understand the levels of complexity. Understanding the levels of complexity provides critical information about the challenges and requirements to effect change in an organization. Schein's model identified assumptions, values, and artifacts as the three fundamental layers of an organization. Hatch (1993) advanced Schein's work with the addition of symbols. The identity of an organizational culture is formed by the underlying assumptions about people, activities, and expectations. This is the deepest layer of an organization and often difficult to discern. Values form the middle layer of organizational culture. Artifacts are considered the superficial layer of an organization such as posters, slogans, directives, and other types of shared information. Symbols, introduced by Hatch, added the interpretive aspect of culture and focus on the relationships linking assumptions, values, and artifacts in a dynamic rather than static model. The dynamics of organizational culture include a fourth element to assess organizational culture—symbols. This addition permits the model to accommodate the influences of both Schein's theory and symbolic-interpretive perspectives (Hatch, 1993). The reformulated model focuses on relationships linking assumptions, values, symbols, and artifacts with a shift from static to dynamic conceptions of culture by looking at interactions between key elements rather than the elements themselves.

As one seeks to advance change or innovation in an organization, the levels of organizational culture and the dynamic relationship among the elements must be considered. Furthermore, alignment of the elements is critical for change to advance. Long-term, lasting change requires firm grounding in organizational culture assumptions. When change or new ideas and expectations are introduced at the artifact level, without agreement on values and assumptions, it is difficult for the change to sustain. Consider the numerous checklists that have been introduced to assure compliance with standards and reporting criteria. If the underlying assumptions are not directly linked to safe patient care, less attention is given to the checklists because there is no perceived quality threat. Thus, the checklist (artifact) becomes ineffective because the expectation for cost-containment is identified as the goal. Quality and economics are perceived to be inconsistent. To effectively change processes, the values for both quality and economics must be clearly articulated at all levels of the culture and in symbolic relationships throughout the organization.

Culture is more about context than content. The context for innovation and EBP has clear requisites and characteristics that affect strategy, tactics, and clinical decisions and actions (Heskett, 2012). The interplay between innovation and patient care demonstrates a seamless and fluid network of interactions, intersections, and relationships. This exemplifies the network's capacity to engage its stakeholders in the essential activities of change, and in advancing and continuously improving service and quality (Anderson & Ackerman-Anderson, 2010). Evidence-based processes represent and demonstrate the character and capacity of a culture of innovation where the ability to adapt and change clinical practices based on the constant generation of evidence is simply an organizational way of life.

IMPACT AND CHANGE: INNOVATION AND EVIDENCE AT WORK

All innovation must at some time create a product or generate an impact. The innovation dynamic and associated processes have no purpose or value if there is no change, product, or outcome. Impact, outcome, or change is a necessary terminal point of the process and, at the same time, the point at which the cyclical, cybernetic dynamic of innovation and evidence cycles back on itself and initiates the cyclic processes at their point of inception. At the end of this process, the impact stage is reached where a combination of evidence and the determination of the metrics and measures prove efficacy (Hoggarth & Comfort, 2010). At the point of impact, the evidence-based process enters the "evaluation zone" where plan, performance, and outcome meet to show the essential character of their interaction and relationship, and the convergence of factors that influence value.

Metrics and measures related to impact and value should be constructed in the earlier stages of the evidentiary process so that they might act as both enumerators and potential predictors of desired outcome. Of course, the outcome must result in some specific change that represents improvement, enhancement, or an effective change in course. Ultimately, the result must be articulated in some measure of difference, as seen in Box 13.1.

It is here that the potential for innovation accelerates. At the point of evaluation, the innovative organization looks carefully at the trajectory and processes associated with evidence-driven activities and determines the challenges, opportunities, insights, and capacity to predict change, alter or adjust processes and practices, shift the trajectory, and incorporate new knowledge and technology (Maddock, Uriarte, & Brown, 2011). Here, they integrate the insight from these factors in a way that contributes to the design and modeling of innovative approaches within the cybernetic process of innovation and evidence.

Assessment and evaluation at the point of impact also lead to reflection and evaluation of both the core of innovation and evidence and the effectiveness of the evidentiary dynamic and

---

BOX **13.1**	*Examples of Innovation and Evidence at Work*

- New knowledge, learning, skills, practices (Note: New knowledge may reflect processes or products that do not positively advance change and are now abandoned.)
- Standards affecting episodes, persons, populations
- Changes in policy, protocol, procedure
- Changes in the capacity of providers, patients, populations, communities
- Changes in patient, provider, community behaviors
- Changes in the organization, systems, community (resources, structures, support systems)
- Changes in capacity, utility, use
- Changes in quality, service, continuity, integrity, viability

its associated processes. The effectiveness and seamlessness of the interface from knowledge creation, practice expertise, clinical values, and care culture to outcome and impact is as important an element of the evaluation as are the clinical dynamics and provider practices. How the gaps were identified, analyzed, accommodated, and addressed and how response to them led to a more seamless interface between the evidentiary stages are important to creating a more seamless evidentiary dynamic (Ouden, 2012). The implications for innovation are exemplified by the degree of intensity of creative approaches that enhanced or advanced evidentiary dynamics and associated processes and validated the utility of the culture of innovation (Figure 13.6).

Evaluation of the environment of innovation (culture) is as important as the embedded components of evaluation in EBP. The key is to observe how the leadership and organizational environment facilitated the creation of a context resulting in openness, responsiveness, timeliness, process-seamlessness, timeliness of response, predictive/adaptive capacity, and the value of essential changes (Goldstein, Hazy, & Lichtenstein, 2010). Leadership and management capacity and skills are also ripe territory for the evaluation of effectiveness of evidence-based processes and practices and the human interaction and dynamics that facilitate and advance them. How open, available, and accessible data and information are demonstrates in the most visible way the culture and action of innovation at work. The point of service capacity to react, deliberate, act, and change also clearly demonstrates the dynamic impact of the culture of innovation. This innovation engine provides the energy within which the dynamics and processes of EBP are generated and supported in a way that assures their relevance and usefulness (Howie, 2011).

The culture of innovation provides the contextual framework that feeds and facilitates all of the structural, organizational, and human infrastructures and capacities that support EBP as a way of doing business in any endeavor. The complementarity between innovation and evidence is the same as that between context and content—one providing the frame, the other providing the processes. This interdependence defines the relationship between innovation and evidence, necessitating a fundamental correlation between each of these dynamics in a way that is generative, supportive, and advances the human experience. Commitment to evidence suggests a corollary commitment to the innovation that supports and enables it. It is the constant work of leadership to advance the integrity of this partnership between innovation and evidence in a way that provides value, sustains quality, and advances the human enterprise in the delivery of effective patient care. In the final section of this chapter,

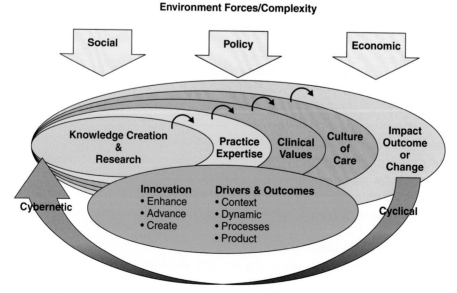

Figure 13.6: Environmental forces: implications for innovation.

an application of the **Cybernetic evidence–innovation dynamic** is presented to further explain the value of the model in analyzing complex situations and identifying specific gaps and potential solutions to close the gaps.

APPLICATION OF CYBERNETIC EVIDENCE–INNOVATION DYNAMIC

The cybernetic evidence–innovation dynamic can be used to increase our understanding of the policy process and advance outcomes. Consider the following example. In 2008, the Robert Wood Johnson Foundation (RWJF) and the IOM launched a 2-year initiative to respond to the need to assess and transform the nursing profession and ultimately recommended that 80% of nurses be prepared at the baccalaureate level by 2020 (Institute of Medicine of the National Academies, 2010).

This recommendation was based on the changing realities of the 21st century, namely the increased complexity of care environments, availability of EBPs not previously considered in nursing education programs, the need to advance and support interdisciplinary collaboration using high-level technology, and the transition to care in communities. Higher levels of education are believed to better prepare nurses to meet these needs. Specifically, research evidence is now available documenting the relationship of baccalaureate nurses to lower mortality, decreases in readmission rates, length of stay, congestive heart failure mortality, pressure ulcers, failure to rescue events, and deep vein thrombosis as well as increased cost savings (American Association of Colleges of Nursing, n.d.).

The environmental forces driving this recommendation are social, political, and economic. The demand for increased quality and lower costs is further documented in the Affordable Care Act and the expectation for value-based care. Knowledge has been created in multiple studies to support this recommendation (Figure 13.7).

Knowledge creation and research continue to emerge supporting the baccalaureate nurse in practice based on multiple studies (American Association of Colleges of Nursing, n.d.). This new evidence is closing the gap in knowledge as to the most effective level of nurse for point of service care.

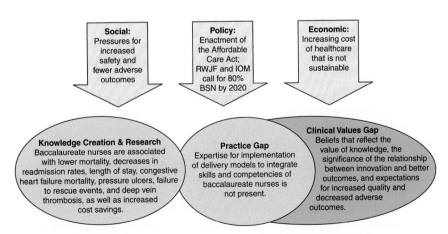

Figure 13.7: Environmental forces: gap identification using the cybernetic interface of innovation and evidence model. IOM, Institute of Medicine; RWJF, Robert Wood Johnson Foundation; BSN, Bachelor of Science in Nursing.

The practice expertise for care delivery currently has gaps in the implementation of delivery models to integrate the skills and competencies of the baccalaureate nurse. New models are needed to utilize the care coordination competencies of baccalaureate nurses as well as to fully integrate all caregivers into care delivery models using the fullest scope of their training and licensure. These gaps must necessarily be addressed from a complex systems perspective that considers interrelationships, uncertainty, and existing evidence. Also, the need for innovative approaches to new models must be recognized and supported by small tests of change to create new standards for care delivery that integrate experience, collective wisdom, and past standards.

Clinical values of all key stakeholders—employers, caregivers, and patients—must now shift to support beliefs that reflect the value of knowledge, the significance of the relationship between innovation and better outcomes, and expectations for increased quality and decreased adverse outcomes as indicated in the new knowledge about the impact of the baccalaureate nurse.

The culture of care for a more educated nurse requires an infrastructure supportive of focused change, course corrections, the value of failures, and the expectations of excellence as the normative standard. The gap between the current healthcare system that focuses on stability and standardization and the inclusion of the leadership of innovation to integrate new research into more robust delivery models must be closed for quality to improve.

Coming full circle, the anticipated outcomes will be congruent with the research; lower mortality, decreases in readmission rates, length of stay, congestive heart failure mortality, pressure ulcers, failure to rescue events, and deep vein thrombosis, as well as increased cost savings.

WANT TO KNOW MORE?

A variety of resources is available to enhance your learning and understanding of this chapter.

- Visit thePoint® to access:
  - Articles from the AJN EBP Step-By-Step Series
  - Journal articles
  - Checklists for rapid critical appraisal and more!

- Lippincott **CoursePoint** combines digital text content with video case studies and interactive modules for a fully integrated course solution that works the way you study and learn.

EBP FAST FACTS

- Innovation does least well in organizations that are rigidly controlled and policy dominated, with a narrow locus of control and an overpowering/overwhelming management authority structure.
- Innovation is not successfully driven from the top of any system; it is generated from the center of the system and enabled by the institutional infrastructures to move in a way that allows the innovation to grow, adapt, and succeed.
- Metrics and measures related to impact and value should have been constructed in the earlier stages of the evidentiary process so that they might act as both enumerators and potential predictors of desired outcome.
- All innovation must create a product or generate an impact; the innovation dynamic and processes associated with it have no purpose or value if there is no change, product, or outcome.

References

Aiken, L. H., Clarke, S. P., Sloane, D., Lake, E. T., & Cheney, T. (2008). Effects of hospital care environment on patient mortality and nurse outcomes. *Journal of Nursing Administration, 38*(5), 223–229.

American Association of Colleges of Nursing. (n.d.). Retrieved from http://www.aacnnursing.org/Portals/42/News/Factsheets/Nursing-Workforce-Fact-Sheet.pdf

Anderson, D. L. (2012). Cases and exercises in organization development & change. Thousand Oaks, CA: SAGE.

Anderson, D., & Ackerman-Anderson, L. S. (2010). Beyond change management: How to achieve breakthrough results through conscious change leadership. San Francisco, CA: Pfeiffer.

Andrews, M. M., & Boyle, J. S. (2012). *Transcultural concepts in nursing care*. Philadelphia, PA: Wolters Kluwer Health/Lippincott Williams & Wilkins.

Baggs, J. G., Ryan, S. A., Phelps, C. E., Richeson, J. F., & Johnson, J. E. (1992). The association between interdisciplinary collaboration and patient outcomes in medical intensive care. *Heart and Lung, 21*, 18–24.

Barton-Burke, M. (2016). Building capacity for evidenced-based practice at the unit level using oncology nursing society putting evidence practice. *Asia-Pacific Journal of Oncology Nursing, 3*(1), 17–20.

Blegen, M., Goode, C. J., Spetz, J., Vaughn, T., & Park, S. H. (2011). Nurse staffing effects on patient outcomes: Safety-net and non-safety-net hospitals. *Medical Care, 49*(4), 406–414.

Braithwaite, J., Hyde, P., & Pope, C. (2010). Culture and climate in health care organizations. Hampshire, UK: Palgrave.

Brown, S. J. (2009). *Evidence-based nursing: The research-practice connection*. Sudbury, MA: Jones and Bartlett.

Brown, V. A., Harris, J. A., & Russell, J. Y. (2010). *Tackling wicked problems: Through the transdisciplinary imagination*. London, UK: Earthscan.

Brynteson, R. (2013). *Innovation at work: 55 activities to spark your team's creativity*. New York, NY: American Management Association.

Burman, M. E., Robinson, B., & Hart, A. M. (2013). Linking evidence-based nursing practice and practice-centered care through patient preferences. *Nursing Administration Quarterly, 37*(3), 231–241.

Burns, L. R. (2012). *The business of healthcare innovation*. Cambridge, UK: Cambridge University Press.

Chan, R. R., & Schaffrath, M. (2017). Participatory action inquiry using baccalaureate nursing students: The inclusion of integrative health care modalities in nursing core curriculum. *Nurse Education in Practice, 22*, 66–72.

Chen, H. T. (2016). Interfacing theories of program with theories of evaluation for advancing evaluation practice: Reductionism, systems thinking, and pragmatic synthesis. *Evaluation and program planning, 59*, 109–118.

Clavelle, J., Porter-O'Grady, T., Weston, M., & Verran, J. (2016). Evolution of structural empowerment: From shared to professional governance. *Journal of Nursing Administration, 46*(6), 308–312.

Cristofoli, D., Markovic, J., & Meneguzzo, M. (2014). Governance, management and performance in public networks: How to be successful in shared governance networks. *Journal of Management and Governance, 18*(1), 77–93.

Cross, B. L. (2013). *Lean innovation: Understanding what's next in today's economy*. Boca Raton, FL: CRC Press.

Curlee, W., & Gordon, R. L. (2011). *Complexity theory and project management*. Hoboken, NJ: Wiley.

Davidson, S. (2017). Recognizing pattern changes as evidence for innovation work. In S. Davidson, D. Weberg, T. Porter-O'Grady, K. Malloch (Eds.), *Leadership for evidence-based innovation in nursing and health* (pp. 303–332). Cambridge, MA: Jones and Bartlett.

Dayer-Berenson, L. (2011). *Cultural competencies for nurses: Impact on health and illness*. Sudbury, MA: Jones and Bartlett.

Dodgson, M., Gann, D., & Salter, A. (2005). *Think, play, do: Technology, innovation, and organization*. New York, NY: Oxford University Press.

Endsley, S. C. (2010). *Putting healthcare innovation into practice*. Chichester, UK: Wiley-Blackwell.

Erickson, J. I., Ditomassi, M., & Adams, J. M. (2012). Attending registered nurse: An innovative role to manage between spaces. *Nursing Economics, 30*(5), 282–287.

Giger, J. N. (2012). *Transcultural nursing: Assessment & interventions*. St. Louis, MO: Elsevier/Mosby.

Goldstein, J., Hazy, J. K., & Lichtenstein, B. B. (2010). *Complexity and the nexus of leadership: Leveraging nonlinear science to create ecologies of innovation*. New York, NY: Palgrave Macmillan.

Gray, M., Coates, J., & Hetherington, T. (2013). *Environmental social work*. Abingdon, UK: Routledge.

Grebel, T. (2011). *Innovation and health: Theory, methodology and applications*. Northampton, MA: Edward Elgar Publishing.

Hast, A. S., DiGioia, A. M., Thompson, D., & Wolf, G. (2013). Utilizing complexity science to drive practice change through patient- and family-centered care. *Journal of Nursing Administration, 43*(1), 44–49.

Hatch, M. J. (1993). The dynamics of organizational culture. *Academy of Management Review, 18*(4), 657.

Heilbron, J. L. (2003). *The Oxford companion to the history of modern science*. New York, NY: Oxford University Press.

Henneman, E. A., Kleppel, R., & Hinchey, K. T. (2013). Development of a checklist for documenting team and collaborative behaviors during multidisciplinary bedside rounds. *Journal of Nursing Administration, 43*(5), 280–285.

Heskett, J. L. (2012). *The culture cycle: How to shape the unseen force that transforms performance.* Upper Saddle River, NJ: FT Press.

Ho, K. (2012). *Technology enabled knowledge translation for eHealth: Principles and practice.* New York, NY: Springer.

Hoggarth, L., & Comfort, H. (2010). *A practical guide to outcome evaluation.* Philadelphia, PA: Jessica Kingsley.

Hook, J. M., Pearlstein, J., Samarth, A., & Cusack, C. (2008). *Using barcode medication administration to improve quality and safety: Findings from the AHRQ Health IT Portfolio.* Rockville, MD: Agency for Healthcare Research and Quality. Retrieved from http://healthit.ahrq.gov/sites/default/files/docs/page/09-0023-EF_bcma_0.pdf

Hovmand, P., & Gillespie, D. (2010). Implementation of evidence-based practice and organizational performance. *The Journal of Behavioral Health Service and Research, 37*(1), 79–84.

Howie, P. J. (2011). *Evolution of revolutions: How we create, shape, and react to change.* Amherst, NY: Prometheus Books.

Institute of Medicine. (2001). *Crossing the quality chasm: A new health system for the 21st century.* Washington, DC: National Academy Press.

Institute of Medicine. (2011). *The future of nursing: Leading change, advancing health.* Washington, DC: National Academies Press.

Institute of Medicine, Committee on Quality Health Care in America. (2000). In L. T. Kohn, M. Corrigan, & M. S. Donaldson (Eds.), *To err is human: Building a safer health system.* Washington, DC: National Academy Press.

Institute of Medicine of the National Academies. (2010). *The future of nursing: Focus on education.* Retrieved from http://www.nationalacademies.org/hmd/~/media/Files/Report%20Files/2010/The-Future-of-Nursing/Nursing%20Education%202010%20Brief.pdf

Kinney, E. D. (2011). Comparative effectiveness research under the Patient Protection and Affordable Care Act: Can new bottles accommodate old wine? *American Journal of Law and Medicine, 37*(4), 522–566.

Kolbasovsky, A., Zeitlin, J., & Gillespie, W. (2012). Impact of point-of-care case management on readmissions and costs. *The American Journal of Managed Care, 18*(8), e300–e306.

Koppel, R., Wetterneck, T., Telles, J. L., & Karsh, B. (2008). Workaround to barcode medication administration systems: Their occurrences, causes, and threats to patient safety. *Journal of the American Medical Informatics Association, 15,* 408–423.

Kuratko, D. F., Hornsby, J. S., & Goldsby, M. G. (2012). *Innovation acceleration: Transforming organizational thinking.* Boston, MA: Pearson.

Lalley, C. (2013). Work-arounds: A matter of perception. *Nurse Leader, 11*(2), 36–40.

Leonard-Barton, D. (2011). *Managing knowledge assets, creativity and innovation.* Hackensack, NJ: World Scientific.

Li, Y., Yu, J., Du, L., Sun, X., Kwong, J. S., Wu, B., . . . Zhang, L. (2015). Exploration and practice of methods and processes of evidence-based rapid review on peer review of WHO EML application. *Journal of Evidence-Based Medicine, 8*(4), 222–228.

Lorenz, J. M., Beyea, S. C., & Slattery, M. J. (2009). *Evidence-based practice: A guide for nurses.* Marblehead, MA: HCPro.

MacGregor, S. P., & Carleton, T. (2012). *Sustaining innovation: Collaboration models for a complex world.* New York, NY: Springer.

Maddock, G. M., Uriarte, L. C., & Brown, P. B. (2011). *Brand new: Solving the innovation paradox—How great brands invent and launch new products, services, and business models.* Hoboken, NJ: Wiley.

Makic, M. B., Rauen, C. A., & VonRueden, K. T. (2013). Questioning common nursing practices: What does the evidence show? *American Nurse Today, 8*(3), 10–13.

Malloch, K. (2010). Innovation leadership: New perspectives for new work. *Nursing Clinics of North America, 45*(1), 1–9.

Malloch, K., & Porter-O'Grady, T. (2009). *Introduction to evidence-based practice in nursing and healthcare.* Boston, MA: Jones & Bartlett.

Malloch, K., & Porter-O'Grady, T. (2010). *The quantum leader: Applications for the new world of work.* Boston, MA: Jones and Bartlett.

Malloch, K., & Porter-O'Grady, T. (2017). Shifting workforce paradigms: From quality to value-driven staffing using evidence and innovation. In S. Davidson, D. Weberg, T. Porter-O'Grady, K. Malloch (Eds.), *Leadership for evidence-based innovation in nursing and health* (pp. 369–397). Cambridge, MA: Jones and Bartlett.

Marshall, E. S. (2011). *Transformational leadership in nursing: From expert clinician to influential leader.* New York, NY: Springer Publishing.

Mattimore, B. W. (2012). *Idea stormers: How to lead and inspire creative breakthroughs.* San Francisco, CA: Jossey-Bass.

Mauk, K. L. (2010). *Gerontological nursing: Competencies for care.* Boston, MA: Jones and Bartlett.

McCarthy, J. A. (2011). *Beyond genius, innovation & luck: The "rocket science" of building high-performance corporations.* Los Altos, CA: 4th Edition Publishing.

Melnyk, B., & Fineout-Overholt, E. (2012). *Evidence-based practice and nursing and healthcare. A guide to best practice* (4th ed.). Philadelphia, PA: Wolters Kluwer/Lippincott Williams & Wilkins.

Merrill, J. A., Yoon, S., Larson, E., Honig, J., & Reame, N. (2013). Using social network analysis to examine collaborative relationships among PhD and DNP students and faculty in a research-intensive university school of nursing. *Nursing Outlook, 61*(2), 109–116.

Nalipay, M. J., Bernardo, A. B., & Mordeno, I. G. (2016). Social complexity beliefs predict posttraumatic growth in survivors of a natural disaster. *Psychological Trauma: Theory, Research, Practice and Policy, 8*(5), 559–567.

Needleman, J., Buerhaus, P., Pankratz, V. S., Leibson, C. L., Stevens, S. R., & Harris, M. (2011). Nurse staffing and inpatient hospital mortality. *The New England Journal of Medicine, 364*(11), 1037–1045.

Ouden, E. D. (2012). *Innovation design: Creating value for people, organizations and society.* London, UK: Springer.

Payne, M. (2011). *Humanistic social work: Core principles in practice.* Chicago, IL: Lyceum Books.

Porter-O'Grady, T., & Malloch, K. (2010). *Quantum leadership: Advancing innovation, transforming healthcare.* Boston, MA: Jones and Bartlett.

Raup, C. M., & Spegman, A. M. (2013). Interprofessional collaboration promotes collaboration. *American Nurse Today, 8*(3), 43–46.

Ridenour, J. (2010). Evidence-based regulation: Emerging knowledge management to inform policy. In K. Malloch & T. Porter-O'Grady (Eds.), *Introduction to evidenced-based practice in nursing and healthcare* (pp. 275–299). Boston, MA: Jones and Bartlett.

Rundquist, J. M. & Givens, P. L. (2013). Quantifying the benefits of staff participation in shared governance. *American Nurse Today, 8*(3), 38–42.

Salas, E., Sims, D. E., & Burke, C. S. (2005). Is there a "big five" in teamwork? *Small Group Research, 36*(5), 555–559.

Schein, E. H. (2004). *Organizational culture and leadership.* San Francisco, CA: Wiley & Sons.

Schultz, A. A. (2009). *Evidence-based practice.* Philadelphia, PA: Saunders.

Sharts-Hopko, N. C. (2013). Tackling complex problems, building evidence for practice, and educating doctoral nursing students to manage the tension. *Nursing Outlook, 61*(2), 102–108.

Smith, M. D, & Institute of Medicine, Committee on the Learning Health Care System in America. (2012). *Best care at lower cost: The path to continuously learning health care in America.* Washington, DC: National Academies Press.

Soriano, R., & Weberg, D. (2017). Incorporating new evidence from big data, emerging technology, and disruptive practices into your innovation ecosystem. In S. Davidson, D. Weberg, T. Porter-O'Grady, K. Malloch (Eds.), *Leadership for evidence-based innovation in nursing and health* (pp. 145–168). Cambridge, MA: Jones and Bartlett.

Stanhope, M., & Lancaster, J. (2010). *Foundations of nursing in the community: Community-oriented practice.* St. Louis, MO: Mosby/Elsevier.

Starr, P. (2011). *Remedy and reaction: The peculiar American struggle over health care reform.* Hartford, CT: Yale University Press.

Straus, S. E., Tetroe, J., & Graham, I. D. (2013). *Knowledge translation in health care: Moving from evidence to practice.* Chichester, UK: John Wiley & Sons.

Tait, A., & Richardson, K. A. (2010). *Complexity and knowledge management: Understanding the role of knowledge in the management of social networks.* Charlotte, NC: Information Age Publishing.

Tocknell, M. D. (2013). *Risk and reward in collaborative care.* HealthLeaders, April, 22–24.

Topol, E. J. (2012). *The creative destruction of medicine: How the digital revolution will create better health care.* New York, NY: Basic Books.

Weberg, D. (2017). Innovation leadership behaviors: Starting the complexity journey. In S. Davidson, D. Weberg, T. Porter-O'Grady, K. Malloch (Eds.), *Leadership for evidence-based innovation in nursing and health* (pp. 43–74). Cambridge, MA: Jones and Bartlett.

Weberg, D., & Davidson, S. (2017). Patient-centered care, evidence, and innovation. In S. Davidson, D. Weberg, T. Porter-O'Grady, K. Malloch (Eds.), *Leadership for evidence-based innovation in nursing and health* (pp. 111–141). Cambridge, MA: Jones and Bartlett.

Deborah Dang, Bernadette Mazurek Melnyk, Ellen Fineout-Overholt, Jennifer Yost, Laura Cullen, Maria Cvach, June H. Larabee, Jo Rycroft-Malone, Alyce A. Schultz, Cheryl B. Stetler, and Kathleen R. Stevens

> **Change is inevitable . . . adapting to change is unavoidable, it's how you do it that sets you together or apart.**
>
> —William Ngwako Maphoto

EBP Terms to Learn

The Advancing Research and Clinical practice through close Collaboration (ARCC) model for implementation and sustainability of EBP
Clinical Scholar Model
Context
Critical Thinking
Data Driven
EBP mentor
Facilitators
Implementation Science
Iowa Model of Evidence-based Practice to Promote Quality Care

Johns Hopkins Nursing Evidence-based Practice Model
Model for Evidence-based Practice Change
Organizational Culture of EBP

Promoting Action on Research Implementation in Health Services (PARIHS) framework
Research Utilization
Stevens Star Model of Knowledge Transformation
Triggers

Learning Objectives

After studying this chapter, learners will be able to:

1. Describe various types of evidence-based practice models that guide implementation and sustainability of evidence-based practice.

2. Discuss how evidence-based practice models can improve healthcare quality and population health outcomes.

Consider the following interventions:

- Home visitation to low-income pregnant women prevents major depressive episodes (Tandon, Leis, Mendelson, Perry, & Kemp, 2013).
- Patient-directed music can reduce anxiety and sedative exposure in critically ill patients who are mechanically ventilated (Chlan et al., 2013).
- A school-based healthy lifestyle intervention program (i.e., COPE [Creating Opportunities for Personal Empowerment] and Healthy Lifestyles TEEN [Thinking, Emotions, Exercise, and Nutrition]) that includes cognitive behavioral skills building can prevent overweight/obesity, improve social skills and academic performance, and reduce depression in severely depressed adolescents (Melnyk et al., 2013).

The clinical interventions described earlier are but a few of many interventions that have been evaluated and shown to have a positive impact on patient outcomes and often on cost savings for the healthcare system. However, are healthcare providers aware of these studies? How do they learn about them? How can healthcare providers keep up-to-date with new knowledge that relates to their practice? Once they acquire new knowledge, how do healthcare providers change their own practices and influence others to change practice behaviors within their organizations? Are evaluations conducted to determine whether evidence-based changes in clinical practice result in beneficial outcomes? All of these questions are important for the effective implementation of evidence-based findings in clinical practice (Box 14.1).

Healthcare providers are highly motivated to be evidence-based practitioners. However, there are many individual and organizational obstacles. At the individual level, clinicians frequently (a) have inadequate skills in searching for and critically appraising research studies (Parahoo, 2000), (b) lack confidence to implement change (Parahoo, 2000), and (c) have misperceptions that evidence-based practice (EBP) takes too much time (Melnyk, Fineout-Overholt, Gallagher-Ford, & Kaplan, 2012).

However, organizational factors often create the most significant barriers to EBP (Parahoo, 2000; Retsas, 2000). Lack of interest, motivation, leadership, vision, strategy, and direction among managers for EBP poses a significant organizational barrier. Findings from a survey of a random sample of nurses across the United States also identified their nurse leaders and managers as a major barrier to EBP (Melnyk et al., 2012). This is especially true for the nursing profession because a change in practice, especially if it involves purchasing new equipment or changing a policy or procedure, requires administrative support (Parahoo, 2000; Retsas, 2000). For example, in the case of pressure sore prevention, nurses have the decision making autonomy to ensure position changes. However, other interventions, such as the purchase of high-specification foam mattresses, require approval of the organization.

Changing clinical practice is complex and challenging. As a result, many models have been developed to systematically guide the implementation of EBP. This chapter begins by describing the components of evidence-based clinical decision making. The chapter then goes on to describe models that are designed to assist clinicians in changing practices on the basis of evidence in their organizations.

BOX 14.1 *Definition of Evidence-Based Practice*

Evidence-based practice is the integration of best research evidence with clinical expertise (including internal evidence) and patient values to facilitate clinical decision making (Sackett et al., 2000).

Evidence-based practice includes the following steps (Melnyk & Fineout-Overholt, 2011):

0. Cultivate a spirit of inquiry.
1. Ask the burning clinical question in PICOT format.
2. Search for and collect the most relevant best evidence.
3. Critically appraise the evidence (i.e., rapid critical appraisal, evaluation, and synthesis).
4. Integrate the best evidence with one's clinical expertise and patient preferences and values in making a practice decision or change.
5. Evaluate outcomes of the practice decision or change based on evidence.
6. Disseminate the outcomes of the EBP decision or change.

EVOLUTION FROM RESEARCH UTILIZATION TO EVIDENCE-BASED CLINICAL DECISION MAKING

In the past, nurses and other healthcare providers used the term **research utilization (RU)** to mean the use of research knowledge in clinical practice. EBP is broader than RU because the clinician is encouraged to consider a number of factors in clinical decision making, one of which is research evidence. Evidence-based practitioners are also encouraged to integrate their clinical expertise with the best available research evidence, **internal evidence** (evidence about the patient's clinical state, setting, and circumstances and evidence generated as a result of outcomes management or quality improvement [QI] and EBP projects), as well as evidence about the patient/family's preferences, and healthcare resources (DiCenso, Ciliska, & Guyatt, 2004; Melnyk & Fineout-Overholt, 2011; Figure 14.1).

Components of Evidence-Based Clinical Decision Making

To illustrate how evidence-based clinical decision making can work consider the following examples.

Research Evidence

It is the clinician's responsibility to identify current, high-quality *research evidence* to inform clinical decisions. Evidence-based practitioners are encouraged to identify the most synthesized research evidence first—online summaries (e.g., Dynamed UpToDate, Best Practice), guidelines, and systematic reviews—through the use of tools and resources such as the 6S Hierarchy of Preprocessed Evidence and the ACCESSSS Federated Search (Agoritsas et al., 2015; DiCenso, Bayley, & Haynes, 2009).

 ACCESSS Federated Search is online at https://plus.mcmaster.ca/ACCESSSS/

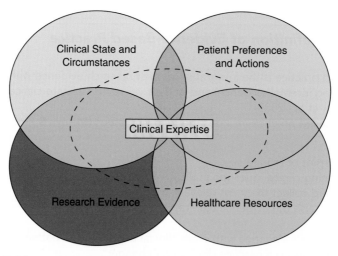

FIGURE 14.1: Evidence-based decision making. (From DiCenso, A., Ciliska, D., & Guyatt, G. [Eds.]. [2004]. *Evidence-based nursing: A guide to clinical practice.* St. Louis, MO: Elsevier.)

Consider an in-hospital example in which nurses are concerned about the high rate of central venous catheter–related bloodstream infections. One nurse, who recently transferred to this setting from another institution, notes that there seemed to be far fewer central venous catheter–related bloodstream infections where she previously worked when chlorhexidine gluconate–impregnated dressings were used. This nurse offers to search for the best available evidence. She finds a systematic review by Ullman et al. (2016) and reviews it with the nurse educator on the unit. Together, they conclude that it is a high-quality systematic review in terms of its methods. With moderate confidence in the findings (**internal validity**) that the true reduction in bloodstream infections with the chlorhexidine gluconate–impregnated dressings is likely to be close to the estimate reported in the systematic review, they feel it is the best available research evidence (Balshem et al., 2011); (Schünemann, Brożek,, Guyatt, & Oxman, 2013). The population and setting of the included studies are sufficiently similar to theirs that they can apply the results in their unit (**external validity**). From the study's findings, the nurses conclude that chlorhexidine gluconate–impregnated dressings on central venous catheter sites may result in fewer catheter-related bloodstream infections. They talk to their nurse manager about chlorhexidine gluconate–impregnated dressings. Their manager agrees but encourages them to evaluate whether the new type of dressing actually results in a reduction in catheter-related infections by recording the number of infections for 3 months before and after switching to chlorhexidine gluconate–impregnated dressings (Hagiwara, Gare, & Elg, 2016). Gathering **internal evidence** on the unit with their own patients will provide further evidence to support their change in practice.

Availability of Healthcare Resources

Another component of clinical decision making is the availability of *healthcare resources*. Sometimes, even the best research evidence cannot be used because the intervention is too resource intensive in terms of financial resources (e.g., cost of the intervention, human re-sources [e.g., personnel/staffing], materials [e.g., workspace]). Take an example of a healthcare organization considering the implementation of home-based primary care interventions involving visits by a primary care provider to a patient's home with longitudinal management to provide comprehensive primary care. A literature search identifies the systematic review by Totten et al. (2016) concluding that although there is research evidence demonstrating that home-based primary care interventions reduce hospitalization and hospital days (especially among patients who are more frail, sicker, or at higher risk for negative outcomes), there is a low level of certainty and insufficient evidence for other important outcomes (e.g., function, symptoms, mortality, hospital readmissions). Considering the research evidence along with limited resources, the organization might decide to implement home-based primary care interventions among patients who are frail, sicker, or at higher risk or decide not to implement home-based primary care interventions at this time. Resources become the dominant element in this decision.

Patient Preferences and Actions

When clinical indications warrant heart valve replacement, patients must often decide between types of valve prosthesis. This choice typically involves weighing the need for long-term anticoagulant therapy and the related risks of bleeding and thromboembolism with a mechanical valve versus the risk of deterioration and potential for reintervention with a bioprosthetic valve (Nishimura et al., 2017). *Patient values and preferences* will be the dominant elements in this decision. Optimally, patient values and preferences are based on careful consideration of information that provides an accurate assessment of the patient's condition and possible treatments as well as the likely benefits, costs, and risks. Shared decision making and the use of decision aids, which are tools to share information and cre-ate a conversation regarding risks and benefits, have emerged to assist clinicians in helping patients make well-informed decisions that also reflect their values and goals (Kunneman, Montori, Castaneda-Guarderas, & Hess, 2016).

 Examples of decision aids can be found online at https://decisionaid.ohri.ca/

Clinical State, Setting, and Circumstances

In addition to patient preferences, clinicians need to consider the patient's *clinical state, setting, and circumstances*. For example, patients who live in remote areas or low-income countries may not have access to the same diagnostic tests or interventions as those who live near a tertiary care medical center or in middle- to high-income countries. Also, the effectiveness of some interventions may vary, depending on the patient's stage of illness or symptoms. Furthermore, outcomes from patients on a specific unit (i.e., internal evidence) might also be integrated into evidence-based decisions.

Clinical Expertise

Evidence-based decision making is influenced by the practitioner's experience and skills. Clinician skills include the expertise that develops from multiple observations of patients and how they react to certain interventions. Because no two clinical decisions are identical, the relative weight and influence of research evidence; healthcare resources; patient preferences and values; and the clinical state, setting, and circumstances varies from decision to decision. In the clinical decision making model, *clinical expertise* is the mechanism that provides for the integration of the other model components and is essential for avoiding the mechanical application of care maps, decision rules, and guidelines.

For example, the practitioner's clinical expertise will influence the following:

- Quality of the initial assessment of the client's clinical state and circumstances;
- Problem formulation;
- Decision about whether the best available research evidence and availability of healthcare resources substantiate a new approach;
- Exploration of patient preferences;
- Delivery of the clinical intervention;
- Evaluation of the outcome for that particular patient.

Integrating Clinical Expertise

The following scenario exemplifies integrating clinical expertise with the other clinical decision making model components. A local school board is concerned about an increase in alcohol use in the high schools in the last year. It asks the school nurses and counselors to implement a brief intervention program, providing in-person information or advice to increase motivation not to use substances and to teach behavior change skills. Parents, teachers, and the school board are very supportive of the program, the school nurses and counselors have the skills to implement this program, and resources are sufficient to mount it. However, the nurses and counselors search the literature and find a high-quality systematic review that shows evidence that these sorts of intervention programs are not any more effective for reducing the frequency and quantity of alcohol consumption than providing information only (Carney, Myers, Louw, & Okwundu, 2016). The school nurses and counselors recommend that the program not be offered but that, instead, the school board participate in offering and evaluating a "healthy school" approach, which provides relevant information about alcohol use to students (e.g., information similar to that provided in the studies included in the systematic review).

In the past, EBP has been criticized for its "cookbook approach" to patient care. Some believe that it focuses solely on research evidence and, in so doing, ignores patient preferences. Figure 14.1 shows that research evidence is only one factor in the evidence-based decision making process and is always considered within the **context** of the other factors. One of the advantages of this model is that healthcare providers have not traditionally considered research evidence in their decision making process, and this model reminds them that such evidence should be one of the factors they consider.

MODELS TO CHANGE PRACTICE IN AN ORGANIZATION

There is increasing recognition that efforts to change practice should be guided by conceptual models or frameworks (Graham, Tetroe, & KT Theories Research Group, 2007). Early in the EBP movement, healthcare scientists, including many nurse scientists, developed models to organize our thinking about EBP and understand how various aspects of EBP work together to improve care and outcomes. These models guide the design and implementation of approaches intended to strengthen evidence-based decision making and help clinicians implement an evidence-based change in practice. Graham et al. conducted a literature review of the many models that exist and identified commonalities in terms of their steps or phases. These include the following:

- Identify a problem that needs addressing;
- Identify stakeholders or change agents who will help make the change in practice happen;
- Identify a practice change shown to be effective through high-quality research that is designed to address the problem;
- Identify and, if possible, address the potential barriers to the practice change;
- Use effective strategies to disseminate information about the practice change to those implementing it;
- Implement the practice change;
- Evaluate the impact of the practice change on structure, process, and outcome measures;
- Identify activities that will help sustain the change in practice.

According to a thematic analysis of theoretical models (Mitchell, Fisher, Hastings, Silverman, & Wallen, 2010), major EBP models can be grouped into three categories:

1. EBP, RU, and Knowledge Transformation Processes;
2. Strategic/Organizational Change Theory to Promote Uptake and Adoption of New Knowledge; and
3. Knowledge Exchange and Synthesis for Application and Inquiry. A thematic analysis of theoretical models for translational science in nursing: Mapping the field.

Each model brings forth strengths and can be selectively applied for a wide array of purposes, including evidence identification, implementation and integration, and educating current and future workforces. The following eight models were created to facilitate integration of EBP for change improvement:

1. The Stetler Model of Evidence-Based Practice;
2. The Iowa Model of Evidence-Based Practice to promote quality care;
3. The Model for Evidence-Based Practice Change;
4. The Advancing Research and Clinical practice through close Collaboration (ARCC) model for implementation and sustainability of EBP;
5. The Promoting Action on Research Implementation in Health Services (PARIHS) framework;

6. The Clinical Scholar Model;
7. The Johns Hopkins Nursing Evidence-Based Practice Model;
8. The Stevens Star Model of Knowledge Transformation.

The Stetler Model of Evidence-Based Practice

The original Stetler/Marram Model for RU was published in 1976 to fill a void regarding realistic application of research findings to practice (Stetler & Marram, 1976). The original model has undergone several revisions to strengthen its underpinnings and usefulness through the following (Stetler, 1985, 1994a, 2001b):

- review of theory, research, and evaluation on knowledge utilization and implementation;
- integration of emerging EBP concepts;
- presentation of the model as an "integrated package of tools and resources for EBP."

Critical thinking and use of research findings remain at the core of the model. However, it has long recognized value in information beyond research and, in 2001, explicitly incorporated additional sources of both external and internal evidence that can influence an ultimate "use" decision. Through work on an organizational model of EBP for a medical center, with the Stetler Model as its underpinning, the 2001 version also formally integrated the concept of EBP: that is, practice that stresses "use of research findings and, as appropriate, QI data, other operational and evaluation data, the consensus of recognized experts and affirmed experience to substantiate practice" (Stetler et al., 1998a, p. 49). Finally, through ongoing work related both to EBP within nursing and the broader field of **implementation science,** the final version (Stetler, 2001b, 2010) was developed with refined assumptions and a "How-to" toolkit.

 See *implementationscience.com* for insights regarding this critical field.

Overview of the Stetler Model

The Stetler Model (Figure 14.2A and B) outlines a series of steps to assess and use research findings to facilitate safe and effective EBP. Over the course of its evolution, the model has grown in complexity in order to provide more guidance around utilization concepts, as well as more detail and options involved in applying research in the real world. In 2009, minor modifications were made to the 2001 model's content, both Parts I and II, to better clarify phases and highlight implementation tools (Stetler, 2010).

The Stetler Model has long been known as a practitioner-oriented model because of its focus on critical thinking and use of findings by the individual practitioner (Kim, 1999; Stetler & Marram, 1976). The 2001 version provided clarification that this guided problem-solving process also applies to groups of practitioners. Yet the model maintains the bottom-line assumption that even prepackaged, research-based recommendations are applied at the skilled practitioner level to individual patients, staff members, or other targets of use.

This model is geared to advanced practitioners, such as CNSs, NPs, and DNP-prepared nurses. These advanced practitioners can use the model in their own practice and in a group setting, facilitating others' use of the phases as appropriate (Stetler, 2010). Multiple examples of the model's use in different settings for numerous topics, from cancer-related protocols to enlightenment of staff regarding patients' psychosocial issues, are provided with the 2010 revision. Ongoing personal communications to the author from advanced practitioner students suggest that the model is currently used to guide capstone projects, dissertation research, clinical projects, and practice innovations.

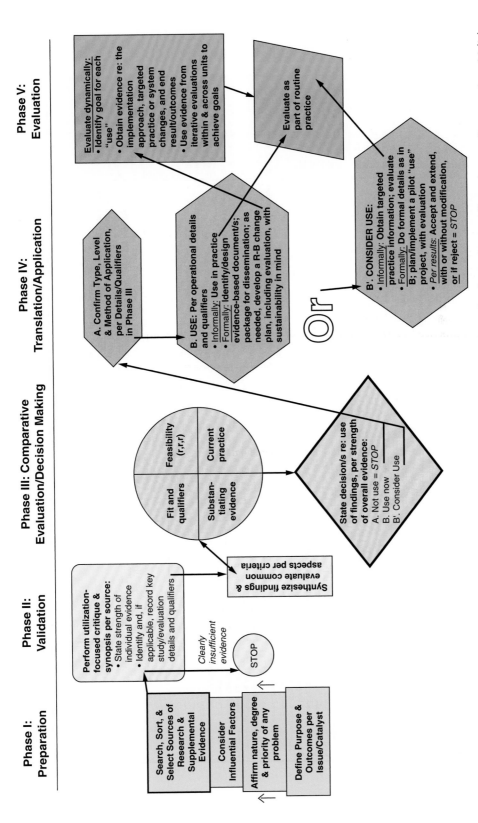

Figure 14.2: The Stetler Model of EBP ©2009 has two parts (**A**, pictured and **B**, described); and it has five phases: Preparation, Validation, Comparative evaluation/Decision making, Translation/Application, and Evaluation. IRB, institutional review board; RU, research utilization. (From Stetler, C. B. [2010]. Stetler Model. In J. Rycroft-Malone & T. Bucknall [Eds.], *Models and frameworks for implementing evidence-based practice: Linking evidence to action.* Oxford, UK: Wiley-Blackwell Publishing.)

Phase I: Preparation	Phase II: Validation	Phase III: Comparative Evaluation/Decision Making	Phase IV: Translation/Application	Phase V: Evaluation
Purpose, Context, & Sources of Evidence:	Credibility of Evidence & Potential for/Detailed Qualifiers of Application:	Synthesis & Decisions/Recommendations per Criteria of Applicability:	Operational Definition of Use/Actions for Change:	Alternative Evaluations:
• **Potential Issues/Catalysts** = *a problem, including unexplained variations; less-than-best practice; routine update of knowledge; validation/routine revision of procedures, etc; or innovative program goal*	• *Critique & synopsize essential components, operational details, and other qualifying factors, per source* ◦ *See instructions for use of utilization-focused review tables,* * *with evaluative criteria, to facilitate this task; fill in the tables for group decision making or potential future synthesis*	• *Synthesize the cumulative findings:* ◦ *Logically organize & display the similarities and differences across multiple findings, per common aspects or subelements of the topic under review* ◦ *Evaluate degree of substantiation of each aspect/subelement; reference any qualifying conditions for application*	• **Types** = *cognitive/conceptual; symbolic &/or instrumental* • **Methods** = *informal or formal; direct or indirect* • **Levels** = *individual; group or department/organization* • **Direct instrumental use:** *change individual behavior (e.g., via assessment tool or Rx intervention options); or change policy, procedure, protocol, algorithm, program, etc.*	• **Evaluation per type, method, level: e.g., consider conceptual use at individual level**[&&] • **Consider cost-benefit of change + various evaluation efforts** • **Use RU-as-a-process to enhance credibility of evaluation data** • **For both dynamic & pilot evaluations, include:**
• **Affirm/clarify perceived problem/s, with internal evidence re: current practice** *[baseline]* • **Consider other influential internal and external factors, e.g., timelines** • **Affirm and focus on high priority issues** • **Decide if need to form a team, involve formal stakeholders, &/or assign project lead/facilitator**	• *Critique* **systematic reviews and guidelines** • **Reassess fit of individual sources** • **Rate the level & quality of each individual evidence source per a "table of evidence"** ◦ *Differentiate statistical and clinical significance* ◦ *Eliminate noncredible sources*	• **Evaluate degree & nature of other criteria:** **feasibility (r,r,r = risk, resources, readiness);** *pragmatic fit, including potential qualifying factors to application; & nature of* **current issues/needs** • **Make a decision whether/what to use:** ◦ *Can be a personal practitioner-level decision or a recommendation to others* ◦ *Judge strength of decision; indicate if*	• **Cognitive use:** *validate current practice; change personal way of thinking; increase awareness; better understand or appreciate condition/s or experience/s* • **Symbolic use:** *develop position paper or proposal for change; or persuade others regarding a way of thinking* • **CAUTION:** *Assess whether translation/product or use goes beyond actual findings/evidence:*	◦ *formative, regarding actual implementation & goal progress* ◦ *summative, regarding identified end goal and end-point outcomes*
• **Determine need for an explicit type of research evidence, if relevant** • **Define desired, measurable outcome/s** • **Seek out systematic reviews/guidelines first** • **Select research sources with conceptual fit**	◦ *End the process if there is clearly insufficient, credible external evidence that meets your need*	*primarily "research-based" (R-B) or, per high use of supplemental info, "E-B"; note level of strength of recommendation/s per related* table*; note any qualifying factors that may influence individualized variations* • **If decision = "Not use" research findings:** ◦ *May conduct own research or delay use till additional research done by others*	◦ *Research evidence may or may not provide various details for a complete policy, procedure, etc.; indicate this fact to users, and note differential levels of evidence therein* • **Formal dissemination & change/implementation strategies should be planned per relevant research and local barriers:** ◦ *Passive education is usually not effective as an isolated strategy. Use Dx analysis** & an*	**NOTE:** Model applies to all forms of practice, i.e., educational, clinical, managerial, or other; to use effectively, read 2001 & 1994 model papers. *Stetler et al, 2006 re: dx analysis
	*Stetler, Morsi, Rucki, et al. *Appl Nurs Res* 1998; 11(4):195–206 for noted tables, reviews, & synthesis process	◦ *If still decide to act now, e.g., on evidence of consensus or another basis for practice, consider need for rigorous planned change and evaluation.* • **If decision = "Use/Consider Use," can mean a recommendation for or against a specific practice**	***implementation framework to develop a plan. Consider multiple strategies: e.g., opinion leaders, interactive education, reminders & audits.* ◦ *Focus on context*[8] *to enhance sustainability of organization-related change* • **Consider need for appropriate, reasoned variation** **WITH B, where made a decision to use in the setting:** ◦ *With formal use, may need a dynamic evaluation to effectively implement & continuously improve/refine use of best available evidence across units & time* **WITH B*, where made a decision to consider use & thus obtain additional, pragmatic information before a final decision** ◦ *With formal consideration, do a pilot project* ◦ *With a pilot project, must assess if need IRB review, per relevant institutional criteria*	***E.g.: Rogers' re: implications of attributes of a change; Rycroft-Malone et al, [&]PARIHS (2002) & Green & Krueter's PRECEDE (1992) models re: implementation [8]Stetler, 2003 on context [&&]Stetler & Caramanica, 2007 on outcomes

Figure 14.2: *(continued)*

Definitions of Terms in the Stetler Model

The term *evidence* first appeared in the model in 1976 and, at that stage, referred only to research findings. However, in 1994, Stetler broadened the concept of "substantiating evidence" to include additional sources of information because research indicates that "experiential and theoretical information are more likely to be combined with research information than they are to be ignored" (Stetler, 1994a, p. 17). By 2001, the concept of evidence—given the evolving nature of the EBP movement across healthcare—had become a key element in "Updating the Stetler Model of Research Utilization to Facilitate Evidence-Based Practice" (Figure 14.2). The following definitions now explicitly underpin the model (Stetler, 2001a, 2001b; Stetler et al., 1998a):

- Evidence, within the context of healthcare, is defined as information or facts that are systematically obtained (i.e., obtained in a manner that is replicable, observable, credible, verifiable, or basically supportable).
- Evidence, within the context of healthcare, can come from different sources and can vary in the degree to which it is systematically obtained and thus the degree to which it is perceived as basically *credible* or supportable for safe and effective use.

Different sources of evidence can be categorized as external or internal. **External evidence** comes primarily from research. However, where research findings are lacking, the consensus opinion/experience of widely recognized experts as well as published program evaluations are considered supportable evidence. These will often be used to supplement research-based recommendations. **Internal evidence** comes primarily from systematically but locally obtained facts or information. It includes data from local performance, planning, quality, outcome, and assessment/evaluation activities, as well as data collected through use of RU/EBP models to assess current practice and measure progress. In addition, internal evidence includes the consensus opinion and experience of local groups, as well as experiential information from individual professionals—*if affirmed*. Although an individual's isolated, unsystematic experience and related opinions alone are not considered to be credible evidence, those experiential observations or ways of thinking that have been reflected on, externalized, or exposed to explorations of truth and verification from various sources of data—and thus *affirmed*—are considered valid evidence in the model (Rycroft-Malone et al., 2002; Rycroft-Malone & Stetler, 2004; Stetler, 2001b; Stetler et al., 1998a).

It is also important to note, as Haynes (2002) did, the need to consider "evidence of patients' circumstances and wishes" (p. 3). Patient wishes are commonly included in EBP definitions, usually labeled as patient preferences. At the individual level, such preferences can be considered internal evidence. These need to be well explored for their origins and related (patient) experiences (Goode & Piedalue, 1999; Haynes, Sackett, Gray, Cook, & Guyatt, 1996), as some patient preferences may be based on ill-informed experiences or information.

Using the Stetler Model

The basic "how to" of EBP using the Stetler Model is divided into five progressive phases of deliberation and action:

1. *Preparation:* Getting started by defining and affirming a priority need, reviewing the context in which use would occur, organizing the work if more than an individual practitioner is involved, and systematically initiating a search for relevant evidence, especially research.
2. *Validation:* Assessing a body of evidence by systematically critiquing each study and other relevant documents (e.g., a systematic review or guideline), with a *utilization* focus in mind, then choosing and summarizing the collected evidence that relates to the identified need.

3. *Comparative evaluation/decision making:* Making decisions about use after synthesizing the body of summarized evidence by applying a set of utilization criteria, then deciding whether, and if so what, to use in light of the identified need and overall set of criteria.

4. *Translation/application:* Converting findings into the type of change to be made/recommended; planning application, most particularly for formal group use, putting the plan into action by using operational details of how to use the acceptable findings, and then enhancing adoption and actual implementation with an evidence-based change plan; and/or incorporating converted findings into one's individual practice.

5. *Evaluation:* Evaluating the plan and actions in terms of the degree to which each was implemented and whether the goal for using the evidence was met.

Figure 14.2A and B, along with related publications, provide specific guidance, case examples, and rationale for each of these steps (Newell-Stokes, Broughton, Giuliano, & Stetler, 2001; Stetler, 1994a, 1999, 2001b, 2010; Stetler, Burns, Sander-Buscemi, Morsi, & Grunwald, 2003; Stetler & Caramanica, 2007; Stetler, Corrigan, Sander-Buscemi, & Burns, 1999; Stetler et al., 1995, 1998b, 2006a, 2006b).

Despite the appearance that the systematic utilization of evidence is a linear, clear-cut process, it is more fluid. Figure 14.2B has serrated lines between the phases to indicate this fluidity and the need to occasionally revisit decisions (e.g., the relevance of specific studies and fit of various findings to the context). Despite the model's complex appearance, its steps and concepts can be integrated into a professional's routine way of thinking about RU and EBP in general. This in turn influences how one reads research and applies related findings (Stetler, 1994b, 1999, 2010; Stetler et al., 1995).

Critical Assumptions and Model Concepts

Key underlying assumptions that generate this model's critical thinking and practitioner orientation must be considered prior to use (Stetler, 1994a, 2001b). For example, the model assumes that both formal and informal use of research findings—with supplemental use of other evidence—can occur in the practice setting. Formal, organization-related RU/EBP activity is most frequently discussed in the nursing literature (e.g., new policies, procedures, protocols, programs, and performance standards [the "Ps"]). After formal documents are disseminated, however, individual, critical-thinking nurses are expected to use these translated and packaged findings. As Geyman (1998) suggests, the use of EBP then "requires the integration, patient by patient, of clinical expertise and judgment with the best available relevant external evidence" in the form of those "Ps" (pp. 46–47). This may require *reasoned variation* or *individualization*, based on a clear rationale (Stetler, 2010), as in the context of a patient's circumstances, status, and preferences. Such reasoned variation is best built into "Ps," where appropriate (Newell-Stokes et al., 2001). Additionally, research and evaluative data usually provide probabilistic information rather than absolutes about each person for whom the evidence is believed to "fit." In light of these assumptions, use of the model requires an RU/EBP-competent individual.

In terms of informal use, individual, RU/EBP-competent practitioners (i.e., those who are knowledgeable and skilled in the process of research/evidence utilization) can use the model's critical-thinking process in their routine practice and interactions with others (Cronenwett, 1994; Stetler, 1994a, 1994b, 1999; Stetler et al., 1995). These practitioners may use evidence to substantiate their decision to institute a new practice or improve a current practice, change their way of thinking about an issue or routine, expand their repertoire of assessment or intervention strategies to be used as needed, or change a colleague's way of thinking about a treatment plan or patient/staff issue (Stetler & Caramanica, 2007). Again, the user must possess a certain level of knowledge and related skills for the safe, appropriate, and effective use of findings (Stetler, 2001b), for example:

- knowledge and affirmed practice behavior regarding the steps of utilization—such as use of tables of evidence and a set of applicability criteria to determine the desirability and feasibility of using guidelines or a credible study;
- knowledge and affirmed practice behaviors regarding the substantive area or clinical practice under consideration.

Advanced-level practitioners are most likely to fulfill such expectations and are also more likely to routinely integrate research findings into their practices (Cronenwett, 1994; Stetler, 1994a, 1994b). Advanced-level clinicians are able to do so because of their critical-thinking skills and advanced knowledge of their specialty area—knowledge that provides them with a *body of evidence* with which to comparatively evaluate any study under consideration for application in their practice. With sufficient education and skill preparation, baccalaureate-prepared providers—**in collaboration with advanced-level clinicians**—can and should participate in the identification of issues and potential solutions, development of formal EBPs, and facilitation of the adoption of affirmed EBPs.

Another of the model's underlying assumptions is that research findings and other credible evidence, such as consensus guidelines, may be used in multiple ways. Practitioners use evidence directly in observable ways to change how they behave or provide care through selected assessments, clinical procedures, and behavioral interventions. They also use evidence indirectly or conceptually, which is not as easy to observe but is extremely important to EBP (Stetler & Caramanica, 2007; Stetler & DiMaggio, 1991). This can involve using evidence to change how one thinks about a patient or an issue. It can also involve adding evidence to one's body of knowledge, merging it with other information, and using it in the future (Stetler, 1994a). Finally, research findings and related evidence can be used symbolically (i.e., strategically) to influence the thinking and behavior of others (Stetler, 1985; Stetler & Caramanica, 2007). A key to safe use in such multiple forms, however, is that competent users understand the strength of evidence underlying targeted uses, as well as the status of applicability criteria.

To thoroughly understand the Stetler Model, it is most useful to read both the 1994 revision—in particular when interested in use of research and related evidence for individual decision making—*and* the 2001 paper, in particular when adding the safe and effective use of research and related evidence for collective, formal decision making. Case examples can make the model's use then come to life (Newell-Stokes et al., 2001; Stetler, 1999, 2010; Stetler & Caramanica, 2007; Stetler et al., 1995, 1998b, 2003).

The Iowa Model Revised: Evidence-Based Practice to Promote Excellence in Healthcare

This model (Iowa Model Collaborative, in press) provides guidance for nurses and other clinicians in making decisions about clinical and administrative practices that affect healthcare outcomes. **The Iowa Model** (Figure 14.3) outlines a pragmatic multiphase change process with feedback loops. The original Iowa Model has been revised and recently updated (Iowa Model Collaborative, in press; Titler et al., 1994, 2001; Watson, Bulechek, & McCloskey, 1987). The model is based on Rogers' (2003) Diffusion of Innovations theory, application of implementation science, and is widely recognized for its applicability and ease of use by interprofessional healthcare teams.

Overview of the Iowa Model

Identify Triggering Issues/Opportunities. The Iowa Model begins by encouraging clinicians to identify questions as an opportunity to improve practice and healthcare. Important issues

The Iowa Model Revised: Evidence-Based Practice to Promote Excellence in Health Care

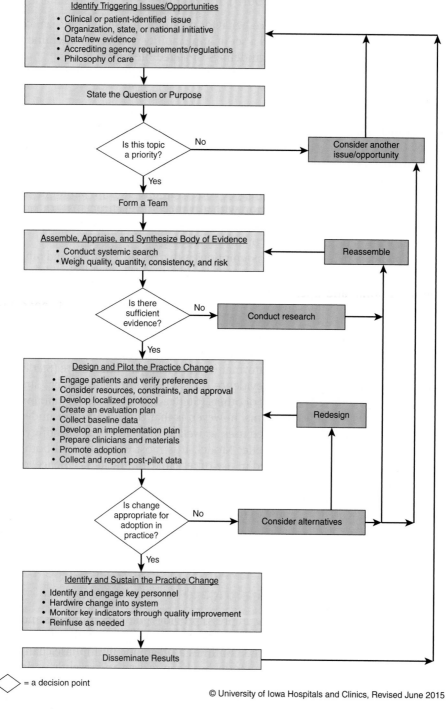

= a decision point

© University of Iowa Hospitals and Clinics, Revised June 2015

Figure 14.3: The Iowa Model of evidence-based practice to promote quality care. (From Iowa Model Collaborative. [2017]. The Iowa model-revised: Development and validation. *Worldviews on Evidence-Based Nursing,* 14[3], 175–182. doi:10.1111/wvn.12223. Used with permission from the University of Iowa Hospitals and Clinics, © 2015/2012. For permission to use or reproduce, please contact the University of Iowa Hospitals and Clinics at UIHCNursingResearchandEBP@uiowa.edu.)

are often identified when questioning current practice. Recent updates combine problem and knowledge-focused triggers and opportunities into a single list. **Triggers** may have existing data that highlight an opportunity for improvement or come from disseminated scientific knowledge (e.g., organizational or national initiatives, data/new evidence), leading clinicians and leaders to question current practice standards. Clinician involvement early in the process is important because different implementation strategies will be required for top-down versus bottom-up EBP changes (Fleiszer, Semenic, Ritchie, Richer, & Denis, 2016b; Kastner et al., 2015; Lau et al., 2016).

Clinical Applications. Nurses identify important and clinically relevant practice questions that can be addressed through the EBP process. A number of clinically important topics have been addressed using the Iowa Model, including managing cancer-related fatigue (Huether, Abbott, Cullen, Cullen, & Gaarde, 2016), early mobility in critically ill pediatric patients (Cullen et al., in press), traditional practices or sacred cows (Hanrahan et al., 2015), use of low-dose ketamine for patients with chronic pain after orthopedic surgery (Farrington, Hanson, Laffoon, & Cullen, 2015), prevention of catheter-associated urinary tract infections for intrapartum women (Hiller, Farrington, Forman, McNulty, & Cullen, in press), and group therapy for adolescent trauma and addiction care (Bougard, Laupola, Parker-Dias, Creekmore, & Stangland, 2016).

Interprofessional and operational topics and educational programs have also been addressed using the Iowa Model (Beinlich & Meehan, 2014; Hosking et al., 2016; Moyers, Finch Guthrie, Swan, & Sathe, 2014; Nayback-Beebe et al., 2013). Important issues have been addressed using the Iowa Model well ahead of regulatory standards or changes in reimbursement (e.g., pain, falls, suicide risk) by supporting clinician-identified important clinical topics. Administrators and nurses in leadership positions can support clinicians' use of EBP by creating a culture of inquiry, clinician ownership, and a system supporting evidence-based care delivery (Harbman et al., 2016; Tistad et al., 2016; Walker-Czyz, 2016; Wocial, Sego, Rager, Laubersheimer, & Everett, 2014).

State the Question or Purpose. Stating a question or purpose is a new addition to the model (Iowa Model Collaborative, in press). Explicit inclusion of a clearly stated purpose reflects the importance this step provides in guiding later steps in the EBP process. Having a clear purpose establishes the charge to the team while defining clear boundaries. Key elements of the purpose statement include the clinical Problem, patient Population, Pilot area, Intervention, Comparison, and desired Outcome. Staying focused on the identified purpose will prevent teams from drifting off target.

Topic Priority. Not every clinical question can be addressed through the EBP process. Identification of issues that are a priority for the organization will facilitate garnering the support needed to complete an EBP improvement. Priority may be given to topics that address patient safety; high-volume, high-risk, or high-cost topics; those that are closely aligned with the institution's strategic plan; or those that are driven by other institutional or market forces (e.g., changing reimbursement). Considering how a topic fits within the organizational priorities can aid in obtaining support from senior leadership and other disciplines as well as in obtaining the resources necessary to carry out the practice change. Discussions determining whether the clinical issue is a priority create early opportunities to connect with stakeholders. If the topic is not an organizational priority, clinicians may want to consider other issues or opportunities. Consider a different focus, outcome, or other triggers for improving practice that better fit organizational needs. This and similar feedback loops within the model highlight the nonlinearity of the work and support continuing efforts for improving quality through evidence-based care delivery.

Form a Team. Once there is commitment to addressing the topic, a team is formed to develop, implement, and evaluate the practice change. The team is composed of stakeholders that may include staff nurse(s), unit managers, advanced practice registered nurses (APRNs), interprofessional colleagues, representatives of shared governance committees (Cullen, Wagner, Matthews, & Farrington, in press), and organizational leaders. Team membership requires several considerations to maximize the use of team members' skills and organizational linkages.

When addressing oral mucositis using the Iowa Model, team membership was designed to capture key linkages clinically and within the governance structure (Cullen et al., 2018; Cullen, Wagner et al., in press). The team included members from pediatric and adult ambulatory and inpatient settings representing staff nurses, nurse managers, APRNs, and interprofessional team members. Committee members also provided active linkages within the governance structure through their membership on or links to nursing quality, hospital dentistry, dietary, hematology–oncology clinicians, radiation oncology, speech pathology, patient education, staff education, the products committee, nursing policy committee, and the nursing management council (Cullen et al., 2018). The team used these linkages to support communication, coordination, and reporting about the initiative. This coordination and collaboration promotes delivery of evidence-based healthcare (Chavez et al., 2015).

Assemble, Appraise, and Synthesize Body of Evidence. Initially, the team selects, reviews, critiques, and synthesizes all available evidence. Collaboration with nursing librarians can be particularly helpful in optimizing yields from online bibliographic databases and other library resources (Koffel, 2015). Librarians' expert knowledge and skills in the functionality of online resources, when matched with clinicians' expertise, will result in yields with the best specificity to address the topic. Appraisal and synthesis of the body of evidence captures best evidence through lower evidence (e.g., local quality data) for consideration and next steps. Weighing the body of evidence helps identify the strength of the recommendation and potential benefit (GRADE Working Group, 2017; U.S. Preventative Services Task Force, 2016).

Sufficient Evidence. Determining whether evidence is sufficient is not a simple process. If high-quality evidence is not available or sufficient for determining practice, the team may recommend using related evidence (e.g., from other patient populations) (Cullen, Hanrahan, Neis, et al., in press; Farrington et al., 2015), lower levels of evidence (Crogan & Dupler, 2014), data mining of local practice data (Dzau et al., 2017), scientific principles, or conduct research to improve the evidence available for practice and operational decisions (Anderson, Kleiber, Greiner, Comried, & Zimmerman, 2016). When the evidence is sufficient or lower levels of evidence are used, a practice change is piloted. The team designs the practice change and pilot evaluation to determine whether the EBP change works in clinical care.

Design and Pilot the Practice Change. Piloting is an essential step in the EBP process. Outcomes achieved in a controlled environment, when research is testing a study protocol in a homogenous group of patients, may be different than those found when the recommendation is used by multiple caregivers in a natural clinical setting without the tight controls of a research study. Thus, trialing the EBP change is essential for identifying issues before instituting in the pilot area or larger rollout/scale-up. Early steps include engaging patients when designing the practice change. Understanding and valuing a partnership with patients is an ongoing priority (Anderson et al., 2016). Patient engagement can take many forms to improve their participation in decisions impacting their health and healthcare (Dzau et al., 2017; Fearns et al., 2016; Stacey et al., 2014).

Establishing an issue as a priority is considered earlier in the Iowa Model. When designing the EBP protocol to pilot, resources and constraints are incorporated in designing the change to ensure feasibility to promote adoption. Evidence-based care delivery is intended to be routine and would not normally require institutional review board approval (Office of Human Research Protections, n.d.; Olsen & Smania, 2016). However, student projects, even if not designed as research, may need organizational approvals (Basol, Larsen, Simones, & Wilson, 2017; Foote, Conley, Williams, McCarthy, & Countryman, 2015).

Designing a draft practice protocol for use in the local setting can take many forms. Frequently, EBP protocols are designed as an evidence-based policy, procedure, care map, algorithm, or other document outlining the practice and decision points for clinician users. The best approach is determined by end users, considering commonly used implementation strategies in that setting, and the complexity of the procedure to be used.

Piloting also involves planning for both implementation and evaluation. Research evidence will provide direction for selecting structure, process, and outcome indicators to use for baseline data measurement. Significant simplification of research measures is needed when evaluating quality indicators for EBP. Pilot evaluation is not replication research and must be narrowed to key indicators needed to provide direction for clinical decision making and implementation. Common process indicators to include in the evaluation for clinicians and patients are their knowledge, attitudes, and practices/health behaviors (Bick & Graham, 2010; Parry, Carson-Stevens, Luff, McPherson, & Goldmann, 2013). Implementation during the pilot requires a phased approach for planning and selection of effective implementation strategies (Figure 14.4; Cullen & Adams, 2012; Esposito, Heeringa, Bradley, Croake, & Kimmey, 2015; Rogers, 2003). Implementation strategies are selected based on prepilot process data.

Evaluation of the structure, process, and outcome indicators is completed before and after implementation of the practice change. Prepilot data is used to design the practice change and implementation plan. A comparison of prepilot and postpilot data will determine the success of the pilot, effectiveness of the EBP protocol, effectiveness of the implementation plan, and need for modification of either the implementation process or the practice protocol before integration or rollout.

Decide if the Change is Appropriate for Practice. Following the pilot, a determination is made regarding appropriateness of adoption in the pilot and beyond. A decision regarding adoption or modification of the practice is based on the evaluative data from the pilot. If the practice change is not appropriate for adoption and rollout, quality or performance improvement monitoring is needed to ensure high-quality patient care. Additional steps for clinicians include redesigning the practice change, watching for new knowledge, collaborating with researchers in the area, or conducting research to guide practice decisions. If the pilot results are positive, rollout and integration of the practice are needed (Cullen & Adams, 2012; Cullen, Hanrahan, Farrington et al., 2018).

Integrate and Sustain the Practice Change. When positive outcomes are achieved, integration of the practice is facilitated through engagement of key stakeholders such as patients and influential leaders. Sustainability is promoted by local champions, opinion leaders, senior leadership support, education, and continuous monitoring of outcomes (Cullen & Adams, 2012; Cullen, Hanrahan, Farrington et al., 2018; Fleiszer, Semenic, Ritchie, Richer, & Denis, 2016a; Fleuren, van Dommelen, & Dunnink, 2015).

EBP changes need ongoing evaluation with information incorporated into quality or performance improvement programs to promote hardwiring or integration of the practice into daily care. Monitoring and reporting trends of key structure, process, and outcomes indicators with actionable feedback to clinicians can promote sustained integration of the practice change (Cullen, Hanrahan, Farrington et al., 2018; Fleiszer et al., 2016a; Fleuren et al., 2015; Hysong, Kell, Petersen, Campbell, & Trautner, 2017).

Implementation Strategies for Evidence-Based Practice

	Create Awareness & Interest	Build Knowledge & Commitment	Promote Action & Adoption	Pursue Integration & Sustained Use
Connecting with Clinicians, Organizational Leaders, and Key Stakeholders	• Highlight advantages* or anticipated impact* • Highlight compatibility* • Continuing education programs* • Sound bites* • Journal club* • Slogans & logos • Staff meetings • Unit newsletter • Unit inservices • Distribute key evidence • Posters and postings/fliers • Mobile 'show on the road' • Announcements & broadcasts	• Education (e.g., live, virtual or computer-based)* • Pocket guides • Link practice change & powerholder/stakeholder priorities* • Change agents (e.g., change champion*, core group*, opinion leader*, thought leader, etc.) • Educational outreach or academic detailing* • Integrate practice change with other EBP protocols* • Disseminate credible evidence with clear implications for practice* • Make impact observable* • Gap assessment/gap analysis* • Clinician input* • Local adaptation* & simplify* • Focus groups for planning change* • Match practice change with resources & equipment • Resource manual or materials (i.e., electronic or hard copy) • Case studies	• Educational outreach/ academic detailing* • Reminders or practice prompts* • Demonstrate workflow or decision algorithm • Resource materials and quick reference guides • Skill competence* • Give evaluation results to colleagues* • Incentives* • Try the practice change* • Multidisciplinary discussion & troubleshooting • "Elevator speech" • Data collection by clinicians • Report progress & updates • Change agents (e.g., change champion*, core group*, opinion leader*, thought leader, etc.) • Role model* • Troubleshooting at the point of care/bedside • Provide recognition at the point of care*	• Celebrate local unit progress* • Individualize data feedback* • Public recognition* • Personalize the messages to staff (e.g., reduces work, reduces infection exposure, etc.) based on actual improvement data • Share protocol revisions with clinician that are based on feedback from clinicians, patient or family • Peer influence • Update practice reminders
Building Organizational System Support	• Knowledge broker(s) • Senior executives announcement • Publicize new equipment	• Teamwork* • Troubleshoot use/ application* • Benchmark data* • Inform organizational leaders* • Report within organizational infrastructure* • Action plan* • Report to senior leaders	• Audit key indicators* • Actionable and timely data feedback* • Non-punitive discussion of results* • Checklist* • Documentation* • Standing orders* • Patient reminders* • Patient decision aides* • Rounding by unit & organizational leadership* • Report into quality improvement program* • Report to senior leaders • Action plan* • Link to patient/family needs & organizational priorities • Unit orientation • Individual performance evaluation	• Audit and feedback* • Report to senior leaders* • Report into quality improvement program* • Revise policy, procedure or protocol* • Competency metric for discontinuing training • Project responsibility in unit or organizational committee • Strategic plan* • Trend results* • Present in educational programs • Annual report • Financial incentives* Individual performance evaluation

* = Implementation strategy is supported by at least some empirical evidence in healthcare

© University of Iowa Hospitals and Clinics/Laura Cullen, MA, RN, FAAN

Figure 14.4: Implementation Strategies for EBP. (Cullen, L., Adams, S. [2012]. Planning for implementation of evidence-based practice. *Journal of Nursing Administration, 42*[4], 222–230. doi: 10.1097/NNA.0b013e31824ccd0a. Used with permission from the University of Iowa Hospitals and Clinics. © 2012. For permission to use or reproduce, please contact the University of Iowa Hospitals and Clinics at UIHCNursingResearchandEBP@uiowa.ed).

Proactive planning for reinfusion is needed to avoid relapsing to old routines. Little research is available to guide timing, but regular, that is, quarterly or biannual, reinfusion until the practice is hardwired may be appropriate. Monitoring data trends will show when reinfusion is needed.

Disseminate Results. Dissemination of results is important for professional learning. Sharing project reports within and outside of the organization through presentations and publications supports growth of an EBP culture in the organization, expands nursing knowledge, and encourages EBP changes in other organizations as well (Cullen, Wagner et al., in press). Project reports can be used to learn the EBP process, learn of practice updates, or to generate additional practice questions. Dissemination of project results is a key step in the cycle promoting adoption of EBPs within the healthcare system (Adams, Farrington, & Cullen, 2012; Saver, 2014; Sigma Theta Tau International Research Scholarship Advisory Committee, 2008; Williams & Cullen, 2016).

This model is a revised version of the model by Rosswurm and Larrabee (1999). The revised steps and schematic (Figure 14.5) were prompted by Larrabee's experience with teaching and leading nurses in the application of the original model since 1999 at West Virginia University Hospitals and prior experience with teaching and leading nurses in RU and QI (Larrabee, 2004).

Model for Evidence-Based Practice Change

The Iowa Model guides clinicians through the EBP process. The model includes several feedback loops, reflecting analysis, evaluation, and modification based on evaluative data of structure, process, and outcome indicators and expertise of team members. These are critical for adapting the evidence to the practice setting, individualizing for patient needs and preferences, and for promoting adoption within the varying healthcare systems and settings within which nurses work. The feedback loops highlight the messy and nonlinear nature of EBP and support teams moving forward. The Iowa Model was designed to support evidence-based healthcare delivery by interprofessional teams (Chavez et al., 2015; Cullen, Hanrahan, Neis et al., in press; Farrington et al., 2015) by following a basic problem-solving approach using the scientific problem-solving process, simplifying the process, and being highly application oriented. The large number of nurses and organizations using the Iowa Model attests to its usefulness in practice. In fact, the Iowa Model has been cited nearly 400 times, and over 1,500 requests have been received to use the updated Iowa Model (unpublished data) since July 2015. The Iowa Model stands the test of time as a pragmatic, application-oriented and theory-based EBP process model.

The title of the revised model was changed to clarify that it was designed for guiding multiple practice change projects because the author thought the original title, "Model for Change to Evidence-Based Practice," could imply a one-time philosophical decision to pursue EBP. The revised model integrates principles of QI, use of teamwork tools, and evidence-based translation strategies to promote adoption of a new practice. The handbook (Larrabee, 2009) describing the revised model includes a number of forms and examples of their use that may be helpful to nurses applying the model. Progression through the six steps is illustrated by a fabricated EBP project focused on improving outcomes for patients with chronic heart failure.

Step 1: Assess the Need for Change in Practice
Key actions consist of identifying a practice problem or opportunity for improvement; creating an EBP team of stakeholders to address the practice problem; collecting internal data about

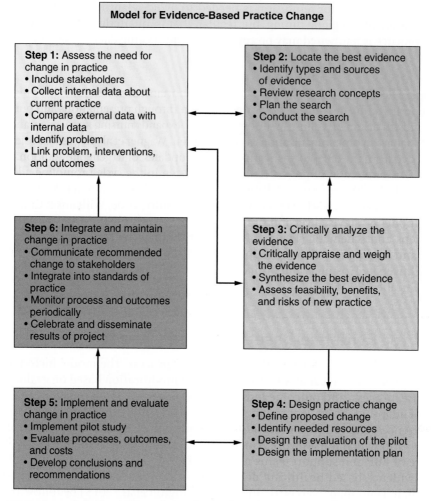

Figure 14.5: A model of evidence-based practice change. (Larrabee, J. H. [2009]. *Nurse to nurse: Practice.* New York, NY: McGraw-Hill. Used with permission of McGraw-Hill Education.)

that practice; collecting external data for benchmarking with the internal data; and refining the practice problem statement by linking the problem with possible interventions and desired outcomes or by developing a PICOT (population-intervention-comparison-outcome-time frame) question.

Often, recognition of a practice problem prompts an EBP project. Practice problems can be identified by members of a clinical unit's RU team or solicited from practicing nurses. Other times, an existing EBP team with the goal of conducting at least one EBP project per year will need to consider what patient outcomes most need improvement. Structured brainstorming and multivoting are teamwork tools that may be helpful during this process. Developing creative avenues for problem identification that increase active involvement from the nurses who will be participating in the implementation stage, such as placing an idea box on the unit for nurses, is crucial for establishing group ownership for the change project.

Once the EBP team has selected a practice problem as the focus of a project, team members should collect internal and external data relevant to that practice problem to confirm that there is an opportunity for improvement. It is important to justify the focus of the EBP project because such projects are resource intensive. Statistical process control tools that may be useful during this activity include histograms and Pareto charts. The EBP team members must prepare a practice problem statement or PICOT question to clarify for themselves and others what the project focus is and to use the statement or question to guide their work during Step 2.

Step 2: Locate the Best Evidence

Key actions are identifying the types and sources of evidence; planning the search for evidence; and conducting the search for the best evidence. Types of evidence include clinical practice guidelines, systematic reviews, single studies, critical appraisal topics, and expert committee reports. Sources of evidence include electronic bibliographic databases, websites, journals, and books. The search for evidence should be planned as a rigorous systematic review, which includes formulating the research question to guide the search, deciding on the search strategy, selecting the inclusion and exclusion criteria, and planning the synthesis. While planning, EBP team members can add rigor to the systematic review by selecting forms for critically appraising evidence sources, for organizing data from the evidence sources in a table of evidence, and identifying key points to use when synthesizing the evidence during Step 3. Critical appraisal forms or checklists are available in journal articles (Rosswurm & Larrabee, 1999) and online, including some that are for systematic reviews and specific research designs (Scottish Intercollegiate Guidelines Network, 2007).The handbook includes examples of forms and completed examples of their use (Larrabee, 2009).

Step 3: Critically Analyze the Evidence

Key actions are critically appraising and judging the strength of the evidence; synthesizing the evidence; and assessing the feasibility, benefits, and risks of implementing the new practice. Critical appraisal of the evidence is conducted using the forms selected during Step 2. Likewise, the forms selected during Step 2 are used to display information about the data sources in an evidence table that is then used to prepare the synthesis worksheet. After synthesizing the evidence, the EBP team members judge whether the body of evidence is of sufficient quantity and strength to support a practice change. If so, EBP team members consider whether or not benefits and risks of the new practice are acceptable and whether the new practice is feasible in their workplace.

Step 4: Design Practice Change

Key actions include defining the proposed practice change; identifying needed resources; designing the evaluation of the pilot; and designing the implementation plan. The description of the new practice may be in the form of a protocol, policy, procedure, care map, or guideline and should be supported by the body of evidence synthesized in Step 3. Needed resources will be specific for the new practice and may include personnel, materials, equipment, or forms. Even if the new practice is specific to just one unit, its use should be pilot tested to evaluate it for any necessary adaptation before making it a standard of care. Therefore, EBP team members need to design the implementation plan and the evaluation plan, considering translation strategies that promote adoption of a new practice. Some strategies include use of change champions, opinion leaders, educational sessions, educational materials, reminder systems, and audit and feedback. After designing the evaluation plan, EBP team members collect baseline data on the process and outcome indicators for which they will collect postpilot data during Step 5.

Step 5: Implement and Evaluate Change in Practice

Key actions include implementing the pilot study; evaluating process, outcomes, and costs; and developing conclusions and recommendations. The EBP team members follow the implementation plan designed during Step 4, obtaining verbal feedback from those expected to use the new practice and from the change champions who are promoting the use of the new practice. That feedback will be used to make minor adjustments in the implementation plan, if necessary. After the pilot phase concludes, the EBP team members collect and analyze the postpilot data, comparing them with the baseline data. Team members use those data together with the verbal feedback to decide if they should adapt, adopt, or reject the new practice. Few teams reach this stage and decide to reject the new practice. More commonly, the new practice needs to be slightly adapted for a better fit with the organization. Once team members make this decision, they prepare conclusions and recommendations to share with administrative leaders during Step 6.

Step 6: Integrate and Maintain Change in Practice

Key actions include sharing recommendations about the new practice with stakeholders; incorporating the new practice into the standards of care; monitoring the process and outcome indicators; and celebrating and disseminating results of the project. Team members provide information about the project and their recommendations to all stakeholders, including administrative leaders who must approve making the new practice a standard of care.

Once that approval is given, the EBP team members can arrange to provide inservice education to all providers expected to use the new practice. It is important to include all stages of the process in the inservice education, such as problem identification and the strength of the evidence, because teams that emphasize only the practice change have higher rates of noncompliance during the implementation phase. They should also make plans for ongoing monitoring of the process and outcome indicators. The frequency of this monitoring can be based on judging how well the indicators are being met. The data from ongoing monitoring can be used to identify the need for further refinements in the new practice or the need for a new EBP project. The handbook (Larrabee, 2009) provides a timeline template for preparing an annual calendar with multiple EBP projects, including ongoing monitoring of completed projects. Finally, EBP team members should consider disseminating information about their project outside the organization through presentation at professional conferences and publication.

The Evidence-Based Advancing Research and Clinical Practice Through Close Collaboration Model: A Model for System-Wide Implementation and Sustainability of Evidence-Based Practice

The purpose of the **ARCC©** Model is to provide healthcare institutions and clinical settings with an organized conceptual framework that can guide system-wide implementation and sustainability of EBP to achieve quality outcomes. Since evidence-based clinicians are essential in cultivating an entire system culture that implements EBP as standard of care, the ARCC© Model encompasses key strategies for individual and organizational change to and sustainability of best practice.

Overview of the ARCC© Model

The original version of the ARCC© Model was conceptualized by Bernadette Melnyk in 1999 as part of a strategic planning initiative to unify research and clinical practice in order to advance EBP within an academic medical center for the ultimate purpose of improving healthcare quality and patient outcomes (Melnyk & Fineout-Overholt, 2002). Shortly following conceptualization of the ARCC© Model, Dr. Fineout-Overholt surveyed advanced practice and point-of-care nurses in the medical center about the barriers and **facilitators** of EBP. The results of this survey along with control theory (Carver & Sheier, 1982, 1998) and cognitive behavioral theory (CBT; Beck, Rush, Shaw, & Emery, 1979) guided the formulation of key constructs in the current ARCC© Model. An important facilitator of EBP identified by nurses who completed the survey was a mentor, which eventually became the central mechanism for implementing and sustaining EBP in the ARCC© Model. For two decades, Melnyk and Fineout-Overholt have further developed the ARCC© Model through empirical testing of key relationships in the model and their extensive work with healthcare institutions across the nation and globe to advance and sustain EBP.

The Conceptual Framework Guiding the ARCC© Model

Control theory (Carver & Scheier, 1982, 1998) contends that a discrepancy between a standard or goal (e.g., system-wide implementation of EBP) and a current state (e.g., the extent to which an organization is implementing EBP) should motivate behaviors in individuals to reach the goal. However, many barriers exist in healthcare organizations that inhibit clinicians from implementing EBP, including (a) inadequate EBP knowledge and skills, (b) lack of administrative support, (c) lack of an EBP mentor, (d) lack of belief that EBP improves patient care and outcomes, (e) perceived lack of authority to change patient care procedures, and (f) nurse leader/manager resistance (Hutchinson & Johnston, 2006; Melnyk, 2007; Melnyk & Fineout-Overholt, 2011; Melnyk, Fineout-Overholt, Gallagher-Ford, & Kaplan, 2012). In the ARCC© Model, EBP mentors (i.e., healthcare providers with in-depth knowledge and skills in EBP as well as individual and organizational change strategies along with mentorship skills) are developed and placed within the healthcare system as a key strategy to remove barriers commonly encountered by practicing clinicians when implementing EBP (Figure 14.6). As barriers diminish, clinicians enhance their implementation of EBP to improve patient outcomes.

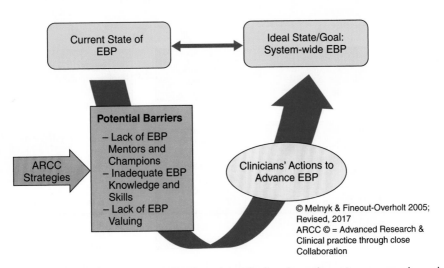

Figure 14.6: Control theory as a conceptual guide for the advancing research and clinical practice through close collaboration (ARCC©) model. EBP, evidence-based practice. (Melnyk, B., & Fineout-Overholt, E., 2005, revised 2017.)

In the ARCC© Model, CBT is used to guide behavioral change in individual clinicians toward EBP. CBT stresses the importance of individual, social, and environmental factors that influence cognition, learning, emotions, and behavior (Beck et al., 1979; Lam, 2005). The basic foundation of CBT is that an individual's behaviors and emotions are, in large part, determined by the way he or she thinks or his or her beliefs (i.e., the thinking–feeling–behaving triangle; Melnyk & Moldenhauer, 2006). Based on CBT, a tenet of the ARCC© Model contends that when clinicians' beliefs about the value of EBP and their ability to implement it are strengthened through strategies such as education and skills building, there will be greater implementation of evidence-based care. In the ARCC© Model, EBP mentors work with point-of-care clinicians to strengthen their beliefs about the value of EBP and their ability to implement it through evidence-based decisions.

> " By changing your thinking, you change your beliefs.
>
> **AUTHOR UNKNOWN**

Central Constructs Within and Evidence to Support the ARCC© Model

Organizational Assessment of Readiness. The first step in the ARCC© Model is an organizational assessment of culture and readiness for system-wide implementation of EBP (Figure 14.7). The culture and environment of an organization can foster EBP or stymie it. If sufficient resources are not allocated to support the work of EBP, progress in advancing EBP throughout the organization will be slow. Leaders, administrators, and point-of-care providers alike must adopt the EBP paradigm for system-wide implementation to be achieved and sustained. Assessment of organizational culture can be determined with the use of the Organizational Culture and

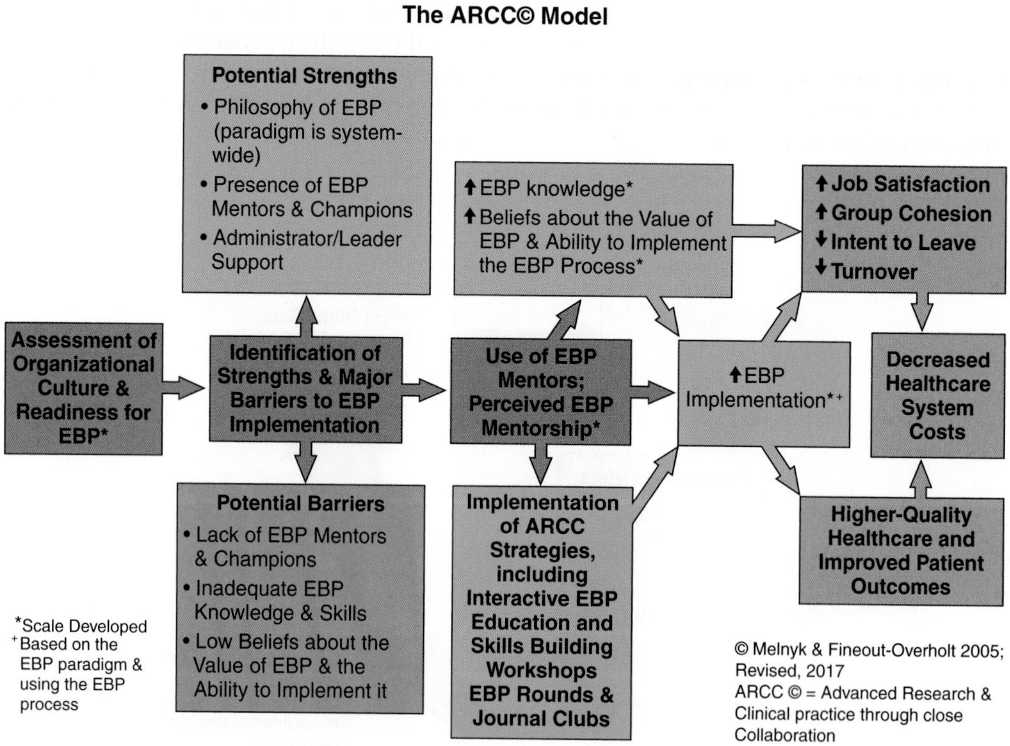

The ARCC© Model

Figure 14.7: Melnyk and Fineout-Overholt's Advancing Research and Clinical Practice Through Close Collaboration (ARCC©) model. EBP, evidence-based practice. (Melnyk, B., & Fineout-Overholt, E., 2005, revised 2017.)

Readiness Scale for System-Wide Integration of Evidence-Based Practice (OCRSIEP) (Fineout-Overholt & Melnyk, 2006). With the use of this 25-item Likert scale, a description of organizational characteristics, including strengths and opportunities for fostering EBP within a healthcare system, is identified. Examples of items on the OCRSIEP include the following:

a. To what extent is EBP clearly described as central to the mission and philosophy of your institution?
b. To what extent do you believe that EBP is practiced in your organization?
c. To what extent is the nursing staff with whom you work committed to EBP?

In the ARCC© Model, higher organizational culture is expected to increase EBP beliefs and implementation, which influence healthcare outcomes. The OCRSIEP scale has established face and content validity, with internal consistency reliabilities consistently greater than 0.85 across many populations (see Appendix K for a sample of the OCRSIEP scale).

EBP Mentors. Once key strengths and opportunities for fostering EBP within the organization are identified with the OCRSIEP scale, a cadre of EBP mentors is developed within the healthcare system. EBP mentors are healthcare providers, typically Advanced Practice Nurses (APNs), transdisciplinary clinicians, or baccalaureate-prepared nurses in health systems that do not have APNs working directly with point-of-care staff to implement EBP. These mentors assist in (a) shifting from a traditional practice paradigm to an EBP paradigm, (b) conducting EBP implementation (EBPI) projects, and (c) generating and integrating practice-based data to improve healthcare quality as well as patient and/or system outcomes. EBP mentors also have knowledge and skills in individual behavior and organizational change strategies to facilitate changes in clinician behavior and spark sustainable changes in organizational culture, which require specific intervention strategies, time, and persistence.

Key components of the EBP mentor role as defined in the ARCC© Model include (a) ongoing assessment of an organization's capacity to sustain an EBP culture; (b) building EBP knowledge and skills by conducting interactive group workshops and one-on-one mentoring; (c) stimulating, facilitating, and educating nursing staff toward a culture of EBP, with a focus on overcoming barriers to best practice; (d) role modeling EBP; (e) conducting ARCC© EBP enhancing strategies, such as EBP rounds, journal clubs, webpages, newsletters, and fellowship programs; (f) working with staff to generate internal evidence (i.e., practice-generated) through outcomes management and EBPI projects; (g) facilitating staff involvement in research to generate external evidence; (h) using evidence to foster best practice; and (i) collaborating with interdisciplinary professionals to advance and sustain EBP. These mentors also have excellent strategic planning, implementation, and outcomes evaluation skills so that they can monitor the impact of their role and overcome barriers in moving the system to a culture of best practice (Melnyk, 2007). Mentorship with direct care staff on clinical units by ARCC EBP mentors© is important in strengthening clinicians' beliefs about the value of EBP and their ability to implement it (Melnyk & Fineout-Overholt, 2002, 2011).

EBP Beliefs Scale. In the ARCC© Model, beliefs about the value of EBP and a clinician's ability to implement it are measured with the EBP Beliefs (EBPB) scale (Melnyk & Fineout-Overholt, 2002). This instrument is a 16-item Likert scale, with responses that range from 1 (strongly disagree) to 5 (strongly agree). Examples of items on the EBPB scale include (a) I am clear about the steps in EBP, (b) I am sure that I can implement EBP, and (c) I am sure that evidence-based guidelines can improve care. The EBPB scale has established face, content, and construct validity, with internal consistency reliabilities consistently greater than 0.85 across multiple studies (Melnyk, Fineout-Overholt, & Mays, 2008; see Appendix K for a sample copy of the scale). In the ARCC© Model, higher beliefs about EBP are expected to increase EBPI and thereby improve healthcare outcomes.

Findings from research indicate that when nurses' beliefs about the value of EBP and their ability to implement it are strong, their implementation of EBP is greater (Melnyk et al., 2004; Melnyk, Fineout-Overholt, Giggleman, & Cruz, 2010). Additionally, findings from a recent randomized controlled pilot study indicated that nurses who received mentoring from an ARCC© EBP mentor, in comparison with those who received mentoring in physical assessment skills, had (a) stronger EBPB, (b) greater implementation of EBP, and (c) stronger group cohesion (Levin, Fineout-Overholt, Melnyk, Barnes, & Vetter, 2011), which is known to be a predictor of nurse satisfaction and turnover rates. Nurses in the ARCC© EBP group also had less attrition/turnover than nurses in the physical assessment group.

A total of eight studies now provide evidence to support the relationships in the ARCC© Model (Levin et al., 2011; Melnyk, 2012; Melnyk et al., 2004, 2008, 2010; Melnyk & Fineout-Overholt, 2002; Melnyk, Fineout-Overholt, Giggleman, & Choy, 2017; Wallen et al., 2010). The role of EBP mentors and their impact on healthcare systems and EBP is also being investigated as they are likely to be the key to sustainability of EBP in organizations (Levin et al., 2011; Melnyk, 2007).

Implementing the Evidence-Based ARCC© Model

EBPI in the ARCC© Model is defined as practicing based on the EBP paradigm. This paradigm uses the EBP process to improve outcomes. The process begins with asking clinical questions and incorporates research evidence and practice-based evidence in point-of-care decision making. However, simply engaging the process is not sufficient. The results of the first three steps of the process (i.e., establishing valid and reliable research evidence) must be coupled with (a) the expertise of the clinician to gather practice-based evidence (i.e., data from practice initiatives such as QI); gather, interpret, and act on patient data; and effectively use healthcare resources and (b) what the patient and family value and prefer (see Figure 13.4). This amalgamation leads to innovative decision making at the point of care with quality outcomes. Although research evidence, practice evidence, and patient/client data as interpreted through expertise and patient preferences must always be present, a context of caring allows each patient–provider encounter to be individualized (see Chapter 1, Figure 1.2). Within an organization and ecosystem or environment that fosters an EBP culture, this paradigm can thrive at the patient–provider level as well as across the organization, resulting in transformed healthcare.

The ARCC© Model is implemented in hospitals and healthcare systems through a 12-month program to prepare a cadre of EBP mentors who work directly with point-of-care clinicians to implement and sustain EBP throughout the entire system or institution. A series of six workshops that consist of 8 days of educational and skills-building sessions are conducted over the 12-month ARCC program©, which is focused on implementing the seven-step EBP process and necessary strategies for building an EBP culture and environment. The content of the ARCC© workshops includes (a) EBP skills building, (b) creating a vision to motivate a change to EBP, (c) transdisciplinary team building and effective communication, (d) mentorship to advance EBP, (e) strategies to build an EBP culture, (f) QI processes, (g) data management and outcomes monitoring/evaluation, and (h) theories and principles of individual behavior change and organizational change.

Before the first workshop, a baseline assessment is conducted to assess the clinicians' EBP beliefs, EBPI, organizational culture and readiness for EBP, job satisfaction, and group cohesion. Data on patient problems identified for improvement by the clinicians in the ARCC program© are also collected and analyzed. Each team who attends the series of workshops implements an EBPI project during the course of the ARCC program©, which is focused on improving quality and reliability (i.e., safety) of care as well as patient outcomes.

Recent implementation of the ARCC© Model at Washington Hospital Healthcare System, a 355-bed community hospital system in the western region of the United States revealed the following findings: (a) Early ambulation in the intensive care unit resulted in a reduction in ventilator days from 11.6 to 8.9 days and no ventilator-associated pneumonias; (b) Pressure ulcer rates were reduced from 6.07% to 0.62% on a medical surgical unit; (c) Education of congestive heart failure patients led to a 14.7% reduction in hospital readmissions, and (d) 75% of patients perceived the overall quality of care as excellent after implementation of an evidence-based family-centered care program compared with 22.2% preimplementation (Melnyk et al., 2017).

EBP implementation in the ARCC© Model is measured with the EBPI scale (Melnyk & Fineout-Overholt, 2002). Clinicians respond to each of the 18 Likert scale items on the EBPI by answering how often in the last 8 weeks they have performed certain EBP initiatives, such as (a) generated a PICOT question about my practice, (b) used evidence to change my clinical practice, (c) evaluated the outcomes of a practice change, and (d) shared the outcome data collected with colleagues. The EBPI has established face, content, and construct validity as well as internal consistency reliabilities greater than 0.85 across multiple studies (Melnyk et al., 2008; see Appendix K for a sample copy of the scale). In the ARCC© Model, it is contended that greater EBPI is associated with higher nurse satisfaction, a trend that will eventually lead to lower turnover rates and healthcare expenditures.

Several healthcare systems and hospitals both across the United States and worldwide have now implemented the ARCC© Model in their efforts to build and sustain an EBP culture and ecosystem in their organizations. As part of the objective of building this culture, groups of nurses and other transdisciplinary healthcare providers have attended a week-long EBP mentorship immersion program, conducted by the authors of the ARCC© Model. These programs have prepared more than 2200 nurses and transdisciplinary clinicians across the nation and the globe as ARCC EBP mentors©. Some of the individuals who have attended these immersion programs have negotiated roles as EBP mentors within their healthcare organizations.

 The EBP mentorship program is now available as an onsite workshop or through an online program offered by the Helene Fuld Health Trust National Institute for Evidence-based Practice in Nursing and Healthcare at The Ohio State University College of Nursing: https://fuld.nursing.osu.edu/

The final step in the ARCC© Model is for EBP mentors and other clinicians who practice according to the EBP paradigm to have an impact on provider, patient, and system outcomes. EBP mentors and those they influence focus on achieving the best outcomes of care, thereby making a difference in patients' lives and the success of the organization.

Using and Evaluating the Evidence-Based ARCC© Model

Because valid and reliable instruments are available to measure key constructs in the ARCC© Model, barriers to and facilitators of EBP along with clinicians' beliefs about and actual implementation of EBP can be readily assessed and identified by organizations. Also available are well-established workshops and online offerings that develop EBP mentors who can work closely with point-of-care staff to strengthen their beliefs about and implementation of EBP. The availability of tools to measure an organization's EBP culture and readiness for EBP as well as clinicians' EBPB and implementation also allow an organization to monitor its progress in the system-wide implementation and sustainability of EBP.

Promoting Action on Research Implementation in Health Services Framework

Overview of the PARIHS Framework

Getting evidence into practice is complex, multifaceted, and dynamic. **The PARIHS framework** was developed in an attempt to reflect these complexities, representing the interdependence and interplay of the many factors that appear to contribute to the successful implementation

(SI) of evidence in practice. Previous research exploring why research evidence is not routinely used in practice has tended to focus at the level of individual practitioners and on barriers to utilization (e.g., Hunt, 1991; McSherry, Artley, & Holloran, 2006; Parahoo, 1999). Although individual factors are important, getting evidence into practice requires more than a focus on addressing individual influencing factors. The PARIHS framework, which provides a conceptual map, is premised on the notion that the implementation of research-based practice depends on the ability to achieve significant and planned behavior change involving individuals, teams, and organizations. SI is represented as a function (f) of the nature and type of evidence (e), the qualities of the context (c) in which the evidence is being introduced, and the way the process is facilitated (f), whereby SI = f(E,C,F). The three elements (i.e., evidence, context, and facilitation) are each positioned on a high-to-low continuum, where in each implementation effort the aim is to move toward *high* in order to optimize the chances of success.

Development and Refinement

The PARIHS framework has developed over time (Kitson, Harvey, & McCormack, 1998; Rycroft-Malone et al., 2002; Rycroft-Malone, Harvey et al., 2004). It was originally conceived inductively from an analysis of practice development, QI, and research project work (Kitson et al., 1998). Theoretical and retrospective analysis of four studies led to the proposal that the most SI seems to occur when evidence is scientifically robust; matches professional consensus and patients' preferences (high evidence); when the context is receptive to change with sympathetic cultures, strong leadership, and appropriate monitoring and feedback systems (high context); and when there is appropriate facilitation of change with input from skilled external and internal facilitators (high facilitation).

Since the framework's conception and publication, it has undergone research and development work. Most notably, this has included a concept analysis of each of the dimensions (Harvey et al., 2002; McCormack et al., 2002; Rycroft-Malone, Seers et al., 2004) and a research study to assess content validity (Rycroft-Malone, Harvey et al., 2004). This enabled some conceptual clarity to be gained about the framework's constituent elements and verification of its content validity. As a result of this work, the framework has been refined over time with the addition, for example, of subelements (Table 14.1).

PARIHS Elements

Evidence. Evidence is conceived in a broad sense within the framework including propositional and nonpropositional knowledge from four different types of evidence (1) research, (2) clinical experience, (3) patients and caregivers' experience, and (4) local context information (see Rycroft-Malone, Seers et al., 2004 for a detailed discussion). For evidence to be considered high, certain criteria have to be met, including that research evidence (qualitative and quantitative) is well conceived and conducted and that there is consensus about it and that clinical experience has been made explicit and verified through critical reflection, critique, and debate. Patient experience is high when patients (and/or significant others) are part of the decision making process and when patient narratives are seen as a valid source of evidence. Finally, local information/data could be considered part of the evidence base if it has been systematically collected, evaluated, and considered. Clearly, this conceptualization indicates the need for an interaction between the scientific and experiential, which requires a dialectical process, that is, a resolution of disagreement through rational and logical discussion.

Context. Context refers to the environment or setting in which the proposed change is to be implemented (see McCormack et al., 2002 for a detailed discussion). Within PARIHS, the contextual factors that promote SI fall under three broad subelements: culture, leadership, and evaluation, which operate in a dynamic, multileveled way. It is proposed that organizations that have cultures that could be described as learning organizations are those that are more

TABLE 14.1   *PARIHS Elements and Subelements*

Elements	Subelements	
Evidence	**Low**	**High**
Research	• Poorly conceived, designed, and/or executed research • Seen as the only type of evidence • Not valued as evidence • Seen as certain	• Well-conceived, designed, and executed research, appropriate to the research question • Seen as one part of a decision • Valued as evidence • Lack of certainty acknowledged • Social construction acknowledged • Judged as relevant • Importance weighted • Conclusions drawn
Clinical experience	• Anecdote, with no critical reflection and judgment • Lack of consensus within similar groups • Not valued as evidence • Seen as the only type of evidence	• Clinical experience and expertise reflected upon, tested by individuals and groups • Consensus within similar groups • Valued as evidence • Seen as one part of the decision • Judged as relevant • Importance weighted • Conclusions drawn
Patient experience	• Not valued as evidence • Patients not involved • Seen as the only type of evidence	• Valued as evidence • Multiple biographies used • Partnerships with healthcare professionals • Seen as one part of a decision • Judged as relevant • Importance weighted • Conclusions drawn
Local data/information	• Not valued as evidence • Lack of systematic methods for collection and analysis • Not reflected upon • No conclusions drawn	• Valued as evidence • Collected and analyzed systematically and rigorously • Evaluated and reflected upon • Conclusions drawn
Context	**Low**	**High**

Culture	• Unclear values and beliefs
	• Low regard for individuals
	• Task-driven organization
	• Lack of consistency
	• Resources not allocated
	• Not integrated with strategic goals
		• Able to define culture(s) in terms of prevailing values/beliefs
		• Values individual staff and clients
		• Promotes learning organization
		• Consistency of individual's role/experience to value:
		  • Relationship with others
		  • Teamwork
		  • Power and authority
		  • Rewards/recognition
		• Resources—human, financial, equipment—allocated
		• Initiative fits with strategic goals and is a key practice/patient issue

(continued)

| TABLE 14.1 | PARIHS Elements and Subelements (continued) |

Elements	Subelements	
Leadership	• Traditional, command and control leadership • Lack of role clarity • Lack of teamwork • Poor organizational structures • Autocratic decision making processes • Didactic approaches to learning/teaching/managing	• Transformational leadership • Role clarity • Effective teamwork • Effective organizational structures • Democratic inclusive decision making processes • Enabling/empowering approach to teaching/learning/managing

Evaluation	• Absence of any form of feedback
	• Narrow use of performance information sources
	• Evaluations rely on single rather than multiple methods
		• Feedback on:
		  • Individual
		  • Team
		  • System
		  • Performance
		• Use of multiple sources of information on performance
		• Use of multiple methods:
		  • Clinical
		  • Performance
		  • Economic
		  • Experience
		  • Evaluations

Facilitation	**Low Inappropriate Facilitation**	**High Appropriate Facilitation**
Purpose Role *Doing for others:*	Task • Episodic contact • Practical/technical help • Didactic, traditional approach to teaching • External agents • Low intensity—extensive coverage	Holistic
Enabling others:	• Sustained partnership • Developmental • Adult learning approach to teaching • Internal/external agents • High intensity—limited coverage	
Skills and attributes	**Task/doing for others** • Project management skills • Technical skills • Marketing skills • Subject/technical/clinical credibility	**Holistic/enabling others** • Cocounseling • Critical reflection • Giving meaning • Flexibility of role • Realness/authenticity

conducive to change (high). Such cultures contain features such as decentralized decision making, a focus on relationships between managers and workers, and management styles that are facilitative. Leaders have a key role to play in creating such cultures. Transformational leaders, as opposed to those who command and control, have the ability to challenge individuals and teams in an enabling, inspiring way (high). Finally, contexts with evaluative mechanisms that collect multiple sources of evidence of performance at the individual, team, and system levels comprise the third element of a high context.

Facilitation. Facilitation refers to the process of enabling or making easier the implementation of evidence into practice (see Harvey et al., 2002, for a detailed discussion). Facilitation is achieved by an individual carrying out a specific role—a facilitator—with the appropriate skills and knowledge to help individuals, teams, and/or organizations apply evidence in practice. With PARIHS, the purpose of facilitation can vary from being task oriented, a prerequisite for which is technical and practical support, to being enabling, a role that calls for a developmental, process-oriented approach. The skills and attributes required to fulfill the role are likely to depend on the situation, individuals, and contexts involved. Therefore, skilled facilitators are those who can adjust their roles and styles to the different stages of an implementation project and the needs of those with whom they are working.

Using the Framework
As each of the elements and subelements are on a continuum of high to low, it is suggested that implementation activities and processes be aimed at moving each of them toward high to increase the chances of success. As such, the framework provides a map of the elements that might require attention and a set of questions that could be asked at the outset of any implementation activity (see Kitson et al., 2008, for examples). This could provide a diagnosis of the current state of readiness to change along with some indication of what needs to be done to move forward (e.g., Brown & McCormack, 2005). Additionally, PARIHS has the potential to be used as an evaluative tool or checklist, which could be used during or after the completion of an implementation project to assess progress, process, or outcome (e.g., Ellis, Howard, Larson, & Robertson, 2005; Hill et al., 2017; Sharp, Pineros, Hsu, Starks, & Sales, 2004). Furthermore, others have used the framework to model and predict the factors involved in RU (Wallin, Estabrooks, Midodzi, & Cummings, 2006).

Future Work
There is a body of evidence from research and practice that shows that the PARIHS framework has conceptual integrity, face, and concept validity. Recently Harvey and Kitson (2016) undertook a revision of PARIHS ("i-PARIHS") where the characteristics of facilitation, innovation, recipients, and context are the core constructs, with facilitation represented as the active element assessing and integrating the other three constructs. As with the original framework, a number of issues still require exploration and further work. These include gaining a clearer understanding of how the constructs interact during implementation and how the framework might be operationalized as both a diagnostic and an evaluative tool. Consistent with the development approach used with PARIHS, users are encouraged to test and evaluate the frameworks in their implementation efforts, particularly through prospective studies.

The Clinical Scholar Model©

Overview of the Clinical Scholar Model©
The Clinical Scholar Model© was developed and implemented to promote the spirit of inquiry, educate direct care providers, and guide a mentorship program for EBP and the conduct of research at the point of care. The words of Dr. Janelle Krueger planted the seeds for the model when she encouraged the conduct and use of research as a staff nurse function and promoted the notion that clinical staff are truly in a position to be able to link research and practice. The philosophy and process used in the Conduct and Utilization of Research in Nursing project, based on the diffusion of innovation theory, formed the early thinking for the model (Horsley, Crane, Crabtree, & Wood, 1983; Rogers, 2003). The concepts presented

in the clinical scholarship resource paper published by Sigma Theta Tau International provided the overarching principles (Clinical Scholarship Task Force, 1999). The innovative ideas cultivated through the curiosity of clinical nurses and the visionary and creative leadership of a nurse researcher combined to flesh out the Clinical Scholar Model©. The model affords a framework for the Clinical Scholar Program©, building the capacity and skills for conducting new research and using evidence at the point of care, thus providing a sustainable solution for changing patterns of thinking, promoting evidence-based care, and improving patient outcomes. The Clinical Scholar Program began as an interactive, outcomes-oriented educational program for nurses but has evolved into an interdisciplinary educational program for direct care providers.

> ❝
> In dwelling upon the vital importance of sound observation, it must never be lost sight of what observation is for. It is not for the sake of piling up miscellaneous information or curious facts, but for the sake of saving life and increasing health and comfort.
>
> **FLORENCE NIGHTINGALE**

Goals of the Model and Program

There are four central goals of the Clinical Scholar Model© and its accompanying educational program:

1. Challenge current practices within direct care.
2. Prepare clinical providers to speak and understand the research language, making day-to-day dialogue featuring discussion of new research findings a common occurrence.
3. Critique and synthesize current research as the core of evidence.
4. Develop clinical scholars to serve as mentors to other staff and to teams who question their practices and seek to improve clinical outcomes.

The structure provided by these goals is important in providing a sense of direction for those whose purpose is creating a center of excellence for patient care.

Components of the Model and Program

The Clinical Scholar Model/Program© is based on clear definitions for research and EBP. The conduct of research is defined as the generation of new, generalizable knowledge using scientific inquiry. Research is conducted when the evidence is not strong enough to support a practice change without potentially creating risk or harm to the recipient of that practice change. EBP is defined as an interdisciplinary approach to healthcare practice that bases decisions and practice strategies to improve patient outcomes on (1) the best available evidence that includes research as the core, national benchmark and QI data and reliable forms of internal evidence; (2) incorporation of clinical expertise; (3) consideration of patient values; and (4) the feasibility of implementation and adoption, the potential risk or harm to the recipient, and the human and material costs.

The Clinical Scholar Model© is grounded in the ideologies of scholarship described in the Clinical Scholarship resource paper published by Sigma Theta Tau International (Clinical Scholarship Task Force, 1999). Although the purpose of the paper was not to describe or define clinical scholarship in terms of research or EBP, the concepts of the clinical scholar provide a sustainable approach to improving patient outcomes: observe and reflect; analyze and critique; synthesize, apply, and evaluate; and disseminate. Each component of the model is further defined within the context of the Clinical Scholar Program (Figure 14.8A).

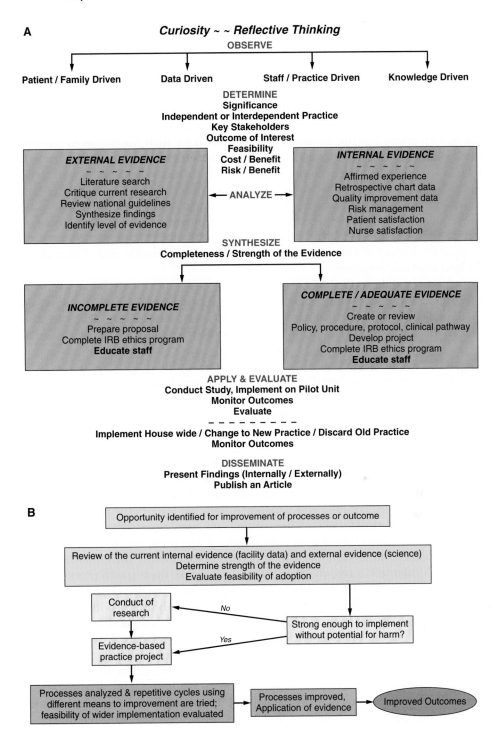

Figure 14.8: **(A)** The Clinical Scholar Model, as further defined within the content of the Clinical Scholar Program. **(B)** Interrelationship between research, EBP, and quality. IRB, institutional review board. **(A**, Used with permission. © Alyce A. Schultz & Associates, LLC [2008]. **B**, From Schultz et al., 2005; used with permission. Courtesy Alyce A. Schultz RN, PhD, FAAN, Bozeman, Montana.)

Clinical Scholar Program Workshops. The Clinical Scholar Program© is based on the Clinical Scholar Model© and is currently utilized in several acute care facilities across the country (Brewer, Brewer, & Schultz, 2009; Honess, Gallant, & Keane, 2009; Mulvenon & Brewer, 2009; Schultz, 2008, 2011a). It is the basis for EBP and research in northern Thailand and northern Philippines (Schultz, 2011b, 2014) and is the framework for at least two nursing EBP collaboratives (Schultz, 2012; Sussong et al., 2009; Weeks, Marshall, & Burns, 2009). English (2016) has recommended the model and program in educating nurses in the Doctorate of Nursing Practice programs in preparation for their leadership as mentors for frontline staff. The program is composed of equal parts of educating, processing, and mentoring in a series of six to eight all-day workshops. The primary goals of the workshops are to (a) challenge the current clinical practices through observation and the spirit of inquiry; (b) speak and understand research language; (c) critique, synthesize, implement, evaluate, and disseminate evidence; and (d) educate direct care providers to serve as mentors to other direct care staff. The ultimate goals are to improve the quality of care provided to patients, to measure the impact of EBP outcomes, and to base administrative and clinical decisions on the best available evidence.

Development and sustainability of an evidence-based culture of excellence requires both an infrastructure where change and innovation are supported and valued by management and staff and a critical mass of direct care providers (i.e., the capacity) who can conduct research, critically synthesize the science, integrate the research findings with internal and other external evidence, and provide leadership to practice change. The infrastructure and capacity must be embedded in a culture where interdisciplinary collaboration is fostered, policies and procedures are based on evidence, and there is a systematic approach to the evaluation of care (Schultz, 2009; Stetler, 2003). Participants selected to attend the Clinical Scholar Programs© are curious, critical thinkers who have either had a research course or are currently enrolled in one and are supported by their clinical supervisors to attend and carry out evidence-based projects or research studies.

The workshops begin with promoting the spirit of inquiry through **observation** and **reflection**. The participants learn to write clear, concise researchable questions, paying particular attention to defining the desired outcomes and the significance of the practice issue to healthcare providers, families, and patients. A librarian teaches the participants how to perform efficient and structured searches on multiple literature databases. Once scientific studies that address the clinical issues are obtained, the participants are taught how to critique the studies and identify the salient outcomes that answer their clinical questions. Evaluation of evidence is a very rigorous process, not unlike the research process; however, the emphasis is clearly on applying the evidence in practice. The principles of synthesis are taught with the use of an evaluation table to delineate the **analysis** and **critique** of each type of research design. During these workshops, published guidelines and systematic reviews are also evaluated for their level of evidence and quality of the science. **Synthesis** is the crux of EBP and the Clinical Scholar Model© (Schultz, 2012; Schultz & Brewer, 2013). It is not a summary of the relevant articles but rather a process of critical thinking built on several principles of synthesis (Box 14.2). There may be several synthesis tables, depending on how the outcomes and/or the interventions are defined. The strength of the evidence is based on levels of research designs, the quality of the studies, the consistency of the relevant findings, the number of studies measuring an independent or dependent variable, and the available internal evidence. Recommendations for practice changes are based on the strength of the evidence and utilized in the development of evidence-based guidelines, policies, procedures, or protocols. APNs and physicians can utilize the synthesized evidence as they develop care plans for their individual patients. Other healthcare providers often have to work through an organizational change process as the new guidelines, policies, or procedures are **applied** to a small sampling of patients and the outcomes are carefully monitored and **evaluated**. Careful adherence to the steps in the new guidelines or procedures or fidelity of the intervention must

> BOX
> **14.2** *Principles of Synthesis*

- Decide which studies to include/exclude
- Arrange studies based on the same or very similar interventions and/or same/similar outcomes measured in the same way
- Thoughtfully analyze inconsistencies across studies
- Establish consensus on major conclusions for each selected outcome variable
- Establish consensus on conclusions drawn from each study
- Establish consensus on clinical implications of findings
- Determine the strength of the findings for pertinent outcomes
- Combine findings into a useful format, with recommendations for implementation in practice if applicable, based on strength of the evidence

also be monitored. If the outcomes for the pilot work are positive, the new guidelines, policies, or procedures are adopted for a broader patient population and outcome measurement continued until the new practices are routinized into daily patterns and positive outcomes are established for the larger group (Schultz, 2007). Finally, the work is **disseminated**, not only to a local audience, but also to a wider audience of direct care providers through poster or podium presentations and publications and through mass media to the general public.

"

To be considered true clinical scholars, nurses must identify and describe their work, making it conscious, so that it can be shared with researchers, colleagues, other health care providers and, perhaps most important, the public.

CLINICAL SCHOLARSHIP TASK FORCE, 1999

Clinical Scholars

Clinical scholars are described as individuals with a high degree of curiosity possessing advanced critical-thinking skills and constantly seeking new knowledge through continuous learning opportunities. They reflect on this knowledge and seek and use a wide variety of resources in implementing new evidence in practice. They never stop asking "Why?" Although most clinical scholars are also highly experienced, experience alone does not assure clinical expertise. Clinical scholarship is not the same as clinical proficiency, where performing a task routinely in a highly efficient manner is deemed proficient. Rather, it requires always questioning whether there is a more efficient and effective way to provide care and whether or not a particular procedure or task needs to be performed at all (Clinical Scholarship Task Force, 1999). These characteristics of clinical scholars are very similar to those of the innovators and early adopters described by Rogers (2003). The Clinical Scholar Model© is inductive using the innovative ideas generated in direct care and driven by the goal of building a community or cadre of scholars who will serve as mentors to other direct care providers in the critique, synthesis, implementation, and evaluation of internal evidence (e.g., QI, risk management, and benchmarking data) and external evidence (i.e., empirical studies).

Clinical scholar mentors are change agents who promote clinical scholarship through the spirit of inquiry and a willingness to challenge and change traditional practice patterns, mentoring other staff in fostering a culture shift. Practicing as a clinical scholar does not require that one always conduct research, but it does require using an intellectual process that is steeped in curiosity and that continually challenges traditional clinical practice through observation, analysis, synthesis of the evidence, application and evaluation, and dissemination (see Figure 14.8B; Schultz et al., 2005). The Clinical Scholar Model© supports the view that if research and other forms of evidence are to be used in practice, both must be understood and valued by direct care providers.

Sustaining the Clinical Scholar Environment

Evaluation of the model is both iterative and cumulative. The research studies and EBP projects developed during the Clinical Scholar Program© must be continually evaluated for achieving their desired outcomes. The environment in which the work is centered must be evaluated for a sustainable change to a culture of inquiry and a breeding ground for innovation.

EBP may initially be encouraged through the application of knowledge to a single intervention or project but, over time, as more staff are educated regarding the critique, synthesis, application, and evaluation of evidence, the culture and the delivery of care will slowly change to the routine use of evidence—both formally and informally—through inquisitive, reflective, critical thinking. Every healthcare provider becomes responsible and accountable for providing care based on the best available evidence; not to do so is unethical. The institutionalization of evidence use in practice requires creative, critical thinkers and the support and flexibility of management to implement and evaluate change.

Through its focus on the development of new clinical scholars who can act as EBP mentors to their colleagues in the future, the Clinical Scholar Model© is self-sustaining. The Clinical Scholar workshops provide a nurturing, rich environment for direct care providers to create and grow extended networks of professional contacts and colleagues to draw upon for future mentoring. The intensity and fast pace of the Clinical Scholar Program© supports a relatively speedy initial adoption of evidence-based care. As the new clinical scholars begin to serve as mentors to new groups, the model is reinforced, and the culture of excellence expands.

In today's environment of limited healthcare budgets, financial support for programs such as the Clinical Scholar Program© can be limited. Financial investment in the program is essential with consideration of the financial implications of any project as an important step in evaluating the probability of adoption of the practice. Evaluating the monetary costs of projects and interventions and including financial outcomes data whenever possible are essential to providing evidence of benefit in this area. Linking the spirit of inquiry to the QI program assures sustainability and financial feasibility (see Figure 14.8B). When the program remains focused on determining what works, for whom, in what situations, with what resources, and with what measurable outcomes, administrative leaders and clinicians alike can find value in and support for the program with the improvement in care that is so central to institutional missions.

The Johns Hopkins Nursing Evidence-Based Practice Model

The Johns Hopkins Nursing Evidence-Based Practice (JHNEBP) Model guides bedside nurses in translating best evidence into practice for clinical, learning, and operational practice. In 2002, the organizational leadership at The Johns Hopkins Hospital (JHH) recognized a gap in the standard for nursing practice of implementing research results. To accelerate the transfer of new knowledge into practice, nursing leadership set a strategic goal to build a culture of nursing practice based on evidence. The tenets of EBP support this goal because (a) nursing is both a science and a profession, (b) the best available evidence is the foundation for nursing practice, (c) a hierarchy of evidence exists, (d) research findings should be translated into practice, and (e) nursing values efficiency and effectiveness (Newhouse, 2007). The desired outcomes were to enhance nurse autonomy, leadership, and engagement with interdisciplinary colleagues.

A team of JHH nurses and faculty from Johns Hopkins University School of Nursing formed a task force to evaluate published EBP models and tools for application by practicing nurses within the clinical setting. A key objective was to select a model that would demystify the EBP process for bedside nurses and embed EBP into nursing practice. For this reason, it was important that bedside nurses were involved in evaluating and piloting the model and process to be used at JHH.

Nurses' evaluation and feedback from the evaluation of published models was clear— nurses wanted a mentored linear process, with accompanying tools to guide them through each step of the EBP process. Based on this feedback, the JHNEBP Model and process were carefully constructed and piloted with a caregiving unit. During the pilot, the team offered EBP educational working seminars in multiple formats, assessed with participants what worked in the pilot as well as the processes that were most challenging. The details of the implementation are reported elsewhere (Dearholt, White, Newhouse, Pugh, & Poe, 2008; Newhouse, Dearholt, Poe, Pugh, & White, 2007). The resulting JHNEBP Model includes a conceptual model, a process, and tools to guide nurses through the critical steps of the process.

The model was then implemented organizationally through standardized education and integration of EBP competencies into job performance expectations. An EBP fellowship was funded by Nursing Administration and external funding obtained to test the model in interprofessional teams. The EBP process was subsequently incorporated into undergraduate and graduate research courses at the Johns Hopkins University School of Nursing.

Overview of the Johns Hopkins Nursing Evidence-Based Practice Model

In the JHNEBP Model, EBP is a problem-solving approach to clinical decision making within a healthcare organization that integrates the best available scientific evidence with the best available experiential (patient and practitioner) evidence, considers internal and external influences on practice, and encourages critical thinking in the judicious application of such evidence to care of the individual patient, patient population, or system.

(Dearholt & Dang, 2018, pp. 4–5)

The JHNEBP Model (Figure 14.9) begins with inquiry sparked by an individual's or team's genuine curiosity about best practices related to a specific problem and/or a particular patient population (Dang & Dearholt, 2018). This inquiry initiates the PET process (Practice Question, Evidence, and Translation), which provides a systematic approach for nurses to develop and refine a practice question, seek out the best evidence, and translate best evidence into practice. Working through the PET process promotes learning as individuals and teams gain new knowledge and insights that impacts practice. Insights gained through practice changes can also lead to additional learning opportunities, making this a continuous, dynamic process. Through the PET process, best practices to answer practice questions are identified, leading to improvements in the areas of clinical, learning, or operational practices. At any point throughout the model, new questions may arise, triggering a new EBP cycle. Because the JHNEBP Model is an open system, it can be influenced by internal organizational (e.g., culture, resources) factors and external factors (e.g., accreditation, licensure, standards, quality measures, legislation, regulations). Internal and external factors can enhance or limit implementation of recommendations, conduct of the process, or the existence of EBP itself within organizations.

As depicted in Figure 14.9, the PET process is the core of the JHNEBP Model. It consists of three phases: *Practice question, Evidence,* and *Translation* (Figure 14.10). Within these phases, there are 19 prescriptive steps. Although the process appears linear, it may be iterative

The Johns Hopkins Nursing Evidence-based Practice Model

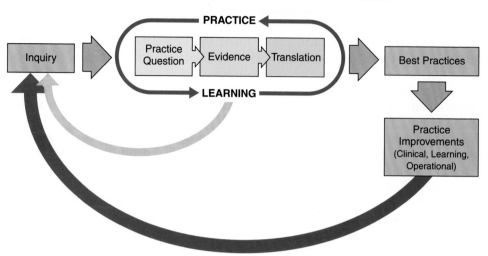

© The Johns Hopkins Hospital/Johns Hopkins University School of Nursing

Figure 14.9: Johns Hopkins nursing evidence-based practice conceptual model. (From Dearholt, S. L., & Dang, D. [2012]. *Johns Hopkins nursing evidence-based practice model and guidelines* [2nd ed.]. Indianapolis, IN: Sigma Theta Tau International. Used with permission.)

as the process evolves. For example, teams may discover other sources of the evidence through their review or hand searching, requiring refinement of the search strategy or PICO, moving them back to the prior step(s).

During the practice question stage, a question is refined in answerable terms, a leader is designated, and an interprofessional team is formed. Next, in the evidence phase, a search for evidence is conducted, and evidence is screened for inclusion criteria, abstracted, appraised using a rating scale, and then summarized. The evidence phase ends with three distinct activities (1) evidence synthesis; (2) recommendations developed by the team based on the level, quality, and quantity of evidence; (3) selection of one of four pathways to translation based on the overall strength of the evidence. There are four pathways for translating evidence into practice:

1. Strong, compelling evidence and consistent results, a prerequisite for a practice change
2. Good and consistent evidence, an indication for considering a pilot of the practice change or need for further investigation
3. Good but conflicting evidence; requires further investigation for new evidence or a research study
4. Little or no evidence; requires further investigation for new evidence, a research study, or discontinuation of the project.

Finally, in the translation stage, a plan is constructed for implementation of appropriate and feasible recommendations. Implementation, evaluation, and dissemination follow. The translation plan is incorporated into the organization's QI framework to communicate effective (and ineffective) changes and engage the organization in adopting those changes.

Ten tools support critical steps in the process: (1) PET and Project Management Guide, (2) Question Development Tool, (3) Stakeholder Analysis Tool, (4) Evidence Level and Quality Guide, (5) Research Evidence Appraisal Tool, (6) Nonresearch Evidence Appraisal Tool, (7) Individual

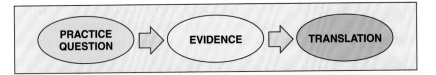

| PRACTICE QUESTION | | EVIDENCE | | TRANSLATION |

PRACTICE QUESTION

Step 1: Recruit interprofessional team
Step 2: Develop and refine the EBP question
Step 3: Define the scope of the EBP question and identify stakeholders
Step 4: Determine responsibility for project leadership
Step 5: Schedule team meetings

EVIDENCE

Step 6: Conduct internal and external search for evidence
Step 7: Appraise the level and quality of each piece of evidence
Step 8: Summarize the individual evidence
Step 9: Synthesize overall strength and quality of evidence
Step 10: Develop recommendations for change based on evidence synthesis
 • Strong, compelling evidence, consistent results
 • Good evidence, consistent results
 • Good evidence, conflicting results
 • Insufficient or absent evidence

TRANSLATION

Step 11: Determine fit, feasibility, and appropriateness of recommendation(s) for translation path
Step 12: Create action plan
Step 13: Secure support and resources to implement action plan
Step 14: Implement action plan
Step 15: Evaluate outcomes
Step 16: Report outcomes to stakeholders
Step 17: Identify next steps
Step 18: Disseminate findings

© The John Hopkins Hospital/The John Hopkins University

Figure 14.10: Johns Hopkins nursing process for evidence-based practice (From Dearholt, S. L., & Dang, D. [2012]. *Johns Hopkins nursing evidence-based practice model and guidelines* [2nd ed.]. Indianapolis, IN: Sigma Theta Tau International.)

Evidence Summary Tool, (8) Synthesis Process and Recommendations Tool, (9) Action Planning Tool, and (10) Dissemination Tool. These tools were developed with input from bedside nurses and include key questions that prompt nurses in the process. The tools were constructed to have high utility with checkbox formats, definitions, and guidelines for use on each form.

After multiple projects using different rating scales, it was clear that many publicly available scales were intended for research evidence based on randomized controlled trials and did not include an approach to evaluate nonresearch sources of evidence. Because the questions proposed by nurses today need an answer tomorrow, the sources of evidence are often found in nonresearch evidence such as integrated reviews, QI data, or expert opinion. Because nursing problems occur in natural settings, they often do not lend themselves to randomized control trials. A rating scale was developed to assess the level and quality of nonresearch evidence to enable nurses to better communicate the strength and quality of evidence on which decisions are made.

The JHNEBP Model applies to clinical, learning, and operational questions in any setting where nursing is practiced, and in academic settings at schools of nursing at the undergraduate and graduate levels. It has also been used for state-level initiatives to review evidence (Newhouse, 2008).

A book is available with the tools to guide teams through the JHNEBP process (Dang & Dearholt, 2018). Bedside nurses can use the model and tools to answer important practice questions using the best available evidence to inform decisions.

Stevens Star Model of Knowledge Transformation

Development of the **Stevens Star Model** was prompted through the work of the Academic Center for Evidence-Based Practice (ACE) at the University of Texas Health Science Center San Antonio during the early phases of the EBP movement in the United States. Uniquely, the Star Model focuses heavily on the relative utility of several *forms* of knowledge in clinical decision making (Stevens, 2004, 2015). From the definition of EBP as *integration of best research evidence with clinical expertise and patient preferences* (Sackett, Straus, Richardson, Rosenberg, & Haynes, 2000, p. ii), it is clear that EBP combines research evidence with clinical expertise and includes individualization of care through incorporation of patient preferences and the circumstances of the setting.

Overview of the Stevens Star Model of Knowledge Transformation

Challenges in moving research into practice emerge from a number of sources. The Star Model explains how to overcome the challenges of (1) the volume of research evidence, (2) the misfit between form and use of knowledge, and (3) integration of expertise and patient preference into best practice. Literature and professional knowledge sources contain a variety of knowledge forms, many of which are not useful for direct practice application. For example, results from a single experiment are not suitable to guide best practices because research results from single studies are often not in harmony. One study demonstrates the effectiveness of an intervention, whereas the next may show no difference. Likewise, the sheer volume of research on a topic presents a challenge for real-time application. At the same time, many *forms* of knowledge are not suited to direct clinical application. The research report is a form of knowledge that, while valuable, is not well suited for directly informing practice. Nor does a single research report account for gaps in knowledge or consideration of patient preferences.

The Star Model explains how specific forms of knowledge, such as the systematic review and the clinical practice guideline, are solutions for moving research into practice. It is a model for understanding the cycles, nature, and characteristics of knowledge that are utilized in various phases of EBP in moving evidence into clinical decision making. The simple, parsimonious Star Model depicts the relationships between various stages of knowledge transformation, from newly discovered knowledge through to best practice and outcomes. It illustrates various *forms* of knowledge in evolutionary sequence, as research evidence is combined with other knowledge and integrated into practice to produce intended outcomes. The Star Model places nursing's previous scientific work within the context of EBP and mainstreams nursing into the formal network of EBP.

Figure 14.11 shows the Star Model configured as a simple 5-point star, illustrating five major stages of knowledge transformation. The Star Model defines the following forms of knowledge: (1) Point 1—Discovery Research, representing primary research studies; (2) Point 2—Evidence Summary, which is the synthesis of all available knowledge compiled into a single harmonious statement, such as a systematic review; (3) Point 3—Translation to Guidelines to inform action, often referred to as evidence-based clinical practice guidelines, combining the evidential base and expertise to extend recommendations; (4) Point 4—Practice Integration into practice is evidence-in-action, in which practice and clinical decision making are aligned to reflect best evidence; and (5) Point 5—Process and Outcome Evaluation, which

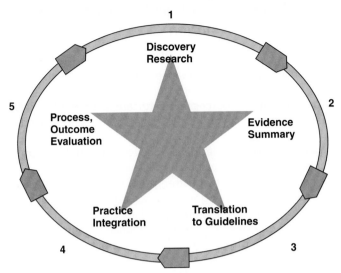

Stevens Star Model of Knowledge Transformation

© 2015 Used with expressed permission

Figure 14.11: Stevens Star Model of Knowledge Transformation. (© Stevens, K. R. [2015]. Stevens Star Model of EBP: Knowledge transformation. *Academic center for evidence-based practice.* San Antonio, TX: The University of Texas Health Science Center. Retrieved from www.acestar.uthscsa.edu. Reprinted with expressed permission.)

is an inclusive view of the impact that the EBP has on patient health outcomes, satisfaction, efficacy and efficiency of care, and health policy. Evidence-informed clinical decisions in healthcare processes and outcomes are the goals of knowledge transformation.

Terms and Premises in the Star Model

A number of basic terms and premises underlie the logic of the Star Model. **Knowledge transformation** is the conversion of research findings from primary research results through a series of stages and forms, to make an impact on health outcomes by way of evidence-based action. Underlying premises of knowledge transformation are described in Box 14.3.

National recommendations have pointed to systematic reviews (Point 2) and clinical practice guidelines (Point 3) as essential forms of knowledge for knowing what works in clinical practice (Institute of Medicine [IOM], 2008, 2011a, 2011b). These two forms of knowledge are identified as the keystones to understanding whether a clinical intervention works. Both must be developed rigorously, to scientific standards, and in efficient ways (IOM, 2008). Evidence-based clinical practice guidelines have the potential to reduce illogical variations in practice by encouraging the use of clinically effective practices.

The Star Model simplifies research evidence for application to clinical decision making. Rather than having practitioners submersed in the volume of research reports, it is better to summarize all that is known on the topic. Likewise, rather than requiring frontline providers to master the technical expertise needed in scientific critique, their point-of-care decisions are better supported by evidence-based recommendations.

Uses of the Stevens Star Model

Integrating EBP Competencies. The Star Model has been widely adopted as nurses strategize to employ EBP. The Star Model, competencies, and Evidence-Based Practice Readiness Inventory (ERI) have been adopted in clinical practice settings. These resources have also been employed

Premises of the Stevens Star Model of Knowledge Transformation

1. Knowledge transformation is necessary before research results are usable in clinical decision making.
2. Knowledge derives from a variety of sources. In healthcare, sources of knowledge include research evidence, experience, authority, trial and error, and theoretical principles.
3. The most stable and generalizable knowledge is discovered through systematic processes that control bias, namely, the research process.
4. Evidence can be classified into a hierarchy of strength of evidence. Relative strength of evidence is largely dependent on the rigor of the scientific design that produced the evidence. The value of rigor is that it strengthens cause-and-effect relationships.
5. Knowledge exists in a variety of forms. As research evidence is converted through systematic steps, knowledge from other sources (expertise, patient preference) is added, creating yet another form of knowledge.
6. The form ("package") in which knowledge exists can be referenced to its use; in the case of EBP, the ultimate use is application in healthcare delivery, services, and policy.
7. The form of knowledge determines its usability in clinical decision making. For example, research results from a primary investigation are less useful to decision making than an evidence-based clinical practice guideline.
8. Knowledge is transformed through the following processes: (a) Summarization into a single statement about the state of the science; (b) Translation of the state of the science into clinical recommendations, with addition of clinical expertise and application of theoretical principles; (c) Integration of recommendations through organizational and individual actions, tailoring care to patient preferences; and (d) Evaluation of impact of actions on targeted actions, care, health outcomes, economic outcomes, and policy.

© Stevens, K. R. (2015). *Stevens Star Model of EBP: Knowledge transformation. Academic center for evidence-based practice.* San Antonio, TX: The University of Texas Health Science Center. Retrieved from www.acestar.uthscsa.edu. Reprinted with expressed permission.

in educational settings as programs are revised to include EBP skills. The Star Model also provides an anchor for the new sciences of improvement and implementation. As an overarching model, it provides quick insight into archiving best practices. Because it drives to the core of EBP, the nature of knowledge, the Star Model is an excellent organizer for more prescriptive detailed EBP models.

As the Institute of Medicine (IOM) urged each profession to develop the details and strategies for integrating EBP competencies into education (National Research Council, 2003), the Star Model was used to develop a national consensus on EBP competencies. With a focus on employing EBP, nurses established a national consensus on competencies for EBP in nursing in 2004 and extended these in 2009 (Stevens, 2009). The Star Model served as the framework for identifying specific competencies needed to employ EBP in a clinical role. Through multiple iterations, expert panels generated, validated, and endorsed competency statements to guide education programs at the basic (associate and undergraduate), intermediate (masters), and doctoral (advanced) levels in nursing. Between 10 and 32 specific competencies are identified for each of four levels of nursing education. Details were published in *Essential Competencies for EBP in Nursing* (Stevens, 2009). These competencies address fundamental skills of knowledge management, accountability for scientific basis of nursing practice, organizational and policy change, and development of scientific underpinnings for EBP (Stevens, 2009).

From these competencies, a measurement approach was developed. The instrument, called the EBP Readiness Inventory (ERI), quantifies the individual's confidence in performing EBP competencies. The ERI exhibits strong **psychometric properties** (reliability, validity, and sensitivity) and is widely used in clinical and educational settings to measure nurses' readiness for employing EBP and assessing the impact of professional development programs (Saunders, Stevens, & Vehviläinen-Julkunen, 2016; Saunders, Vehviläinen-Julkunen, & Stevens, 2016; Stevens, Puga, & Low, 2012). Available as an online survey, the ERI reports on an individual's confidence in their ability (self-efficacy) in their EBP competency.

Organizing and Interpreting Evidence for Clinical Application. As new knowledge resources are developed, the Star Model can be used to organize and interpret relevance to clinical application. For example, systematic reviews from the Cochrane Library can be organized on to Point 2, indicating that the next step is to locate evidence-based clinical practice guidelines. There are many sources of evidence-based guidelines for Point 3 of the Star Model. Critical appraisal of guidelines is important to complete to ensure that they are best available evidence. Ideas for integration of EBP into practice (Point 4) can be accessed from the Agency for Healthcare Research and Quality (AHRQ) Health Care Innovations Exchange. Finally, Point 5 quality indicators are provided by AHRQ.

 Find helpful resources for Point 4 online:
The AHRQ Health Care Innovations Exchange is at http://www.innovations.ahrq.gov/
Quality indicators can be found at: http://www.qualityindicators.ahrq.gov/

Research on the Science of EBP. The Star Model also guides research on the *science of EBP*. Point 4 of the Star Model provides a reference for the new fields of improvement and implementation science. Once knowledge is available in sound clinical practice guidelines, the task of actually changing practice is faced. These new scientific fields focus on the study of improvement strategies to increase our understanding of factors that facilitate or hinder integration and implementation of EBP. The aim of improvement science is to determine which improvement strategies work as we strive to assure EBP through safe and effective care; a key feature is that these fields focus primarily on the healthcare delivery system and microsystem (Improvement Science Research Network, 2013). As a key component in the translational science movement, implementation research is important to EBP improvement in that it assesses ways to link evidence into practice, systems, and clinical decision making (Stevens, 2013); it adds to our understanding of the effectiveness of strategies to "adopt and integrate evidence-based health interventions and change practice patterns within specific settings" (Mittman, Weiner, Proctor & Handley, 2015; National Institutes of Health, 2013).

CONCLUSIONS

Recognizing the challenges inherent in changing practice at an individual or organizational level, numerous models have been created. Common to these models is the recognition of the need for a systematic approach to practice change. Many of the models include common steps such as identification of change agents (e.g., APNs, champions, and practice facilitators) to lead organizational change; identifying problems engaging stakeholders to assist with the practice change; comprehensive searching of the literature to find high-quality evidence to inform the practice change; attention to potential organizational barriers to practice change; using effective strategies to disseminate information about the practice change to those implementing it; and evaluating the impact of the practice change.

More research is needed to confirm the advantages of using particular models and how these models could work in tandem. Those who use the models described in this chapter or other models should document their experiences to better understand the models' usefulness in facilitating EBP and to provide information to others who might use the model in the future (Graham et al., 2007).

Once the EBP change is implemented, sustainability of the change can be a challenge. Davies et al. (2006) collected data from 37 organizations that had implemented nursing best practice guidelines and found that after 3 years, 59% of the organizations were sustaining implementation of these guidelines. Most of those organizations also expanded their use by implementing the guidelines in more units or agencies, engaging more partners, encouraging multidisciplinary involvement, and integrating the guidelines with other QI initiatives. Top facilitators for sustaining and expanding the use of guidelines were leadership champions, management support, ongoing staff education, integration of the guidelines into policies and procedures, staff buy-in and ownership, synergy with partners, and multidisciplinary involvement. Sustained practice change involves those at the front line as well as at the executive levels. An important element to ensure sustainability is an **organizational culture supportive of EBP.** Changing nursing practice to be more evidence informed is a dynamic, long-term, and iterative process.

EBP FAST FACTS

- Models can guide clinicians and healthcare systems in the implementation and sustainability of EBP.
- The original Stetler Model for RU was published in 1976 to help fill a void regarding the realistic application of research findings into clinical practice; it has five phases, including (1) preparation, (2) validation, (3) comparative evaluation/ decision making, (4) translation/application, and (5) evaluation.
- The Iowa Model of Evidence-Based Practice to Promote Quality Care describes a multiphase change process with feedback loops that provides guidance in making decisions about clinical and administrative practices that affect patient outcomes.
- The Model for Evidence-Based Practice Change guides clinicians through six steps, namely, (1) assess the need for change in practice, (2) locate the best evidence, (3) critically analyze the evidence, (4) plan the practice change, (5) implement and evaluate change in practice, and (6) integrate and maintain change in practice.
- The Advancing Research and Clinical practice through close Collaboration (ARCC©) Model is an evidence-based system-wide implementation and sustainability model for EBP, which uses ARCC© EBP mentors as a key strategy in facilitating evidence-based care with clinicians and creating a culture and environment that support EBP.
- The PARIHS framework emphasizes that EBPI activities and processes should be targeted toward moving the three main elements of evidence, context, and facilitation on a continuum from low to high in order to increase chances of success.
- The Clinical Scholar Model© was developed and implemented to promote the spirit of inquiry, educate direct care providers, and guide a mentorship program for EBP and the conduct of research at the point of care.
- The JHNEBP Model facilitates bedside nurses in translating evidence to clinical, administrative, and educational nursing practice.
- The Stevens Star Model of Knowledge Transformation explains how to overcome the challenges of (1) the volume of research evidence; (2) the misfit between form and use of knowledge in decision making; and (3) integration of expertise and patient preference into best practice.

> ## WANT TO KNOW MORE?
>
> A variety of resources are available to enhance your learning and understanding of this chapter.
>
> - Visit thePoint® to access:
>   - Articles from the AJN EBP Step-By-Step Series
>   - Journal articles
>   - Checklists for rapid critical appraisal and more!
> - Lippincott CoursePoint combines digital text content with video case studies and interactive modules for a fully integrated course solution that works the way you study and learn.

References

Adams, S., Farrington, M., & Cullen, L. (2012). Evidence into practice: Publishing an evidence-based practice project. *Journal of PeriAnesthesia Nursing, 27*(3), 193–202. doi:10.1016/j.jopan.2012.03.004

Agoritsas, T., Vandvik. P. O., Neumann, I., Rochwerg, B., Jaeschke, R., Hayward, R., . . . McKibbon, A. K. (2015). Chapter 5: Finding current best evidence. In G. Guyatt, D. Rennie, M. O. Meade, & D. J. Cook (Eds.), *Users' guides to the medical literature: A manual for evidence-based clinical practice* (3rd ed., pp. 29–50). New York, NY: McGraw-Hill Education.

Anderson, R., Kleiber, C., Greiner, J., Comried, L., & Zimmerman, M. (2016). Interface pressure redistribution on skin during continuous lateral rotation therapy: A feasibility study. *Heart and Lung, 45*(3), 237–243. doi:10.1016/j.hrtlng.2016.02.003

Balshem, H., Helfand, M., Schünemann, H., Oxman, A. D., Kunz, R., Brożek, J., . . . Guyatt, G. H. (2011). GRADE guidelines: 3. Rating the quality of evidence. *Journal of Clinical Epidemiology, 64*, 401–406. doi:10.1016/j.jclinepi.2010.07.015

Basol, R., Larsen, R., Simones, J., & Wilson, R. (2017). Evidence into practice: Hospital and academic partnership demonstrating exemplary professional practice in EBP. *Journal of PeriAnesthesia Nursing, 32*(1), 68.e7–71.e7. doi:10.1016/j.jopan.2016.11.002

Beck, A., Rush, A., Shaw, B., & Emery, G. (1979). Cognitive therapy of depression. New York, NY: The Guilford Press.

Beinlich, N., & Meehan, A. (2014). Resource nurse program: A nurse-initiated, evidence-based program to eliminate hospital-acquired pressure ulcers. *Journal of Wound, Ostomy, and Continence Nursing, 41*(2), 136–141. doi:10.1097/WON.0000000000000001

Bick, D., & Graham, I. D. (2010). *Evaluating the impact of implementing evidence-based practice.* Chichester, UK: Wiley-Blackwell Publishing and Sigma Theta Tau International.

Bougard, K. G., Laupola, T. M., Parker-Dias, J., Creekmore, J., & Stangland, S. (2016). Turning the tides: Coping with trauma and addiction through residential adolescent group therapy. *Journal of Child and Adolescent Psychiatric Nursing, 29*(4), 196–206. doi:10.1111/jcap.12164

Brewer, B. B., Brewer, M. A., & Schultz, A. A. (2009). A collaborative approach to building the capacity for research and evidence-based practice in community hospitals. *Nursing Clinics of North America, 44*(1), 11–25.

Brown, D., & McCormack, B. (2005). Developing postoperative pain management: Utilising the Promoting Action on Research Implementation in Health Services (PARIHS) framework. *Worldviews on Evidence-Based Nursing, 3*(2), 131–141.

Carney, T., Myers, B. J., Louw, J., Okwundu, C. I. (2016). Brief school-based interventions and behavioural outcomes for substance-using adolescents. *Cochrane Database of Systematic Reviews,* (1), CD008969. doi:10.1002/14651858.CD008969.pub3

Carver, C. S., & Scheier, M. F. (1982). Control theory: A useful conceptual framework for personality-social, clinical, and health psychology. *Psychological Bulletin, 92*, 111–135.

Carver C. S., & Scheier, M. F. (1998). *On the self-regulation of behavior.* Cambridge, UK: Cambridge University Press.

Chavez, J., Bortolotto, S. J., Paulson, M., Huntley, N., Sullivan, B., & Babu, A. (2015). Promotion of progressive mobility activities with ventricular assist and extracorporeal membrane oxygenation devices in a cardiothoracic intensive care unit. *Dimension of Critical Care Nursing, 34*(6), 348–355. doi:10.1097/DCC.0000000000000141

Chlan, L. L., Weinert, C. R., Heiderscheit, A., Tracy, M. F., Skaar, D. J., Guttormson, J. L., & Savick, K. (2013). Effects of patient-directed music intervention on anxiety and sedative exposure in critically ill patients receiving mechanical ventilator support: A randomized clinical trial. *JAMA, 309*(22), 2335–2344.

Clinical Scholarship Task Force. (1999). *Clinical scholarship resource paper.* Retrieved from http://alpha.nursingsociety.org/aboutus/aboutus

Crogan, N. L., & Dupler, A. E. (2014). Quality improvement in nursing homes: Testing of an alarm elimination program. *Journal of Nursing Care Quality, 29*(1), 60–65. doi:10.1097/NCQ.0b013e3182aa6f86

Cronenwett, C. (1994). Using research in the care of patients. In G. LoBiondo-Wood & J. Haber (Eds.), *Nursing research: Methods, critical appraisal, and utilization* (pp. 89–90). St. Louis, MO: Mosby.

Cullen, L., & Adams, S. L. (2012). Planning for implementation of evidence-based practice. *The Journal of Nursing Administration, 42*(4), 222–230. doi:10.1097/NNA.0b013e31824ccd0a

Cullen, L., Hanrahan, K., Farrington, M., Deberg, J., Tucker, S., & Kleiber, C. (2018). *Evidence-based practice in action: Comprehensive strategies, tools, and tips from the University of Iowa Hospitals and Clinics.* Indianapolis, IN: Sigma Theta Tau International.

Cullen, L., Hanrahan, K., Neis, N., Farrington, M., Laffoon, T., & Dawson, C. (in press). Evidence-based practice: Strategies for nursing leaders. In D. Huber (Ed.), *Leadership and nursing care management* (6th ed.). Philadelphia, PA: Elsevier.

Cullen, L., Wagner, M., Matthews, G., & Farrington, M. (in press). Evidence into practice: Optimizing dissemination within an organizational infrastructure. *Journal of PeriAnesthesia Nursing.*

Davies, B., Edwards, N., Ploeg, J., Virani, T., Skelly, J., & Dobbins, M. (2006). *Determinants of the sustained use of research evidence in nursing: Final report.* Ottawa, ON, Canada: Canadian Health Services Research Foundation & Canadian Institutes for Health Research.

Dearholt, S., White, K., Newhouse, R. P., Pugh, L., & Poe, S. (2008). Educational strategies to develop evidence-based practice mentors. *Journal for Nurses in Staff Development, 24*(2), 53–59.

Dearholt, S. L., & Dang, D. (2018). Johns Hopkins nursing evidence-based practice: model and guidelines (3rd ed.). Indianapolis, IN: Sigma Theta Tau International.

DiCenso, A., Bayley, L., & Haynes, R. B. (2009). Accessing preappraised evidence: Fine-tuning the 5S model into a 6S model. *ACP Journal Club, 151*(3), JC3-1–JC3-3.

DiCenso, A., Ciliska, D., & Guyatt, G. (2004). Introduction to evidence-based nursing. In A. DiCenso, D. Ciliska, & G. Guyatt (Eds.), *Evidence-based nursing: A guide to clinical practice* (pp. 3–19). St Louis, MO: Elsevier.

Dzau, V. J., McClellan, M. B., McGinnis, J. M., Burke, S. P., Coye, M. J., Diaz, A., . . . Zerhouni, E. (2017). Vital directions for health and health care: Priorities from a National Academy of Medicine initiative. *JAMA. 317*(14), 1461–1470. doi:10.1001/jama.2017.1964

Ellis, I., Howard, P., Larson, A., & Robertson, J. (2005). From workshop to work practice: An exploration of context and facilitation in the development of evidence-based practice. *Worldviews on Evidence-Based Nursing, 2*(2), 84–93.

English, R. (2016). Evidence-based teaching tactics for Frontline Saff using the Clinical Nurse Scholar Model. *The Journal of Nurse Practitioners, 12*(1), e1–e5.

Esposito, D., Heeringa, J., Bradley, K., Croake, S., & Kimmey, L. (2015). *PCORI dissemination and implementation framework.* Retrieved from http://www.pcori.org/sites/default/files/PCORI-Dissemination-Implementation-Framework.pdf

Farrington, M., Hanson, A., Laffoon, T., & Cullen, L. (2015). Low-dose ketamine infusions for postoperative pain in opioid-tolerant orthopaedic spine patients. *Journal of PeriAnesthesia Nursing, 30*(4), 338–345. doi:10.1016/j.jopan.2015.03.005

Fearns, N., Kelly, J., Callaghan, M., Graham, K., Loudon, K., Harbour, R., . . . Treweek, S. (2016). What do patients and the public know about clinical practice guidelines and what do they want from them? A qualitative study. *BMC Health Services Research, 16,* 74. doi:10.1186/s12913-016-1319-4

Fineout-Overholt, E., & Melnyk, B. M. (2006). *Organizational culture and readiness scale for system-wide integration of evidence-based practice.* Gilbert, AZ: ARCC, LLC.

Fleiszer, A. R., Semenic, S. E., Ritchie, J. A., Richer, M. C., & Denis, J. L. (2016a). A unit-level perspective on the long-term sustainability of a nursing best practice guidelines program: An embedded multiple case study. *International Journal of Nursing Studies, 53,* 204–218. doi:10.1016/j.ijnurstu.2015.09.004

Fleiszer, A. R., Semenic, S. E., Ritchie, J. A., Richer, M. C., & Denis, J. L. (2016b). Nursing unit leaders' influence on the long-term sustainability of evidence-based practice improvements. *Journal of Nursing Management, 24*(3), 309–318. doi:10.1111/jonm.12320

Fleuren, M. A., van Dommelen, P., & Dunnink, T. (2015). A systematic approach to implementing and evaluating clinical guidelines: The results of fifteen years of Preventive Child Health Care guidelines in the Netherlands. *Social Science & Medicine, 136–137,* 35–43. doi:10.1016/j.socscimed.2015.05.001

Foote, J. M., Conley, V., Williams, J. K., McCarthy, A. M., & Countryman, M. (2015). Academic and Institutional Review Board collaboration to ensure ethical conduct of doctor of nursing practice projects. *Journal of Nursing Education, 54*(7), 372–377. doi:10.3928/01484834-20150617-03

Geyman, J. (1998). Evidence-based medicine in primary care: An overview. *Journal of the American Board of Family Practice, 11*, 46–56.

Goode, C., & Piedalue, F. (1999). Evidence-based clinical practice. *Journal of Nursing Administration, 29*, 15–21.

GRADE Working Group. (2017). *Why rate certainty in evidence and strength of the recommendations?* Retrieved from http://www.gradeworkinggroup.org/

Graham, I. D., Tetroe, J., & KT Theories Research Group. (2007). Some theoretical underpinnings of knowledge translation. *Academic Emergency Medicine, 14*(11), 936–941.

Hagiwara, M. A., Gare, B. A., & Elg, M. (2016). Interrupted time series versus statistical process control in quality improvement projects. *Journal of Nursing Care Quality, 31*(1), E1–E8.

Hanrahan, K., Wagner, M., Matthews, G., Stewart, S., Dawson, C., Greiner, J., . . . Williamson, A. (2015). Sacred cow gone to pasture: A systematic evaluation and integration of evidence-based practice. *Worldviews on Evidence-Based Nursing, 12*(1), 3–11. doi:10.1111/wvn.12072

Harbman, P., Bryant-Lukosius, D., Martin-Misener, R., Carter, N., Covell, C. L., Donald, F., . . . Valaitis, R. (2016). Partners in research: Building academic-practice partnerships to educate and mentor advanced practice nurses. *Journal of Evaluation in Clinical Practice, 12*(1), 3–11. doi:10.1111/jep.12630

Harvey, G., & Kitson, A. (2016). PARIHS revisited: from heuristic to integrated framework for the successful implementation of knowledge into practice. *Implementation Science,* 11:33. doi:10.1186/s13012-016-0398-2

Harvey, G., Loftus-Hills, A., Rycroft-Malone, J., Titchen, A., Kitson, A., McCormack, B., & Seers, K. (2002). Getting evidence into practice: The role and function of facilitation. *Journal of Advanced Nursing, 37*(6), 577–588.

Haynes, R. (2002). What kind of evidence is it that evidence-based medicine advocates want health care providers and consumers to pay attention to? *BMC Health Services Research, 2,* 3.

Haynes, R., Sackett, D., Gray, J., Cook, D., & Guyatt, G. (1996). EBM notebook: Transferring evidence from research into practice: 1. The role of clinical care research evidence in clinical decisions. *Evidence Based Medicine, 1,* 196–198.

Hill, J. N., Guihan, M., Hogan, T. P., Smith, B. M., LaVela, S., Weaver, F. M., . . . Evans, C. T. (2017). Use of the PARIHS framework for retrospective and prospective implementation evaluation. *Worldviews on Evidence-Based Nursing, 14*(2), 99–107.

Hiller, A., Farrington, M., Forman, J., McNulty, H., & Cullen, L. (in press). Evidence into practice: Evidence-based nurse-driven algorithm for intrapartum bladder care. *Journal of PeriAnesthesia Nursing.*

Horsley, J. A., Crane, J., Crabtree, M. K., & Wood, D. J. (1983). *Using research to improve nursing practice: A guide.* Orlando, FL: Green & Stratton.

Honess, C., Gallant, P., & Keane, K. (2009). The Clinical Scholar Model: Evidence-based practice at the bedside. *Nursing Clinics of North America, 44*(1), 116–130.

Hosking, J., Knox, K., Forman, J., Montgomery, L. A., Valde, J. G., & Cullen, L. (2016). Evidence into practice: Leading new graduate nurses to evidence-based practice through a nurse residency program. *Journal of PeriAnesthesia Nursing, 31*(3), 260–265. doi:10.1016/j.jopan.2016.02.006

Huether, K., Abbott, L., Cullen, L., Cullen, L., & Gaarde, A. (2016). Energy through motion®: An evidence-based exercise program to reduce cancer-related fatigue and improve quality of life. *Clinical Journal of Oncology Nursing, 20*(3), E60–E70. doi:10.1188/16.CJON.E60-E70

Hunt, J. (1991). Barriers to research utilisation. *Journal of Advanced Nursing, 23*(3), 423–425.

Hutchinson, A. M., & Johnston, L. (2006). Beyond the barriers scale: Commonly reported barriers to research use. *The Journal of Nursing Administration, 36*(4), 189–199.

Hysong, S. J., Kell, H. J., Petersen, L. A., Campbell, B. A., & Trautner, B. W. (2017). Theory-based and evidence-based design of audit and feedback programmes: Examples from two clinical intervention studies. *BMJ Quality & Safety, 26*(4), 323–334. doi:10.1136/bmjqs-2015-004796

Improvement Science Research Network. (2013). *What is improvement science?* Retrieved from http://www.isrn.net/about/improvement_science.asp

Institute of Medicine. (2008). *Knowing what works: A Roadmap for the nation.* In J. Eden, B. Wheatley, B. L. McNeil, & H. Sox (Eds.). Washington, DC: National Academies Press.

Institute of Medicine. (2011a). *Clinical guidelines we can trust [Committee on Standards for Developing Trustworthy Clinical Practice Guidelines].* Washington, DC: National Academies Press.

Institute of Medicine. (2011b). *Finding what works in health care: Standards for systematic reviews [Committee on Standards for Systematic Reviews of Comparative Effective Research; Board on Health Care Services].* Washington, DC: National Academies Press.

Iowa Model Collaborative. (in press). Revised Iowa Model of evidence-based practice: Development and validation. *Worldviews on Evidence-Based Nursing.*

Kastner, M., Bhattacharyya, O., Hayden, L., Makarski, J., Estey, E., Durocher, L., . . . Brouwers, M. (2015). Guideline uptake is influenced by six implementability domains for creating and communicating guidelines: A realist review. *Journal of Clinical Epidemiology, 68*(5), 498–509. doi:10.1016/j.jclinepi.2014.12.013

Kim, S. (1999). *Models of theory-practice linkage in nursing.* Paper presented at the International Nursing Research Conference: Research to Practice, University of Alberta, Edmonton, Canada.

Kitson, A., Harvey, G., & McCormack, B. (1998). Enabling the implementation of evidence based practice: A conceptual framework. *Quality in Health Care, 7*(3), 149–158.

Kitson, A., Rycroft-Malone, J., Harvey, G., McCormack, B., Seers, K., & Titchen, A. (2008). Evaluating the successful implementation of evidence into practice using the PARIHS framework: Theoretical and practical challenges. *Implementation Science, 3*(1), 1–12.

Koffel, J. B. (2015). Use of recommended search strategies in systematic reviews and the impact of librarian involvement: A cross-sectional survey of recent authors. *PLoS One, 10*(5), e0125931. doi:10.1371/journal.pone.0125931

Kunneman, M., Montori, V. M., Castaneda-Guarderas, A., & Hess, E. P. (2016). What is shared decision making? (and what it is not). *Academic Emergency Medicine, 23*(12), 1320–1324. doi:10.1111/acem.13065

Lam, D. (2005). A brief overview of CBT techniques. In S. Freeman & A. Freeman (Eds.), *Cognitive behavior therapy in nursing practice* (pp. 29–47). New York, NY: Springer Publishing Company.

Larrabee, J. H. (2004). Advancing quality improvement through using the best evidence to change practice. *Journal of Nursing Care Quality, 19*(1), 10–13.

Larrabee, J. H. (2009). *Nurse to nurse: Evidence-based practice.* New York, NY: McGraw-Hill.

Lau, R., Stevenson, F., Ong, B. N., Dziedzic, K., Treweek, S., Eldridge, S., . . . Murray, E. (2016). Achieving change in primary care—Causes of the evidence to practice gap: Systematic reviews of reviews. *Implementation Science, 11*, 40. doi:10.1186/s13012-016-0396-4

Levin, R. F., Fineout-Overholt, E., Melnyk, B. M., Barnes, M., & Vetter, M. J. (2011). Fostering evidence-based practice to improve nurse and cost outcomes in a community health setting: A pilot test of the advancing research and clinical practice through close collaboration model. *Nursing Administration Quarterly, 35*(1), 21–33.

McCormack, B., Kitson, A., Harvey, G., Rycroft-Malone, J., Titchen, A., & Seers, K. (2002). Getting evidence into practice: The meaning of 'context.' *Journal of Advanced Nursing, 38*(1), 94–104.

McSherry, R., Artley, A., & Holloran, J. (2006). Research awareness: An important factor for evidence based practice. *Worldviews on Evidence-Based Nursing, 3*(3), 103–115.

Melnyk, B. M. (2007). The evidence-based practice mentor: A promising strategy for implementing and sustaining EBP in health care systems. *Worldviews on Evidence-Based Nursing, 4*(3), 123–125.

Melnyk, B. M. (2012). Achieving a high-reliability organization through implementation of the ARCC model for systemwide sustainability of evidence-based practice. *Nursing Administration Quarterly, 36*(2), 127–135.

Melnyk, B. M., & Fineout-Overholt, E. (2002). Putting research into practice. *Reflections on Nursing Leadership, 28*(2), 22–25.

Melnyk, B. M., & Fineout-Overholt, E. (2011). *Evidence-based practice in nursing and health care: A guide to best practice.* Philadelphia, PA: Lippincott, Williams & Wilkins.

Melnyk, B. M., Fineout-Overholt, E., Feinstein, N., Li, H. S., Small, L., Wilcox, L., & Kraus, R. (2004). Nurses' perceived knowledge, beliefs, skills, and needs regarding evidence-based practice: Implications for accelerating the paradigm shift. *Worldviews on Evidence-Based Nursing, 1*(3), 185–193.

Melnyk, B. M., Fineout-Overholt, E., Gallagher-Ford, L., & Kaplan, L. (2012). The state of evidence-based practice in US nurses: Critical implications for nurse leaders and educators. *Journal of Nursing Administration, 42*(9), 410–417.

Melnyk, B. M., Fineout-Overholt, E., Giggleman, M., & Choy, K. (2017). A test of the ARCC© model improves implementation of evidence-based practice, healthcare culture, and patient outcomes. *Worldviews on Evidence-Based Nursing, 14*(1), 5–9.

Melnyk, B. M., Fineout-Overholt, E., Giggleman, M., & Cruz, R. (2010). Correlates among cognitive beliefs, EBP implementation, organizational culture, cohesion and job satisfaction in evidence-based practice mentors from a community hospital system. *Nursing Outlook, 58*(6), 301–308.

Melnyk, B. M., Fineout-Overholt, E., & Mays, M. (2008). The evidence-based practice beliefs and implementation scales: Psychometric properties of two new instruments. *Worldviews on Evidence-Based Nursing, 5*(4), 208–216.

Melnyk, B. M., Jacobson, D., Kelly, S., Belyea, M., Shaibi, G., Small, L., . . . Marsiglia, F. F. (2013). Promoting healthy lifestyles in high school adolescents. *American Journal of Preventive Medicine, 45*(4), 407–415.

Melnyk, B. M., & Moldenhauer, Z. (2006). *The KySS guide to child and adolescent mental health screening, early intervention and health promotion.* Cherry Hill, NJ: NAPNAP.

Mitchell, S. A., Fisher, C. A., Hastings, C. E., Silverman, L. B., & Wallen, G. R. (2010). A thematic analysis of theoretical models for translational science in nursing: Mapping the field. *Nursing Outlook, 58*(6), 287–300.

Mittman, B. S., Weiner, B. J., Proctor, E. K., & Handley, M. A. (2015). Expanding D&I science capacity and activity within NIH Clinical and Translational Science Award (CTSA) Programs: Guidance and successful models from national leaders. *Implementation Science, 10*(1), A38.

Moyers, P. A., Finch Guthrie, P. L., Swan, A. R., & Sathe, L. A. (2014). Interprofessional evidence-based clinical scholar program: Learning to work together. *American Journal of Occupational Therapy, 68* (Suppl. 2), S23–S31. doi:10.5014/ajot.2014.012609

Mulvenon, C., & Brewer, M. K. (2009). From the bedside to the boardroom: Resuscitating the use of nursing research. *Nursing Clinics of North America, 44*(1), 145–152.

National Institutes of Health. (2013). *Dissemination and implementation research in health*. PAR 10-038. Retrieved from http://grants.nih.gov/grants/guide/pa-files/PAR-10-038.html

National Research Council. (2003). *Health professions education: A bridge to quality*. Washington, DC: The National Academies Press.

Nayback-Beebe, A. M., Forsythe, T., Funari, T., Mayfield, M., Thoms, W., Jr., Smith, K. K., . . . Scott, P. (2013). Using evidence-based leadership initiatives to create a healthy nursing work environment. *Dimensions of Critical Care Nursing, 32*(4), 166–173. doi:10.1097/DCC.0b013e3182998121

Newell-Stokes, V., Broughton, S., Giuliano, K. K., & Stetler, C. (2001) Developing an evidence-based procedure: Maintenance of central venous catheters. *Clinical Nurse Specialist, 15*, 199–206.

Newhouse, R. P. (2007). Creating infrastructure supportive of evidence-based nursing practice: Leadership strategies. *Worldviews on Evidence-Based Nursing, 4*(1), 21–29.

Newhouse, R. P. (2008). Evidence driving quality initiatives: The Maryland hospital association collaborative on nurse retention. *Journal of Nursing Administration, 38*(6), 268–271.

Newhouse, R. P., Dearholt, S., Poe, S., Pugh, L. C., & White, K. (2007). Organizational change strategies for evidence-based practice. *Journal of Nursing Administration, 37*(12), 552–557.

Nishimura, R. A., Otto, C. M., Bonow, R. O., Carabello, B. A., Erwin, J. P., Fleisher, L. A., . . . Thompson, A. (2017). AHA/ACC focused update of the 2014 AHA/ACC guideline for the management of patients with valvular heart disease: A report of the American College of Cardiology/American Heart Association Task Force on Clinical Practice Guidelines. *Circulation, 135*(25), e1159–e1195. doi:10.1161/CIR.0000000000000503

Office of Human Research Protections. (n.d.). *Quality improvement activities FAQs*. Retrieved from https://www.hhs.gov/ohrp/regulations-and-policy/guidance/faq/quality-improvement-activities/

Olsen, D. P., & Smania, M. A. (2016). Determining when an activity is or is not research. *American Journal of Nursing, 116*(10), 55–60. doi:10.1097/01.NAJ.0000503304.52756.9a

Parahoo, K. (1999). A comparison of pre-project 2000 and project 2000 nurses' perceptions of their research training, research needs and their use of research in clinical areas. *Journal of Advanced Nursing, 29*, 237–245.

Parahoo, K. (2000). Barriers to, and facilitators of, research utilization among nurses in Northern Ireland. *Journal of Advanced Nursing, 31*, 89–98.

Parry, G. J., Carson-Stevens, A., Luff, D. F., McPherson, M. E., & Goldmann, D. A. (2013). Recommendations for evaluation of health care improvement initiatives. *Academic Pediatrics, 13*(6 Suppl.), S23–S30. doi:10.1016/j.acap.2013.04.007

Retsas, A. (2000). Barriers to using research evidence in nursing practice. *Journal of Advanced Nursing, 31*, 599–606.

Rogers, E. M. (2003). *Diffusion of innovations* (5th ed.). New York, NY: The Free Press.

Rosswurm, M. A., & Larrabee, J. (1999). A model for change to evidence-based practice. *Image: Journal of Nursing Scholarship, 31*(4), 317–322.

Rycroft-Malone, J., Harvey, G., Seers, K., Kitson, A., McCormack, B., & Titchen, A. (2004). An exploration of the factors that influence the implementation of evidence into practice. *Journal of Clinical Nursing, 13*, 913–924.

Rycroft-Malone, J., Kitson, A., Harvey, G., McCormack, B., Seers, K., Titchen, A., & Estabrooks, C. (2002). Ingredients for change: Revisiting a conceptual framework. *Quality & Safety in Health Care, 11*, 174–180.

Rycroft-Malone, J., Seers, K., Titchen, A., Harvey, G., Kitson, A., & McCormack, B. (2004). What counts as evidence in evidence-based practice. *Journal of Advanced Nursing, 47*(1), 81–90.

Rycroft-Malone, J., & Stetler, C. (2004). Commentary on evidence, research, knowledge: A call for conceptual clarity. *Worldviews in Evidence-Based Nursing, 1*(2), 98f.

Sackett, D. L., Straus, S. E., Richardson, W. S., Rosenberg, W. M. C., & Haynes, R. B. (2000). *Evidence-based medicine: How to practice and teach EBM*. London, England: Churchill Livingstone.

Saunders, H., Stevens, K. R., & Vehviläinen-Julkunen, K. (2016). Nurses' readiness for evidence-based practice at Finnish university hospitals: a national survey. *Journal of Advanced Nursing, 72*(8), 1863–1874.

Saunders, H., Vehviläinen-Julkunen, K., & Stevens, K. R. (2016). Effectiveness of an education intervention to strengthen nurses' readiness for evidence-based practice: A single-blind randomized controlled study. *Applied Nursing Research, 31*, 175–185.

Saver, C. (2014). *Anatomy of writing for publication for nurses* (2nd ed.). Indianapolis, IN: Sigma Theta Tau International.

Scottish Intercollegiate Guidelines Network. (2007). *Critical appraisal: Notes and checklists*. Retrieved from http://www.sign.ac.uk/methodology/checklists.html

Schultz, A. A. (2007). Implementation: A team effort. *Nursing Management, 38*(6), 12, 14.

Schultz, A. A. (2008). The clinical scholar program: Creating a culture of excellence. *RNL, Reflections on Nursing Leadership*. Retrieved from http://www.nursingsociety.org/pub/rnl/pages/vol34_2_schultz.aspx

Schultz, A. A. (Guest Editor). (2009). Evidence-based practice. *Nursing Clinics of North America, 44*(1), xv–xvii.

Schultz, A. A. (2011a). *Practical strategies for EBP and clinical research collaboration*. Minot, ND: Minot State University, Presentation.

Schultz, A. A. (2011b, November 2). *The clinical scholar program: A Fulbright Collaboration in Northern Thailand*. Grapevine, TX: Sigma Theta Tau International.

Schultz, A. A. (2012) *Basics of synthesis. Planning evidence-based practice and research projects.* Minot, ND: Trinity Health Care System.

Schultz, A. A. (2014). *Introduction to the Fulbright Scholars Workshops on developing and implementing clinical practice guidelines.* Presentation to Deans and Chief Nurses. Cordillera Administrative Region, Bontoc, Mountain Province Philippines, August 31, 2014.

Schultz, A. A. & Brewer, B. B. (2013). Synthesis, not summary: The core of evidence-based decision making for the direct care nurse. Unpublished manuscript.

Schultz, A. A. (Guest Editor), Honess, C., Gallant, P., Kent, G., Lancaster, K., & Sepples, S. (2005). Advancing evidence into practice: Clinical scholars at the bedside [Electronic version]. *Excellence in Nursing Knowledge.*

Schünemann, H., Brożek, J., Guyatt, G., & Oxman, A., (2013, October). *GRADE Handbook: 5. Quality of evidence.* Retrieved from http://gdt.guidelinedevelopment.org/app/handbook/handbook.html#h.9rdbelsnu4iy

Sharp, N., Pineros, S. L., Hsu, C., Starks, H., & Sales, A. (2004). A qualitative study to identify barriers and facilitators to the implementation of pilot intervention in the Veterans Health Administration Northwest Network. *Worldviews on Evidence-Based Nursing, 1*(4), 129–139.

Sigma Theta Tau International Research Scholarship Advisory Committee. (2008). Sigma theta tau international position statement on evidence-based practice February 2007 summary. *Worldviews on Evidence-Based Nursing, 5*(2), 57–59. doi: 10.1111/j.1741-6787.2008.00118.x

Stacey, D., Legare, F., Col, N. F., Bennett, C. L., Barry, M. J., Eden, K. B., . . . Wu, J. H. (2014). Decision aids for people facing health treatment or screening decisions. *Cochrane Database of Systematic Reviews,* (1), CD001431. doi:10.1002/14651858.CD001431.pub4

Stetler, C. (1985). Research utilization: Defining the concept. *Image: The Journal of Nursing Scholarship, 17,* 40–44. doi:10.1111/j.1547-5069.1985.tb01415.x

Stetler, C. (1999). Clinical scholarship exemplars: The Baystate Medical Center. In *Clinical Scholarship Task Force's Clinical Scholarship White Paper: Knowledge work, in service of care, based on evidence.* Indianapolis, IN: Sigma Theta Tau International.

Stetler, C., Burns, M., Sander-Buscemi, K., Morsi, D., & Grunwald, E. (2003) Use of evidence for prevention of work-related musculo-skeletal injuries. *Orthopaedic Nursing, 22,* 32–41.

Stetler, C., Corrigan, B., Sander-Buscemi, K., & Burns, M. (1999). Integration of evidence into practice and the change process: A fall prevention program as a model. *Outcomes Management for Nursing Practice, 3*(3), 102–111.

Stetler, C. & DiMaggio, G. (1991). Research utilization among clinical nurse specialists. *Clinical Nurse Specialist, 5,* 151155.

Stetler, C., Legro, M., Rycroft-Malone, J., Bowman, C., Curran, G., Guihan, M., . . . Wallace, C. (2006a). Role of "external facilitation" in implementation of research findings: A qualitative evaluation of facilitation experiences in the Veterans Health Administration. *Implementation Science, 1,* 22.

Stetler, C., Legro, M., Wallace, C. M., Bowman, C., Guihan, M., Hagedorn, H., . . . Smith, J. L. (2006b). The role of formative evaluation in implementation research and the QUERI experience. *Journal of General Internal Medicine, 21*(Suppl. 2), S1–S8.

Stetler, C., Morsi, D., Rucki, S., Broughton, S., Corrigan, B., Fitzgerald, J., . . . Sheridan, E. A. (1998b). Utilization-focused integrative reviews in a nursing service. *Applied Nursing Research, 11*(4), 195–206.

Stetler, C. B. (1994a). Refinement of the Stetler/Marram model for application of research findings to practice. *Nursing Outlook, 42,* 15–25.

Stetler, C. B. (1994b). Using research to improve patient care. In G. LoBiondo-Wood & J. Haber (Eds.), *Nursing research: Methods, critical appraisal, and utilization* (pp. 1–2). St. Louis, MO: Mosby.

Stetler, C. B. (2001a). *Evidence-based practice and the use of research: A synopsis of basic strategies and concepts to improve care.* Washington, DC: Nova Foundation.

Stetler, C. B. (2001b). Updating the Stetler model of research utilization to facilitate evidence-based practice. *Nursing Outlook, 49,* 272–278.

Stetler, C. B. (2003). Role of the organization in translating research into evidence-based practice. *Outcomes Management, 7,* 97–103.

Stetler, C. B. (2010). Stetler model. In J. Rycroft-Malone & T. Bucknall (Eds.), *Evidence-based practice series. Models and frameworks for implementing evidence-based practice: Linking evidence to action.* Oxford, England: Blackwell Publishing Limited.

Stetler, C. B., Bautista, C., Vernale-Hannon, C., Foster, J. (1995). Enhancing research utilization by clinical nurse specialists. Nursing Clinics of North America, 30(1), 457–473

Stetler, C. B., Brunell, M., Giuliano, K., Morsi, D., Prince, L., & Newell-Stokes, G. (1998a). Evidence based practice and the role of nursing leadership. *Journal of Nursing Administration, 8,* 45–53.

Stetler, C. B., & Caramanica, L. (2007). Evaluation of an evidence-based practice initiative: Outcomes, strengths and limitations of a retrospective, conceptually-based approach. *Worldviews on Evidence-Based Nursing, 4*(4), 187–199.

Stetler, C. B., & Marram, G. (1976). Evaluating research findings for applicability in practice. *Nursing Outlook, 24,* 559–563.

Stevens, K. R. (2004). *ACE Star Model of EBP: Knowledge transformation.* Academic Center for Evidence-based Practice. The University of Texas Health Science Center at San Antonio. Retrieved from www.acestar.uthscsa.edu

Stevens, K. R. (2009). *Essential evidence-based practice competencies in nursing* (2nd ed.). San Antonio, TX: Academic Center for Evidence-Based Practice (ACE) of University of Texas Health Science Center.

Stevens, K. R. (2013). The impact of evidence-based practice in nursing and the next big ideas. *Online Journal of Nursing Issues, 8*(2), 4.

Stevens, K. R. (2015). *Stevens Star Model of EBP: Knowledge transformation.* Academic Center for Evidence-based Practice. The University of Texas Health Science Center at San Antonio. Retrieved from www.acestar.uthscsa.edu

Stevens, K. R., Puga, F., & Low, V. (2012). *The ACE-ERI: An instrument to measure EBP readiness in student and clinical populations.* Retrieved from http://www.acestar.uthscsa.edu/institute/su12/documents/ace/8%20The%20 ACE-ERI%20%20Instrument%20to%20Benchmark.pdf

Sussong, A. E., Cullen, S., Theriault, P., Stetson, A., Higgins, B., Roche, S., . . . Patillo, D. (2009). Renewing the spirit of nursing: Embracing evidence-based practice in a rural state. *Nursing Clinics of North America, 44*(1), 32–42.

Tandon, S. D., Leis, J. A., Mendelson, T., Perry, D. F., & Kemp, K. (2013). Six-month outcomes from a randomized controlled trial to prevent perinatal depression in low-income home visiting clients. *Maternal Child Health Journal.*

Tistad, M., Palmcrantz, S., Wallin, L., Ehrenberg, A., Olsson, C. B., Tomson, G., . . . Eldh, A. C. (2016). Developing leadership in managers to facilitate the implementation of national guideline recommendations: A process evaluation of feasibility and usefulness. *International Journal of Health Policy and Management, 5*(8), 477–486. doi:10.15171/ijhpm.2016.35

Titler, M. G., Kleiber, C., Steelman, V., Goode, C., Rakel, B., Barry-Walker, J., . . . Buckwalter, K. (1994). Infusing research into practice to promote quality care. *Nursing Research, 43*(5), 307–313.

Titler, M. G., Kleiber, C., Steelman, V., Rakel, B. A., Budreau, G., Everett, L. Q., . . . Goode, C. J. (2001). The Iowa model of evidence-based practice to promote quality care. *Critical Care Nursing Clinics of North America, 13*(4), 497–509.

Totten, A. M., White-Chu, E. F., Wasson, N., Morgan, E., Kansagara, D., Davis-O'Reilly, C., & Goodlin, S. (2016). *Home-based primary care interventions (Prepared by the Pacific Northwest Evidence-based Practice Center under Contract No. 290-2012-00014-I.) AHRQ Publication No. 15(16)-EHC036-EF.* Rockville, MD: Agency for Healthcare Research and Quality. Retrieved from www.effectivehealthcare.ahrq.gov/reports/final.cfm

Ullman, A. J., Cooke M. L., Mitchell, M., Lin, F., New, K., Long, D. A., . . . Rickard, C. M. (2016). Dressing and securement for central venous access devices (CVADs): A Cochrane systematic review. *International Journal of Nursing Studies, 59*, 177–196. doi:10.1016/j.ijnurstu.2016.04.003

U.S. Preventative Services Task Force. (2016). *Methods and processes.* Retrieved from https://www.uspreventiveservice staskforce.org/Page/Name/methods-and-processes

Walker-Czyz, A. (2016). The impact of an integrated electronic health record adoption on nursing care quality. *Journal of Nursing Administration, 46*(7–8), 366–372. doi:10.1097/NNA.0000000000000360

Wallen, G. R., Mitchell, S. A., Melnyk, B., Fineout-Overholt, E., Miller-Davis, C., Yates, J., & Hastings, C. (2010). Implementing evidence-based practice: Effectiveness of a structured multifaceted mentorship programme. *Journal of Advanced Nursing, 66*(12), 2761–2771.

Wallin, L., Estabrooks, C. A., Midodzi, W. K., & Cummings, G. G. (2006). Development and validation of a derived measure of research utilization by nurses. *Nursing Research, 55*(3), 149–160.

Watson, C. A., Bulechek, G. M., & McCloskey, J. C. (1987). QAMUR: A quality assurance model using research. *Journal of Nursing Quality Assurance, 2*(1), 21–27.

Weeks, S. M., Marshall, J., & Burns, P. (2009). Development of an evidence-based practice & research collaborative among urban hospitals. *Nursing Clinics of North America, 44*(1), 26–31.

Williams, J. L., & Cullen, L. (2016). Evidence into practice: Disseminating an evidence-based practice project as a poster. *Journal of PeriAnesthesia Nursing, 31*(5), 440–444. doi:10.1016/j.jopan.2016.07.002

Wocial, L. D., Sego, K., Rager, C., Laubersheimer, S., & Everett, L. Q. (2014). Transforming the image of nursing: The evidence for assurance. *Health Care Manager, 33*(4), 297–303. doi:10.1097/HCM.0000000000000028

Creating a Vision and Motivating a Change to Evidence-Based Practice in Individuals, Teams, and Organizations

Bernadette Mazurek Melnyk and Ellen Fineout-Overholt

Shoot for the moon because even if you miss, you will land among the stars.

—Les Brown

EBP Terms to Learn
SCOT (strengths, character-builders, opportunities, and threats) analysis
SMART (specific, measurable, achievable, relevant, and time-bound) goals
Strategic plan

Learning Objectives

After studying this chapter, learners will be able to:

1. Identify important elements for successful organizational change.
2. Discuss four models of organizational change.
3. Identify barriers to organizational change and strategies to overcome them.

In today's rapidly changing healthcare environment in which health professionals are often confronted with short staffing, cost reductions, and heavy patient loads, the implementation of a change to evidence-based practice (EBP) to meet the quadruple aim in healthcare can be a daunting or "character-building" endeavor. Individual, team, and organizational changes are often a complex and lengthy process. Cultures also take years to change and leaders often get frustrated during the process if they do not see things moving fast enough in a positive direction. Leaders must realize that change efforts fail about 50% of the time and culture change efforts have an average success rate of only 19% (Gibbons, 2015). However, there are general principles at the individual, team, and organizational levels that will expedite the process of change when an exciting vision is created and a well-thought-out strategic plan is carefully executed.

Most organizational change theories are conceptual rather than evidence-based (Gibbons, 2015). As a result, leaders are often left with making decisions about strategy without solid research to guide their planning. In addition, many organizational change initiatives fail because leaders and teams (a) lose sight of their vision; (b) get steeped in challenging barriers; and (c) forget the stages of change that are a normal part of the process, which can lead to abandoning the change initiative.

This chapter discusses critical principles and steps for implementing change in individuals, teams, and organizations, with an emphasis on four unique non-healthcare models of organizational change that are useful in guiding successful change efforts in healthcare institutions. Strategies to enhance team functioning as well as the cooperation of individuals with various personality styles are highlighted. The major intent is to stimulate innovative "out-of-the-box" or nontraditional thinking in motivating a change to best practice within individuals, teams, and organizations.

Although it is imperative to consider the structure, culture, and environment when designing strategy for change within a system, it is also critical that the leaders and individual(s) implementing the change have a clear vision, belief in that vision, and persistence to overcome the many difficult or "character-building" experiences along the journey to bring that change to fruition. Experiences, beliefs, and action constitute the culture of an organization and when they work in harmony with one another, results are achieved; this is referred to as The Results Pyramid (Connors & Smith, 2011).

ESSENTIAL ELEMENTS FOR SUCCESSFUL ORGANIZATIONAL CHANGE

Important elements that must be present for change to be accomplished successfully are vision, belief, and a well-formulated strategic plan. Agility, action, persistence, and patience are additional key elements necessary for successful change.

Vision

The first essential element for implementing change, whether it is at the macro (i.e., large scale) or micro (i.e., small scale) level, is a crystal clear, exciting vision or dream of what is to be accomplished because nothing happens unless it is a dream first. Leaders often forego this step in strategic planning and it is a fatal flaw in organizational change. A clear vision of the desired outcome is needed to unify stakeholders, keep them excited, and outline a plan for implementing success strategies. In numerous biographies of highly successful people, a recurrent theme is that those individuals had big dreams and a clear vision of what they wanted to accomplish in their lives. Although it is important to have a well-planned process for execution, without vision the dream is unlikely to come to fruition.

For example, Dr. Robert Jarvik, the man who designed the world's first artificial heart, was rejected at least three times by every medical school in the United States. However, he also had a large dream that was not going to be denied. He was finally accepted into the University of Utah School of Medicine in 1972, and a decade later, he achieved a medical breakthrough that has gone down in history. Dr. Jarvik had none of the conventional assets (e.g., superior grades, a high score on the medical entrance examination), but he possessed important intangibles (e.g., a big dream, passion, and persistence to achieve his dream).

Dr. William DeVries, the chief surgeon who inserted the first artificial heart in a human patient, commented about how he had the vision of performing this procedure for years. Dr. DeVries repeatedly rehearsed that procedure in his mind in terms of what and how he was going to accomplish it so that when the opportunity finally presented itself, he was ready to perform.

Walt Disney visualized a dream of an amusement park where families could spend quality time together long before that dream became a reality. His strong visualization prompted him to take action and persist in his efforts, despite many character-building experiences. Most individuals do not realize that Walt Disney was bankrupt when he traveled across the country, showing his drawing of a mouse to bankers, investors, and friends. He faced countless rejections and tremendous mockery for his ideas for years before his dream started to become a reality. However, Disney stayed focused on his dream and thought about it on a daily basis. This intense daily focus facilitated a cognitive plan of a series of events that led him to act on that dream. He believed that once you dream or visualize what it is that you want to accomplish, the things you need to accomplish it will be attracted to you, especially if you think about *how you can do it* instead of *why you will not be able to accomplish it*. Walt Disney died before Disney World was completed and, in the park opening ceremony, a reporter commented to his brother that it was too bad that Walt never had the opportunity to see the wonderful idea come to fruition. His brother, however, commented emphatically that the reporter was incorrect and, in fact, that Walt had seen his dream for many years.

Mark Spitz dreamed of becoming an Olympic gold medalist for many years. He prepared himself by swimming many hours a day looking at a black line on the bottom of the pool. As he swam and looked at the black line, he kept the vision of standing on the Olympic podium and receiving a gold medal. It was that dream that kept him persisting through many character-building days of grinding practice.

If you knew it were impossible to fail, what would be the vision that you have for a change to EBP in your organization? Both within yourself and in your organization, how you think is everything. It is important to *think success* at the outset of any new individual or organizational initiative and to keep your vision larger than the fears of and obstacles associated with implementation.

> **❝**
> What will you do in the next 3–5 years
> if you know you cannot fail?
>
> **BERNADETTE MAZUREK MELNYK**

Establishing an exciting shared dream or vision with the team of individuals who will lead organizational change to EBP is important for buy-in and success of the project. Top-down dictates without involvement of a team is often a formula for failure. However, when a team of leaders and individuals share a common vision for which everyone has had the opportunity for input, there is greater ownership and investment by the team members to facilitate organizational change.

Belief

Belief in one's ability to accomplish the vision is a key element for behavior change and success. Too often, individuals have excellent ideas, but they lack the belief and confidence necessary to successfully spearhead and achieve their initiatives. Thus, many wonderful initiatives do not come to fruition.

A change to EBP in individuals requires a change in their behaviors, which is not easy. Individuals typically do not change behavior because they are provided with information or didactic education. Most individuals change when a crisis happens (e.g., a sibling who did not take his antihypertensive medication as prescribed or engage in regular physical activity dies young of a heart attack) or their emotions are raised. Use of emotional stories can be a powerful facilitator of change in individuals and organizations (Gibbons, 2015). Furthermore, behavior change in clinicians requires education and repeated skills-building activities. In their educational programs, clinicians are usually taught models to assist patients with behavior change (e.g., smoking cessation, healthy eating). However, those same models are rarely considered when working with clinicians on behavior change and should be incorporated into behavior change strategies within organizational change efforts.

Cognitive behavior theory is a useful framework to guide individual behavioral change toward EBP, because it contends that an individual's behaviors and emotions are, in large part, determined by the way he or she thinks or his or her beliefs (i.e., the thinking–feeling–behaving triangle; Beck, Rush, Shaw, & Emery, 1979; Lam, 2005; Melnyk & Jensen, 2013). Research findings support that cognitive beliefs affect emotions and behaviors, including the ability to successfully function or attain goals (Melnyk et al., 2006, 2013). For example, if an individual does not believe or have confidence in the ability to achieve an important goal, he or she is likely to feel emotionally discouraged and not take any action toward accomplishing that goal. Study findings also support that when clinicians' beliefs about the value of EBP and their ability to implement it are high, they have greater implementation of evidence-based care than when their beliefs are low (Melnyk, Fineout-Overholt, Giggleman, & Cruz, 2010; Melnyk, Fineout-Overholt, Giggleman, & Choy, 2017).

> **"**
> Anything that the mind can conceive and believe, it can achieve.
>
>
> NAPOLEAN HILL

Goals and a Well-Formulated Strategic Plan

Once the vision and beliefs are well established, the next essential element required for successful change is a well-defined and written strategic plan. A **strategic plan** is a road map with well-delineated goals, implementation strategies or action tactics, outcomes, and timelines. Many initiatives fail because individuals and teams do not carefully outline implementation strategies for each established goal. As part of the strategic planning process, it is important to accomplish a **SCOT (Strengths, Character-Builders, Opportunities, and Threats) analysis**, which will

- assess and identify the Character-Builders or challenges in the system that will facilitate the success of a new project;
- assess and identify the Challenges in the system that may hinder the initiative;
- outline the Opportunities for success;
- delineate the Threats or barriers to the project's completion, with strategies to overcome them.

Written goals with designated time frames for how that vision will be accomplished are essential for the vision and strategic plan to be achieved. Individuals with written goals are usually more successful in attaining them than those without written goals. For example, findings from a classic Harvard Business School study indicated that 83% of the population did not have clearly defined goals; 14% had goals that were not written; and 3% had written goals. This landmark study also found that the 3% of individuals with written goals were earning 10 times more than the individuals without written goals (McCormack, 1986).

A helpful acronym for setting goals is **SMART (Specific, Measurable, Achievable, Relevant, and Time-bound)**.

Agility, Action, Persistence, and Patience

Other elements for the success of any organizational change project are agility, action, persistence, and patience. Agile organizations innovate and are nimble in every function (Gibbons, 2015). They cannot be steeped in a culture of "that's the way we do it here." They must base decisions on the best available evidence, and when evidence is not available or of high quality, fresh innovations must be launched and tested to gather evidence behind them. Innovations with evidence to support them are more likely to sustain. Action is a key element of success because vision without execution or action will not lead to success.

All too often, projects are terminated early because of the lack of persistence and patience and faulty execution, especially when challenges are encountered or the results of action are not yet seen. An analogy to this scenario may be seen in an Asian tree, the giant bamboo.

The tree has a particularly hard seed. The seed is so difficult to grow that it must be watered and fertilized every day for 5 years before any portion of it breaks the soil. At the end of the fifth year of watering, the tree shows itself. Once the plant breaks the surface, it is capable of growing as fast as 4 feet a day to a height of 90 feet in less than a month. The question that is often asked is whether the tree grew 90 feet in under a month or if it grew to its height over the 5 years. Of course, the answer is that it took 5 years to grow. It is critical to stay persistent until your dream and outcomes are realized.

> **"**
>
> Nurse your dreams and protect them through the bad times and tough times to the sunshine and light which always come.
>
> WOODROW WILSON

Thomas Edison tried 9,000 different ways to invent a new type of storage battery before he found the right combination. His associate used to laugh at him, saying that he had failed 9,000 times. However, Edison kept his dream in front of him and persisted, commenting that at least he found 9,000 ways that it would not work. What would have happened if Edison had stopped his efforts to invent a storage battery on his 8,999th attempt?

The bottom line is that vision and a well-executed strategic plan that is acted on and executed with persistence and patience are key elements for success in accomplishing any new initiative.

FOUR MODELS OF ORGANIZATIONAL CHANGE

Chapter 14 outlined several models that have been used to stimulate EBP in the health professions. However, four organizational change models are presented here because they take different elements and strategies into consideration. These models were selected because they are based either on hundreds of interviews and real-life experiences by highly qualified change experts who have worked to facilitate change in business organizations for a number of years (Duck, 2002; Kotter & Cohen, 2012; Rogers, 2003), or they are based on a behavior change model that has been empirically supported for a number of years as effective in producing behavior change in high-risk patient populations (e.g., smokers, people who engage in risky sexual behavior). The principles of these models add unique perspectives and could easily be applied to healthcare organizations interested in motivating a change to EBP. Empirical testing of these models could move forward the field of organizational change in healthcare organizations.

The Change Curve Model

Although published in the early 2000s, Duck's (2002) Change Curve model emphasizes basic assumptions for change in an organization that still apply today (Box 15.1). In addition, it emphasizes the stages of organizational change with potential areas for failure.

Stage I: Stagnation

The first stage of organizational change in the Change Curve model is *stagnation*. The causes of stagnation are typically a lack of effective leadership, failed initiatives, and too few resources. The emotional climate in the stage of stagnation is one in which individuals feel comfortable, there is no sense of threat, depression occurs, and/or hyperactivity exists and individuals become stressed and exhausted. Stagnation ends when action is finally taken.

| BOX **15.1** | *Basic Assumptions for Change in an Organization* |

- Changing an organization is a highly emotional process.
- Group change requires individual change.
- No fundamental change takes place without strong leadership.
- The leader must be willing to change before others are expected to change.
- The larger and more drastic the change, the more difficult the change.
- The greater the number of individuals involved, the tougher the change will be to effect.

From Duck, J. D. (2002). *The change monster. The human forces that fuel or foil corporate transformation and change.* New York, NY: Crown Business.

Stage II: Preparation

The second stage of the Change Curve model is *preparation*. In this stage, the emotional climate of the organization is one of anxiety, hopefulness, and/or reduced productivity. Buy-in from individuals is essential at this stage when people must ask themselves what they are willing to do. The opportunity that exists at this stage is getting people excited about the vision. The danger at this stage of change is the length of preparation: the project may fail if it is too short or too long.

Stage III: Implementation

The third stage of the Change Curve model is *implementation*. In this stage, it is essential to assess individuals' readiness for the change as well as to increase their confidence in their ability to help make the change happen.

In the implementation stage, Duck (2002) emphasizes that individuals must see "what is in it for them" if they are going to commit to making a change. In addition, she asserts that when emotion is attached to the reason, individuals are more likely to change.

Stage IV: Determination

The fourth stage of the Change Curve model is *determination*. If results are not being experienced by now, individuals begin to experience change fatigue. The opportunity in this stage of organizational change is to create small successes along the way to change. The danger is that this is the stage in which the initiative has the highest chance of failure.

Stage V: Fruition

The fifth and final stage in the Change Curve model is *fruition*. In this stage, the efforts are coming to fruition, and positive outcomes can be seen. The opportunity in this stage is to celebrate and reward individuals for their efforts as well as to seek new ways to change and grow. This stage is in danger when individuals revert to a level of complacency and begin to stagnate again.

"

I have learned that success is to be measured not so much by the position that one has reached in life as by the obstacles which he has overcome while trying to succeed.

BOOKER T. WASHINGTON

Kotter and Cohen's Model of Change

Based on evidence gathered during interviews from more than 100 organizations in the process of large-scale change, Kotter and Cohen (2012) proposed that the key to organizational change lies in helping people feel differently (i.e., appealing to their emotions). They assert that individuals change their behavior less when they are given facts or analyses that change their thinking than when they are shown truths that influence their feelings. In other words, there is a seeing, feeling, and changing pattern if successful behavioral change is going to occur. Evidence from Kotter and Cohen's work with organizations to change the behavior of professionals has indicated that change agents must communicate their vision and make their points in compelling and emotionally engaging ways. It is this type of communication that enables individuals to identify a problem or the solution to a problem, prompts them to experience different feelings (e.g., passion, urgency, hope), and changes behavior (i.e., they see, feel, and change). In their book *The Heart of Change* (2012), Kotter and Cohen outline eight steps for successful change in an organization (Table 15.1).

Step 1: Urgency

According to Kotter and Cohen, the first step in changing an organization is creating a *sense of urgency*. This is especially important when individuals in an organization have been in a rut or a period of complacency for some time.

Step 2: Team Selection

The second step is carefully selecting a strong team of individuals who can guide change. Members of the team should possess the needed knowledge, skills, respect, and trust with other individuals in the organization as well as a commitment to the project. They should also show enthusiasm for the project, because enthusiasm, like stress, is contagious. In some prior studies that have implemented interventions to facilitate a change to EBP, opinion leaders (e.g., individuals with the ability to influence others) and EBP champions have been a critical element in a change to EBP. It is important to remember that informal leaders (i.e., those individuals without a formal title with a positive influence over others) can often be

TABLE **15.1**	*Eight Steps for Successful Change*
Action	**New Behavior**
Step 1: Increase urgency.	"Let's go."; "We need to change."
Step 2: Build the guiding team.	A group forms to guide the change and work together.
Step 3: Get the vision right.	The team develops the right vision and strategy for the change effort.
Step 4: Communicate for "buy-in."	People begin to see and accept the change as worthwhile.
Step 5: Empower action and remove barriers.	People begin to change and behave differently.
Step 6: Create short-term wins.	Momentum builds. Fewer people resist the change.
Step 7: Do not let up.	The vision is fulfilled.
Step 8: Make change stick.	New and winning behavior continues.

Adapted from Kotter, J. P., & Cohen, D. S. (2012). *The heart of change: Real-life stories of how people change their organizations* (table entitled "The Eight Steps for Successful Large-Scale Change," p. 6). Boston, MA: Harvard Business School Press.

as or more effective than formal titled leaders. Therefore, look for informal leaders within the environment to place on the team.

Step 3: Vision and Strategy

In step 3, the team guiding the project creates a clear vision with realistic implementation strategies for accomplishing that vision. In this step, it is important that the strategies are implemented in a reasonable time frame because very slow implementation may lead to the initiative's failure.

Step 4: Communicating the Vision

Step 4 of Kotter and Cohen's organizational change model emphasizes the importance of communicating the vision and strategies with "heartfelt messages" that appeal to people's emotions. For example, instead of telling individuals that EBP results in better patient outcomes, stories of real-life examples where EBP really made a difference need to be shared with them. For instance, some examples might be that thousands of low birth weight infants were saved from dying because of a systematic review of randomized controlled trials, which indicated that dexamethasone injections to women in premature labor enhanced lung surfactant production in the fetus; or, mortality rates in intensive care units dropped because of a change in endotracheal suctioning procedures. Repetition is also key so that everyone is clear on the strategies that need to be implemented.

Step 5: Empowerment

In step 5, individuals need to be empowered to change their behaviors. Barriers that inhibit successful change (e.g., inadequate resources or skills) should be removed. If not, individuals will become frustrated and change will be undermined.

Step 6: Interim Successes

Step 6 in Kotter and Cohen's model consists of establishing short-term successes. If individuals do not experience some degree of early success in their attempts to change, they will soon become frustrated and the initiative will falter.

Step 7: Ongoing Persistence

In step 7, continued persistence is essential to make the vision a reality. Organizational change efforts often fail because individuals try to accomplish too much in a short time or they give up too early, especially when the going gets tough.

Step 8: Nourishment

In step 8, it is important to nourish the new culture to make the change last, even if the leadership team experiences transitions. This nourishment is essential if the new culture and behaviors are to be sustained.

Rogers's Diffusion of Innovations

Concepts in Everett M. Rogers's (2003) landmark theory of diffusion of innovations can be very useful when rolling out an organizational change to EBP. In this theory, a bell-shaped curve is used to describe the rate of adoption of fresh innovations by individuals (Figure 15.1).

Innovators comprise 2.5% of the innovation curve in Rogers's theory. They are out-of-the-box thinkers and readily recognize innovative opportunities. Next are the early adopters or opinion leaders, who comprise 13.5% of the curve. These individuals are highly influential in organizations and encourage others to adopt innovations. The next group of individuals, comprising approximately 34% of the innovation curve, is the early majority. This group

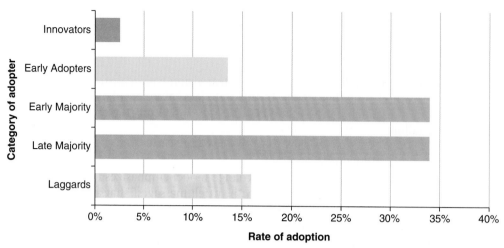

Figure 15.1: How individuals adopt innovation: innovators to laggards. (Data from Rogers, E. M. (1995). *Diffusion of innovations* (4th ed.). New York, NY: The Free Press.)

of individuals follows the lead of the early adopters in implementing the innovation. The late majority also comprises 34% of the innovation curve. This group of individuals spends additional time watching how the innovation is progressing and are more cautious in its adoption. Finally, the last 16% of individuals are the laggards, or the individuals fairly steeped in tradition and have much difficulty with change. They eventually adopt the innovation, but not until it becomes the standard practice. According to the theory, there needs to be a critical mass of 15% to 20% of innovators, early adopters, and early majority before innovative change really begins to take hold (Rogers, 2003).

If leaders embarking on an innovative change to EBP do not expect this pattern of diffusion, they can easily be frustrated and relinquish the initiative prematurely. According to the theory, it is important to target the early adopters in the change effort because they help facilitate a change to EBP in the organization. Many change efforts fail because focus and energy are placed on the late majority as well as on the laggards who are much slower to adopt change, instead of targeting the individuals who welcome and/or are receptive to it.

The Transtheoretical Model of Health Behavior Change

For the past two decades, the Transtheoretical Model of Health Behavior Change with its five stages (i.e., precontemplation, contemplation, preparation, action, and maintenance) has been empirically supported as being useful in precipitating and explaining behavior change in patients (Velicer, Brick, Fava, & Prochaska, 2013).

In the stage of precontemplation, the individual does not intend to take action in the next 6 months. In contemplation, the individual intends to take action in the next 6 months. In preparation, the individual plans to take action in the next 30 days. The stage of action is when overt changes were made less than 6 months ago. Finally, the stage of maintenance is when overt changes were made more than 6 months ago (Prochaska, Prochaska, & Levesque, 2001).

Research indicates that approximately 40% of individuals in a specific population (e.g., smokers) are in the precontemplation stage, 40% are in the contemplative stage, and 20% are in the preparation phase (e.g., Laforge, Velicer, Richmond, & Owen, 1999). In applying these statistics, if only approximately 20% of the staff in an organization are preparing (preparation stage) to take action in implementing EBP, it will be challenging for the initiative to succeed because many of these individuals will likely view a change to EBP as imposed and resist the idea (Prochaska et al., 2001).

The Transtheoretical Model is now beginning to be applied in the field of organizational change and, specifically, to guide healthcare systems in change efforts (Bentley et al., 2016; Prochaska et al., 2001). The extension of this model to healthcare providers when a change to EBP is desired could continue to extend the theory's pragmatic efficacy. For example, when attempting to stimulate a change to EBP in individuals in the precontemplative and contemplative stages, the focus should be on making a connection with them and assisting them to progress to the next stage of readiness (e.g., from precontemplative to contemplative), rather than working with them on actual behavior change strategies.

Strategies to assist individuals to move from the precontemplative or contemplative stages to a stage of readiness to change might include strengthening their belief that EBP results in the best patient outcomes and highest quality of care, and supporting their self-efficacy or confidence (i.e., they can indeed make the shift to EBP).

For individuals planning to implement EBP (i.e., in the preparation stage) or those who are actively changing their practices to EBP (i.e., in the action stage), assisting them with EBP strategies (e.g., how to search for the best evidence, how to conduct efficient critical appraisal) would be an appropriate course of action. By matching the intervention strategies to the stage in which individuals are currently engaged, the model proposes that resistance, stress, and the time needed to implement the change will diminish (Prochaska et al., 2001). Matching the intervention to the stages of change will also allow individuals to participate in the initiative, even if they are not ready to take action.

OVERCOMING MAJOR BARRIERS TO IMPLEMENTATION OF EBP

Even the best-written strategic plans can go awry because of a number of barriers to implementation. Therefore, it is critical to conduct an organizational analysis prior to starting the change effort to identify these barriers as well as strategies for their removal. Some of these barriers and recommended strategies for removing are discussed in the following sections.

Dealing With Skepticism and Misperceptions About EBP

Any time a change is introduced in a system, there will be some degree of skepticism about it. Individuals tend to be skeptical about a change if they do not clearly understand the reason for it, if they are fearful about it, or if they have misperceptions about why the change is needed. The best strategy for overcoming this barrier to change in implementation of EBP is to allow individuals to express their skepticism, fears, and anxieties about the change as well as to clarify any misperceptions that they may have about EBP (e.g., that it takes too much time). Educating clinicians about EBP in a way that appeals to their emotions and enhances their beliefs about their ability to implement it will enhance the change process.

Knowing Individual Personality Styles and How Best to Motivate Individuals

Any time that change is introduced in a system, it is important to be sensitive to the personality styles of individuals. Knowing the four major personality styles will assist in the change effort by facilitating strategies to work successfully with each of them.

Rohm and Carey (1997), seasoned psychologists who have written books on the different personality styles, use a DISC model (see descriptions in the following sections) for working with individuals who possess different personality styles. Although a particular style tends to predominate, individuals often are in combinations of two or more styles.

D Personality Styles: Drivers

Individuals with **D** personality styles like to take charge of projects and are highly task oriented. They are dreamers, dominant, driving, and determined. An excellent strategy for working with individuals with this type of personality style is to create excitement by giving them opportunities to lead the way by spearheading specific tasks or initiatives (Rosenberg & Silvert, 2015).

I Personality Styles: Inspired

Individuals who possess predominantly **I** personalities are typically people who are social and like to have fun. They are inspirational, influencing, impressive, and interactive. As such, they usually get excited about a new initiative when shown that it can be a fun and exciting process. Ask them to help you integrate fun into the plan and help spearhead recognition events.

S Personality Styles: Supportive and Steady

Individuals with predominantly **S** personalities are typically reserved and like to be led. They tend to be supportive, steady, submissive, and shy. The best strategy for working with these individuals is to lead the way, telling them that they will be important to help the project succeed but that they themselves do not need to spearhead the effort.

C Personality Styles: Contemplators

Individuals with predominantly **C** personality styles are very analytical and detail oriented. They tend to be competent, cautious, careful, and contemplative. At one extreme, they can experience "analysis paralysis," to a point where initiatives never get launched. These individuals, although they mean well, may prolong the planning stage of a new initiative so much that others lose enthusiasm for embarking on the change process. The best way to deal with these individuals is to show them all of the details of the specific action plan that will be used to accomplish the change to EBP. Also, consider giving them a leadership role in ensuring that process is being followed and tracking outcomes.

Formulating a Well-Written Strategic Plan With Set Goals

Again, it is essential to have a written strategic plan with clearly established goals for a change to EBP to occur. Lack of a detailed plan is a major barrier to implementing a change to EBP within a system. The goals established should be SMART (Feldman, 2016). The established goals also should be high enough to facilitate growth in individuals and the organization, but not so high that people get easily frustrated by their inability to reach them.

Communicating the Vision and Strategic Plan

Communication is key to any successful organizational change plan. Individuals in the system need to be very clear about the vision and their role in the strategic planning efforts. Repetition and visual reminders of the vision and plan are important for the project's success. Involving individuals in creating the vision and plan will facilitate their buy-in and commitment to the project. Top-down directives typically do not sustain.

> "

Change is stressful enough even when people are well prepared
for its demands. Action imposed on people who are not
adequately prepared can become intolerable.

PROCHASKA ET AL., 2001, P. 258

Interprofessional Teamwork

Interprofessional team building and teamwork are essential for successful organizational change to EBP. Research supports the fact that successful implementation of new best practices is a multilevel process involving healthcare delivery teams and their effectiveness, not just individual clinicians, with the strongest link being team knowledge and skills to make the desired improvements (Lukas, Mohr, & Meterko, 2009). Research has shown that interprofessional teams demonstrate higher quality of patient care and better outcomes than individual professions functioning in silos (Institute of Medicine [IOM], 2013). Therefore, forming teams consisting of individuals from multiple disciplines will further accelerate the change effort and facilitate a higher quality of safe, patient-centered care.

It is important to understand that the team-building process is dynamic and that it requires creativity and flexibility. In addition, knowing the typical stages of team development (i.e., forming, storming, norming, and performing) will promote successful development of the team and prevent the early termination of a project owing to typical team struggles, especially in the storming phase (Table 15.2).

Organizational Context, Including Resources and Administrative Support

Organizational context (i.e., the environment), including resources and administrative support, has been linked to the diffusion of EBPs throughout an organization (Rycroft-Malone et al., 2004). When leaders visibly express support for change or innovation and provide the resources and tools needed to succeed, the change is more likely to occur (Lukas et al., 2009). In addition, effective leaders adopt innovation early and view change as an opportunity to learn, adapt, and improve (Rogers, 2003).

TABLE 15.2	*Stages of Team Development With Associated Characteristics*
Forming	Anxiety, excitement, testing, dependence, exploration, and trust
Storming	Resistance to different approaches; attitude changes; competitiveness and defensiveness; tension and disunity
Norming	Satisfaction increases; trust and respect develops; feedback is provided to others; responsibilities are shared; decisions are made.
Performing	Level of interaction is high; performance increases; team members are comfortable with one another; there is optimism and confidence.

Source: Egolf, D. B., & Chester, S. L. (2013). *Forming, storming, norming & performing. Successful communication in groups and teams* (3rd ed.). Bloomington, IN: iUniverse.

Assessment of resources in the organization and the level of readiness for system-wide change is an important step in the change process (e.g., web access and data bases for searching, assistance from a librarian, EBP mentors, educational and skills-building programs, shared governance model that encourages clinicians to routinely question their practices; Ogiehor-Enoma, Taqueban, & Anosike, 2010). Although a large number of resources is not necessary to begin a change to EBP, there is no doubt that having ample resources as well as support and EBP role modeling from leaders and managers will expedite the process (van der Zijpp et al., 2016). Findings from a recent study revealed that nurses named leaders and managers as the one thing that prevented them from implementing EBP (Melnyk, Fineout-Overholt, Gallagher-Ford, & Kaplan, 2012). Therefore, it is critical that leaders and managers be targeted in change efforts because their role modeling and support is necessary if point-of-care clinicians are going to consistently engage in evidence-based care. Leaders and managers also must be clear about their expectations for clinicians, including that healthcare professionals must meet the EBP competencies, yet provide the support needed to achieve them (Melnyk, Gallagher-Ford, Long, & Fineout-Overholt, 2014).

Systems also can begin to introduce small initiatives to implement a change to EBP, such as conducting journal clubs or EBP rounds. It is important to remember that small changes throughout the grass roots of an organization can have substantial impact (MacPhee, 2007).

> **"**
> ## What is the smallest change that you can make based on evidence that will have the largest impact?
> **BERNADETTE MAZUREK MELNYK**

Placing PICOT boxes and EBP posters visibly in clinical settings can spark a spirit of inquiry in clinicians to consistently ask themselves what the evidence is behind the care practices that are being implemented with their patients. These have been used successfully as part of the Advancing Research and Clinical Practice through Close Collaboration (ARCC) model; (Melnyk & Fineout-Overholt, 2002; Melnyk et al., 2017; see Chapter 14). Effective teams also can be instrumental for sparking a change to EBP when there is a weak organizational context (Lukas et al., 2009).

In EBP rounds, the staff generate an important practice question. Then, they are assisted with searching for and critically appraising the evidence, followed by a presentation to other staff, where findings and implications for practice are discussed.

In systems without administrative support for a change to EBP, it is challenging but not impossible to ignite change. Assisting administrators to understand how a change to EBP can improve the quality and cost effectiveness of patient care, and appealing to their emotions with concrete examples of how a lack of evidence-based care resulted in adverse outcomes can help secure their support. Sharing of important documents that herald EBP as the standard for quality care and health professional education (e.g., Greiner & Knebel, 2003; IOM, 2001) will support the position of implementing a change to EBP in the organization as well as demonstrating the return on investment with EBP.

Overcoming Resistance

Resistance in an organization is frequently the result of poorly planned implementation and is the major reason that organizational change initiatives often fail (Prochaska et al., 2001). Individuals who display resistance to change are often not clear about the benefits of change and/or they have fears and anxiety about their role in implementing change or how it will affect them.

When confronted with individuals resisting a change to EBP, it is essential to facilitate conversations that will help them express their thoughts, hesitations, fears, and misperceptions. Listening to these individuals' perspectives on change with respect and acceptance is essential to overcoming resistance (Corey & Corey, 2002; Prochaska et al., 2001). Once concerns and fears are expressed, strategies to overcome them can be implemented.

Organizational Culture and Mentorship: Key Elements for Sustaining Organizational Change

It is one thing to begin implementation of EBP in a healthcare organization, but a whole other entity to sustain the momentum. Organizational culture is the attitudes, beliefs, experiences, and values of the organization. It is defined as "the specific collection of values and norms that are shared by people and groups in an organization that control the way they interact with each other and with stakeholders outside the organization" (Hill & Jones, 2001). In order to sustain EBP, adoption of the EBP paradigm by a critical mass of administrators and managers, leaders, and individual clinicians is essential. This paradigm should be reflected in the vision, mission, and goals of an organization as well as in its standards of practice, clinical ladder promotion systems, and new employee orientations.

The paradigm shift to an EBP culture does not happen overnight; it typically takes years as well as consistent and persistent effort to build and sustain. Unfortunately, many leaders give up prematurely when they do not see the outcomes of their efforts materialize in the time frame that they believe the change should occur. Therefore, having a mechanism for support and regular recognition within the organization for individuals facilitating this shift to an EBP paradigm is important.

EBP mentors are another key ingredient for the sustainability of EBP as first described in the ARCC model by Melnyk and Fineout-Overholt (2002); see Chapter 14 for a full description of ARCC. These healthcare professionals typically have (a) a master's degree; (b) in-depth knowledge and skills in EBP; and (c) knowledge and skills in individual, team, and organizational change strategies. EBP mentors work directly with point-of-care staff on shifting from a traditional paradigm to an EBP paradigm, which includes (a) assisting clinicians in gaining EBP knowledge and skills; (b) conducting EBP implementation projects; (c) integrating practice-generated data to improve healthcare quality as well as patient and/or system outcomes; and (d) measuring outcomes of EBP implementation (Melnyk, 2007). Findings from a study in the Visiting Nurse Service indicated that nurses who received mentorship from an ARCC EBP mentor, compared with those who received instruction in physical assessment (i.e., the attention control group), had higher EBP beliefs, greater EBP implementation, and less attrition/turnover. In addition, there was no significant difference between the ARCC and attention control groups on the outcome variable of nurses' productivity, indicating that nurse involvement in learning how to integrate EBP into their daily practice along with implementing an EBP project during work time did not affect the number of home visits made by the nurses (Levin, Fineout-Overholt, Melnyk, Barnes, & Vetter, 2011). Findings from another recent study showed that having a critical mass of ARCC EBP mentors within a hospital led to improvements in organizational culture, EBP beliefs, and implementation along with patient outcomes (Melnyk et al., 2017). In other studies, mentors or EBP facilitators have been noted as critical for advancing EBP (Dogherty, Harrison, Graham, Vandyk, & Keeping-Burke, 2013; Melnyk & Fineout-Overholt, 2002). For further evidence on the outcomes of mentoring and additional information on the specific role of the EBP mentor, see Chapter 18.

Preventing Fatigue

The barrier of fatigue typically presents itself when the implementation phase of a project is exceedingly long. An excellent strategy for preventing and/or decreasing fatigue in a system is to create small successes along the course of the change project and to recognize (reward) individuals for their efforts. Recognition and appreciation are very important in demonstrating the value of individuals' efforts and sustaining enthusiasm along the course of a project.

The road to implementing a change to EBP will be challenging but extremely rewarding. Essential elements for success include a clear shared vision, strong leadership, and a well-defined written strategic plan as well as knowledge and skills regarding the process of organizational change, team building, and working with individuals with different personality styles. Finally, an ability to persist through the multiple challenges or "character-builders" that will be confronted along the course of an organization's change is essential for success.

Never, never, never, never, never, never, never quit!

WINSTON CHURCHILL

EBP FAST FACTS

- The first step in moving toward an organizational change to EBP is to create an exciting team vision of what is to be accomplished and belief that it can be accomplished.
- A well-formulated strategic plan is necessary with strategies to overcome potential barriers.
- Vision without execution in the form of action will not result in the desired outcomes.
- Knowing the stages of change and what to expect in each stage will enhance the chances of success.
- An organizational culture and environment and a critical mass of EBP mentors are necessary to sustain the change to EBP.
- Persistence through the "character-builders" is necessary for success, so do not give up!

WANT TO KNOW MORE?

A variety of resources is available to enhance your learning and understanding of this chapter.

- Visit thePoint® to access:
  - Articles from the AJN EBP Step-By-Step Series
  - Journal articles
  - Checklists for rapid critical appraisal and more!
- Lippincott CoursePoint combines digital text content with video case studies and interactive modules for a fully integrated course solution that works the way you study and learn.

References

Beck, A., Rush, A., Shaw, B., & Emery, G. (1979). *Cognitive therapy of depression*. New York, NY: The Guilford Press.

Bentley, T., Rizer, M., McAlearney, A. S., Mekhijan, H., Siedler, M., Sharp, K., . . . Huerta, T. (2016). The journey from precontemplation to action: Transitioning between electronic medical record systems. *Health Care Management Review, 41*(1), 22–31.

Connors, R., & Smith, T. (2011). *Change the culture. Change the game*. New York, NY: The Penguin Group.

Corey, M. S., & Corey, G. (2002). *Groups: Process and practice* (6th ed.). Pacific Grove, CA: Brooks/Cole.

Dogherty, E., Harrison, M. B., Graham, I. D., Vandyk, A. D., & Keeping-Burke, L. (2013). Turning knowledge into action at the point-of-care: The collective experience of nurses facilitating the implementation of evidence-based practice. *Worldviews on Evidence-Based Nursing, 10*(3), 129–139.

Duck, J. D. (2002). *The change monster: The human forces that fuel or foil corporate transformation and change*. New York, NY: Crown Business.

Feldman, S. (2016). *Smart goal setting. How to set smart goals*. CreateSpace Independent Publishing Platform.

Gibbons, P. (2015). *The science of successful organizational change. How leaders set strategy, change behavior, and create an agile culture*. New York, NY: Pearson Education.

Greiner, A., & Knebel, E. (2003). *Health professions education: A bridge to quality*. Washington, DC: National Academy Press.

Hill, C. W. L., & Jones, G. R. (2001). *Strategic management*. New York, NY: Houghton Mifflin.

Institute of Medicine. (2001). *Crossing the quality chasm: A new health system for the 21st century*. Washington, DC: National Academy Press.

Institute of Medicine. (2013). *Interprofessional education for collaboration: Learning how to improve health from interprofessional models across the continuum of education to practice: Workshop summary*. Washington, DC: The National Academies Press.

Kotter, J. P., & Cohen, D. S. (2012). *The heart of change: Real-life stories of how people change their organizations*. Boston, MA: Harvard Business School Press.

LaForge, R. G., Velicer, W. F., Richmond, R. L., & Owen, N. (1999). Stage distributions for five health behaviors in the USA and Australia. *Preventive Medicine, 28*, 61–74.

Lam, D. (2005). A brief overview of CBT techniques. In S. Freeman & A. Freeman (Eds.), *Cognitive behavior therapy in nursing practice* (pp. 29–47). New York, NY: Springer Publishing.

Levin, R. F., Fineout-Overholt, E., Melnyk, B. M., Barnes, M., & Vetter, M. J. (2011). Fostering evidence-based practice to improve nurse and cost outcomes in a community health setting: A pilot test of the advancing research and clinical practice through close collaboration model. *Nursing Administration Quarterly, 35*(1), 21–33.

Lukas, C. V., Mohr, D. C., & Meterko, M. (2009). Team effectiveness and organizational context in the implementation of a clinical innovation. *Quality Management in Health Care, 18*(1), 25–39.

MacPhee, M. (2007). Strategies and tools for managing change. *Journal of Nursing Administration, 37*(9), 405–413.

McCormack, M. H. (1986). *What they don't teach you at Harvard Business School: Notes from a street smart executive*. New York, NY: Bantam.

Melnyk, B. M. (2007). The evidence-based practice mentor: A promising strategy for implementing and sustaining EBP in healthcare systems [Editorial]. *Worldviews on Evidence-Based Nursing, 4*(3), 123–125.

Melnyk, B. M., & Fineout-Overholt, E. (2002). Putting research into practice, Rochester ARCC. *Reflections on Nursing Leadership, 28*(2), 22–25.

Melnyk, B. M., Fineout-Overholt, E., Giggleman, M., & Cruz, R. (2010). Correlates among cognitive beliefs, EBP implementation, organizational culture, cohesion and job satisfaction in evidence-based practice mentors from a community hospital system. *Nursing Outlook, 58*(6), 301–308.

Melnyk, B. M., Fineout-Overholt, E., Gallagher-Ford, L., & Kaplan, L. (2012). The state of evidence-based practice in US nurses: Critical implications for nurse leaders and educators. *Journal of Nursing Administration, 42*(9), 410–417.

Melnyk, B. M., Gallagher-Ford, L., Long, L. A., & Fineout-Overholt, E. (2014). The establishment of evidence-based practice competencies for practicing registered nurses and advanced practice nurses in real world clinical settings: Proficiencies to improve healthcare quality, reliability, patient outcomes and costs. *Worldviews on Evidence-Based Nursing, 11*(1), 5–15. doi:10.1111/wvn.12021

Melnyk, B. M., Fineout-Overholt, E., Giggleman, M., & Choy, K. (2017). A test of the ARCC© model improves implementation of evidence-based practice, healthcare culture, and patient outcomes. *Worldviews on Evidence-Based Nursing, 14*(1), 5–9.

Melnyk, B. M., Jacobson, D., Kelly, S., Belyea, M., Shaibi, G., Small, L., . . . Marsiglia, F. F. (2013). Promoting healthy lifestyles in high school adolescents: A randomized controlled trial. *American Journal of Preventive Medicine, 45*(4), 408–416.

Melnyk, B. M., & Jensen, P. (2013). *A practical guide to child and adolescent mental health screening, early intervention and health promotion* (2nd ed.). New York, NY: National Association of Pediatric Nurse Practitioners.

Melnyk, B. M., Small, L., Morrison-Beedy, D., Strasser, A., Spath, L., Kreipe, R., . . . Van Blankenstein, S. (2006). Mental health correlates of healthy lifestyle attitudes, beliefs, choices & behaviors in overweight teens. *Journal of Pediatric Health Care, 20*(6), 401–406.

Ogiehor-Enoma, G., Taqueban, L., & Anosike, A. (2010). 6 steps for transforming organizational culture. *Evidence-Based Nursing, 41*(5), 14–17.

Prochaska, J. M., Prochaska, J. O., & Levesque, D. A. (2001). A transtheoretical approach to changing organizations. *Administration and Policy in Mental Health, 28*(4), 247–261.

Rogers, E. M. (2003). *Diffusion of innovations* (5th ed.). New York, NY: The Free Press.

Rohm, R. A., & Carey, E. C. (1997). *Who do you think you are . . . anyway? How your personality style acts, reacts, and interacts with others.* Atlanta, GA: Personality Insights.

Rosenberg, M., & Silvert, D. (2015). Taking flight! *Master the DISC styles to transform your career, your relationships . . . your life.* Upper Saddle River, NJ: FT Press.

Rycroft-Malone, J., Harvey, G., Seers, K., Kitson, A., McCormack, B., & Titchen, A. (2004). An exploration of the factors that influence the implementation of evidence into practice. *Journal of Clinical Nursing, 13*, 913–924.

van der Zijpp, T. J., Niessen, T., Eldh, A. C., Hawkes, C., McMullan, C., Mockford, C., . . . Seers, K. (2016). A bridge over turbulent waters: Illustrating the interaction between managerial leaders and facilitators when implementing research evidence. *Worldviews on Evidence-Based Nursing, 13*(1), 25–31.

Velicer, W. F., Brick, L. A., Fava, J. L., & Prochaska, J. O. (2013). Testing 30 predictions from the Transtheoretical model again, with confidence. *Multivariate Behavior Research, 48*(2), 220–240.

16 Teaching Evidence-Based Practice in Academic Settings

Ellen Fineout-Overholt, Susan B. Stillwell, Kathleen M. Williamson, and John F. Cox III

> **The meaning of "knowing" has shifted from being able to remember and repeat information to being able to find and use it.**
>
> —*National Research Council, 2007*

EBP Terms to Learn
Educational prescription (EP)
Evidence-based decision making (EBDM)
Evidence user
Informatics
Internal evidence
Quality improvement

Learning Objectives
After studying this chapter, learners will be able to:

1. Explain a conceptual framework for teaching EBP.
2. Discuss leveled educational expectations and strategies for teaching EBP.
3. Integrate EBP across BS, MS, and doctoral programs in health professions education.

Evidence-based decision making (EBDM) is required for all clinicians, and the traditional paradigm of authority is shifting to the background in healthcare decision making (Porter-O'Grady & Malloch, 2016). This permanent shift begins with cultivating the transition to EBDM for clinicians as learners and students. Educators may sometimes find this shift challenging because they did not necessarily have this content in their education programs (Felicilda-Reynaldo & Utley, 2015). However, it is clear from accrediting bodies, healthcare professionals, policy makers, and payers that evidence-based practice (EBP) is essential to providing effective patient care (American Association of Colleges of Nursing [AACN], 2006, 2008, 2011; American Nurses Credentialing Center, 2014; Centers for Medicare and Medicaid Services, 2014; Joint Commission, 2013). Early in the 21st century, the Institute of Medicine (IOM, 1999, 2001, 2002) set forth a vision that all healthcare professionals would be educated to practice patient-centered care as members of an interdisciplinary team, who, utilizing **quality improvement** approaches and **informatics** (i.e., data collection, storage, and use), would base their decision making on valid, reliable evidence (Greiner & Knebel, 2003). The core healthcare education competencies required to meet the needs of the healthcare system in this century continue to be

- Provide patient-centered care
- Work in interdisciplinary teams
- Employ EBP
- Apply quality improvement
- Utilize informatics (Greiner & Knebel, p. 46)

The Health Professions Educational Summit recommended that everyone involved in education address these competencies from an oversight perspective, in essence from leadership downward. Professional organizations and accrediting bodies have used these competencies as standards for criteria that define successful curricula for academic programs (AACN, 2006; 2008, 2011; Association of American Medical Colleges, 2007). Futhermore, there are now specific EBP competencies for nurses, both basic and advanced, that apply to all clinicians who claim to be evidence based (Melnyk, Gallagher-Ford, & Fineout-Overholt, 2017; Melnyk, Gallagher-Ford, Long, & Fineout-Overholt, 2014). Accordingly, to meet the expectations of today's healthcare organizations, clinicians need knowledge, skills, and language that enable them to look past the traditional focus of the conduct of research to the use of this important resource in practice (Fineout-Overholt, 2015). Twenty-first-century clinicians are expected to bring the best and latest evidence to bear on their decision making with patients. As such, the primary role of 21st-century health professions faculty is to teach learners how to think like evidence-based clinicians, using language that incorporates into daily practice the appraisal and application of research and practice-based data (i.e., data generated from clinical practice) and evaluation of outcome. These faculty will assist learners to shift their primary focus from clinical tasks to a lifelong approach of mastery of knowledge and skills for improving outcomes for patients, providers, and systems. Clinical decisions made on expert opinion alone are no longer satisfactory; rather, learners need to develop evidence synthesis skills that value and require up-to-date complete knowledge of best care treatments and delivery modalities. Transformation of the health industry is dependent on learners solidifying their EBP decision making as they embrace inquiry and an in-depth way of thinking and doing in the classroom and associated clinical practica that incorporates valid scientific and theoretical evidence; their own expertise and practice-based data; and their patients' choices, concerns, and values to achieve best outcomes (i.e., EBP). To help faculty achieve this goal, this chapter provides a conceptual framework designed to assist on how they can integrate EBP into existing curricula. Each aspect of the framework is discussed with suggestions for actualizing the framework in readers' educational organizations.

ARCC-E: A CONCEPTUAL FRAMEWORK FOR EVIDENCE-BASED EDUCATORS

The Advancing Research and Clinical Practice through Close Collaboration in Education (ARCC-E; Fineout-Overholt & Melnyk, 2011) provides educators with a comprehensive approach to meeting learners' needs for understanding daily decision making based on the EBP paradigm. This framework assists educators in academic settings to strategically craft their approach to achieve evidence-based educational outcomes. First, faculty and administrators must have expressed belief in the EBP paradigm and process. To implement these in education, as in clinical practice, educators' first strategic step is to begin with the end in mind by considering the following tips: (a) identify the program outcomes you desire in your graduates; (b) identify the milestones students must meet during their educational progression and how these are measured; and (c) describe the strategies within your organization that are influenced by the culture and used by faculty colleagues and within your own teaching approach to achieve these important results. Once you have written these down (i.e., a to c), begin to draw lines to connect the outcomes to the strategies in place to achieve them. You have just taken the first step to understand the current state of your educational institution's culture and to evaluate whether or not there are sufficient supports for integrating EBP into curricula, which is also the first initiative for implementing the ARCC-E model. The ARCC-E model frames this chapter's discussion of education to prepare evidence-based decision makers, offering insights into the necessary considerations for fully engaging EBP in educational settings. The discussion will include such important issues as ensuring sufficient financial resources for educators to build foundational knowledge and skills that they can share as they integrate EBP into their courses.

Building a Culture and Support of EBP

Simply having knowledge and/or skills in EBP does not necessarily ensure their use; however, researchers have repeatedly demonstrated that those with knowledge and *beliefs* in EBP were more likely to share their knowledge with their colleagues (Melnyk et al., 2004; Melnyk, Fineout-Overholt, Feinstein, Sadler, & Green-Hernandez, 2008; Melnyk, Fineout-Overholt, Giggleman, & Cruz, 2010; Wallen et al., 2010; Orta, Messmer, Valdes, Turkel, Fields, & Wei, 2016). Building student and collegial beliefs is therefore imperative for evidence-based educators. Part of building beliefs is diffusely integrating the EBP paradigm (for further information on the EBP paradigm, see Chapter 1) and principles across curricula, both in clinical and in academic settings. This in-depth thinking lays the foundation for integration of EBP in daily decisions. Without the EBP paradigm and process along with diffuse integration, there may be a perceived "disconnect" by learners between the paradigm and process and their clinical practice. Learners may view EBP as academic and unrelated to clinical skills they are learning. Furthermore, the EBP paradigm and process must be valued by faculty. For example, faculty must make no distinction regarding the rigor of the foundational courses in which EBP principles and concepts are initially taught and other courses with more clinical content that, ideally, use those foundational principles. This disparity in rigor and faculty expectation can be subtle, as in shallow engagement in EBP principles or lack of clinical connection, or it can be overt, as in faculty informally agreeing that students will not fail foundational EBP courses. Either of these approaches sends a message to other faculty and students that these courses and their content are "less than" clinical courses (e.g, medical/surgical courses). Rather, EBP principles and concepts must be the foundation of *every* course in the curriculum. Once foundational principles of the paradigm and process are learned, each course thereafter reinforces EBDM by using those principles and expecting evidence of integration of the paradigm, including use of language, the steps of the EBP process, and evaluation of expected outcomes. This approach to learning fosters students' realization that clinical skills are tools to be used within the context of delivering evidence-based care and problem solving using the EBP paradigm—a shift that focuses learning on achieving an outcome versus simply mastering a skill.

More broadly, for learners to grasp the need for integrating EBP principles, their relevance must be evident, and the culture must be saturated with EBP. The product of academic educational endeavors must be learners who have fully engaged the paradigm shift and foster a culture and mindset underpinned by EBP principles. Furthermore, educators need to be mentored to set their own evaluation goals and be encouraged to take time to self-reflect on the extent to which they are meeting them. As an initial step, it is helpful to consider how the organization as a whole embraces integration of EBP across its decision making and curricula. The process for curricula-wide integration of EBP using the Advancing Research and Clinical Practice through Close Collaboration in Education (ARCC-E) model (Fineout-Overholt & Melnyk, 2011) is graphically represented in Figure 16.1. Consider the graphic model as you read through the chapter.

> Without change there is no innovation, creativity, or incentive for improvement. Those who initiate change will have a better opportunity to manage the change that is inevitable.
>
> **WILLIAM POLLARD**

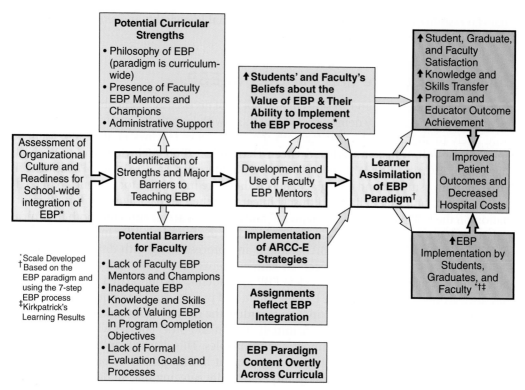

Figure 16.1: Advancing Research and Clinical Practice through Close Collaboration in Education (ARCC-E). EBP, evidence-based practice. (Copyright © Fineout-Overholt & Melnyk, 2011.)

ASSESSMENT OF ORGANIZATIONAL CULTURE

The first step in establishing a successful program for teaching EBP, be it large or small, is to assess the organization and its capacity for moving toward school-wide integration of EBP into its curriculum and culture. This includes, among other concerns, the institutional support, resources allotted, and the commitment and engagement in EBP by the educators and learners. Palaima (2010) discovered that organizational factors influenced learners' roles in the organization as well as their use of EBP. Furthermore, learners who practice EBP positively influence the organizational culture. These findings emphasize the importance of conducting an organization assessment prior to any intervention. The assessment questions in this chapter are drawn from EBP scales that were developed to assist in assessment of organizations' efforts to embrace EBP as the foundation of their educational efforts (Fineout-Overholt & Melnyk, 2005; Fineout-Overholt & Melnyk, 2010a, 2010b, 2011; Fineout-Overholt & Melnyk, 2017, see Appendix J). The Organizational Culture and Readiness for School-Wide Integration of EBP (OCRSIEP-E; Fineout-Overholt & Melnyk, 2010, see Appendix J) was specifically developed to provide the initial assessment of this important paradigm shift in education. OCRSIEP-E has been used reliably across multiple educational settings with reliability coefficients of >0.80. The sections that follow discuss what is necessary for an educational organization to demonstrate a culture of EBP.

Institutional Support for Evidence-Based Practice

For school-wide integration of EBP, it is essential for EBP language and intent to be present in the philosophy and mission of the organization. For example, the words evidence, synthesis, outcomes, and dissemination should be considered where appropriate. In addition, there are some underlying questions to help determine the extent to which EBP is a basic tenet of an organization (Box 16.1). If the philosophy or culture is less than supportive of EBP (i.e., fully integrated into all curricula and culture), primary efforts may need to focus on demonstrating to the organization the effectiveness of EBP through the success of small initiatives by the committed champions of EBP (e.g., demonstration that courses are taught from an EBP paradigm, including small changes such as changing simple language of assignments to include EBP language [e.g., change "provide the rationale" to "provide the evidence"]).

The goals and objectives of an educational organization need to be congruent with a mission to produce evidence-based clinicians. Evaluation of the role of varied goals and competing agendas needs to be conducted to assist faculty with full integration of EBP concepts across the curricula. The first step toward building an evidence-based curriculum is to obtain buy-in and support from all levels of administration. From this support will flow other necessary resources for a successful EBP program, such as committed, qualified personnel; continuing education; evidence databases; and full-access computers. Another evaluation of buy-in is assessment of the resources available that are or could be dedicated to EBP. Box 16.2 contains important secondary questions that can assist in evaluating the support needed to shift to a school-wide culture of EBP.

Commitment of Educators and Administrators

Demonstrated commitment to the EBP paradigm and process among educators and administrators that results in practice excellence is imperative for EBP to be fully integrated across academic curricula. One way to ascertain whether educators are committed to EBP is to observe their educational practices (e.g., observe whether they teach based on evidence or on tradition [i.e., "we have always done it that way"]; observe how they integrate current scientific and practice-based evidence into their teaching). Other facets of evaluating this commitment may involve what educators read, how they seek to enhance their database-searching skills, their receptivity to discussing supporting evidence for decision making, their willingness to discuss EBP, and their involvement in EBP initiatives. Because commitment is not a tangible outcome, this can be a challenging requirement to demonstrate; however, it is no less

BOX 16.1 *Questions for Evaluating the Environmental Readiness for Teaching Evidence-Based Practice (EBP) Successfully*

- Does the philosophy and mission of my institution support EBP?
- What is the personal commitment to EBP and practice excellence among educators and administration?
- Are there educators who have EBP knowledge and skills?
- Do all educators have basic computer skills?
- Do all students and educators have ready access to quality computers (e.g., that will support Internet access)?
- Do educators have skills in using databases to find relevant evidence?
- Are there librarians who have EBP knowledge and skills and who can be involved in teaching EBP?

Adapted from Fineout-Overholt, E., & Melnyk, B. M. (2011). *Organizational culture and readiness for school-wide integration of evidence-based practice.* Marshall, TX: ARCC Publishing.

BOX
16.2
Secondary Questions: Does the Philosophy and Mission of My Institution Support Evidence-Based Practice (EBP)?

1. How is EBP taught in my organization, throughout all mediums (e.g., inservices, formal classroom offerings, one-on-one mentoring)?
2. Is it a goal of the institution or practice to promote EBP?
3. If so, how is this mission "lived out" in the atmosphere/curriculum of the institution or practice?
4. Are there champions for EBP at my institution? If so, how would I describe them (having responsibility and authority)?
5. What kind of physical resources are available to practitioners, educators, and students to support reaching EBP goals?
6. What incentives are in place for practitioners and educators to incorporate EBP into practice, curriculum, and courses for which they are responsible?
7. What are the EBP assignments throughout the educational objectives or curriculum that evaluate the integration of EBP concepts?

Adapted from Fineout-Overholt, E., & Melnyk, B. M. (2011). *Organizational culture and readiness for school-wide integration of evidence-based practice.* Marshall, TX: ARCC Publishing.

important than the latest technological resources, such as computers and databases. According to change theorists (Duck, 2002; Kotter & Schlesinger, 2008), it is strategically wise advice to invite those who are the biggest resistors to assist you in advancing the change, because this may facilitate movement toward a unified commitment among faculty to foster learning through the EBP paradigm. Purposefully engaging those who are not committed to EBP may be what it takes for them to join in the journey toward integration of EBP into the curriculum.

Unfortunately, lack of commitment to EBP by educators or administrators is not easily remedied. However, persistent exposure of administrators, faculty, and learners to the benefits of EBP and how it improves outcomes in education and practice will, hopefully, reap the naysayers' involvement in building the foundation needed to move EBP forward in academic organizations.

Qualities of Evidence-Based Educators and Learners

Champions for EBP are committed to excellent patient care, whether they are educators or learners. These individuals continually strive for excellence and want to understand their students' or patients' problems thoroughly and apply the current best evidence appropriately to all aspects of work—they are evidence based. Box 16.3 lists the essential qualities that characterize evidence-based educators and learners. Desiring excellence in patient care is foundational to fostering clinicians who seek after relevant information to address patient issues, just as achieving the highest quality of care requires those who teach EBP to be committed to excellence in education.

Excellent Clinical Skills. Excellent clinical skills in patient interviewing and physical examination are needed for clinicians to accurately understand the clinical problem, the patient's unique situation and values, and the evidence-based management options related to the identified problem. In addition, excellent communication skills are essential so that clinicians and educators of EBP can clearly explain to patients and learners the risks and benefits of the available options and evidence-based recommendations.

BOX
16.3

**BOX
16.3**

*Essential Qualities for Evidence-Based Practice
Educators and Learners*

Commitment to:

1. Excellent patient care
2. Excellent clinical skills
3. Excellent clinical judgment
4. Diligence
5. Perspective

Excellent Clinical Reasoning and Judgment. Excellent clinical reasoning and judgment are of paramount importance because they enable clinicians to weigh the risks and benefits targeted by the available research evidence in light of the patient's values and preferences and apply it appropriately. Time, exposure, and experience are essential elements for developing clinical reasoning and clinical judgment. Faculty will be expected to have highly developed clinical reasoning and judgment, whereas early learners will grow in these qualities. Intentional cultivation of clinical reasoning and judgment would be wisely integrated across healthcare curricula as well as woven into educator development plans.

Diligence. Diligence is another desirable educator and learner quality. Educators and learners of EBP must be consistently willing to work hard, to search the ever-expanding array of available healthcare information resources to find the best evidence for a given clinical question, and to return to the clinical scenario and apply the evidence appropriately. Diligence is needed to communicate and hone the other essential clinical skills as well as clinical reasoning and judgment.

Perspective. Perspective rounds out the essential characteristics for an EBP teaching/learning culture. Perspective allows for incorporating newly appraised evidence appropriately into a greater body of healthcare knowledge and accepted practice, with a particular focus on integration with student or patient preference. Gaining perspective comes from the extensive study required to become proficient in the practice of healthcare and requires tolerance of uncertainty. If an educator or learner has an "all-or-nothing" attitude, evidence is usually categorized as either good or bad, and this is seldom beneficial to the student or patient. Most of the evidence that exists today is in the in-between category, neither perfectly valid nor worthy of rejection. The more mature perspective of educators will cultivate openness to uncertainty that will benefit learners.

Educator efforts to cultivate desirable learner qualities must be tailored to the learner's proficiency in the steps of the EBP process. For example, learners without much experience asking questions about their patients should be encouraged to start asking questions, then coached to refine those questions into more searchable, answerable questions. In the process, learners will start to see the benefit of walking through the stages of the EBP process and that careful formulation of the question leads to a more fruitful search for information. Only after learners have developed some proficiency in asking the searchable, answerable question does it make sense to focus teaching efforts on improving searching efficiency.

In the early stages, learners typically are excited about finding out information relevant to their patients in clinical practicums. These early learners may use textbooks to answer most of their questions. This is appropriate because many questions of early learners are background questions (i.e., those questions that ask for general information about a clinical issue). As learners gain knowledge and experience in asking pertinent questions about their patients' care, questions shift from background questions answered by a textbook to foreground questions that require more up-to-date information to answer them. Chapter 2 has an excellent discussion of foreground and background questions. Determining which type of question the learner is asking has implications for how the educator directs the learning.

For various reasons, early learners may often neglect to report the source of their information for their clinical decision. It is necessary for faculty to prompt learners explicitly to provide their rationale for their choice of information resources used in clinical decision making. Furthermore, educators who are at this early stage need to query their learners consistently about which resources they used to find their information and their opinion of the validity of the information they found, as well as the ease of use—or lack thereof—of the resource. Such discussion is useful for all involved because those resources that are updated regularly; are easy to search; and provide clear, evidence-based recommendations are likely to emerge as the favorites.

This discussion sets the stage for the expectation that learners will critically appraise primary articles from the literature when they progress to the point that they are using the research evidence for the purpose of answering their own questions versus performing an academic exercise. This is a shift from traditional education where learners simply received information passively. In EBP, learners must actively formulate clinical questions, search out evidence to answer them, determine the validity of the evidence, and decide how to use it in practice (Fineout-Overholt, 2015; Fineout-Overholt & Johnston, 2007).

SHIFT IN EDUCATIONAL PARADIGM: FROM TRADITIONAL TO EVIDENCE-BASED PRACTICE

Traditional research education focuses on preparing research generators (i.e., learning to design studies and generate hypotheses) or critiquing research for strengths and weaknesses. EBP education focuses on preparing the learner to be an **evidence user**. The learner is taught to think of issues in the clinical area in a systematic fashion and to formulate questions around the issues in a searchable, answerable way. Teaching learners to find evidence quickly that can answer their clinical questions and critically appraise it, not only for strengths and weaknesses (validity) but also for applicability to the given patient situation, is integral to EBP education. This decision cannot be made solely on the scientific evidence itself but must include consideration of the patient's values and preferences, as well as the clinician's expertise, which incorporates **internal evidence**. If the scientific evidence is useful to the practitioner, the next step in learning is to understand how to apply the evidence and evaluate the outcomes of the intervention. Assisting learners to understand how the EBP process flows is essential to success in teaching EBP concepts. There are many models for implementing EBP (see Chapter 14 for more information) that have at their core the EBP paradigm, which underpins the models as well as the EBP process. Indeed, most of the EBP models follow the EBP process specifically. Others add an integrated approach to implementing EBP, focusing also on system elements, such as culture and sustainability. Integrating the EBP models as well as the system models into healthcare professions curricula is an imperative if there is to be an operational shift in the paradigm that drives education.

The Evidence-Based Practice Paradigm

To understand the EBP paradigm, faculty must understand what is considered evidence. In this book, evidence has been described as internal evidence (i.e., practice-generated evidence) and external evidence (i.e., research). When using evidence (i.e., external and internal) for decision making along with patient preferences and clinician expertise, faculty and students must realize that a new responsibility comes with this broadened EBP scope: lifelong problem solving that integrates (a) a systematic search for, critical appraisal, and synthesis of the most relevant and best research (i.e., external evidence) to answer a clinical question; (b) clinicians' expertise, which includes abilities to interpret information generated from practice (i.e., internal evidence), from patient assessment, and from the evaluation and subsequent careful use of resources available to improved outcomes; and (c) the values and preferences of patients (see Chapter 1, Figure 1.2).

In the EBP paradigm, how the three EBP components meld together when making a clinical decision is dependent on each patient–clinician interaction. Students practicing from this paradigm have a better sense of why they are learning about urinary catheter insertion or turning every 2 hours. The variability of the weight of each component is directly related to the characteristics of the patient–clinician encounter. Clinical expertise involves how clinicians integrate knowledge of research and what they know about their work and population. Use and development of clinical reasoning and judgment is part of building clinical expertise. Faculty have the unique opportunity to help learners reflect on their life experience and how those experiences enhance their expertise. Furthermore, discussion around the innate talents of each learner can enlighten students' perspectives on what they bring to clinical decision making. Students' understanding of what they know about their patients' preferences rounds out some of the contributors that make up clinical expertise. The best clinical decisions come when all of these factors are actively contributing to the role of clinical expertise in the decision making process.

In the same way, patient preferences are not uninformed preferences. Clinicians have the responsibility to provide needed information in a manner that the patient can appreciate so that patients expectations best meet the clinical situation. Once informed, patients determine how they choose to proceed with the decision. For example, evidence from research might support the efficacy of one naturopathic supplement over another in treating gastrointestinal irritation. However, if the patient is likely to experience financial hardship from the preferred supplement because it is so expensive and will likely refuse to take it, and if there is another supplement with similar efficacy, the clinician has a responsibility to discuss these options with the patient. The patient can then decide which supplement works best for him or her. In this case, patient preference will outweigh the evidence from research and perhaps from clinical expertise, and the healthcare provider and the patient will choose an alternative supplement with similar efficacy and tolerable financial burden that will resolve the gastrointestinal irritation.

This important foundational paradigm underpins student and faculty understanding and practice of the EBP process and helps EBP models make sense. Otherwise, the EBP process and models simply become following steps. The bottom line for educators is to help students grasp why they are learning and what outcome they are striving to achieve. This clarity helps students put their energies into learning to improve outcomes versus studying to pass a test or procedural check-off.

Knowledge of Evidence-Based Practice

In teaching EBP, one of the key aspects for faculty and students is knowledge of EBP language, processes, and outcomes. Faculty cannot teach what they do not have knowledge about—they can teach only what they know. An evidence-based academic organization needs to have educators who have considerable comfort with EBP knowledge and skills. Knowledge of the EBP paradigm and use of the EBP processes are imperative for teaching EBP. This knowledge and its use must be transparently evaluated and any deficits filled with learning opportunities provided by the organization. For example, some evaluation questions could be: To what extent do educators construct their educational learning experiences based on the EBP paradigm framework? How well do they know how to construct a searchable, answerable clinical question in proper format? Can they convey what distinguishes clinical from research questions? How well can they communicate how to systematically search for relevant evidence? How well do they know how to critically appraise (i.e., rapidly critically appraise, evaluate, synthesize, and recommend) all levels of evidence? How well can they apply the evidence to a clinical situation? How well can they guide learners in evaluating outcomes? After it has been determined how well educators are prepared to teach about EBP, the challenge then becomes one of providing development opportunities to gain the information needed to close the gaps in knowledge and skills (Malik, McKenna, & Griffiths, 2017).

A caveat is warranted here in that sometimes faculty may exhibit a high commitment to teaching EBP, but may not be able to discern the gaps in their knowledge. In a survey of nurse practitioner faculty, Melnyk et al. (2008) found that of the sample of 79 graduate educators, 97% indicated they taught EBP in their curricula; however, the top-cited teaching strategy was supporting clinical practice with a single study. The EBP paradigm focuses on what we know (i.e., a body of evidence) versus basing practices on a single study. These findings allude to faculty's commitment to teaching EBP and identify gaps in their knowledge of the EBP paradigm and what teaching EBP requires (Melnyk et al., 2008). Furthermore, Stichler, Fields, Kim, and Brown (2011) found that faculty's traditional research knowledge did not necessarily translate into support of EBP; thus, faculty knowledge of EBP must be assessed and educational sessions on how to teach EBP may be warranted. Faculty development must be relevant and focused. For example, Zelenikova, Beach, Ren, Wolff, and Sherwood (2014) found that graduate faculty perceived to be most competent in asking clinical questions, considering patient preferences, and appraising a body of evidence were also perceived as least competent in assessing EBP readiness and the EBP barriers and facilitators in the clinical environment, communicating best evidence, and mentoring/teaching evidence-based practice to others. Conducting assessment of EBP knowledge and skills and subsequently providing faculty development that shores up identified gaps, as well as integration of use of EBP into annual evaluations, may help with uptake of ongoing, relevant educational offerings.

Gaining Knowledge

There are numerous mechanisms available to assist faculty in gaining EBP knowledge and skills. There are formal, expert-led workshops that present basic and advanced EBP concepts, as well as more flexible online tutorials that can be accessed easily at one's convenience to learn about EBP. Box 16.4 also contains resources that can help educators learn more as well as use to teach others about EBP.

After determining the level of EBP knowledge of the key people in your institution, consider whether the workloads of those individuals can accommodate a new endeavor. Administrative involvement is essential to this preliminary evaluation step. Organization support, resources, and time have been identified as barriers to teaching EBP (Stichler et al., 2011). Without administrative support of an endeavor to initiate EBP, success will be difficult to achieve (Fineout-Overholt, 2015; Fineout-Overholt & Melnyk, 2005; Melnyk, Fineout-Overholt, Gallagher-Ford, & Kaplan, 2012).

Integration of Technology Into Strategies to Teach EBP

Integrating technology to foster meaningful learning experiences can help healthcare professions' schools shift their paradigms to EBP. Selecting and incorporating technological tools that make retrieving evidence easier helps successfully support learning and is essential to overcome challenges inherent in supporting the innovative delivery of content and use of technology by faculty and students. Barriers arising from the costs, compatibility, technical issues, and the culture of the use of technology need to be evaluated to successfully integrate essential technology into the curriculum (Mann, Medves, & Vandenkerkhof, 2015;

BOX **16.4**	*Resources for Educating About Evidence-Based Practice (EBP)*

There are many articles about the basic knowledge of EBP, including:
- The widely used EBP Step-by-Step Series in the *American Journal of Nursing* by Fineout-Overholt et al. (2010–2012)
- The *Users' Guides to the Medical Literature: A Manual for Evidence-Based Clinical Practice* (http://jamaevidence.mhmedical.com/Book.aspx?bookId=847)
- The *Tips for Teaching EBP* series (e.g., Kennedy et al., 2008; McGinn et al., 2008; Prasad, Jaeschke, Wyer, Keitz, Guyatt, & Evidence-Based Medicine Teaching Tips Working Group, 2008; Richardson, Wilson, Keitz, Weyer, & EBM Teaching Scripts Working Group, 2008; Williams & Hoffman, 2008)
- The current recurring column *Tactics for Teaching EBP* in *Worldviews on Evidence-Based Nursing*, along with the prior *Teaching EBP* column (e.g., Fineout-Overholt & Johnston, 2005; Johnston & Fineout-Overholt, 2005; Kent & Fineout-Overholt, 2007; O'Mathuna, Fineout-Overholt, & Kent, 2008)

Strandell-Laine, Stolt, Leino-Kilpi, & Saarikoski, 2015; Zayim & Ozel, 2015). Determining the basic informatics and computer literacy of educators is an important step in building the foundation for teaching EBP. Without educators who are knowledgeable in informatics (e.g., adequate computer skills, ability to use databases to find relevant evidence), teaching EBP will be challenging. Before technology to enhance teaching EBP can be considered, basic skills in informatics must be assessed. Faculty with excellent informatics knowledge and skills can use technology to increase access to information in order to promote efficient clinical decision making skills (Zayim & Ozel, 2015). Faculty can also improve learning opportunities by expanding the methods available to disseminate the necessary curricular information to engage learners (Mann et al., 2015).

When determining the fiscal resources needed to teach EBP, funding for computers and access to evidence-based clinical decision support resources (e.g., UpToDate, ClinicalKey, and/or AHRQ's ePSS©) need to be recognized as essential budget items. Foundationally, updated, fast computers with Internet access are a must for educators and learners who will be learning about EBP. Administrators will need to commit to campus-wide WiFi access points to support student devices or on-site computer access for all students, clinicians, and educators. With increasing online programs, seamless remote access to full databases and desktops (e.g., from home) is an imperative. In addition, administrative commitment to ensuring that all learners and educators are computer literate at a basic level is essential. Administrators, faculty, and students must realize that the presence of technology alone does not determine success (Zayim & Ozel, 2015). Healthcare educators must ensure that students understand the connection between the available technology with its associated resource and its role in actively and efficiently delivering curricular content to guide their preparation as evidence-based decision makers.

Availability of Medical or Health Sciences Librarians
A medical or health sciences librarian who is knowledgeable about EBP is an invaluable resource on the EBP teaching team. It is imperative that these librarians be involved in the plan to initiate and sustain EBP in the academic courses across levels of education (i.e., undergraduate to doctoral). They can provide perspective and expertise in systematically searching databases as well as facilitate aspects of information literacy needed by students and faculty who strive to successfully teach and learn about EBP. Medical or health sciences librarians are

indispensable to the EBP process and can help learners and educators accomplish the goal of informatics and computer literacy. Often, librarians offer classes on computer basics and database-searching techniques, among other helpful topics. Faculty–librarian collaboration has been shown to contribute to building student EBP competencies (Dorsch & Perry, 2012).

Many university librarians have access to a platform called LibGuides©. This web-based platform allows for faculty to collaborate with their librarian to publish specialized EBP content, resources, and subject material in an organized fashion using an indexed, tabbed system. By creating library guides, faculty and students can have access to this information on and off campus, although they may need to log in to the university library for full access. This is particularly helpful when remote access to evidence is restricted, because faculty can synopsize articles, provide synthesis tables for students to peruse and respond to, or use other creative strategies to engage student learners by making content available that is on-campus access only. LibGuides© also help faculty and librarians use resources available more effectively and efficiently, as well as build an infrastructure to support integration of EBP across disciplines, which is an imperative for 21st-century health professions education.

 See an example of EBP content on LibGuides© at http://libguides.mwsu.edu/c .php?g=340604&p=2293006

Online tutorials are available for faculty and students to increase their EBP knowledge and can be found through any search engine (e.g., Google or Bing). Online tutorials about basic computer function are also helpful resources.

 An online tutorial on basic computer functions is available at: http://tech.tln.lib.mi.us/tutor/

Tell me and I will forget.
Show me and I will remember.
Involve me and I will understand.
Step back and I will act.

OLD CHINESE PROVERB

ARCC-E STRATEGIES FOR TEACHING/ENHANCING EBP IN ACADEMIC SETTINGS

Once the organizational culture and context are evaluated, the areas found to be the weakest provide guidance as to where to invest time and energy, building creative strategies to best enhance educators' ability to teach EBP as well as its integration across the curricula. These strategies include ensuring that necessary human, fiscal, and technological resources are available to faculty and students. Human resources can include EBP champions and evidence-based librarians who have knowledge of EBP and time to accomplish the goal. Fiscal resources include committed funds for ongoing development of the teaching program to educate the educators and for purchasing the best technology available to enhance the program and ease the workload of faculty. Technological resources are vast and always changing. Considering how best to use them to enhance EBP is an imperative.

According to a 2004 systematic review conducted by Coomarasamy and Khan, knowledge, skills, attitude, and behavior were improved with the clinical integration of EBP; however, stand-alone EBP courses only improved knowledge. The need for integrated curricula to improve knowledge, skills, and attitudes toward EBP has been confirmed in further systematic reviews (Ahmadi, Baradaran, & Ahmadi, 2015; Ilic & Mahoney, 2014). Thus, EBP must be incorporated across all settings in healthcare education, to parallel learners' daily experiences (e.g., ambulatory care and inpatient experiences, direct patient care, patient rounds, change-of-shift meetings, and unit-to-unit report when a patient is being transferred).

Teaching EBP should not be restricted to one instructor or to a stand-alone course (e.g., academic or clinical course). Rather, it should be so woven into the fabric of academic programs' overall curricula that it becomes part of the culture. Learners need to see EBDM used and have the opportunity to learn in every setting to which they are exposed. This ever-present implementation and learning of EBP concepts serves to model for the learners that EBP is not merely an academic exercise but an actively used tool in clinical practice. Furthermore, it is important that EBP knowledge and skills of clinical faculty be assessed and development opportunities made available. Upton, Scurlock-Evans, Williamson, Rouse, and Upton (2015) found that academic faculty reported greater EBP knowledge and skills in EBDM than clinical staff, which can set up dissonance for students. If students are to value integration of evidence into practice, there must be congruency among academic faculty and staff in role modeling the use of evidence to inform clinical practice.

Human Resources

Technological support for integration of EBP into curricula is imperative. Administrators, educators, librarians, and learners are key stakeholders in this initiative. Administrators, for the purposes of this chapter, are defined as persons who provide fiscal and managerial support to an EBP program (e.g., university presidents, vice presidents for academic affairs, academic deans, residency directors, department chairs, chief financial officers, chief executive officers). Administrators exhibit their belief in EBP and its impact on outcomes when they include designated fiscal resources for EBP in their strategic plans and prospective budgets (e.g., for ongoing education, technology, evidence databases, librarian involvement, and recognition of experts' time in training and compensation) and when integration of EBP is reflected in their strategic planning. Further evidence of administrative belief in EBP is the actualization of cultural expectations for integration of EBP within the annual performance appraisal criteria as well as promotion and tenure guidelines. Program directors and senior faculty role model integration of EBP by proposing a plan outlining the integration of EBP throughout the curricula and the potential benefits and costs, which will assist in obtaining support from administration.

Involve the Librarian Early

In preparing for integration of EBP across the curriculum, early involvement of the librarian is crucial. It is an evidence-based medical/health sciences librarian's job to be proficient in knowing where and how to get information. Librarians' knowledge of databases, informatics resources, and information retrieval is integral to successful EBP teaching programs. Librarians can assist educators in developing database and Internet searching skills as a means of finding relevant evidence to answer clinical questions. In addition, librarians can set up direct search mechanisms in which the faculty or students pose their PICOT (population–intervention–comparison–outcome–time frame) question electronically and the librarian then scours the databases for the answer and sends at minimum the citations and abstracts for the body of evidence to the inquirer. If the articles are available full text, the librarian is responsible for sending them along to the clinician. This approach to evidence retrieval can save enormous amounts of time and use some of the many talents of medical/health sciences librarians well.

Develop and Cultivate EBP Champions

Educators support teaching EBP by being knowledgeable and skilled in EBP and able to meaningfully articulate the concepts to students. A preliminary investment is required to ensure that educators teaching EBP have the necessary expertise for meaningful and successful delivery and role modeling of EBP concepts. For example, assigning faculty to teach a fundamental critical appraisal methods course when their primary focus is generating evidence and they are novices at using evidence in practice is likely to be frustrating to the faculty member and students. Helping the faculty to become more proficient in understanding the EBP paradigm and how it blends with their research paradigm can facilitate their transition from frustration to being a champion of EBP. Despite faculty having a positive attitude about EBP, they may not rate their EBP knowledge and skills positively (Stichler et al., 2011). Educators need to be familiar with the concepts of EBP to be able to assist students in determining whether observed practice is built on solid evidence or solely on tradition (Fineout-Overholt, 2015). Educators role modeling EBP concepts (e.g., addressing a student question at the time it is asked with a search of the literature and a discussion of findings and outcomes) can assist learners to integrate EBP concepts into their own practice paradigms.

Additional champions required for successful communication of EBP concepts are the learners themselves. There are always different levels of learners. Those who quickly absorb the concepts of EBP can become champions who assist other learners in integrating EBP principles into their practices. Integration of EBP concepts into one's practice is essential for learners to both see and do. Without learner champions, educating other learners will be less successful. Often in venues such as journal clubs, the learners are the ones who create an environment that encourages the less-than-enthusiastic learner to join in the process. Using ideas such as learning EBP can be analogous to making a quilt, building piece by piece, and may help learners to see the EBP process as wholly integrated. Educators, clinical preceptors, and other learners using EBP concepts are the "patches" in the quilt. When learners see EBP concepts integrated by these patches, there is implied agreement among faculty that integration of EBP is a valued tenet for education. Furthermore, the EBP paradigm and process take on perspective and purpose, much as patches put together make a pattern that can be seen only in the completed quilt. Without faculty and learner champions, broad valuing of the EBP paradigm and process, and implementation of EBP into educational practices (Fineout-Overholt, 2015; Fineout-Overholt, Melnyk, Stillwell, & Williamson, 2010a, 2010b) school-wide integration of EBP is unlikely.

Technological Resources

Technological resources are imperative for educators as they develop curricula using multiple instructional technologies to provide varied learning opportunities for students to improve their information literacy skills required to engage the 21st-century workplace (Stephens-Lee, Lu, & Wilson, 2013). Furthermore, these skills are required to effectively and efficiently access resources to answer clinical questions (Melnyk et al., 2012; Pravikoff, Pierce, & Tanner, 2005; Schutt & Hightower, 2009). According to the AACN (2000, 2008), technology affords an increased collaboration among faculties in teaching, practice, and research. In addition, technology in education may enhance the professional ability to educate clinicians for practice, prepare future healthcare educators, and advance professional science.

The Summit on Health Professions Education (Greiner & Knebel, 2003) identified the use of informatics as one of the core competencies for 21st-century health education. Through the use of informatics, medical errors can be avoided as students learn in a safe environment from experiences enhanced by technology such as simulation, thereby ensuring that their mistakes do no harm to the patient (IOM, 1999, 2001). In the IOM report, Educating Health Professionals to Use Informatics (2002), informatics is described as an enabler that may enhance patient-centered care and safety, making possible EBP, continuous improvement in quality of care, and support for interdisciplinary teams. When teaching organizations assume a leadership role in enhancing learning with technology, clinical organizations also benefit (IOM, 2001). To bring these transformative, foundational goals to fruition, organizations such as the American Medical Informatics Association (2013) offer virtual courses to help healthcare professionals gain knowledge and skill above their clinical education to ensure proper guidance and use of technology in healthcare. Selecting and incorporating technological tools such as e-books, virtual simulations, handheld devices, evidence-based clinical reference software, interactive whiteboards, and simulation experiences requires an understanding of how the tool will assist in the learning process. To successfully support learning, it is essential to overcome challenges and find the fiscal and physical support to ensure the innovative delivery of content and development of EBP competencies.

Information technology (IT) provides students and faculty with access to evidence-based resources that are necessary for learning about evidence-based care (Technology Informatics Guiding Education Reform [TIGER], 2007). Furthermore, the TIGER (2007) initiative leadership put forward the recommendation that all nurses, and other healthcare providers, develop informatics competencies and learn to use evidence and research to inform practice decisions. To bring this recommendation to fruition, it is necessary for all types of technology to be integrated in healthcare professions curricula. Through IT support, students can collect practice-based evidence (e.g., quality improvement data), combined with external evidence (i.e., research), to make evidence-based decisions at the bedside in their clinical practica (Hinton-Walker, 2010; TIGER Summit Report, 2007). Infusing educational technologies should sustain lifelong learning, promote active collaboration among learner and faculty, and expand interprofessional learning opportunities (Josiah Macy Jr. Foundation, 2015). Faculty need to acquire expertise in selecting the most appropriate technologies that would facilitate engaging educational strategies, meeting educational expectations, and assessing educational outcomes (Josiah Macy Jr. Foundation, 2015). These chosen technologies should transform education as a bridge for clinicians and educators to improve the delivery of care (Josiah Macy Jr. Foundation, 2015).

Technology provides virtual environments, tools, and tasks for students to engage in simulations, problem solving, collaborations, and other learning activities that require students to use higher order thinking skills. Finding creative ways to integrate the use of technology tools and removing barriers to deliver course content in an engaging way will help mitigate the potential for technology to be viewed as a distraction. Consideration by faculty of the value-added element of technology will enable students to do the same. Value added can be realized through adoption of a framework for implementation, which also helps decrease the distractors and supports appropriate curriculum integration of technology. One educational technology framework is the SAMR model that was developed by Dr. Ruben Puentedura.

 Learn more about the progression of the SAMR model at the following sites:

- **2006** http://hippasus.com/resources/tte/
- **2009** http://www.hippasus.com/rrpweblog/archives/000025.html
- **2012** http://www.youtube.com/watch?v=NemBarqD6qA

Puentedura's SAMR model consists of the Substitution, Augmentation, Modification, and Redefinition levels and is designed to articulate levels of educational technology that lead to transformational learning (Figure 16.2). Considering each of these levels and faculty's use of technology can enable thoughtful consideration of the student outcome of that use. The first two, Substitution and Augmentation, are expected to lead to *enhancement* of the learning

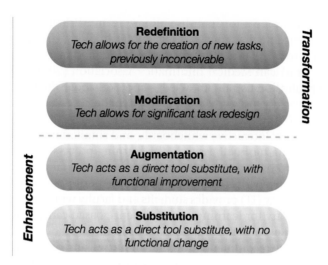

Figure 16.2: Ruben Puentedura's SAMR (Substitution-Augmentation-Modification-Redefinition) Model (2006, 2009, 2015).

experience. At the Substitution level, technology is a direct substitute for traditional educational practices; however, there is no meaningful improvement. For example, a substitute-level technology use could be an e-book instead of a print book. At the Augmentation level, again, technology is a direct substitute for traditional educational practices; however, there is some improvement. For example, an augmentation-level technology could be using Google Earth compared to a printed map. The second two levels, Modification and Redefinition, are expected to contribute to *transformation* of the learning experience.

At Modification, faculty use technology to significantly (functionally) redesign task. For example, faculty may use the FlipBoard application on a smartphone or tablet rather than the printed newspaper. The final level, Redefinition, allows for technology to be used for creation of a new task or activity that otherwise would not be possible without it; for example, using an iMovie versus role-play to illustrate a point in one's teaching. Faculty development programs that prepare faculty to integrate pedagogy with technology at increasingly sophisticated levels to achieve corresponding levels of deeper learning are essential for helping faculty meet 21st-century healthcare professions' students' learning needs.

Opportunities abound to infuse technology into the curriculum. Although students use technologies in their everyday lives, they can sometimes revert backward when in the educational milieu, preferring a less technical approach to education. Therefore, many instructional technologies should be included in curriculum planning and delivery, including (a) simulation technology; (b) mobile devices; (c) Internet-accessed social networking sites, such as Facebook, Twitter, Instagram, and Snap Chat; (d) Learning Management Systems, such as Brightspace created by Desire2Learn, Canvas©, Blackboard, and Moodle, provide a flexible delivery for course content to be delivered in an interactive way in any learning platform that enables faculty to administer, document, and connect digital tools to seamlessly integrate content; (e) audio and video conferencing through Internet-based programs such as WebEx, Adobe Connect, Zoom©, and Skype; FaceTime and GoToMeeting; and (f) electronic health record (EHR) software, such as SimChart, Cerner, and Lippincott DocuCare©, provides faculty with the opportunity to prepare students for the demand to use technology for documentation within the practice setting.

Simulation, mobile devices, EHRs, and the Internet to access social networking sites via the World Wide Web are expected to be the most used and important technologies in healthcare and healthcare education. These products have the potential to enable students to access data and information for point-of-care decision making and support healthcare clinicians with workflow, continuing education, collaboration, and access to EBP resources. Innovative technologies are being developed and applied daily to enhance patient care delivery and provider productivity that can and should be incorporated at all levels across the curriculum. Faculty support through creative instructional design and the development of realistic scenarios is essential to successful integration of technology into nursing education. Faculty development that encourages integration of technology into the teaching and learning process will enhance the nursing curriculum. Subsequent thoughtful evaluation of the impact through measurement of the skill set students use within the practice setting will enable support for continuing such development. Furthermore, implementing a curriculum that integrates EBP through incorporating technology can offer opportunities to increase students' information literacy skills. Bloom's Domains of Learning and Digital Taxonomy and Society of College, National and University Libraries' Seven Pillars of Information Literacy can be helpful to developing students' information literacy skills (Skiba, 2013; Springer, 2010). Educational agencies continue to use technology to foster collaborative learning communities to move toward knowledge development, dissemination, and implementation of best practices based on evidence (Hinton-Walker, 2010; TIGER, 2009).

With technology changing the landscape of education, there is concern over copyright and ensuring protection of intellectual property. For the purposes of this chapter, the U.S. copyright law indicates that a work may be used for the purpose of critique, scholarship, and for teaching, among other uses, which may be considered fair use (U.S. Copyright Law, section #107).

Find the applicable copyright law at: http://www.copyright.gov/title17/92chap1.html#107

Additional copyright information can be found at http://www4.law.cornell.edu/uscode/17/.

Information about the TEACH Act, including a checklist for use, can be found in the TEACH Act Toolkit at http://atkinsapps.uncc.edu/copyright/teach

---

One way of dealing with the copyright issue, which can sometimes be difficult and time consuming, is to use only links to full-text study reports as teaching tools. This places the responsibility on learners to obtain information straight from the source. The disadvantage to this practice is that there are many good teaching tools that are not provided as full text. Despite the challenges that come with electronic information, resources such as the Internet, electronic journals, and other computer databases are essential to a successful EBP teaching program.

There are many strategies that can assist in teaching EBP in academic settings. The key to all of them is to keep it simple. Focusing on the EBP paradigm and how it is being lived or exemplified in course documents and teaching will facilitate this simplicity. A common language and the steps of the EBP process are areas of course curricula that are readily incorporated into existing courses without a tremendous upheaval.

Curricular Resources

There are specific elements that must be considered when developing a curriculum that is underpinned by EBP, beginning with fostering a common language across courses (see EBP Terms to Learn at the beginning of each chapter and the glossary). Teaching clinicians that they must rigorously adhere to the iterative EBP process enables learners to embrace the imperative of the EBP paradigm and process as the foundation for best practice.

Introduce EBP Language Into Every Course

The goal of integrating EBP into the curriculum is to do so without faculty getting overwhelmed. A good place to begin is to review course syllabi and related course documents for the opportunity to use language that reflects EBP. For example, something as simple as changing the word "rationale" to "evidence" or "improve client care" to "improve client outcomes" can facilitate learning and shifting of paradigms for learners. These small steps reflect the EBP paradigm, and students and faculty will begin to speak the language. The purpose of learning a new language is to communicate. Without understanding EBP language, students will find it much more difficult to blend the best evidence (i.e., research studies shown to be valid and reliable through appraisal), clinical expertise (including practice data and personal experiences), with patient preferences and values to make the best clinical decision that will impact their patients' outcomes of care.

Another simple step that can be taken is to review the current learning activities and course assignments and reframe them to reflect EBP. For example, in an undergraduate nursing program, learning activities could be reviewed and altered, for example by adding EBP-related criteria for the assignments. A simple change could be adjusting the existing literature search assignment requirements to include a systematic search based on a developed PICOT question, with instructions for students to search library databases for all the evidence available versus cherry-picking a few articles. The focus is on the method of searching AND the yield. Another example is requiring students to develop aesthetic projects that represented their first nursing experience and incorporating peer review of these projects. Peer review is essential to EBP and can be important for both the learner and the evaluator. Evaluation questions such as "How did this project (either yours or your peers) help you understand the EBP process?" can be added to the peer review form used by students to reflect on the EBP process. Another example of language adaptation is the existing literature evaluation assignment. Often, learners are asked to evaluate studies, but are given a *Critique Form*—an old approach. Simply retitling it to *Appraisal Form* guides learners to reframe the activity and look for the value or worth of the project to clinical practice. One final simple example is to add patient preferences to an existing clinical encounter tool that students use to obtain assessment data. In this almost effortless way, existing assignments may become framed within the EBP paradigm, making doable the integration of EBP into courses.

Consider the best place to introduce the theoretical underpinnings of EBP and additional courses into which it can be integrated throughout the curriculum. An imperative approach for making EBP real for students is relevance—it must be important enough to them to integrate into their learning. In particular, because new healthcare professional students may not have sufficient clinical reference points to make examples clear, using current exemplars of how they make decisions, such as purchasing iPods, automobiles, or flight tickets, can make the connection.

Use the steps in the EBP process for problem solving across all courses. It is important for faculty to use the EBP process across courses as the chosen process for problem solving. When there are EBP abstainers (i.e., those who choose not to embrace and use the EBP process), students can get a mixed message about the importance of this paradigm for their learning and clinical decision making. When this occurs, it becomes something like "that's the way that professor wants to do it, but I like this professor's approach that is not so challenging—let's do it this way." Fully embracing the EBP process as the problem-solving approach for the school will require that the resources listed earlier be available, and it will help ensure that students do not consider EBP a course-specific rhetoric; rather, they will use the principles to make daily decisions with and for their patients.

Ask Clinical Questions

Faculty must keep in mind that the EBP process is a means for making clinical decisions to improve patient, provider, and organizational outcomes. Improving clinical practice requires asking clinical questions and challenging the status quo. However, faculty also must keep in mind that Step 0 of the EBP process is fostering a spirit of inquiry. Assigning students to write a clinical question without first fostering inquiry will not lead to student engagement. Once Step 0 is achieved, students can focus on Step 1. Faculty may need to practice writing foreground (PICOT) questions before they feel confident teaching students; however, it is easily mastered with practice (see Chapter 2). Creative use of interactive instructional methods can assist students in learning how to frame their inquiry, particularly the use of terminology for formulating the question. The language of the PICOT question does not indicate a direction for the desired outcome (e.g., *increased* glucose, *decreased* falls). For example, a PICOT question would be framed as "In women with back pain, how does yoga compared to simple stretching *affect* back pain?" However, research questions use different language, based on the theoretical approach of the investigator and the expected effectiveness of the intervention or issue; for example, "Do(es) specific interventions have an *increased/decreased effect* on an outcome?" Specific examples of research questions could be "What is the effect of yoga on back pain?" or "Does yoga *decrease* back pain?" Clinical questions are not research questions. Faculty need to incorporate teaching strategies to help students distinguish these two prevalent questioning methods. Teaching–learning strategies for understanding how to formulate a PICOT question may vary depending on the student's clinical experience or educational level. For a better understanding of these strategies across levels of education, please review Table 16.1.

Systematically Search for Evidence

Step 2 of the EBP process is systematically searching for the evidence. This step begins with a well-formulated clinical question. Searching for the evidence involves multiple competencies (for more information, see Chapter 3). Addressing searching from an EBP perspective will help eliminate some of the reported barriers to finding answers to the clinical question (Ebell, 2009; Hartzell & Fineout-Overholt, 2017; Melnyk et al., 2012). Although undergraduate and graduate students may report they have experience "searching" databases, this experience is typically the "as you like it" activity with no systematic approach to searching. Strategies to teach how to systematically search for the evidence include formal classes on effectively using electronic databases. This content cannot be left to librarians alone. All faculty must be able to role model systematic searching and collaborate with librarians to ensure students understand the difference between simple searching and systematic searching guided by the PICOT question. There are resources that faculty can use to improve their skills as well as students' skills, such as online searching PubMed tutorial (Winters & Echeverri, 2012) as well as faculty/librarian-led workshops (Ilic, Tepper, & Misso, 2012). Collaboration with librarians, whether they are from academic or clinical settings, is essential for consistency in introducing students to library resources, including access to available electronic databases. In the Internet-mediated classroom, faculty have the real-time opportunity to demonstrate systematic searching techniques that may be perceived as challenging to students, such as using subject headings, Boolean connectors, and limits (see Chapter 3 for more information). In the clinical setting, student and preceptor can collaborate on clinical questions and searching the databases (Winters & Echeverri, 2012).

Laptops in the classroom or using a teaching-friendly computer lab can serve as learning tools for the immediate retrieval of evidence to answer questions generated by case studies or making the activity relevant when connecting EBP to concurrent course assignments (e.g., systematically search for the evidence to support pharmacological decision making). Role modeling proper searching techniques helps learners understand their importance. Requiring search histories as part of written papers (e.g., students capture their search using screenshots that are pasted into their papers) demonstrates the quality of students' searching skills.

TABLE
16.1

Strategies for Teaching the Difference Among Clinical, Research, and QI Questions

Educational Level	Teaching Strategy	Learning Activity Example
Undergraduate	• Engage in a discussion of how students make decisions on purchasing an item; and have students provide examples. • Provide an example of internal evidence and outcome (QI); active research and EBP with appropriate use, special focus on kinds of questions. Introduce methods and outcomes for each. • Students work in small groups to complete the learning activity.	• Students share examples of the decision making process related to a purchased item. • Provide a worksheet with examples of research questions, and instruct students to formulate a PICOT question and a QI question. • Provide a clinical scenario and instruct students to formulate a clinical question using PICOT format. • Ask students to present their patient and formulate a clinical question using PICOT format.
Master's	• Discussion on differences and similarities among research, EBP, and QI. • Student shared example QI, active research, and EBP. • Present with question, methods and outcomes for their exemplar.	• Group discussion with a focus on their experiences with EBP, QI, and research. Discuss relevant clinical outcomes that need improvement, and have students develop PICOT questions. • Have students share clinical issues currently being addressed in their agencies; what questions are being asked; and what methods are used to answer them. • Discuss how EBP is visible in their agencies.
Doctorate	• Discuss EBP Process: role of question that drives process from inquiry and uncertainty to dissemination. • Substantiate clinical issue through internal evidence (epidemiology) to establish exemplar. • Students work in small groups to complete the learning activity.	Require students to sequentially: • Systematically search the literature on inquiry and uncertainty. • Using an exemplar, present what they have learned. • Group members formulate various questions that could come from the clinical exemplar, depending on what is found in the search (should be able to generate clinical, research, and QI questions from exemplar). • Use a reflective approach to the discussion.

EBP, evidence-based practice; PICOT, population, intervention or issue of interest, comparison, outcome, and time; QI, quality improvement.

 A tutorial on how to capture a screenshot is available at: http://graphicssoft.about.com/cs/general/ht/winscreenshot.htm

When a student engages a librarian or faculty with this information, it can reinforce successful skill building through evaluative feedback as well as provide an opportunity for peer review and learner self-assessment of efficiency with searching (Hartzell & Fineout-Overholt, 2017; Stillwell, Fineout-Overholt et al., 2010). For a better understanding of strategies for teaching systematic searching across levels of education, please review Table 16.2.

TABLE 16.2	Examples of Teaching Strategies for Systematically Searching Across Educational Levels	
Educational Level	**Strategy**	**Learning Activity Example**
Undergraduate	• Invite the librarian to provide an interactive session on resources for searching for evidence and the purpose of each healthcare database. • Use modules or other interactive demonstrations of systematically searching each database (at least three). • Assign students into groups and assign each group a PICOT question. • Students work in their small groups to systematically search three databases for evidence to answer their PICOT questions. Groups report back to larger class about lessons learned.	• Guided skill-building • Access three databases • Use provided PICOT questions to systematically construct search • Group participation/roles reported as well as results of student-conducted searches of multiple databases • Present to class with screenshots of systematic search strategy • Discuss how to narrow search using PICOT question and inclusion/exclusion criteria.

Master's	• Invite librarian to provide refresher on how to systematically search.
	• Add to resources:
	  • Alternate spellings
	  • Grey literature
	  • Saved searches software, such as Refworks
	• Discuss use of professional organization websites, Listservs, and other sources of evidence
		• Same group project with adding more resources (see strategy column).
		• Have groups report on the new resources that graduate students are now responsible for successfully searching.

Doctoral	• Invite librarian to provide refresher on how to systematically search at the graduate level. • Have doctoral student groups create tutorials on how to systematically search. • Discuss the role of leadership in systematic searching for doctoral students.	• Same group project as graduate students. • Have doctoral students create their systematic searching tutorials to share with the other groups. • Have other groups follow their tutorial and evaluate it for effective instruction on how to search at an undergraduate level. • Discuss the role of systematic searching in forming a body of evidence. • Discuss pitfalls and common errors that hinder successful systematic searching.

PICOT, population, intervention or issue of interest, comparison, outcome, and time.

Critically Appraise Research

Step 3 of the EBP process is critical appraisal. The key to teaching critical appraisal is for faculty to understand and use it in their educational practices. Critical appraisal is comprised of four phases: (1) rapid critical appraisal (RCA) to determine keeper studies (e.g., those studies retained for further appraisal; for RCA checklists, see Appendix B and Word versions available on thePoint®); (2) evaluation, in which data are extracted from keeper studies and entered into one table for comparison (for an evaluation table template, see Appendix C); (3) synthesis, in which data are compared and conclusions drawn from agreement or disagreement across studies (for more on synthesis, see Chapter 5); and (4) recommendations, in which conclusions from synthesis are reformulated into definitive recommendations for practice (e.g., all patients needing peripheral intravenous catheters should be prepped ahead of time with subcutaneous lidocaine). Teaching strategies should address each of these four phases of critical appraisal. If one of the phases is left out, students have a skewed view of the scope and purpose of critical appraisal as well as suspect recommendations.

There are a variety of teaching strategies that have been reported in the literature to teach critical appraisal. The better methods include the opportunity for all four phases to be addressed, including journal clubs and letter writing (Edwards, White, Gray, & Fischbacher, 2001; Fineout-Overholt et al., 2010a, 2010b, 2010c; Laaksonen, Hannele, von Schantz, Ylönen, & Soini, 2013; Purnell & Majid, 2017). Researchers have found that the majority of clinicians and students found journal clubs satisfactory learning opportunities to increase their EBP skills overall and, in particular, their critical appraisal skills (Laaksonen et al., 2013; Purnell & Majid, 2017). An example of journal clubs to enhance critical appraisal skills may include a small-group structure in which the participants present the four phases of critical appraisal of a preselected paper to their peers. Advanced learners may choose to compose a letter to the article author that outlines the complete appraisal, including the recommendation of its use in practice.

To address different learners, at different levels of learning and having different desired outcomes, it is recommended that faculty use a blend of various strategies to teach critical appraisal versus just one or two. For example, in a mixed-methods study, Ilic, Hart, Fiddes, Misso, and Villanueva (2013) found that teaching EBP with the blended-learning approach compared to the traditional lecture-type approach significantly improved the confidence students reported in their critical appraisal skills. Zwickey et al. (2014) found that EBP competencies are helpful for ensuring integration of EBP across the curriculum and provide guidance for faculty development (for more on EBP competencies, see Chapter 11).

Another essential for teaching critical appraisal to students is delineating the processes of EBP, research and quality improvement (Fineout-Overholt, 2013, 2015; Shirey et al., 2011). Although these are complementary processes, they are distinct, with distinct outcomes. In academic settings, there may be an intellectual assent that undergraduate nursing programs need to move away from the traditionally emphasized critiques of research, and in the development of a research proposal or conducting research, there is still a focus on heavy research methods; however, faculty are increasingly reporting redesigning the traditional research course to an EBP approach (Melnyk et al., 2012). Simple interventions to integrate EBP are required to move from traditional approaches to teaching research methods within critical appraisal as a basis for health professions students' decision making. First, consider restructuring and refocusing existing research courses into incremental experiential EBP learning opportunities in which students learn about research methods for the purpose of laying an EBDM foundation that clinical educators can build on in clinical courses. Educators can use levels of evidence as the framework for discussing the appropriate research design to answer clinical question as well as critical appraisal of evidence. To fully integrate the concepts of EBP into the curriculum requires that faculty be educated about critical appraisal, participate in curriculum revisions to incorporate this important step in the EBP process, and demonstrate buy-in by actively using critical appraisal in their teaching, no matter what course they teach.

Incorporating critical appraisal into various courses helps students realize the importance of the use of research in clinical decision making. Foundational to using an evidence-based approach is clinicians understanding which methods lead to valid and reliable research. For faculty to teach critical appraisal effectively, their outcomes must be refocused to producing evidence users versus evidence generators. The how-tos of conducting research are not the imperative; however, knowing the markers of good research is imperative, which includes the language of research and critical appraisal. All research designs must be included in the discussion of available evidence. Furthermore, for EBP to be a lived experience, there must be an active engagement of EBP initiatives at the educational institution.

In an example, faculty who teach traditional research courses were the champions charged with integration of EBP into the curriculum, and an EBP expert sanctioned by the curriculum committee to lead the integration of EBP in the curriculum strategically planned how to best begin the integration of EBP into each course. The sample objectives and learning activities from the redesigned course clearly show the shift from producing a research proposal to using concepts and principles of EBP and can be found in Box 16.5. In addition, faculty must consider that teaching–learning strategies for appraising the evidence may vary depending on students' clinical experience or educational level. To understand more about leveling of critical appraisal assignments, see Table 16.3.

Incorporate Clinical Expertise and Patient Preferences

In Step 4 of the EBP process, along with evidence, clinical expertise and patient values and preferences play an integral part in clinical decision making. Realization of their impact on patient outcome is an essential of EBDM. Students' confidence in decision making and

---

 BOX
16.5

Sample Overall Course Objectives and Learning Assignments

Course Objective	Example Assignment
• Formulate searchable, answerable questions from clinical issues	• Generate PICOT questions for written assignment
• Examine clinical questions in relation to levels of evidence	• Groups share and give feedback on PICOT questions
• Find the best evidence to answer the clinical question through searching existing healthcare databases and other sources of evidence	• Search two types of questions and post search strategies/results • Groups share and give feedback to peers • Paper on search for the evidence to a clinical question
• Critically appraise best evidence (i.e., evaluating research methodologies for validity, reliability, and applicability) to answer selected clinical questions	• Conduct a rapid critical appraisal of a quantitative study • Groups share and give feedback to peers • Paper on appraisal of the evidence
• Discuss strategies for implementing evidence into daily practice	• Paper on proposed change in practice

PICOT, population, intervention or issue of interest, comparison, outcome, and time.

TABLE 16.3	*Examples of Critical Appraisal Across Levels of Education*	
Educational Program	**Strategy Examples**	**Learning Activity Examples**

Under-graduate	• Class on appraisal would include discussion of:
	  • what appraisal means
	  • using EBP language (appraising the value or worth to practice; avoid "critique")
	  • EBP terms
	  • types of research and associated research methods
	  • common research statistics for interpretation of study findings
	• Select preappraised literature and use a critical appraisal checklist (e.g., appraisal tools are available at Joanna Briggs website http://joannabriggs.org/research/critical-appraisal-tools.html or Appendix B)
		• Students complete worksheets consisting of components of an appraisal.
		• Students work in small groups guided by faculty member.
		• Provide students with a preappraised study and critical appraisal checklist that they use to appraise study and report to the class.
		• Faculty leads an appraisal of a full study relevant to the area of the discipline (study assigned to students to read prior to class).
		• Conduct appraisals throughout didactic and clinical courses.
		• Create an evaluation table entry after appraising each study (one evaluation table).
		• Use evaluation table to form a synthesis table for making decisions.
		• Discuss the decision within the small group.
		• Discuss current practices noted in practica compared to what the evidence indicates is best practice.

Master's	• Emphasize the difference between critique and appraise. • Compare and contrast research and EBP language. • Discuss levels of evidence. • Discuss research designs and methods. • Discuss common statistical analyses by research design to interpret study results. • Create examples of different appraisal checklists by research design and discuss associated concepts of validity and reliability. • Discuss principles of evaluation and synthesis. • Provide examples of evaluation and syntheses tables with associated recommendations.	• Begin with preappraised literature and progress to published primary studies. • Students begin their work in groups to mirror clinical practice. • Use the journal club approach for weekly appraisals to develop the appraisal skills as a group. • In a parallel process, individual master's students create an evaluation table with at least 8–10 studies, including systematic reviews. • Data from evaluation table are extracted to create at least two synthesis tables (a level of evidence and an outcome synthesis table). • Recommendations are made for clinical practice that are implemented in a capstone project. • Begin capstone with educational interventions to make agency staff aware of current evidence. • Use evaluation and synthesis tables as the basis of capstone planning. • Begin capstone with educational interventions to make agency staff aware of current evidence. • Appraise clinical practice guidelines for applicability and compare to observed practice.

TABLE 16.3	Examples of Critical Appraisal Across Levels of Education (continued)	
Educational Program	**Strategy Examples**	**Learning Activity Examples**
Clinically focused Doctorates (e.g., DNP, MD, PharmD, DPT)	• All Master's strategies apply to doctoral study. In addition: • Dig deeper into research methods and associated statistical analyses for interpretation of study results. • Emphasize ownership of a body of evidence—that is, ALL the evidence we have on the topic. Students in clinical doctorates must be the experts in both the current evidence and what is done in the clinical setting (current practice). • Discuss integration of internal and external evidence in decision making. • Explain the expectation of leading critical appraisal for undergraduate and master's prepared clinicians.	• All Master's expectations apply to doctoral students. In addition: • Explain impact of organizational culture within body of evidence (all that we know). • Consider role of evidence in policy-making. • Consider evidence review and need for publishing appraisal. • Consider leadership in updating clinical practice guidelines. • Consider the use of clinical practice guidelines in observed practice.
Research-focused Doctorates (e.g., PhD)	• Emphasize the need for critical appraisal of evidence versus literature review. • Emphasize the benefits of evaluation and synthesis to answer an unbiased clinical question over literature review of cherry-picked studies or a biased review of directional outcomes.	• Appraise a body of evidence • Evaluation and synthesis tables of what we currently know • Synthesis table with a focus on identification of gaps in: • Knowledge • Research design or methods issues • Proposal to address the appraised issues.

evaluation of outcomes is dependent on their healthcare knowledge and their clinical reasoning (Tauzon, 2017). Faculty must create learning opportunities for students to explore the importance of clinical expertise, reasoning, and judgment in their decision making, with the goal of making a firm connection to their use of evidence in practice. Without intentional efforts to make these connections, there may be a misperception by students about their impact on patient, provider, and system outcomes.

Similarly, faculty assessment of where learners are taught about the importance of understanding the role of patient preferences is critical. Learning activities focused on heightening health professions students' awareness of the importance of patient preferences can be intentionally designed around students' day-to-day experiences with patient-centered care. For example, a learning activity with beginning students can include clinical experiences in which students are obtaining patient histories. This experience can provide a rich forum for discussing patients' preferences, desires, and values about their health and their expectations of healthcare and how those preferences are being integrated into the care received. For more advanced learners, discussion of strategies to actively include the role of patient preferences in care interventions would be appropriate. As with clinical expertise, intentional learning activities are needed so that healthcare students can explore the connection between their incorporation of patient preferences in their decision making about the use of evidence in practice and outcomes. Otherwise, this connection may be less apparent to students (Tauzon, 2017).

Lectures, Group Learning, Journal Clubs, and More. Methods used to teach EBP should emphasize active participation by the learners as much as possible. Examples of potential strategies include lectures, discussion groups, small- and large-group presentations, journal clubs and competitive journal clubs, critically appraised topics (CATs), elective rotations, grand rounds, unit rounds, multimedia, and change-of-shift discussions for practica. Educators are best to act in the facilitator role while learners take front stage in working through the concepts, much like the flipped classroom described by Bergmann and Sams (2012). That being said, learners expect educators to have credibility and an expertise in their field (Johnston et al., 2016).

Presentations Integrated With Clinical Practicum. A good way to begin any type of educational presentation on EBP is to provide a short synopsis on the definition and EBP process with examples. When teaching EBP in a classroom setting, an interactive teaching style is preferred (e.g., Socratic questioning and group work), because the students can get lost in the content if not engaging the material. If you want to engage the flipped classroom approach, you will need to prepare 10-minute interactive videos that provide the essential content, post them online, and spend class time exploring the concepts of EBP and how they relate to clinical care. However you choose to conduct your class, choose methods to facilitate student engagement.

Clinically integrated teaching–learning activities aimed at improving knowledge, attitude, and behavior are superior to classroom teaching alone. However, classroom teaching that incorporates activities (e.g., case studies, group work, role-play, hands-on learning) can increase educational effectiveness. Clinical teaching can include didactic information by the educator who directly applies the content to patient situations. Using interactive teaching strategies at a clinical site can make learning more effective. Didactic teaching without interactive teaching strategies is less effective and leads to rote memory. A landmark hierarchy of teaching and learning activities related to educational effectiveness was suggested by Khan and Coomarasamy (2006) some time ago, but healthcare educators can still benefit from this list (see Box 16.6).

Small-Group Seminars. Research evidence has supported the benefits of seminars targeting specific EBP skills for some time (Novak & McIntyre, 2010; Shuval et al., 2007; West & McDonald, 2008; Yew & Reid, 2008); however, small-group work requires creativity on the

BOX
16.6   *Hierarchy of Teaching and Learning Activities*

Level 1	Interactive and clinically integrated activities
Level 2(a)	Interactive but classroom-based activities
Level 2(b)	Didactic but clinically integrated activities
Level 3	Didactic classroom or stand-alone teaching

part of the educator and engagement from learners (Morris, 2016). If you are in doubt about what sort of topic would be of interest for small-group work, ask for suggestions from the participants. Suggestions can be offered either before the group work seminar so that pre-digested or preappraised examples can be used or at the time of the seminar in more of an "on-the-fly" setup. These more spontaneous sessions tend to be risky, because if the example is too difficult, the learners can quickly become lost and disheartened, potentially viewing EBP as a tedious and difficult process. A skillful educator can build confidence in the learner by crafting or framing the issue in a way that easily guides the learner to a clinical question that can be formulated rather easily, then to an available answer that can be found from a relatively simple search, and then to the evidence that can be easily critically appraised. This is an initial engagement step, and each group work seminar could build in difficulty and ambiguity of the EBP process. Beginning this way will enable the group to feel that the process is not only learnable but also useful and doable, because they have participated in it and accomplished many of the steps themselves.

When moving toward seminars more focused in EBP skills, remember to orient your group of learners to how the skill you are teaching fits into the greater context of the EBP process. For example, if you are teaching a seminar on how to search the healthcare literature, it is important to stress that searching is simply a tool to be used to find the most relevant, valid research evidence and not the only—or even the most important—skill that needs to be learned in the EBP process. Whetting their appetites about the focus of the search and prompting them on to the next steps of critical appraisal and application of evidence to the clinical problem can help learners to realize the broader scope of the EBP process rather than focus on an isolated skill.

Another practical suggestion when establishing small, focused group seminars on EBP concepts is to provide time and means of hands-on practice. For example, when teaching a session on composing and formatting answerable, searchable questions, ask the partici-pants to individually think of clinical questions from their own experience. Provide ample time for them to share their questions with the group and then determine whether they are foreground or background questions (see Chapter 2 for more information on formulating clinical questions). If the question was foreground, the group would decide what type of question it was (e.g., treatment, diagnosis, harm, meaning) and construct it in the PICOT format. Then the group would access computers to search for relevant scientific evidence to answer their questions.

Alternatively, the leader could present a case to the group members, asking them to write down questions they generate during the presentation. Then the leader asks each member of the group to share the questions phrased in the PICOT format with their group. This sort of individual practice and skill building as a group is quite powerful as a teaching and learning method. All participants are working actively, not passively, to learn the concepts, and their peers in the group provide immediate feedback and "reality testing" for each individual.

Whether the learning is in a seminar or classroom, learning searching skills led by a medical librarian knowledgeable in EBP should include hands-on practice in searching for evidence to answer their own questions. This combines the principle of relevance to the learner with the evidence-based method of skill-building workshops and thereby fosters more active participation and learning.

For teaching critical appraisal skills, it is useful to work with three small groups, each group focusing on a specific appraisal criterion. (Chapters 4 to 7 have more information on critical appraisal of evidence.) For example, one small group would report back to the larger group on the results of the study. Another group would discuss the validity of the study, and the third group would discuss the applicability of the study findings to the given patient scenario. This process assists the learners to view the critical appraisal process as a coherent whole.

Incorporating small-group work in a classroom setting provides learners with more opportunities to discuss EBP content in a less threatening atmosphere. Small groups can be a successful forum to formulate PICOT questions from a provided clinical scenario, critically appraise studies, and report back to the class.

Journal Clubs. Another option for teaching EBP is the journal club. A journal club has many benefits, including improved critical appraisal skills (Lachance, 2014) and demonstrating a professional behavior to promote lifelong learning. Consider that a journal club is not a gathering of faculty or students to passively discuss topics. Rather, a journal club is an active group discussion in which all people involved participate. When establishing a journal club in an academic setting, to optimize attendance it is important to begin by being explicit about the purpose, who should participate, the timing, and the format. The participants can be those interested in learning and teaching EBP or students in a course. Although the leader of the group can rotate among the members, an educator–mentor knowledgeable in EBP is essential to validate the journal club's importance and to provide mentoring when the group needs her or his expertise to ask facilitating questions about each step of the EBP process.

The timing of a journal club should be amenable to participants' schedules. Scheduling journal clubs over the lunch hour may work well for some; others can attend those held in the early evening. Whatever the time, food and camaraderie are great incentives to increase attendance. Instituting a competitive journal club has been shown to increase attendance and participation in a pediatric hospital (McKeever, Kinney, Lima, & Newall, 2016). Box 16.7 contains the essential elements of a journal club, which were supported in systematic review of how to run an effective journal club (Deenadayalan, Grimmer-Somers, Prior, & Kumar, 2008).

Journal Club Teaching Formats: Grazing or Hunting. In journal clubs, determining which teaching format will work best for your participants is crucial. Consider first whether a "grazing" format or a "hunting" format would best meet learners' needs. The grazing format has been the most common to this point and typically begins with a group of individuals, such as faculty wanting to learn more about EBP or students postconference, dividing the relevant journals in their field among themselves. Each individual is then responsible for perusing— or grazing on—one to three journals for recent publications of interest to the group. At the small-group meeting, members of the group take turns presenting the information they have found to the rest of the group members.

BOX 16.7	*Characteristics of a Successful Journal Club*

- Regular and anticipated meetings
- Mandatory attendance
- Clarity of purpose
- Appropriate times to meet
- Incentives for meeting
- A leader to choose articles and lead the discussion
- Having articles circulated before the meeting
- Internet use for dissemination and storing data
- Applying established critical appraisal criteria
- Providing a summary of the club's findings

Unless it is a required component during clinical experiences for students, the grazing process has its inherent inefficiencies. First, in this format, the number of journals reviewed tends to be a function of the number of individuals in the group. Thus, the group is likely to leave several journals unreviewed and therefore miss evidence. Second, the group effect is further complicated by members' abilities to make it to the meetings. Third, there are many citations in given journals that are of poor quality. Wading through several journals looking for quality research evidence can be quite tedious. Fourth, the time required by the group members to accomplish the given goal tends to be quite high. In view of these inefficiencies of grazing, many members may relegate the small-group meeting to just another thing on their already full to-do lists.

Despite the inherent inefficiencies, grazing is still an essential activity in keeping up with the latest information. Fortunately, there are now secondary publications that do the grazing, cutting down the time it takes to find quality research evidence. The editorial boards of these resources systematically survey the existing literature. Any relevant studies that meet certain methodological criteria are abstracted in a quickly readable format. Examples of sources for predigested or preappraised evidence are the *Evidence-Based Nursing Journal, Evidence-Based Medicine Journal, Worldviews on Evidence-Based Nursing, American College of Physicians Journal Club, Clinical Evidence, POEMS,* and *American Academy of Pediatrics Grand Rounds.* Thus, grazing is very helpful in keeping current, especially when grazing in these greener pastures.

An alternative to grazing is a hunting format. This format begins with a clinical issue and the question of interest to the individual or group. A question is posed from a concern about a clinical issue. The question is then converted into a PICOT question, one that is answerable and searchable. A systematic search to find relevant research evidence is performed. Finally, any relevant studies are brought back to the group to critically appraise and discuss application to clinical decision making.

The hunting format has two distinct advantages. First, it is by definition relevant to the group because its own members posed the original question, rather than relying on whatever happened to be published since the last meeting. Second, it includes the question and search components of the EBP process, which are left out of the grazing format. The hunting format can easily be adapted for use in formal coursework. Simply assign group members the task of presenting the results of their question, search, and critical appraisal at the various meetings on a rotating basis.

It is important to make a distinct link between the applicable clinical scenario; the searchable, answerable search question; the systematic search findings; and the subsequent critical appraisal and application of research evidence to allow the group to see the process as a coherent whole. Otherwise, because so much time is spent in learning critical appraisal, learners can quickly equate EBP with only critical appraisal instead of seeing it as a comprehensive process.

MAKE EVIDENCE-BASED CLINICAL DECISIONS ACROSS LEVELS OF EDUCATION

Recognizing that learners across the continuum in healthcare education need varying approaches to teaching EBP is likely acknowledged by most faculty; however, guidance for how these approaches vary is lacking, particularly for graduate students. In a search in CINAHL using the focused and exploded subject headings of *professional practice, evidence-based* OR *nursing practice, evidence-based* combined with the focused subject heading *education, nursing baccalaureate* yielded 97 hits; *education, nursing master's* yielded 18 hits; *education, nursing doctorate* yielded 19 hits; *education, occupational therapy* yielded 38 hits; and *education, physical therapy* yielded 47 hits. A search in PubMed MeSH database using the advanced search for the terms *evidence-based practice* OR *evidence-based medicine* AND *medical education, undergraduate* yielded 173 hits, and *medical education, graduate* yielded 125 hits. There was no effort to review these yields for relevance; however, these results clearly indicate that we need more guidance on how to incorporate EBP into health professions' education. In an attempt to help in this area, Table 16.4 provides guidance about reasonable EBP expectations of students at the

TABLE 16.4	Leveled EBP Expectations Across Educational Levels
Educational Level	**EBP Expectations**
Undergraduate	• Competent use of EBP language • Competent in using PICOT format for asking clinical questions • Novice systematic searching skills • Novice knowledge of critical appraisal of research methods and findings • Novice skills in integrating evidence into practice while blending with clinical expertise and patient preferences • Novice skills in evaluation of clinical outcomes • Novice skills in dissemination of project findings
Master's	• Expert use of EBP language • Expert in using PICOT format for asking clinical questions • Expert systematic searching skills • Leads staff in critical appraisal of external evidence • Leads staff in internal evidence evaluation and integration with external evidence • Leads staff in integration of evidence into practice while blending with clinical expertise and patient preferences • Leads staff in evaluation of clinical outcomes • Actively disseminates project findings, including others in the process • Actively mentors/coaches staff in EBP
Clinical Doctorate	• Collaborates with interprofessional healthcare team • Leads healthcare team in use of EBP language • Leads healthcare team in using PICOT format for asking clinical questions • Leads healthcare team in systematic searching skills • Leads healthcare team in critical appraisal of external evidence • Leads healthcare team in internal evidence evaluation and integration with external evidence • Leads healthcare team in integration of evidence into practice while blending with clinical expertise and patient preferences to resolve organizational issues • Leads healthcare team in evaluation of organizational outcomes • Actively disseminates project findings, including others in the process • Actively mentors/coaches healthcare team in EBP • Integrate evidence with clinical expertise and organizational preferences.
Research Doctorates	• Competent in use of EBP language • Competent in using PICOT format for asking clinical questions • Expert systematic searching skills • Expert in critical appraisal of existing evidence • Expert in asking research questions from evidence appraisal • Expert in dissemination of research studies • Leads DNP/PhD collaboration to address clinical issues

EBP, evidence-based practice; PICOT, population, intervention or issue of interest, comparison, outcome, and time.

completion of undergraduate, master's, and clinical as well as research doctoral programs. Content and assignments would follow these expectations. There is a need for faculty to consider conducting research as they engage students in learning EBP across the educational continuum to help improve our understanding of what works best.

EDUCATORS AS EBP MENTORS/STUDENTS AS EBP MENTORS

The final champion for successfully teaching EBP is the EBP mentor, sometimes called a coach, information broker, or confidant (see Chapter 18). This individual's job is to provide one-on-one mentoring of educators, providing them with on-site assistance in problem solving about how to teach EBP. Mentoring has been a long-standing tradition in academia. It is important that these efforts are supported by administration, purposeful and focused, to maximize success. Faculty who believe in EBP and desire to teach students to be evidence-based clinicians may find that competing priorities within an academic environment must be overcome in order that they may provide the amount of guidance they would like to their fellow educators. An EBP mentor's primary focus in the academic setting is on improving the student's and faculty's understanding and integration of EBP in practice and educational paradigms. This is often accomplished by providing the right information at the right time that can assist not only the student to provide the best possible care to the patient but also the faculty to provide the best evidence-based education to the student. These mentorships need to be formal, paid positions with time dedicated for teaching EBP. Through mentored relationships, students and faculty have the opportunity to reflect on how well they are achieving their learning goals and advancing EBP.

EVALUATING SUCCESS IN TEACHING EVIDENCE-BASED PRACTICE

Evaluation of outcomes based on evidence is an essential step in the EBP process and in teaching EBP. Effective outcome evaluation of EBP teaching programs is as imperative as their existence. Evaluation involves an assessment of (a) learners, (b) educators/preceptors, (c) curricula, and (d) the program (Fineout-Overholt, 2013). Most instruments used to evaluate educational programs measure the self-efficacy of EBP skills, knowledge, behaviors, outcome expectation, and attitudes of the learners (Bernhardsson & Larsson, 2013; Chang & Crowe, 2011; Hart et al., 2008; Ireland et al., 2009; Shaneyfelt et al., 2006; Sherriff, Wallis, & Chaboyer, 2007; Varnell, Haas, Duke, & Hudson, 2008; Wallin, Bostrom, & Gustavsson, 2012). Shaneyfelt et al. conducted a systematic review evaluating EBP in education and found that a number of instruments were used to evaluate some dimension of EBP and could be used to evaluate individuals as well as educational programs. These studies did not measure the outcome of the impact EBP has on patient outcomes. A systematic review by Leung, Trevena, and Waters (2014) measured the psychometric properties of 24 instruments measuring EBP knowledge, skills, and attitudes; however, these were still not measured for the outcome of the impact of EBP on patient outcomes. In addition to evaluating how EBP is integrated into courses and curricula, a deliberate focus on evaluating how evidence-based teaching strategies and practices are used in courses is imperative. Kalb, O'Conner-Von, Brockway, Rierson, and Sendelbach (2015) reported that faculty strongly agreed it was important to use evidence in nursing education; however, some faculty were not aware that it was essential to use evidence in their teaching to promote learning outcomes. This provides support for incorporating the use of evidence-based teaching strategies and practices in faculty performance evaluation and student course evaluation criteria.

Evaluation of Learner Assimilation of EBP

The outcome of ARCC-E strategies is learner assimilation of the EBP paradigm. This means that learners' clinical decisions inherently include external evidence, internal evidence, their expertise, and patient preferences. The role of the health professions educator is to transfer the EBP paradigm to new healthcare providers as the basis of their practice. This ensures that the mantle of health professions will be thoughtfully handed down to clinicians who will uphold their profession with the honor, pride, commitment, dedication, and determination of their predecessors.

Learner Evaluation by Educational Level

Evaluating learners' integration of EBP concepts into their thinking, problem solving, and practice is not an easy task. However, several mechanisms are discussed that can assist in determining how well learners have integrated EBP concepts into their practices.

Classroom Learning. Depending on the educational delivery program (e.g., formal classroom, online, seminars), there are many options for evaluating the specific levels of the cognitive domain related to EBP concepts. Formal testing or specific EBP assignments can assist the learners to identify areas in the process that need remedial work. However, synthesis is a higher cognitive level, and synthesis papers or presentations seem to be a common option that educators use to determine the learner's ability to comprehend, synthesize, and apply EBP concepts and principles in formal educational settings and can be assigned as a group, individual, or combined assignment (see Box 16.8 for examples of synthesis assignment criteria).

In a systematic review of nine studies that explored which teaching format was best suited to teach EBP, three studies showed differences in learning outcomes based on format. The most effective teaching formats included didactic compared to problem-based learning; librarian presence compared to no librarian presence; and online learning plus work-based experience compared to work-based experience alone (Dragan & Maloney, 2014). The authors of the review noted that a limitation of the study was that all studies used different outcome measurement tools, and educational researchers should recognize this as a call to consider existing evidence and measurement when planning their studies. Furthermore, Kyriakoulis et al. (2016) conducted a systematic review of 20 studies to evaluate the effectiveness of a range of strategies for teaching EBP to undergraduate health professions students (e.g., workshops, journal clubs, online, lectures, with varying frequency and length) or a combination of strategies. The authors categorized the strategies into single or multifaceted interventions and found that seven studies reported higher EBP competence with multifaceted interventions.

Clinical Experiences. Traditionally, clinical experiences in nursing programs have used care plans, care maps, and logs to evaluate clinical knowledge and application. Alternate evaluation methods include the objective structure clinical examination (OSCE) and other simulated evaluations, such as a case study. The Fresno Test for evidence-based medicine (Ramos, Schafer, & Tracz, 2003) offers another objective evaluation method for determining how well clinicians assimilate EBP into their daily decisions. Another evaluative method, depending on the level of the student, is to have the learner find and critically appraise the scientific evidence to support a chosen intervention, then describe in an EBP application paper how this evidence influenced decision making, taking into consideration the clinical team's expertise and the patient's preferences and values.

| BOX 16.8 | *Examples of Synthesis Assignments* |

Combined Group and Individual Synthesis

- Learning Outcome: Find the best evidence to answer a clinical question through the search of existing healthcare databases and other sources of valid and reliable evidence: The purpose of this assignment is for students to enhance their skills in evidence synthesis and communication of best practice to the professional nursing community.
- Groups will be assigned a clinical scenario from which a PICOT question can be formulated that has a known body of evidence. **Each person in the group must have a specific part of the presentation to be responsible for, complete their part of the appraisal, create the slides and present the information during the presentation (see "Criteria for Creative PowerPoint Presentation" below).** Group evaluation will be a part of this process.

Criteria for Creative PowerPoint Presentation

- Clinical issue, background and significance; statistics that demonstrate there is a significant issue required
- PICOT question in PICOT format (appropriate template)
- Search strategy with resultant cohort of studies found, screenshots of search required
- Appraisal of evidence: evaluation and synthesis tables required (evaluation table may be as handout, but synthesis is required in the presentation)
- Applicability for practice and recommendations for evidence-based decision making
- American Psychiatric Association (APA) for citations and reference slide

Note: Each student is responsible for writing a three-page paper that reflects this project, using the criteria above. Screenshots of the group search will be included as a figure in the paper and will be in the appendix along with any other tables or figures students choose to use. The culminating paragraphs will be the conclusion from the evidence and recommendations for clinical practice change based on the evidence.
PICOT, population, intervention or issue of interest, comparison, outcome, and time.

In addition, a checklist to assist in evaluation of students' clinical skills can be helpful. Table 16.5 contains an EBP skills inventory that may be used to assess learners' self-perceived strengths and weaknesses with regard to the essential skills of EBP. Informal assessment has demonstrated that learners as well as educators have gained valuable perspectives from this self-assessment. Using this type of questionnaire, EBP educators can discover learners' comfort with learning to be an evidence-based practitioner. In addition, educators can discern the importance they attach to improving their EBP skills.

Making learning relevant is one of the most important strategies for developing learners' enthusiasm for and skill in practicing EBP. The examples, assignments, and concepts used in teaching must be based on real patients. In addition, applying the results of the process to learners' current or future practice helps to cement the concepts for them. In the academic setting, if students are given assignments that are not relevant to practice, all but the most highly motivated EBP students will perceive it as busy work and lose enthusiasm.

An effective reflection tool is the **educational prescription (EP)**. Though it was originally described by Sackett, Haynes, Guyatt, and Tugwell (1991) as a mechanism to teach people

TABLE 16.5	EBP Skills Inventory

To help your preceptor improve your skills in EBP, please indicate your experience by checking the appropriate box.

	No Experience	Some Experience	Much Experience
Asking answerable questions about my patients	☐	☐	☐
Performing efficient searches for evidence that answers my clinical questions	☐	☐	☐
Selecting the best evidence from what is found in the search	☐	☐	☐
Critically appraising the evidence	☐	☐	☐
Applying the evidence to my practice	☐	☐	☐

EBP, evidence-based practice.

how to "do" critical appraisal, it is easily applicable to clinical practica. The educator writes an EP for an early learner when a learner does not know the answer to a question that is pertinent to the evaluation or management of his or her patient. Given that the hope is that learners eventually start to identify their own knowledge deficits and write their own EPs, this tool can become an evaluation method for clinical postconference. Asking learners to report how the evidence they find will alter the management of their patients teaches them perspective. Fundamental to the successful use of EPs is educators' willingness to admit they do not know everything, write their own EPs, and present them to the learners, thereby modeling the desirable qualities of commitment to excellence in patient care, diligence, and perspective.

 More can be learned about traditional critical appraisal EPs from the toolbox on the website for the Centre for Evidence-Based Medicine: https://ebm-tools.knowledgetranslation.net/educational-prescription

A different use of the EPs is for learners to conduct a self-assessment of how they will approach learning about the EBP process, including reflecting on what they currently know, what they need to learn, and how they plan to learn the information. Initiating the learner EP (LEP) at the beginning of an educational term allows students to reflect on their upcoming learning and on their engagement and outcome of their learning at the end of the term. This approach also offers faculty an opportunity to evaluate their effectiveness in how well students performed in assignments across the term and their reflection journaling about the effectiveness of the LEP (i.e., how effective was their EP for what they needed to do to gain the knowledge they identified as lacking at the beginning of the term). Box 16.9 contains an example of the elements of an LEP.

> What is experienced and seen in the clinical area is what will likely predict future behavior.
>
> **BOB BERENSON**

Educator and Preceptor Evaluation

Preparing educators and preceptors for teaching EBP to learners is imperative. It is known that learners emulate what they see modeled in their preceptors and educators. Berenson (2002)

Example of an Learner Education Prescription (LEP): Beginning and End of the Term

LEP (beginning of term)

Student Name and Date

- My Assessment of where I am right now:
  - What do I know about EBP?
- What I have identified as what I need to know after reviewing the syllabus and course calendar: Write as measurable objectives (action verb and measurable outcome).
- What I have identified as specific actions that I believe will help me reach the goals previously mentioned.
- Explain briefly why you think this LEP will work for you.

Reflection and Evaluation (end of term; reflecting on the LEP above)

Student Name and Date

- My Reflection of where I am now at the end of the course compared to at the beginning:
  - What do I know now about basing practice change on evidence?
- My Reflection on the program course content or learning activities that were facilitators of my success in this course, please identify the course(s) and activities.
- My Reflection on what I identified as specific LEP actions at the beginning of or during this course to set myself up for successful engagement and learning within the course.
- What I believe helped me reach my goals, and what I experienced as barriers along my learning journey.
- EVALUATION: Explain briefly why you think this LEP worked for you. Describe how reflection on your learning influenced your success this semester and how it will inform your future role as a health professional.

© Fineout-Overholt, 2016.

made that point very clear when he articulated, in a discussion about healthcare professionals' education, that even if the benefits of EBP are clearly presented in a didactic venue, what is experienced and seen in the clinical area is what will likely predict future behavior.

Whether the educational program is nursing, physical therapy, or medicine, or the level of education is baccalaureate, graduate, or postgraduate, educators/preceptors should clarify the course objectives and expectations of the learning about EBP. Knowledge of EBP should be evident in the educators'/preceptors' clinical discussions with learners and should be central to the teaching–learning process. An example of a great opportunity for demonstrating the operation of the EBP process is preceptors asking advanced practice nurses questions about why a particular treatment option was chosen or a care trajectory decided. For instance, during the clinical experience of a student at a large southeast university, the healthcare team was discussing the appropriateness of the common practice of prescribing multiple tests for those who test negative for *Clostridium difficile*. One of the preceptors indicated that current evidence supports single assay testing and that routine use of multiple testing increases the likelihood that a false-positive test would occur (Bobo, Dubberke, & Kollef, 2011). Further discussion focused on the cost savings, avoidance of inappropriate treatment, and patient comfort by implementing current evidence. Another clinician in the group described how difficult it was for clinicians to accept the variation from traditional practice. A discussion ensued, in which the combined use of science, expertise, and patient concerns and choices to make the best clinical decision was reflected on. The role of uncertainty in clinical practice and the benefits of clinical inquiry were also discussed. Subsequently, the student was asked to design a project that would apply EBP principles to this clinical situation and evaluate the plan, including measurement of practice outcomes. This kind of preceptor interaction to foster the application of EBP principles in the clinical area is invaluable to the learner. Gerrish et al. (2011) found that advanced practice nurses who were committed to facilitating EBP in the clinical setting used a knowledge broker approach. These nurses facilitated EBP in clinical nurses through role modeling, teaching, clinical problem solving, and facilitating change. These principles and roles used are also the ones by which they would be evaluated. Evaluation forms delineating these principles can be prepared that students and preceptors complete to indicate the extent to which they perceive the principles were present in the learning experience.

An additional measure to evaluate educator/preceptor teaching is peer review. Course syllabi, teaching materials, lesson plans, or case studies, as well as peer observation of the educator/preceptor in the clinical or classroom setting can be one source of evaluation data to assess teaching effectiveness. Student evaluations of teaching can also assist the educator/preceptor to reflect on aspects of teaching that are helpful or can be improved to foster student learning. Establishing a peer review rubric assists with consistency of evaluation. There are many online sources of such rubrics. For example, Google results for *peer review rubric* elicited more than a dozen readily available peer review rubrics, ranging from paper rubrics to team work rubrics.

Curricula Evaluation

The design of the curriculum guides the content and activities that are implemented in a health professions educational program. Competence as an outcome must be clearly linked with the expected learner outcomes. EBP as the foundation of a curriculum should be sequenced logically, allowing for incremental learning of the depth and breadth of all essential content. One way to determine this is to develop a grid or matrix that identifies EBP program outcomes and course objectives reflecting Bloom's taxonomy (http://www.nwlink .com/~donclark/hrd/bloom.html). The EBP content, the learning activities that relate to the objectives, and the evaluative methods that measure the learner outcomes can be entered into the matrix to determine internal consistency and vertical organization. The curricular design should mirror the institution's mission and philosophy statements, which should actively reflect EBP. Specific courses can be reviewed to determine the internal consistency of course objectives, content, learning activities, and evaluative methods and their placement in the curriculum and how they reflect EBP knowledge, skills, and attitudes. In informal workshop or seminar formats, it is equally important to evaluate the objectives, content, learning activities, and outcomes to foster successful learning about EBP.

Program Evaluation

To evaluate the program, careful consideration of what to evaluate, when to evaluate, and whom to evaluate is imperative. Evaluating learners' ongoing absorption of EBP concepts throughout an educational program is integral to knowing the success of the program. However, other outcomes of the overall program that need to be examined include program goal(s) and environmental outcomes. Some of these outcomes may be evaluated on a continual basis (e.g., graduates' application of EBP in daily practice), and some may be a one-time assessment (e.g., number of attendees from different locations to measure scope of attendance).

Continual monitoring of the environment and outcomes (goals) is necessary for either teaching or implementing EBP. Periodically, the educator/preceptor champions of EBP need to determine where they are in reaching the goals of the EBP program. This first requires a commitment to setting measurable program goals that can be monitored on an ongoing basis. Evaluation of the program's foundation (environment) can be obtained by examining the questions raised in the first part of this chapter. If there are insufficient answers (e.g., educators' knowledge of up-to-date EBP concepts is lacking), the program has not been completely successful in that area. Steps would then be taken to address the areas that lack support (e.g., send the educators to an EBP conference or hold an EBP conference on the program site). The learners can provide feedback on the courses and learning experiences at the conclusion of the courses. This input can be analyzed and used to make decisions about the courses.

Program goals should address the subject of whether learners can formulate a searchable, answerable clinical question; efficiently find relevant evidence; discern what is best scientific evidence; and apply the best scientific evidence with clinical expertise and patient input to clinical decision making. Part of the Summit on Health Professions Education (Greiner & Knebel, 2003) competency regarding practicing using evidence stated that across and within disciplines, efforts must be focused on the development of a scientific evidence base. The final goal for a teaching program must be for learners to actively evaluate outcomes based on evidence.

In addition, the Summit recommended that funding sources such as the Agency for Healthcare Research and Quality (AHRQ) support ongoing clinical and education research that evaluates care based on the five specified competencies. An example of this type of research could be a study to evaluate educational outcomes for an EBP teaching program across two or more disciplines (e.g., nursing and medicine).

Final Assessment

There is usually some type of cumulative assessment for learners completing a degree program, such as comprehensive exams. However, not every discipline uses this form of outcome evaluation. National licensure and certifying exams may provide outcome evaluation for some disciplines and some levels of education. Whatever form of final assessment a teaching program in EBP employs (e.g., EBP implementation project; see Appendix I), it must address the EBP paradigm, particularly application and evaluation. These are the most challenging steps of the EBP process to evaluate. Without evaluating the EBP process in a final evaluation, educators cannot know whether learners are prepared to apply principles they have learned in their daily practices.

Program Effectiveness

The overall EBP program is effective if the learners are successful in integrating EBP concepts into their thinking and practice. Integration of EBP concepts into daily practice can be discerned by periodic follow-up with graduates to ask them about the integration of EBP in their practices. Although self-report has its drawbacks, querying what EBP initiatives learners have been involved in during the past 12 months can assist the educator in obtaining more objective information on how they have applied EBP knowledge to practice.

An example could be that EBP concepts and principles are integrated throughout the health professions major. Evaluation of the impact of EBP integration on students' EBP beliefs and implementation of concepts and principles would be planned and executed before the first introduction to EBP content. Foundational concepts for EBP should be introduced in the first semester while learning about the healthcare professions, with specific learning activities placed in specific courses in that semester. An introduction to the evaluation of research and its use in practice are the focus of the second semester. A foundational course focuses on the underpinnings of the EBP paradigm with at least two other courses providing the incremental learning. These courses would replace any traditional research generation course. As students progress in their learning, no further didactic information would be presented; however, building skills in critical appraisal and application of evidence to practice would be emphasized in all clinical settings. Competence in effecting change and improving outcomes through the integration and amalgamation of evidence, clinician expertise, and patient preference would be demonstrated through a culmination capstone project in the final semester of their healthcare education.

Box 16.10 contains tools to determine the impact of EBP in education by comparing total beliefs, implementation and organizational culture scores, as well as individual educator and student beliefs and implementation. Data from these assessments can provide information about the curriculum in terms of strengths and areas to focus EBP learning. A full assessment of the environment is imperative for moving forward.

To know if the change to evidence-based curricula was effective, the transition requires focused evaluation. This could be part of ongoing quality improvement of the EBP integration, during which students' beliefs about EBP and use of EBP principles were measured. Students who had a more traditional approach could be compared with those who used an EBP approach. Evaluating the impact of EBP programs on learners and healthcare providers' performance may involve various approaches, such as tests, papers, EPs, and self-report, to evaluate various outcomes (e.g., knowledge, attitude, and behaviors). In more formal academic settings, to facilitate ease of evaluation, a portfolio may be used to capture the integration of the EBP paradigm.

BOX
16.10 Tools to Determine the Impact of an EBP-Integrated Curriculum: Evaluating Evidence-Based Practice (EBP) in Education

- Evidence-Based Practice Beliefs for Educators scale (EBPB-E; Fineout-Overholt & Melnyk, 2010a)
- Evidence-Based Practice Beliefs for Students scale (EBPB-S; Fineout-Overholt & Melnyk, 2017)
- Evidence-Based Practice Implementation for Educators (EBPI-E; Fineout-Overholt & Melnyk, 2010b)
- Evidence-Based Practice Implementation for Students (EBPI-S; Fineout-Overholt & Melnyk, 2010c)
- Organizational Culture and Readiness for School-wide Integration of Evidence-based Practice for Educators (OCRSIEP-E; Fineout-Overholt & Melnyk, 2011)
- Organizational Culture and Readiness for School-wide Integration of Evidence-based Practice in Education for Students (OCRSIEP-ES; Fineout-Overholt & Melnyk 2011)

see Appendix J for samples

BARRIERS TO TEACHING/ENHANCING EBP IN ACADEMIC SETTINGS: LESSONS LEARNED

Reflection offers the opportunity to learn from our life's journey. Among the lessons learned about the structure and content of an EBP integration curriculum, five are noted here: ensure incremental learning, set clear deadlines, carefully assess skill levels, ensure education has meaning, and foster learning and growth.

First Lesson: Ensure Incremental Learning

Building knowledge and skills in EBP can be overwhelming. Teaching EBP to undergraduates with no or minimal clinical experience requires offering opportunities to learn the language of EBP, its principles, and the EBP paradigm over time and in small doses. Heavier doses may lead to discontent with learning and may be perceived as competitive versus complementary (i.e., foundational) to learning the clinical tasks associated with health professions. Furthermore, advanced learners will appreciate the opportunity to incrementally assimilate knowledge and skills into their practice as well.

Second Lesson: Set Clear Deadlines

Deadlines for any product of learning are crucial. Clinicians, both educators and learners, are very busy in a complex clinical setting. Because there are many distractions, it is important to be explicit about the goals and timeline of any assigned learning experience. Examples of this are a 2-day return on search results for a question generated by both educator and learner, assigning an EP on a question to be presented the next day on rounds or in report, and breaking up a large project into smaller ones with shorter deadlines (e.g., divide an EBP paper assignment into three stages due 1 month apart: question and search strategy, critical appraisal, and application of evidence). In short, it is important to keep the learning experience on the learner's radar screen within the context of the experience, workshop, seminar, or coursework.

Third Lesson: Carefully Assess Skill Levels

The third lesson learned is that learners begin an educational program with widely varied skills in informatics and EBP. Determining learners' skills prior to starting the teaching program is essential. Because becoming an evidence-based provider is a complex task, much like becoming a licensed practitioner, the program should be broken down into reasonable parts that learners can accomplish. It is important to meet learners where they are and to foster growth in knowledge and skills from that point. Any bar to reflect learner growth should be flexible enough to be angled upward or downward for a specific learner. This avoids the frustration that sets in when learners are overwhelmed with the material or process. Setting realistic expectations for each experience and providing formative feedback along the way in addition to summative information at the end of the experience will encourage learners' growth.

Fourth Lesson: Ensure Education Has Meaning

The fourth lesson learned is to make the content, settings, formats, and methods meaningful to learners. This shows learners firsthand that EBP is applicable and useful to them in their particular practice setting. Use relevant examples and scenarios. This is best accomplished by beginning the process with a question generated by the learner. It is incredibly powerful to learn the EBP process by working through a clinical issue that the learner actually cares about and that the learner can imagine herself or himself using in the future. One teaching–learning experience that can assist students to synthesize the EBP process and make it relevant is developing a shared partnership between academia and clinical agency where students would engage in best practice and improve patient outcomes in real time (Odell & Barta, 2011).

Fifth Lesson: Foster Learning and Growth

The fifth lesson learned is to foster learning and growth in those you teach, with the goal that they, in turn, will share their EBP knowledge with their colleagues. Focusing on getting a particular grade or checking off a required assignment will not produce lifelong learners who will improve outcomes. Learners who do not readily understand PICOT questions, patient preferences, effect size, or intention-to-treat will improve their knowledge and comfort with the subject matter if they experience mentored learning. According to Thomas, Saroyan, and Dauphinee (2011), a cognitive apprenticeship approach can provide students with opportunities to learn EBP from clinicians and faculty.

WHAT'S ON THE HORIZON FOR TEACHING EBP IN ACADEMIC SETTINGS

A challenge to teaching EBP remains having faculty and students who understand and embrace that EBP is about advancing the practice of evidence in patient care as opposed to teaching to the "project" and improving organizational metrics (e.g., when you go back to school, be sure you solve this problem). Students learning the EBP process are consumed with the how-tos to complete required assignments for courses. Guest speakers frequently speak to students about the EBP projects that have been implemented in their clinical agencies as opposed to what paradigm underpins patient care at their organization, and it is patient-centered. Discovering the best strategies that promote clinicians' ownership of the EBP process as a clinical decision making approach at the point of care is key to the faculty role in teaching EBP. Taylor, Priefer, and Alt-White (2016) referred to integration of EBP as an underdeveloped, though integral concept to teaching EBP. Studies have focused on healthcare professionals' knowledge, skills, and attitudes of EBP with little attention to how healthcare professionals carry out clinical decisions based on patient preferences and clinician expertise. Because each patient encounter is different, and not all patients will be accepting of the evidence, amalgamating the evidence, patient preferences, and the clinician's expertise is critical (Fineout-Overholt, Stillwell, Williamson, Cox, & Robbins, 2015). Perhaps next steps include incorporating patient–provider clinical decision simulation and OSCEs in healthcare provider curricula to evaluate student assimilation of the EBP paradigm and process (Taylor et al., 2016). These evaluative mechanisms may help in identifying champions and those who need further help to become the evidence-based clinicians needed for 21st-century healthcare.

As faculty consider how to embrace the upcoming challenges for teaching EBP, they must consider how expectations for learning and assimilation are leveled by degree. Exemplars offer insights as to how to proceed, so the next section contains leveled exemplars across degree programs.

EXEMPLARS OF TEACHING EVIDENCE-BASED PRACTICE IN ACADEMIC SETTINGS

Degree programs need to integrate EBP so that knowledge and skills are built upon throughout the program. The leveling of EBP courses throughout the program focuses on building an understanding of the EBP paradigm and principles of critical appraisal and theory in the first few semesters while students are gaining expertise in clinical specialty. This sequencing enables learners to incrementally engage the EBP paradigm as they integrate it into their practices. Capstone experience, whether in undergraduate or graduate programs, offers a wonderful opportunity for students to bring to culmination what they have learned in courses across the curriculum. Furthermore, across courses within the curriculum, faculty could integrate building blocks for their capstone project, thus enabling students to avoid the need to complete the entire project in one semester. For example, students could complete a synthesis of a body of evidence to answer a clinical question in their first or second semester (e.g., graduate: exhaustive; undergraduate: guided). As they engage in clinical experiences, they can work with clinicians to build a plan for implementing that evidence and determining outcomes to demonstrate the impact of the evidence. As a culmination of their learning, within their capstone course students can engage evidence implementation and outcome evaluation. Finally, learners can reflect on their projects and their impact on local organizations with whom they partnered and choose a method of dissemination that matches their project. As faculty plan for incremental learning, it would be important for a clinical component to be planned, outlining specific EBP milestones that assist learners with benchmarking where they are in the process and evaluating their progress. Boxes 16.11 and 16.12 contain some suggested educational evaluation methods that help health professions students assimilate EBP concepts as they learn their craft.

BOX 16.11 *Example of Outcomes Management Project Assignment Criteria*

- Background and significance of project are clear. (Support that there is insufficient evidence to answer the clinical question.)
- Clinically meaningful question is clear. (Use PICOT to identify question components.)
- Sources and process for identifying outcomes for project are clear. (The outcomes flow from the question. All possible outcomes are considered and addressed to answer the question.)
- Sources and process for collecting data are clear. (How approval was obtained, collection tool, who is collecting data, and from whom or what.)
- Data analysis approach assists in answering the clinical question. (Was the right statistical test for the level of data collected?)
- Proposed presentation of data is clear. (Graphs are readable on slide/handout. All data are synthesized and presented to audience in written form, slide/handout.)
- Implications for practice changes based on the data are clear. (What the data indicate that needs to be different in practice.)
- Plan for change is clear. (Specific steps for change.)
- Anticipated barriers, facilitators, and challenges to plan are clear.
- Outcomes for evaluation of plan are clear and measurable.
- Dissemination plan is clear and feasible. (What is going to be done with the information gathered in the project?)
- PowerPoint presentation and supporting documents enhance presentation.
- Overall argument is compelling and worthy of change in practice.

PICOT, population, intervention or issue of interest, comparison, outcome, and time.

Example of Requirements for an Evidence-Based Implementation Project

Purpose

This small-group project (two people per group) has been designed to assist students in searching for the best evidence and appraising it so that scholarly, up-to-date care for patients can be provided.

Instructions

1. Identify a clinical question of interest from a patient you have cared for in your clinical experiences. Topics must be preapproved by the course faculty.
2. Briefly describe the background to the problem, its clinical significance, and how you searched for the best evidence to answer your question.
3. Present the best evidence to answer this clinical question.
4. Critically appraise the evidence.
5. Discuss implications for practice and future research.
6. Include a glossary of all research terms used in your paper.
7. All studies appraised must accompany paper submission (paper must be in hard and disk copy).

Academic Teaching EBP Exemplar: Undergraduate

The purpose of EBP in the baccalaureate program is to introduce the concepts of EBP early in the program and thread it into courses so students learn to use the process and it becomes part of the decision making process they use to provide evidence-based care. Integrating EBP throughout the curriculum provides students and faculty with the opportunity to share research findings and learn the process for using the best evidence to inform practice (such as finding evidence to support interventions on a care plan). Building a foundation that allows for a culture of inquiry, the use of research, and the opportunity to appraise evidence, leads to preparing students that understand the steps of the EBP process. Engaging students in the exploration of the EBP process will help them to be active team members to assist in the translation of the best evidence into practice.

The AACN Baccalaureate Essentials (2008) II identifies that Bachelor of Science in Nursing (BSN) students should learn how to identify a practice issue, appraise and integrate the evidence, and evaluate outcomes. Integrating the EBP process into all courses in the BSN curriculum enables students to build competencies in EBDM.

Core Courses

Interprofessional Practice Course. Students learn the role of research in interprofessional practice decision making. In this course, students learn how to evaluate the research process for quality indicators and apply valid research findings to practice issues. The key assignment is an online PowerPoint presentation on a selected practice problem in which students share the PICOT question, search process, and the recommendation from the evaluation and synthesis of the evidence appraised. The recommendation includes an explanation of whether there is enough evidence to warrant a practice change or a need for further research to build a body of evidence to guide practice.

Introduction to Nursing Course. To build the student knowledge about research and scholarly activity, students interview a nurse scholar and examine their program of scholarship. Through a search of the nurse scholar, students learn searching techniques, reading research articles authored by the nurse scholar, and professional organizations that they may be involved in. Once they investigate the nurse scholar and read the articles, they connect to interview the person. During the interview, they learn about the nurse scholar's interest, career goals, and advice on beginning a nursing career. On completion of the interview, students write a paper based on the interview questions and reflect on the contribution that this person has made to the nursing profession and/or society.

Nursing Leadership Course. In a leadership course, students learn the management of nursing care, healthcare delivery, and strategies of implementing change. A common objective in this type of course is to utilize problem-solving and decision making processes. This helps develop the students' ability to use critical thinking skills, apply their knowledge, and work in an interdisciplinary fashion to accomplish improvements in care. Assignments include working on PICOT questions, locating the evidence, and sharing the results in order to contribute to safe, quality patient care.

EBP Course. Build competency with the EBP process to understand the steps of the evidence-based practice process and identify various EBP models to translate evidence into practice. This course could focus on enhancing the student's ability to read, comprehend, critically appraise, and apply the best evidence to practice. Assignment could include interviewing various groups of people (such as nurses, physical therapists, medical doctors, patients, social workers, nurse managers) in practice to determine the significance of nursing research and EBP. Once the interviews are complete, the student writes a paper comparing and contrasting the responses to the questions asked. They then reflect on their responses, and with the support of references they defend or debate the responses to the questions and their reflection.

Ideas for Integration Across the Curriculum

By integrating EBP into undergraduate clinical and simulation experiences, students are offered the opportunity to assimilate the EBP competencies into their practice. Simulation is essential to the development of critical thinking and to the development of clinical skills in a supporting environment. Faculty are key to creating such an environment in which students are encouraged to ask questions about practice decisions made during simulation experiences. Incorporating evidence as the basis for pre- and post-debriefing sessions models further supports how it underpins decision making. Clinical examples of how EBP can be integrated across courses could be through the care planning process or observation of care provided during their time on a clinical unit. Students can create PICOT questions based on a clinical issue that they observed during a clinical rotation or as it relates to the patient care they provided. As they create the care plan for the patient, they can include the evidence that supports the care they provided or locate evidence to support a change in practice.

Academic Teaching EBP Exemplar: Master's Degree

Master's education provides the foundation for healthcare professionals to transform healthcare. Given the rapid and uncertain change in healthcare, master's-prepared healthcare providers are well positioned to advance healthcare practices and bring about change based on evidence. According to the American Association of Colleges of Nursing (AACN, 2011), the expected role of master's-prepared nurses is to translate evidence into practice and lead change to improve patient, provider, and healthcare systems outcomes. This preparation requires an understanding of how to evaluate the usefulness of research, quality improvement methods, and evidence-based implementation strategies along with opportunities to fuse the knowledge, processes, and skills into the health provider role.

To enable master's-prepared clinicians to translate evidence into practice, core courses are vital for creating a robust knowledge base to establish, advance, and sustain an evidence-based approach to healthcare delivery.

Core Courses

Quality Improvement, Evidence-based Practice, and Research Course. This foundational course explores the similarities and differences among quality improvement, evidence-based practice, and research. The purpose, components, and tools for each of the three processes are examined, compared, and exemplified in the context of healthcare.

Key assignments include: (a) Interview a researcher, quality improvement coordinator, and evidence-based practice mentor/educator about their role, responsibilities, and accomplishments. Search the literature for articles describing these three roles, and (b) Compare and contrast the individuals' responses with the descriptions in the literature. Create position descriptions for each role that delineate their varying responsibilities.

Interpreting Statistics for Evidence-Based Practice Course. This course examines the role of statistics in the translation of research into practice. Interpreting statistics is emphasized, and determining the reliability of results for applying evidence in practice is underscored.

Key assignments: (a) Select a clinical unit that admits a specific population. Your staff want to learn more about the individuals and families to whom they provide care. What data would you collect, and how would you present the data to your staff. Include an informational sheet that explains the statistic(s); (b) Create a chart comparing characteristics of and reasons why the following study designs would be appropriate: randomized controlled trial, cohort study, meta-analysis, and case-control study; and (c) Appraise a randomized control trial using Melnyk and Fineout-Overholt Rapid Critical Appraisal checklist or Joanna Briggs Critical Appraisal checklist. Create a one-page synopsis of the study. Interpret the results addressing the statistic(s) used and the definition of the statistic, and discuss the appropriateness of the statistic(s) and what the statistic(s) mean.

Evidence for Clinical Decision Making Course. EBP process is the focus of this course. The EBP steps are applied with an emphasis on appraising, evaluating, and synthesizing evidence for clinical decision making. Influencing positive patient, provider, and systems outcomes through leadership is proposed.

Key assignments include: (a) Identify a PICOT question, search the databases for three studies to answer the question; (b) Appraise the validity, reliability, and applicability of the three studies. Create an evaluation table extracting key elements from the studies. Construct a synthesis table to include population, intervention, and outcomes of the three studies. Based on the synthesis of the evidence, what recommendation would you make? Defend your decision; and (c) Select a protocol or policy from your agency. Search databases for evidence to support the protocol or policy. Update the protocol/policy.

Ideas for Integration Across the Curriculum

Integration across master's courses is imperative so that students have an integrated approach to learning how to lead in EBDM. Clinical, education, administration, leadership courses can easily incorporate an evidence requirement to substantiate practice choices into their assignments. Using synthesized knowledge from the body of evidence to implement and evaluate a practice change is a must for master's-level learners.

Academic Teaching EBP Exemplar: Clinical Doctorate

The clinical doctorate is the pinnacle of clinician preparation. Nursing, medicine, pharmacy, and other professions have clinical doctorates that prepare expert leaders for the healthcare team. The role of the clinical doctorate is leading healthcare delivery change to ensure excellence in outcome—patient, provider, and systems. The curricular programs that prepare these leaders must include a heavy emphasis on translation of evidence into practice through the assimilation of the EBP paradigm and acquiring expert skills in the use of the EBP process.

Core Courses

Doctorally Prepared Clinical Expert Role. This course prepares the master's-educated clinician to assimilate the doctorally prepared expert role. Offers opportunity for transitioning their thinking thinking to leadership, excellence, and expert EBDM. Students focus on the EBP paradigm as the decisions making framework for doctorally prepared clinical experts.

Guiding Systems Change Through EBP. This course focuses on providing opportunities for students to engage the EBP process by defining clinical issues and using evidence to determine what is best practice. The course is accompanied by clinical hours in which the clinical doctorate student implements system-wide change.

Evidence-Based Quality Improvement. This course focuses on the role of the data in decision making, from staff to organization. Sources of data, evaluation and analysis of data, and subsequent decisions based on the analysis results are engaged by the student. Emphasis is laid on moving from data to solutions.

Sustainable Policy for Healthcare Outcomes. This course focuses on the results of the EBP process and accompanying translation of evidence into practice, which is sustainable change. Mechanisms for ensuring sustainability are discussed, including social media and outcome delivery methods within organizations, such as dashboards. Systems theory guides discussion within this course, and students become well-versed in negotiation and communication.

Ideas for Integration Across the Curriculum

Understanding EBP and using the process is the focus of a clinical doctorate as it applies to the discipline. All courses should be integrated so that the clinician becomes owner of the expert knowledge about a clinical issue and applies that knowledge to a population to improve outcomes that are currently known to be subpar. All clinical skills and knowledge are interpreted through the EBP paradigm. Growth in clinical expertise is framed as essential to decision making with patients to achieve their best outcomes.

Academic Teaching EBP Exemplar: Research Doctorate

The research doctorate is focused on preparing scientists who provide sound, reliable information to guide clinical practice through rigorous research methodology. Interprofessional and intraprofessional collaboration is an imperative to meet 21st-century healthcare goals. Research doctorate students must understand generation of research and how research is translated. Research doctorates are the only degree programs in which integration of EBP across the curriculum is not required.

Core Course

Evidence Synthesis and Translation. This course is focused on students gaining knowledge and skills in evidence synthesis for the purpose of identifying gaps in methodology to best frame the scientists' work. This provides context for how the scientists' work fits within what we currently know about clinical issues. The second half of the course focuses on how the scientists' work will be translated into practice. Strategies for writing for clinicians are emphasized, including guidance for understanding statistical results and tips for translation. Scientists write an evidence synthesis and a plan for translation of their work in this course.

Academic Teaching EBP Exemplar: Postdoctoral Residency

Postdoctoral residency is quite common in some clinical doctorates and less common in others. The purpose of a postdoctoral residency is not engaging formal courses, but to experientially actualize the potential of learners as they actively contribute to daily EBDM.

This exemplar features the University of Rochester Internal Medicine, Pediatrics, and Medicine-Pediatrics residency experience. The postdoctoral residency offers a variety of teaching–learning methods in both clinical *practicum* and academic *courses* as part of residents' learning experiences (e.g., morning report, journal club, ambulatory conferences, skills blocks, and an EBP elective). During morning report, participants are required to present an EP once every month as they rotate among different patient units. The clinical questions are to be drawn from their practice experiences, with the search, critical appraisal, and application discussed among the group. This 1-hour teaching conference usually consists of two cases being presented and discussed, each for half an hour. Once per week, an EP is presented and discussed instead of a case. The group in attendance (including a seasoned mentor) gives immediate feedback to the resident.

Journal club meets once per week. During this noon conference, a hunting format is used, and the group is divided into smaller groups, each with the task of analyzing one aspect of a systematic review or study and presenting back to the large group. Skills blocks are specific 2-week rotations set aside for nonclinical, classroom learning of clinical concepts, with a large portion of these sessions being devoted to the teaching of EBP concepts. These skill block minicourses are quite successful in bringing beginners to a common place of facility with EBP. Table 16.6 illustrates a workable skill block minicourse schedule.

TABLE 16.6	*Example of Workable Skill Block Minicourse Schedule*
Session	**Topic**
1. 3 hours	Introduction of principles of evidence-based practice (large group)
	Session on asking answerable questions (large group)
	Break into small groups of 8–10 and select project topics
2. 2 hours (large group)	Search tutorial by medical librarian
3. 1 hour (small groups)	Critically appraise and discuss an article on therapy—preselected article
4. 1 hour (small groups)	Critically appraise and discuss an overview (meta-analysis). This overview optimally contains the article on therapy from the previous session
5. 1 hour (small groups)	Critically appraise and discuss an article on diagnostic testing—preselected article
6. 1 hour (small groups)	Critically appraise and discuss an article on prognosis—preselected article
7. 2 hours	Small group—participants present their project (educational prescription)
	Large group—wrap up and answer any overall questions

For the more advanced learner, an EBP elective is offered. This is a 2-week course that consists of two 2-hour sessions daily. Attendance is limited to 8 to 10 participants for optimizing individual participation. In an introductory session where individual and group goals are set, learning needs are identified. Following the introductory session are a session on asking an answerable and searchable question; a search tutorial with a medical librarian; and sessions on the critical appraisal and application of articles of therapy, diagnosis, prognosis, overview, and harm using preselected articles. The remainder of the elective is left open for the group to decide what to present and discuss. Individuals are required to take turns leading these open sessions, teaching the group something they did not know beforehand. This program is designed to address the three ingredients of optimal adult learning:

1. A pretest that reveals a knowledge deficit
2. A learning phase to fill the knowledge deficit
3. A posttest where the learner presents what she or he has learned

To conclude the elective, group members individually present a project of their choosing, ranging from an appraisal of related single studies to formulating a complete EP.

CHARGE TO HEALTH PROFESSIONS EDUCATORS

Health professions educators are the key to a strong workforce in the future. We have the distinct opportunity to prepare those clinicians who will care for us and our loved ones. Although there are many considerations when planning to integrate EBP into a curriculum, it is keeping this outcome in mind that can help us be successful. The ARCC-E framework provides guidance for the critical elements that will foster learners' integration of EBP into their practices. Techniques and interventions abound here and elsewhere, and, in addition, educators will have ideas of their own for how to address the mandate of evidence-based education. The key is for educators to move, not stand still. Be brave—know that you will not always do things perfectly, and you may get results you didn't desire; however, that is an opportunity to put your knowledge to the test and replan so that the next time your results are different—then share what you have discovered about what worked and what did not. Above all else, as educators and learners alike embrace integration of EBP into current healthcare professions' curricula, we would do well to keep in mind and share with our students the perspective of Dr. Charles Swindoll, a noted theologian:

Words can never adequately convey the incredible impact of attitude toward life [integration of EBP]. The longer I live the more convinced I become that life is 10% what happens to us and 90% how we respond to it. I believe the single most significant decision I can make on a day-to-day basis is my choice of attitude. It is more than my past, my education, my bankroll, my successes or failures, fame or pain, what other people think of me or say about me, my circumstances, or my position. Attitude keeps me going or cripples my progress. It alone fuels my fire or assaults my hope. When my attitudes are right, there's no barrier too high, no valley too deep, no dream too extreme, no challenge too great for me.

CHARLES S. SWINDOLL—ELLEN PURSUING PERMISSION

EBP FAST FACTS

- A systematic approach is necessary to teaching EBP in academic settings (e.g., using the ARCC-E framework).
- Offering plenty of step-by-step learning opportunities facilitates learning EBP incrementally.
- Teaching EBP requires a leveled approach across educational degrees.
- Reflection, ongoing evaluation, and data-driven improvements are essential elements of teaching EBP in academic settings.
- Never give up!

WANT TO KNOW MORE?

A variety of resources are available to enhance your learning and understanding of this chapter.

- Visit thePoint˚ to access:
  - Articles from the AJN EBP Step-By-Step Series
  - Journal articles
  - Checklists for rapid critical appraisal
  - Sample for instruments to evaluate integration of EBP into curricula and more!
- Lippincott **CoursePoint** combines digital text content with video case studies and interactive modules for a fully integrated course solution that works the way you study and learn.

References

Ahmadi, S., Baradaran, H., & Ahmadi, E. (2015). Effectiveness of teaching evidence-based medicine to undergraduate medical students: A BEME systematic review. *Medical Teacher, 37*(1), 21–30.

American Association of Colleges of Nursing. (2000). Distance technology in nursing education: Assessing a new frontier. AACN white paper. *Journal of Professional Nursing, 16*(2), 116–122.

American Association of Colleges of Nursing. (2006). *The essentials of doctoral education for advanced nursing practice.* Retrieved from http://www.aacnnursing.org/DNP/DNP-Essentials

American Association of Colleges of Nursing. (2008). *The essentials of baccalaureate education for professional nursing practice.* Retrieved from http://www.aacnnursing.org/Portals/42/Publications/BaccEssentials08.pdf

American Association of Colleges of Nursing. (2011). *The essentials of master's education in nursing.* Retrieved from http://www.aacnnursing.org/Portals/42/Publications/MastersEssentials11.pdf

American Medical Informatics Association. (2013). *AMIA 10X10 programs.* Retrieved from http://www.amia.org/education/10x10-courses

American Nurses Credentialing Center. (2014). *ANCC Magnet Recognition Program.* Retrieved from https://www.nursingworld.org/organizational-programs/magnet/

Association of American Medical Colleges. (2007). *Advancing educators and education: Defining the components and evidence of educational scholarship.* Retrieved from https://members.aamc.org/eweb/upload/Advancing%20Educators%20and%20Education.pdf

Berenson, B. (2002). *Crossing the quality chasm: Next steps for health professions education. Major stakeholders comment on key strategies and action plans.* Retrieved from https://www.med.unc.edu/cmep.html/about/quality/documents/crossing-the-quality-chasm

Bergmann, J., & Sams, A. (2012). *Flip your classroom: Reach every student in every class, every day.* Eugene, OR: International Society for Technology in Education (ISTE).

Bernhardsson, S., & Larsson, M. E. (2013). Measuring evidence-based practice in physical therapy: Translation, adaptation, further development, validation, and reliability test of a questionnaire. *Physical Therapy, 93*(6), 819–832.

Bobo, L., Dubberke, E., & Kollef, M. (2011). *Clostridium difficile* in the ICU: The struggle continues. *Chest, 140*(6), 1643–1653.

Centers for Medicare and Medicaid Services. (2014). *Quarterly provider updates*. Retrieved from http://www.cms.gov/Regulations-and-Guidance/Regulations-and-Policies/QuarterlyProviderUpdates/index.html

Chang, A., & Crowe, L. (2011). Validation of scales measuring self-efficacy and outcome expectancy in evidence-based practice. *Worldviews on Evidence-Based Nursing, 8*(2), 106–115.

Coomarasamy, A., & Khan, K. (2004). What is the evidence that postgraduate teaching in evidence-based medicine changes anything? A systematic review. *British Medical Journal, 329*, 1017–1022.

Deenadayalan, Y., Grimmer-Somers, K., Prior, M., & Kumar, S. (2008). How to run an effective journal club: A systematic review. *Journal of Evaluating Clinical Practice, 14*(5), 898–911.

Dorsch, J. L., & Perry, G. (2012). Evidence-based medicines at the intersection of research interests between academic health science librarians and medical educators: A review of the literature. *Journal of Medical Library Association, 100*(4), 251–257.

Dragan, I., & Maloney, S. (2014). Methods of teaching medical trainees evidence-based medicine: A systematic review. *Medical Education, 48*, 124–135.

Duck, J. D. (2002). *The change monster: The human forces that fuel or foil corporate transformation and change*. New York, NY: Crown Business.

Ebell, M. H. (2009). How to find answers to clinical questions. *American Family Physician, 79*(4), 293–296.

Edwards, R., White, M., Gray, J., & Fischbacher, C. (2001). Use of a journal club and letter writing exercise to teach critical appraisal to medical undergraduates. *Medical Education, 35*, 691–694.

Felicilda-Reynaldo, R. D., & Utley, R. (2015). Reflections of evidence-based practice in nurse educators' teaching philosophy statements. *Nursing Education Perspectives, 36*(2), 89–95.

Fineout-Overholt, E. (2013). Outcome evaluation for programs teaching EBP. In R. F. Levin & H. R. Feldman (Eds.), *Teaching evidence-based practice in nursing* (2nd ed., pp. 205–224). New York, NY: Springer.

Fineout-Overholt, E. (2015). Getting best outcomes: Paradigm and process matter. *Worldviews on Evidence-Based Nursing, 12*(4), 183–186.

Fineout-Overholt, E., & Johnston, L. (2005). Teaching EBP: A challenge for educators in the 21st century. *Worldviews on Evidence-Based Nursing, 2*(1), 37–39.

Fineout-Overholt, E., & Johnston, L. (2007). Evaluation: An essential step to the EBP process. *Worldviews on Evidence-Based Nursing, 4*(1), 54–59.

Fineout-Overholt, E., & Melnyk, B. M. (2005). Building a culture of best practice. *Nurse Leader, 3*(6), 26–30.

Fineout-Overholt, E., & Melnyk, B. M. (2010a). *Evidence-based practice beliefs for educators*. Gilbert, AZ: ARCC Publishing.

Fineout-Overholt, E., & Melnyk, B. M. (2010b). *Evidence-based practice beliefs for students*. Gilbert, AZ: ARCC Publishing.

Fineout-Overholt, E., & Melnyk, B. M. (2010c). *Evidence-based practice implementation for students*. Gilbert, AZ: ARCC Publishing.

Fineout-Overholt, E., & Melnyk, B. M. (2011). ARCC evidence-based practice mentors: The key to sustaining evidence-based practice. In *Evidence-based practice in nursing and healthcare: A guide to best practice* (2nd ed., pp. 344–352). Philadelphia, PA: Lippincott, Williams & Wilkins.

Fineout-Overholt, E., & Melnyk, B. M. (2011). *Organizational culture and readiness for school-wide integration of evidence-based practice for educators*. Marshall, TX: ARCC Publishing.

Fineout-Overholt, E., & Melnyk, B. M. (2011). *Organizational culture and readiness for school-wide integration of evidence-based practice for students*. Marshall, TX: ARCC Publishing.

Fineout-Overholt, E., & Melnyk, B. M. (2017). *Evidence-based practice beliefs for students*. Hallsville, TX: ARCC Publishing.

Fineout-Overholt, E., Melnyk, B. M., Stillwell, S. B., & Williamson, K. M. (2010a). Evidence-based practice step by step: Critical appraisal of the evidence: part I. *American Journal of Nursing, 110*(7), 47–52.

Fineout-Overholt, E., Melnyk, B. M., Stillwell, S. B., & Williamson, K. M. (2010b). Evidence-based practice, step by step: Critical appraisal of the evidence: part II. *American Journal of Nursing, 110*(9), 41–48.

Fineout-Overholt, E., Melnyk, B. M., Stillwell, S. B., & Williamson, K. M. (2010c). Evidence-based practice, step by step: Critical appraisal of the evidence: part III. *American Journal of Nursing, 110*(11), 43–51.

Fineout-Overholt, E., Melnyk, B. M., Stillwell, S. B., & Williamson, K. M. (2010–2012). *EBP Step-by-Step Series*. Retrieved from the American Journal of Nursing Collections: http://journals.lww.com/ajnonline/pages/collectiondetails.aspx?TopicalCollectionId=10

Fineout-Overholt, E., Stillwell, S. B., Williamson, K. M., Cox, J. F., & Robbins, B. W. (2015). Teaching evidence-based practice in academic settings. In B. M. Melnyk & E. Fineout-Overholt (Eds.), *Evidence-based practice in nursing and healthcare: A guide to best practice* (3rd ed., pp. 330–362). Philadelphia, PA: Lippincott, Williams & Wilkins.

Gerrish, K., McDonnell, A., Nolan, M., Guillaume, L., Kirshbaum, M., & Tod, A. (2011). The role of advanced practice nurses in knowledge brokering as a means of promoting evidence-based practice among clinical nurses. *Journal of Advanced Nursing, 67*(9), 2004–2014.

Greiner, A., & Knebel, E. (Eds.). (2003). *Health professions education: A bridge to quality*. Washington, DC: National Academy Press.

Hart, P., Eato, L., Buckner, M., Morrow, B., Barrett, D., Fraser, D., . . . Sharrer, R. L. (2008). Effectiveness of a computer-based educational program on nurses' knowledge, attitude, and skill level related to evidence-based practice. *Worldviews on Evidence-Based Nursing, 5*(2), 75–84.

Hartzell, T., & Fineout-Overholt, E. (2017). The evidence-based practice competencies related to searching for best evidence. In Melnyk, Gallagher-Ford, & Fineout-Overholt, *Implementing the EBP competencies in health-care: A practice guide for improving quality, safety & outcomes* (pp. 55–76). Indianapolis, IN: Sigma Theta Tau International.

Hinton-Walker, P. (2010). The TIGER initiative: A call to accept and pass the baton. *Nursing Economics, 28*(5), 352–355.

Ilic, D., Hart, W., Fiddes, P., Misso, M., Villanueva, E. (2013). Adopting a blended learning approach to teaching evidence based medicine: a mixed methods study. *BMC Medical Education, 13*, 169.

Ilic, D., & Maloney, S. (2014). Methods of teaching medical trainees evidence-based medicine: A systematic review. *Medical Education, 48*(2), 124–135.

Ilic, D., Tepper, K., & Misso, M. (2012). Teaching evidence-based medicine literature searching skills to medical students during the clinical years: A randomized controlled trial. *Journal of the Medical Library Association, 100*(3), 190–196.

Institute of Medicine. (1999). *To err is human: Building a safe health system*. Washington, DC: National Academy Press.

Institute of Medicine. (2001). *Crossing the quality chasm: A new health system for the 21st century*. Washington, DC: National Academy Press.

Institute of Medicine. (2002). *Educating health professionals to use informatics*. Washington, DC: National Academy Press.

Ireland, J., Martindale, S., Johnson, N., Adams, D., Eboh, W., & Mowatt, E. (2009). Blended learning in education: Effects on knowledge and attitude. *British Journal of Nursing, 18*(2), 124–130.

Johnston, B., Coole, C., Feakes, R., Whitworth, G., Tyrell, T., Hardy, B. (2016). Exploring the barriers to and facilitators of implementing research into practice. *British Journal of Community Nursing, 21*(8), 392–398.

Johnston, L., & Fineout-Overholt, E. (2005). Teaching EBP: "Getting from zero to one." Moving from recognizing and admitting uncertainties to asking searchable, answerable questions. *Worldviews on Evidence-Based Nursing, 2*(2), 98–102.

The Joint Commission. (2013). *Revised requirements for the hospital accreditation program*. Retrieved from http://www.jointcommission.org/assets/1/6/PrepublicationReport_CMS_HAP.pdf

Josiah Macy Jr. Foundation. (2015). *Enhancing health professions education through technology: Building a continuously learning health system*. Arlington, VA: Author. http://macyfoundation.org/docs/macy_pubs/JMF_Exec-Summary_Final.pdf

Kalb K. A., O'Conner-Von S., Brockway C., Rierson C. L., & Sendelbach, S. (2015). Evidence-based teaching practice in nursing education: Faculty perspectives and practices. *Nursing Education Perspectives, 36*(4), 212–219.

Kennedy, C. C., Jaeschke, R., Keitz, S., Newman, T., Montori, V., & Wyer, P. C.; Evidence-based medicine teaching tips working group. (2008). Tips for teachers of evidence-based medicine: Adjusting for prognostic imbalances (confounding variables) in studies on therapy or harm. *Journal of General Internal Medicine, 23*(3), 337–343.

Kent, B., & Fineout-Overholt, E. (2007). Teaching EBP: Clinical practice guidelines: Part 1. *Worldviews on Evidence-Based Nursing, 4*(2), 106–111.

Khan, K. S., & Coomarasamy, A. (2006). A hierarchy of effective teaching and learning to acquire competence in evidence-based medicine. *BMC Medical Education, 6*, 59.

Kotter, J. P., & Schlesinger, L. A. (2008). Choosing strategies for change. *Harvard Business Review, 86*(7/8), 130.

Kyriakoulis, K., Patelarou, A., Laliotis, A., Wan, A., Matalliotakis, M., Tsiou, C., & Patelarou, E. (2016). Educational strategies for teaching evidence-based practice to undergraduate health students: Systematic review. *Journal of Educational Evaluation in Health, 13*, 34.

Laaksonen, C., Hannele, P., von Schantz, M., Ylönen, M., & Soini, T. (2013). Journal club as a method for nurses and nursing students' collaborative learning: A descriptive study. *Health Science Journal, 7*(3), 285–292.

Lachance, C. (2014). Nursing journal clubs: A literature review on the effective teaching strategy for continuing education and evidence-based practice. *The Journal of Continuing Education in Nursing, 45*, 559–565.

Leung, K., Trevena, L., & Waters, D. (2014). Systematic review of instruments for measuring nurses' knowledge, skills and attitudes for evidence-based practice. *Journal of Advanced Nursing, 70*(10), 2181–2195.

Mann, E., Medves, J., & Vandenkerkhof, E. (2015). Accessing best practice resources using mobile technology in an undergraduate nursing program: a feasibility study. *Computers, Informatics, Nursing: CIN, 33*(3), 122–128.

Malik, G., McKenna, L., & Griffiths, D. (2017). Using pedagogical approaches to influence evidence-based practice integration—processes and recommendations: Findings from a grounded theory study. *Journal of Advanced Nursing, 73*(4), 883–893.

McKeever, S., Kinney, S., Lima, S., Newall, F. (2016). Creating a journal club competition improves paediatric nurses' participation and engagement. *Nurse Education Today. 37*, 173–7.

McGinn, T., Jervis, R., Wisnivesky, J., Keitz, S., & Wyer, P. C.; Evidence-based Medicine Teaching Tips Working Group. (2008). Tips for teachers of evidence-based medicine: Clinical prediction rules (CPRs) and estimating pretest probability. *Journal of General Internal Medicine, 23*(8), 1261–1268.

Melnyk, B., & Fineout-Overholt, E. (2003a). *Evidence-based practice beliefs scale*. Rochester, NY: ARCC Publishing.

Melnyk, B., & Fineout-Overholt, E. (2003b). *Evidence-based practice implementation scale*. Rochester, NY: ARCC Publishing.

Melnyk, B. M., Fineout-Overholt, E., Feinstein, N., Li, H. S., Small, L., Wilcox, L., & Kraus, R. (2004). Nurses' perceived knowledge, beliefs, skills, and needs regarding evidence-based practice: Implications for accelerating the paradigm shift. *Worldviews on Evidence-Based Nursing, 1*(3), 185–193.

Melnyk, B. M., Fineout-Overholt, E., Feinstein, N. F., Sadler, L. S., & Green-Hernandez, C. (2008). Nurse practitioner educators' perceived knowledge, beliefs, and teaching strategies regarding evidence-based practice: Implications for accelerating the integration of evidence-based practice into graduate programs. *Journal of Professional Nursing, 24*(1), 7–13.

Melnyk, B. M., Fineout-Overholt, E., Gallagher-Ford, L., & Kaplan, L. (2012). The state of evidence-based practice in US nurses: Critical implications for nurse leaders and educators. *Journal of Nursing Administration, 42*(9), 410–417.

Melnyk, B. M., Fineout-Overholt, E., Giggleman, M., & Cruz, R. (2010). Correlates among cognitive beliefs, EBP implementation, organizational culture, cohesion and job satisfaction in evidence-based practice mentors from a community hospital system. *Nursing Outlook, 58*(6), 301–308.

Melnyk, B. M., Gallagher-Ford, L., & Fineout-Overholt, E. (2017). *Implementing the evidence-based practice (EBP) competencies in healthcare: A practical guide for improving quality, safety, and outcomes.* Indianapolis, IN: Sigma Theta Tau International.

Melnyk, B. M., Gallagher-Ford, L., Long, L. E., & Fineout-Overholt, E. (2014). The establishment of evidence-based practice competencies for practicing registered nurses and advanced practice nurses in real-world clinical settings: Proficiencies to improve healthcare quality, reliability, patient outcomes, and costs. *Worldviews on Evidence-Based Nursing, 11*(1), 5–15.

Morris, J. (2016). The use of team-based learning in a second year undergraduate pre-registration nursing course on evidence-informed decision making. *Nurse Education in Practice, 21*, 23–28.

Novak, I., & McIntyre, S. (2010). The effect of education with workplace supports on practitioners' evidence-based practice knowledge and implementation behaviours. *Australian Occupational Therapy Journal, 57*, 386–393.

Odell, E., & Barta, K. (2011). Teaching evidence-based practice: The bachelor of science in nursing essentials at work at the bedside. *Journal of Professional Nursing, 27*, 370–377.

O'Mathuna, D. P., Fineout-Overholt, E., & Kent, B. (2008). How systematic reviews can foster evidence-based clinical decisions: part II. *Worldviews on Evidence-Based Nursing, 5*(2), 102–107.

Orta, R., Messmer, P. R., Valdes, G. R., Turkel, M., Fields, S. D., & Wei, C. C. (2016). Knowledge and competency of nursing faculty regarding evidence-based practice. *The Journal of Continuing Education in Nursing, 47*(9), 409–419.

Palaima, M. (2010). *Evidence based practice: Clinical experiences of recent doctor of physical therapy graduates.* Presented at Combined Sections Meeting, American Physical Therapy Association, New Orleans, LA.

Porter-O'Grady, T., & Malloch, K. (2016). *Leadership in nursing practice: Changing the landscape of health care.* Sudbury, MA: Jones and Bartlett.

Prasad, P., Jaeschke, R., Wyer, P., Keitz, S., & Guyatt, G.; Evidence-Based Medicine Teaching Tips Working Group. (2008). Tips for teachers of evidence-based medicine: Understanding odds ratios and their relationship to risk ratios. *Journal of General Internal Medicine, 23*(5), 635–640.

Pravikoff, D. S., Pierce, S. T., & Tanner, A. (2005). Evidence-based practice readiness study supported by academy nursing informatics expert panel. *Nursing Outlook, 53*(1), 49–50.

Puentedura, R. R. (2006). *Transformation, technology, and education*. Retrieved from http://hippasus.com/resources/tte/

Puentedura, R. R. (2012). *Technology in education: The first 200,000 years. The NMC Perspective Series: Ideas that Matter. NMC Summer Conference.* Retrieved from http://www.youtube.com/watch?v=NemBarqD6qA

Puentedura, R. R. (2015). *SAMR: A brief introduction.* Retrieved from http://hippasus.com/rrpweblog/archives/2015/10/SAMR_ABriefIntro.pdf

Purnell, M., & Majid, G. (2017). A paediatric nurses' journal club: Developing the critical appraisal skills to turn research into practice. *Australian Journal of Advanced Nursing, 34*(4), 34–41.

Ramos, K., Schafer, S., & Tracz, S. (2003). Validation of the Fresno test of competence in evidence based medicine. *British Medical Journal, 326*, 319–321.

Richardson, W. S., Wilson, M. C., Keitz, S. A., & Weyer, P. C.; EBM Teaching Scripts Working Group. (2008). Tips for teachers of evidence-based medicine: Making sense of diagnostic test results using likelihood ratios. *Journal of General Internal Medicine, 23*(1), 87–92.

Sackett, D. L., Haynes, R. B., Guyatt, G. H., & Tugwell, P. (1991). *Keeping up to date—The educational prescription in clinical epidemiology* (2nd ed.). Boston, MA: Little Brown.

Schutt, M. S., & Hightower, B. (2009). Enhancing RN-to-BSN students' information literacy skills through the use of instructional technology. *Journal of Nursing Education, 48*(2), 101–105.

Shaneyfelt, T., Baum, K. D., Bell, D., Feldstein, D., Houston, T., Kaatz, S., . . . Green, M. (2006). Instruments for evaluating education in evidence-based practice: A systematic review. *American Medical Association, 296*(9), 1116–1127.

Sherriff, K. L., Wallis, M., & Chaboyer, W. (2007). Nurses' attitudes to and perceptions of knowledge and skills regarding evidence-based practice. *International Journal of Nursing Practice, 13*, 363–369.

Shirey, M. R., Hauck, S. L., Embree, J. L., Kinner, T. J., Schaar, G. L., Phillips, L. A., . . . McCool, I. A. (2011) Showcasing differences between quality improvement, evidence-based practice, and research. *Journal of Continuing Education in Nursing, 42*(2), 57–68.

Shuval, K., Berkovits, E., Netzer, D., Hekselman, I., Linn, S., Brezis, M., & Reis, S. (2007). Evaluating the impact of an evidence-based medicine educational intervention on primary care doctors' attitudes, knowledge and clinical behaviour: A controlled trial and before and after study. *Journal of Evaluation in Clinical Practice, 13*(4), 581–598.

Skiba, D. J. (2013). Bloom's digital taxonomy and word clouds. *Nursing Education Perspectives, 34* (4): 277–80. http://dx.doi.org/10.5480/1536-5026-34.4.277

Springer, H. (2010). Learning and teaching in action. *Health Information and Libraries Journal, 27*, 327–331.

Stephens-Lee, C., Lu, D., & Wilson, K. (2013). Preparing students for an electronic workplace. *Online Journal of Nursing Informatics (OJNI), 17*(3). Retrieved from http://ojni.org/issues/?p=2866

Stichler, J., Fields, W., Kim, S. C., & Brown, C. (2011). Faculty knowledge, attitudes and perceived barriers to teaching evidence-based nursing. *Journal of Professional Nursing, 27*(2), 92–100.

Stillwell SB, Fineout-Overholt E, Melnyk BM, Williamson KM. (2010). Evidence-based practice, step by step: asking the clinical question: a key step in evidence-based practice. *American Journal of Nursing, 110*(3), 58–61

Strandell-Laine, C., Stolt, M., Leino-Kilpi, H., Saarikoski, M. (2015). Use of mobile devices in nursing student–nurse teacher cooperation during the clinical practicum: An integrative review. *Nurse Education Today, 35*(3), 493–499.

Taylor, M., Priefer, B., & Alt-White, A. (2016) Evidence-based practice: Embracing integration. *Nursing Outlook, 64*, 575–582.

Technology Informatics Guiding Education Reform. (2007). *The TIGER initiative: Evidence and informatics transforming nursing: 3-year action steps toward a 10-year vision.* Retrieved from http://www.tigersummit.com/uploads/TIGERInitiative_Report2007_Color.pdf

Technology Informatics Guiding Education Reform. (2009). *The TIGER initiative: Collaborating to integrate evidence and informatics into nursing practice and education: An executive summary.* Retrieved from http://www.tigersummit.com/uploads/TIGER_Collaborative_Exec_Summary_040509.pdf

Thomas, A., Saroyan, A., & Dauphinee, W. D. (2011). Evidence-based practice: A review of theoretical assumptions and effectiveness of teaching and assessment interventions in health professions. *Advances in Health Sciences Education: Theory and Practice, 16*(2), 253–276.

Tuazon, N. (2017). A case study of the meaning of evidence-based practice among ICU staff nurses. *Journal of Nursing Practice Applications and Review of Research, 7*(1), 4–13.

Upton, P., Scurlock-Evans, L., Williamson, K., Rouse, J., & Upton, D. (2015). The evidence-based practice profiles of academic and clinical staff involved in pre-registration nursing students' education: A cross sectional survey of US and UK staff. *Nurse Education Today, 35*(1), 80–85.

Varnell, G., Haas, B., Duke, G., & Hudson, K. (2008). Effect of an educational intervention on attitudes toward and implementation of evidence-based practice. *Worldviews on Evidence-Based Nursing, 5*(4), 172–181.

Wallen, G. R., Mitchell, S. A., Melnyk, B. M., Fineout-Overholt, E., Miller-Davis, C., Yates, J., & Hastings, C. (2010). Implementing evidence-based practice: Effectiveness of a structured multifaceted mentorship programme. *Journal of Advanced Nursing, 66*(12): 2761–2771.

Wallin, L., Bostrom, A., & Gustavsson, J. P. (2012). Capability beliefs regarding evidence-based practice are associated with application of EBP and research use: Validation of a new measure. *Worldviews Evidence-Based Nursing, 9*(3), 139–148.

West, C. P., & McDonald, F. S. (2008). Evaluation of a longitudinal medical school evidence-based medicine curriculum: A pilot study. *Journal of General Internal Medicine, 23*(7), 1057–1059.

Williams, B. C., & Hoffman, R. M. (2008). Teaching tips: A new series in JGIM. *Journal of General Internal Medicine, 23*(1), 112–113.

Winters, C. A., & Echeverri, R. (2012). Teaching strategies to support evidence-based practice. *Critical Care Nurse, 32*(3), 49–54.

Yew, K. S., & Reid, A. (2008). Teaching evidence-based medicine skills: An exploratory study of residency graduates' practice habits. *Family Medicine, 40*(1), 24–31.

Zayim, N. & Ozel, D. (2015). Factors Affecting Nursing Students' Readiness and Perceptions Toward the Use of Mobile Technologies for Learning. *Computers, Informatics, Nursing: CIN, 33*(10), 456–464.

Zelenikova, R., Beach, M., Ren, D., Wolff, D., & Sherwood, P. (2014). Faculty perception of the effectiveness of EBP courses for graduate nursing students. *Worldviews on Evidence-Based Nursing, 11*(6), 401–413.

Zwickey, H., Schiffke, H., Fleishman, S., Haas, M., Cruser, D. A., LeFebvre, . . . Gaster, B. (2014). Teaching evidence-based medicine at complementary and alternative medicine institutions: strategies, competencies, and evaluation. *Journal of Alternative & Complementary Medicine, 20*(12), 925–31.

17 Teaching Evidence-Based Practice in Clinical Settings

Ellen Fineout-Overholt, Martha J. Giggleman, Katie Choy, and Karen Balakas

You must unlearn, what you have learned.

—*Yoda*

EBP Terms to Learn

EBP mentors
Evidence-based intervention
Fidelity of the evidence-based intervention
Point-of-care clinicians
Senior leadership

Learning Objectives

After studying this chapter, learners will be able to:

1. Explain the importance of teaching evidence-based practice (EBP) in clinical settings.
2. Describe the barriers and facilitators of EBP in clinical settings.
3. Discuss strategies for teaching EBP in clinical settings.

It is critically important for all healthcare clinicians and leadership to consider how and why evidence-based practice (EBP) is a part of the culture of any organization. For best practice to thrive, the EBP paradigm must be a core value held by leadership and **point-of-care clinicians**, versus just an edict from the top-down. Despite decades of advances in teaching EBP in clinical settings and subsequent reports of highly valuing evidence-based decision making, clinicians still do not implement EBP (Warren et al., 2016), and healthcare leaders do not place a high value on EBP (Melnyk et al., 2016). Educators in healthcare are essential facilitators for a cultural shift that embraces EBP at the point of care (Rickbeil & Simones, 2012). Furthermore, designating educators as **EBP mentors** formally recognizes their role in fostering a culture of EBP within an organization (Gawlinski & Becker, 2012).

One method that healthcare educators can employ to shift the thinking of point-of-care clinicians to EBP is to document how others have changed outcomes through the implementation of EBP. There are many examples in the literature of how clinicians use the EBP process to improve patient outcomes. Despite this progress, full integration into daily decision making is ongoing. For example, hourly rounding has been documented for some time as an effective intervention to reduce fall rates in acute care settings (Goldsack, Bergey, Mascioli, & Cunningham, 2015; Mitchell, Lavenberg, Trotta, & Umscheid, 2014; Tucker, Bieber, Attlesey-Pries, Olson, & Dierkhising, 2012), but not all organizations use this important **evidence-based intervention**. We need to discover why the lack of evidence-based intervention uptake exists. Evidence-based change may be seen as temporary, unless all clinicians are aware of the purpose and the process for each evidence-based initiative. For example, Tucker et al. (2012) had an unexpected clinical situation emerge at the time the hourly rounding was being implemented that resulted in a mandate from administration for hourly rounding rather than the planned approach that began with staff-based training. Subsequently, the

fidelity of the evidence-based intervention (i.e., how well the intervention was followed as it was described in the research) was quite variable, with nursing staff reporting that they felt a lack of decision making. Real-life examples such as these are very helpful to educators who are working with clinicians who daily experience the competing priorities of "getting the work done" and of ensuring evidence-based care.

Not only is EBP the right thing to do, because it improves healthcare outcomes (Goldsack et al., 2015; Jeffs et al., 2013; Kim et al., 2016; Linton & Prasun, 2013; Lusardi, 2012; Melnyk, Fineout-Overholt, Giggleman & Choy, 2017; Mitchell et al., 2014; Murphy, Wilson, & Newhouse, 2013), but also regulatory and accrediting agencies have indicated that, from a safety standpoint as well as a reimbursement standpoint, organizations that are practicing based on evidence will reap rewards. Patient safety is an imperative. Organizations are accountable to ensure that the best initiatives are being implementing so that they can reliably produce the safest environments. Part of this accountability lies with educators' ability to translate, for clinicians, the evidence that demonstrates expected safety outcomes. The context for this accountability lies in the awareness that lives are lost every year because of preventable errors by clinicians and systems (Institute of Medicine [IOM], 2001). The National Patient Safety Goals (The Joint Commission, 2013) clearly indicated that evidence-based initiatives are to be put into place to achieve best outcomes for patients. Furthermore, the Centers for Medicare & Medicaid Services (Department of Health and Human Services, 2015) mandated that preventable, nosocomial infections (e.g., urinary tract infections), and other complications (e.g., pressure injury/ulcers), will no longer be reimbursed and that evidence-based care must be manifest. Such a mandate is an opportunity to bring the evidence to the clinician that supports why these clinical issues are so important to address. EBP offers a partnership that enables innovative decision making between the patient and the provider that can bring about outcomes that will be best for the patient. This partnership also can impact potential disengagement by the point-of-care provider, which, as a matter of course, will foster the accountability that will fulfill the mandate.

Evidence-based care makes sense from a safety perspective and from a best care perspective; however, best care cannot be distilled down into safe-only care. There are issues such as cost-effectiveness, quality, and satisfaction that are also important to consider. The American Nurses Credentialing Center's (ANCC) Magnet program has become a driver in the EBP movement by setting standards of clinical excellence (Schreiber, 2013). These standards hinge on the EBP paradigm as the underpinning philosophy for healthcare, from care delivered at the bedside to decisions made in the executive boardroom. Healthcare educators have the privilege of making these standards meaningful to point-of-care clinicians as well as leadership. Although this may sound simple, there are challenges to bringing EBP alive in clinical settings.

CHALLENGES IN THE CLINICAL SETTING

EBP is now recognized as a necessary component of quality patient care, prompting many healthcare organizations to invest resources into the creation of a culture that sustains the integration of evidence into direct care decision making. Nurses at the point of care are essential to the implementation of EBP; therefore, it is important to ascertain factors that may hinder its adoption by these clinicians. Identification of barriers to achievement of EBP has been studied extensively (De Pedro-Gomez et al., 2011; Grant, Janson, Johnson, Idell, & Rutledge, 2012; Johnston et al., 2016; Sadoughi, Azadi, & Azadi, 2017). Among the most cited barriers remain individual clinicians' EBP skill level and the time needed to find sufficient research (Dalheim, Harthug, Nilsen, & Nortvedt, 2012; Johnston et al., 2016; Maaskant, Knops, Ubbink, & Vermeulen, 2013; Sadoughi et al., 2017).

Challenges With Changing Healthcare Provider Characteristics

Today's clinicians are increasingly being challenged by patients and healthcare organizations to demonstrate high-quality and measurable patient care outcomes. However, clinicians report that they continue to use experience-based knowledge collected from their own observations and input from colleagues (Dalheim et al., 2012). Thus, because clinicians most often practice guided by what they learned in school and their clinical experiences, evaluating how age and educational preparation of the healthcare providers affect their decision making may offer insights.

One prime example is the 2015 National Sample Survey of Registered Nurses (NSSRN; Budden, Moulton, Harper, Brunell & Smiley, 2016), which stated that the median age of the nurse remained steady at 48.8 years, reflecting an increase since 2004, but a slight decrease since 2013. There continues to be a rise in nurses reporting bachelor of nursing (BSN) programs as their foundational education, and EBP, by the Institute of Medicine (IOM) and the American Association of Colleges of Nursing essentials mandate, is part of BSN education. However, it is important to note that almost 40% of the nursing workforce is either nearing or at retirement age (Budden et al., 2016).

Educational preparation is an important factor that needs to be considered when planning strategies to teach EBP. Budden et al. (2016) reported that about 39% of RNs obtained their primary nursing education in an associate degree program and would have had little formal education in research or EBP. From 2004 to 2015, the percentage of nurses whose highest initial nursing preparation was a baccalaureate degree increased only slightly, whereas the number of diploma prepared nurses continued to steadily decline (Budden, Moulton, Harper, Brunell, & Smiley, 2016). Although these figures reflect a slight change in initial nursing preparation and, therefore, an expectation of foundational knowledge of EBP, there is some evidence to support that today's nursing population will still require education specific to EBP in the clinical environment (Kim et al., 2016).

Challenges With Attitudes Toward Use of Research in Practice

According to Kim et al. (2016), nurses have difficulty interpreting and applying study findings, and knowledge resulting from research continues to be challenging to use in practice. Gallegos and Sortedahl (2015) found that pediatric nurses reported that they perceived themselves as participants in research and protectors of human subjects, but there was no assessment of the understanding of how these nurses perceived their knowledge and skills to translate research into practice. The possible limited ability of clinicians to understand how research translates into practice is of great concern, because nurses are expected to evaluate research to determine which findings produce better outcomes before they apply it. Kelly et al. (2011) reported that nurses are aware of the importance of research to guide practice; however, often it is implemented through a top-down hierarchy that eliminates the point-of-care clinician from the process. Addressing these organizational issues is imperative for EBP to be actualized system-wide.

Nurses report that although they believe that practice should be based on all evidence, including research, they rarely consult with healthcare librarians or use nursing research. Nurses often lack the skills and the time needed to locate research information and indicate that they feel much more confident asking colleagues or searching the Internet (e.g., Google Scholar) than using bibliographic databases such as PubMed or CINAHL (Linton & Prasun, 2013; Rickbeil & Simones, 2012). Heavy patient loads and outdated policies and procedures were additional factors that decreased the application of evidence among nurses (Barako, Chege, Wakasiaka, & Omondi, 2012). Melnyk et al. (2016) found that nursing leadership perceived EBP as less important than any other priorities, while also indicating quality and safety ranked at the top. These are just several of the issues that educators must address as they strive to help clinicians be adequately prepared to understand how to evaluate research methods and apply reliable findings to practice to deliver evidence-based, safe, and quality care.

In addition to education preparation requirements for nurses, the NSSRN (HRSA, 2010; Budden et al., 2016) also demonstrated that although there had been substantial changes in the healthcare delivery system, hospitals still remain the primary setting in which nurses are employed. Stressors related to shortages in the RN workforce and the demands associated with long shifts and increased patient loads have been well documented for some time (American Association Colleges of Nursing, 2012; Zinn, Guglielmi, Davis, & Moses, 2012). It is not surprising that a lack of time continues to be frequently cited as one of the major barriers to the implementation of EBP (Barako et al., 2012; Hauck, Winsett, & Kuric, 2012; Heaslip, Hewitt-Taylor, & Rowe, 2012; Johnston et al., 2016; Linton & Prasun, 2013; Sadoughi et al., 2017). Nurses reported that they had little time either during scheduled working hours or during their personal time to engage in activities required for EBP. For many clinicians, there was no time not only to search for evidence, but also to read or appraise research.

Challenges With Environment and Workplace

Prior to current initiatives to incorporate EBP into the workplace, staff nurses and other healthcare clinicians may have had no expectation to question current practice. Adherence to institutional policies and procedures and following physician orders were anticipated behaviors by nurses and other clinicians. Nurses, for example, incorporated safety into their practice, such as checking medication doses and interactions, but may not have sought information to support or change patient care interventions. Within the current, changing healthcare environment, clinicians are being asked to formulate clinical questions and translate research findings to ensure cost-efficient, clinically effective patient care, and they need educators to help them meet these expectations.

Despite clear regulatory support and mandates, clinicians have reported that managers do not always support the implementation of EBP and that there is a lack of organizational commitment to engage in EBP as well as research (Hauck et al., 2012; Melnyk et al., 2016; Rickbeil & Simones, 2012). These studies support that there may be a discrepancy between a stated goal for EBP implementation and competing organizational as well as leadership priorities. Healthcare agencies that focus on achieving and maintaining a balance that considers patient and staff safety, productivity, improved clinical outcomes, hospital financial viability, enhanced patient satisfaction, and increased staff satisfaction must do so with EBP as the foundation for these goals. Support from immediate managers and unit educators is critical to facilitate change toward evidence-based care (Hauck et al., 2012; Melnyk et al., 2016; Sandstrom, Borglin, Nilsson, & Willman, 2011; Wilkinson, Nutley, & Davies, 2011). It is also necessary for **senior leadership** to provide support and training for the unit managers as they are expected to play an essential leadership role in EBP implementation at the unit level; otherwise it will be an impediment to implementation (Hauck et al., 2012; Melnyk et al., 2016; Warren, Montgomery, & Friedmann, 2016; van der Zijpp et al., 2016).

Challenges With Clinical Education About Evidence-Based Practice

For bedside clinicians to engage in EBP, they must have the necessary tools; therefore, teaching EBP has become an imperative for healthcare organizations. Because bedside clinicians directly influence patient care outcomes, it is essential for organizational leadership to understand their ability to implement EBP in the real practice environment (for more information, see Chapter 12). This understanding drives the design of educational initiatives to meet point-of-care clinicians' learning needs. The introduction of EBP education must be carefully planned and executed so that clinicians can truly incorporate EBP into their everyday practice. The manager plays a role in influencing, empowering, facilitating, and providing autonomy for clinicians to engage in EBP (Stetler, Ritchie, Malone, & Charns, 2014; Wilkinson, Nutley, & Davies, 2011; van der Zijpp et al., 2016).

According to Melnyk, Fineout-Overholt, Stillwell, and Williamson (2010), the key to teaching nurses and other healthcare clinicians about EBP is *buy-in*. Buy-in may not be strong enough—perhaps ownership is truly the key to successful integration of EBP into an organizational culture. When teaching point-of-care clinicians or healthcare administrators about EBP, the first place to start is with what motivates daily care decisions. For true EBP ownership to occur, it must be part of the organizational strategic plan developed by senior leadership. Otherwise, EBP becomes just another process improvement idea, and it will not be taken seriously by clinicians. The relational aspects between the managerial staff and clinical leaders need consideration as well when implementing any new process, and communication is key (van der Zijpp et al., 2016).

The traditional practice paradigm often embraces the comfort of "we've always done it that way." This is the sacred cow approach to practice that dies a hard death and can remain, even with the best organizational support for EBP healthcare practices (Hanrahan et al., 2015). Although most of those reading this chapter would agree that this is not the best paradigm to follow, we also would likely admit that it is reassuring to be able to predict how things are going to be done. However, the difficulty with this paradigm is that tradition does not guarantee predictable outcomes. Rather, the outcomes vary with every clinician's interpretation of the norm.

Practicing based on the EBP paradigm (see Figure 1.2) enables variation of care processes with some standardization regarding the inclusion of the external evidence (i.e., research), patient preferences, clinical expertise, and internal evidence. This paradigm focuses on patient outcomes, which, for all clinicians and administrators, is the unifying factor. When initiating care practices, the outcome is the driver of decisions. Consider teaching all those involved in healthcare about why they engage in care practices such as inserting an intravenous line, administering a medication, or performing a diagnostic test. Often clinicians may indicate that processes are the goal of care initiatives; however, processes lead to outcomes. The outcomes are bottom-line drivers for fiscal and resource allocation, and other decisions that establish priorities in healthcare. Some may see EBP as a burden, a challenge, or a disturbance of the status quo; however, without this kind of disruption, transformation of healthcare will not occur (Ubbink, Guyatt, & Vermeulen, 2013). Educators, particularly as EBP mentors, are the key to this paradigm shift at the bedside.

ORGANIZATIONAL READINESS FOR TEACHING EVIDENCE-BASED PRACTICE

Teaching EBP in clinical settings is not an option; it is a necessity and, therefore, a leadership responsibility. Although the individual point-of-care clinicians may lack the skills for EBP, it is the healthcare leaders who must establish a culture for EBP (Fitzsimons & Cooper, 2012), which includes providing the resources and leadership needed to transform the culture to one that uses EBP on a daily basis. The ANCC's Magnet program has long indicated that transformational leadership is a requirement for an evidence-based organization. Through this leadership, the vision and value for EBP are communicated to clinicians and an appeal for their active involvement is clearly conveyed. Leaders must be innovative and challenge assumptions. They need to partner with point-of-care clinicians to achieve outcomes. Transformational leaders demonstrate their commitment by setting forth the vision and providing resources necessary to establish an EBP culture (Everett & Sitterding, 2011; Hauck et al., 2012). Although the incorporation of EBP into health professions' curricula has occurred in most undergraduate programs, the culture must be present to support these new clinicians to ask the clinical questions and seek the answers. Leaders are challenged to ensure that the organization is structured to provide the supportive environment needed for EBP to flourish. Doctorally prepared leaders, such as nurse scientists, doctors of nursing practice, and advanced practice nurses, need to be accessible and responsive to the point-of-care clinicians who provide direct care (Pierce, 2011).

One method for achieving mutual goals is through shared governance. Establishing a councilor structure in an EBP organization includes an EBP Research/EBP Council to address clinical issues with evidence. This becomes part of an EBP culture. Clinicians begin to rely on this council for tackling the clinical issues that are important to bedside staff and providing guidance for applying the evidence to their organization. A Practice Council can be a partner that takes the evidence compiled and synthesized by the EBP Council and operationalizes plans for putting standards of care and other policies into place across the organization to address the given clinical issue based on evidence. Commitment to shared governance is key to providing a voice for point-of-care providers so that they are able to actively participate in evidence-based initiatives and improve outcomes (Fitzsimons & Cooper, 2012; Ubbink et al., 2013). Having an EBP Council provides an opportunity to have an impact on the spread of evidence-based decision making. When all councils begin to use evidence-based thinking, the EBP process becomes the norm for making decisions in the organization. An Education Council can make sure that programs offered are evidence based and that EBP is an essential component of orientation and continuing education for all clinical staff. A Leadership Council can ensure that essential resources are provided for clinicians to practice based on evidence and for educators to facilitate a culture of EBP.

> Do.
> Or do not.
> There is no try.
>
> **YODA**

ESSENTIAL RESOURCES FOR TEACHING EVIDENCE-BASED PRACTICE

Essential resources needed for teaching EBP include an organizational plan for EBP implementation, a theoretical basis to plan change, education from the board room to the bedside to increase support, and emphasis on the benefits such as improved outcomes, quality improvement, and cost reduction through spending limited resources wisely. An IOM aim is that 90% of clinical decisions will be evidence based by 2020 (IOM, 2010). Organizational leadership must be trained on the benefits of EBP, to support and develop a strategic plan for EBP and a budget for implementation (Wilson et al., 2015). Diffusion of Innovation Theory has been used by some organizations to plan change that will occur to the culture (Hanrahan et al., 2015). A successful change theory will be one that fits the organizational cultural of the institution the best. Magnet-designated hospitals have successfully implemented EBP through their empowering structures and processes and, through transformational leadership at all levels, a higher number of RNs with higher education levels and certifications. Clinicians that have increased education have increased experience with EBP, and studies have indicated that patients experience better outcomes resulting in cost reduction (Wilson et al., 2015).

Over time, EBP should become embedded into the professional practice of healthcare organizations. The American Nurses Association charged nurse administrators with the responsibility for integrating research findings into practice and providing an environment for EBP to flourish (Gallagher-Ford, 2014). However, Melnyk et al. (2016) demonstrated that there are still growth opportunities in healthcare leadership support of EBP. These findings make Gallagher-Ford's (2014) imperative for the chief executive officer and all senior leadership support for an EBP transformational culture to develop and persist extremely poignant. Supportive and effective EBP leaders are dynamic and use a range of integrated and transparent leadership behaviors that are strategic, functional, multifaceted, both formal and informal, and reach all levels of the organization (Stetler et al., 2014). Moreover, leadership must continuously be vision driven, deliberate, and role model on a day-to-day basis how EBP integrates into practice at all levels to support nurses in sustaining the culture (Melnyk et al., 2016; Stetler et al., 2014). Otherwise, EBP is a flavor of the month process change that is soon forgotten, when new and competing organizational priorities emerge as they always do. Therefore, leaders should see themselves as not only facilitators, but also active participants engaging with interprofessional teams and ensuring that EBP implementation strategy is clear and resources and education are available and ongoing, giving nurses the willingness to learn, implement, and sustain EBP (Warren, Montgomery, et al., 2016).

Assess Available Resources

One of the first steps in establishing an educational program for EBP in the clinical setting is to assess the resources that are available or could be dedicated to EBP. Challenges to the implementation of EBP can occur at the institutional level as well as with individuals. Competing priorities, difficulty with recruiting and sustaining a workforce, and insufficient funds to purchase database subscriptions have been found to be some of the institutional barriers to implementing EBP in organizations (Sadoughi et al., 2017; Solomons and Spross, 2011). Leadership in the development of educational strategies is contingent upon the human resources within the healthcare organization. A doctorally prepared clinical expert (i.e., Doctor of Nursing Practice) is key to supporting and guiding the development of an EBP program. A doctorally prepared clinical expert who is dedicated to the vision of EBP also can provide insight and support as a program is developed. Teaching the EBP process and its associated skills requires the ability to pose searchable, answerable questions; assist in searching for relevant evidence; critically appraise and synthesize evidence; apply evidence in the clinical setting; and guide clinicians in evaluating outcomes based on evidence (Pierce, 2011; Sawin et al., 2010). If an individual with in-depth knowledge of EBP and research is not available within the organization, establishing a partnership with an academic institution can help to facilitate the development of a program (Linton & Prasun, 2013; Schreiber, 2013).

Assess Educators' Knowledge of Evidence-Based Practice

The next step is to assess the knowledge level about EBP among educators within the organization to determine whether additional education may be needed. Building a team of EBP educators and mentors is a crucial component of any educational strategy and EBP culture (Aitken et al., 2011; Fitzsimons & Cooper, 2012; Kim et al., 2016, Magers, 2014). Interdisciplinary teams are an essential factor for building an evidence-based framework in the clinical setting (Sibbald, Wathen, Kothari, & Day, 2013). Once the gaps are identified regarding knowledge and skills needed to teach EBP, there are numerous workshops, courses, and online programs that are available throughout the country to assist team members in gaining basic and advanced EBP knowledge and skills. Some of the more established programs are listed in Box 17.1, and online tutorials that can be easily accessed are listed in Box 17.2.

BOX
17.1 *A Sampling of Available Educational Programs to Learn About Evidence-Based Practice (EBP)*

- **Duke University Medical Center** offers a 4-day EBP workshop for educators and champions of "Evidence-Based Medicine" that is focused on developing EBP knowledge and skills, including a mentor guiding small groups to achieve workshop goals (https://sites.duke.edu/ebmworkshop).
- **The Johanna Briggs Institute** offers a 6-month workplace, evidence-based, implementation program involving two 5-day intensive training residencies (http://joannabriggs.org/education/short-courses/clinical-fellowship). In addition, there are other courses available to help build EBP knowledge and skills (http://joannabriggs.org/education).
- **Johns Hopkins Center for Evidence-based Practice** offers a 5-day EBP workshop that focuses on mastery of the EBP process (http://www.hopkinsmedicine.org/evidence-based-practice/boot-camp.html).
- **McMaster University** offers a 5-day course that is designed to help participants advance their critical appraisal skills, improve their skills in acknowledging and incorporating patient values and preferences in clinical decision making, and learn how to teach EBP using a variety of educational models (http://ebm.mcmaster.ca/).
- **The Ohio State University Center for Transdisciplinary Evidence-Based Practice** offers a 5-day immersion program targeted at clinicians to develop effective strategies to integrate and sustain EBP within their organization as well as change the organizational culture, as well as online programs to learn about EBP (http://nursing.osu.edu/sections/ctep/).

BOX
17.2 *A Sampling of Online Resources for Learning About Evidence-Based Practice (EBP; some require a fee)*

- **Centre for Evidence-Based Medicine** from the Mt. Sinai Hospital and University Health Network (Toronto, Ontario, Canada)—this website offers comprehensive and detailed materials on EBP (https://ebm-tools.knowledgetranslation.net).
- **Johns Hopkins Nursing Evidence-Based Practice** online course can be accessed at https://www.ijhn-education.org/content/jhn-evidence-based-practice-series.
- **The University of Texas Health Science Center's** EBP modules for basics and intermediate learners can be accessed at http://nursing.uthscsa.edu/onrs/starmodel/index.asp under learning about EBP.
- **Users' Guides to Evidence-Based Practice** from the Canadian Centre for Health Evidence (http://www.cche.net/main.asp).

Assess Computer Literacy

Determining the basic informatics and computer literacy of educators and clinicians is necessary in developing the groundwork for teaching EBP in clinical settings. Without educators who are knowledgeable in informatics, including adequate computer skills and the ability to use databases to find relevant evidence, teaching EBP will be challenging. Chapter 3 provides in-depth information for developing effective search strategies for finding relevant evidence in multiple databases to answer clinical questions.

Include Knowledgeable Medical Librarian

Another important issue in the preliminary evaluation of resources is to ensure that you have a clinical (i.e., on the unit) or medical librarian on the teaching team who is knowledgeable about EBP. It is imperative that medical librarians be involved in the plan to initiate EBP. It is important to plan for early involvement of librarians in preparing an EBP teaching program. If your organization does not have an on-site librarian, it would be important to work toward a partnership with a librarian in a nearby agency or educational institution. As active partners, evidence-based librarians can provide perspective and expertise in search strategy development as well as access to databases and other sources of evidence. In addition, healthcare librarians are experts in informatics and information literacy and can facilitate teaching the skills needed by nurses, physicians, and other healthcare clinicians who strive to be successful at EBP. Evidence-based librarians foster a culture of EBP within an organization.

An essential resource that facilitates the work of EBP mentors and educators to teach about and sustain EBP implementation is ready access to databases and evidence to support changes in practice. Both PubMed and the Cochrane Library offer free access to search and read abstracts, but clinicians need full-text articles to appraise and apply the evidence. Subscriptions to databases such as CINAHL and online resources such as Nurse or MD Consult can be very helpful for obtaining clinical information. Many hospitals have healthcare libraries and can include vital resources in their holdings that are necessary for clinicians to provide evidence-based care to their population of patients. If a hospital does not have a library, there are online resources that clinicians can join for a fee. DynaMed is an online reference developed for point-of-care clinicians that contains thousands of summaries. This resource is updated daily and monitors the content of more than 500 medical journals and systematic review databases. The literature is critically appraised, integrated into existing content, and synthesized to deliver the best available evidence. Another tool is *Isabel*, a decision-support tool that helps clinicians expand their differential diagnosis at the point of care providing evidence-based critical information. Another online peer-reviewed resource providing evidence-based reviews is UpToDate, which contains thousands of articles in over 30 categories and provides the user with synthesized recommendations upon which to make treatment decisions. Point-of-care clinicians can also subscribe to the Nursing Reference Center to obtain relevant clinical information. All of these resources can help clinicians model and teach the critical value of EBP to provide improved patient outcomes. Chapter 3 contains more information on sources of evidence.

Information on UpToDate can be found at: http://www.uptodate.com/home

Information on DynaMed and a free trial can be found at: https://store.dynamed.com/subscribe/free-trial

Information on the Nursing Reference Center can be found at: https://www.ebscohost.com/nursing/products/nursing-reference-center

Information on *Isabel* can be found at: http://www.isabelhealthcare.com/home/default

---

Financial Support

A final crucial element required to teach EBP is financial support. Clinicians need protected time to participate in classes, develop clinical questions, locate evidence, read and appraise the evidence, plan for application of the evidence and implementation of practice changes, and determine evaluation strategies to assess outcomes. This means that administrators and unit-level managers must include time for EBP in their budgets. This time must be reflected as valuable on the schedule as well as the budget. Terms such as "nonproductive time" do not facilitate valuing of EBP among staff, managers, or agency leadership. A budget that provides for dedicated time to engage in evidence-based project work demonstrates to point-of-care clinicians that the education for and implementation of EBP is valued by leadership (Schifalacqua & Soukup, 2012; Strusowski et al., 2017; Ubbink et al., 2013).

EDUCATIONAL STRATEGIES FOR TEACHING EVIDENCE-BASED PRACTICE

Teaching EBP requires a tiered educational approach. It is not enough to just offer classes to bedside clinicians without first engaging direct-line managers in the process. Managers, unit educators, and clinicians in advanced practice serve as models of change for point-of-care staff. They can foster the implementation of EBP if they understand its value and their role in the process and can see the link between the use of external and internal evidence and improved patient outcomes. One way to accomplish this undertaking is to first determine the model(s) upon which to base the program. The next step is to schedule one or several meetings to introduce the EBP model(s), discuss the steps of EBP, and present the clinicians' unique role in developing and sustaining EBP on the unit. An example from the authors' experiences with organizations includes one pediatric hospital's professional practice department's decision to host a luncheon meeting for unit managers and administrators prior to launching an educational program for staff nurses. This preliminary step proved to be a crucial one, because each nurse manager was needed to identify a staff nurse whose leadership skills might grow from being involved in an EBP program. In another institution, the Nursing Research/EBP Committee developed a strategic plan that specifically addressed establishment of a culture to support EBP. The role of nursing leadership in promotion of an EBP culture was listed among the plan's objectives. It is vital to the success of an EBP project that it is fully supported by managers with clearly identified benefits for each unit's population. Similar meetings to present EBP to supervisors, case managers, and clinical educators also are needed to sustain adoption of EBP.

Strategy One: Evidence-Based Practice Workshop Format

Once a team of educators and EBP mentors has been developed, additional intensive efforts can begin to educate bedside caregivers. Numerous EBP educational programs for clinical staff have been documented in the literature for several years (Bromirski, Cody, Coppin, Hewson, & Richardson, 2011; Gawlinski & Becker, 2012; Grant et al., 2012; Kelly et al., 2011; Kim et al., 2016; Lusardi, 2012; Rickbeil & Simones, 2012). The length and depth of each program vary, but the basic content is consistent and includes a comprehensive overview of EBP, a presentation for each step in the process, a discussion of change theory, and often an opportunity to complete a project using what has been taught. Some of the programs are offered in a workshop format that may range from 1 day to 7 days and are presented at one point in time or over several months. Some of these programs include a formal application process and are delivered in a combination of didactic classes, discussion groups, and mentored projects. Classes within these programs provide the clinician with intensive guidance on the development of a PICOT question, building searching skills to locate and retrieve evidence, learning critical appraisal skills, and application of evidence for practice change. Requiring the identification of a clinical question or area of interest prior to participation in a program is very helpful, as it makes it easier for the clinicians to quickly focus on their thinking about evidence-based decision making and applying the steps of EBP. Using clinicians' PICOT questions and providing computers for interactive sessions while teaching searching skills is very effective. If a computer lab is not available, securing laptop computers and encouraging participants to work as partners can help to facilitate learning. Given that most hospitals have clinical guidelines readily available, some programs incorporate critical review and updating of the guidelines as a component of the EBP course. This exercise provides the learner with a relevant example to illustrate one aspect of applying the principles of EBP. These programs serve to not only educate clinical staff but also build a cadre of EBP mentors to lead and promote EBP initiatives within the organization. An outline of potential class topics and exercises is listed in Box 17.3.

Because not all clinicians are able to commit to a mentoring role, classes that introduce the concepts of EBP and highlight its potential for improving patient care outcomes can support continued adoption of EBP. For example, educators who have adequate EBP knowledge and skills could partner with a medical librarian to offer a workshop for bedside staff to deliver an overview of the EBP process. The staff who participate in the workshops would then be eligible to apply for a longer EBP fellowship that includes more in-depth classes

---

BOX 17.3 *Sample Topical Outline for an Evidence-Based Practice (EBP) Program*

1. Introducing the principles of the EBP framework and process
   a. Incorporating the vision for EBP in the organization
   b. Explaining the use of the institutional EBP model in daily decision making
   c. Developing focused clinical questions
      i. Defining the clinical problem based on quality data
      ii. Developing a clinical question using PICOT format
2. Recruiting an interdisciplinary team that is relevant to the question
3. Systematically searching for relevant external evidence using the PICOT question
   a. Using all healthcare databases and EBP databases
   b. Finding clinical guidelines that contain recommendations that answer the PICOT question
   c. Exploring EBP websites
   d. Benchmarking with like institutions
4. Searching for internal evidence such as quality data that informs about the current state of practice
5. Determining performance improvement indicators
6. Critically appraising the evidence
   a. Explain the research designs in the body of evidence
   b. Use rapid appraisal forms that are appropriate for the research design
   c. Understanding how to interpret statistics
7. Synthesizing evidence
   a. Using an evaluation table
   b. Using a synthesis table
   c. Making a recommendation for use of evidence in practice
8. Translating evidence into practice: Execute a plan
   a. Recommendation to practice change
   b. Defining and evaluating outcomes from the research
   c. Piloting the change with an eye on organizational diffusion
9. Evaluating the outcomes to sustain the change
10. Crafting policy based on evidence
11. Disseminating the evidence

and individual mentoring to complete a project. Teaching smaller classes can adapt content for relevance to the participant's clinical background and prepare a significant number of caregivers who embrace inquiry and value EBP for best practice.

Self-directed learning has been a part of healthcare education for several decades, and the benefits have been documented in the literature for more than 25 years. Self-directed learning incorporates adult learning principles and encourages participants to take an active role in the learning process. This approach may be helpful for motivated clinicians who are not able to attend face-to-face classes or conferences and wish to learn the principles of EBP. Through self-directed learning, participants have the opportunity to set their own priorities and determine their own timeframe for learning.

 Joanna Briggs Institute offers extensive EBP resources and continuing education http://joannabriggs.org/education. You can also consider one of the library guides such as Duke University's http://guides.mclibrary.duke.edu/c.php?g=158201&p=1036002.

Additional initiatives can be created within the work environment to provide staff with opportunities for learning EBP outside of more traditional methods. One hospital, intent on creating a supportive culture for EBP, conducted an educational needs assessment and discovered inconsistent use of EBP principles by staff. To stimulate consistent integration of EBP, nursing administration partnered with an academic institution to provide several introductory EBP lectures that were open to all staff. Following this fundamental education, they developed a competitive EBP award program to fully engage staff in the integration of EBP. After an application process and critical review by nurse representatives from administration, education, performance improvement, research, and frontline staff, three teams were awarded $5,000 to conduct their projects. Postaward mentoring and seminars were provided to help participants overcome barriers and complete their projects (Kelly et al., 2011; Magers, 2014).

Educational offerings have increasingly moved from local 1-day hands-on workshops to full week immersions and cohort-based residencies that culminate in achievable organizational-focused projects, such as the exemplar in Box 17.4. Residencies blend what traditionally has been considered an EBP fellowship that helped staff nurses professionally develop and improve their skills in evidence-based decision making with a systems-focused and operationalized program that includes mentoring through dissemination of the project. Kim et al. (2016) found that a mentored residency resulted in improved beliefs and implementation of EBP by staff nurses.

Another venue for teaching EBP is the committee structure of the organization. Increasingly acute care organizations are moving from traditional support for a committee dedicated to the development and review of policies and procedures that impart guidance for the care frontline staff provide to patients and families to shared governance structures that allow staff to have an active voice in policies and procedures, patient education, and implementation and evaluation of innovative interventions to improve patient outcomes. Establishing a process that supports the integration of evidence into daily decisions as well as policies, procedures, and guidelines can ensure safe care. EBP models can help staff nurses actualize the EBP process as the chosen organizational problem-solving approach. To accomplish the goal of evidence-based decision making expectation of everyone from staff to administration, EBP knowledge and skills need to be a part of orientation, all continuing education, all committee structures, and all documentation within the organization, including performance appraisals. Incorporating evidence in the development of organizational documents guides committees' work and sets the context for care delivery and outcome evaluation.

<table>
<tr><td>

BOX

17.4

</td><td>

Exemplar of a Cohort Workshop Format to Teach Evidence-Based Practice (EBP) in a Clinical Setting

</td></tr>
</table>

Using both hospital and grant funding, an acute care hospital on the West Coast implemented the Advancing Research and Clinical Practice Through Close Collaboration model to train nurses and other interdisciplinary team members on EBP to change culture and improve patient care outcomes. Nursing and interdisciplinary staff were selected to participate by their managers based on interest, ability, and availability. All staff were paid to participate in training and to develop and implement their unit projects. The project took place over 12 months, with all staff demonstrating a positive affinity for embracing EBP. Senior management ensured that resources were available for project implementation, training on EBP knowledge and skills, and the support for care delivery using EBP. EBP project teams were implemented to work on a chosen and approved problem area. Each team formulated their PICOT question, plans were developed based on literature review and research, and outcomes were measured after project implementation. All teams were encouraged to submit their project results at a local, regional, national, or international conference. The hospital honored the staff by paying to send staff to the conferences and meetings to present and disseminate their work. Most importantly, by immersing many staff into the EBP process, staff supported each other and created momentum for culture change (Melnyk, Fineout-Overholt, Giggleman, & Choy, 2016).

A next phase of training and immersion was planned and implemented to train selected staff to be EBP mentors for the hospital. This training required a deeper dive into all aspects of EBP to provide the skills and support for the mentors to lead team projects as needed in the future to keep the EBP culture alive and thriving as a way of providing the best care and outcomes for patients. Through embracing EBP in a cohort workshop format, nurses grew in their professional role and increased the body of knowledge for the nursing profession.

Strategy Two: Journal Club Format

There are several additional approaches to helping staff gain knowledge and skills in actualizing the EBP process. One of those approaches is a journal club, which has been used effectively for decades in the clinical setting to assist clinicians who want to improve the translation of research into practice. Traditionally, journal clubs that have been either *topic-based* or *teaching-based* provided a forum for healthcare clinicians to discuss clinical issues, the current research available on the topic, and the recommended basis for clinical decisions related to treatment options. They have also been used as a teaching/learning strategy to help clinicians learn about EBP and how evidence can be used for clinical decision making. EBP skills-focused journal clubs teach participants the steps needed for EBP from development of a PICOT question through application of evidence and evaluation of clinical outcomes.

Active participation in a journal club is frequently dependent on some knowledge of the research appraisal process. Providing classes about the critical appraisal of research, including evaluating the validity of research methods, can support bedside clinicians to become involved in unit-based journal clubs. However, participation in such classes may seem daunting for some clinical staff. Also, the additional time commitment for another meeting may compete with other hospital committees and the daily demands of patient care needs. Incorporating a modified journal club format into existing unit committee meetings is an effective teaching strategy to teach appraisal skills and engender interest in the use of research to guide practice. The EBP mentor/teacher can locate an article relevant to the unit's patient population and either post it on the unit's bulletin board or distribute it electronically prior to the meeting. The beginning of the meeting can then be used to role model appraisal of the article and brainstorm with the group potential applications for practice. This strategy has been used successfully in one hospital during unit practice committee meetings to implement bedside reporting, a new tube-feeding protocol, fall-prevention rounds, family presence during resuscitation, the effective use of capnography, and the use of noninvasive technology to assess tissue oxygenation and stroke volume. Committee members have learned the steps of EBP and can clearly articulate why they chose specific practices. It is reasonable to expect that as clinical staff become educated about EBP, they are able to communicate more effectively with other disciplines and engage more frequently in scholarly discussions.

Strategy Three: Academic-Service Partnerships

Teaching EBP in the clinical setting can also be enhanced through partnerships with academic institutions. For example, faculty from two nursing programs and a clinical nurse specialist at one institution collaboratively developed two EBP projects. The first project was 20 nursing students developing a comprehensive oral hygiene program for adult and pediatric patients in critical care and acute care settings. The second project centered on best practices for sleep apnea patients. Both projects involved frontline nurses along with students in the EBP process as policies were developed and education was delivered to hospital committees and staff. The EBP collaboration involved staff nurses identifying significant problems and guiding students through hospital processes, while students brought their expertise in searching the literature and appraising the study findings to the projects (Rickbeil & Simones, 2012).

As clinicians become skilled in the steps of EBP and complete projects, they will need guidance in learning how to share their work through oral and poster presentations. Some staff will be required to deliver a presentation following the completion of an educational program, whereas others will want to communicate the results of their endeavors internally and externally. In addition to individual guidance, classes in how to develop presentations can be very helpful. Promotion of attendance and presentations at local, state, and national conferences by the EBP leadership team supports previous teaching efforts and strengthens the clinician's knowledge base. One example from my work with organizations includes nurses from one community and one academic hospital participating in a 12-month EBP Fellowship program that produced 12 completed projects. When a call for abstracts from the state university was issued, the staff nurses were encouraged to submit their projects. EBP mentors helped them write and submit the abstracts and then helped them develop their posters. Hospital administration from both institutions financially supported the nurses' attendance at the regional EBP conference where they expanded their knowledge of EBP and returned with increased enthusiasm and commitment to EBP.

Teaching EBP in a clinical setting requires commitment, diligence, enthusiasm, creativity, and teamwork. It is not accomplished through one program, one committee or council, or one project. It requires an ability to set goals and then evaluate progress toward the attainment of those goals. Teaching EBP is a continuous process that will result in improved patient care outcomes, professional growth, and an empowered clinical staff. Teaching EBP can be a personally and professionally rewarding experience.

EBP FAST FACTS

- EBP is essential for optimal patient outcomes and clinical educators must be able to promote and sustain its everyday implementation.
- Although nurses state they believe practice should be based on research, nurse leaders still do not value EBP as a high priority.
- Barriers to EBP implementation remain in the clinical setting, most often reported as the skill level of the individual nurse, lack of time, and lack of managerial support.
- For bedside nurses to engage in EBP, they must have the necessary tools, thus teaching EBP has become an imperative for healthcare organizations.
- Teaching EBP is a leadership responsibility and requires organizational commitment to provide the resources needed to support a cultural change for EBP.
- Following assessment of organizational readiness, financial support, and available resources, a tiered educational approach is needed to engage managers, educators, and point-of-care clinicians in EBP.

WANT TO KNOW MORE?

A variety of resources are available to enhance your learning and understanding of this chapter.

- Visit thePoint˚ to access:
  - Articles from the AJN EBP Step-by-Step Series
  - Journal articles
  - Checklists for rapid critical appraisal and more!
- Lippincott CoursePoint combines digital text content with video case studies and interactive modules for a fully integrated course solution that works the way you study and learn.

References

Aitken, L. M., Hackwood, B., Crouch, S., Clayton, S., West, N., Carney, D., & Jack, L. (2011). Creating an environment to implement and sustain evidence based practice: A developmental process. *Australian Critical Care: Official Journal of the Confederation of Australian Critical Care Nurses, 24*(4), 244–254. doi:10.1016/j.aucc.2011.01.004

American Association Colleges of Nursing. (2012). *Nursing shortage.* Retrieved from http://www.aacn.nche.edu/media-relations/fact-sheets/nursing-shortage

Barako, T. D., Chege, M., Wakasiaka, S., & Omondi, L. (2012). Factors influencing application of evidence-based practice among nurses. *African Journal of Midwifery and Women's Health, 6*(2), 71–77.

Bromirski, B. H., Cody, J. L., Coppin, K., Hewson, K., & Richardson, B. (2011). Evidence-based practice day: An innovative educational opportunity. *Western Journal of Nursing Research, 33*(3), 333–344.

Budden, J. S., Moulton, P., Harper, K. J., Brunell, M. L., Smiley, R. (2016). The 2015 national nursing workforce survey. *Journal of Nursing regulation, 7*(1): s1–s92.

Dalheim, A., Harthug, S., Nilsen, R. M., & Nortvedt, M. W. (2012). Factors influencing the development of evidence-based practice among nurses: A self-report survey. *BMC Health Services Research, 12*, 367. doi:10.1186/1472-6963-12-367

Department of Health and Human Services, Centers for Medicare and Medicaid Services. (2015). *Hospital Acquired Conditions (HAC) in Acute Inpatient Prospective Payment System (IPPS) hospitals.* Retrieved on August 19, 2017, from http://www.cms.gov/Medicare/Medicare-Fee-for-Service-Payment/HospitalAcqCond/downloads/hacfactsheet.pdf, https://www.cms.gov/Medicare/Medicare-Fee-for-Service-Payment/HospitalAcqCond/Hospital-Acquired_Conditions.html

De Pedro-Gomez, J., Morales-Asencio, J. M., Bennasar-Veny, M., Artigues-Vives, G., Perello-Campaner, C., & Gomez-Picard, P. (2011). Determining factors in evidence-based clinical practice among hospital and primary care nursing staff. *Journal of Advanced Nursing, 68*(2), 452–459. doi:10.1111/j.1365-2648.2011.05733.x

Everett, L. Q., & Sitterding, M. C. (2011). Transformational leadership required to design and sustain evidence-based practice: A system exemplar. *Western Journal of Nursing Research, 33*(3), 398–426. doi:10.1177/0193945910383056

Fitzsimons, E., & Cooper, J. (2012). Embedding a culture of evidence-based practice. *Nursing Management, 19*(7), 14–19.

Gallagher-Ford, L. (2014). Implementing and sustaining EBP in real world healthcare settings: A leader's role in creating a strong context for EBP. *Worldviews on Evidence-Based Nursing, 11*(1), 72–74.

Goldsack, J., Bergey, M., Mascioli, S., Cunningham, J. (2015). Hourly rounding and patient falls: what factors boost success? *Nursing, 45*(2), 25–30.

Gawlinski, A., & Becker, E. (2012). Infusing research into practice. *Journal for Nurses in Staff Development, 28*(2), 69–73. doi:10.1097/NND.0b013e31824b418c

Grant, M., Janson, J., Johnson, S., Idell, C., & Rutledge, D. N. (2012). Evidence-based practice for staff nurses. *The Journal of Continuing Education in Nursing, 43*(3), 117–124. doi:10.3928/00220124-20110901-02

Hauck, S., Winsett, R. P., & Kuric, J. (2012). Leadership facilitation strategies to establish evidence-based practice in an acute care hospital. *Journal of Advanced Nursing, 69*(3), 664–674. doi:10.1111/j.1365-2648.2012.06053.x

Health Resources and Services Administration. (2010) *The registered nurse population: Findings from the 2008 national sample survey of registered nurses.* Retrieved on August 19, 2017, from https://bhw.hrsa.gov/sites/default/files/bhw/nchwa/rnsurveyfinal.pdf

Heaslip, V., Hewitt-Taylor, J., & Rowe, N. E. (2012). Reflecting on nurses' views on using research in practice. *British Journal of Nursing, 21*(22), 1341–1346.

Institute of Medicine. (2001). *Crossing the quality chasm.* Washington, DC: National Academies Press.

Jeffs, L., Sidani, S., Rose, D., Espin, S., Smith, O., Martin, K., . . . Ferris, E. (2013). Using theory and evidence to drive measurement of patient, nurse and organizational outcomes of professional nursing practice. *International Journal of Nursing Practice, 19*(2), 141–148. doi:10.1111/ijn.12048

Johnston, B., Coole, C., Feakes, R., Whitworth, G., Tyrell, T., & Hardy, B. (2016). Exploring the barriers to and facilitators of implementing research into practice. *British Journal of Community Nursing, 21*(8), 392–398.

Kelly, K. P., Guzzetta, C. E., Mueller-Burke, D., Nelson, K., DuVal, J., Hinds, P. S., & Robinson, N. (2011). Advancing evidence-based nursing practice in a children's hospital using competitive awards. *Western Journal of Nursing Research, 33*(3), 306–332. doi:10.1177/0193945910379586

Kim, S. C., Stichler, J. F., Ecoff, L., Brown, C. E., Gallo, A., & Davidson, J. E. (2016). Predictors of evidence-based practice implementation, job satisfaction, and group cohesion among regional fellowship program participants. *Worldviews on Evidence-Based Nursing, 13*(5), 340–348.

Linton, M. J., & Prasun, M. A. (2013). Evidence-based practice: Collaboration between education and nursing management. *Journal of Nursing Management, 21,* 5–16. doi:10.1111/j.1365-2834.2012.01440.x

Lusardi, P. (2012). So you want to change practice: Recognizing practice issues and channeling those ideas. *Critical Care Nurse, 32*(2), 55–63. doi:10.4037/ccn2012899

Maaskant, J. M., Knops, A. M., Ubbink, D. T., & Vermeulen, H. (2013). Evidence-based practice: A survey among pediatric nurses and pediatricians. *Journal of Pediatric Nursing, 28,* 150–157. doi:10.1016/j.pedn.2012.05.002

Magers, T. L. (2014). An EBP mentor and unit-based EBP team: A strategy for successful implementation of a practice change to reduce catheter-associated urinary tract infections. *Worldviews on Evidence-Based Nursing, 11*(5), 341–343.

Melnyk, B., Fineout-Overholt, E. Giggleman, M., & Choy, K. (2017). A Test of the ARCC© model improves implementation of evidence-based practice, healthcare culture, and patient outcomes. *Worldviews on Evidence-Based Nursing, 14*(1), 5–9.

Melnyk, B., Fineout-Overholt, E., Stillwell, S., & Williamson, K. (2010). Transforming healthcare quality through innovations in evidence-based practice. In T. Porter-O'Grady & K. Malloch (Eds.), *The leadership of innovation: Creating the landscape for healthcare transformation* (pp. 167–194). Sudbury, MA: Jones & Bartlett.

Melnyk, B. M., Fineout-Overholt, E., Giggleman, M., & Choy, K. (2016). A Test of the ARCC© Model Improves Implementation of Evidence-Based Practice, Healthcare Culture, and Patient Outcomes. *Worldviews on Evidence-based Nursing, 14*(1), 5–9.

Melnyk, B. M., Gallagher-Ford, L., Thomas, B. K., Troseth, M., Wyngarden, K., & Szalacha, L. (2016). A study of chief nurse executives indicates low prioritization of evidence-based practice and shortcomings in hospital performance metrics across the United States. *Worldviews in Evidence-Based Nursing, 13*(1), 6–14.

Mitchell, M., Lavenberg, J., Trotta, R., & Umscheid, C. (2014). Hourly rounding to improve nursing responsiveness: A systematic review. *Journal of Nursing Administration, 44*(9), 462–472.

Murphy, L. S., Wilson, M. L., & Newhouse, R. P. (2013). Improving care transitions through meaningful use stage 2: Continuity of care document. *Journal of Nursing Administration, 43*(2), 62–65. doi:10.1097/NNA.0b013e31827f2076

Pierce, C. J. (2011). Establishing a methodology for development and dissemination of nursing evidence-based practice to promote quality care. *U.S. Army Medical Department Journal*, 41–44.

Rickbeil, P., & Simones, J. (2012). Overcoming barriers to implementing evidence-based practice: a collaboration between academics and practice. *Journal of Nurses Staff Development, 28*(2), 53–6.

Sadoughi, F., Azadi, T., & Azadi, T. (2017). Barriers to using electronic evidence based literature in nursing practice: A systematised review. *Health Information & Libraries Journal, 34*(3), 187–199.

Sandstrom, B., Borglin, G., Nilsson, R., & Willman, A. (2011). Promoting the implementation of evidence-based practice: A literature review focusing on the role of nursing leadership. *Worldviews on Evidence-Based Nursing, 8*(4), 212–223. doi:10.1111/j.1741-6787.2011.00216.x

Sawin, K. J., Gralton, K. S., Harrison, T. M., Malin, S., Balchunas, M. K., Brock, L. A., . . . Schiffman, R. F. (2010). Nurse researchers in children's hospitals. *Journal of Pediatric Nursing, 25*(5), 408–417. doi:10.1016/j.pedn.2009.07.005

Schifalacqua, M. M., & Soukup, M. (2012). Does evidence-based nursing increase ROI? *American Nurse Today, 7*(1), Retrieved from https://www.americannursetoday.com/does-evidence-based-nursing-increase-roi/

Schreiber, J. A. (2013). Beyond evidence-based practice: Achieving fundamental changes in research and practice. *Oncology Nursing Forum, 40*(3), 208–210. doi:10.1188/13.ONF.208-210

Sibbald, S. L., Wathen, C. N., Kothari, A., & Day, A. M. B. (2013). Knowledge flow and exchange in interdisciplinary primary health care teams (PHCTs): An exploratory study. *Journal of the Medical Library Association, 101*(2), 128–137. doi:10.3163/1536-5050.101.2.008

Solomons, N. M., & Spross, J. A. (2011). Evidence-based practice barriers and facilitators from a continuous quality improvement perspective: An integrative review. *Journal of Nursing Management, 19*(1), 109–120. doi:10.1111/j.1365-2834.2010.01144.x

Stetler, C., Ritchie, J. A., Malone, J. R., & Charns, M. P. (2014). Leadership for evidence-based practice: Strategic and functional behaviors for institutionalizing EBP. *Worldviews on Evidence-Based Nursing, 11*(4), 219–226.

Strusowski, T., Sein, E., Johnston, D., Gentry, S., Bellomo, C., Brown, E., . . . Messier, N. (2017). Standardized evidence-based oncology navigation metrics for all models: A powerful tool in assessing the value and impact of navigation programs. *Journal of Oncology Navigation & Survivorship, 8*(5), 220–243.

The Joint Commission. (2013). *Hospital: National patient safety goals*. Retrieved from http://www.jointcommission.org/standards_information/npsgs.aspx

Tucker, S. J., Bieber, P. L., Attlesey-Pries, J. M., Olson, M. E., & Dierkhising, R. A. (2012). Outcomes and challenges in implementing hourly rounds to reduce falls in orthopedic units. *Worldviews on Evidence-Based Nursing, 9*(1), 18–29. doi:10.1111/j.1741-6787.2011.00227.x

Ubbink, D. T., Guyatt, G. H., & Vermeulen, H. (2013). Framework of policy recommendations for implementation of evidence-based practice: A systematic scoping review. *BMJ Open, 3*, e001881. doi:10.1136/bmjopen-2012-001881

Warren, J. I., McLaughlin, M., Bardsley, J., Eich, J., Esche, C. A., Kropkowski, L., & Risch, S. (2016).The strengths and challenges of implementing EBP in healthcare systems. *Worldviews on Evidence-Based Nursing, 13*(1), 15–24.

Warren, J. I., Montgomery, J. L., & Friedmann, E. (2016). Three-year pre–post analysis of EBP integration in a magnet-designated community hospital. *Worldviews on Evidence-Based Nursing, 13*(1), 50–58.

Wilkinson, J. E., Nutley, S. M., & Davies, H. T. O. (2011). An exploration of the roles of nurse managers in evidence-based practice implementation. *Worldviews on Evidence-Based Nursing, 8*(4), 236–246. doi:10.1111/j.1741-6787.2011.00225.x

van der Zijpp, T. J., Niessen, T., Eldh, A. C., Hawkes, C., McMullan, C., Mockford, C., . . . Seers, K. (2016). A bridge over turbulent waters: Illustrating the interaction between managerial leaders and facilitators when implementing research evidence. *Worldviews on Evidence-Based Nursing, 13*(1), 25–31.

Zinn, J. L., Guglielmi, C. L., Davis, P. P., & Moses, C. (2012). Addressing the nursing shortage: The need for nurse residency programs. *AORN Journal, 96*(6), 652–657. doi:10.1016/j.aorn.2012.09.011

ARCC Evidence-Based Practice Mentors: The Key to Sustaining Evidence-Based Practice

Ellen Fineout-Overholt and Bernadette Mazurek Melnyk

Mentors change lives. . .
—*Richie Norton*

EBP Terms to Learn
EBP mentor

Learning Objectives
After studying this chapter, learners will be able to:

1 Explain the role of the evidence-based practice (EBP) mentor.

2 Discuss the importance of the EBP mentor role to sustainability of an EBP culture.

3 Describe evidence that supports EBP mentor role impact.

OVERVIEW OF THE ARCC MODEL AND EVOLUTION OF EVIDENCE-BASED PRACTICE MENTORS

A mentor is a trusted coach or teacher, whether in evidence-based practice (EBP) or any other endeavor. In his blog, Maxwell (2015) shared three defining characteristics of mentors: (1) "mentors know the way"; (2) "mentors show the way"; and (3) "mentors go the way." These characteristics actualize the trusted coach/teacher definition. In a landmark work, Tobin (2004) described seven mentor roles: (1) teacher, (2) sponsor, (3) advisor, (4) agent, (5) role model, (6) coach, and (7) confidante. Through these roles mentors demonstrate the characteristics of *know, show,* and *go.* Fleming et al. (2013) crafted a measure of mentor competence that spanned six domains: (1) effective communication, (2) aligning expectations, (3) assessing understanding, (4) fostering independence, (5) addressing diversity, and (6) promoting development. Mentees also have the characteristics they must exhibit as well, which include leadership, self-awareness, creative thinking, receptiveness to constructive feedback, good judgment, integrity, and political awareness (Abedin et al., 2012). Based on these characteristics, role responsibilities and competencies, all of which apply to Advancing Research and Clinical practice through close Collaboration (ARCC) mentors and Advancing Research and Clinical practice through Close Collaboration in Education (ARCC-E) EBP mentors (see Appendix H on thePoint'), the mentor–mentee relationship is not engaged lightly; rather, it is usually enduring and dynamic. Note that within this chapter, ARCC and ARCC-E EBP mentors, while different in concept, function similarly in their work; therefore, hereafter will simply be referred to as ARCC EBP mentors. The ARCC EBP mentor–mentee relationship is synergistic. This synergy is intentionally focused on improving the organizational culture and healthcare outcomes as a result of the relationship (Figure 18.1).

This chapter provides a foundational overview of the role and purpose of the ARCC EBP mentor. Primary to the ARCC EBP mentor–mentee relationship is the knowledge that

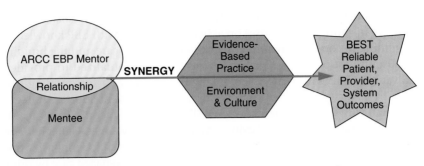

Figure 18.1: Unique relationship between ARCC EBP mentor and mentee.

implementation of EBP improves quality of care and patient outcomes. Third-party payers are incentivizing organizations to deliver evidence-based care, and healthcare systems are still having challenges sustaining a culture of EBP. *Sustainability* has become a buzzword in today's world and, in its broadest sense, means an emphasis on cultivating a high quality of life for generations to come by promoting and maintaining security, clean air, and health (Fineout-Overholt, Williamson, Gallagher-Ford, Melnyk, & Stillwell, 2011; Gallagher-Ford, Fineout-Overholt, Melnyk, & Stillwell, 2011); however, for healthcare organizations, sustainability is far more than security, clean air, and health. To sustain EBP in healthcare systems, there needs to be a key mechanism that is inherent in organizations for the purpose of promoting the continued system-wide advancement of evidence-based care, once it is initiated. As first proposed in the ARCC model (Melnyk & Fineout-Overholt, 2002; Melnyk, Fineout-Overholt, Gallagher-Ford, & Stillwell, 2011), this key mechanism is an **EBP mentor**. Typically, an EBP mentor is an advanced practice clinician with in-depth knowledge and skills in EBP, individual and organizational growth, individual behavioral as well as healthcare systems change, and organizational culture shift. An EBP mentor, however, can be any clinician with expert knowledge of EBP and a desire to assist others in advancing excellence through evidence-based care. Other terms that have been used to describe those who have advanced EBP are facilitator and champion. A facilitator works with individuals, teams, and organizations to prepare, guide, and support them through the evidence implementation process. **Champions** hold expertise in EBP and are able to bring about evidence-based change, disseminate how they do their work, and improve the uptake of EBP (Frantsve-Hawley & Meyer, 2008; Shifaza, Evans, Bradley, & Ullrich, 2013). While facilitators, champions, and EBP mentors are focused on successful evidence implementation, its context and the subsequent change in patient, provider, and system outcomes, an EBP mentor is also concerned with the growth and development of individual clinicians caring for patients (Christenbery, Williamson, & Wells, 2016). Individual clinical growth and development, in EBP and otherwise, leads to sustainable changes in the organizational environment and culture that reap benefits beyond simply improved patient outcomes.

As with other mentoring relationships, careful consideration of role expectations of both the EBP mentor and those receiving mentorship should include building rapport between mentor and mentee; selecting mechanisms for regular communication in which feedback is shared between mentor and mentee; advocating for a supportive environment in which administrative as well as overall psychosocial support is evident; striving for work–life balance while maximizing career progression options; and fostering social networking (Nick et al., 2012). Both mentor and mentee require clear expectations. The ARCC EBP mentor role should be a formal role outlined in an organization's role description as well as performance appraisal criteria. These specialized roles require continued opportunities to learn about how to be an EBP mentor, such as seminars or workshops that include how to negotiate and effectively leverage release time for this role.

The ARCC model is a guide for system-wide implementation and sustainability of EBP in healthcare organizations that focuses on assisting clinicians with EBP knowledge, beliefs, and skills-building to consistently implement evidence-based care and the building of EBP cultures to sustain best practices. The model was first conceptualized to provide a framework for advancing EBP within an academic medical center and surrounding community (see Chapter 14). Nurses identified mentorship as an important success strategy to assist point-of-care staff with the implementation of EBP (Melnyk, & Fineout-Overholt, 2002, 2010; Levin et al., 2011; Fineout-Overholt, Levin, & Melnyk, 2013; Melnyk, Gallagher-Ford, Long, & Fineout-Overholt, 2014). Thus, the term *EBP mentor* was coined to emphasize the key role of mentorship in promoting and sustaining the use of evidence-based care by point-of-care staff and in building cultures that support EBP (Melnyk & Fineout-Overholt, 2010).

In the ARCC and ARCC-E Models, EBP mentors use findings from an assessment of the readiness and culture of an organization for system-wide implementation of EBP to guide them in developing a strategic plan to enhance clinicians' knowledge and skills in EBP and to foster a culture of best practice. Evidence from research demonstrates that EBP mentors enhance point-of-care providers' beliefs about the value of EBP and their ability to implement it, which in turn leads to greater EBP implementation (EBPI; Kim et al., 2017; Levin et al., 2011; Mariano et al., 2011; Melnyk et al., 2004; Saunders & Vehviläinen-Julkunen, 2016; Wallen et al., 2010). Research further shows that when EBP Beliefs and EBPI are enhanced, job satisfaction and group cohesion are strengthened (Kim et al., 2017; Levin et al., 2011) and turnover rates are less (Levin et al., 2011). A key outcome of reduced staff turnover is substantial cost savings for healthcare organizations. For more specific information about the ARCC model, see Chapter 14; and about the ARCC-E model, see Chapter 16.

THE ARCC EVIDENCE-BASED PRACTICE MENTOR ROLE

EBP mentors first ensure that those they mentor and others with whom they work have a common understanding of the definition of EBP and its language. For these mentors, EBP is defined as a problem-solving approach to clinical practice that integrates the *best evidence* (after systematic appraisal of both internal and external evidence) with a *clinician's expertise* and *patient preferences and values* to make decisions about the type of care that is provided in their setting and that are the most appropriate outcomes to be evaluated to demonstrate sustainable best care. The language of EBP is an essential for clinicians who advocate best practice to learn prior to full assimilation of EBP. For example, EBP mentors must convey that use of research methodology terms such as randomized controlled trial, sample size, and informed consent are for critical appraisal only and do not have a place in evidence implementation. Terms such as internal evidence, sustainability, and impact are commonly used for implementation. There are crossover terms that are used in both research and EBP, such as intervention, evaluation, and measurement; however, the focus of these terms may be different.

In addition, EBP mentors ensure that the rigor and the progression of the seven-step EBP process is well understood by point-of-care providers as well as managers or administrators (see Chapter 1 for more on the seven-step EBP process). The spirit of inquiry is an important focus for the EBP mentor. Without this initial element of an EBP culture, the EBP mentor role is less effective and often can be perceived as nothing more than another bureaucratic role established by administration to support their agenda. EBP mentors can serve both as catalysts for change toward best practice and as stability factors that foster sustainable outcomes through consistent delivery of evidence-based care.

In the ARCC and ARCC-E Models, there are important components of the EBP mentor role (Box 18.1) that enable these mentors to engage in strategic planning, implementation, and outcomes evaluation that are focused on monitoring the impact of their role and overcoming

---

BOX
18.1

Components of the Evidence-Based Practice (EBP) Mentor Role

- Ongoing assessment of an organization's capacity to sustain an EBP culture
- Building EBP knowledge and skills through conducting interactive group workshops and one-to-one mentoring
- Stimulating, facilitating, and educating clinicians toward a culture of EBP, with a focus on overcoming barriers to best practice
- Role modeling EBP
- Conducting Advancing Research and Clinical practice through close Collaboration and Advancing Research and Clinical practice through Close Collaboration in Education strategies to enhance the implementation of EBP, such as journal clubs, EBP rounds, web pages, newsletters, fellowship programs, or integration of EBP into curricula
- Working with staff to generate internal evidence (i.e., practice-generated) through quality improvement, outcomes management, and EBP implementation projects
- Facilitating staff involvement in research to generate external evidence
- Using evidence to foster best practice
- Collaborating with interdisciplinary professionals to advance and sustain EBP

barriers in moving the system to a culture of best practice (Melnyk, 2007; Wallen et al., 2010). Evidence continues to demonstrate that a determined purpose in the mentoring of direct care staff, from primary care practice to public health, is to strengthen clinicians' beliefs about the value of EBP and their ability to implement it (see Figure 18.1; Fineout-Overholt & Melnyk, 2015; Holliman, Resler, Edmunds, & Child Life Council, 2010; Kim et al., 2017; Levin et al., 2011; Melnyk & Fineout-Overholt, 2002; Olson Keller, Strohschein, & Schaffer, 2011; Saunders & Vehviläinen-Julkunen, 2016; Spiva et al., 2017; Wallen et al., 2010).

Each agency can craft the role of the EBP mentor by first attending to the imperative components of the role that are found in Box 18.1, and can then individualize the other components that would be necessary to reap reliable best outcomes in their environments. Often, healthcare has been focused on processes, such as measurement of time from door to discharge in the emergency department or sign-in to exit for a primary care practice. EBP mentors are focused on both the outcomes of these processes and the processes themselves. These mentors assist with refining processes for the purpose of improving outcomes (Melnyk, Fineout-Overholt, Giggleman, & Cruz, 2010; Roe & Whyte-Marshall, 2011).

As systems strategists, EBP mentors (a) strategically plan, implement, and monitor/evaluate outcomes; (b) evaluate the impact of their role as EBP mentors; and (c) overcome barriers in moving to a culture of best practice (Table 18.1). These mentors play a strategic role in sustaining an EBP culture (Ervin, 2005; Fineout-Overholt & Melnyk, 2015; Fineout-Overholt, Melnyk, & Schultz, 2005; Levin et al., 2011; Melnyk & Fineout-Overholt, 2002; Melnyk et al., 2010; Morgan, 2012; Saunders & Vehviläinen-Julkunen, 2016; Wallen et al., 2010). Mentorship makes a difference (Sambunjak, Straus, & Marušic, 2006). Drs Rona Levin and Linda Olson-Keller indicated that they had taught clinicians about EBP for many years, but not until the mentor was introduced into their respective groups did the clinicians embrace the use of evidence (Levin et al., 2011). The problem was not a knowledge deficit that could not be resolved by teaching alone. What was missing was the

TABLE 18.1	Identified Barriers and Facilitators of the Evidence-Based Practice (EBP) Mentor Role	

Barriers	Facilitators
• Competing clinical priorities	• Continued contact with the mentorship program faculty
• Time	• The ability to ask questions
• Allocated resources	• The availability of assistance with data analysis
• Existing politics in the organization	• Assistance with project development
• Lack of administrative support	• A supportive chief nursing officer or director of EBP or nurse researcher
• No accountability for EBP	• A network of fellow EBP mentors
• Lack of knowledge about EBP	• EBP as an expectation of The Joint Commission and Magnet

mentoring component that moved EBP into the realm of the everyday, the expected norm for professional practice (Levin et al., 2011).

> What is experienced and seen in the clinical area is what will likely predict future behavior.
>
> **BOB BERENSON**

EVIDENCE TO SUPPORT THE POSITIVE IMPACT OF MENTORSHIP ON OUTCOMES

There is a growing body of evidence that supports the positive impact that mentors have on individual and system outcomes (Table 18.2; Abdullah et al., 2014; Bruheim, Woods, Smeland, & Nortvedt, 2014; Fineout-Overholt & Melnyk, 2015; Kim et al., 2017; Magers, 2014; Melnyk et al., 2010; Melnyk, Fineout-Overholt, Giggleman, & Choy, 2017; Roe & Whyte-Marshall, 2011; Spiva et al., 2017; Varkey et al., 2012). Findings of the 2006 systematic review of 42 mainly cross-sectional descriptive studies that evaluated the evidence about the prevalence of mentorship and its impact on career development (Sambunjak et al., 2006) continue to be relevant. This review indicated that less than 50% of medical students and, in some fields, less than 20% of faculty had mentors. Overall, individuals with mentors had significantly higher career satisfaction scores than those without mentors. Eight studies from this systematic review reported

TABLE 18.2	Evidence-Supported Outcomes of Mentoring	

Outcome	Impact
Satisfaction	⇑
Career progression/development	⇑
Self-confidence	⇑
Publications	⇑
Research	⇑
Grants	⇑

the positive influence that mentorship had on personal development and career guidance. Furthermore, 21 studies in the review described the impact of mentoring on research development and productivity. Findings indicated that mentors increased mentees' self-confidence and provided resources and support for their activities. Mentees were more productive in the number of publications and grants than those individuals without mentors. They were also more likely to complete their theses. A lack of mentorship was reported as a barrier to completing scholarly projects and publications. Mentors were viewed as an important motivating factor in pursuing a research career. Overall, the studies from this systematic review indicated that mentorship was perceived to be important for career guidance, personal development, career choice, and productivity. Despite these compelling studies, mentorship programs are not necessarily commonplace in education of health professionals (Harrington, 2011).

Adding to this body of evidence, Abdullah et al. (2014) conducted a systematic review evaluating the effectiveness of EBP mentorship on uptake and impact of EBP. These researchers found that efforts to advance EBP worked better with mentors in place. Although some studies reported EBP mentorship aided in improvement of patient outcomes, the researchers reported this was an inconsistent result across studies. Furthermore, Kim et al. (2017) found that EBP mentors who completed a fellowship program had sustained EBP Beliefs and subsequent implementation 6 months after completing the program. Mentorship is key to sustainability of EBP in organizations.

> ## Mentoring is a brain to pick, an ear to listen, and a push in the right direction.
>
> **JOHN CROSBY**

To support the benefits of mentoring in nursing, The Academy of Medical Surgical Nurses (AMSN) developed a mentoring program entitled Nurses Nurturing Nurses (N3; Grindel & Hagerstrom, 2009; Reeves, 2004). Some of the benefits of mentoring for mentors outlined by the Academy included

- development of professional colleagues, self-awareness, and interpersonal relationships;
- professional development;
- stimulation to question practice; and
- improved political skills.

In addition, benefits for those being mentored proposed within N3 included

- recipient of one-to-one nurturing;
- insight into unwritten rules and politics;
- assistance with career development;
- increased network of contacts; and
- development of self-confidence and problem-solving skills.

This program demonstrated that mentorship, as with EBP, must be part of the organizational culture. The impact of mentoring is lessened with unsustained mentorship. The AMSN continues to offer a mentoring program, complete with a mentor guide, mentee guide, and site coordinator guide to facilitate smooth program delivery (American Medical Surgical Nurses, 2017). The Institute of Medicine (2010) recommended mentorship programs for nurses as part of their recommendations for building leaders to advance health. The American Nurses Association (2017) responded by crafting a mentoring program for nurses. These initiatives dovetail with the process that hospitals must embark upon to seek Magnet status from the American Nurses Credentialing Center, which is considered the gold standard for nursing practice, and includes mechanisms for mentoring and professional development of nurses as well as succession planning (e.g., mentoring nurses into leadership roles). In the application process, examples must be provided that speak to mentoring for these purposes (American Nurses Credentialing Center, 2019). Mentorship is part of becoming a contributing member of the nurse profession. The connection between mentoring in nursing and mentoring for EBP must be made to sustain best practice.

ARCC EVIDENCE-BASED PRACTICE MENTORS: MAKING A DIFFERENCE?

Ideally, every healthcare organization would have ARCC EBP mentors who could assist staff and others to practice based on evidence to achieve better outcomes. However, some organizations, healthcare educators, and providers continue to practice as they always have—without attention to the evidence, inclusion of the patient's preferences, and with little recognition of the role of clinical expertise. Programs have been put in place to prepare staff nurses, advanced practice nurses, nurse researchers, and other healthcare providers to serve as leaders and mentors in changing organizational cultures through the promotion, implementation, and sustainability of EBP from administration to the bedside (Fineout-Overholt & Melnyk, 2015; Freisen, 2017; Gawlinski & Becker, 2012; Kim et al., 2017; Melnyk, Fineout-Overholt, Giggleman, & Choy, 2017; Spiva et al., 2017; Saunders & Vehviläinen-Julkunen, 2016; Underhill, Roper, Siefert, Boucher, & Berry, 2015). Although some of these programs evaluated three outcomes, EBP Beliefs (EBPB), EBP Implementation (EBPI), Organizational Culture & Readiness for System-wide Integration of EBP (OCRSIEP), to compare results across these programs, only EBPB and EBPI will be discussed.

These educational intervention programs fostered a shift to the EBP paradigm and had the seven-step EBP process as their basis:

1. cultivate a spirit of inquiry;
2. ask the clinically relevant question in PICOT format;
3. search for the best evidence;
4. critically appraise and synthesize the evidence;
5. plan and implement evidence;
6. evaluate the outcomes; and
7. disseminate the outcome.

Additional program foci included the implementation of what is known from a body of evidence and development of the EBP mentor role. The EBP mentors either crafted a strategic project plan for implementation back at their home organization or implemented an EBP project as part of a longitudinal, onsite mentorship program.

All of the five programs evaluated outcome of evidence-based practice beliefs (EBPB) using the 16-item EBP Beliefs (EBPB) scale (Melnyk & Fineout-Overholt, 2003a). EBPB scale responses range from 1 (strongly disagree) to 5 (strongly agree) on each of the 5-point Likert scale items. Examples of the items on the EBPB scale include (a) "I believe that EBP results in the best clinical care for patients," (b) "I am clear about the steps of EBP," and (c) "I am sure that I can implement EBP." Scoring consists of a sum for beliefs, after two negatively phrased items are reverse-scored (i.e., "I believe EBP takes too much time"; "I believe EBP is difficult"). A total score for the EBPB ranges between none (16), marginal (32), some (48), moderate (64), and very strong beliefs (80; Melnyk, Fineout-Overholt, & Mays, 2008). Each of the 16 items can be evaluated to help discern where the largest strengths and deficits are within those responding (item means less than 2.5 would require intervention). The Cronbach's alpha (i.e., reliability coefficient) across multiple groups has been consistently above 0.80.

All five programs evaluated the outcome of evidence implementation using the 18-item EBPI scale (Melnyk & Fineout-Overholt, 2003b). Program participants responded to each of 18 items on the 5-point frequency scale by indicating how often in the past 8 weeks they performed the item. Sample items include (a) used evidence to change my clinical practice, (b) shared an EBP guideline with a colleague, (c) promoted the use of EBP to my colleagues, and (d) shared the outcome data collected with colleagues. Scoring of the instrument consists of summing all 18 items with a range between 0 and 72, with none equal to 0 times within the past 8 weeks; 18 equal to *1 to 3 times* within the past 8 weeks; 36 equal to *4 to 5 times* within the past 8 weeks; 54 equal to *6 to 8 times* within the past 8 weeks; and 72 equals *greater than 8 times* within the past 8 weeks (Melnyk et al., 2008). Each of the 18 items can be evaluated to help discern the aspects of EBP that were most frequently implemented and those that were rarely implemented within the EBP mentor program (i.e., given that EBP mentors would be expected to frequently engage in evidence implementation, item means less than three would provide insight into potential opportunities to bolster knowledge and skills in EBP). The reliability coefficient of the EBPI has been consistently greater than 0.85.

All but one program had improvement in EBPI, whereas three programs showed improvement in EBPB (see Table 18.3). Fineout-Overholt and Melnyk (2015) reported that ARCC EBP mentors achieved outcomes over and above the measured EBPB and EBPI (Box 18.2), further demonstrating that EBP mentor impact can extend beyond the program completion.

One EBP mentor program (Fineout-Overholt & Melnyk, 2015) measured organizational culture using the 25-item Organizational Culture & Readiness for System-wide Integration of EBP Scale (OCRSIEP; Fineout-Overholt & Melnyk, 2006). Examples of scale items include (a) To what extent is EBP clearly described in the mission and philosophy of your institution? (b) To what extent do practitioners model EBP? and (c) To what extent are fiscal resources used to support EBP? The range of summed scores was between 25 and 125, with 25 representing *not much EBP organizational support for an EBP culture*; 50 representing *marginal organizational support for an EBP culture*; 75 representing *some organizational support for an EBP culture*; 100 representing *moderate organizational support for an EBP culture*; and 125 representing *full (system-wide) organizational support for an EBP culture*. The EBP mentors' OCRSIEP scores were compared with a similar sample of EBP workshop participants and found to have a slightly higher mean (83 [SD = 16] and 80 [SD = 18], respectively). The EBP mentors perceived their organizations to fall between some and moderate organizational support for EBP. This is an expected finding in that organizations that already support the formal role of EBP mentor would reasonably provide organizational support for system-wide EBP. Although it is encouraging to find that organizations with EBP mentors have moderate support for EBP, these findings indicate that healthcare systems in which these EBP mentors work still have room for growth to establish a sustained culture of EBP.

Findings from the evaluation of these ARCC EBP mentor programs indicated that mentors were able to strengthen and sustain their EBP Beliefs and increase EBPI, despite some organizational challenges. With a strong focus on education and skills-building during the educational interventions, the participants were equipped to implement into clinical practice the EBP knowledge and skills that they learned. These programs have done a great job of careful documentation of outcomes, which role models for their EBP mentors how to demonstrate their impact on patient care, system outcomes, and the care practices of their colleagues. Given the results from this educational intervention across these four programs designed specifically for developing EBP mentors to operationalize the ARCC model, and the other evidentiary support for mentoring clinicians, the charge is for all healthcare settings to determine how best they can actualize EBP mentors in their environments to foster best outcomes for patients, providers, and systems.

TABLE
18.3 *Evidence Demonstrates Impact of Evidence-Based Practice (EBP) Mentor Programs*

Home Area	No. in Project or Study	Program Contents*	Evaluation Measures	Findings	Study
Northeast	112	• EBP process with exemplars • EBP language • Offered 20 minute sessions on units (as you go) and online educational module • Involvement in ongoing EBP projects • Time frame unreported	EBPB EBPI	• EBPB • T1 median = 56.5 • T2 median = 57 • EBPI: • T1 median = 11 • T2 median = 12 • Time between T1 & T2 unreported	Underhill et al. (2015)
Southwest	38	• EBP Process • EBP Language • EBP Culture • EBP Mentor Network • EBP Project Plan • Personal Growth • 5-day Program	EBPB EBPI OCRSIEP	• EBPB • T1 = 61 (SD = 7.4) • T2 = 68 (SD = 6.2) • EBPI • T1 = 19 (SD = 13.2) • T2 = 55 (SD = 18.6) • Time between T1 & T2 = at least 1 year	Fineout-Overholt Melnyk (2015)
Midwest	83	• EBP Process • EBP Project Implementation • EBP Model operationalized • 16-week program	EBPB EBPI	• EBPB • T1 (N = 83) = 64.54 (SD = 7.72) • T2 (N = 57) = 65.89 (SD = 9.8) • EBPI • T1 (N = 83) 32.9 (12.5) • T2 (N = 57) 36.9 (17.39)† • Time between T1 & T2 = 16 weeks	Friesen, Brady, Milligan, and Christensen (2017)

West	120	• EBP Process • EBP Project Implementation • 9-month program (3 cohorts across 2 years)	EBPB EBPI	EBPB • T1 = 61.7 (SD = 7.12) • T2 = 67.3 (SD = 6.01)† EBPI • T1 = 15.0 (SD = 12.7) • T2 = 24.8 (SD = 13.7)† • Time between T1 & T2 = 9 months	Kim et al. (2017)
West	45	• EBP Process • EBP Project Implementation • 12-month program • Interprofessional project teams	EBPB EBPI OCRSIEP	EBPB • T1 = 60.7 (SD = 7.6) • T2 = 64.9 (SD = 6.7)† EBPI • T1 = 17.8 (SD = 10.3) • T2 = 51.9 (SD = 16.8)† • Time between T1 & T2 = 12 months	Melnyk et al. (2017)

* Not all programs listed called their programs EBP mentor programs, but did foster same outcomes and used similar methods.

† Statistically significant.

EBPB, EBP Beliefs; EBPI, EBP implementation; OCRSIEP, Organizational culture & readiness for system-wide integration of EBP.

BOX
18.2

Impact of Evidence-Based Practice (EBP) Mentor Educational Intervention

EBP mentors reported that they were able to:

- Become more influential
- Speak more intelligently about evidence
- Improve outcomes
- Formulate the question and find the evidence
- Read research
- Lead EBP initiatives (e.g., through gaining promotions that facilitated their influence on organizational change)
- Advance their education through returning to school
- Provide valued contributions to care
- Serve as sought-after consultants/resources for EBP

Southwest EBP Mentorship Program

EBP FAST FACTS

- EBP mentors are central to a sustainable EBP culture.
- Engaging in specific education designed to prepare EBP mentors can demonstrate a return on the investment through improved organizational patient, provider, and system outcomes.
- Evidence supports preparation and impact of EBP mentors.

WANT TO KNOW MORE?

A variety of resources are available to enhance your learning and understanding of this chapter.

- Visit thePoint° to access:
  - Appendix H: System-Wide ARCC Model EBP Mentor Role Description
  - Articles from the AJN EBP Step-By-Step Series
  - Journal articles
  - Checklists for rapid critical appraisal and more!
- Lippincott CoursePoint combines digital text content with video case studies and interactive modules for a fully integrated course solution that works the way you study and learn.

References

Abdullah, G., Rossy, D., Ploeg, J., Davies, B., Higuchi, K., Sikora, L., & Stacey, D. (2014). Measuring the effectiveness of mentoring as a knowledge translation intervention for implementing empirical evidence: A systematic review. *Worldviews on Evidence-Based Nursing, 11*(5), 284–300.

Abedin, Z., Biskup, E., Silet, K., Garbutt, J., Kroenke, K., Feldman, M. D., . . . Pincus, H. A. (2012). Deriving competencies for mentors of clinical and translational scholars. *Clinical Translational Science, 5*(3), 273–280. doi:10.1111/j.1752-8062.2011.00366.x

American Medical Surgical Nurses. (2017). *AMSN mentoring program.* Retrieved on January 2, 2018, from https://www.amsn.org/professional-development/mentoring

American Nurses Association. (2017). *ANA mentoring program.* Retrieved on January 3, 2018, from http://www.ananursespace.org/pages/mentorprogram?ssopc=1

American Nurses Credentialing Center. (2019). *The magnet application manual.* Silver Spring, MD: Author.

Bruheim, M., Woods, K. V., Smeland, S., & Nortvedt, M. V. (2014). An educational program to transition oncology nurses at the Norwegian Radium Hospital to an evidence-based practice model: Development, implementation, and preliminary outcomes. *Journal of Cancer Education, 29,* 224–232.

Christenbery, T., Williamson, A., & Wells, N. (2016). Immersion in evidence-based practice fellowship program: A transforming experience for staff nurses. *Journal of Nurses Professional Development, 32*(1), 15–20.

Ervin, N. E. (2005). Clinical coaching: A strategy for enhancing evidence-based nursing practice. *CNS, 19*(6), 296–301.

Fineout-Overholt, E., Levin, R., & Melnyk, B. (2013). Defining mentorship for EBP. In R. Levin & H. Feldman's (Eds.) *Teaching Evidence-based Practice in Nursing: A Guide for Academic & Clinical Settings.* New York, Springer.

Fineout-Overholt, E., & Melnyk, B. (2006). *Organizational culture & readiness for system-wide integration of evidence-based practice.* Gilbert, AZ: ARCC Publishing.

Fineout-Overholt, E., & Melnyk, B. M. (2015). ARCC evidence-based practice mentors: The key to sustaining evidence-based practice. In B. Melnyk & E. Fineout-Overholt (Eds.), *Evidence-based practice in nursing & healthcare: A guide to best practice* (3rd ed.). Philadelphia, PA: Wolters Kluwer.

Fineout-Overholt, E., Melnyk, B. M., & Schultz, A. (2005). Transforming healthcare from the inside out: Advancing evidence-based practice in the 21st century. *Journal of Professional Nursing, 21*(6), 335–344.

Fineout-Overholt, E., Williamson, K. M., Gallagher-Ford, L., Melnyk, B. M., & Stillwell, S. B. (2011). Following the evidence: Planning for sustainable change. *American Journal of Nursing, 111*(1), 54–60.

Fleming, M., House, S., Hanson, V. S., Yu, L., Garbutt, J., McGee, R., . . . Rubio, D. M. (2013). The Mentoring Competency Assessment: Validation of a new instrument to evaluate skills of research mentors. *Academic Medicine: Journal of the Association of American Medical Colleges, 88*(7), 1002–1008.

Frantsve-Hawley, J. & Meyer, D. (2008).The Evidence-Based Dentistry Champions: A Grassroots Approach to the Implementation of EBD. *Journal of Evidence-based Dental Practice, 8,* 64–69.

Friesen, M. A., Brady, J. M., Milligan, R., & Christensen, P. (2017). Findings from a pilot study: Bringing evidence-based practice to the bedside. *Worldviews on Evidence-Based Nursing, 14*(1), 22–34.

Gallagher-Ford, L., Fineout-Overholt, E., Melnyk, B. M., & Stillwell, S. (2011). Implementing an evidence-based practice change: Beginning the transformation from an idea to reality. *American Journal of Nursing, 111*(3), 54–60.

Gawlinski, A., & Becker, E. (2012). Infusing research into practice: A staff nurse evidence-based practice fellowship program. *Journal for Nurses in Staff Development, 28*(2), 69–73.

Grindel, C. G., & Hagerstrom, G. (2009). Nurses nurturing nurses: Outcomes and lessons learned. *MEDSURG Nursing, 18*(3), 183–194.

Harrington, S. (2011). Mentoring new nurse practitioners to accelerate their development as primary care providers: A literature review. *Journal of the American Academy of Nurse Practitioners, 23*(4), 168–174.

Holliman, J., Resler, R., Edmunds, T., & Child Life Council. (2010). *The leaders of the pack: Three EBP models used in pediatric settings.* Retrieved from http://citeseerx.ist.psu.edu/viewdoc/download;jsessionid=D9DD77BDADEBCB311FFFC5919EDC6468?doi=10.1.1.689.5561&rep=rep1&type=pdf

Institute of Medicine. (2010). *The future of nursing: Leading change, advancing health.* Washington, DC: Institute of Medicine of the National Academies Press.

Kim, S. C., Ecoff, L., Brown, C. E., Gallo, A. M., Stichler, J., & Davidson, J. (2017). Benefits of a regional evidence-based practice fellowship program: A test of the ARCC model. *Worldviews on Evidence-Based Nursing, 14*(2), 90–98.

Levin, R. F., Fineout-Overholt, E., Melnyk, B. M., Barnes, M., & Vetter, M. J. (2011). Fostering evidence-based practice to improve nurse and cost outcomes in a community health setting: A pilot test of the advancing research and clinical practice through close collaboration model. *Nursing Administration Quarterly, 35*(1), 21–33.

Magers, T. L. (2014). An EBP mentor and unit-based EBP team: A strategy for successful implementation of a practice change to reduce catheter-associated urinary tract infections. *Worldviews on Evidence-Based Nursing, 11*(5), 341–343.

Mariano, K., Caley, L., Eschberger, L., Woloszyn, A., Volker, P., Leonard, M., & Tung, Y. (2011). Building evidence-based practice with staff nurses through mentoring. *Journal of Neonatal Nursing, 15,* 81–87.

Maxwell, J. (2015, July 1). *3 ways my mentors have changed my life.* [Web log post]. Retrieved on January 1, 2018 from http://www.johnmaxwell.com/blog/3-ways-my-mentors-have-changed-my-life

Melnyk, B. M. (2007). The evidence-based practice mentor: A promising strategy for implementing and sustaining EBP in healthcare systems. *Worldviews on Evidence-Based Nursing, 4*(3), 123–125.

Melnyk, B., & Fineout-Overholt, E. (2003a). *Evidence-based practice beliefs scale.* Rochester, NY: ARCC Publishing.

Melnyk, B., & Fineout-Overholt, E. (2003b). *Evidence-based practice implementation scale.* Rochester, NY: ARCC Publishing.

Melnyk, B., & Fineout-Overholt, E. (2010). ARCC (Advancing Research and Clinical practice through close Collaboration): A model for system-wide implementation & sustainability of evidence-based practice. In J. Rycroft-Malone & T. Bucknall (Eds.), *Models and frameworks for implementing evidence-based practice*. Indianapolis, IN: Wiley-Blackwell & Sigma Theta Tau International.

Melnyk, B. M., & Fineout-Overholt, E. (2002). Putting research into practice. *Reflections on Nursing Leadership, 28*(2), 22–25.

Melnyk, B. M., Fineout-Overholt, E., Feinstein, N., Li, H. S., Small, L., Wilcox, L., & Kraus, R. (2004). Nurses' perceived knowledge, beliefs, skills, and needs regarding evidence-based practice: Implications for accelerating the paradigm shift. *Worldviews on Evidence-Based Nursing, 1*(3), 185–193.

Melnyk, B. M., Fineout-Overholt, E., Gallagher-Ford, L., & Stillwell, S. (2011). Evidence-based practice, step by step: Sustaining evidence-based practice through organizational policies and an innovative model. *American Journal of Nursing, 111*(9), 57–60.

Melnyk, B. M., Fineout-Overholt, E., Giggleman, M., & Choy, K. (2017). Test of the ARCC model improves implementation of evidence-based practice, healthcare culture, and patient outcomes. *Worldviews on Evidence-Based Nursing, 14*(1), 5–9.

Melnyk, B. M., Fineout-Overholt, E., Giggleman, M., & Cruz, R. (2010). Correlates among cognitive beliefs, EBP implementation, organizational culture, cohesion and job satisfaction in evidence-based practice mentors from a community hospital system. *Nursing Outlook, 58*(6), 301–308.

Melnyk, B. M., Fineout-Overholt, E., & Mays, M. (2008). The evidence-based practice beliefs and implementation scales: Psychometric properties of two new instruments. *Worldviews on Evidence-Based Nursing, 5*(4), 208–216.

Melnyk, B. M., Gallagher-Ford, L., Long, L. E., & Fineout-Overholt, E. (2014). The establishment of evidence-based practice competencies for practicing registered nurses and advanced practice nurses in real-world clinical settings: Proficiencies to improve healthcare quality, reliability, patient outcomes, and costs. *Worldviews on Evidence-Based Nursing, 11*(1), 5–15.

Morgan, L. (2012). A mentoring model for evidence-based practice in a community hospital. *Journal for Nurses in Staff Development, 28*(5), 233–237.

Nick, J., Delahoyde, T., Del Prato, D., Mitchell, C., Ortiz, J., Ottley, C., . . . Siktberg, L. (2012). Best practices in academic mentoring: A model for excellence. *Nursing Research and Practice, 2012*, 937906, 9. doi:10.1155/2012/937906

Olson Keller, L., Strohschein, S., & Schaffer, M. (2011). Cornerstones of public health nursing. *Public Health Nursing, 28*(3), 249–260.

Reeves, K. A. (2004). Nurses nurturing nurses: A mentoring program. *Nurse Leader, 2*(6), 47–54.

Roe, E., & Whyte-Marshall, M. (2011). Mentoring for evidence-based practice: A collaborative approach. *Journal for Nurses in Staff Development, 28*(4), 177–181.

Sambunjak, D., Straus, S. E., & Marušic, A. (2006). Mentoring in academic medicine: A systematic review. *The Journal of the American Medical Association, 296*(9), 1103–1115.

Saunders, H., & Vehviläinen-Julkunen, K. (2016). Nurses' evidence-based practice beliefs and the role of evidence-based practice mentors at University Hospitals in Finland. *Worldviews on Evidence-Based Nursing, 14*(1), 35–45.

Shifaza, F., Evans, D., Bradley, H., Ullrich, S. (2013). Developing evidence-based practice champions in the Maldives. *International Journal of Nursing Practice, 19*, 596–602.

Spiva, L. A., Hart, P. L., Patrick, S., Waggoner, J., Jackson, C., & Threatt, J. L. (2017). Effectiveness of an evidence-based practice nurse mentor training program. *Worldviews on Evidence-Based Nursing, 14*(3), 183–191.

Tobin, M. J. (2004). Mentoring: Seven roles and some specifics. *American Journal of Respiratory and Critical Care Medicine, 170*, 114–117.

Underhill, M., Roper, K., Siefert, M. L., Boucher, J., & Berry, D. (2015). Evidence-based practice beliefs and implementation before and after an initiative to promote evidence-based nursing in an ambulatory oncology setting. *Worldviews on Evidence-Based Nursing, 12*(2), 70–78.

Varkey, P., Jato, A., Williams, A., Mayer, Al., Ko, M., Files, J., . . . Hayes, S. (2012). The positive impact of a facilitated peer mentoring program on academic skills of women faculty. *BMC Medical Education, 12*, 14.

Wallen, G. R., Mitchell, S. A., Melnyk, B. M., Fineout-Overholt, E., Miller-Davis, C., Yates, J., & Hastings, C. (2010). Implementing evidence-based practice: Effectiveness of a structured multifaceted mentorship programme. *Journal of Advanced Nursing, 66*(12), 2761–2771.

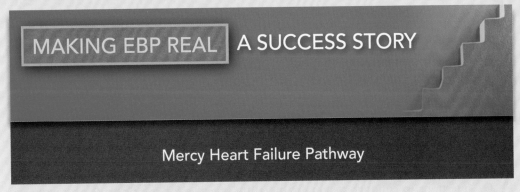

Mercy Heart Failure Pathway

Robin Kretschman, H.C.-M.B.A., M.S.N., R.N., N.E.A.-B.C

The Impetus for Designing Pathways as a New Care Delivery Strategy

The national vital statistics report lists heart disease as the leading cause of death in 2015 (CDC, 2016). Heart failure represents a large segment of this population and was therefore chosen as the pilot for the Mercy pathway strategy.

The challenges facing healthcare today demand innovations and operational diligence. The cost per capita amount spent on healthcare in America is $10,345 (PBS, 2016). Although we spend more money on healthcare than do other nations, we "die sooner and experience more illness than residents in many other countries" (IOM Committee on Population, Division of Behavioral and Social Sciences and Education, 2013, p. 20). Healthcare reform is a challenge to develop a more efficient and effective healthcare process.

The current healthcare environment is the impetus for this change. From a healthcare reform perspective, the Affordable Care Act, Value-Based Purchasing, Readmission Reduction, Healthcare-Associated Conditions reduction, Hospital Compare measures, Accountable Care organizations, Medical and Health Homes, and Meaningful Use were all designed to challenge healthcare organizations and providers to redesign care delivery.

Setting

The setting for the pathway work is Mercy, the sixth largest Catholic healthcare system in the United States at the time of this project, a complex system spanning four states and the entire healthcare continuum with 32 hospitals (4,571 beds) and over 300 outpatient facilities, 5,320 physicians on the medical staff, 1,900 clinic physicians, and over 12,000 nurses. Pathways support each of these clinicians.

STEP 0 — Cultivate a Spirit of Inquiry & EBP Culture

The work begins with an evaluation of diagnosis-related groupings (DRGs). Pathways chosen for development meet specific criteria: populations with high patient volumes, similar treatment needs, and foreseeable benefits. These are evaluated in conjunction with the cost of care.

Once a patient population is selected for the pathway approach, nurse and physician specialists are identified from across the organization to serve as pathway leads. Master's-prepared nurses with specialty and clinical workflow expertise are selected as pathway leads and then equipped with EBP mentor skills and lean training. These coworkers assemble the evidence, define patient outcomes and daily goals, and then partner with physician leads to make evidence-based recommendations. Comprehensive pathways are then built into the electronic health record (EHR).

STEP 1 Ask the PICO(T) Question

The target audience for Mercy Heart Failure Pathways is the 35,000 patients in the Mercy service area with heart failure. Competencies for the pathway lead role include being able to define the clinical questions associated with a population, using PICOT questions to conduct systematic literature searches for components of a pathway. The question arises, In heart failure patients, how does system-wide implementation of an interprofessional care pathways compared to having no pathways affect patient outcomes, such as include length of stay, readmission rates, direct care variable costs, and compliance/utilization of pathways within the first quarter after implementation?

STEP 2 Search for the Best Evidence

Nurses participate in an EBP immersion that allows them to hone the skills required to assemble the pathway content. A key tactic used for pathway development is a 14-16 week production cycle. Leveraging lean methodologies and the manufacturing discipline, Mercy has invested in a performance acceleration department dedicated to supporting the pathway leads. Time is allocated to develop EBP knowledge, skills, and competencies. Time is also allocated to compile the evidence. Nurses' positions in patient care units are backfilled to free them up for the production cycle.

STEP 3 Critically Appraise the Evidence

The EBP immersion focus includes critically appraising the research, including evaluation, synthesizing, and crafting recommendations from the body of evidence. The work to be done is mapped out in flow sheets, and all resources are brought to bear to create the most efficient and effective process.

STEP 4 Integrate the Evidence with Your Clinical Expertise and Patient Preferences to Make the Best Clinical Decision

Nurses, physicians, librarians, pharmacists, ancillary leaders, administrative assistants, clinical informatics specialists, and information technology specialists are all identified as members of a collaborative team: the right people with the right expertise doing the right work at the right time. Many of the typical barriers associated with implementing EBP are eliminated using this approach.

STEP 5 Evaluate the Outcomes(s) of the EBP Practice Change

Mercy's own analysis of supply cost trends, the cost of providing care trends, avoidable costs, and projections of shifts in payer mixes clearly articulate a need to create systems that address the key clinical drivers of optimal outcomes.

Between June 2012 and September 2013, 24 pathways were deployed using this strategy.

As the pathway is constructed, the team identifies the appropriate clinical, operational, and financial outcomes associated with each pathway. A data warehouse and real-time feeds are then used to provide the most up-to-date measures.

Measures tracked for all pathways include length of stay, readmission rates, direct care variable costs, and compliance/utilization of pathways. Unique, critical-to-process, and specialty-specific measures are also tracked. For heart failure, this includes hours to first order, hours to a diuretic, severity index, and mortality risk.

Achieving a standard of care across a large population will enable us to conduct regression studies, determine key clinical drivers, and utilize feedback loops to improve the interventions included on the pathway.

STEP 6　　## Disseminate the Outcome(s)

Communication and information flow are crucial to the project's success. In addition to the EHR, an intranet site houses a pathway library and pathway dashboards. The library provides detailed information about each pathway, including the EBP references used to determine physician orders, nursing interventions, daily patient goals, documentation requirements, and tasks associated with the care.

Dashboard reporting tracks outcomes and provides a mechanism for Mercy benchmarking, providing valuable information. Pathway measures are reviewed by executives, operations teams, and physicians. Additionally, leaders are incentivized to assure pathway success.

In the heart failure population, this process has reduced length of stay and cost of care as well as successfully reduced variation in care. As the first organization to leverage electronic pathway functionality for complex conditions and chronic progressive diseases, there are many opportunities to publish.

Strategy for Sustainable EBP Integration

Evidence-based pathways built into the EHR is the strategy Mercy has adopted to meet the challenges of the future. Between June 2012 and September 2013, 24 pathways were deployed using this strategy.

Pathways typically focus on stable, predictable conditions. Mercy pathways go beyond stable conditions to address complex conditions and chronic progressive diseases. The Mercy pathway development process combines EBP, electronic functionality, and lean and manufacturing discipline with collaborative specialty teams that integrate evidence into practice.

The EHR has become so much more than a longitudinal record of patient health information for one or more encounters. It is the basis of healthcare business intelligence, providing the data required for clinical and financial analysis.

As the primary vehicle for interdisciplinary communication, decision support, and care planning, the EHR is a key component in the Mercy strategy for EBP integration. To assure that decision support within the EHR is current best practice, a team responsible for content development makes up the second major component in this strategy.

As a national leader in EHR implementation, physician integration, and adoption of Meaningful Use measures, Mercy was in a perfect position to integrate EBP through technology.

No longer viewed apart from our work, technology is core to the work of healthcare; the EHR automates portions of the clinicians' workflow, provides communication channels and information flow, captures discrete data, and generates the legal medical record. Decisions support based on the evidence is embedded in the electronic system to direct clinicians to needed interventions.

Pathways are only one component of the larger effort to create care paths across the continuum. The principles used to identify evidence and create lean clinical and electronic workflow are being used in emergency departments, care management, ambulatory settings, and the chronic disease center. An interactive patient portal completes the tools used to coordinate care across the continuum.

References

Centers for Disease Control and Prevention, National Center for Health Statistics. (2016, December). Multiple cause of death 1999-2015 on CDC WONDER online database. Data are from the Multiple Cause of Death Files, 1999-2015, as compiled from data provided by the 57 vital statistics jurisdictions through the Vital Statistics Cooperative Program. Retrieved from http://wonder.cdc.gov/mcd-icd10.html

IOM Committee on Population, Division of Behavioral and Social Sciences and Education. (2013). *U.S. health in international perspective: Shorter lives, poorer health.* Washington, DC: The National Academies Press.

PBS. (2016, July 13). $10,345 per person: U.S. health care spending reaches new peak. Retrieved from https://www.pbs.org/newshour/health/new-peak-us-health-care-spending-10345-per-person

Step Six: Disseminating Evidence and Evidence-Based Practice Implementation Outcomes

You see, in life, lots of people know what to do, but few people actually do what they know. Knowing is not enough! You must take action.

—*Tony Robbins*

EBP Terms to Learn
BOPPS model
Evidence-based practice
  competencies
Elevator speech
Evidence-informed health
  policy
Health policy
Health policy making
Journal clubs
Organizational policies
Policy

UNIT OBJECTIVES

Upon completion of this unit, learners will be able to:

1 Discuss how to use evidence to influence organizational and health policy.

2 Describe key strategies for disseminating evidence through oral and poster presentations, publications, the media, and health policy briefs.

MAKING CONNECTIONS: AN EBP EXEMPLAR

The interprofessional team who worked on the successful implementation of the evidence-based fall prevention program was ecstatic to see the outcomes of its work, including a substantial reduction in falls, an increase in patient satisfaction rates, and major cost savings for its hospital. Members of the team were determined to ensure sustainability of the new evidence-based protocol by disseminating the outcomes to the interprofessional collaborative organizational policy committee so that a change in hospital policy on fall prevention would be made (*Step 6: Disseminate Project Outcomes*). The group had another planning meeting to determine who would be responsible for making an oral presentation of the outcomes to the policy committee. During this meeting, team members also discussed other routes for dissemination of their project's outcomes. These included grand rounds at their hospital; statewide, regional, and national conferences held by their professional associations; and a manuscript that would be submitted for publication. Lei, the project coordinator, suggested that their project might also get some local media attention, so the group decided to talk with their hospital's marketing and communication team about writing a press release about the project and its impactful outcomes that could be disseminated to local media.

The group decided that Lei and the hospital's chief qualify officer, Dr. Ayita, would make the presentation to the policy committee. Lei contacted the chair of the policy committee, who agreed to place them on the agenda for the next monthly policy meeting. Lei and Dr. Ayita made an outline of their 20-minute presentation and decided that Lei would deliver the background, aims, PICOT question, and the evidence that was found to answer the PICOT question. Dr. Ayita agreed to present the project's outcome data, which would provide strong rationale for the change in hospital policy that they would recommend to conclude the presentation. Dr. Ayita offered to create their PowerPoint presentation, which would be comprised of 20 slides (1 minute of presentation per slide). They asked the rest of the team if they would be willing to listen to a "practice presentation" and give constructive feedback to improve it before the meeting with the policy committee. The team enthusiastically agreed.

Lei and Dr. Ayita's presentation to the policy committee was a smashing success. Members of the policy committee were impressed at the quality of the body of evidence that was presented by Lei that substantiated the project's practice change and the outstanding outcomes that were described by Dr. Ayita. The committee unanimously agreed that a policy change was warranted and committed themselves to making that happen in the next few months.

The group then strategized on who would take the lead in developing abstracts for upcoming statewide, regional, and national conferences. They decided that all the members of the team who were responsible for developing, implementing, and evaluating the project would be included as authors on all conference abstracts and a paper for publication. Dr. Reyansh volunteered to take the lead in writing a manuscript of the project's outcomes with the team's hearty approval, because she was an accomplished writer with several publications to her credit. After the discussion, the group decided to target the "Implementing EBP in Real World Practice Settings" column in the journal *Worldviews on Evidence-Based Nursing* for their publication. Dr. Reyansh drafted an outline for the paper; some team members volunteered to write sections, and others agreed to review it and provide constructive feedback. They also made a commitment to write and submit the paper in the next 90 days. A week after contacting the hospital's marketing and communication department, a press release was issued, and, to the team's delight, one of the local TV stations picked up the story and featured their project on the local news channel. One year later, a total of five presentations had been delivered at professional conferences by the team members, and their paper was accepted for publication in *Worldviews on Evidence-Based Nursing!*

The C-Suite executives were so pleased with this practice change and its resultant return on investment that a decision was made to provide additional funds to the EBP committee to continue focusing on evidence-based quality improvement projects that would improve outcomes. The entire experience so enthused all the team members that they decided to immediately tackle another important project within their hospital—the high readmission rates for patients with heart failure. The interprofessional team learned firsthand that EBP really does make a difference in enhancing the patient experience and quality of healthcare, improving population health outcomes, decreasing costs, and empowering clinicians so that they are fully inspired and engaged to make a positive impact—in other words, achieving the quadruple aim in healthcare.

Jacqueline M. Loversidge and Cheryl L. Boyd

> Pretending that politics and science do not coexist is foolish, and cleanly separating science from politics is probably neither feasible nor recommended.
>
> —Madelon Lubin Finkel

EBP Terms to Learn

Evidence-based practice competencies (EBP)

Evidence-informed health policy (EIHP)

Health policy

Interprofessional collaboration

Organizational policy

Learning Objectives

After studying this chapter, learners will be able to:

1. Identify the differences between the clinical environment and the health policy environment relative to the evidence-based practice (EBP) process, focusing on the dissemination of evidence.

2. Describe two methods to prepare evidence for dissemination to influence health policy makers.

3. Discuss leadership strategies that support application of the EBP process in the development of organizational policies.

The use of evidence-based practice (EBP) as the preeminent process for addressing clinical problems has been the major emphasis of this book. However, there are times when the reach of clinical problems and their real or potential evidence-based solutions extends beyond the immediate clinical setting. This chapter focuses on dissemination from the perspective of using health science–related evidence to influence policy—at both the macro and the micro levels.

Content in the first part of this chapter covers the use of evidence to influence health policy-making. This requires some modification of the EBP process, because of the differences between clinical settings and health policy settings. The differences necessitating these modifications are explained, and an Evidence-informed Health Policy (EIHP) model, adapted from the Melnyk and Fineout-Overholt EBP Model (2015) to meet the unique challenges of the health policy milieu, is outlined. Then, using the EIHP model, methods for disseminating evidence to influence policy makers (e.g., in policy briefs and in testimony) are described.

The second half of this chapter dwells on using evidence to effect change in organizational policy. Utilization of interprofessional evidence-based hospital policy committee structures and processes, involving an emphasis on EBP competency and effective interprofessional teamwork, is described. The role of an organization's policy and procedure committee, to develop and disseminate patient care policies that improve patient care through the conscientious use of best evidence in combination with a clinician's expertise as well as patient preferences and values, is explained. In that venue, policy committee leaders are responsible for assessing the EBP competency of the members and advancing the committee's EBP knowledge, skills, and attitudes that form the foundation of policy committees' enculturation; methods for accomplishing this are described.

USING EVIDENCE TO INFLUENCE HEALTH POLICY

Traditionally, legislators have looked to a variety of sources of information to inform policy-making. Their own opinions influence how they write policy and how they vote. However, they must listen to appeals from constituents, professional associations, and business-related organizations, in addition to keeping their own counsel. Solid evidence can serve as a fulcrum for stakeholders involved in the policy-making process and provide essential information to guide decision making.

What Is Health Policy?

Both the healthcare and policy environments in which health professionals function are rapidly changing. **Health policy** can have profound effects on healthcare consumers, practice, and organizations. Therefore, it is incumbent on health professionals to understand the health policy process and how evidence can be used to influence health policy-making.

The term *policy* is often used as an umbrella term to describe both the *entity* and the *process*. As an *entity*, policy is a tangible result. At the government level, it is often the outcome of lawmaking (e.g., federal law, state law, or municipal code), rulemaking (e.g., executive-branch government agency regulation), or other governmental process and can include judicial decrees, position statements, resolutions, and budget priorities (Milstead, 2016). Government-established policy is enforceable by law. Other kinds of broad health policies may be published by nongovernmental organizations (e.g., national evidence-based clinical guidelines); these are not enforceable by law but have tremendous effects on the healthcare environment. At the organizational level, formal documented directives become "policy" for the organization.

As a *process*, policy-making is the series of actions and activities taken to bring a problem to the attention of (generally) government actors who work to address the problem (Milstead, 2016). When policy refers to health policy specifically, these products and courses of action have historically been thought of as those targeting improvements for the health of populations (Niessen, Grijseels, & Rutten, 2000).

Challenges Unique to the Relationship Between Evidence and Health Policy

Policy-making is a notoriously nonlinear process and often relies more on politics than evidence. Policy-making is influenced by social and political factors, including partisanship, diverse stakeholder values, public opinion, media coverage, timing of congressional and legislative cycles, budget restraints, strategy and skill of the players, and a host of other factors (Lanier, 2016; Milstead, 2016; Shamian & Shamian-Ellen, 2011). Because the policy-making environment is so complex, gaps are evident between scientific evidence to inform policy and policy as enacted. However, the stakes in healthcare policy are high; therefore, it is essential to disseminate policy-relevant evidence by methods that capture policy makers' attention.

It is equally important to be realistic about the boundaries of the uses of evidence in policy-making. Whereas in clinical settings, it is essential, and often possible, to press for practice based on evidence, in political environments this approach may result in less favorable outcomes. There has been a trajectory in the development of the term *evidence-informed* policy-making since the turn of the millennium, by both American and international authors; this is the term that is used now, rather than evidence-based policy-making, for three reasons (Loversidge, 2016b). First, it acknowledges that the use of evidence in health policy is indirect; it is best used to inform, influence, or mediate dialogue between policy makers and stakeholders (Campbell et al., 2009; Elliott & Popay, 2004; Lavis et al., 2009; Morgan, 2010). Second, it recognizes the rapidly changing and often inflexible policy milieu, which may be influenced by factors such as legislative cycle timing or budget limits (Bowen & Zwi, 2005; Jewell & Bero, 2008). Third, the use of *evidence-informed* in reference to policy-making is the emerging global standard term (Lavis et al., 2009; World Health Organization, 2016).

ADAPTING THE EBP MODEL FOR IMPACT IN HEALTH POLICY: AN EVIDENCE-INFORMED HEALTH POLICY MODEL

Policy makers need credible evidence to make sound policy; they are more likely to respond positively to evidence when it is presented in a way that is *compelling, understandable, and conveyed in the context of citizen/constituent needs* (Loversidge, 2016a). EBP models are useful to prepare a body of evidence to disseminate to policy makers, in principle, because EBP models are process models and are therefore adaptable. However, some adjustments need to be made for EBP to be useful in policy settings. This is because of the unique environment in which policy is made. In addition, the *problem* is one of policy, not a clinical problem. As a result, the way the question is asked, the focus of evidence retrieval and appraisal, and how evidence is integrated with the other two components of the model (see Table 19.1) affect dissemination of findings to policy makers and other stakeholders.

The Melnyk and Fineout-Overholt EBP Model (2015) is readily adaptable for use in policy settings with some modifications because (1) the three EBP components are transferable from the clinical experience to the political experience; and (2) the seven process-focused steps are comparable. This modified model, an **Evidence-informed Health Policy (EIHP)** model, "... *combines the use*

TABLE 19.1	*Comparison of Evidence-Based Practice and Evidence-Informed Health Policy Components*
Evidence-Based Practice Components	**Evidence-Informed Health Policy Components**
External evidence	External evidence
• Research, evidence-based theories, and best evidence from opinion leaders and expert panels	• Adds best evidence from *relevant government and private data sources*
Clinical expertise (i.e., Internal evidence)	*Issue* expertise (Internal evidence)
• Outcomes management, or evidence-based quality improvement project data, patient or staff survey data, etc.	• Adds data from *professional associations, healthcare organizations, professions' understanding or experience with the health policy issue, etc.*
Patient values and preferences	*Stakeholder* values and *ethics*
• Patients and care partners	• Includes *policy shapers/makers, healthcare providers, consumers, consumer protection groups, government agencies responsible for implementation, etc.*

Source: Components of EIHP adapted from The Components of EBP used with permission from: Melnyk, B. M., & Fineout-Overholt, E. (2015). *Evidence-based practice in nursing and healthcare: A guide to best practice* (3rd ed., p. 4). Philadelphia, PA: Lippincott Williams & Wilkins; Table adapted from Loversidge, J. M. (2016). An evidence-informed health policy model: Adapting evidence-based practice for nursing education and regulation. *Journal of Nursing Regulation, 7*(2), 29. doi:10.1016/S2155-8256(16)31075-4

of the best available evidence and issue expertise with stakeholder values and ethics to inform and leverage dialogue toward the best possible health policy agenda and improvements" (Loversidge, 2016a, p. 27).

Comparing the Three Components

Like the EBP model, the EIHP model consists of three components. Both models rely on *external evidence*, but in the EIHP model, external evidence may be additionally enhanced by relevant government or private data sources. Modifications to the second component are more apparent; *internal evidence* focuses on expertise around the *policy issue* and may come from individual healthcare providers, their associations/organizations, or from government agencies (e.g., executive-branch agencies), as well as other available internal data sources. Finally, rather than patient values and preferences, the EIHP model relies on the *values and ethics of stakeholders*. Stakeholders may include healthcare providers, policy makers or shapers, healthcare consumers or interest groups, government executive-branch agencies responsible for implementation, and others (Loversidge, 2016a). Table 19.1 compares the major elements of the three components, with differences italicized.

Comparing the Steps of EBP and EIHP

The seven steps of EBP are found in Chapter 1 (p. 10). The eight steps of the EIHP process are comparable to the steps of EBP. The eight steps, with differences in italics, are as follows:

Step 0: Cultivate a spirit of inquiry *within the policy culture/environment.*

Step 1: Identify the *policy problem* and *ask the policy question* in PICOT format.

Step 2: Search for and collect the most relevant best evidence.

Step 3: Critically appraise the evidence.

Step 4: Integrate the best evidence *with issue expertise, and stakeholder values and ethics* in making a *health policy decision or change.*

Step 5: *Contribute to the health policy development and implementation process.*

Step 6: *Frame policy change for appropriate dissemination to affected parties.*
Step 7: *Evaluate effectiveness of the policy change and disseminate findings.*

(Loversidge, 2016a, p. 30).

Two aspects of the EIHP model are noteworthy when preparing evidence to inform dialogue and leverage outcomes of policy development; both aspects ultimately bear relationships to dissemination. The first is how the PICOT question is used. The second is how the term "dissemination" is considered in policy, because there are two relevant time frames and audiences: (1) the first time frame is the policy development stage, and the audience policy makers with whom the evidence will be used as leverage for policy development; and (2) the postimplementation and/or postevaluation stage, when constituents who will be the eventual consumers affected by the policy change are notified of the policy's substance, or when the public is apprised of policy evaluation findings. The rest of the discussion on dissemination focuses on the first time frame and audience.

Using the PICOT

As in the EBP model, the PICOT format is used to formulate the question; the difference is that a **health policy** *question* is being asked, rather than a clinical problem, and is derived after identifying a *health policy problem or issue*. Because the problem focus is different, the (P), the population of interest, is often the representative consumer population that will be the focus of the health policy. This PICOT question drives the literature search, as in EBP.

However, it is not uncommon for problems in health policy to emerge around questions of existing policy, or during formulation of policy (e.g., a bill that has been introduced may become problematic). In the EIHP model, the PICOT question can also be used for deconstructing pending or existing policy to facilitate deep analysis of the policy's elements. The PICOT format is used in this way to parse out the policy's component parts for deeper understanding (Loversidge, 2016a). In either case, asking the right PICOT question provides focus. If used in Step 2 to drive the literature search, the result will be a more effective exploration of existing evidence that can inform the next steps of the process; if used for retrospective analysis, the result will be a more thorough scrutiny of the pending or enacted policy.

Government websites for sources of evidence.

Access to government documents, including bills, laws, regulations, or hearing testimony, may be needed to inform the policy-making process. Documents available from these websites may be the very policies that are being analyzed or may constitute part of a body of "internal" evidence for another purpose. Three important sources are U.S. Congress, your state legislature, and state boards of nursing (BONs):

- Tracking the U.S. Congress: Govtrack.us is the official source of information on bills, resolutions, and members of congress: https://www.govtrack.us/
- State legislature websites: From the home page it is common to be able to access legislators, senate and house committees, legislation, legislative summaries, and often testimony provided during hearings. Begin by searching for your home state legislature website.
- Boards of Nursing: Search for your own state/territory BON, or go to NSCBN.org and click on "Contact a Member Board": https://www.ncsbn.org/contact-bon.htm

Timing: Two Opportunities for Dissemination

In EBP, dissemination generally comes as the last step. However, in health policy, there are at least two major opportunities for "dissemination." One comes early in the process, during Steps 4 and/or 5. Recall that the health policy process is never linear, so the placement in the process must be thought of as flexible. The last opportunities come during the final steps, Steps 6 and 7.

Dissemination in Steps 4 and 5

In Steps 4 and 5, the work of dissemination is to make the body of scientific evidence clear and unambiguous so it can be effectively considered as a part of influencing policy development (i.e., considered as one of the three components of EIHP). In Step 4, the best evidence is integrated with issue expertise and stakeholder values and ethics in making a health policy decision or change. This is more likely to happen during behind-the-scenes negotiation/planning or task force meetings, with bill sponsors (legislators) or regulatory agency staff, and perhaps other stakeholders and interested parties, rather than during public hearings. This is when, and where, it is most likely the body of evidence will be most helpful for leveraging dialogue and reaching a positive policy solution. However, legislators may ask for evidence during hearings, particularly if testimony does not provide sufficient information for them to make a sound policy decision. This example occurred during a state legislative committee hearing, during which a state nurses' association provided proponent testimony for a bill that would prevent employers from requiring nurses to work mandatory overtime when suffering from significant fatigue:

> *The testimony included accounts of nurses mandated to work half shifts beyond their 12-hour shift, then return on schedule, stories about threats to nurses' employment status, and note of the literature on risk of medical error related to provider fatigue. The testimony was compelling; however, legislators requested stronger evidence and innovative solutions, including staffing models: (1) incorporating the evidence on fatigue working 8 hour vs. 12 hour shifts; (2) comparable to other high-reliability organization-based professions, e.g., aviation; and (3) assuring patient care coverage as the priority. Legislators also requested evidence of employer threats in the form of redacted letters or emails.*

Congress has heard the report of The President's Commission on Evidence-Based Policy-making (2017), and a national imperative to assure evidence is employed in policy-making is being legislated. That state legislators are following suit is promising.

In Step 5, stakeholders contribute to the health policy development and implementation process. The hoped-for progression would be that the body of evidence, and integration with the other EIHP components that occurred during Step 4, would continue into Step 5. Recall, though, that the health policy process is typically nonlinear. As a result, one should expect that evidence redissemination will need to occur.

Dissemination in Steps 6 and 7

In Step 6, the policy change is framed for appropriate dissemination to affected parties, and in Step 7, the effectiveness of the policy change is evaluated and findings are disseminated. Dissemination in this step is consistent with the steps of EBP, in that it is a final part of the process, following implementation of the policy. The outcome of an enacted policy must be made public to the stakeholders and consumers it will affect and in a form that can be understood. The acute pain prescribing regulations that were recently promulgated in Ohio, as a response to the opioid crisis, provide an example of appropriately framed dissemination of evidence-informed policy-making:

> *The Joint Commission introduced organizational standards for improving the care of patients in pain, including use of the quantitative 10-point scale to assess pain, in 2001 (Baker, 2017). Around the same time, the U.S. Veterans Health Administration began referring to pain as The Fifth Vital Sign (U.S. Department of Veterans Affairs, 2000). Providers increased prescribing of both non-opioid and opioid drugs, for both chronic and acute pain, accordingly. However, the escalating opioid crisis has created an awareness of the problems associated with overprescribing, and evidence-based practice guidelines call for reductions in opioid prescribing for acute pain (National Academy of Sciences, Engineering, and Medicine, 2017). Ohio's Governor responded by calling for the state BONs, medicine, pharmacy and dentistry to cooperate by generating profession-specific regulations to limit opioid prescribing for acute pain. Advanced practice registered nurse (APRN) prescriber limits include such restrictions as a 7 day maximum opioid prescription for adults, to be exceeded only if a specific reason is documented in the health care record, and a maximum total morphine equivalent dose (MED) that cannot exceed an average of 30 MED per day (Ohio Administrative Code, Rule 4723-9-10).*

In addition, policy evaluation may (or may not) be conducted, either by the government or private agencies that have adopted the policy or by public interest groups; the results of these policy evaluations should be disseminated to the public, in reports or by other appropriate methods.

PREPARING EVIDENCE FOR DISSEMINATION TO POLICY MAKERS

Preparing an effective means to disseminate evidence, in particular to the policy-maker audience, is extraordinarily important. It is essential to follow two basic principles for preparing evidence consistent with the components of EIHP: (1) the body of evidence is clear, compelling, unambiguous, and relevant in terms of making your case (external evidence); and (2) it is prepared with sensitivity to the policy makers' values, ethics, and their constituent's needs (stakeholder values and ethics). Preparing evidence in this way is discussed in detail in Chapter 20.

In general, two options, or methods, are used. Both described here are necessarily brief; both *can* be used as one-way dissemination/communication methods. The first is the *"Elevator Speech" one-page policy brief*, which typically consists of bulleted talking points. These may be used in meetings with policy makers and their legislative aide(s). One's *role* in such meetings might be as a constituent, or as a representative of a professional organization. Meetings may include other members of the professional organization and are sometimes inclusive of "opposing" organizational representatives. Therefore, the method and tone of evidence dissemination is important. In addition to talking points, tables, charts, and other visuals can often have the desired impact. Box 19.1 presents suggestions on how to focus on evidence dissemination in a one-page elevator-speech policy brief. The same policy briefs should be kept handy for impromptu meetings with other policy makers who may influence decision making. Although these policy briefs are designed to

BOX 19.1 *How to Focus on Evidence in a One-page "Elevator Speech" Policy Brief*

- Keep it *brief*; the rule of thumb is one page, one-sided, with bullet points.
- Add another page if you have compelling visuals (tables, graphs, charts, etc.).
- The title on the brief should clearly identify the policy being addressed and the representative organization (if appropriate; if it is a personal statement, make that clear).
- State the organization's position if established (proponent, opponent, or interested party).
- Introduce the *body of evidence*, and describe how it informs the direction of the policy.
- Summarize the major points using clear language; stay focused on how use of the evidence would make a positive difference in the policy for citizens/constituents.
- Do not use medical terminology or jargon; explain clearly using lay terminology.
- Be clear, succinct, logical, and express the information without exaggeration or emotion.
- Conclude with contact information and a statement indicating willingness to provide any additional information or respond to any questions. *Note: If policy makers ask questions during meetings that you cannot answer, let them know when they can expect a response.*
- Provide a separate page with a reference list. Include live URL links if available.
- Add an evidence table as an appendix only if the body of evidence is complex and you believe it is essential information.

TABLE 19.2	Dos and Don'ts of Using Evidence During Testimony

Dos

- Analyze the policy-maker "audience," likely lawmakers or regulators.
- Know committee membership, i.e., who is the Chair? Minority leader? Any healthcare professionals?
- Know lawmakers' concerns, particularly those with the greatest power to influence the policy decision.
- Analyze current level of policy makers' understanding regarding evidence relevant to the issue.
- Address how evidence is relevant.
- Be specific about how you/your organization propose/s the evidence be used to change the proposed policy.
- Use examples from your own clinical expertise to bridge evidence-to-practice reality.
- Respond professionally to questions. If you do not have an immediate answer, indicate you will seek out the answer.
- Include a reference page as an appendix to your testimony with URL links.

Don't

- Use medical jargon or research terms.
- Go into testimony unprepared; do your homework—know the evidence, and know the lawmakers' ideas and values.
- Cite individual research studies—focus on the relevant *body* of evidence.
- Make your description of evidence too technical or complex; get to the point.
- Become defensive or emotional during testimony delivery or questioning.
- Express evidence in ways that could be misinterpreted as an example of a "turf" battle (e.g., scope of practice issues).
- Digress from the purpose of lobbying for the body of evidence to improve the quality and direction of the policy.
- Respond to a question you do not know the answer to with a simple "I don't know." Say, "That's a great question. I will be happy to find out and get back to you." Follow through—within 24 hours.

provide for one-way dissemination, when used in meetings, they are useful springboards for dialogue.

A second, more formal, opportunity to disseminate evidence with policy makers is to *provide testimony during a hearing*, for example, a congressional or state legislative committee meeting, or a regulatory board hearing. Individuals may be asked to testify as representatives of an organization or may provide testimony as citizens/constituents. Although testimony is usually time-limited, it may be appropriate to add examples using stories from clinical practice to bring a sense of reality to the body of evidence. Table 19.2 contains a list of dos and don'ts of using evidence during testimony.

Since policy-making often follows a nonlinear and convoluted pathway, think of these occurrences as opportunities rather than parts of any one step, and the elevator speech and testimony as dissemination "delivery methods."

> **"**
> The fact that an opinion has been widely held is no evidence
> whatever that it is not utterly absurd.
>
> BERTRAND RUSSELL

USING EVIDENCE TO INFLUENCE ORGANIZATIONAL POLICY

Patient care can be enhanced by embracing EBP as the foundation for policy-making and patient care decisions. Leaders have an opportunity to role model EBP and create policy-making, team-based committee work environments that integrate and sustain EBP. To respond appropriately to complex patient needs and deliver high-quality, evidenced-based care, the Institute of Medicine (IOM) set a goal that 90% of clinical decisions be evidence-based by 2020 (Institute of Medicine [US] Roundtable on Evidence-Based Medicine, 2009). However, organizations and leaders find that effective mechanisms to change their cultures and practice environments to an EBP culture is challenging. These concepts are discussed in greater detail in Chapters 12 and 15. **EBP competencies** help organizations establish expectations for clinicians, develop mechanisms to build EBP knowledge and skills, measure achievement of each competency, and hold clinicians accountable to this professional expectation; EBP competencies are discussed in detail in Chapter 11 (Melnyk & Gallagher-Ford, 2014; Melnyk, Gallagher-Ford, Long, & Fineout-Overholt, 2014).

An early step necessary to embed EBP in organizations is to create successful change in policy committee practice. This entails establishing EBP-focused visionary leadership, identifying internal and external resources, nurturing academic partner relationships, and developing time- and cost-efficient methods to incorporate EBP education and mentoring. Improving the **organizational policy** and the EBP knowledge and skills of procedure committee members by integrating EBP education into committee meetings will ensure a greater level of EBP process in patient care policy development, and focus professional interactions among the interprofessional members on safe patient care. The systematic step-by-step approach to improve the integration of evidence into patient care policies, over time, can be cost effective. Committee engagement in project planning and evaluation is essential to participant buy-in and facilitates EBP utilization in organizational policy committees.

PATIENT CARE DECISION MAKERS: ORGANIZATIONAL POLICY AND PROCEDURES COMMITTEES

Patient care practices and procedures used by nurses, respiratory therapists, pharmacists, social workers, and other disciplines are usually managed by a hospital policy committee that oversees clinical practice. Regular review is required; however, a strategic committee approach should be developed to engage in review and incorporate new evidence whenever it is available (McKeever et al., 2016). Reviews should attend to alerts and new information gleaned from current literature reviews and professional organization publications.

EBP is an effective **organizational policy** committee strategy that contributes to improved patient care, reductions in morbidity, and reduced costs. Quality clinical decisions should be based on the systematic search, critical appraisal, and synthesis of research, along with internal evidence from quality improvement or management projects (Melnyk & Fineout-Overholt, 2015). Organizational policies and procedures are the major clinical practice resources guiding staff clinical practice; yet policy committee members' competencies in using evidence to guide practice may be limited. However, the literature offers little guidance for integrating EBP into interprofessional policy-making, or for guiding effective organizational process relative to evidence-based policy and procedure committee work.

Successful Policy Committee Structures and Processes

Several structural components and processes should be in place for organizational policy committees to succeed in incorporating EBP into their policy and procedure work. These include a sound committee infrastructure, establishing strong committee leadership, an assessment of committee members' EBP competency level, and establishing a framework and strategy for committee EBP education and development.

Committee Infrastructure: Charter, Checklists, and Membership

Organizational policy committees should review and agree on committee purpose, which is usually found in a charter, bylaws, or guidelines. Often, EBP is mentioned in the committee's scope or charge, but may not be consistently implemented. Committee process checklists can be adopted that clearly communicate expectations to include the steps of EBP in the review of all policies. Process checklists can be accompanied by a cover letter explaining expectations, their importance, and consistency with organization mission and values. The checklist and cover letter can also be distributed to staff expressing interest in a new policy or policy change (McKeever et al., 2016).

Committee members should see themselves as EBP champions with the mission to serve on an **interprofessional collaborative** team to influence the evidence-based culture and environment of the organization (Aarons et al., 2016). Members should be representative of various areas and disciplines to which the policies apply. Most often, committee membership includes individuals who represent staff, practitioners, and leadership.

Policy Committee Leadership

Successful integration and sustainability of an organizational EBP environment can be accomplished only with visible, tangible leadership engagement. Leaders who embrace EBP as the foundation of decision making and care decisions, and who are EBP-positive role models, can create supportive EBP cultures and work environments. A critical leadership position is the **organizational policy** committee chair. Key administrative activities navigated by that position include engagement of committee members in enhancing their EBP competency and promoting and sustaining an effective EBP culture in the committee.

Leadership plays a vital role in promoting an environment supportive of EBP. New policy committee leaders benefit from transformational and EBP education, and supervision and mentoring from upper level leadership. Policy committee leaders who learn transformational leadership skills are better able to positively negotiate compromise, resolve disagreements, and move the project forward. Transformational leaders establish a milieu where mutual respect supports optimal team function (McKibben, 2017). Aarons et al. (2016) found that transformational leaders are more likely to establish a mission, vision, and strategic plan to ensure EBP project success. In addition, they discovered that leaders who are proactive in problem solving and use transformational leadership style are more likely to be a positive influence with regard to sustaining EBP practices.

Competency Assessment for Policy Committees

To support the committee culture necessary to promote efficacious use of the EBP process in **organizational policy** committees, a competency assessment can be designed and aimed toward policy committee development education programming. External EBP experts can be sought to advise program and project planning, to promote integration of EBP into the organization's policy-making processes (Hanrahan et al., 2015). Most academic, teaching, and community hospitals have affiliations with academic nursing. Partnering with EBP expert consultants/faculty is a practical, cost-effective way to approach EBP education and skills building.

Operationalizing a Collaborative Interprofessional Policy Committee

Although educating for collaboration between nurses and other healthcare disciplines may not be typical in most organizations, **interprofessional collaboration** can be improved by educating physicians, nurses, and other health professionals together, and by collaborating on quality improvement projects focused on improving patient outcomes. Regan, Lashinger, and Wong (2016) reported that nursing leaders can enhance interprofessional collaboration by creating work environments that empower teamwork and providing ample opportunity to promote understanding of the roles and responsibilities of colleagues from other disciplines.

Aasekjaer, Waehle, Ciliska, Nordtvedt, and Hjalmhult (2016) studied successful implementation of the EBP steps and identified challenges associated with creating a compelling learning environment. Allowing members time to work on projects as they learn the steps supports successful implementation of a program of EBP education. Using an external EBP expert to teach the steps of EBP in a systematic education program and using real-world examples keeps committee members interested and helps them recognize that learning an EBP process will provide positive and fulfilling results.

Policy committees should follow the Advancing Research and Clinical Practice through Close Collaboration (ARCC) model to develop EBP mentors (Melnyk, Fineout-Overholt, Stillwell, & Williamson, 2010). EBP competencies become tools to guide the development of a committee's EBP knowledge and skills. Table 19.3 shows a step-by-step policy committee

TABLE 19.3	Systematic Step-by-Step Policy Committee EBP Education/Enculturation
EBP Step	**Action Tactics for Policy Committees**
0: Cultivate a spirit of inquiry.	Stimulate ongoing curiosity for clinical decision making; practice examples needing updated evidence. Create a safe environment for asking "why?"
1: PICOT question	Formulate clinical questions in PICOT format. Critique each other's PICOT questions. Provide individual coaching as needed.
2: Search for the best evidence.	Secure a librarian to teach literature search skills and library services. Select key words from PICOT questions. Determine levels of evidence and practice clinical examples.
3: Critical appraisal	Build critical appraisal skills by sharing studies and using critical appraisal checklists. Determine the highest quality of evidence to guide policies. Create synthesis tables. Practice with policies in need of change.
4: Integrate the evidence.	Determine if there is patient/family population-specific evidence. Include stakeholders' opinion and regulatory concerns.
5: Evaluate the outcomes.	Incorporate EBP into QI processes. Compare data outcomes to preproject data and research databases, peer organizations, and national practice standards.
6: Disseminate the outcomes.	Provide information to professional stakeholders, use plain talk with consumers; publish/present to a wide audience. Use various dissemination methods (e.g., electronic posting on org. websites, staff meetings, and quality and safety committees).

EBP, evidence-based practice; QI, quality improvement.

EBP education and enculturation program designed to refocus an interprofessional policy committee to more effectively implement and sustain evidence-based clinical practice policies.

CHALLENGES AND CHANGE MANAGEMENT

Barriers to the implementation of EBP include factors such as a lack of resources, manager and leader resistance, peer and colleague resistance, embedded organizational culture, and time constraints (Melnyk & Fineout-Overholt, 2015; Melnyk, Fineout-Overholt, Gallagher-Ford, & Kaplan, 2012). These are likely experienced during an EBP enculturation committee project. Other challenges likely encountered include organization-set timelines, or situations where committee members and other stakeholders express conflicting ideas or exhibit a broad range of levels of knowledge about and competency in EBP. Once the EBP process is under way, multiple PICOT questions within one policy/procedure might be identified, or evidence might be minimal on specific topics, particularly in pediatrics or other specialties, necessitating a shift to research mode; also, access to EBP mentors/ resources in the organization might be limited. Additionally, shifts in committee membership present their own set of challenges. Three major committee management challenges—time, differences in committee member competency and confidence, and shifting committee membership—are addressed here.

Time

Timely processing of practice change policies requires tight review schedules. Most practice committees oversee multitudes of policies; most organizational policy committees generally require, at a minimum, a review of each policy every 3 years. However, many policies are reviewed more often when practice or regulations change. Considering the workload volume, expecting the committee to compress business to make room for EBP education requires efficiency on the part of the chair and committee cooperation. Flexibility and consensus around the value of EBP and EBP competency education are needed for process enculturation to occur. Learning **EBP competencies** and effective implementation requires many months. An additional constraint is the time required for literature searches. Although committee meeting time is supported by the organization, search time is not; committee members often report that this complicates their work. Members may also have difficulty managing the meeting and education/practice session schedules because their positions often require them to multitask in multiple meetings or clinical areas that overlap with committee meetings.

Committee Member Variation in Skill and Confidence

Health professionals with the experience to qualify as a policy committee chair or as a member may not have learned about EBP during their educational programs of study. Of all the EBP steps, developing skill and confidence in critical appraisal provides the greatest challenge. Leading discussions with stakeholders outside the committee can also be challenging. Organizational policy committees frequently need clinical expertise from outside the committee structure, as a part of internal evidence. Eliciting the involvement of clinical experts requires skilled communication and an ability to impart the importance of their contribution to the policy work. Finally, it is imperative that committee members gain the requisite skills and abilities, and have a sense of the committee leader's support, so they are able to confidently comport themselves in the committee role as a full contributor.

Changes in Committee Membership

Healthcare policy committee members may serve terms of one or more years or may be in the position until they resign from the committee. Members may also leave the organization, requiring the committee chair to find and orient a new member, who may need to begin an EBP development program. Managing incoming new members requires a formal process for orientation. When existing members leave, continuing without introducing a new member to the committee who is not competent in EBP should be considered (Aasekjaer et al., 2016)

EBP FAST FACTS

- Health policy is both an entity (e.g., governmental law or rules, or organizational policy) and a process (i.e., policy-making).
- The use of evidence in policy-making is affected by numerous social and political factors.
- In governmental policy-making, the realistic use of evidence is to inform and leverage dialogue.
- EBP should, and can, be followed closely in organizational policy making—patient outcomes depend on it.
- Interprofessional organizational policy committees can learn to use EBP processes effectively with education, time, and support.

WANT TO KNOW MORE?

A variety of resources are available to enhance your learning and understanding of this chapter.

- Visit thePoint° to access:
  - Articles from the AJN EBP Step-By-Step Series
  - Journal articles
  - Checklists for rapid critical appraisal and more!
- Lippincott CoursePoint combines digital text content with video case studies and interactive modules for a fully integrated course solution that works the way you study and learn.

References

Aarons, G. A., Green, A. E., Trott, E., Willging, C. E., Torres, E. M., Ehrhart, M. G., & Roesch, S. C. (2016). The roles of system and organizational leadership in system-wide intervention sustainment: A mixed-method study. *Administration and Policy in Mental Health and Mental Health Services Research, 43*(6), 991–1008.

Aasekjaer, K., Waehle, H. V., Ciliska, D., Nordtvedt, M. W., & Hjalmhult, E. (2016). Management involvement—A decisive condition when implementing evidence-based practice. *Worldviews on Evidence-Based Nursing, 13*(1), 32–41.

Baker, D. W. (2017, May 5). *The Joint Commission's pain standards: Origins and evolution.* Oakbrook Terrace, IL: The Joint Commission. Retrieved from https://www.jointcommission.org/assets/1/6/Pain_Std_History_Web_Version_05122017.pdf

Bowen, S., & Zwi, A. B. (2005). Pathways to "evidence-informed" policy and practice: A framework for action. *PLoS Medicine, 2*(7), 0600–0605.

Campbell, D. M., Redman, S., Jorm, L., Cooke, M., Zwi, A. B., & Rychetnik, L. (2009). Increasing the use of evidence in health policy: Practice and views of policy makers and researchers. *Australia and New Zealand Health Policy, 6*, 21–31.

Commission on Evidence-Based Policymaking. (2017). *The promise of evidence-based policymaking: Report of the commission on evidence-based policymaking.* Retrieved from https://www.cep.gov/cep-final-report.html

Elliott, H., & Popay, J. (2004). How are policy makers using evidence? Models of research utilization and local NHS policy making. *Journal of Epidemiology and Community Health, 54*(6), 461–468.

Hanrahan, K., Wagner, M., Matthews, G., Stewart, S., Dawson, C., Greiner, J., . . . Williamson, A. (2015). Sacred cow gone to pasture: A systematic evaluation and integration of evidence-based practice. *Worldviews on Evidence-Based Nursing, 12*(1), 3–11.

Institute of Medicine (US) Roundtable on Evidence-Based Medicine. (2009). *Leadership commitments to improve value in healthcare: Finding common ground: Workshop summary.* Washington, DC: National Academies Press. Retrieved from https://www.ncbi.nlm.nih.gov/books/NBK52847/

Jewell, C. J., & Bero. L. A. (2008). "Developing good taste in evidence": Facilitators of and hindrances to evidence-informed health policymaking in state government. *The Milbank Quarterly, 86*(2), 177–208.

Lanier, J. K. (2016). Government response: Legislation. In J. A. Milstead (Ed.), *Health policy & politics: A nurses guide* (5th ed., pp. 69–97). Burlington, MA: Jones & Bartlett.

Lavis, J. N., Oxman, A. D., Souza, N. M., Lewin, S., Gruen, R. L., & Fretheim, A. (2009). SUPPORT tools for evidence-informed health policymaking (STP) 9: Assessing the applicability of the findings of a systematic review. *Health Research Policy and Systems, 7*(Suppl. 1), 1–7.

Loversidge, J. M. (2016a). An evidence-informed health policy model: Adapting evidence-based practice for nursing education and regulation. *Journal of Nursing Regulation, 7*(2), 27–33. doi:10.1016/S2155-8256(16)31075-4

Loversidge, J. M. (2016b, November 11). A call for extending the utility of evidence-based practice: Adapting EBP for health policy impact. *Worldviews on Evidence-based Nursing, 13*(6), 399–401. doi:10.1111/wvn.12183

McKeever, S., Twomey, B., Hawley, M., Lima, S., Kinney, S., & Newall, F. (2016). Engaging a nursing workforce in evidence-based practice: Introduction of a nursing clinical effectiveness committee. *Worldviews on Evidence-Based Nursing, 13*(1), 85–88.

McKibben, L. (2017). Conflict management: Importance and implications. *British Journal of Nursing, 26*(2), 100–103.

Melnyk, B. M., & Fineout-Overholt, E. (2015). *Evidence-based practice in nursing and healthcare: A guide to best practice* (3rd ed.). Philadelphia, PA: Lippincott Williams & Wilkins.

Melnyk, B. M., Fineout-Overholt, E., Gallagher-Ford, L., & Kaplan, L. (2012). The state of evidence-based practice in US nurses: Critical implications for nurse leaders and educators. *Journal of Nursing Administration, 42*(9), 410–417.

Melnyk, B. M., Fineout-Overholt, E., Stillwell, S. B., & Williamson, K. M. (2010). The seven steps of evidence-based practice. *American Journal of Nursing, 110*(1), 51–53.

Melnyk, B. M., & Gallagher-Ford, L. (2014). Evidence-based practice as mission critical for healthcare quality and safety: A disconnect for many nurse executives. *Worldviews on Evidence-Based Nursing, 11*(3), 145–146. doi:10.1111/wvn.12037

Melnyk, B. M., Gallagher-Ford, L., Long, L. E., & Fineout-Overholt, E. (2014). The establishment of evidence-based practice competencies for practicing registered nurses and advanced practice nurses in real-world clinical settings: Proficiencies to improve healthcare quality, reliability, patient outcomes, and costs. *Worldviews on Evidence-Based Nursing, 11*(1), 5–15.

Milstead, J. A. (2016). Advanced practice registered nurses and public policy, naturally. In J. A. Milstead (Ed.), *Health policy & politics: A nurses guide* (5th ed., pp. 1–43). Burlington, MA: Jones & Bartlett.

Morgan, G. (2010). Evidence-based health policy: A preliminary systematic review. *Health Education Journal, 69*(1), 43–47. doi:10.1177/0017896910363328

National Academy of Sciences, Engineering, and Medicine. (2017). *Pain management and the opioid epidemic: Balancing societal and individual benefits and risks of prescription opioid use.* Washington, DC: The National Academies Press. doi:10.17226/24781

Niessen, L. W., Grijseels, E. W. M., & Rutten, F. F. H. (2000). The evidence-based approach in health policy and health care delivery. *Social Science and Medicine, 51*, 859–869.

Ohio Administrative Code. *Rule 4723-9-10 Formulary; standards of prescribing for advanced practice registered nurses designated as clinical nurse specialists, certified nurse-midwives, or certified nurse practitioners.* Retrieved from http://codes.ohio.gov/oac/4723-9-10v1

Ohio Board of Nursing. (2018). *Rule 4723-9-10, OAC: CNPs, CNSs, CNMs prescribing opioid analgesics for acute pain.* Retrieved from http://www.nursing.ohio.gov/PDFS/AdvPractice/4723-9-10_OAC%20Overview_Acute_Pain_Prescribing-3.pdf

Regan, S., Lashinger, H. K. S., & Wong, C. A. (2016). The influence of empowerment, authentic leadership, and professional practice environments on nurses' perceived interprofessional collaboration. *Journal of Nursing Management, 24*(1), E54–E61. doi:10.1111/jonm.12288

Shamian, J., & Shamian-Ellen, M. (2011). Shaping health policy: The role of nursing research—Three frameworks and their application to policy development. In A. S. Hinshaw & P. A. Grady (Eds.), *Shaping Health Policy Through Nursing Research* (pp. 35–51). New York, NY: Springer.

U. S. Department of Veterans Affairs (2000). *Pain as the 5th vital sign toolkit.* Retrieved from https://www.va.gov/PAINMANAGEMENT/docs/Pain_As_the_5th_Vital_Sign_Toolkit.pdf

World Health Organization. (2016). *Evidence-informed policy network: What is EVIPNet?* Retrieved from http://www.who.int/evidence/about/en/

Disseminating Evidence Through Presentations, Publications, Health Policy Briefs, and the Media

Cecily L. Betz, Kathryn A. Smith,
Bernadette Mazurek Melnyk, and Timothy Tassa

The best preparation for tomorrow is doing your best today.

—H. Jackson Brown Jr

EBP Terms to Learn
BOPPPS model
Evidence-based clinical
  rounds
Journal clubs
News embargo

Learning Objectives

After studying this chapter, learners will be able to:

1. Describe effective strategies for presenting high-quality oral and poster presentations.
2. Discuss success tips for publishing papers and health policy briefs.
3. Identify best approaches for dealing with the media.

The seven-step evidence-based practice (EBP) process is a major emphasis of this book, along with implementation of the best evidence to improve clinical practice and patient outcomes. However, new evidence will not achieve its maximum value to practice and improve patient outcomes unless it is communicated and disseminated effectively. While clinicians communicate constantly with patients, peers, and colleagues in their work, many are not familiar with or confident in the use of the intricacies, tools, processes, and opportunities to professionally communicate evidence-based findings.

Despite the many changes driven by communication technology advances, best practices for disseminating evidence and evidence-based information have remained relatively stable across time. To speak before an audience, present a poster, publish a paper, write a health policy brief, or place a story with the media requires sufficient preparation, planning, and, in most cases, the use of the same communications principles. Excellent preparation reduces performance anxiety, builds confidence, and enhances the success of any communications initiative. The primary goal of disseminating evidence, whatever the channel or tool as described in this chapter, is to facilitate the transfer and adoption of research findings into clinical practice or to disseminate evidence-based quality improvement projects (Majid et al., 2011). For the majority of clinicians in advanced practice and leadership roles, enrollment in some type of instructional program (e.g., a continuing education course, staff development class, or college course) to learn the knowledge and skills to successfully make presentations or publish manuscripts is readily available (Lannon, Gurak, & Daemon, 2012). Moreover, many websites have helpful information for creating and delivering professional oral presentations, and online courses exist as well. However, most learning to obtain advanced professional skills is gained through practical experience, mentoring by experienced colleagues, and modeling the observable behavior and materials demonstrated by leading professionals (Marble, 2009; Tinkham, 2013).

This chapter presents information on the strategies and communication tools that can be used by healthcare professionals to disseminate evidence. Content covered includes podium/oral, panel, roundtable, poster, and small group presentations as well as community meetings, hospital-based and professional committees, and journal clubs. This is followed by a detailed look at professional publishing and dissemination of evidence to influence policy and enhance healthcare. Finally, suggestions are provided for disseminating evidence through the media.

DISSEMINATING EVIDENCE THROUGH PODIUM/ORAL PRESENTATIONS

Conference presentations offer rich and dynamic opportunities to share and learn knowledge and enhance clinical expertise pertaining to EBP, evidence-based quality improvement, case studies, program evaluation, and research. Whether the presenter has been invited or submitted an abstract that has been accepted, the process for developing the oral presentation is similar (Billings & Kowalski, 2009a).

An effective evidence-based presentation begins with an understanding of audience characteristics and needs, conference characteristics and presentation guidelines, and topical focus. It would be incorrect to make unwarranted assumptions about the presentation to be given; each conference will be uniquely different from others. In preparing for a podium or oral presentation, it is important to know the audience composition, the context of the presentation, the desired length and format, and any special considerations (Blome, Sondermann, & Augustin, 2017; Sawatzky, 2011). Therefore, the first step toward developing an effective oral presentation is to conduct a thorough analysis of the expectations and guidelines. This can be accomplished by gathering the necessary information from the conference announcements, speaker handbook, and contact with the conference representative, be it the conference manager, public relations contact, or member of the organizing committee. Professional organizations often use conference planning organizations, and communication regarding conference requirements will take place through these entities.

> "
> Whether you think you can or think you can't, you're right.
>
> **HENRY FORD**

Analyzing Audiences for Presentations

As you begin preparing the presentation, ask the following substantive questions:

- What are the educational level and practice specialties of the audience?
- What is the audience's current knowledge of the material to be presented?
- Is the content meant for an audience with limited knowledge of the evidence-based topic?
- Why is the audience interested in the presentation?
- Is the audience expected to use evidence-based approaches in providing clinical care?
- What other information, if any, will the audience be receiving?
- What previous exposure has the audience had to the content of the presentation?

- How might the members of the audience use the information from the presentation to improve their practices, teaching, or other aspects of their work?
- How many people are expected to attend the presentation?
- How will participants use the information presented?

Additional logistical questions to consider include:

- What is the availability of audiovisual equipment (e.g., LCD projector for PowerPoint presentations), and are there any charges that may be incurred?
- Are there live-streaming or remote viewing options for the presentation, and will it be archived (recordings may limit podium mobility)?
- Is there a hashtag or social media component that can be incorporated into the presentation that is reflective of the overarching theme of the conference?
- Is there the capacity to incorporate multimedia into the presentation?
- Does the room have Internet/Wi-Fi access?
- What type of microphone is available (i.e., podium, lavaliere [personal/clip microphone])?
- How long is the presentation? Are their time constraints or parameters?
- What is the format of the presentation? Is there time for questions and answers from the audience or moderator?
- What are the expectations regarding handouts?

Developing the Presentation

Once these questions are answered, development of the presentation can begin. The first step is the development of learner objectives. If this is an invited presentation, the objectives may be defined by the organizer. Otherwise, objectives are developed by the presenter. The development of the objectives will be further facilitated following the conversation with the conference representative using the analysis format for determining the needs of the audience and conference purpose (Rogoschewsky, 2011). For presenters whose conference abstract was accepted, the objectives are to be closely aligned with it. For presentations to disseminate evidence from a study, the following topical outline is suggested:

1. Introduction to the clinical problem (e.g., depression affects approximately 25% of adults in the United States)
2. The purpose/primary aim of the study (e.g., to determine the short- and long-term effects of cognitive behavior therapy [CBT] on depressive symptoms in young adults)
3. The theoretical framework used to guide the study
4. Hypotheses (e.g., young adults who receive CBT will have less depressive symptoms than young adults who do not receive CBT) or study questions (what are the effects of CBT on depressed adults?)
5. The design (e.g., a randomized controlled trial)
   a. A description of the interventions used if an experimental study is being presented
   b. A description of the sample with inclusion and exclusion criteria (e.g., the sample included 104 depressed adults between the ages of 21 and 30 years; potential subjects were excluded if they had a mental health problem with psychotic features), as well as a concise description of the demographics of the sample
   c. The dependent variables and instruments used to measure the study's outcomes, along with validity and reliability information of each instrument (e.g., the Beck Depression Inventory was used to measure depressive symptoms; construct validity of the Beck Inventory has been supported in prior work, and internal consistency reliability is reported as consistently higher than 0.80)

6. Findings from the study
   a. Approach to statistical analyses (e.g., types of statistical tests used [an independent *t*-test was used to test the study hypothesis])
   b. Findings (it is best to represent the findings in easy-to-read graphs, tables, or infographics, which are visually creative and impactful representations of data)
7. Discussion of the findings, along with major strengths and limitations of the study (e.g., substantial attrition rate, difficulties in recruitment)
8. Implications
   a. Implications for future research (e.g., what was learned from this study that can guide future research in the area)
   b. Implications for clinical practice (e.g., how this evidence can be used to improve practice). Key messages and the content for each section of the outline can be developed along with the time allocation for each component of the presentation. Many conferences limit research/evidence-based presentations to 20 minutes or less, some as few as 5 minutes, with it being commonplace for three to four individuals to deliver related talks in the same session. For presentations with short time frames, it is critical to deliver only nuts-and-bolts information. Because many beginning presenters often go beyond the allocated time limit, it is valuable to hold a practice presentation with colleagues who can time and critique it.

Other more lengthy presentations will require a more thoughtful approach to the allocation of time to each section. Although the objectives will guide the development of the presentation, the extent to which each section is developed is based on the audience analysis and conference purpose. The interdisciplinary **BOPPPS model** (*B*ridge, *O*bjectives, *P*retest, *P*articipatory learning, *P*ost-test, and *S*ummary) provides a template for developing a presentation.

 The BOPPPS model can be accessed at http://hlwiki.slais.ubc.ca/index.php/BOPPPS_Model

---

Whether a novice or an experienced presenter, rehearsal of the presentation is recommended. Practicing the presentation will enable the speaker to become not only familiar with the content and its sequencing but also confident with the task of presenting. Practice enables the speaker to edit, refine, and reorganize the presentation to a degree of satisfaction and comfort needed to be effective. A well-rehearsed presentation generates speaker confidence, enabling a more energetic, enthused presentation while lessening the anxiety and jitters associated with public speaking. A speaker who is not reliant on presentation notes or slides is able to maintain better eye contact with the audience with a greater potential to engage the audience with the subject matter discussed (Blome et al., 2017; Stuart, 2013). A well-prepared speaker should be able to provide the information by simply glancing at the slides or notes as a reminder and at the same time maintain a relationship with the audience. Voice modulation is another important element with successful presentations. The speaker's volume, pitch, and intensity need to vary during the presentation to avoid speaking too quickly or monotonously (Blome et al., 2017; Campbell, 2011; Stuart, 2013). A rehearsed presentation will enable the speaker to feel more confident about his or her presentation.

Excellent resources to assist speakers to be more effective with their presentations can be downloaded from the Burroughs-Welcome Fund website: https://www.scribd.com/doc/34887738/Communicating-Science-Giving-Talks-Second-Edition#download

---

Slides to Enhance the Presentation

When presentation content is completed, slides should be developed to enhance delivery and hold the attention of the audience. A rule of thumb is that a minimal amount of information/text should be contained on each slide and that the total number of slides presented should not distract from the flow of the presenter's remarks. Slides with photos and figures help to capture the participants' attention and should be used liberally. The tempo for slides is no more than one slide every 30 to 60 seconds (Billings & Kowalski, 2009b). However, it may be that far fewer slides are needed as the presenter uses the slide as a prompt for expanding upon the bullet points presented on the slide. The use of slides is not a substitute for the oral presentation. That is, the speaker's remarks should not be restricted to the slide content, because this approach would become one-dimensional and stilted. PowerPoint slides have a notes section available at the bottom of the slide, not seen by the audience but allowing the speaker to include additional information or prompts for the presentation.

If presenting at a conference, first talk with a contact or the person who is liaising with speakers, because they may have an existing PowerPoint template and corresponding PowerPoint design guidelines that must be followed. If creating an original slide deck, a helpful guideline is to create simple slides in terms of the colors, graphics, and fonts used. A dark or medium background (e.g., navy blue or maroon) with light color lettering (e.g., yellow or white) is most readable by viewers, although it may not photocopy well if copies are to be distributed. White, light grey, or pale-colored backgrounds should be complemented with other compelling visual features, like borders or logos. Individuals in the back of a room should be able to read all text, not forgetting members of the audience who may be color-blind. Fonts should be modern and simple, font size between 24 and 32 points, and sans serif fonts, such as Arial or Calibri. Font and background color should be consistent throughout the slide presentation, and important points should appear in boldface. Excessive use of bolding, italics, and underlining can be distracting for the reader. Underlining can be problematic because it may be misconstrued as a hyperlink (Blome et al., 2017; Grand Valley State University, Office of Undergraduate Research and Scholarship, 2016; Stuart, 2013; Sawatzky, 2011). In addition, images enhance presentations, hold the audience's attention, and help emphasize major points (see this book's companion website at http://thepoint. lww.com/Melnyk4e for an example of a slide presentation for a 20-minute research report). If multimedia is to be incorporated into the slide presentation, the feasibility of using it will be dependent on the conference technical capacity and costs, because the presenter may be expected to incur the additional costs associated with Internet and electronic linkages. The presenter needs to have absolute confidence that the integration of multimedia into the presentation will not cause technical problems. A dry run or rehearsal of the slide presentation may be available at the conference just before the presentation in the speakers' preparation room. Avoid the use of comics, slide animations, and entertaining sound effects to maintain a professional tone. When acronyms are used, they should be defined by the speaker when first referenced, enabling tremendous convenience for presenters (Coumoyer, 2012).

Epson Presenters Online has excellent tutorials on creating PowerPoint slides, as well as downloadable templates and clip art at www.presentersonline.com/

A useful resource developed by the Division of Information of Technology, Eastern Michigan University, for creating a poster using Microsoft PowerPoint 2010 can be found at http://www.emich.edu/apc/guides/apcposterpowerpoint2010.pdf

Browse other effective PowerPoint templates and themes at https://templates.office.com or use a search engine, such as Google and Bing, to find examples of effective presentations and visual supplements.

Other Types of Evidence-Based Oral Presentations

The following guidelines for presenting evidence from a study also apply to delivering evidence-based implementation projects. The format for presenting *systematic reviews* of evidence should include:

- Introduction to the clinical problem
- Purpose of the systematic review or the clinical question addressed
- Methods (e.g., search strategy)
- Results (i.e., presentation and critical appraisal of the evidence)
- Implications for future research and practice

It is important to be aware that conference presentation materials can be converted into a manuscript for publication with additional effort. The information communicated at a conference would also be appropriate and timely for an audience targeted by print and/or electronic media (Cleary, Happell, Lau, & Mackey, 2013).

Converting the Presentation to Publication

Acknowledgment of work expended in presenting a poster or podium presentation has fostered the appreciation and recognition that the next phase of this scholarly process should include the publication of the investigation/project (Hicks, 2015). The initial poster/presentation abstract submission provides the groundwork for converting this work into a manuscript, although additional effort will be needed as the requirements for a poster submission differ from those for a manuscript submission. However, the extra effort involved in developing a manuscript for publication from a poster abstract is an example of smartly leveraging the preceding work in creating a poster for a scientific/healthcare conference into a potentially publishable manuscript. Obviously, the author will need to adapt, write, and possibly re-write the content and/or make format changes with tables and perhaps add new ones that weren't presented in the abstract with a manuscript submission. Nevertheless, the amount of work expended in converting the poster abstract into a manuscript submission is far less than would be expected with a manuscript with no antecedent work drafts or compositions.

A good rule of thumb is to submit a manuscript within 90 days of an oral or poster presentation, because the work used to create the presentation can be used to facilitate the writing of a paper (Melnyk, 2016).

DISSEMINATING EVIDENCE THROUGH PANEL PRESENTATIONS

Panel presentations are an effective strategy to convey divergent perspectives on evidence-based topics. This type of presentation format is especially effective to convene colleagues from various clinical settings or professions to disseminate evidenced-based information. For example, during a panel presentation, clinicians or relevant researchers or analysts can discuss their various evidence-based approaches to promoting spiritual support services on their hematology–oncology units. Listening to different views enriches the session for the audience. The style and purpose of panel presentations vary according to the roles of the moderator and panelists. The moderator may serve as the coordinator, meaning that this individual manages the agenda of the panel by first giving background or introductory information and commentary on the subject matter to be discussed. Then, the moderator directs the discussion and asks questions of the panel members to elicit their opinions on the topic. Questions from the audience are taken to delve further into particular areas of interest or offer other points of view for panelists' reaction.

Another panel model takes a more formalized approach, in which members of the panel present prepared remarks, with the moderator serving as a discussion facilitator by offering commentary for panel response and encouraging audience questions. The panel format is dependent on a number of factors, including panelist expertise, public speaking experience, organizational practices, and the moderator's competence in the role. Participation in a panel requires close adherence to the allotment of time given to each panel member in order to assure that each is able to present their material. If questions will be taken from the audience, inform them as to whether they will be taken after each presenter, or at the end of all the presentations.

Panelist Preparation

Serving as a panelist requires knowing the expectations for participation (e.g., delivering a prepared presentation or sharing expert opinions with the audience). The panel format will dictate the type of preparation necessary for the presentation. Whatever the format, it is necessary to know the context in which the information is to be presented.

First, the prospective panelist must know the theme of and rationale for the panel, as well as session objectives. For example, is the panelist expected to provide a clinically based or theoretically oriented presentation? Coupled with this information, it is important to know the backgrounds of the other panelists, their areas of expertise, and the topics that the other panelists will address, along with their particular biases or perspectives. It is also necessary to know the time frame for the entire panel, including time allotted for audience questions, each panelist's prepared remarks, and the moderator's commentary (Griffin, Buccino, Klein, & Thaler-Carter, 2010).

In addition, the following strategies will ensure success of the panel presentation:

- Limit the number of slides to prevent distraction from the presentation. It is helpful to have a brief conversation or initiate e-mail contact with the other panelists and agree on a number of slides and time frames so that none of the panelists dominate. Much of this organization may be directed by the moderator.
- If possible, the sharing of PowerPoint slides before the panel presentation, particularly panels that are based upon a thematic presentation involving all panelists, is helpful to avoid overlap or repetition of content and to be aware of the information provided by the other panelists.
- Develop a time clock system (e.g., set a timepiece in front of the speaker or have the moderator invoke the time with signage or some other method; often, a staff member of the organization that is hosting the event may provide timing assistance).
- Use an active voice that holds the audience's attention, and illustrate content with real-life examples.
- Maintain eye contact with the audience that fosters the speaker's engagement with the audience.
- Identify the major theme of the presentation, and add three to five major points to support the thrust of the theme.

If a panelist is expected to offer expert opinions in response to questions, the following preparatory steps are needed:

- Similarly to preparing for presentations, panelists need to gather information on their audience and gear responses to the needs of the group. Consulting with colleagues before the panel presentation is also useful.

- Anticipate audience questions; colleagues can be asked to contribute to a potential list of questions for advance preparation.
- Paraphrase questions asked from the audience before responding; this allows everyone in the audience to hear the questions and allows the presenter time to organize his or her thoughts.
- Treat all questions with the same importance so as not to display a bias or preference for certain individuals in the audience.

During the session, panelists are expected to conduct themselves professionally, with sensitivity to the fact that each of them is only one of several experts sharing the stage from whom the audience wants to hear new information and practice ideas. Box 20.1 lists suggestions for panelist dos and don'ts.

Moderator Preparation

The moderator's role during a panel presentation is to ensure that the session objectives are met, that the panelist presentations are pulled together in a cohesive fashion, and that all participants fulfill their duties without dominating the presentation. The moderator will begin the session by providing introductory remarks that include an overview of the panel's purpose, a brief biographical introduction, and the evidence-based topic of each panelist. The moderator's role is to ensure the even flow of the panel discussion and questions from the audience. Throughout the panel, the moderator may ask follow-up questions to hone in on key messages or points. At the conclusion of the panel, the moderator should provide summary statements of the major themes of each evidence-based presentation; therefore, note-taking during the session will be necessary while being attentive to coordinating questions from the audience and panelist responses. Box 20.2 presents specific responsibilities of the moderator during a panel presentation.

Before the panel session, the moderator should contact all panelists individually to obtain sufficient information about their presentation and area of expertise. An exchange of information about the other panel members should also occur, including contact information (i.e., e-mail address) so that coordination by panel members can be made before the presentation. In addition, the moderator can serve as a liaison for exchanging logistic information (e.g., panel schedule, audiovisual needs, room setup, projected number of individuals attending the presentation for distribution of handouts, and confirmation of

BOX **20.1**	*A Panelist's Dos and Don'ts*

Do

- Be sensitive to time limitations for both prepared and spontaneous remarks.
- Make notations of other speakers' comments for response and essential points for an organized, well-thought-out reply.

Don't

- "Jump" on the remarks of other speakers (i.e., enable them to speak without interruption).
- Look at another panelist when responding to his or her comments; rather, speak directly to the audience.
- Express political or partisan opinions.

BOX
20.2

Responsibilities of the Moderator During a Panel Presentation

- Provide a brief introduction of each panelist, emphasizing his or her expertise or experience with the evidence-based topic.
- Select audience members who have questions to ask of panelists.
- Repeat questions (or have panelists do it) for the audience's benefit.
- Remind the audience members or panelists of time constraints if too much time is used.
- Redirect the panelists' comments as needed to ensure that one or two panelists do not dominate the session.

the meeting time and place). These tasks also may be performed by the organization that is hosting the panel or event. The moderator also needs to ensure that the panel conforms to time constraints and clearly conveys to panelists time remaining in their speaking slots.

DISSEMINATING EVIDENCE THROUGH ROUNDTABLE PRESENTATIONS

Roundtable presentations are a third way to "narrowcast" EBP data. They are an informal way to share information with a small group of people—literally, the number of individuals that fit around a table. Roundtable presentations offer the opportunity to share specific information with a group but also to allow the group to discuss the practical application of the content.

Room size and the arrangement of table and chairs are pivotal in convening roundtable presentations that enable full involvement of all participants. A room that is not adequate for the size of the group is problematic because it can contribute to presentation delays, unnecessary distractions with participants (i.e., locate and retrieve chairs from other rooms), and cramped and awkward seating arrangements (i.e., squeezing participants uncomfortably around a table that is too small). A functioning room thermostat set at a comfortable temperature contributes to the proper environmental climate of the room.

Because the group for a roundtable is generally small—6 to 12 persons—it is appropriate to introduce group members first, which will make them more comfortable to engage in discussion. The use of audiovisual equipment is often not possible in this setting, but printed handouts of slides can be used to identify key points or provide supplemental information (slides with a light background with dark print photocopy better). As in the case of a formal lecture, it is important to understand the needs of the audience and their reasons for attending the roundtable (Larkin, Griffith, Pitler, Donahue, & Sbrolla, 2012).

Preparation for a Roundtable Discussion

In planning the presentation, it is important to allow ample time for discussion. Anticipate that one half to one third of the allotted time will be spent in discussion related to the prepared evidence-based material. Advance discussion questions distributed by the presenter help to facilitate dialogue among the participants, should conversation lapse.

Content for a roundtable is prepared in the same way as for a lecture presentation. Delivery of the material will be different, given the small group size and intimate setting in which the roundtable takes place. After introductions, the goals of the evidence-based presentation are stated. Any handouts are distributed and described in terms of their utility and relevance to the EBP topic. The content of the presentation is then delivered. Because the group is small, it is important to scan the group regularly, making eye contact with each person, in order to engage all present. Questions can be answered either during the presentation or at the end. If questions are taken and discussion allowed during the delivery of the content, it is important to watch the time to ensure that all content will be covered (Blome et al., 2017; Griffin et al., 2010).

Concluding the Roundtable

At the end of a roundtable session, participants should be thanked for attending, and any final questions that require additional clarification should be answered. The group may wish to exchange business cards or other identification or information (e.g., e-mail addresses) so that dialogue among the members may continue. The presenter should offer his or her business card to allow future follow-up and may stay in the vicinity of the roundtable for some time after the session to answer individual questions.

DISSEMINATING EVIDENCE THROUGH POSTER PRESENTATIONS

Poster presentations provide an alternative option for presenting evidence-based information to professional audiences, but they are different in a number of ways from those given from a podium. Podium presentations are more formal in both style and format. There are several types of poster presentations: display, easel, and table top (DeSilets, 2010). More recently, laptop and electronic poster presentations, wherein the poster is displayed via computer or wide-screen monitors, have been introduced at conferences as more economical, "green," and space saving (Beamish, Ansell, Foster, Foster, & Egan, 2014; Health Care Transition Research Consortium [HCTRC], 2013). The presenter typically provides more information from the podium as contrasted with the poster, wherein only the most essential aspects of information about a study or evidence-based project are given. The podium presenter adheres to a fairly standard format for providing information, with little or no time allowed to take audience questions. The poster presenter also adheres to a defined format for displaying information; however, this type of presentation allows for more interaction between colleagues in the area of clinical interest, enabling the sharing and learning that otherwise would not have been possible with a podium presentation (Billings & Kowalski, 2010). If projected, it is important that the material be large enough to be legible.

Typically, the presenter stands near his or her poster during the times designated by conference planners. Standing to the side of the poster will enable participants to read, and reflect on, the poster content without feeling intruded upon or intimidated by the presenter's presence (Beamish et al., 2014; Billings & Kowalski, 2010). When the participant is ready, the poster presenter is available to answer questions or discuss key points. Individuals displaying posters can explore any number of issues that are not possible with podium presentations. For example, colleagues might discuss in greater detail the clinical implications of the evidence presented, such as implementation challenges in a community-based setting compared with those in a tertiary care setting. Poster presentations also enable the dissemination of preliminary research data or evidence reviews (Miracle, 2008). Having business cards available for conference attendees facilitates additional consultation and conveys the message of accessibility.

Podium presentations have time limits of usually 15 to 20 minutes, whereas posters are displayed for longer periods, allowing the presenter more time to speak directly with colleagues about his or her work. A poster presentation is less intimidating than a podium presentation because public speaking can be uncomfortable for professionals who are not accustomed to presenting before large numbers of people (Christenbery & Latham, 2013). Displaying information also may be preferable to giving an oral presentation for individuals who process information better in visual rather than verbal format.

The key to developing an effective visual poster is to construct it in a way that captures the attention of the conference participants. It is useful to think about the attractive characteristics of poster presentations seen at various professional conferences (see http://thepoint .lww.com/Melnyk3e for two well-designed posters that were displayed at national/international conferences). Notable aspects of these posters include their design and symmetry, the logical sequencing of content, evident navigational direction of content, the contrast of colors used, use of key words or phrases to emphasize important content, and use of graphs/figures to present study findings. As with PowerPoint presentations, a poster composed of a light background with darker print has been identified as preferable. The use of color accents and graphics pertinent to the topic can be effective (Siedlecki, 2017). A poster that is content dense is not an effective poster because it obscures the essence of the messaging and is visually unattractive and difficult to read (Billings & Kowalski, 2010; DeSilets, 2010; Illic & Rowe, 2013). Posters that are poorly designed often present content in a disorganized format, contain too much or too little information, use colors that clash, and do not use figures/graphs to display content. Oftentimes, organizations have poster templates for their employees or faculty members to use, including appropriate logos. Consider other creative ways to convey information. Recently, presenters have learned to embed tablets, like an iPad, within their poster design, offering a more interactive component to the viewing experience.

However, the display of graphics and organization of a poster are not enough. Knowing how to present information to colleagues in succinct, scholarly, and precise terms is just as important. Substance and design, when combined effectively in a poster, can serve as an effective vehicle for conveying information to colleagues. The poster becomes a magnet for attracting colleagues, not only to read about one's work but also to provide a comfortable setting for additional discussion with sharing of information that is the cornerstone of collegial discourse and "reciprocal dialogue" (DeSilets, 2010; Illic & Rowe, 2013, p. 10; Miracle, 2008; Siedlecki, 2017).

If resources are available, it is useful to consult with a graphic design expert when developing a poster. Consulting with an expert certainly makes it easier, but the designer has limitations as well because this individual's area of expertise is limited to graphic design, not the poster content (Sherman, 2010). If consulting with a designer is not an option, then accessing examples of posters from print resources or the Internet or from colleagues is an alternative. Several software programs are available for developing posters, which include Microsoft PowerPoint, Adobe Illustrator, and InDesign (Billings & Kowalski, 2010). Another useful resource to consult when developing a poster is ePoster. This is an open-access journal containing nearly 2000 scientific and healthcare posters that have been developed for presentations at international scientific and healthcare conferences.

Poster examples on ePoster can provide creative inspiration for constructing a professional poster: http://www.eposters.net/posters/

The University of North Carolina Graduate School webpage on poster and presentation resources serves as a gateway portal to other website links and offers valuable assistance with developing effective posters: http://gradschool.unc.edu/academics/resources/postertips.html

When a poster is accepted for presentation at a conference, authors typically receive size guidelines for construction and display of their posters from a conference organizer and/ or an association. These guides are critical to the presenter before beginning the poster's design so that time is not lost in preparing a product that does not meet the requirements of the poster session.

The Pragmatics of Constructing a Poster: Getting Started

The first step in developing a poster presentation is to translate ideas and images into graphic form. Sketching out or developing a mock-up of the poster with self-sticking notes or using a computer template may be useful (Hamilton, 2008).

Evidence-Based Poster Presentations

The content of an evidence-based poster presentation is similar to other EBP presentation forms and generally includes the following sections:

- **Background/significance:** Provide background as to the nature or status of the clinical problem (e.g., prevalence data or other statistics demonstrating the growing importance of the problem; professional association's position statements).
- **Clinical question:** Specifically identify what clinical problem or question was investigated.
- **Search for evidence/accepted practice:** Identify briefly the methods and sources used to collect evidence (e.g., search strategy for the review of literature, focus groups, and surveys of institutional practices).
- **Presentation and critical appraisal of the evidence:** Provide a succinct summary of the conclusions drawn from evaluating the scope of evidence available.
- **Clinical practice implications:** Describe clinical practice implications, based on the process of collecting and evaluating the evidence.

It is also important to obtain and carefully review poster guidelines received, such as the poster size that is standard for the conference (e.g., the typical size is 4 × 6 feet) so that the poster text and graphics are readable from a distance of 4 feet. Keeping the following principles in mind will enhance the readability of the poster:

- Remember that English-speaking participants will read the poster from left to right and from top to bottom.
- Number the order of the poster presentation to assist the reader in information sequencing.
- Vary the font size on the poster according to the type of information being presented, for example, 100 point (pt.) or larger for the poster title (readable from 20 feet), 72 pt. or larger for authors' names and affiliations, 36 to 48 pt. or larger for poster headings and subheadings, and 24 pt. for poster text.
- Use infographics or illustrations in lieu of text when appropriate, such as when reporting findings.
- Limit the use of special effects.
- Avoid designing a monotone poster.
- Keep headings and subheadings brief (fewer than five words).
- Use bulleted phrases or short sentences of seven words or less.
- Use high contrast between lettering and background (i.e., dark text and light background).

- Use familiar fonts (e.g., Calibri, Times New Roman, Courier New, and Arial) and the same font style throughout the poster (some recommend a different font for the title). Keep in mind that sans serif fonts (without ascenders or descenders, like Arial and Calibri) are more readable.
- Avoid using shadowing and underlines; use bold instead for areas of emphasis.
- Use active tense (e.g., "Findings reveal. . .") and plain language.
- Organize the poster in four sections: background information, methodology, findings, and implications; *or*
- Organize the poster in three sections: purpose/methods; findings, implications.
- Limit the number of references cited on the poster by listing them on the handout or at the end of a corresponding section.
- Limit text blocks to 50 or fewer words.
- Insert institutional branding logo at the top of the poster.
- Have supplemental materials available as appropriate.
- Have business cards available.

The presentation of content should follow a logical sequence from beginning to end—the same format used for publishing research papers. The presentation of research content, although dependent on the specifications of the conference, typically includes:

- **Introduction/Background:** The focus of the introduction section is to attract the attention of colleagues about the significance of the project by emphasizing the need, prevalence of the problem, or clinical issue.
- **Objectives(s):** This section should be brief in that it states the focus of the study.
- **Design/Methods:** Brevity is the key unless there is something of interest about the methods or design that warrants emphasis (e.g., recruiting and training interviewers for culturally diverse populations).
- **Data Analysis:** This section should be concise in terms of listing analyses conducted.
- **Study Findings:** The emphasis in this section is on presenting graphs or tables with limited explanatory text to accompany them.
- **Conclusions:** Brief statements are made regarding the most significant findings as well as the clinical implications for practice.
- **Acknowledgment:** When appropriate, it is important to recognize the names of other colleagues on the project and/or the funding source.

Expectations of Poster Presenters

Poster presenters are expected to stand beside their posters in accordance with the designated display times. It is disappointing for colleagues to walk among posters without the authors or investigators present, because one of the primary purposes of a poster presentation is to facilitate scholarly and clinical dialogue among colleagues. Having PowerPoint handouts of the poster presentation or other supplemental materials available for distribution is also helpful (Bingham & O'Neal, 2013; Illic & Rowe, 2013). PowerPoint handouts are more readable with light-colored background with dark text (Grand Valley State University, Office of Undergraduate Research and Scholarship, 2016). The handouts may contain additional information that was not possible to include in the poster display (e.g., more detail on the review of pertinent literature, the theoretical framework, research instruments, and references). In lieu of handouts, presenters may create flash drives containing PDF versions of the display or supporting materials, allowing visitors to reference the information at their convenience. Contact information with e-mail address for later correspondence is helpful as well (Billings & Kowalski, 2010; Hamilton, 2008).

Helpful Resources for Constructing Posters

The Internet has many excellent resources to help with constructing posters, and these resources provide practical details (e.g., durable poster materials, display layout and format, logistics of color selection, photos, and graphics). Some sites provide information on using PowerPoint and creating posters for online purposes. These sites are contained in Box 20.3.

Listed below are some fail-safe suggestions to avoid poster presentation mistakes.

- Develop a timeline that accommodates unexpected delays in processing over which one has no control (e.g., use of graphic designer, photography).
- Back up files as the poster is being developed so that no data are lost through computer malfunctioning or as a result of a virus. Consider storing data on a cloud service that can be accessed remotely, such as iCloud, Dropbox, or Google Drive.
- Determine the best method for transporting the poster while traveling because it may have to be carried to the passenger section and stored overhead. Shipping the poster in advance risks not having it arrive for your presentation.
- Consider constructing poster using fabrics rather than paper as more portable; many commercial vendors are now producing posters in cloth.
- Bring a flash drive or upload the file onto the laptop computer of the poster in case it gets lost, damaged, or destroyed in transit.
- Locate the business office at the conference site or nearby copy center if needed prior to leaving, in case the poster needs to be reprinted.
- Label the poster to ensure its security if staying at a hotel to prevent loss in transit.

BOX 20.3 *Helpful Websites for Creating Poster Presentations*

1. *Creating Effective Poster Presentations: An Effective Poster.* This website provides succinct information on the construction of posters akin to listing of "helpful hints." Background information is presented on the rationale and benefits for considering poster sessions as an option for professional presentation. http://www.ncsu.edu/project/posters/

2. *Creating Medical Poster Presentations.* This website provides information about poster sessions for medical and scientific presentations using PowerPoint software. http://www.free-power-point-templates.com/articles/create-poster-powerpoint-2010/

3. *Designing Effective Posters.* This website provides the most comprehensive and detailed information about poster sessions of any website. Jeff Radel, Department of Occupational Therapy Education, University of Kansas Medical Center, provides detailed information on every aspect of creating a poster, from formatting the poster title to transport and storage. This website is really a must. http://www.kumc.edu/SAH/OTEd/jradel/Poster_Presentations/PstrStart.html

4. *American College of Physicians.* This website provides "how to" information on developing a poster for a scientific presentation. The website content includes a poster production timeline, tips on creating effective posters, and the poster format. https://www.acponline.org/membership/residents/competitions-awards/abstracts/preparing/poster

5. *MakeSigns Scientific Posters.* An online self-paced, self-instructional tutorial is provided for users who will be creating a poster. This is a commercial site that produces both paper and cloth posters. http://www.makesigns.com/tutorials/scientific-poster-parts.aspx

- Remember to bring materials (e.g., masking tape, double-sided tape, push pins) to display the poster, although they will often be provided.
- Have handouts available for colleagues who want additional information on the literature review, methodology, and references.
- Bring sufficient numbers of business cards.

Laptop Poster Presentations

Laptop poster presentations are an electronic iteration of the hard copy poster. The content of the laptop poster is similar to the hard copy version; however, its appearance and format are similar to a PowerPoint presentation. The laptop poster is composed of a limited number of slides (five to six). The poster presenter engages actively with one or more individuals while providing a brief oral commentary as the slides are shown. The attendees are encouraged to ask questions and make comments as the poster presentation is given (HCTRC, 2013).

DISSEMINATING EVIDENCE TO SMALL GROUPS

Disseminating evidence also can be accomplished in small group formats, such as in evidence-based grand rounds and evidence-based clinical rounds.

Evidence-Based Grand Rounds

Grand rounds can serve as a major forum for evidence-based presentations. Departments within tertiary care and academic settings often host grand rounds or forums designed for clinicians to speak directly to their colleagues on topics that are innovative or that call for new approaches to care. Usually, speakers present empirically based answers to clinical practice questions, typically findings from their own or others' studies or policy updates with clinical implications for staff. Grand rounds usually consist of formal oral presentations accompanied by audiovisual slides or video presentations. Generally, a question-and-answer period follows the speaker's presentation.

Just as there are journal club websites (discussed in more detail later in the chapter), grand rounds presentations can be found on websites. Internet-based grand rounds are another setting for experts to share evidence-based information with colleagues on topics of mutual interest. Internet grand rounds topics may be presented or reviewed by several clinical experts, enabling users to e-mail questions that can later be posted on the website. The advantages of Internet usage are the widespread access that is available to users, the ability to combine the perspectives and expertise of many clinical specialists, and the convenience for the users. Additionally, users are not bound by the time constraints of real-time meetings, enabling them to participate at their convenience.

Evidence-Based Clinical Rounds

Evidence-based clinical rounds, smaller in scope than grand rounds, are another effective medium to present evidence to guide clinical practice changes, as well as meaningfully involve clinical staff in the process. Evidence-based clinical rounds have been used very successfully as part of the Advancing Research and Clinical Practice through Close Collaboration (ARCC) model. One or a few clinicians will do the following in preparation for these rounds:

- Identify a clinical question (e.g., What is the most effective medication to decrease pain in postsurgical cardiac patients?).
- Conduct a systematic search for the evidence to answer the clinical question.
- Critically appraise the evidence found.
- Recommend guidelines for practice changes based on the evidence.

These clinicians then present the information that they gathered and make recommendations for clinical practice to their colleagues, based on the evidence, in the form of an oral presentation during a more casual session than the more formal, larger grand rounds.

Brief Consultations

The ultimate goal of excellence in clinical care is to integrate evidence into clinical practice as a standard of care for *all* patients under *all* circumstances. This level of practice can be achieved only by fostering the organizational environment to support it. As one expert has stated, "hallway consultations," which occur informally between colleagues in the hallways about patients, are an on-the-ground approach to facilitate discussion about nursing care interventions that are evidence-based. These are excellent opportunities for collegial consultation and instruction (Van Soeren, Hurlock-Chorostecki, & Reeves, 2011).

Digitizing Evidence Communications

Technological advances have enabled the use of podcasts, videocasts, webinars, social media, and other digital tools to communicate information to targeted audiences (Savel, Goldstein, Perencevich, & Angood, 2007). A *podcast* is "a digital audio file" made available on the Internet for downloading to a computer or mobile device, typically available as a series, new installments of which can be received by subscribers automatically (https://en.oxforddictionaries.com/definition/podcast). A video cast—also known as a *video podcast* or a *vodcast*—refers to "the online delivery of video on demand, video clip content via Atom or RSS enclosures" (Vodcast, 2009). A *webinar* is an interactive synchronous online presentation that allows participants to ask questions or make comments.

The advantage of these electronic tools is that the presentation, whether in audio or video format, can be archived on a specific website for later convenient use by the learner (Abe, 2007; Skiba, 2006). For example, journal clubs and presentations can be recorded and videotaped for later use for those unable to attend at the scheduled time. Podcasts and vodcasts are relatively simple to access by users and inexpensive to produce (Rowell, Corl, Johnson, & Fishman, 2006). PowerPoint presentations can be integrated into podcasts as a means of accompanying the audiotapes (Jham, Duraes, Strassler, & Sensi, 2008). Both podcasts and vodcasts can be downloaded to the user's own mobile device (e.g., iPods, BlackBerry, MP3 players; Abe, 2007).

Disadvantages of these web-based tools are that every user may not have the technology hardware and software and/or the experience to use it. Additionally, unless an interactive feature is integrated into the podcast, the learning is primarily a passive instructional approach (Jham et al., 2008). Refer to Box 20.4 for a listing of websites that provide information on the development of podcasts and vodcasts.

DISSEMINATING EVIDENCE AT COMMUNITY MEETINGS

Recognized experts in a geographic area may be asked to present evidence-based information in a community setting. This type of presentation can be particularly challenging because community groups may include laypersons and the media, in addition to professionals. This requires that the speaker be able to address all segments of the group in a way that they understand. Before making the presentation, it is important to collaborate with community leaders about the nature of the content to be presented as well as to be culturally sensitive to the potential attendees. Tips for presenting to a mixed audience include the following:

Helpful Websites for Podcasts

The following websites provide guidance for developing podcasts:

- How to create your own podcasts—A step by step tutorial
  https://www.lifewire.com/how-to-create-your-own-podcast-2843321
- Learning in hand with Tony Vincent—Create podcasts
  https://learninginhand.com/podcasting/
- Online tools and software for creating podcast feeds and posts
  https://www.emergingedtech.com/2017/02/10-great-tools-creating-quality-educational-podcasts/
- How to create a podcast
  https://www.digitaltrends.com/how-to/how-to-make-a-podcast/

Jackson, C., Jones, A., & Kemp., K. (2017). ProfHacker: 10 Things We Learned Producing a Podcast at a University. The Chronicle of Higher Education. Retrieved from: https://www.chronicle.com/blogs/profhacker/10-things-we-learned-producing-a-podcast-at-a-university/64262 on May 27, 2018

- Begin the presentation with a general overview of its purpose, followed by a review of the major points or findings.
- If the group is small enough, it is helpful to ask for introductions so the presentation can be more closely tailored to the group.
- Define all abbreviations and acronyms (e.g., the American Academy of Nurse Practitioners, rather than AANP).
- Provide definitions as you speak (e.g., ". . . risk pool, that is, a group of individuals brought together to purchase insurance in order to spread the risk, or cost, among a larger group of people . . .").
- Avoid offhand remarks that could be misinterpreted or misquoted by any media present. Stick with the facts as you know them or offer your professional, educated opinion when asked.
- Offer to answer questions personally after the session for those who might be reluctant to ask a question before a large group.
- When offering examples, consider the potentially mixed nature of the audience and cite cases that all members can understand.
- Allow ample time for questions and answers as well as general discussion.

The use of slides and corresponding handouts is also useful in keeping all participants interested and focused on the presentation (Bingham & O'Neal, 2013). Refer to the earlier discussion on *Slides to Enhance the Presentation* for guidance on the development of PowerPoint slides. Providing information on relevant websites and articles is also helpful.

DISSEMINATING EVIDENCE AT HOSPITAL/ORGANIZATIONAL AND PROFESSIONAL COMMITTEE MEETINGS

Presenting evidence-based information to a committee of fellow professionals can be a stressful experience. Adequate preparation is again the key to ensure success (Blome et al., 2017; Stuart, 2013). Anticipate questions that may reflect not only the information that is being presented but also historical information, because not everyone in the group will be aware of all of the relevant history surrounding a particular issue. Consider the following:

- Why is the group interested in the topic?
- What is the history of the issue in the particular institution?
- Has there been any controversy surrounding the issue that may interfere with the presentation? If so, should it be openly addressed before the presentation begins?
- Are there some members of the group who may be more critical than others with regard to the information presented? If it is possible to learn more about concerns ahead of time, they can be addressed more readily during the meeting.
- If one member of the group appears to have a particular concern that is impacting the agenda, offer to have a private conversation at the conclusion of the meeting.
- Is there any related information that may need to be discussed during the presentation, and does the presenter have adequate knowledge in the related area?
- Is this a group whose meetings are informal, or does the group maintain formal meeting rules?

The most important pieces of information needed before beginning to prepare for a committee presentation are:

- What is the composition of the audience? What do they know about the topic at hand?
- How much time will there be to share information and answer audience questions?

Whoever invites the presenter to the meeting or is responsible for serving as chairperson should be able to describe the expected attendance, the disciplines represented, and the relevance of the information for the group.

Committee meetings are usually tightly scheduled, with little opportunity to go beyond the allotted time for the agenda items. Therefore, it is important to be able to provide key information within the time frame allowed. In addition, if the meeting is held in a hospital or similar facility, staff members may come in and out of the meeting when they are answering pages or attending to patient care responsibilities. This movement in and out of the room can be distracting and unnerving for the speaker, so it is important to prepare mentally for this possibility. In addition, anticipate that some latecomers will ask for information that has already been presented. The best approach is to provide the information in a brief manner and offer to discuss it more fully after the meeting.

After a brief introduction as to its relevance for the group, the presentation can generally follow the format for a journal article on an EBP topic:

- Clinical question
- Search for evidence
- Critical appraisal
- Implications for practice
- Evaluation (if the practice change had been implemented)

This should be followed by a discussion period as to the utility of the information for the committee or the facility.

DISSEMINATING EVIDENCE THROUGH JOURNAL CLUBS

The concept of journal clubs has evolved considerably over the years, especially with the use of the Internet as a vehicle for scholarly exchange. A quick online search of "journal club" will reveal multiple sites by various healthcare disciplines and national professional associations, most of which are evidence-based in focus and which appreciate their roles as conduits for the dissemination of clinical care knowledge. Whether journal clubs are offered in person—in the clinical setting or in a more relaxed off-site setting—or via the Internet, they serve as another mechanism for disseminating the best evidence on which to base healthcare practice by physicians, nurses, and other providers to improve their clinical practice and patient outcomes (Marble, 2009; Moonan, Bukoye, Clapp, Shermont, & Oliveira, 2015, 2016; Silversides, 2011; Steele-Moses, 2013). For example, journal clubs may be used as a strategy to foster the goal of a healthcare organization's nursing department to obtain Magnet status or create linkages to clinicians who work in isolation, such as school nurses (McLaughlin, Speroni, Patterson, Guzzetta, & Desale, 2013; Sortedahl, 2012; Tinkham, 2013).

On-site Journal Clubs

Journal clubs provide an opportunity for clinicians to share and learn about evidence-based approaches in their work settings. The success of the journal club will depend on several factors:

- Expertise of the advanced-level clinician in selecting an appropriate review article and other supporting articles that provide substantial sources of evidence
- Organizational resources to facilitate the activities of the journal club, such as access to online bibliographic resources that include evidence-based reviews (e.g., Cochrane Controlled Trials Register)
- Participation by motivated colleagues or staff
- Application to practice, resulting in practice changes
- Provision of nursing continuing education units
- Topics that are of clinical interest and relevance
- Nursing administrative resources and support (i.e., research consultation available to journal club facilitators to host journal club)

A journal club is typically led by an advanced-level clinician who understands research design, methods, and statistics, or sometimes by a trainee with his or her faculty mentor (Gelling, 2011; Marble, 2009; McKeever, Kinney, Lima, & Newall, 2016; Steele-Moses, 2013; Tinkham, 2013). This clinician serves not only as the discussion facilitator but also as an educator because it is likely that colleagues will ask for additional contextual information (McLeod, Steinert, Boudreau, Snell, & Wiseman, 2010). Questions from journal club participants typically focus on the type of research design used, sample selection criteria, instrumentation, and statistical analyses. Therefore, it is essential that the journal club leader have the knowledge to answer these types of questions adequately. Additionally, in order to be effective, the journal club leader needs facilitator skills to encourage members of the club to participate as well as to feel comfortable and supported in sharing input. The facilitation skills for an effective journal club leader include:

- Actively listening to questions asked
- Using open-ended questions to facilitate discussion
- Avoiding the appearance of preference or bias in responding to questions by stating that a particular question is "good," unless equivalent affirming comments are made about all questions
- Clearly communicating messages about the purpose and expectations for the club
- Coming to the meeting well prepared and organized to conduct the meeting professionally (e.g., ensuring room availability and setup, as well as a sufficient number of handouts and other materials)
- Monitoring the flow of discussion to ensure that it is focused on the topic

- Interceding when conversation "drift" occurs, redirecting the conversation back to the topic (e.g., "getting back to our point," "as was said before," and "we were talking about . . .")
- Reinforcing responses to questions asked by members with affirming comments in order to encourage group participation ("good question," "interesting point," etc.)
- Summarizing major points at the end of the session before concluding the meeting
- Demonstrating application to practice

The journal club leader will most likely have the responsibility for selecting the journal article to be discussed by the group participants (Johnson, 2016; McKeever et al., 2016; O'Nan, 2011). This article should meet the journal club criteria for an evidence-based presentation and should be relevant to the clinical practice of the staff. Selected articles should be on current studies or evidence reviews, use valid and reliable instrumentation, have an adequate number of subjects, and use a research design appropriate for the research question or purpose. Although there may be variations in the format for the journal club, such as including content on the "how to's" for critiquing research articles (Christenbery, 2011; McKeever et al., 2016; Moonan et al., 2015, 2016), the standard process for the discussion of articles, focusing on the key points and not a reread of the articles, is as follows:

- Study objectives/hypotheses
- Design and methods, including the setting in which the study was conducted (e.g., the community, the intensive care unit, outpatient clinic, or the home) as well as instruments used along with their validity and reliability for the sample studied
- Data analyses, with rationale for the specific tests used
- Findings, specifically in terms of the relative significance of the findings, paying careful attention to whether the study had a large enough sample size with power to detect significant findings
- Conclusions of the study with clinical implications, such as the clinical procedure related to aseptic management of long-term gastrostomy tubes
- Efficient critical appraisal of the study, including its strengths and limitations as well as applicability to practice (e.g., clinicians might be hesitant to change their practice based on the findings from one study that had a very small number of subjects)

Journal clubs are held at regularly scheduled times and locations, enabling participants to plan for meetings. Some journal clubs, held in off-site locations, incorporate social time for members to network (Silversides, 2011). Articles for the journal club should be distributed to members well in advance so that members can read and digest the material. Distribution of forthcoming meetings and identification of the topic to be discussed by e-mail via the institution's targeted mailing list is a convenient and time-efficient method (Christenbery, 2011).

Online Journal Clubs

The Internet provides additional resources and opportunities for developing other types of journal clubs for healthcare professionals (Moonan et al., 2015, 2016). There are numerous online bibliographic databases that can be accessed for obtaining evidence-based answers to questions or accessing substantive articles for a journal club.

For example, an advanced-level clinician on a pediatric unit of a major tertiary medical center wants to find a high-quality article on pediatric pain for next month's journal club. The most effective strategy for finding this article is to access one of several online evidence-based review databases because the most current and rigorously reviewed studies can be found there. These databases include the ACP Journal Club, Evidence-Based Medicine Reviews,

BOX
20.5

Results of a Search on "Pediatric Pain" in Evidence-Based Review Databases

1. Beecham, E., Candy, B., Howard, R., McCulloch, R., Laddie, J., Rees, H., . . . Jones, L. (2015). Pharmacological interventions for pain in children and adolescents with life-limiting conditions. *Cochrane Database of Systematic Reviews*, (3), CD010750. doi:10.1002/14651858.CD010750.pub2
2. Bradt, J., Dileo, C., Magill, L., Teague, A. (2016). Music interventions for improving psychological and physical outcomes in cancer patients. *Cochrane Database of Systematic Reviews*, (8), CD006911. doi:10.1002/14651858.CD006911.pub3
3. Martin, A. E., Newlove-Delgado, T. V., Abbott, R. A., Bethel, A., Thompson-Coon, J., Whear, R., Logan, S. (2017). Pharmacological interventions for recurrent abdominal pain in childhood. *Cochrane Database of Systematic Reviews*, (3), CD010973. doi:10.1002/14651858.CD010973.pub2
4. Ohlsson, A., Shah, P. S. (2015). Paracetamol (acetaminophen) for patent ductus arteriosus in preterm or low-birth-weight infants. *Cochrane Database of Systematic Reviews*, (3), CD010061. doi:10.1002/14651858.CD010061.pub2
5. Tighe, M., Afzal, N. A., Bevan, A., Hayen, A., Munro, A., Beattie, R. M. (2014). Pharmacological treatment of children with gastro-oesophageal reflux. *Cochrane Database of Systematic Reviews*, (11), CD008550. doi:10.1002/14651858 .CD008550.pub2

Cochrane Database of Systematic Reviews, Cochrane Controlled Trials Register, and Database of Abstracts of Reviews of Effectiveness (DARE). Searching these databases for "pediatric pain" reveals the five citations listed in Box 20.5. Based on the needs of the clinical staff, a clinician selects an article published by Martin et al. in 2017 because it addresses specific clinical practice issues related to pediatric pain.

There are online **journal clubs** that incorporate the technological advantages available with the Internet. This format enables individual users to access the journal club website at times convenient to personal work schedules, interests, and learning style. Website journal clubs, although highly individualized, are similar to the group meeting format in that an article is reviewed for its applicability for clinical practice (Moonan et al., 2015; Steenbeek et al., 2009). The difference with the online format is the process, which varies from site to site (e.g., a critical review of a clinical trial initiated by a contributing author and reviewed by website editors, individual efforts of a website editor with feedback from its users). Several online evidence-based websites are listed in Box 20.6.

Additionally, online professional journals may offer a journal club feature enabling feedback from readers. For example, the *American Journal of Critical Care* offers a supplemental section at the end of selected articles for the reader, enabling the review and critique of the study as a preliminary step in considering its application to practice. Discussion of its applicability with other journal readers is available through an online discussion using electronic letters, as demonstrated in the Smith and Grami article (2017).

Institution-related journal clubs benefit from incorporating an evaluation process. This can be done informally at the conclusion of each of the on-site meetings or at a predetermined end of the online sessions. Evaluation forms can also be used to evaluate the perceived benefit of journal clubs.

There are disadvantages and advantages in using online journal clubs. The user does not have the benefit of hearing the views of colleagues, which may limit learning regarding others' own clinical areas of expertise, critical thinking, and professional attitudes and values. Having

BOX
20.6
Examples of Websites Containing Evidence-Based Practice Information

1. **Oncology Nursing Society, Evidenced-Based Practice (EBP) Research Center.** This website provides a number of resources on EBP and its application to the specialty of oncology nursing practice. PowerPoint presentations on EBP can be easily accessed.
http://www.ons.org/Research/PEP/
2. **Johns Hopkins Center for Evidence-Based Practice.** This website contains exemplars of EBP practice projects and other resources.
http://www.hopkinsmedicine.org/evidence-based-practice
3. **The Helene Fuld Health Trust National Institute for Evidence-based Practice in Nursing and Healthcare at The Ohio State University College of Nursing.** This website contains a variety of resources on implementing EBP in healthcare organizations and institutions of higher learning as well as disseminating evidence.
https://nursing.osu.edu/sections/fuld-institute-ebp/

the opportunity to participate in open discussion of professional issues is an important activity that promotes group cohesiveness and understanding, often fostering teamwork and group morale. Some learners may benefit more from the group discussion format because it is more suitable to their learning style. Likewise, other staff members may prefer the online format because it is more convenient and accessible. Technical problems associated with security firewall software, problems with the user's computer capacity and connecting to networks are potential barriers (Moonan et al., 2015, 2016; Sortedahl, 2012; Steenbeek et al., 2009).

Journal club meetings enable the moderator to demonstrate professional behavior for other staff members. Professional development is an ongoing process, and the journal club is yet another opportunity for leaders to model the importance of using evidence for nursing practice, to demonstrate ways of discussing practice issues in a nonthreatening venue, and to create expectations for professional practice (Johnson, 2016; Marble, 2009; McKeever et al., 2016; Steele-Moses, 2013).

DISSEMINATING EVIDENCE THROUGH PUBLISHED ARTICLES

Many publishing options are available for individuals who are interested in sharing evidence-based information with colleagues. Typically, writing a journal article or contributing a chapter to a book is the first idea that comes to mind when publishing is considered. Publications of this magnitude may appear overwhelming in terms of time, effort, and lack of prior writing experience. However, there are many other opportunities and options available for individuals who are considering publishing.

Publishing experience can be gained by taking on less ambitious projects, such as serving on a publication committee at work or through a professional organization. Serving on these committees enables professionals to network and learn from each other about the methods and mechanics of publishing. Although the specific purpose of the committee may vary slightly (e.g., a newsletter committee, a publication committee), these committees are not necessarily designed for creating or fostering collective writing efforts. Publication committees may serve as panels to review publication content submitted by prospective authors to an association's newsletter or journal. Other committees may provide oversight to the production of professional materials to ensure that the association or organization's affiliation is properly represented.

Regardless of the specific type of publication committee, membership helps aspiring authors to learn a variety of skill-enhancing efforts on how to write and professionally publish. Ideally, seasoned committee members mentor less experienced committee members in acquiring these skills. For example, reviewing the written work of other colleagues enables one to learn, through the editing process, the difference between a well-written manuscript and a poorly written one. Writing a manuscript is not only about sharing expertise concerning evidence-based approaches, but also about learning how to present information in a manner that enhances readability and understanding by professional audiences. Reading drafts in process is an indirect method of learning to write.

Committee discussions of evidence-based issues and approaches provide an understanding of the processes involved in writing an EBP manuscript that include:

- Posing the burning clinical question
- Searching for the best and latest evidence
- Critically appraising and synthesizing the evidence
- Clinically implementing a practice change
- Evaluating the change

Also, working with colleagues who have published professionally can influence those who are learning by building their confidence.

Finding a Mentor

Finding a mentor is beneficial for professionals who have had limited publishing experience. This mentor might be found at school or work, on the Internet, with a professional organization, and, in some cases, by asking a nursing journal editor for suggestions. A mentor can guide the novice writer through the process, starting with an idea for a topic and leading to the actual writing and submission process. It is important that the mentor selected be an individual who possesses sufficient publication experience and the willingness to help (Costello, 2012; Oermann et al., 2015).

There may also be opportunities to collaborate on a joint writing project with a colleague with publication experience. The optimal circumstance for convening a writing team is to locate a cowriter in the same or geographically convenient community. Although the Internet has facilitated working with colleagues in distant locations, the first foray into a writing project with another colleague is best achieved with someone in close proximity. Real-time meetings involving personal contact are a prerequisite for the teaming of professionals with disparate writing experiences. This is yet another form of mentoring with extended hands-on involvement (Baker, 2013; Horstman & Theeke, 2012).

There are advantages to working with a team of colleagues to write and submit a manuscript for publication. The synergistic energy of collective efforts in brainstorming not only the proposed manuscript outline and its development but also the organizational process for its completion is significant. Collective and collaborative efforts can be a boon to generating the manuscript in a less burdensome and timelier process. Essential to productive, collaborative publishing efforts is the documented agreement among the authorship team of the roles and responsibilities of each of the members of the writing team. This predetermined agreement involves the specification of individual contribution of each author together with identified benchmarks of progress/completion as well as identification of consequences in the event the author team member does not meet the terms of the agreement. The process of clearly explicating each team members' responsibilities is a critical step to moving forward with the collective publishing endeavor (Baker, 2013). In addition, many journals now require that the roles of the authors in the development of the manuscript be described.

Two excellent resources pertaining to authorship issues are the International Academy of Nursing Editors (INANE; https://nursingeditors.com/) and the International Committee of Medical Journal Editors (ICMJE; http://www.icmje.org/)

Although experience and expertise are important, so is compatibility (e.g., writing style, temperament, and personality). A colleague who interacts uncomfortably or arrogantly with a novice writer is a significant detriment. Those who publish must devote extra time and effort beyond their usual workloads; therefore, engaging in an effort that is unpleasant and literally painful is likely to be short lived. Persistence with a specific publishing effort is likely to be brief if these types of negative circumstances exist. Publishing should be both a professionally rewarding and a fun experience (Fowler, 2013; Price, 2014; Yoder-Wise & Vlasses, 2012).

Generating the Idea

The first step in getting started with publishing an evidence-based paper is determining the topic. Generating the topic for publication is based on an individual's area of expertise, the clinical question that arises from clinical practice, and the availability of resources to support the initial curiosity and attention to the idea. An idea for an evidence-based publication may have been germinating for some time before it is fully acknowledged as a potential publication topic. For example, a clinician may have noticed that older adult residents in assisted living facilities have extended periods of confusion following hospital admissions. This clinical interest may lead the clinician to search the literature for information on the phenomenon and to find evidence for instituting new interventions. The experience prompts the clinician to believe that other colleagues would benefit from learning about these practices. As a result, the clinician decides to write an article for a gerontology journal.

Brainstorming with other colleagues, including your mentor and/or those with publishing experience, is another approach to generate ideas through a free-association process. The momentum achieved through a rapid exchange of ideas can result in many more ideas that would otherwise not have been identified (Phillips, Sweet, & Blythe, 2009).

The conviction that current practice is inadequate to meet patient needs is another generator of evidence-based publication ideas. For example, health outcome data may demonstrate the need for improvement in selected patient outcomes. A manuscript describing an evidence-based intervention to improve a particular set of patient outcomes is an example of a publication designed to improve both professional practice and patient outcomes (Brennan, Mattick, & Ellis, 2011). Providing the reader with a different slant not previously found in the literature, such as addressing long-term management in community settings, is yet another example of generating ideas for manuscripts (Fowler, 2013).

As mentioned previously, a presentation and/or a poster given at a scientific/professional meeting can serve as the basis for extended development as a manuscript. The advantages of having done a considerable amount of research and planning for a conference presentation/poster lends itself to an opportunity for publication (Hicks, 2015).

Planning the Manuscript

Once an idea or a set of ideas has been decided, the prospective author needs to sketch out a plan on how this initial idea or concept can be developed into a manuscript. For evidence-based papers, the formats for writing them do not vary significantly because there is a specified order for presentation of the content; the differences are based more on style rather than substance. Although publication formats vary according to technical specifications and editorial policy of each journal, the standard format for an evidence-based manuscript is title page, abstract, introduction, narrative, and conclusions and clinical applications. Prospective authors are encouraged to access the websites of prospective journals for additional guidance in preparing the manuscript.

Title Page

The title page is the first page of the manuscript and contains the article's title and all of the authors' names, job titles, affiliations, and contact information. If there are many authors, the corresponding author is indicated. The manuscript title should be succinct, and the key words in the title should be well known and accessible for content bibliographic searches. For example, if the author intends to write an evidence-based manuscript about adolescents, having the term "children" in the title might mislead readers.

Abstract

An abstract is a brief summary or synopsis of the article. Summaries indicate to the reader whether it is a research or clinical article. The abstract also identifies the major themes or findings and clinical implications. It is important that the abstract adheres to the technical specifications of the journal in terms of word limit and format (Costello, 2012; Happell, 2008). Technical specifications for manuscript abstracts are typically available in the journal's "Information for Authors" guidelines.

Introduction

The introduction of the manuscript should be written in a succinct manner and should not be longer than a few paragraphs. It contains information about the purpose of the article, the importance of the topic for the professional audience, and brief supporting evidence as to why this topic is important. Supporting evidence might include prevalence data or demonstration of need. A well-written introduction that is organized and informative will create more interest and motivation for the individual to pursue reading the article (Costello, 2012).

Manuscript Narrative

The narrative, or "middle section" of the manuscript, will differ according to the type of evidence-based paper that is written, journal guidelines, and editorial policy. It is useful to select a couple of examples of articles published in the journal targeted for the submission to obtain a clear idea of how the narrative can be developed. Tables and/or boxes that highlight essential concepts of the narrative are enhancements that improve the readability of the manuscript.

Conclusions and Clinical Implications

The conclusions of the research evidence are presented in a summary form to emphasize the essence or the important "take home" message of the narrative discussion (Costello, 2012; Price, 2014). For professionals who are accustomed to reading clinically oriented articles, the format of evidence-based papers may be unfamiliar and more difficult to follow. The conclusion enables the reader to locate the information succinctly if the previous discussion has not been sequenced clearly. The clinical implications section informs the reader about how this evidence can be applied to clinical practice and substantiates the rationale for its use in clinical practice.

Adopting a Positive Attitude

"

Your living is determined not so much by what life brings to you as by the attitude you bring to life; not so much by what happens to you as by the way your mind looks at what happens.

JOHN HOMER MILLER

Having a positive attitude toward professional publishing, especially for beginning authors, is an absolute must. When an individual decides to write professionally, she or he needs to develop a resolute attitude that the publication task will be completed regardless of what problems and how many challenges are encountered. First-time authors have the unusual experience of engaging in a very solitary activity that is undertaken by literally hundreds of thousands of people. Yet, there are very few opportunities that enable authors to communicate with one another about the highs and lows of the writing experience (Heinrich, 2007). In 2001, Stephen King wrote a book entitled simply *On Writing* that provides insight into his life as a writer and what he has learned along the way. Most times authors toil at their computers, writing and deleting what they have written and rewriting until the words on the page seem to accurately convey their ideas to their readers.

It is also important for writers to remember that their receipt of request for revisions and rejection letters is the norm for all authors. It is essential not to take the comments personally and put aside the emotional reaction to scholarly criticism. An objective perspective of reviewing comments both negatively and positively is important to writing the revised manuscript draft (Happell, 2011). Reviewer feedback can be very helpful in clarifying portions of the manuscript that are unclear and suggesting additional information to be included. For novice writers, uncertainty about the scope of comments received is best dealt with by reviewing the comments with the mentor or colleagues, who have publication experience.

"

You measure the size of the accomplishment by the obstacles you had to overcome to reach your goals.

BOOKER T. WASHINGTON

For many authors, uncertainty and self-doubt can interfere with their writing, resulting in an unfinished manuscript that languishes on the computer's hard drive. For others, perhaps a harsh critique is mailed to them after the review has been completed, releasing feelings of disappointment or anger. For these individuals, the feedback is traumatic and demoralizing. Regrettably, some become unwilling to subject themselves to this harrowing experience again. However, it is important to know and appreciate that even the most successful and prominent authors have been subjected to their fair share of rejections. A major difference between those who are successful and those who are not is *persistence*—one of the keys to getting work published (Fowler, 2013).

Sharing the writing responsibilities with other colleagues can mitigate the disappointment of an unfavorable review. Collective review of the manuscript will evoke a more diffuse and divergent response to negative criticism of the paper as compared to the solo author. Having a cohesive team of authors, rather than just one, is more likely to generate the motivation needed to promptly revise the paper. Friction and conflict among members of the author team experienced during the first submission may make it more problematic for writing subsequent drafts (Baker, 2013).

> ❝
>
> Criticism, like rain, should be gentle enough to nourish a man's growth without destroying his roots.
>
> **FRANK A. CLARK**

Being Organized

Organization is another major factor that contributes to writing success. That is, the process of getting an evidence-based publication submitted and accepted is dependent on creating the circumstances for it to occur. The organizational approach to getting thoughts down on paper in an acceptable professional format will require allocation of time periods for writing and achievement of the steps described in this section on publishing. Therefore, it is useful to remember the following (Baker, 2013; Fowler, 2013; Kiefer, 2010; Price, 2014):

- Work on eliminating destructive thinking (e.g., "I can't do this" or "This paper will never get published").
- Remember that every author at some point in his or her career had to start at the beginning.
- Negative manuscript reviews should never be taken personally and often serve as an opportunity to improve the manuscript.
- Some individuals should not serve as reviewers because their critical perspectives are demeaning rather than helpful.
- Manuscript reviews may reflect mixed views wherein one reviewer evaluates the paper favorably whereas another is critical of the manuscript.
- There is a collective experience of feeling confident, unsure, hesitant, weary, excited, bored, and tired that all authors can relate to when writing for publication.
- Authors who are successful do not easily take *no* for an answer. They are able to accept criticism, look at it objectively, and revise the paper accordingly, resulting in an improved document that meets the publication readers' needs.
- Setting realistic goals for initiating and completing a writing task is essential to prevent the disappointment of unrealistic expectations and possibly abandoning the project entirely.
- Setting aside incremental amounts of uninterrupted time for writing on a consistent basis will facilitate the progress needed to achieve the writing goal less painfully.
- Developing a plan that specifies a concrete course of action with attainable milestone accomplishments enables an author to feel satisfied that he or she is achieving the goal.
- Goal setting is especially important for the collaborative team, including specification of consequences when a member of the team does not meet delegated writing benchmarks.
- Be clear as to the purpose for writing the manuscript.

Deciding What to Publish

Professional publications on EBP can be found everywhere. The extent of its influence is demonstrated by the number of publications that can be found through bibliographic searches, the number of professional journals that regularly feature columns on EBP, and other publications that address the topic exclusively, such as this book and the journals *Worldviews on Evidence-Based Nursing* and *Evidence-Based Nursing*. Many funders are moving to the reimbursement of EBPs exclusively or preferentially; therefore, it is essential that clinicians are able to identify and interpret such information.

One of the first decisions an author makes in beginning the writing process is the choice of what to write and how it will be written. There are numerous opportunities for publishing that vary from something as straightforward as a letter to the editor to authoring a major nursing textbook. Here is a listing of the wide range of publishing options:

- Letters to the editor
- Op-eds (traditionally refers to guest editorials appearing opposite the editorial page)
- Commentaries
- Books
- Continuing education reviews
- Chapters
- NCLEX questions
- Articles
- Evidence-based clinical practice guidelines
- Newsletter inserts
- Standards of care
- Book and media reviews
- Policy briefs

Authors with limited publishing experience may want to begin with a more manageable writing project, such as a letter to a journal editor, a review of another's work, or a brief article in an organization's newsletter.

Selecting a Journal

The format and content of a manuscript targeted for an article submission will be dictated by the editorial guidelines and technical specifications of the journal. The author must first target a journal that corresponds to the subject content of the manuscript and reaches the appropriate audience for the information. In today's publishing environment, with the emergence of open-access journals, it is incumbent upon prospective authors to assess the journal's credibility, which is discussed in greater detail below under the topic of predatory journals. Authors intending to submit evidence-based papers will need to learn the following typical criteria before making the decision to submit to a particular journal (Price, 2014):

- Is the journal peer reviewed?
- What is the journal's impact factor?
- What is the profile of the journal's readership?
- What is the turnaround cycle for review?
- What is the "in press" period (i.e., from time of acceptance to publication)?
- What are the technical specifications?
- Is this an open or closed access journal or a combination of both?
- Are manuscripts published in print, online, or both?
- Are there specific reporting guidelines for selected manuscripts (i.e., quality improvement projects, systematic reviews, research studies) that the journal has adopted?

Manuscripts submitted to peer-reviewed journals are critiqued by a team of reviewers who have expertise in the subject matter of the paper. Any identification of the manuscript's author(s) is removed, and likewise, the anonymity of the reviewers is maintained during the review process. This type of review process is known as the *blind review*. It is believed that the blind review process is the most objective and fair way of judging the significance, technical competence, and contribution to professional literature.

Peer-reviewed journals publish more rigorously reviewed manuscripts than those reviewed by editorial staffs alone. Generally, most authors prefer to have their manuscripts published in peer-reviewed journals for this reason. Manuscripts published in regularly featured columns of peer-reviewed journals may not be peer reviewed, however. Authors need to ascertain this fact before submission. Another useful criterion to use in considering the choice for journal submission is the readership profile. Although the style and format of articles published by journals will be obvious to the author in terms of the type of article (e.g., data-based, clinical, or policy-oriented papers), having other editorial information is useful in terms of understanding the need to insert additional narrative on research methodology or clinical implications (Carroll-Johnson, 2013; Price, 2014).

In most instances, information on the review process (e.g., the review period time frame and technical specifications) can be found in the "information for authors" section in each journal or online at the journal's website. Many authors are concerned about the timeliness in which manuscripts are published. Authors may worry that a research paper that has undergone a lengthy review process will not then be published in a timely manner. Concerns also exist regarding the delay in publishing an in-press manuscript because a lengthy time frame will substantially slow the dissemination and implementation of research findings. In response to these concerns, several developments in publishing have occurred to facilitate the dissemination of scientific and clinical information. Many journals, including nursing journals, will post manuscripts online on the journal's website as uncorrected or corrected proofs prior to publication as a hard copy version. Each in-press manuscript is assigned a Digital Object Identifier (DOI) number until it is published in the journal issue. This digital string is the unique identification number assigned to electronic versions of manuscripts. The trend in citing references is to continue to include the DOI number after the paper has been published (American Psychological Association [APA], 2013a). The term *in press* in this electronic age of publishing now has several different connotations:

- *in press*, accepted manuscript papers that have been accepted by the review panel and journal editor.
- *in press*, uncorrected proof manuscripts that have been copyedited as a PDF file by the journal copyeditor; however, the author or team of authors have not reviewed, made necessary corrections, responded to queries from the copyeditor (i.e., missing references) or approved the PDF. A DOI number has been assigned, and the uncorrected proof is available online.
- *in press*, corrected proof—all corrections have been made and approved by the authors, and the electronic version is available online and will be assigned to a journal issue and number. The manuscript has the same DOI number as assigned as an uncorrected proof.

Answers to these questions can be easily obtained from journal editors. Numerous websites for nursing journals list technical specifications, editorial philosophy, and hyperlinks available to the journal's publisher or editor for convenient access (APA, 2013b). **It is critical to follow the journal's guidelines in preparation of the manuscript.** If the journal's word limit is 5,000 words, it is important not to exceed it. The journal's technical specifications include the following:

- Manuscript format depending on type of paper submitted (i.e., research, clinical, column)
- Page length, word limits
- Reference style format (e.g., American Psychological Association)
- Abstract format and word limit

- Declaration of conflict of interests
- Acknowledgment that the manuscript is not currently under review by another journal
- Margins, font style, and size
- Use of graphics, tables, photos, and figures
- Face page and author identifying information
- Electronic version and software

A noteworthy development with journal publication is the *open access* of electronic journals (Stuber, 2013). These journals are freely available to individuals, in contrast to subscription journals that are based on an annual subscription rate. As with subscription journals, there are peer-reviewed and non–peer-reviewed open-access journals. In some circumstances, an author may be asked to pay a fee to have an article published in an open-access journal, which can run from a nominal fee to several thousand dollars. Open-access journals, which have the institutional support of a university or organization, may not need to charge a fee. It is important for the author to be fully informed as to the reputation of the open-access journal, as with any subscription journal. *Directory of Open Access Journals* (DOAJ) and *Open J-Gate* are online directories of open-access journals.

Directory of Open Access Journals is online at http://www.doaj.org/

Open J-Gate is online at http://openj-gate.org/

Authors who may consider submitting to an open-access journal need to be fully aware and informed about the prospective journal. Unfortunate and disturbing developments have unfolded in the open access-journal environment—the emergence of predatory journals (Betz, 2016). These journals are not legitimate publishing entities and are operated by individuals who have nefarious motivations. There are a number of "warning signs" a prospective author needs to be aware of, including an editorial board composed of individuals without recognizable affiliations or prominence in the field, no identifiable journal editor, an unrealistic review turnaround of just a few days, and a questionable listing of articles previously published. Authors are encouraged to engage in "due diligence," fully vetting potential journals that have not been accessed to retrieve previously published articles. The International Academy of Nursing Editors (2014) has led the effort to inform the nursing community and beyond of the challenges and problems associated with predatory publishing, with the 2014 initiative, *Open Access, Editorial Standards and Predatory Publishing*.

An INANE resource, *Best Practices for Journal Websites*, is an excellent tool for authors to assist them with determining the credibility of the journal: https://nursingeditors.com/inane-initiatives/best-practices-for-journal-websites-2/

Reporting Guidelines

In the effort to promote excellence in science and practice, expert groups have formed to develop reporting guidelines for the publication of research, quality improvement projects, and systematic reviews. According to the Enhancing the Quality and Transparency of Health Research Network (EQUATOR), which serves as a repository and clearinghouse for reporting guidelines, the goal is "to improve the reliability and value of published health research literature by promoting transparent and accurate reporting and wider use of robust reporting guidelines."

EQUATOR is online at http://www.equator-network.org/about-us/t

Examples of reporting guidelines available on EQUATOR include:

- Randomized Control Trials: CONSORT
- Case Reports: CARE
- Qualitative Research: SRQR
- Systematic Reviews: PRISMA
- Quality Improvement Projects: SQUIRE

In addition to the compilation of reporting guidelines available on EQUATOR, other resources of use to writers are available. These resources include publication tool kits, courses, and pertinent updates on reporting guidelines.

Developing the Manuscript Concept

Developing the manuscript concept depends on the author's area of clinical expertise and a lack of accessible information on which to base clinical practice. A clinician may want to share information with colleagues about an innovative intervention or implementation of a program improvement or may report the findings of testing a new approach to provide clinical services. There is an urgent need to publish articles on the search for and critical appraisal of evidence, because healthcare providers increasingly desire to base their practices on empirically tested approaches, and payers are beginning to demand it.

As the author proceeds with the process of refining the concept for writing an article on EBP, a literature review will assist in organizing the topic into an outline. Reviewing the literature will enable the author to gain an understanding of how to develop this publication uniquely and in a manner that contributes to the body of evidence-based nursing literature (*Science Direct*, n.d.).

Review of the Literature

Throughout this chapter, the Internet has been identified as a technology resource. This is also true for publishing efforts. Use of online bibliographic databases enables writers to conduct more comprehensive and better literature searches. The following bibliographic databases will be useful when proceeding with the literature search for writing evidence-based articles and reports:

- Cochrane Database of Systematic Reviews (interdisciplinary)
- Cochrane Controlled Trials Register (interdisciplinary)
- ACP Journal Club (interdisciplinary)
- Evidence-Based Medicine Reviews (interdisciplinary)
- DARE (interdisciplinary)
- Cumulative Index of Nursing and Allied Health Literature (CINAHL, a nursing and allied health literature database that contains international journals from these disciplines)
- MEDLINE (a medical literature database of international medical, nursing, and allied health journals that contains primarily medical journals and selected nursing and allied health journals that have met the criteria for inclusion)
- Google Scholar
- Directory of Open Access Journals
- Open J-Gate

A few guidelines need to be considered before starting to write a manuscript. First, a literature review must be conducted to cite references that should be recent, or within the past 3 to 5 years. In some professions, it may be difficult to find current citations from the literature, thereby necessitating accessing the interdisciplinary literature representing not only health-related disciplines but also other disciplines (e.g., education, job development, and rehabilitation). There are also classic references, older than the 3 to 5 years' time frame, from any field that should be included in a publication because these are seminal works on which subsequent publications are based and cannot be ignored.

An author will have completed his or her search for evidence when the author cannot find any new references and is familiar and knowledgeable with the existing literature. Clinicians who write evidence-based articles will rely heavily on empirically based articles because they are searching for evidence. Authors will be less likely to include clinically oriented articles other than to demonstrate the relevance to clinical practice, such as the prevalence of falls among older adults. Textbooks should be referenced sparingly in evidence-based publications unless the books are written on highly specialized topics and are a compilation of perspectives from experts in the field (Heinrich, 2002).

A literature search will inform an author as to the scope of the topic and the evident gaps in the literature. As the literature search proceeds, the author's thinking will be further shaped with new insights and fortified with expert opinion and evidence-based articles that may result in modifications and enhancements of the purpose of the original article. Uncovering the body of literature in a field of science and practice is a dynamic and evolving intellectual and practice-focused endeavor.

Developing a Timeline

Healthcare professionals are well acquainted with developing and adhering to a work plan that identifies benchmarks of achievement. Having a work plan specifies in a concrete form the necessary tasks the author must undertake to complete the writing goal. The greater the level of specificity, the better the chance the author will have to reach his or her goal. Together with the identified tasks, *realistic* timelines should be listed along with strategies for keeping on track with accomplishing the steps of the writing project. A writing project timeline might look like the one listed below:

- Operationalize the idea/select a topic—June 1
- Develop the outline—June 15
- Locate journals/author guidelines—July 15
- Survey the literature—September 15
- Develop the first draft—November 15
- Review/proofread—December 10
- Make revisions—January 8
- Submit—January 20

Writing Strategies

Content outlines for articles will vary according to the type of manuscript. The generic outline for an evidence-based article, as used in the ongoing evidence-based column in the journal *Pediatric Nursing*, follows this format:

- Introduction to the clinical problem
- The clinical question
- Search for the evidence (i.e., the search strategy used to find the evidence and the results)

- Presentation of the evidence
- Critical appraisal of the evidence with implications for future research
- Application to practice (i.e., based on the evidence reviewed, what should be implemented in clinical practice settings)
- Evaluation (includes outcomes of the practice change if they were measured)

Obviously, writing an article for publication involves much more than just following an outline. The writing process is a slow and tedious effort that is characterized by stops and starts, cutting and pasting, and the frequent use of the delete key. However, writers use several pragmatic tips to help them complete their writing projects. Writing begins with following the manuscript outline at whatever section that can be written, even if it means first writing the simpler portions of the manuscript (e.g., the conclusion and introduction). Placing words on paper is important to "getting words down on paper," meaning to write anything, even if initially the words are awkward sounding and stilted. Inspiration will not necessarily happen spontaneously and requires trial and error and much mental perspiration. Start with any sentence for which there is inspiration; the beginning or the ending of the section can be written later.

Creativity is dependent on discipline and organizational techniques (Issa et al., 2013). These organizational techniques include the following:

- The manuscript outline should be followed as written. If the author discovers the narrative would be better written otherwise, the outline needs revision.
- Writing something is preferable to writing nothing. Awkward-sounding statements can always be edited and/or deleted. Initially, generating loose ideas that are difficult to couple with words can lead to more fluid thinking and word composition.
- Before completing a writing session, leave notes within the document that can be used as prompts for the next writing period. Leaving author notes ensures continuity with the train of thought from the last writing session and helps to facilitate recall and ease with the writing process.
- Write the paper anonymously, meaning there is no self-identification, although there may be exceptions in discussing particular programs. Use the same verb tense throughout, and avoid the use of the passive voice. Note the major themes of paragraphs in the margins of the manuscript to discern the discussion sequencing, highlighting potential problems with organization.
- Avoid the use of *should, must,* and other words that are opinionated. Insert information that can be replicated and applied by others by avoiding the use of jargon.

Proofreading the Manuscript

If possible, the optimal proofreading strategy is to have colleagues or friends read the manuscript draft, including individuals who have expertise in the content area as well as those who possess no content expertise. Those without content expertise are specifically helpful in reading the manuscript for clarity, style, and grammatical errors (Fowler, 2013; Price, 2014). However, it is essential that whoever proofreads the draft be a good writer with the capacity to provide specific suggestions for editing purposes. Very often, faculty members whose students are writing for publication outside of their course assignments are willing to serve as proofreaders. It is important to provide colleagues with the targeted journal's guidelines for manuscript submission so that they can review the paper with those guidelines in mind (e.g., formatting, length).

Authors, of course, also serve as their own proofreaders. Setting the manuscript draft aside for a week or two will create the distance needed to read it again with a set of fresh eyes. In this manner, the author can read his or her own work more objectively and potentially pick out flaws with sentence structure, spelling, organization, and content. Once proofreading is completed, the draft is revised based on collegial feedback and the author's own proofing.

In addition to attention to content, the document needs to be well written. A fact-filled manuscript that is choppy or does not flow well, or in which there is poor grammar, will result in a poor review. Reviewers who are distracted by typos or poor writing will not be able to focus adequately on the technical content, and this will be reflected in the review. Students may have access to the writing center of their university to help improve their basic writing skills. Writing is more art than science, and professionals should not be embarrassed to seek out assistance to improve their writing, irrespective of the subject matter.

Spell checking the document is an absolute must in proofing manuscripts. However, automatic spell checking is not enough because it is not capable of detecting problems with some misspellings. The numbering of tables, graphics, and figures will need to be double-checked to ensure that they are properly matched with the sequence identified in the article. The citation of references in the text is checked with those in the reference list for correct spelling, dates of publication, and referencing format. Other technical specifications (e.g., pagination, use of headers, margins, fonts) are reviewed to ensure conformity to those listed in the author guidelines. Permissions and transfer of copyright are included with the packet of materials that will be sent to the editorial office.

Once this process is completed, the manuscript can be submitted for review. The information for authors and/or the receipt from the editorial office will indicate the expected turnaround period for the manuscript review. If no feedback has been received after six to eight weeks, it is appropriate to e-mail or call the editorial office to inquire about the status of the review. As mentioned previously, it is important not to take feedback personally. An impassive approach will serve the author well by moving beyond what might be stinging criticisms to revising the draft based on the reviewers' recommendations. It is at this juncture that the author needs to keep focused on what was and continues to be the original goal—to publish the article and contribute to the professional literature on EBP (Mee, 2013).

"

Remember that you never get a second chance to make a great first impression, so make the first submission of the manuscript as flawless as possible.

BERNADETTE MELNYK

For additional interdisciplinary and nursing resources on publishing, refer to Box 20.7.

BOX 20.7	*Transdisciplinary and Nursing Publishing Resources*

BioMed Central: This website provides prospective authors with comprehensive information pertaining to publishing from selecting the appropriate journal to actual writing of the manuscript. http://www.biomedcentral.com/getpublished/writing-resources

COBWEB: A free online tool to assist with the writing of a randomized control trial. http://cochrane.fr/cobweb/

EQUATOR Toolkit: Writing Research. This tool kit provides the author with specific information in writing a research manuscript. http://www.equator-network.org/toolkits/writing-research/

Nicoll, L. (2012). *Manuscript success.* Portland, ME: Bristlecone Pine Press.

Nicoll, L., & Chinn, P. L. (2015). *Writing in the digital age: Savvy publishing for healthcare professionals.* Philadelphia, PA: Lippincott, Williams & Wilkins.

Oermann, M. H., & Hays, J. (2015). *Writing for publication in nursing* (3rd ed.). New York, NY: Springer.

Saver, C. (2014). *Anatomy of writing for publication for nurses* (2nd ed.). Indianapolis, IN: Sigma Theta Tau.

DISSEMINATING EVIDENCE TO INFLUENCE HEALTH POLICY

Healthcare providers are in an enviable position to advocate for change because they are highly regarded and trusted by the American public. As a leading politician remarked to a colleague, "Political endorsements from state nursing organizations are one of the most important endorsements a politician seeks to obtain." In essence, such a testimonial is *evidence* of the potential influence that healthcare providers, individually and collectively, have to impact changes in policy and to be engaged in policy making. The key is not only recognizing this potential but also actively taking advantage of opportunities that arise to be engaged in policy making at all levels of government and within professional organizations and service agencies. See Chapter 19 for a full discussion of how to use evidence to influence health policy.

Writing Health Policy Issue Briefs

There is an urgent need for healthcare professionals to write compelling policy briefs based on findings from sound research that legislators can readily understand. A legislator cannot bring forward legislation without having the necessary substantiation to establish the need or problem. However, findings from a survey of a random sample of legislators indicate that they are often overwhelmed by the huge volume of information they receive and any information provided to them should be concise and relevant to current debates (Sorian & Baugh, 2002). Unfortunately, research is often not published in readily digestible form for policy makers and their staff (Health Affairs, 2012). In addition, legislators often rely on their staff to gather information about a topic and provide an overview to them, making legislative staffers a potential audience for evidence-based literature.

One avenue for providing policy makers with sound evidence is by developing issue briefs (see Appendix E available on thePoint˚ for a brief developed by the American Association of Colleges of Nursing to assist policy makers in drafting a bill to enhance the nursing work force). A policy brief is a powerful communication tool that provides current evidence, based on prevalence reports and research by scientists, and/or the opinion of experts that can lead to successful decision making about key policy issues (Health Affairs, 2012).

The key to developing issue briefs is to be succinct and direct in communicating with the intended audience. A well-written issue brief summarizes and clearly communicates to the reader the scope of the policy issue. The reader should be able to scan the document quickly and be able to comprehend the major aspects of the policy issue that is featured. Tips for organizing an issue brief include the following:

- Lead with a title on the masthead that clearly conveys the purpose.
- Identify the policy issue in the first sentence so that by the end of the opening paragraph, the reader knows the policy issue.
- Include background information that highlights the major features of the issue.
- Indicate the historical pattern of response to the problem in subsequent statements.
- Identify the inherent limitations as well as the problem and why it is still a problem.
- Include common opposing views and refute them as well.

Another format for writing policy briefs includes the following components:

- Clear statement of the issue
- Context and background of the issue/problem, most effectively captured in bullet format
- Options: Pros and cons of each recommendation listed
- Resources used to prepare the policy brief (Health Affairs, 2012)

An issue brief provides a systematic review and synthesis of literature based on the selected topic addressing the demonstrated clinical outcomes of interventions, cost-effectiveness, and applicability. As the supporting evidence is presented, the reader is led in a logical sequence through the presentation of information that enables a clear understanding of the need for policy change. The concluding remarks of this section provide the links between research, clinical practice, and policy making. It distills for the reader what has been done and how it can be applied to policy making, which may be difficult for elected representatives or stakeholders if they do not have the expertise to "point the way" (Box 20.8).

A review of the literature should be conducted differently for policy makers than for a research audience. The analysis is conducted not only with clinical knowledge in the area but also with an understanding of the practical implications for policy makers. Where the information was obtained (i.e., the type of research studies reviewed and synthesized in the paper; expert opinion of researchers, clinicians, and experts) is incorporated in the brief. Once the strength of the available evidence has been analyzed, conclusions are made about where gaps in the literature exist for which further research is needed. The conclusion will be much briefer than those written for research or review of literature articles.

The healthcare provider who is involved in constructing a policy issue brief will emphasize the application for policy and practice. That is, what is being advocated for policy

---

BOX 20.8 — Typical Topics and Components of a Health Policy Issue Brief

Issue briefs are developed to address issues of interest to policy makers:

Typical Topics
Healthcare financing
Quality and safety of patient outcomes
Risk/benefit analysis of cost reduction alternatives
Lower rates of mortality and improved morbidity
The role of technology in healthcare
Human resource needs
System change to improve services

Typical Components
Title
Background of the issue
Historical pattern of response to the problem
Inherent limitations and problems
Why it remains a problem
Review and synthesis of the literature
Clinical outcomes of interventions
Cost-effectiveness
Applicability
Patient privacy (Health Insurance Portability and Accountability Act)
Policy implications
System changes
Services proposed
Population outcomes and health disparities

change? How will the policy result in a change for services, such as treatments, assessment approaches, and evaluation of intervention outcomes (e.g., What clinical outcomes for the target population are expected, such as improved health as evidenced by better cardiovascular status and a higher level of daily functioning)? Policy conclusions should define in detail the possible clinical implications. For example, implications would recommend:

- Funding priorities in the treatment of chronic conditions
- Projected effects of funding cutbacks (e.g., a decrease in access to care and treatment)
- Longitudinal studies of various treatment approaches (e.g., hormone replacement therapy [HRT])
- Identification of actual and anticipated population outcomes

In this way, issue briefs assist policy makers in understanding the evidence so that they can create legislation founded on the premise that policy change is based on good science and knowledge.

Design layout of policy briefs helps convey the message to the audience. Obvious requirements in design layout of policy briefs are to ensure that there are graphics to highlight the major propositions, problems, facts, and recommendations. Boxes that contain bulleted, succinct statements are effective. A pullout that defines terminology may be useful if the language or medical terms are unfamiliar to readers. It is important to ensure the graphics are not too busy to be a distraction from the material presented. A case example to illustrate the nature of the problem or the implications of recommendations may be helpful. In a nutshell, policy makers are more likely to use information and evidence from a policy brief if:

- The issue is clearly stated.
- The research evidence in the brief is focused.
- The document can be skimmed quickly for salient points.
- It is synthesized, conclusion-oriented, and succinct (i.e., no more than 2 to 4 pages)

Use of graphics and visual pointers also enables the reader to navigate through the material easily. To add depth, briefs can be accompanied by other tools, such as slides, spreadsheets, links to articles, websites, and a list of key contacts.

Understanding the Target Audience

Consumers are bombarded daily with new information about healthcare that includes promising medications and treatments, hope for medical cures, and new treatment approaches. The barrage of information can be confusing for consumers. The conflicting information on HRT is an excellent example of the confusion women have experienced in understanding what might be the long-term effects of taking hormones. Policy experts have noted that the public seeks information that will enable them to better understand the disease pathophysiology and clinical application of that knowledge. In writing for a particular audience, the author needs to have an awareness of what type of information the audience is looking for and what would be considered most helpful.

Thoughtful and well-referenced issue briefs will be used by professional associations to assist them in the development of critical paths and practice guidelines. For example, the Agency for Healthcare Research and Quality (AHRQ) sponsored the former National Guidelines Clearinghouse, which contained more than 1,000 clinical practice guidelines. AHRQ was involved in supporting the implementation efforts of the Affordable Care Act. Additionally, policy makers and other stakeholders can work with clinicians in suggesting topics for evidence review and development.

Writing in Understandable Language

The content and format of a policy brief will vary depending on the knowledge and interest of the intended audience and whether the readers are primarily consumers, policy makers, or professionals. To illustrate, if an issue brief is written for a professional audience, the summary of the research evidence can be presented using research terminology. If issue briefs are written for non–health professional audiences (e.g., legislators), research terminology is presented in more general terms to aid comprehension. Generally speaking, the reading level for widespread consumer distribution should be for a sixth-grade reading level (using the Flesch Kineard Reading Level found in software tools to assess reading level is most helpful). For policy makers, the format needs to emphasize practical information that is easy to read, free of health jargon, although the content may also be adapted to the interests of individual legislators.

> **❝**
> "Don't write so that you can be understood . . . write so you can't be misunderstood."
>
> **PRESIDENT WILLIAM HOWARD TAFT**

Health literacy is now recognized as a major public health concern affecting Americans. The U.S. digital brochure entitled *Healthy People 2020* identifies the following objective to increase health awareness among Americans: Increase public awareness and understanding of the determinants of health, disease, and disability, and the opportunities for progress (U.S. Department of Health and Human Services, 2013). As national surveys and research studies demonstrate, the majority of the U.S. public have limited and inadequate understanding of the health information they receive to care for themselves and their families (Flores, Abreu, & Tomany-Korman, 2005; Kutner, Greenberg, Jin, & Paulsen, 2006; Leyva, Sharif, & Ozuah, 2005).

It is the writer's responsibility to apply or translate for the reader the synthesis of research for policy (i.e., how a particular practice can be improved and what the expected outcomes are for the targeted underserved populations). Authors need to keep in mind the targeted readership and the change that is being advocated. Based on these two primary criteria, the issue brief will be written in the style and format appropriate for the audience. All knowledge must have local application in order to be used. Briefs that are effective need to be written in a manner that policy makers can see the relevance and impact for application at the local, state, and/or national levels. Lastly, the constant stream of information available today can lead to overload and be a barrier to accessing and using evidence. Having an existing relationship or intending to develop one with policy makers is important. It was found that seeking the advice and expertise of colleagues related to medical issues was preferable to seeking information from the literature. This model would likely apply to working with policy makers as well. Relationships and other methods of contact will strengthen the ties with policy makers, such as bulletins for decision makers that focus on a particular issue. Additionally, healthcare provider experts aware of the organizational barriers of workload, time constraints, and authority to implement change associated with projected change will be in a position to address these concerns directly through personal contacts with policy makers (Fatemah, 2012). Policy briefs are designed to inform readers with analyses of research results that have policy relevance. Issue briefs are effective tools for use by nursing professionals to describe, discuss, and recommend the need for policy changes.

WORKING WITH THE MEDIA TO DISSEMINATE EVIDENCE

Healthcare professionals and researchers need to think realistically about reasons the news media may want to report about their evidence-based story. Professionals who are serious about disseminating evidence need to understand how to work best with news media and what attracts their interest to writing or producing a story. The knowledge may mean the difference between a successful or a fruitless effort.

This section provides general guidance for talking to the media about findings from research and evidence-based implementation projects. Emphasis is placed on the dynamic nature of news, factors influencing why reporters cover certain stories, and information about how to influence the process for the best chances of success.

The Basics

The Internet and other online and mobile tools have changed how content is consumed. Web-based or digital media outlets have increased exponentially with the various delivery technologies, such as Twitter, Facebook, Instagram, Snapchat, blogs, and other social media, which is evolving constantly. The control over news by the established mass media, especially metropolitan newspapers, broadcast outlets, and consumer magazines, has been reduced. While opportunities abound, competition for media space, spanning healthcare and other newsworthy topic areas, has increased.

Consumers of media are often overwhelmed with information and the 24/7 news cycle. At any instant, people can choose from hundreds of channels from a cable provider, receive on-demand content from Netflix or Amazon, select from millions of websites, read news from a multitude of specialty professional publications, and obtain byte-size news from social media, such as Pinterest, Instagram, Facebook, and Twitter, as well as blogs and wikis. Breaking through this noise is a challenge for many healthcare professionals trying to leverage media to promote their research.

The first step in gaining media attention is to have a clear and newsworthy message that is easy to understand. What is the importance of your message to the public? Have you developed a new method for identifying children at risk of abuse? Does your work inspire young people to explore education and careers in research or the healthcare professions? Have you developed a new method to prevent obesity and cardiovascular disease? Are there new statistics that may align with your findings (e.g., medical errors are the third-leading cause of death), helping your topic seem more relevant to reporters?

Second, knowing the audience you need to reach is essential to disseminating your information effectively. You need to identify the media outlet's readers, viewers, and listeners, as well as get a sense for whether the publication has covered research or study results in the past. Relatedly, because you want a reporter to listen to what you have to say about the evidence on a particular topic, it does not mean the reporter will be interested in writing a story or article. This may be the most common mistake healthcare professionals make when working with media.

When contacting media by e-mail or phone, first formulate a plan and develop a media pitch, summarizing the key messages and findings of the research in a few short sentences. For an e-mail pitch, consider using a concise subject line that articulates the most compelling research findings. When interacting with reporters, know that they are often already informed on the topic and that they are working at a frenetic pace because of multiple deadlines and time pressures. If you reach a reporter on the phone, be prepared to state your message confidently and quickly, and be ready to move quickly if the reporter deems the content interesting and worthy of a story. However, keep your expectations in check; yours is likely one of dozens of media pitches that the reporter has received throughout that day or week, and they may be in the middle of completing other demanding tasks that need to be accomplished on deadline.

Make your case quickly for why a reporter should cover your story, and place yourself and your story through scrutiny that mirrors a review from a top journal. You should know who has done or is doing similar work to yours and how your work differs. Be prepared to justify why funding was provided for your research or project. Be ready to explain the significance of your work in a way that the reporter can understand, which may result in an explanation unlike one you have ever given to other colleagues. It is important to first ask yourself this question: Why should my story be published on a day when many major health news stories are also breaking?

News Is Dynamic

Once you have refined your story pitch and defined the audience that you would like to reach, you need to recognize the inherent power of the media. Once people turn to the Internet, cable TV, radio, or apps on their phones, they are hit with a burst of information. Most people simply tend to listen to what they hear, see, or follow on social media. For example, people turn on the radio, hear the day's top news, and retain the stories that most resonated with them. On platforms like Twitter, people may see only the news that involves subjects that they deliberately choose to follow.

However, there is no central repository of developments and events deemed to be "news" from which the media selects systematically. Instead, editors make fast intuitive decisions on the news they think interests the majority of their readers. Consequently, the public's interest, current events, and a health professional's efforts to tell their story, in part, determine what gets covered.

As a consumer of news, you permit your views to be influenced by a journalist or editor based on the content decisions they make. Whether it is a radio announcer in Albuquerque, a TV news producer shouting across a newsroom in Los Angeles, or a blogger writing content from his or her computer in their home office, you are subjecting yourself to their decisions about what is news and what isn't. As a result, you may often tell your peers about the stories that most interested you on a given day, either through traditional conversation or on social media.

For members of the media, deciding the news is an incredibly dynamic and intuitive process, and for health professionals, becoming aware of this is a huge step toward working with reporters (Figure 20.1). Prepare carefully first, then pursue your share of media attention

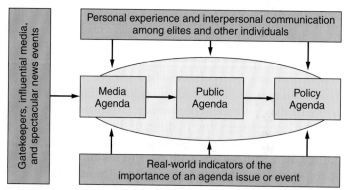

Figure 20.1: The many components of deciding what is the news. (Public Relations Society of America, Study Guide for the Examination for Accreditation in Public Relations, 2011.)

because there are certainly many competitors trying to "pitch" their messages or stories on any given day. The winner of the race is often the one who is proactive and convincing in "messaging" the value of their story to the media.

In addition to the specifics of your story, there are a multitude of factors that will decide whether your news is relevant on any given day (Box 20.9). Being aware of these and other factors is important if your story is to make the news.

- What categories of news does the media outlet cover most often?
- Consider the reporter's deadline time when contacting him or her.
- What else is happening in the community, state, nation, or world today? Has there been a big layoff locally? A major accident with fatalities? Is there a major vote in Congress?
- Which other staff reporters cover your healthcare evidence topic when the regular beat writer is unavailable? Who is the health editor at the publication or outlet?
- What is the editorial approach or policy of the news outlet? Aggressive or conservative?
- What are the reader/viewer/listener demographics of the media outlet?
- Can you quickly provide or offer the best opportunity for artwork or videotape or a visually interesting angle?
- In the case when a journalist reaches out to request information for a story he or she is writing, which source answered most quickly?

You cannot control most of the answers to the above questions, but they often determine coverage of stories. For example, a public relations specialist prepared publicity about a

---

BOX
20.9   *Factors That Help Determine the News Value of Research Evidence*

- *Interest*—Is it interesting and newsworthy?
- *Relevance*—Is it relevant? How could the findings make a difference in anyone's life and health?
- *Other events*—What else is happening in the nation, state, or local community this day or week (e.g., a hospital closing, impeachment proceedings, a war)?
- *Availability*—How available or reachable is the healthcare provider?
- *Exceptionality*—Is the evidence-based research extraordinary in a measurable sense? Is the research funding an unusually large amount?
- *Compatibilities*—How does the development fit into the overall strategy of the institution?
- *Quotability*—Is the healthcare provider quotable? Does he or she speak in a relatable, nontechnical language? Is the spokesperson experienced and/or comfortable talking with news media?
- *Visual appeal*—Are good photos or graphic artwork available quickly?
- *High-profile affiliations*—Are the study's findings being announced through a major journal or at a major conference?
- *Human interest*—Is a patient who was included in the study available so that human experience can be included in the story?
- *Clarity and applicability*—Is the take-home message clear and applicable to people's lives?
- *Cost*—What is the total amount of funding involved?

research finding published in a top scientific journal (i.e., a fossil of a tropical beast known as a "champsosaur" that was found in the Arctic Circle) that included a global warming theme, a well-executed color sketch of an interesting beast, an animal whose name sounded like "champsosaurus," an accessible and engaging scientist, and a top-notch publication. All of these aligned to promise tremendous coverage. That same day, however, the U.S. House of Representatives voted to impeach President Clinton. As a result, the "champosaurus" story was not published, owing to a development over which the researcher or reporter had no control.

The point to remember is that news is a fluid, unpredictable medium. There are all sorts of people influencing events to determine what is read, heard, viewed, or tweeted. You can compete successfully for media attention if you follow the above points, take a realistic approach, and have a positive attitude.

You also will find that many others may attempt to communicate about your evidence or research findings. Box 20.10 provides some examples. Your graduate student may seek to turn the findings into a job offer. The public relations (PR) department may tout the results to the media, seeking positive publicity for the institution. The fundraising office may meet with a prominent donor who might give millions of dollars, based on work just like yours. Your competitors will comb through the article, seeking weak spots. The company funding your pharmaceutical research may be thrilled with the results and will promote them to investors. Also, politicians may claim credit for approving the funding that resulted in such important knowledge. The list goes on and on.

Much of the competition for news coverage and its interpretation is invisible to the typical healthcare professional, who usually spends years immersed in his or her work, rather than crafting compelling "pitches" to reporters. Thus, many healthcare professionals approach the media with overconfidence or naivety, expecting coverage in top-tier publications or guest appearances on major news programs. Although anyone who works with the media

---

BOX 20.10 *Who Can Help Disseminate Evidence?*

- Your graduate students
- Your postdoctoral fellows
- Your department chair
- Your dean
- Your colleagues
- Public relations (PR) staff
- Development office
- Technology-transfer office
- Alumni office
- Funding organization/agency
- Journals that publish findings
- Professional organizations/associations
- Manufacturer of the product you tested
- PR firm hired by manufacturer
- PR firm hired by journal
- Political leaders in states and cities impacted most
- Patient advocacy groups
- Collaborators at other institutions

ought to be prepared for a negative response, healthcare providers seem to be particularly vulnerable to being caught off-guard when a supposedly straightforward process of communication goes poorly.

The Up- and Downsides of Working With Media

Working with the media to advance your evidence story may produce many surprises. There are a great many pitfalls about working with the media, so a cost-versus-benefit analysis needs to be done before deciding to pursue this avenue of dissemination.

Media may really scrutinize your claim that your project is the first or only one with certain findings, as you sincerely believed to be the case. Researchers at other universities may dispute your findings to protect their proprietary evidence-based research data. Your colleagues down the hall in the college may be jealous of your work because prospective graduate students want to visit your team, not theirs. Simply put, working with the media may consume large amounts of time and energy, with minimal returns.

However, media attention can be extremely beneficial as well. You might be invited to speak at a national conference based on an organizer's topic-based online search results. After reading about your work, a representative from a large company may contact you about funding your work. The article may help fuel perceived momentum around an expansion of research or a healthcare topic, resulting in a spike in donations that will fund future initiatives. There may also be a boost in coverage by other media that helps strengthen your institution's reputation or brand and recruit and retain the best and brightest individuals. News coverage about the findings from a clinical trial can also speed research and fuel initiatives to better health outcomes for the public. Researchers and clinicians who promote their research findings have witnessed all these results and more. News coverage about a nurse's study of rocking-chair therapy to treat dementia was covered by major publications around the world and is now used by dozens of nursing homes, thanks to some basic PR. Before that story was widely publicized, it was rejected by dozens of reporters.

However, a single news story by a reporter at *The Boston Globe* launched the story into popularity and the research into use worldwide. Publicity about a finding on vaccines and thimerosal resulted in editorials in *The New York Times* and *The Wall Street Journal*. Also, research shows that coverage in the general press has a positive impact on the number of times a research article is cited in the scientific press. Increased citations in the scientific press, more funding, greater collaboration, jobs for students, and research making a difference in public health—these are all important outcomes to healthcare providers.

Frequently, the first step toward the realization of these media outcomes is simply calling or e-mailing a reporter. Many healthcare professionals are hesitant to take this simple action for fear that the mere act of informing a person outside of their communities may be construed as "hyping" or bragging about the results. However, many individuals forget that much of the funding for their work came from taxpayers and that they have an obligation to report back to the people who paid for their work.

Some Sound Advice

Many organizations have a PR department that tracks newsworthy events, including publications, of employees and faculty members. Department staff can assist in making your material available to media outlets and provide guidance in avoiding pitfalls. Even if you are reluctant to call or e-mail reporters, chances are strong that you will have contact with a reporter about your study's findings eventually, especially if the data are groundbreaking. When this occurs, you might want to have Box 20.11 posted nearby as a starting point or

BOX 20.11	*When a Reporter Calls: A Quick Guide to Action*

- Call your public relations person for advice, background information on the journalist, support, and backup.
- Relax and talk with the reporter in a calm and confident tone.
- Think of the messages that you want to communicate in advance? Focus on two or three main messages that you want to convey, and be ready to work those into your answers to the reporter's questions.
- Before the interview, have background materials ready, and offer to provide them to the reporter.
- Think before you answer and do not be pressured to provide immediate answers. Offer to call the reporter back, and use time to collect your thoughts. In many cases, when a person claims to have been misquoted, they are simply unhappy about what they said to the reporter.
- Give the reporter your phone numbers (including home number), and say you would be happy to take calls anytime if he or she has any more questions or would like further clarification.
- Do not ask to see the story in advance, because you are not the reporter's boss; do not own the publication, station or online news site; and do not determine what is covered and how. Instead, offer to be a resource and encourage the reporter to contact you with further questions.

simply have handy the phone number of your PR person, who should work as your advocate. Frequently, a PR representative can provide you with a reporter's background and identify any red flags that may indicate a reporter may be looking into a different news angle. It is common for a local reporter to have limited knowledge about research or the health area one's research or evidence affects. On the other hand, journalists at prestigious outlets might have extensive subject-matter expertise and the knowledge and ability to talk in depth about your evidence findings. A PR staff member can also redirect a call or interview request to someone else in the organization who is more appropriate or skilled in a particular research area. Occasionally, a PR representative might also help you to provide minimal information and be cautious working with certain reporters because of their editorial biases or negative experiences. In general, however, reporters are fair and are held to high standards of accuracy.

If a PR professional supports your work, you must remain aware that he or she is also interpreting the story to some extent and placing your work in a particular context to have the best chance of media coverage and to present the supporting institution in the best possible manner. For instance, after a PR specialist receives background on the study and performs necessary follow-ups, he or she attempts to write a news release of the healthcare professional's work in approximately 600 words (see Appendix F available on thePoint® for an example of a news release draft provided for review). Typically, a physician, nurse, or researcher will review and provide minor changes while offering insights about the research that PR professionals may not know. During this review process, it rarely occurs to many professionals that they have left the entire interpretation of their work (e.g., the context, the emphasis, the key messages) up to the PR specialist. Often, PR specialists represent the data accurately, and a release is quickly approved (it is great when that happens!). But healthcare professionals should consider whether the PR person's version is accurate or in context before approving and disseminating.

A PR practitioner who specializes in supporting research can also advise you about a host of other issues that may arise when disseminating evidence to the media. Some of these issues include the following.

Embargoes

A **news embargo** (i.e., a restriction on the reporting of findings from a study before they are published in a journal or released by an institution or organization) is a PR technique used to give reporters time to develop a story on a complex or exciting topic. However, not all reporters agree to embargoes; many see them as authorized or misguided attempts to "manage" the news. To be safe, if you are pitching an embargoed story, you need to clarify this up front with the reporter before you say anything of substance. Hundreds of research stories are embargoed every week, and most often, embargoes are honored. If you and the reporter agree on the embargo, it is fine to speak to the reporter, and the story will appear once the embargo lifts.

Off-the-Record Comments

Do not go there. Unless agreed upon beforehand by both the interviewee and the reporter, anything you say is on the record. If you have started an interview, and then say afterward, "That was off the record," the reporter has no obligation to honor that request. You have to establish that *before* the interview. Even then, it is risky and better to avoid.

Peer Review

Peer review is crucial to experienced research reporters. If you are making a claim, you need to have evidence that has been reviewed by other experts in the field. Stories claiming any type of medical or scientific progress in detail usually rely on a publication in a journal or at least a presentation at a professional meeting. Even so, the rules are not always clear. A journal article almost always has much more detailed evidence and has been more rigorously reviewed than an abstract for a poster presentation, so the timing can be delicate. So, too, can the news about a paper or presentation. For instance, some journals reject manuscripts if you or your institution has actively promoted the results in other media, but they might accept them if you can prove that other media initiated the coverage.

News Conferences

Professionals from most health disciplines tend to be nervous when speaking or being interviewed during a news conference. It's a challenging forum for even the best public speakers. If participating in a news conference, consider using charts and images that can help to emphasize or better explain major or complex points and reduce anxiety. Keeping comments short also puts the speaker at ease. Do not joke or make offhand comments that can be taken out of context. When planning a news conference, select speakers with exemplary subject-matter expertise and experience in presenting. If you are talking about research results, make sure you have already presented them at a meeting or published in a journal before the conference. Healthcare professionals who make claims and present study findings at a news conference without supporting evidence that has been peer-reviewed place their careers at risk.

It is also important to remember technology-transfer issues. In other words, contact your technology-transfer department and consider filing a patent application on any research/program products *before* you publish or present your results.

Never argue with anyone who buys ink by the barrel.

CONGRESSMAN BRUCE BROWNSON, 1964

Reporters come with a variety of interests and abilities, but all have the power to reach more people with your message than you can possibly reach without them. When dealing with a reporter on a deadline, spending 5 minutes explaining a complex point will save the journalist 45 minutes to conduct research on their own as well as lessen the risk of errors. Avoiding the temptation to send them to the library, along with the other "don'ts" listed in Box 20.12, will go a long way toward building your effectiveness as a reliable media source.

You may not want to work with certain reporters because of their reputation for inaccuracy or bias on certain topics. This information may be ascertained from the background information you receive from a PR specialist or from your own research efforts. Unfortunately, there are reporters who have no interest in looking objectively at news and who instead are seeking a human face to place on a story already written. Additionally, there are reporters who will try to lead you in a direction that reflects their bias or predetermined story angle. In a story about why people were volunteering to be vaccinated against smallpox, a representative

---

| BOX 20.12 | *Some "Don'ts" When Working With Reporters* |

- Don't use scientific jargon.
- Don't assume you are a media expert.
- Don't wait hours to return a call; call back immediately.
- Don't expect a story to name every contributor or collaborator.
- Don't assume the reporter is familiar with the details of your project or discipline—ask.
- Don't dictate the "proper" questions or the story angle.
- Don't talk about just the positive aspects of your research findings; also discuss the limitations.
- Don't ask to see a copy of the story before it is published.

Fast Facts to Communicating EBP to Media

- Inform your public relations staff of your plan to contact the media and ask for relevant information and advice.
- Establish a relationship of mutual respect when working with journalists.
- Research what stories or articles the reporter has written recently to increase your credibility in working with them.
- Be ready to define EBP when working with general reporters who do not cover healthcare stories regularly.
- Develop three major messages or points about why your EBP story is of interest to the news outlet's readers, viewers, or listeners; write them on an index card before you talk with the reporter or editor. Tell the reporter that you will call back in 5 to 10 minutes if you do not have these points prepared.
- Always respect journalists' time and preferences for communicating with them.
- Never demand that an "error" be corrected; explain that you would like to provide more accurate information for future coverage of the topic.
- Avoid arguing with a journalist during an interview or after a story is published; always discuss points of disagreement in a professional manner.

EBP, evidence-based practice.

from a major TV network was not satisfied with the answer provided by one participant. The answer did not match the producer's preconceived notion of why people were volunteering, so he instructed the participant to use the word *patriotism* in his answer. Because the young man had been prepared for the pressure exerted by reporters, he disregarded the advice and provided an honest answer. The story was a success, in addition to being truthful.

The payoff from working effectively with print and digital media can be enormous, but the work to accomplish it can be daunting. It is important to prepare thoroughly, seek the assistance of an experienced PR advisor, be patient and persistent, and do your best. Although it would be simpler if quality work attracted attention on its own, the reality is that news is a competitive game and you should prepare a game plan and practice to play your best.

Do-It-Yourself (DIY) Opportunities

So reporters were not interested in a breaking news piece regarding your research findings? That is OK and fairly common. As has been reaffirmed in this chapter, demands on reporters and competition for space can negatively impact your chances for an article in a local or national outlet. However, this does not mean it is the end of the road to earn some well-deserved visibility. In fact, there are various opportunities to consider:

Write an Op-ed Or Commentary

A reporter may not have time to write about your research, but there are other forums that can be leveraged to convey your work. Most newspapers and various online outlets or blogs offer opportunities to submit guest commentaries or op-eds. These pieces usually have to follow editorial guidelines that are listed on the website, and they are often published if the content is relevant to a reader or aligns with other current events or new statistics. In general, op-eds/commentaries are 500 to 800 words, demonstrate thought leadership and expertise, and are offered exclusively to the publication. Op-eds are valuable because they afford health professionals their own by-lines and convey their findings using their voice and interpretation. For example, medical errors were recently reported as the third-leading cause of death in the United States. Sensing an opportunity to react to the news, Dr. Bernadette Melnyk, from The Ohio State University, published an op-ed in Modern Healthcare, communicating her findings on the lack of adoption of evidence-based practice in hospital settings as a contributor to medical errors and how the increased implementation of EBP may lead to fewer errors and better outcomes. While the original release of the research had already come and gone, she was able to keep her EBP findings in the public view by crafting a well-timed editorial for a respected publication.

Because of the volume of submissions and the range of competing topics, it is challenging to publish commentaries in top-tier outlets, such as *The New York Times, The Washington Post, The Wall Street Journal,* and *USA Today.* However, consider other local or regional newspapers or reputable online sources like Modern Healthcare, Kaiser Health News, STAT News, Morning Consult, and Medscape, which have a dedicated healthcare readership. Articles published by these outlets often get residual coverage when they are curated in newsletters, blogs, or posted on social media by other influencers.

When you submit an op-ed or commentary to an editor, it may take 3 to 5 days for a response, if you receive one at all. If an editor declines or does not respond, don't get discouraged. Move on to the next outlet that has a similarly relevant audience or consider reframing your piece if you feel it needs to be modified or strengthened. If your commentary is ultimately not accepted by any outlet, you may decide to post it on your institution's blog. Work with the institution's PR specialists to ensure the content is further promoted in newsletters and on social media, particularly on Twitter and Facebook.

Social Media Tips

Social media is ever evolving, and its capabilities are increasingly beneficial for researchers and health professionals to sidestep traditional media and amplify research using some fun, creative methods. There are a plethora of ways to engage on social media, and it's important that you work with PR specialists in your organization to complement important external communications with robust social media promotion.

After you have published your research, you may find that your work reflects themes from a particular annual health observance, such as National Recovery Month, Breast Cancer Awareness Month, Childhood Obesity Awareness Month, or National Nurses Week. There are a host of ways to participate in an observance, many of which have dedicated websites with resources and tool kits to get involved.

 Use the website https://healthfinder.gov/NHO to find a calendar of health observances. In addition, the online resource Symplur (https://www.symplur.com) is an effective tool to find social media events that may be relevant to your topic.

One such event may be a Twitter Chat or Tweet Chat, where participants can openly discuss topics and answer questions posed by a moderator account, all using a specific #hashtag that organizes the topic-based discussion. If you are participating in a chat, be prepared to link to your published study or share helpful images or infographics that convey the most compelling data.

Lastly, if you are using social media to promote your work, coordinate with the social media manager at your organization or institution to ensure that they are also sharing or retweeting your messages. Organizational accounts usually have more followers than individual accounts, so their partnership can extend the reach of your message and also help you pick up more followers.

As you ponder the myriad ways to communicate about your research, remember that traditional media coverage, although still among the most reputable ways to have your work recognized and disseminated, is not your only option. Always work with other communications professionals to establish the best integrated PR strategy to effectively announce your work.

EBP FAST FACTS

- New evidence will not achieve its maximum value to clinical practice and better patient outcomes unless it is communicated and disseminated effectively.
- The primary goal of disseminating evidence, whether it is presentations or publications, is to facilitate the transfer and adoption of research findings and evidence-based quality improvement projects into clinical practice.
- Excellent preparation for dissemination reduces performance anxiety, builds confidence, and enhances the success of any communications initiative. Remember, you never get a second chance to make a great first impression.
- An effective presentation begins with an understanding of audience characteristics and needs, conference characteristics, and topical focus.
- Follow journal guidelines meticulously when submitting a manuscript because you never get a second chance to make a great first impression.
- Set a goal to turn a presentation into a manuscript for publication within 90 days of the presentation.
- Target the media and policy makers as outstanding venues for evidence dissemination in addition to more traditional routes of dissemination (presentations and publications).

WANT TO KNOW MORE?

A variety of resources are available to enhance your learning and understanding of this chapter.

- Visit thePoint® to access:
  - Appendix E: Example of a Health Policy Brief; and Appendix F: Example of a Press Release
  - Articles from the AJN EBP Step-By-Step Series
  - Journal articles
  - Checklists for rapid critical appraisal and more!
- Lippincott CoursePoint combines digital text content with video case studies and interactive modules for a fully integrated course solution that works the way you study and learn.

References

Abe, D. (2007). Teacher upgrade: Podcasts uploading your childbirth class. *International Journal of Childbirth Education, 22,* 38.

American Psychological Association. (2013a). *What is a digital object identifier, or DOI?* Retrieved from http://www.apastyle.org/learn/faqs/what-is-doi.aspx

American Psychological Association. (2013b). *Publication manual of the American Psychological Association* (6th ed.). Washington, DC: Author.

Baker, J. D. (2013). Collaborative writing. *AORN Journal, 97*(1), 4–6.

Beamish, A. J., Ansell, J., Foster, J. J., Foster, K. A., & Egan, R. J. (2014). Poster exhibitions at conferences: Are we doing it properly? *Journal of Surgical Education, 72,* 278–282. doi:10.1016/j.surg.2014.08.011/

Betz, C. L. (2016). Authors beware: Open access predatory journals. *Journal of Pediatric Nursing, 31*(3), 233–234. doi:10.1016/j.pedn.2016.02.006

Billings, D. M., & Kowalski, K. (2009a). Strategies for making oral presentations about clinical issues: Part 1. At the workplace. *The Journal of Continuing Education in Nursing, 40*(4), 152–153.

Billings, D. M., & Kowalski, K. (2009b). Strategies for making oral presentations about clinical issues: Part 1. At professional conferences. *The Journal of Continuing Education in Nursing, 40*(5), 198–199.

Billings, D. M., & Kowalski, K. (2010). Don't ignore that call for posters! *The Journal of Continuing Education in Nursing, 41*(9), 392–393.

Bingham, R., & O'Neal, D. (2013). Developing great abstracts and posters: How to use the tools of science communication. *Nursing Women's Health, 17*(2), 131–138.

Blome, C., Sondermann, H., & Augustin, M. (2017). Accepted standards on how to give a medical research presentation: a systematic review of expert opinion papers. *GMS Journal for Medical Education, 34*(1), Doc11. doi:10.3205/zma001088

Brennan, N., Mattick, K., & Ellis, T. (2011). The map of medicine: A review of evidence for its impact on healthcare. *Health Information Library Journal, 28*(2), 93–100.

Campbell, R. (2011). *Communication science: Giving talks* (2nd ed.). Retrieved from https://www.scribd.com/doc/34887738/Communicating-Science-Giving-Talks-Second-Edition#download

Carroll-Johnson, R. M. (2013). Submitting a manuscript for review. *Clinical Journal of Oncology Nursing, 5*(3 Suppl.), 13–16. Retrieved from http://www.ons.org/Publications/CJON/AuthorInfo/WritingSupp/Submitting/

Christenbery, T. (2011). Manuscript peer review: A guide for advanced practice nurses. *Journal of the American Academy of Nurse Practitioners, 23*(1), 15–22.

Christenbery, T. L., & Latham, T. G. (2013). Creating effective scholarly posters: A guide for DNP students. *Journal of the American Academy of Nurse Practitioner, 25*(1), 16–23.

Cleary, M., Happell, B., Lau, S. T., & Mackey, S. (2013). Student feedback on teaching: Some issues for consideration for nurse educators. *International Journal of Nursing Practice, 19*(Suppl. 1), 62–66.

Costello, J. (2012). Publish or perish: Getting yourself published. *British Journal of Cardiac Nursing, 7*(11), 549–551.

Coumoyer, B. (2012). *How to project PowerPoint slides via iPad, iPhone or iPod touch.* Retrieved from https://www.brainshark.com/ideas-blog/2012/September/project-powerpoint-slides-ipad-iphone-ipod

DeSilets, L. D. (2010). Poster presentations. *The Journal of Continuing Education in Nursing, 41*(10), 437–438.

Fatemah, R. (2012). Evidence-informed health policy making: The role of the policy brief. *International Journal of Preventive Medicine, 3*(9), 596–598.

Flores, G., Abreu, M., & Tomany-Korman, S. C. (2005). Limited English proficiency, primary language at home, and disparities in children's health care: How language barriers are measured matters. *Public Health Reports, 120,* 418–430.

Fowler, J. (2013). Advancing practice: From staff nurse to nurse consultant. Part 8 publication. *British Journal of Nursing, 22*(8), 490.

Gelling, L. (2011). Welcome to the club. *Nursing Standard, 26*(1), 61.

Grand Valley State University. Office of Undergraduate Research and Scholarship. (2016). *Oral Presentation Tips.* Retrieved from https://www.gvsu.edu/ours/oral-presentation-tips-30.htm

Griffin, I., Buccino, R., Klein, D., & Thaler-Carter, R. E. (2010). Profession speaking: 10 Tips on moderating a panel discussion. *Executive communications.* Retrieved from http://www.exec-comms.com/blog/2010/08/02/10-tips-on-moderating-a-panel-discussion/

Hamilton, C. W. (2008). At a glance: A stepwise approach to successful poster presentations. *Chest, 134,* 457–459.

Happell, B. (2008). Conference presentations: A guide to writing the abstract. *Nurse Researcher, 15,* 79–87.

Happell, B. (2011). Responding to reviewers' comments as part of writing for publication. *Nurse Researcher, 18*(40), 23–27.

Health Affairs. (2012). *Health policy brief: Basic health programs.* Retrieved from https://www.healthaffairs.org/do/10.1377/hpb20121115.215619/listitem/healthpolicybrief_80.pdf

Health Care Transition Research Consortium. (2013). *Health Care Transition Research Consortium 5th Annual Research Symposium.* Retrieved from https://sites.google.com/site/healthcaretransition/presentations

Heinrich, K. T. (2002). Manuscript development. Slant, style, and synthesis: 3 keys to a strong literature review. *Nurse Author and Editor, 12*(1), 1–3.

Heinrich, K. T. (2007). Dare to share: A unique approach to presenting and publishing. *Nurse Educator, 32,* 269–273.

Hicks, R. W. (2015). Transforming a presentation to a publication: Tips for nurse practitioners. *Journal of the American Association of Nurse Practitioners, 27*(9), 488–496.

HLWIKI International. (2013). *BOPPPS model.* Retrieved from http://hlwiki.slais.ubc.ca/index.php/BOPPPS_Model

Horstman, P., & Theeke, L. (2012). Using a professional writing retreat to enhance professional publications, presentations, and research development with staff nurses. *Journal of Nurse Staff Development, 28*(2), 66–68.

Illic, D., & Rowe, N. (2013). What is the evidence that poster presentations are effective in promoting knowledge transfer? A state of the art review. *Health Information and Libraries Journal, 30,* 4–12.

International Academy of Nursing Editors. (2014). *Open access, editorial standards and predatory publishing.* Retrieved from https://nursingeditors.com/2015/02/09/inane-initiative-on-predatory-publishers-is-well-underway/

Issa, N., Mayer, R. E., Schuller, M., Wang, E., Shapiro, M. B., & DaRosa, D. A. (2013). Teaching for understanding in medical classrooms using multimedia design principles. *Medical Education, 47*(4), 388–396.

Jham, B. C., Duraes, G. V., Strassler, H. E., & Sensi, L. G. (2008). Joining the podcast revolution. *Journal of Dental Education, 72,* 278–281.

Johnson, J. A. (2016). Reviving the journal club as a nursing professional development strategy. *Journal for Nurses in Professional Development, 32,* 104–106. doi:10.1097/NND.0000000000000241

Kiefer, J. C. (2010). Science communications: Publishing a scientific paper. *Developmental Dynamics, 239*(2), 723–726.

King, S. (2001). *On writing.* New York, NY: Pocket Books.

Kutner, M., Greenberg, E., Jin, Y., & Paulsen, C. (2006). *The health literacy of America's adults: Results from the 2003 National Assessment of Adult Literacy (NCES 2006-483).* Washington, DC: National Center for Education Statistics.

Lannon, J., Gurak, L., & Daemon, D. (2012). *Technical communication* (12th ed.). Boston, MA: Longman.

Larkin, M. E., Griffith, C. A., Pitler, L., Donahue, L., & Sbrolla, A. (2012). Building communities of practice: The research nurse round table. *Clinical and Translational Science, 5*(5), 428–431.

Leyva, M., Sharif, I., & Ozuah, O. (2005). Health literacy among Spanish-speaking Latino parents with limited English proficiency. *Ambulatory Pediatrics, 5,* 56–59.

Majid, S., Foo, S., Luyt, B., Zhang, X., Theng, Y., Chang, Y., & Mokhtar, I. (2011). Adopting evidence-based practice in clinical decision making: Nurses' perceptions, knowledge, and barriers. *Journal of the Medical Library Association, 99*(3), 229–236.

Marble, S. G. (2009). Five-step model of professional excellence. *Clinical Journal of Oncology Nursing, 13*(3), 310–315.

Martin, A. E., Newlove-Delgado T. V., Abbott, R. A., Bethel, A., Thompson-Coon, J., Whear, R., Logan, S. (2017). Pharmacological interventions for recurrent abdominal pain in childhood. *Cochrane Database of Systematic Reviews,* (3), CD010973. doi:10.1002/14651858.CD010973.pub2

McKeever, S, Kinney, S., Lima, S., & Newall, F. (2016). Creating a journal club competition improves paediatric nurses' participation and engagement. *Nurse Education Today, 37,* 173–177. doi:10.1016/j.nedt.2015.11.017

McLaughlin, M. K., Speroni, K. G., Patterson, K., Guzzetta, C. E., & Desale, S. (2013). National survey of hospital nursing research, part 1: Research requirements and outcomes. *The Journal of Nursing Administration, 43*(1), 10–17. doi:10.1097/01.NNA.0000435148.24090.ea

McLeod, P., Steinert, Y., Boudreau, D., Snell, L., & Wiseman, J. (2010). Twelve tips for conducting a medical education journal club. *Medical Teaching, 32*(5), 368–370.

Mee, C. L. (2013). Ten lessons on writing for publication. *Clinical Journal of Oncology Nursing*, Retrieved from http://www.ons.org/Publications/CJON/AuthorInfo/WritingSupp/TenLessons/

Melnyk, B. M. (2016). Disseminating evidence by turning presentations into publications: Key strategies for success. [Editorial]. *Worldviews on Evidence-Based Nursing, 13*(4), 259–260.

Miracle, V. A. (2008). Effective poster presentations. *Dimensions of Critical Care Nursing, 27*, 122–124.

Moonan, M., Bukoye, B., Clapp, A., Shermont, H., & Oliveira, J. O. (2015). Charting the Course for a nursing online journal club: Part I. *Journal of Continuing Education in Nursing, 46*, 546–548. doi:10.3928/00220124-20151112-05

Moonan, M., Bukoye, B., Clapp, A., Shermont, H., & Oliveira, J. O. (2016). Charting the Course for a nursing online journal club: Part II. *Journal of Continuing Education in Nursing, 47*, 14–16. doi:10.3928/00220124-20151230-05

O'Nan, C. L. (2011). The effect of a journal club on perceived barriers to the utilization of nursing research in a practice setting. *Journal for Nurses in Staff Development, 27*(4), 160–164. doi:10.1097/NND.0b013e31822365f6

Oermann, M. H., Leonardelli, A. K., Turner, K. M., Hawks, S. J., Derouin, A. C., & Hueckel, R. M. (2015). Systematic review of educational programs and strategies for developing students' and nurses' writing skills. *Journal of Nursing Education, 54*, 28–34.

Phillips, W. L., Sweet, C. A., & Blythe, H. R. (2009). Collaborating on writing. *Academe, 95*(5), 31. Retrieved from http://www.aaup.org/article/collaborating-writing#.U4Uq_vldXOM

Price, R. (2014). Writing a journal article: Guidance for nursing authors. *Nursing Standard, 28*, 35, 40–47.

Rogoschewsky, T. L. (2011). Developing a conference presentation: A primer for new library professionals. *Partnership: The Canadian Journal of Library and Information Practice and Research, 6*(2). Retrieved from https://journal.lib.uoguelph.ca/index.php/perj/article/view/1573/2284

Rowell, M. R., Corl, F. M., Johnson, P. T., & Fishman, E. K. (2006). Internet-based dissemination of educational audiocasts: A primer in podcasting-How to do it. *American Journal of Radiology, 186*, 1792–1796.

Savel, R. H., Goldstein, E. B., Perencevich, E. N., & Angood, P. B. (2007). The critical care podcast: A novel medium for critical care communication and education. *Journal of American Medical Informatics Association, 14*, 94–99.

Sawatzky, J. V. (2011). My abstract was accepted, now what? A guide to effective conference presentations. *Canadian Journal of Cardiovascular Nursing, 21*(2), 37–41.

Science Direct. (n.d.) *Articles in press*. Retrieved from http://www.sciencedirect.com/science/journal/aip/08825963#FCANote

Sherman, R. O. (2010). How to create an effective poster presentation. *American Nurse Today, 5*(9), 13.

Siedlecki, S. L. (2017). Original research: How to create a poster that attracts an audience. *American Journal of Nursing, 117*, 48–54.

Silversides, A. (2011). Journal clubs: A forum for discussion and professional development. *The Canadian Nurse, 107*(2), 19–23.

Skiba, D. J. (2006). Emerging technologies center: The 2005 word of the year: Podcast. *Nursing Education Perspectives, 27*, 54–55.

Smith, C. D., & Grami, P. (2017). Feasibility and effectiveness of a delirium prevention bundle in critically ill patients. *American Journal of Critical Care, 26*, 19–27. doi:10.4037/ajcc2017374

Sorian, R., & Baugh, T. (2002). Power of information: Closing the gap between research and policy. *Health Affairs, 21*(2), 264–268.

Sortedahl, C. (2012). Effect of online journal club on evidence-based practice knowledge, intent, and utilization in school nurses. *Worldviews on Evidence-Based Nursing, 9*(2), 117–125. doi:10.1111/j.1741-6787.2012.00249.x

Steele-Moses, S. K. (2013). Developing a journal club at your institution. *Clinical Journal of Oncology Nursing, 13*(1), 109–112.

Steenbeek, A., Edgecombe, N., Durling, J., LeBlanc, A., Anderson, R., & Bainbridge, R. (2009). Using an interactive journal club to enhance nursing research knowledge acquisition, appraisal, and application. *International Journal of Nursing Education Scholarship, 6*(1), 1–8. doi:10.2202/1548-923X.1673

Stuart, A. C. (2013). Engaging the audience: Developing presentation skills in science students. *The Journal of Undergraduate Neuroscience Education, 12*, A4–A10.

Stuber, P. (2013). *Open access overview: Focusing on open access to peer-reviewed research articles and their preprints*. Retrieved from http://legacy.earlham.edu/~peters/fos/overview.htm

Tinkham, M. R. (2013). The road to magnet: Implementing new knowledge, innovations, and improvements. *AORN Journal, 97*(5), 579–581.

U.S. Department of Health and Human Services. (2013). *Healthy People 2020: Understanding and improving health* (2nd ed.). Washington, DC: U.S. Government Printing Office.

Van Soeren, M., Hurlock-Chorostecki, C., & Reeves, S. (2011). The role of nurse practitioners in hospital settings: Implications for interprofessional practice. *Journal of Interprofessional Care, 25*(4), 245–251.

Vodcast. (2018). Cambridge Advanced Learner's Dictionary & Thesaurus (2018). Retrieved from https://dictionary.cambridge.org/us/dictionary/english/vodcast

Yoder-Wise, P. S., & Vlasses, F. R. (2012). Pathways to a leadership legacy: Pursuing professional publication. *Nurse Leader, 10*(5), 36–38.

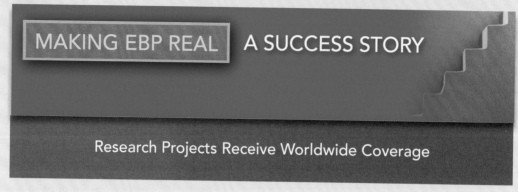

MAKING EBP REAL | A SUCCESS STORY

Research Projects Receive Worldwide Coverage

Emily Caldwell, MS
Reprinted with permission from The Ohio State University.

Two research projects by Dr. Bernadette Melnyk of The Ohio State University and Dr. Linda Chlan of Mayo Clinic have been covered by media outlets from all over the globe and continue to generate interest. What follows is an account of the studies' research findings and examples of the attention following their papers being published in major medical journals.[1]

Example 1: The COPE Program[2]

Adding a mental health component to school-based lifestyle programs for teens could be key to lowering obesity, improving grades, alleviating severe depression, and reducing substance use, a new study suggests.

As a group, high-school students who participated in an intervention that emphasized cognitive behavioral skills building in addition to nutrition and physical activity had a lower average body mass index (BMI), drank less alcohol, and had better social behaviors and higher health class grades than did teenagers in a class with standard health lessons.

Symptoms in teens who were severely depressed also dropped to normal levels at the end of the semester compared with the control group, whose symptoms remained elevated. Most of the positive outcomes of the program, called COPE, were sustained for 6 months.

Thirty-two percent of youths in the United States are overweight or obese, and suicide is the third leading cause of death among young people aged 14 to 24 years, according to the Centers for Disease Control and Prevention. Yet most school-based interventions don't take on both public health problems simultaneously or measure the effects of programs on multiple outcomes, said Bernadette Melnyk, PhD, RN, APRN-CNP, FAANP, FNAP, FAAN, creator of the COPE program, dean of The Ohio State University College of Nursing, and lead author of the study. "This is what has been missing from prior healthy lifestyle programs with teens—getting to the thinking piece. We teach the adolescents that how they think directly relates to how they feel and how they behave," says Melnyk, also Ohio State's chief wellness officer. The study is published in the *American Journal of Preventive Medicine*.

A total of 779 high-school students aged 14 to 16 years in the Southwestern United States participated in the study. Half attended a control class that covered standard health topics such as road safety, dental care, and immunizations. The others were enrolled in the intervention Melnyk et al. were testing for its effectiveness—a program called COPE (Creating Opportunities for Personal Empowerment) Healthy Lifestyles TEEN (Thinking, Emotions, Exercise, Nutrition).

---

[1]The National Institute of Nursing Research supported this research (#1R01NR012171; Principal Investigator—Bernadette Melnyk). Coauthors include Diana Jacobson, Stephanie Kelly, Michael Belyea, Gabriel Shaibi, Leigh Small, Judith O'Haver, and Flavio Marsiglia.
[2]This research was funded by a grant from the National Institute of Nursing Research.

Melnyk began developing COPE more than 20 years ago while she was a nurse practitioner at an inpatient psychiatric unit for children and adolescents. The program is based on the concepts of cognitive behavioral therapy, with an emphasis on skills building.

It's not counseling in the classroom, however. The entire COPE curriculum, a blend of weekly 50-minute behavioral skills sessions, nutrition information, and physical activity over the course of 15 weeks, is spelled out for instructors in manuals and PowerPoint presentations.

"These are skills that I can teach a variety of professionals how to deliver, and they don't have to be certified therapists," says Melnyk, also a professor of pediatrics and psychiatry in the College of Medicine.

At its core, the COPE program emphasizes the link between thinking patterns, emotions, and behavior as well as the ABCs of cognitive behavioral skills building: activator events that trigger negative thoughts, negative beliefs teens may have about themselves on the basis of the triggering event, and the consequences of feeling bad and engaging in negative behavior as a result.

"We teach kids how to monitor for activator events and show them that instead of embracing a negative belief, they can turn that around to a positive belief about themselves," Melnyk says. "Schools are great at teaching math and social studies, but we aren't giving teens the life skills they need to successfully deal with stress, how to problem-solve, and how to set goals, and those are key elements in this healthy lifestyle intervention."

COPE includes also nutrition lessons on such topics as portion sizes and social eating and 20 minutes of movement—dance, dodge ball, taking a walk—anything to keep the students out of their seats.

Immediately after the programs ended, and 6 months afterward, COPE students' outcomes exceeded the control group's, on average, in several areas: 4,061 more steps per day; a significantly lower average BMI; better scores in cooperation, assertion, and academic competence; and a trend toward lower alcohol use among the COPE teens. In addition, 97.3% of COPE teens who started at a healthy weight remained in that category.

Melnyk noted that it's not possible to tease out exactly which component of the program has the most profound effect on teens, but it's likely to be the combination of all of them together.

Six school districts and a YMCA chapter in Ohio have already adopted COPE. Melnyk plans to continue testing an adapted version of the program for younger children in schools and community settings. See Box 1 for a list of publications in which stories about COPE have appeared.

Example 2: Anxiety and ICU Patients on Mechanical Ventilators[3]

Chlan, a research scientist at Mayo Clinic, led this study while a member of the faculty at the University of Minnesota. Coauthors include Craig Weinert, Annie Heiderscheit, Mary Fran Tracy, Debra Skaar, and Kay Savik, all of the University of Minnesota and Jill Guttormson of Marquette University.

New research suggests that for some hospitalized intensive care unit (ICU) patients on mechanical ventilators, using headphones to listen to their favorite types of music could lower anxiety and reduce their need for sedative medications.

In a clinical trial, the option to listen to music lowered anxiety, on average, by 36.5%, and reduced the number of sedative doses by 38% and the intensity of sedation by 36% compared with ventilated ICU patients who did not receive the music intervention. These effects were seen, on average, 5 days into the study.

The research is published online in the *Journal of the American Medical Association*.

Researchers first assessed the patients' musical preferences and kept a continuous loop of music running on bedside CD players. When patients wished to listen to music, they were

BOX 1	**COPE Study Media Coverage**

Stories about Bernadette Melnyk's research originally published in the *American Journal of Preventive Medicine* have appeared in or on the following:

TIME Health
U.S. News & World Report
Reuters Health
WTOP 103.5FM DC
KPTV Fox12 Oregon
Health.com
dailyRx
MedicalXpress
Philly.com
KVVU Fox5 Las Vegas
Guardian Express
National Post
Counsel & Heal
eNews Park Forest
WOSU 89.7 FM—All Sides with Ann Fisher
National Academies of Practice newsletter
American Association of Nurse Practitioners
RedOrbit
WTTG Fox5 DC
PsychCentral
Phoenix Health News Examiner
EmpowHER
The Globe and Mail
NIH Medline
Medicine Online
MedCity News

able to put on headphones that were equipped with a system that time- and date-stamped and recorded each use.

Professional guidelines recommend that pain, agitation, and delirium be carefully managed in the ICU, with the goal of keeping mechanically ventilated patients comfortable and awake. However, the researchers acknowledged that oversedation is common in these patients, which can lead to both physiologic problems linked to prolonged immobility and psychological issues that include fear and frustration over not being able to communicate, and even posttraumatic stress disorder.

"We're trying to address the problem of oversedation from a very different perspective, by empowering patients. Some patients do not want control, but many patients want to know what is going on with their care," says Linda Chlan, PhD, RN, FAAN, associate dean for nursing research at the Mayo Clinic and lead author of the study.

"But I'm not talking about using music in place of the medical plan of care. These findings do not suggest that clinicians should place headphones on just any ICU patient. For the intervention to have the most impact and to have the desired effect of reducing anxiety, the music has to be familiar and comforting to the patient—which is why tailoring the music collection for the patient to listen to was key to the success of this study."

Chlan et al. conducted the study with 373 patients in 12 ICUs at 5 hospitals in the Minneapolis-St. Paul area. Of those, 126 patients were randomized to receive the patient-directed music intervention, 125 received usual care, and 122 were in an active control group and could self-initiate the use of noise-canceling headphones. All patients had to be alert enough to give their own consent to participate.

A music therapist assessed each patient in the music group to develop a collection that met the patient's preferences. This was no easy task because the patients are not able to speak when they are on a ventilator.

Researchers instructed patients to use the intervention if they were feeling anxious, wanted to relax, or needed quiet time. Nurses were asked to prompt patients twice during each shift about their interest in listening to music.

In all patients, researchers performed daily assessments of anxiety and two measures of sedative exposure to any of eight commonly used medications. Anxiety was measured with a visual analog scale that asked patients to describe their anxiety by pointing to a chart anchored by the statements "not anxious at all" and "most anxious ever." Patients remained in the study as long as they were on ventilators, up to a maximum of 30 days.

A complex statistical analysis of the data showed that significant reductions in anxiety and sedation could be seen in patients in the music intervention within 5 days when they were compared with patients who received usual care. Patients using noise-canceling headphones showed some improvements in anxiety and lower sedation intensity, but the effects were not as strong as those seen in the music group.

BOX
2
Music Study Media Coverage

Media placements about Linda Chlan's research originally published in the *Journal of the American Medical Association* have appeared in or on the following:

CBS Radio
The Globe and Mail
MedPage Today
State of Health blog
AACN Critical Care
American Thoracic Society News
UPI wire services
MDLinx
U.S. News & World Report
Philadelphia Inquirer
Huffington Post
Nurse Practitioner News
Critical Care SmartBrief
WOSU—Music in Mid-Ohio
WOSU—All Sides with Ann Fisher
MENAFN News (Middle East North Africa Financial Network)
American College of Physicians Hospitalist magazine
Psychiatric News
Reader's Digest
Chlan also served as an expert source in a story about music reducing the amount of stress children have over IV needles, which was covered in the *Chicago Tribune*, *Baltimore Sun*, and Fox News.

"There is something there with noise-canceling headphones, but the music is so much more powerful. With the music, we were able to show a simultaneous reduction in anxiety and in sedation," Chlan said. "When we listen to music, our entire brain lights up. We want to capitalize on the pleasant, comforting memories associated with music because it occupies brain channels that otherwise would be occupied by an anxiety-producing stimulus. That's why music is so much more than just something nice to listen to."

A former medical ICU nurse, Chlan now leads a research program that emphasizes testing treatment strategies that complement traditional medical approaches to ICU care.

"I think about tackling the modifiable risk factors. And sedation is directly modifiable because it is controlled by the clinician. Nonpharmacologic, integrative interventions like music bring in a piece that does not induce adverse side effects and does not contribute to ICU-acquired problems," she says.

She and her colleagues now are working on making the highly controlled research protocol more friendly to standard hospital practices. "If this is going to have wide clinical impact, that really has to be done," she says. See Box 2 for a list of publications in which stories about the music study have appeared.

Generating External Evidence and Writing Successful Grant Proposals

> Nothing in the world can take the place of persistence. Talent will not; nothing is more common than unsuccessful men with talent. Genius will not; unrewarded genius is almost a proverb. Education will not . . .. Persistence and determination alone are omnipotent. The slogan Press On! has solved and always will solve the problems of the human race.
>
> — *Calvin Coolidge*

EBP Terms to Learn

Attention control group
Beneficence
Booster interventions
Confounding/extraneous variable
Construct validity
Content validity
Correlational descriptive and predictive designs
Cross-sectional designs
Data safety and monitoring plan
Effectiveness trial
Efficacy trial
Face validity
Institutional review board/ research subjects review board
Internal consistency reliability
Interrater reliability
Justice
Manipulation checks
Maturation
Mediating variable
Nonexperimental design
Nonmaleficence
Participatory action research
Pilot research
Principle of fidelity
Random sampling
Randomized block design
Scalability
Solomon four group design
"So what" factor
Stratification
Test–retest reliability

UNIT OBJECTIVES

Upon completion of this unit, learners will be able to:

1. Describe important elements of quantitative and qualitative studies.

2. Discuss various types of quantitative and qualitative study designs.

3. Identify specific steps in writing a successful grant proposal.

4. Describe attributes of successfully funded grant proposals.

MAKING CONNECTIONS: AN EBP EXEMPLAR

As part of the roll-out for their evidence-based fall prevention project, Lei and the evidence-based practice (EBP) Council members planned to address one of the identified barriers to successful EBP implementation: recognition of successes, small and large. They chose an innovative way to recognize contributions by staff, patients, families, and all those involved in care of the patient joining in innovation: As a project success indicator was observed, a paper drop would be completed and taped to paper buckets that were placed on the doors of the unit. There were one for families, one for patients, and one for personnel. Because this was an innovation and not part of what was done in the studies, Dr. Ayita, the DNP-prepared clinical expert, and Dr. Reyansh, the nurse scientist for the organization, partnered in exploring the feasibility of this initiative through a pilot study. The pilot was not intended to be generalizable to a wider population, but was intended to offer some insight into the effectiveness of this innovation and its impact on the staff. Drs. Ayita and Reyansh decided that a mixed methods design was best for their pilot. After reviewing the literature and writing a brief on the background and significance of project recognition programs, they formulated the following research questions:

1. Is it feasible for families, patients, and staff to complete drops to recognize contributions to the hourly rounding fall prevention program?
2. Do staff, families, and patients perceive the drops recognition initiative as helpful to the process of implementation?
3. Do staff, families, and patients who completed the drops recognition initiative perceive better outcomes (FRisk assessment, call light use, fall rates, and patient satisfaction)?

The intervention protocol was presented in a booklet, and the staff, families, and patients attended an educational session on how to use the drops and buckets. DeAndre, the EBP mentor, videotaped the session for future education of new staff, families, and patients to keep everyone informed about the intervention. Additionally, the booklet and video offered an opportunity to maintain the fidelity of the intervention. After the educational session, either in-person or by video, there was a short knowledge quiz and each of the participants who completed a drop within 3 days of their session qualified for a completion certificate. The drops completed were reviewed for congruence with how the intervention was taught.

The pilot study was submitted to the ethics review board of the organization for ethical review and approval. In this organization, the ethics review board is called the institutional review board (IRB). In compliance with the IRB approval, each of the staff, families, and patients who were potential participants in the pilot was provided a consent form that described the study and its potential benefits. Those who chose to participate in the pilot were scheduled for the education session.

Data collection consisted of project outcomes; a questionnaire that asked staff, families, and patients about their perceptions of the feasibility and helpfulness of the drop recognition initiative; and focus groups to discuss the impact of the initiative on project outcomes. The feasibility and helpfulness questionnaire was modeled after prior studies in which helpfulness of intervention components was evaluated (Dalcin et al., 2015). The questionnaire had a 5-point Likert response ranging from 1: not at all helpful to 5: extremely helpful. There were three questions: (1) How helpful was the drop recognition program to the effectiveness of the hourly rounding fall prevention program? (2) How easy was it to engage in the drop recognition program? and (3) How effective was the drop recognition program in reducing falls, improving call light usage, and improving patient satisfaction? The pilot was conducted for 3 months, across which data were collected.

Once these data were analyzed, focus groups were held. Participants were shown the quantitative data and asked to provide their perceptions/insights about the data, particularly in relationship to the project outcomes. The focus groups were recorded and transcribed. Themes were extracted from the data and presented to staff, families, and patients who had participated in the project in a poster that hung on the target unit's main area.

Drs. Ayita and Reyansh discussed the findings with the EBP Council. The project team agreed that the drop initiative was an added bonus to the project implementation and included it in their dissemination plans, discussing it with their presentation audiences. Administration and nursing leadership were fully supportive of the team and their contribution to excellent patient care and anticipated the EBP Council's next project.

Reference

Dalcin, A. T., Jerome, G. J., Fitzpatrick, S. L., Louis, T. A., Wang, N-Y., Bennett1, W. L., ...Coughlin, J. W. (2015). Perceived helpfulness of the individual components of a behavioural weight loss program: results from the Hopkins POWER Trial. *Obesity Science & Practice*, 1(1), 23-32.

Bernadette Mazurek Melnyk, Dianne Morrison-Beedy, and Denise Cote-Arsenault

Man's mind, stretched to a new idea, never goes back to its original dimensions.

—*Oliver Wendell Holmes*

EBP Terms to Learn

Attrition
Basic research
Blocking
Categorical data
Ceiling effect
Cohort study
Comparative effectiveness trial (CET)
Confounding/extraneous variable
Correlational descriptive design
Correlational predictive design
Covary
Cross-sectional
Dependent variable
Descriptive studies
Effectiveness trial
Efficacy trial
Ethnography
Exclusion criteria
Experimental design
External validity
Factorial design
Feasibility
Floor effect
Generalizability
Grounded theory
History
Homogeneity
Inclusion criteria
Independent variable
Institutional review board (IRB)/research subjects review board (RSRB)

Integrity of the intervention
Internal consistency reliability
Internal validity
Interrater reliability
Manipulation checks
Maturation
Mediating variable
Nonexperimental design
Ordinal data
Participatory action research
Phenomenology
Pilot research
Power
Pragmatic trial
Pre-experiment
Principal investigator (PI)
Qualitative research
Quantitative research
Quasi-experiment

Quasi-experimental design
Random sampling
Randomized controlled trials
Randomization/random assignment
Randomized block design
Reliable
Research design meeting
Scalability
Solomon four-group design
"so what" factor
Stratification
Test-retest reliability
Theoretical or conceptual framework
True experiment
Valid
Validity

Learning Objectives

After studying this chapter, learners will be able to:

1. Describe the purposes of quantitative and qualitative research.

2. Discuss various types of quantitative research, including descriptive and experimental studies.

3. Identify the strongest design for supporting cause-and-effect relationships.

4. Describe various types of sampling designs.

5. Discuss various types of qualitative research methodologies.

6. Describe the steps in designing a quantitative and qualitative study.

When there is a lack of research reported in the literature to guide clinical practice, it becomes necessary to design and conduct studies to generate **external evidence** (i.e., evidence generated through rigorous research that is intended to be used outside of one's own clinical practice setting). There are many areas in clinical practice that do not have a sufficient evidence base (e.g., care for dying children; interventions for family caregivers of critically ill patients). As a result, there is an urgent need to conduct studies so that healthcare providers can base their treatment decisions on sound evidence from well-designed studies instead of continuing to make decisions that are steeped solely in tradition or opinion.

THE IMPORTANCE OF GENERATING EXTERNAL EVIDENCE

This chapter provides a general overview and practical guide for formulating clinical research questions and designing quantitative and qualitative studies to answer these questions. It also includes suggestions on when a quantitative versus qualitative approach would be more appropriate to answer a specific question. A variety of quantitative research designs are discussed, from **descriptive studies** to **randomized controlled trials (RCTs)**. Descriptive studies are designed to explore or predict relationships between variables. RCTs are rigorous studies designed to test the effect of interventions or treatments. Descriptive studies serve as the building blocks for RCTs. Techniques to enhance the rigor of quantitative research designs are highlighted, including strategies to strengthen **internal validity** (i.e., the ability to say that it was the independent variable or intervention that caused a change in the dependent variable or outcome, not other extraneous variables) as well as **external validity** (i.e., generalizability, which is the ability to generalize findings from a study's sample to the larger population). Specific principles of conducting **qualitative research** also are described in this chapter.

Getting Started: From Idea to Reality

"

We are told never to cross a bridge until we come to it,
but the world is owned by men who have 'crossed bridges'
in their imagination far ahead of the crowd.

SPEAKERS LIBRARY

Many ideas for studies come from clinical practice settings in which questions arise regarding best practices or evolve from a search for evidence on a particular topic (e.g., Is music or relaxation therapy more effective in reducing the stress of patients after surgery? What are the major variables that predict the development of posttraumatic stress disorder in adults after motor vehicle accidents? What are the stages of grief that parents experience after the death of a child?). However, these ideas are often not studied by clinicians because of competing demands or inadequate knowledge, skills, or resources to undertake research and complete the project successfully. However, clinical ideas or research questions can be shared with PhD-prepared researchers who can partner with clinicians to launch and conduct a study. Thus, the person who had the idea or question can assume an active role on the study team but need not take on the role of the lead person, or **principal investigator (PI)**, who is responsible and accountable for overseeing all elements of the science and research project.

After an idea is generated for a study and a search for and critical appraisal of the literature have been conducted to get an understanding of the available body of evidence,

"

The greatest successful people of the world have used their
imagination . . .. They think ahead and create their mental picture,
and then go to work materializing that picture in all its details,
filling in here, adding a little there, altering this a bit and that a bit,
but steadily building—steadily building.

ROBERT COLLIER

a collaborative team can be established to be part of the research planning process from
the outset. Because clinicians often have many crucial clinical questions but typically need
assistance with details of study design, methods, and analysis, formulating a team comprised
of seasoned interprofessional clinicians and research experts (e.g., PhD-prepared researchers)
will usually lead to the best outcomes. Increasingly, teams of transdisciplinary professionals
are brought together, adding value to the project by broadening perspectives and approaches
applied, especially during the study design and interpretation of findings. Many funding
agencies often expect transdisciplinary collaboration on research projects. Convening this
collaborative team for a **research design meeting** at the outset of a project is exceedingly
beneficial in developing the study's design and methods.

Approximately 1 to 2 weeks before the research design meeting is conducted, a concise,
two-page draft of the study should be prepared and disseminated. This draft acts as an outline
or overview of the clinical problem and includes the research question and a brief description of the proposed methods (see Box 21.1 for an example of a study outline and Boxes
21.2 and 21.3 for completed examples of study outlines for different types of studies). As
the study outline is developed, a list of questions related to the project should be answered:

- Is this idea feasible and clinically important?
- What is the **"so what" factor**? (i.e., the conduct of research with high-impact po-
  tential to improve outcomes that the current healthcare system is focused on,
  such as patient complications, readmission rates, length of stay, cost; Melnyk &
  Morrison-Beedy, 2012)
- What is the aim of the study, along with the research question(s) or hypotheses?
- What is the best design to answer the study question(s) or test the hypotheses?
- What are the "so what" outcomes (e.g., rate of various complications, cost) that are
  important to measure and potential sources of data?
- Are there valid and reliable instruments to measure the desired outcomes?
- What should be the **inclusion** and **exclusion criteria** for the potential study
  participants?
- What are the essential elements of the intervention, if applicable, and how will
  integrity of the intervention be maintained (i.e., assurance that the intervention is being delivered exactly in the manner in which it was intended to be
  delivered)?

The research design planning session needs to foster an environment in which constructive
feedback and candid discussion will promote a finely tuned study design. It is important to
define the roles for each of the study team members (e.g., percentage of effort on the study,
specific functions, availability, and order of authorship once the study is published). In addition, potential funding sources for the study should be discussed as well as who will assume
specific responsibilities in writing a grant proposal if funding is necessary to conduct the
project (see Chapter 22 for specific steps in writing a successful grant proposal and Box 21.4
for a summary of initial steps in designing a study).

Outlining Important Elements of a Quantitative Study

Before developing a study protocol, it is extremely beneficial to develop a one- to two-page outline of the elements of a study.
I. Significance of the problem and the "so what?" factor
II. Specific aim(s) of the study
   A. Research Question(s) or
   B. Hypotheses
III. Theoretical/conceptual framework
IV. Study design
V. Subjects
   A. Sampling design
   B. Sampling criteria
      1. Inclusion criteria
      2. Exclusion Criteria
VI. Variables
   A. Independent variable(s) (in an experimental study, the intervention being proposed)
   B. Dependent variable(s) (the "so what" outcomes) and Measures
   C. Mediating Variable, if applicable (e.g., the variable through which the intervention will most likely exert its effects)
   D. Confounding or extraneous variable(s) with potential control strategies
VII. Statistical issues
   A. Sample size
   B. Approach to analyses

Example of a Completed Study Outline for a Descriptive Correlational Study

A nonexperimental study entitled "Relationship between Depressive Symptoms and Motivation to Lose Weight in Overweight Teens."
I. Significance of the problem
Data from the Centers for Disease Control indicate that 33% of adolescents are overweight or obese. The major negative consequences associated with obesity in adolescence include premature death, type 2 diabetes, hyperlipidemia, hypertension, and depression. It is known that motivation to lose weight is a key factor in weight loss, but the relationship between depressive symptoms and motivation to lose weight in adolescence has not been studied.
II. Specific aim of the study with research question(s) or hypotheses
The aim of this study is to answer the following research question: What is the relationship between depressive symptoms and motivation to lose weight in overweight/obese adolescents?
III. Theoretical/Conceptual framework
Control theory contends that when there is a discrepancy between a standard or goal (e.g., perceived ideal weight), this discrepancy should motivate individuals to initiate behaviors (e.g., exercise, healthy eating) that allow them to achieve their

goal. However, there are often barriers that may inhibit an individual in being motivated to initiate these behaviors. In this study, depression is viewed as a barrier to motivation and behaviors that would allow teens to achieve their ideal weight.

IV. Study design

A descriptive correlational design will be used.

V. Subjects

    A. *Sampling design*: A random sample of 80 overweight/obese adolescents will be drawn from two randomly selected high schools in Columbus, Ohio; one from the city school district and the other from the suburban area.

    B. *Sampling criteria*

        1. *Inclusion criteria*: Adolescents with a body mass index of 25 or greater enrolled in the two high schools.

        2. *Exclusion criteria:* Adolescents with a current diagnosis of major depression and/or suicidal ideation.

VI. Variables

    A. *Independent variable(s):* Depressive symptoms will be measured with the well-known, valid, and reliable Beck Depression Inventory (BDI-II).

    B. *Dependent variable(s):* Motivation to lose weight will be measured with a newly constructed scale that has been reviewed for content validity with experts in the field. This new scale has been pilot tested with 15 overweight teens and found to have a Cronbach's alpha of 0.80.

    C. *Mediating variable, if applicable*: Not applicable.

    D. *Confounding or extraneous variable(s) with potential control strategies*: Gender is a potential confounding variable, because there is a higher incidence of depression in adolescent females than in males documented in the literature. Therefore, stratified random sampling will be used so that an equal number of males and females will be drawn for the sample.

VII. Statistical issues

    A. *Sample Size*: To obtain a power of 0.8 and medium effect size at the 0.05 level of significance, a total of 80 adolescents will be needed.

    B. *Approach to analyses*: A Pearson's r correlation coefficient will be used to determine whether a relationship exists between the number of depressive symptoms and motivation to lose weight in this sample.

BOX 21.3

Example of a Completed Study Outline for a Randomized Controlled Trial

A Randomized Clinical Trial entitled "Maintaining HIV Prevention Gains in Female Adolescents" (Morrison-Beedy, D., funded by the National Institutes of Health/National Institute of Nursing Research, R01-NR008194-01A1)

  I. Significance of the problem

Reducing the number of HIV infections in adolescents is a critical adolescent objective in *Healthy People 2020* and the highest priority on the national HIV agenda. Adolescents, persons 13 to 19 years of age, are the only age category where the number of females infected with HIV or with AIDS exceeds the number of males. The majority of these cases were a result of transmission of HIV through heterosexual contact. STIs such as chlamydia and gonorrhea also facilitate the transmission

(continued)

BOX
21.3   *Example of a Completed Study Outline for a Randomized Controlled Trial* **(continued)**

of HIV, and young women aged 15 to 18 years have higher reported rates of these diseases than adolescent males or older persons of either gender. Prevention interventions to reduce risk behaviors remain the foremost means to curtail the AIDS epidemic, yet very few RCTs are targeted at adolescent females.

II. Specific aim with research question/hypothesis
The purpose of this randomized controlled trial is to test the short- and long-term efficacy of a theoretically based, manualized HIV-prevention intervention in sexually active adolescent girls aged 15 to 19. We hypothesized that participants of the theoretically based intervention will increase (a) HIV-related knowledge, (b) motivation to reduce risk, (c) HIV-preventive behavioral skills, and (d) decrease the frequency of risky sexual practices as compared to control participants *in a structurally equivalent health promotion intervention at postintervention, and at 3, 6, and 12 months.*

III. Theoretical/Conceptual framework
The theoretical framework for this study is derived from Fisher and Fisher's Information-Motivation-Behavioral Skills Model (IMB). The IMB combines elements from several health behavior models to specify several critical determinants of HIV-related behavioral change. They posit that initiating and maintaining these behaviors result from **information** about HIV prevention and transmission, the **motivation** to reduce risk, and the **behavioral skills** specific to HIV prevention. Using the IMB to guide intervention development for adult women, we have extended information-only and information-and-skills-based programs by enhancing the motivational components of an HIV risk reduction program for women. We included aspects of both immediate (behavior-focused) motivation and broader-based motivation related to life goals, personal and community values, and other transsituational influences. Designed to increase the participant's collaboration and avoid resistance to change, this client-centered but directive style differs from purely didactic or confrontational approaches. Our team subsequently conducted elicitation research with sexually active girls 15 to 19 years and modified the intervention to address the needs of this age group. A pilot test of this intervention suggests that this approach may be particularly useful when developing HIV-prevention interventions for adolescent females as well. *The study allows us to explore important gender-related moderators of behavior change in adolescent girls (e.g., sexual assertiveness, self-management skills),* an important omission in prior studies of adolescent girls.

IV. Study design
An RCT will be used with random assignment of subjects to either the experimental intervention group or the control group.

V. Participants
A. *Sampling criteria:* Adolescent girls who meet the following criteria will be eligible for study participation:
1. Aged 15 to 19
2. Neither pregnant nor actively trying to become pregnant
3. No births within the past 3 months
4. Heterosexually active within the past 3 months
5. English-speaking

   B. *Sampling design:* A convenience sample of adolescent girls who meet the inclusion criteria and agreed to participate in the study.
VI. Variables
   A. *Independent variable(s):* The experimental and control group both participated in interventions that were theoretically and empirically guided, gender-focused, and developmentally appropriate for adolescents aged 15 to 19 and included content that addressed the following variables:
      1. Information regarding HIV in the experimental group or health information in the control group
      2. Motivation to change behaviors improve health
      3. Behavioral skills such as assertive communication in both groups
   B. *Dependent variable(s):* The frequency of unprotected and protected vaginal, oral, and anal intercourse in the past 3 months will be assessed at baseline, postintervention, and at 3, 6, and 12 months. Number and type of sexual partner(s) will also be assessed (i.e., steady vs. nonsteady partner).
   C. *Confounding or extraneous variable(s) With Potential Control Strategies:* Results could be confounded if participants brought up topics within the control group that were related to the experimental intervention. However, facilitators were trained, and the manual provided specific instructions on how to steer the conversation back to control topics. Other concerns were that there might be "crosstalk," that is, cross-contamination between girls randomized to different groups who might come together in social or school settings. However, researchers believed that as the trained interventionists used motivational interviewing strategies, the content could not be duplicated simply by conversations between the groups.
VII. Statistical issues
   A. *Sample size:* The sample size of 738 was based on the expected small effect size anticipated for change in STI rates (biologically documented) lab tests.
   B. *Approach to analyses:* Cronbach's alpha will be used to determine internal consistency reliability of the study instruments. Baseline characteristics of the intervention groups will be tabulated, and any significant differences between groups and between sites will be noted. Additionally, we will conduct analyses to identify the correlates of program attendance to determine whether any baseline characteristic is associated with program completion or attrition. Formal analyses will use the intent-to-treat principle, that is, keeping all study subjects in their assigned randomization group for analysis and will require a two-sided alpha level of 0.05 for statistical significance. To test the study hypotheses, we will use zero-inflated Poisson (ZIP) regression analyses for frequency of sexual behavior. We will also analyze the impact of the intervention on the number of sex partners, by categorizing the number of partners and then modeling using generalized logit regression to assess differences between participants based on the number of partners. The ZIP model will be evaluated with 3-, 6-, and 12-month postintervention outcome data.

Designing a Quantitative Study

Box 21.5 identifies several factors to consider in developing a quantitative study. Understanding prior work in the area of study builds the initial case for need. This is followed closely by significance of the problem and feasibility of investigating the issue. Once an important question has been identified and it is likely that a study to investigate the problem can be carried out, the building blocks have been laid for designing the study.

BOX
21.4 *Initial Steps in Designing a Quantitative Study*

- Cultivate a spirit of inquiry as you deliver care to patients in your practice setting.
- Ask questions about best practices for specific clinical problems.
- Develop a "creative ideas" file as thoughts for studies emerge.
- Pursue a clinical research question that you care about and that is an important "so what?" factor.
- Search for, critically appraise, and synthesize systematic reviews and prior studies in the area of interest.
- Establish a potential collaborative team for the project.
- Plan a research design meeting.
- Prepare and disseminate a concise two-page study outline.
- Conduct the research design meeting to plan specific details of the clinical study, decide on the roles of team members, and plan the writing of a grant proposal for funding if needed.
- Incorporate feedback and input from team members and other experts to improve the study design.

BOX
21.5 *Major Factors to Consider When Designing a Quantitative Study*

- Prior studies in the area
- Significance of the problem and the "so what" factor
- Innovation of the project
- Feasibility
- Setting for the study and access to potential subjects
- Study team
- Ethics of the study

Search for, Critical Appraisal and Synthesis of Prior Evidence

If the search for, critical appraisal and synthesis of prior research reveal numerous studies that describe a particular construct or phenomenon, such as stressors of family caregivers of hospitalized elders as well as studies that identify the major predictors of caregiver stress during hospitalization (e.g., uncertainty regarding the caregiving role in the hospital, lack of knowledge regarding how best to enhance outcomes in the hospitalized elder), another descriptive study in the field is probably not needed. Instead, the next logical step in this example (based on the descriptive and predictive evidence already generated from prior studies) would be to design and test an educational intervention that informs family caregivers of the functions they can perform to improve their hospitalized elder's health outcomes. In contrast, if the phenomenon of caregiver stress is not well understood or inadequately measured in the literature, conducting a qualitative or descriptive study may be the most appropriate next step. This type of study might begin with open-ended questions to allow participants to respond in their own words to such questions as: "How would you describe what it is like for you to care for your partner or parent?" or "How have things changed for you

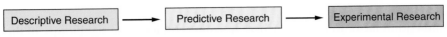

Figure 21.1: Progression of quantitative research.

now, while your family member is in the hospital?" Research in a particular area frequently begins with qualitative work in which a phenomenon or construct is explored with heavy emphasis on interview or observation data. When more is known about the nature of the phenomenon through qualitative work, quantitative research is usually undertaken in which the construct of interest is described using measurement scales, test scores, and statistical approaches (Figure 21.1). Oftentimes, descriptive, quantitative, qualitative, and formative work is conducted in parallel or alternating steps, and these findings build the case for, and ultimately design of, interventions that impact health outcomes.

As Figure 21.1 shows, quantitative research designs range from descriptive and correlational descriptive/predictive studies to RCTs. **Correlational descriptive** and **correlational predictive designs** examine the relationships between two or more variables (e.g., What is the relationship between smoking and lung cancer in adults? or What maternal factors in the first month of life predict infant cognitive development at 1 year of age?). These designs are the study of choice when the **independent variable** cannot be manipulated experimentally because of some individual characteristic or ethical consideration (e.g., individuals cannot be assigned to smoke or not smoke). The goal in correlational descriptive or correlational predictive studies is to provide an indication of how likely it is that a cause-and-effect relationship *might* exist (Powers & Knapp, 2010). Correlational studies assess relationships among variables and cannot establish cause and effect like experimental studies.

Although RCTs, or *experiments*, are the strongest designs for testing cause-and-effect relationships (i.e., testing the effects of certain clinical practices or interventions on patient outcomes), only a small percentage of studies conducted in many of the health professions are experimental studies or clinical trials. Additionally, of those intervention studies reported in the literature, many have limitations that weaken the evidence that is generated from them. Such limitations include:

- Lack of random assignment to study groups
- Lack of or underdeveloped theoretical frameworks to guide the interventions
- Small sample sizes that lead to inadequate **power** to detect significant differences in outcomes between the experimental and control groups
- Limited attention to maintaining the fidelity of the intervention so that all participants receive a similar treatment
- Omission of **manipulation checks**, which are assessments verifying that subjects have actually processed the experimental information that they have received or followed through with prescribed intervention activities, such as physical activity
- Failure to limit **confounding** or **extraneous variables** (i.e., those factors that interfere with the relationship between the independent and dependent variables)
- Lack of more long-term follow-up to assess the sustainability of the treatment or intervention

Therefore, because a **true experiment** (i.e., one that has an intervention, a comparison or attention control group, and random assignment) is the strongest design for the testing of cause-and-effect relationships and provides strong, or **Level II evidence** (i.e., evidence generated from an RCT, the next strongest evidence behind systematic reviews of RCTs; see Chapter 1) on which to change or improve practice, there is an urgent need for healthcare professionals to move beyond descriptive and correlational studies in order to build higher level evidence.

Significance of the Question

A second critical factor to consider when designing studies is the significance of the problem or research question, otherwise known as the "so what?" factor. There may be research questions that are interesting (e.g., Do pink or blue scrubs worn by intensive care unit nurses have an impact on the mood of unit secretaries?), but answering them will not significantly improve care or patient outcomes. Therefore, a funding agency is not likely to rate the significance of the problem as important. Problems that are significant for study are usually those that affect a large percentage of the population or those that frequently affect the process, outcomes, or cost of patient care.

Feasibility

The third factor to consider when designing a study is **feasibility**. Before embarking on a study, important questions to ask regarding feasibility are

- Can the study be conducted in a reasonable amount of time?
- Are there an adequate number of potential subjects to recruit into the study?
- Have the settings for recruitment been identified, and is accessibility a concern?
- Does the lead person (PI) have sufficient time and expertise to spearhead the effort?
- Are there major ethical or legal constraints to undertaking this study?
- Are there adequate resources available at the institution or clinical site to conduct the study? If the answer is no, what is the potential for obtaining funding?

If the answer to any of these questions is no, further consideration should be given to the feasibility of the project.

As a general rule, it typically takes more time to carry out a clinical study than is originally projected. Even when participant numbers are projected to be sufficient for the time allotted for data collection when planning a study, it is wise to incorporate a buffer period (i.e., extra time) in case **institutional review board (IRB)** approval is delayed, access to recruitment settings is more time consuming, or subject recruitment takes longer than anticipated. Also, certain times of the year are more conducive for data collection than others (e.g., in conducting a study with elementary school students, data collection will be possible only when school is in session). Certain settings are more conducive to the conduct of clinical research than others. Settings that tend to facilitate research are those in which there is administrative approval and staff "buy-in" regarding clinical studies. Settings in which staff members perceive research as burdensome to them or their patients may confound study results as well as hamper a study's progress. Obtaining administrative approval to conduct a study and getting a sense of staff support for a project are an early and critical preparatory step for a clinical research project.

> " Alone we can do so little; together we can do so much.
>
> **HELEN KELLER**

It is important to consider the experience, skills, interest, and commitment of each member of the team. Study team members should possess the skills needed to plan, implement, analyze, and interpret the research data. For a novice researcher, the addition of seasoned researchers to the project will be important for its success, especially as challenges are encountered in the course of the study.

Ethical considerations include the need to assess the burden to study participants as well as whether the benefits of participation in the study will exceed the risks. Serious consideration also must be given to the gender, age, and racial/ethnic composition of the sample. For federal grant applications, a strong rationale must be provided if women, children, and minority subjects will be excluded from the research project. All study team members need to be knowledgeable regarding the ethics of conducting the study and the rights of participant subjects. Further discussion about obtaining research subjects' review approval for a clinical study appears later in this chapter and in Chapter 23.

Ultimately, feasibility rests on the financial support available for conducting the study. Even the smallest of studies requires resources, even if only in the time and energy of the person serving as PI. The study can be supported by grants through internal or external agencies or by in-kind support of personal efforts and materials. Careful attention to various factors affecting study feasibility sets the stage for successful research investigations.

> **It is literally true that you can succeed best and quickest by helping others to succeed.**
>
> **NAPOLEON HILL**

SPECIFIC STEPS IN DESIGNING A QUANTITATIVE STUDY

When designing a quantitative study, there is a specific series of orderly steps that are typically followed (Box 21.6). This is referred to as the *scientific approach to inquiry*.

Step 1: Formulate the Study Question

The first step in the design of a study is developing an innovative yet answerable study question. Feasibility is an important issue when formulating a research question. Although a research question may be interesting (e.g., What is the effect of a therapeutic intervention program on depression in women whose spouses have been murdered?), it could take years to collect an adequate number of participants to conduct the statistical analysis to answer the question.

On the other hand, if a research question is not interesting to the investigator, there is a chance that the project may never reach completion, especially when challenges arise that make data collection difficult. Other feasibility issues include the amount of time and funding needed to conduct the project as well as the scope of the study. Studies that are very broad and that contain too many goals are often not feasible or manageable.

BOX 21.6 — *Specific Steps in Designing a Quantitative Study*

1. Formulate the study question.
2. Establish the significance of the problem and the "so what?" factor.
3. Search for, critically appraise, and synthesize available evidence.
4. Develop the theoretical/conceptual framework.
5. Generate hypotheses when appropriate.
6. Select the appropriate research design.
7. Identify the population/sampling plan and implement strategies to enhance external validity.
8. Determine the measures that will be used.
9. Outline the data collection plan.
10. Apply for human subjects' approval.
11. Implement the study.
12. Prepare and analyze the data.
13. Interpret the results.
14. Disseminate the findings.
15. Incorporate the findings in EBP and evaluate the outcomes.

Research questions should be novel, meaning that obtaining the answer to them should add to, confirm, or refute what is already known, or they should extend prior research findings. Replication studies (studies that use the same methods but with different subjects) are important, especially if they address major limitations of prior work, and are necessary for systematic reviews, which are the strongest level of evidence to guide clinical practice.

Research questions should be ethical in that they do not present unacceptable physical or psychological risks to the subjects in the study. Risks cannot exceed the benefits of participation in a study. Before a research study is conducted, review of the entire protocol by a **research subjects review board (RSRB)**, sometimes referred to as an IRB, is necessary.

 Many universities and clinical agencies have websites that provide comprehensive information on (a) how to submit studies for review; (b) answers to frequently asked questions; and (c) information about regulations regarding research, including specific details related to HIPAA (Health Insurance Portability and Accountability Act) (see http://orrp.osu.edu/irb/)

In institutions where a formal RSRB is not in existence, there should be some type of ethics committee that reviews and approves research proposals.

Finally, research questions should be relevant to science and/or clinical practice. They should also have the potential to have an impact on health policy and guide further research (Box 21.7).

Step 2: Establish Significance of the Problem and the "So What?" Factor

The problem of interest should be one that is clinically important or that will extend the science in an area and have an impact on important outcomes (Melnyk & Morrison-Beedy, 2012). When embarking on a study, it is imperative to ask questions about why the clinical problem is important, including:

- What is the prevalence of this particular problem?
- How many individuals are affected by this problem?
- Will studying this problem potentially improve the quality and/or cost of care that is delivered to patients?
- Will studying this problem potentially influence health policy?
- Will studying this intervention lead to better health outcomes in patients?

BOX
21.7   *Characteristics of a Good Study Question*

F = Feasible
I = Interesting
N = Novel
E = Ethical
R = Relevant

Based on Hulley, S. B., Cummings, S. R., Browner, W. S., Grady, D., & Newman, T. B. (2006). *Designing clinical research* (3rd ed.). Philadelphia, PA: Lippincott Williams & Wilkins.

- Will studying this problem assist clinicians in gaining a better understanding of the area so that more sensitive clinical care can be delivered?
- "So what" will be the end outcome of the study?

Step 3: Search for, Critically Appraise, and Synthesize Evidence

A thorough search for, critical appraisal of, and synthesis of all relevant studies in the area are essential (see Chapters 3 to 6) before the study design is planned. It is beneficial to begin with a search for **systematic reviews** on the topic. A systematic review is a summary of evidence in a particular topic area that attempts to answer a specific clinical question using methods that reduce bias, usually conducted by an expert or expert panel on a particular topic (Melnyk & Fineout-Overholt, 2015). When it is conducted properly, a systematic review uses a rigorous process for identifying, critically appraising, and synthesizing studies for the purpose of answering a specific clinical question and drawing conclusions about the evidence gathered (e.g., How effective are educational interventions in reducing sexual risk-taking behaviors in teenagers? What factors predict osteoporosis in women?). In using a rigorous process to determine which types of studies will be included in a systematic review, author bias is usually eliminated, and greater credibility can be placed in the findings from the review.

In systematic reviews, methodological strengths and limitations of each study included in the review are discussed, and recommendations for clinical practice as well as further research are presented. The availability of a systematic review in a particular topic area can provide quick access to the status of interventions or clinical studies in a particular area as well as recommendations for further study. If a systematic review in the area of interest is not available, the search for and critical appraisal of individual studies should begin. In reading prior studies, it is helpful to develop a table of the following information so that a critical analysis of the body of prior work can be conducted:

- Demographic characteristics and size of the sample
- Study setting
- Research design used (e.g., descriptive correlational study, RCT), including the type of intervention (if applicable)
- Outcome variables measured, including instruments used
- Major findings
- Strengths and limitations

Once a table such as this is developed, it will be easier to identify strengths as well as gaps in prior work that could be addressed by the proposed study.

Step 4: Identify a Theoretical/Conceptual Framework

A **theoretical** or **conceptual framework** is comprised of a number of interrelated statements that attempt to describe, explain, and/or predict a phenomenon. Identifying a conceptual or theoretical framework is an important step in designing a clinical study. Its purpose is to provide a framework for selecting the study's variables, including how they relate to one another, as well as to guide the development of the intervention(s) in experimental studies. Without a well-developed theoretical framework, explanations for the findings from a study may be weak and speculative.

As an example, for decades, self-regulation theory (Johnson, Fieler, Jones, Wlasowicz, & Mitchell, 1997) has long provided an excellent theoretical framework for providing educational interventions to patients undergoing intrusive procedures (e.g., endoscopy) and chemotherapy/radiation. The basic premise of this theory is that the provision of concrete objective information to an individual who is confronting a stressful situation or procedure will facilitate a cognitive schema or representation of what will happen that is similar to the real-life event. As a result of an individual knowing what he or she is likely to experience, there is an increase in understanding, predictability, and confidence in dealing with the situation as it unfolds (Johnson et al., 1997), which leads to improved coping outcomes.

Through a series of experimental studies, Melnyk et al. (2006) extended the use of self-regulation theory to guide interventions with parents of critically ill children (Melnyk et al., 2004; Melnyk, Crean, Feinstein, & Fairbanks, 2008) and with parents of low-birth-weight premature infants. Extensive evidence in the literature from descriptive studies indicated that a major source of stress for parents of critically ill children is their children's emotional and behavioral responses to hospitalization. Thus, it was hypothesized that parents who receive the Creating Opportunities for Parent Empowerment (COPE) intervention program, which contains educational information about children's likely behavioral and emotional changes during and following hospitalization, would have stronger beliefs about their children's responses to the stressful event. It was also hypothesized that the COPE program would work through parental beliefs about their children and their role—the proposed **mediating variable** (i.e., the variable or mechanism through which the intervention works)—to positively influence parent and child outcomes. As a result of them knowing what to expect of their children's emotions and behaviors during and following hospitalization, it was predicted that parents who receive the COPE program would have better emotional and functional coping outcomes (i.e., a decreased negative mood state and increased participation in their children's care) than would parents who did not receive this information. Ultimately, because the emotional contagion hypothesis contends that heightened parental anxiety leads to heightened child anxiety, it was expected that the children of parents who received the COPE program would have better coping outcomes than would those whose parents did not receive this educational information. Thus, through this series of clinical trials, empirical support for the effectiveness of the COPE program was generated in addition to data that explain how the intervention actually works to affect patient and family outcomes (Figure 21.2).

Step 5: Generate Hypotheses When Appropriate

Hypotheses are predictions about the relationships between study variables. For example, when using self-regulation theory, a hypothesis that would logically emerge from the

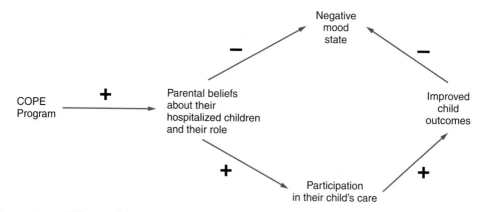

Figure 21.2: Effects of the Creating Opportunities for Parent Empowerment (COPE) program on maternal and child outcomes during and following critical care hospitalization.

theory would be that parents who receive concrete objective information about their children's likely responses to hospitalization (i.e., the independent variable) would report less anxiety (i.e., the **dependent** or **outcome variable**) than would parents who do not receive this information. To include hypotheses in a clinical study, there should be either a theory or conceptual framework to guide the formulation of these predictions or enough evidence from prior work to provide a sufficient foundation on which to make predictive statements. In situations where the evidence on which to base predictive statements is insufficient or where an investigator chooses not to use a theoretical or conceptual framework to guide his or her work (which is not advised), research questions should be developed so that the problem might be more fully understood rather than predicting how variables will change.

Step 6: Select the Appropriate Research Design

The **design** of a clinical study is its foundation. It is the overall plan (i.e., the study protocol for testing the study hypotheses or questions) that includes the following:

- Strategies for controlling confounding or extraneous variables
- Strategies for when and how the intervention will be delivered (in experimental studies)
- How often and when the data will be collected

A good quantitative design is one that

- Appropriately tests the hypotheses or answers the research questions
- Lacks bias (i.e., objectivity)
- Controls extraneous or confounding variables (i.e., factors that interfere with the relationship between the independent and dependent variables).
- Has sufficient **power** (i.e., the ability to detect statistically significant findings)

If the research question or hypothesis concerns itself with testing the effects of an intervention or treatment on patient outcomes, the study calls for an **experimental design**. In contrast, if the hypothesis/research question is interested in quantitatively describing a selected variable or is interested in the relationship between two or more variables (e.g., What is the relationship between the average amount of sleep and test performance in college students? What presurgery demographic variables predict successful recovery from open heart surgery?), a **nonexperimental study design** would be the most appropriate. The next section of this chapter reviews the most common designs for nonexperimental as well as experimental studies.

Nonexperimental Study Designs

Typically, nonexperimental designs are used to describe, explain, or predict a phenomenon. These types of designs also are undertaken when it is undesirable or unethical to manipulate the independent variable or, in other words, to impose a treatment. For example, it would be unethical to assign underage teenagers randomly to drink alcohol in order to study its effects on sexual risk-taking behaviors. Therefore, an alternative design would be a nonexperimental study in which sexual risk-taking behaviors are measured in a group of adolescents who report alcohol use, compared with a group that does not report use.

Descriptive Studies. The purpose of descriptive studies is to describe, observe, or document a phenomenon that can serve as a foundation for developing hypotheses or testing theory.

For example, a descriptive study design would be appropriate to answer each of the following clinical questions:

- What is the incidence of complications in women who are on bed rest with preterm labor?
- What is the average number of depressive symptoms experienced by teenagers after a critical care hospitalization?
- In adults with type 2 diabetes, what are the most common physical comorbidities?

Survey Research. Surveys provide a way to obtain descriptive information using self-report data and are typically collected to assess a certain condition or status. Most survey research is **cross-sectional** (i.e., all measurements are collected at the same point in time) versus research that is conducted over time (e.g., **cohort studies**, which follow the same sample longitudinally).

Survey data can be collected via multiple strategies; in addition to personal or telephone interviews and mailed or in-person questionnaires, data can also be obtained using technology such as computers or cell phones. For example, a group of healthcare providers might be surveyed with a questionnaire designed to measure their knowledge and attitudes about evidence-based practice (EBP). Data gained from this survey might then be used to design in-service education workshops to enhance the providers' knowledge and skills in this area.

Major advantages of survey research include rapid data collection and flexibility. Disadvantages of survey research include low response rates—especially if the surveys are mailed—and gathering information that is fairly superficial.

Correlational Studies. Correlational research designs are used when there is an interest in describing the relationship between or among two or more variables. In this type of design, even when there is a strong relationship that is discovered between the variables under consideration, it is not substantiated to say that one variable caused the other to happen. For example, if a study found a positive relationship between adolescent smoking and drug use (e.g., as smoking increases, drug use increases), it would not be appropriate to state that smoking causes drug use. The only conclusion that could be drawn from these data is that these variables **covary** (i.e., as one changes, the other variable changes as well).

Correlational Descriptive Research. When there is interest in describing the relationship between two variables, a correlational descriptive study design would be most appropriate. For example, the following two research questions would be best answered with correlational designs:

- What is the relationship between number of days that a person is on bed rest after a severe motor vehicle accident (the independent variable) and the incidence of decubiti ulcers (the dependent variable)?
- What is the relationship between smoking marijuana (the independent variable) and the incidence of sexually transmitted infections in female adolescents (the dependent variable)?

Correlational Predictive Research. When an investigator is interested in whether one variable that occurs earlier in time predicts another variable that occurs later in time, a correlational predictive study should be undertaken. For example, the following research questions would best lend themselves to this type of study (Figure 21.3):

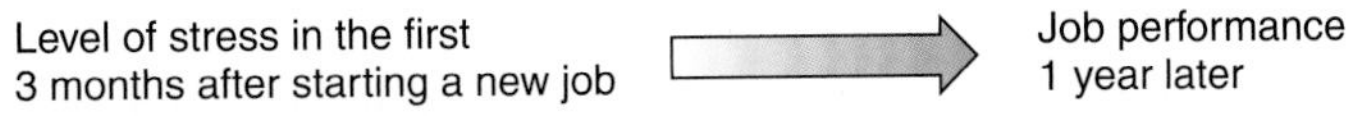

| Level of stress in the first 3 months after starting a new job | → | Job performance 1 year later |

Figure 21.3: A correlational predictive study.

- Does maternal anxiety shortly after a child's admission to the intensive care unit (the independent variable) predict posttraumatic stress symptoms 6 months after hospitalization (the dependent variable)?
- Does the level of stress during the first 3 months after starting a new job (the independent variable) predict performance 1 year later?

Establishing a strong relationship between variables in correlational predictive studies provides evidence for the need to influence the independent variable in a future intervention study. For example, if findings from research indicated that job stress in the initial months after starting a new position as a practitioner predicted later job performance, a future study might evaluate the effects of a training program on reducing early job stress with the expectation that a successful intervention program would improve later job performance. Although it should never be stated that a cause-and-effect relationship is supported with a correlational study, a predictive correlational design is stronger than a descriptive one with regard to making a causal inference because the independent variable occurs before the dependent variable in time sequence (Polit & Beck, 2016).

Case-Control Studies. Case-control studies are those in which one group of individuals (i.e., cases) with a certain condition (e.g., migraine headaches) is studied at the same time as another group of individuals who do not have the condition (i.e., controls) to determine an association between one or more predictor variables (e.g., family history of migraine headaches, consumption of red wine) and the condition (i.e., migraine headaches). Case-control studies are usually retrospective or *ex post facto* (i.e., they look back in time to reveal predictor variables that might explain why the cases contracted the disease or problem and the controls did not).

Advantages of this type of research design include an ability to determine associations with a small number of subjects, which is especially useful in the study of rare types of diseases, and an ability to generate hypotheses for future studies. One of the major limitations to using this study design is **bias** (i.e., an inability to control confounding variables that may influence the outcome). For example, the two groups of individuals previously presented (i.e., those with migraines and those without migraines) may be different on certain variables (e.g., amount of sleep and stress) that may also influence the development of migraine headaches. Another limitation is that because case-control studies are usually retrospective, one is limited to data available at a prior time. Often, data on interesting variables were not thought to be important and not collected.

Cohort Studies. A cohort study follows a group of subjects longitudinally over a period of time to describe the incidence of a problem or to determine the relationship between a predictor variable and an outcome. An example would be finding out whether daughters of mothers who had breast cancer have a higher incidence of the disease versus those whose mothers did not have breast cancer. Two groups of daughters (i.e., those with and without a mother with breast cancer) would be studied over time to determine the incidence of breast cancer in each group. A major strength (advantage) of prospective cohort studies includes being able to determine the incidence of a problem and its possible cause(s). A major limitation (disadvantage) is the lengthy nature of this type of study, the costs of which often become prohibitive.

Experimental Study Designs

A true experiment, or RCT, is the strongest design for testing cause-and-effect relationships (e.g., whether an intervention or treatment affects patient outcomes) and provides strong evidence on which to change and improve clinical practice. For evidence to support causality (i.e., cause-and-effect relationships), three criteria must be met:

1. The independent variable (i.e., the intervention or treatment) must precede the dependent variable (i.e., the outcome) in terms of time sequence.
2. There must be a strong relationship between the independent and dependent variables.
3. The relationship between the independent and dependent variables cannot be explained as being due to the influence of other variables (i.e., all possible alternate explanations of the relationship must be eliminated).

Although true experiments are the best designs to control for the influence of confounding variables, it must be recognized that control of potential confounding or extraneous variables is very challenging when conducting studies in the real world—not in the laboratory. Other limitations of experiments include the fact that they are usually time consuming and expensive.

Intervention studies or clinical trials typically follow a five-phase development sequence:

- **Phase I: Basic research** that is exploratory and descriptive in nature and that establishes the variables that may be amenable to intervention or in which the content, strength, and timing of the intervention are developed, along with the outcome measures for the study.
- **Phase II: Pilot research** (i.e., a small-scale study in which the intervention is tested with a small number of subjects so that the feasibility of a large-scale study is determined and alternative strategies are developed for potential problems).
- **Phase III: Efficacy trials** in which evaluation of the intervention takes place in an ideal setting and clinical efficacy is determined (in this stage, much emphasis is placed on internal validity of the study and preliminary *cost-effectiveness* of the intervention).
- **Phase IV: Effectiveness trials** in which analysis of the intervention effect is conducted in clinical practice and clinical effectiveness is determined, as is cost-effectiveness (in this stage, much emphasis is placed on external validity or generalizability of the study).
- **Phase V: Effects on public health** in which wide-scale implementation of the intervention is conducted to determine its effects on public health (Whittemore & Grey, 2002).

Many clinicians assume a leadership role in Phases I and II of this sequence and more of a collaborative role as a member of a research team in Phases III through V.

Randomized Controlled Trial or True Experiment. The best type of study design or gold standard for evaluating the effects of a treatment or intervention is an RCT or true experiment because it is the strongest design for testing cause-and-effect relationships. True experiments or RCTs possess three characteristics:

1. An experimental group that receives the treatment or intervention
2. A control or comparison group that receives standard care or a comparison intervention that is different from the experimental intervention
3. **Randomization** or **random assignment**, which is the use of a strategy to randomly assign subjects to the experimental or control groups (e.g., tossing a coin)

R	O_1	X_1	O_2
R	O_1	X_2	O_2

Figure 21.4: Two-group randomized controlled trial with pretest/posttest design and structurally equivalent comparison group. R, random assignment; X, intervention/ treatment, with X_1 being the experimental intervention and X_2 being the comparison/ control intervention; O, observation/measurement, with O_1 being the first time the variable is measured (at baseline) and O_2 being the second time that it is measured (after the intervention).

Random assignment is the strongest method to help ensure that the study groups are similar on demographic or clinical variables at baseline (i.e., before the treatment is delivered). Similarity between groups at the beginning of an experiment is very important in that if findings reveal a positive effect on the dependent variable, it can be concluded that the treatment, not other extraneous variables, is what affected the outcome. For example, results from an RCT might reveal that a cognitive behavioral intervention reduced depressive symptoms in adults. However, if the adults in the experimental and control groups were not similar on certain characteristics prior to the start of the intervention (e.g., level of social support, number of current stressful life events), it could be that differences between the groups on these variables accounted for the change in depressive symptoms at the end of the study, instead of the change being due to the positive impact of the intervention itself.

Examples of true experimental designs along with advantages and disadvantages of each are presented in Figures 21.4 through 21.9. The symbol designations in the figures have been used for decades in the literature since the publishing of a landmark book on experimental designs by Campbell and Stanley (1963). Note that time moves from left to right, and subscripts can be used to designate different groups if necessary.

Two-Group RCT With Pretest/Posttest Design and Structurally Equivalent Comparison Group. The major advantage of the design illustrated in Figure 21.4 is that it is a true experiment, the strongest design for testing cause-and-effect relationships. As seen in Figure 21.4, the inclusion of a comparison group in the design that receives a different or "attention control" intervention similar in length to the experimental intervention is important. This control group helps to provide evidence that any effects of the experimental intervention are not just the result of giving participants "something" instead of "nothing" but are actually due to the effect of the experimental intervention itself. At the same time, including a comparison intervention may dilute some of the positive effects of the experimental intervention. This is especially true if a study outcome being measured is tapping a psychosocial variable, such as anxiety (e.g., giving participants something instead of nothing, as would be the case with a pure control group, might reduce anxiety simply because someone spent time with the participant). The benefits of this design (i.e., including an attention control or comparison intervention) outweigh the risk of diluting the positive effects of the experimental intervention. Although pretesting the subjects on the same measure that is being used as the outcome for the study (e.g., state anxiety) may, in itself, sensitize them to respond differently when answering questions on the anxiety measure the second time, this approach allows the investigator to determine whether subjects are similar on anxiety at the beginning of the study. A disadvantage of this design, as with all experiments, is that it is typically more expensive and time consuming than nonexperimental designs.

R	X_1	O_1
R	X_2	O_1

Figure 21.5: Two-group randomized controlled trial with posttest design only. R, random assignment; X, intervention/treatment, with X_1 being the experimental intervention and X_2 being the comparison/control intervention; O_1, observation/ measurement.

Two-Group RCT With Posttest-Only Design. The advantage of conducting a two-group RCT with a posttest-only design is that there is no pretesting effect (Figure 21.5). For example, if you were interested in evaluating the effects of a human immunodeficiency virus/sexually trans- mitted infection (HIV/STI) educational program on adolescent girls' knowledge of sexual-risk reduction, you may not want to pretest the participants by asking them questions such as "Can a person get HIV from a toilet seat?" or "Can using a latex condom or rubber lower a person's chance of getting HIV?" Despite the fact that they did not receive the educational program, the administration of a pretest itself may lead the girls in the control group to ask their healthcare providers about HIV risk. As a result, findings may reveal no difference in knowledge between the two study groups at the end of the study—not necessarily because the intervention did not work but because the pretesting effects strongly influenced the outcome.

The main disadvantage of a posttest-only design is that baseline differences on the study groups are unknown. Even though random assignment is used (see Figure 21.5), to control for extraneous or confounding variables, there is still a chance that the two groups may be unequal or different at the start of the study. Differences in important baseline study measures between experimental groups may then negatively affect a study's outcomes or interfere with the ability to say that it was the intervention itself that caused a change in the dependent variable(s). For example, in an intervention to control postoperative pain in patients following surgery, differing levels of anxiety prior to the intervention between both groups may alter the impact of the pain-reduction intervention. Without assessing these differences before the intervention, the investigator will be limited in the ability to say whether posttest data provide support for the utility of the intervention.

Two-Group RCT With Long-Term Repeated Measures Follow-up. If an investigator is interested in whether an intervention produces both short-term and long-term effects on an outcome, it is important for a study to build into its design repeated measurements of the outcome variable of interest (Figure 21.6). The advantage of this type of design is that repeated as- sessments of an outcome variable over time allow an investigator to determine the sustain- ability of an intervention's effects. A disadvantage of this type of design is that *study attrition* (i.e., loss of subjects) may be a threat to the internal validity (control) of the study. Another disadvantage of this design is that it is costly to follow subjects for longer periods of time.

R	X_1	O_1	O_2	O_3
R	X_2	O_1	O_2	O_3

Figure 21.6: Two-group randomized controlled trial with long-term repeated measures follow-up. R, random assignment; X, intervention/treatment, with X_1 being the experimental intervention and X_2 being the comparison intervention; O, observation/ measurement, which will occur at three different time points (i.e., O_1, O_2, and O_3) after the intervention/treatment is delivered.

| R | X_1 | O_1 |
| R | | O_1 |

Figure 21.7: Two-group RCT with true control group that receives no intervention. R, random assignment; X, intervention/treatment, with X_1 being the experimental intervention; O, observation/measurement.

In addition, repeated follow-up on the same measures may also have the disadvantage of introducing testing effects that influence the outcome. For example, individuals may think about their answers and change their beliefs as part of the repeated follow-up sessions, not as the result of the intervention. Also, subjects may learn how repeated follow-up assessments work, and, if the study entails extensive questioning when individuals admit to certain things (e.g., being depressed or taking drugs), they may learn to respond in a way to avoid these lengthy follow-up questions or interviews.

Two-Group RCT With True Control Group That Receives No Intervention. The real disadvantage to conducting an RCT with a true control group that receives no attention or intervention whatsoever (Figure 21.7) is that any positive intervention effects that are found may be solely related to participants in the intervention group "receiving something versus nothing." For example, if a healthcare provider was studying the effects of a stress reduction program on college students experiencing test anxiety, simply having someone spend extra time with the students could reduce their anxiety, regardless of whether the intervention itself was helpful.

Three-Group RCT. The inclusion of a third group, as shown in Figure 21.8, allows an investigator to separate the effects of giving something (i.e., a comparison or attention control intervention) from a pure control group (i.e., a group that receives nothing or standard care)—a very strong experimental design. Disadvantages typically include the need to recruit additional subjects for the three conditions and increased costs to conduct the study.

Solomon Four-Group Design. The main advantage to conducting an experimental study that employs a **Solomon four-group design** (i.e., an experiment that uses a before–after design for the first experimental and control groups and an after-only design for the second experimental and control groups; Polit & Beck, 2016) is that it can separate the effects of pretesting the subjects (i.e., gathering baseline measures) on the outcome measure(s) (Figure 21.9). Disadvantages include the need for additional participants as well as costs for increasing the size of the sample.

R	X_1	O_1
R	X_2	O_1
R		O_1

Figure 21.8: Three-group randomized controlled trial (i.e., one group that receives one type of experimental intervention, one group that receives a different or comparison intervention, and a pure control group that receives no intervention or standard care). R, random assignment; X, intervention/treatment, with X_1 being the experimental intervention and X_2 being the comparison intervention; O, observation/measurement, which occurs only once (i.e., postintervention).

R	O_1	X_1	O_2
R		X_1	O_2
R	O_1	X_2	O_2
R		X_2	O_2

Figure 21.9: Solomon four-group design in which a pair of experimental and control groups receive pretesting, as depicted by O_1, and a pair do not receive pretesting. R, random assignment; X, intervention/treatment, with X_1 being the experimental intervention and X_2 being the comparison/control intervention; O, observation/measurement, with O_1 being the pretest (i.e., measured at baseline) and O_2 being the posttest (i.e., measured after the intervention is delivered).

EDUCATIONAL INFORMATION

		Yes	No
EXERCISE	Yes	Education and exercise	Exercise only
	No	Education only	Neither education nor exercise

Figure 21.10: 2 × 2 factorial experiment that generates four study groups. (**A**) A group that receives both education and exercise. (**B**) A group that receives education only. (**C**) A group that receives exercise only. (**D**) A control group that receives neither education nor exercise.

Factorial Design. A **factorial design** (Figure 21.10) is an experiment that has two or more interventions or treatments. A major advantage of this type of design is that it allows an investigator to study the separate and combined effects of different types of interventions. For example, if a healthcare provider were interested in the separate and combined effects of two different interventions (i.e., educational information and an exercise program) on reducing blood pressure in adults with hypertension, this type of design would result in four groups:

1. A group of subjects who would receive educational information only
2. A group of subjects who would receive an exercise program only
3. A group of subjects who would receive both educational information and an exercise program
4. A group of subjects who would receive neither information nor exercise

A major strength of this design is that it could be determined whether education or exercise alone positively affects blood pressure or whether a combination of the two treatments is more effective than either intervention alone. Disadvantages to this design typically include additional subjects and costs.

Quasi-Experimental Studies. Designs in which the independent variable (i.e., a treatment) is manipulated or introduced but where there is a lack of random assignment or a control group are called **quasi-experimental designs.**

Although **quasi-experiments** may be more practical and feasible, they are weaker than true experimental designs in the ability to establish cause-and-effect inferences (i.e., to say that the independent variable or treatment was responsible for a change in the dependent variable and that the change was not because of other extraneous factors).

| O_1 | X_1 | O_2 |
| O_1 | X_2 | O_2 |

Figure 21.11: A quasi-experiment with pretest and posttest design and a comparison/control group but lacking random assignment. X, intervention, with X_1 being the experimental intervention and X_2 being the comparison/control intervention; O, observation, with O_1 indicating measurement at baseline and O_2 indicating measurement after the intervention is delivered.

There are times when quasi-experiments need to be conducted because random assignment is not always possible. For example, individuals cannot be assigned to smoking and nonsmoking conditions. Even when it is ethically feasible to use random assignment, the study setting might prevent it. For example, school principals frequently resist assigning children to programs based on random assignment. In addition, random assignment can be disruptive in schools (e.g., taking children out of their regular classrooms for special programs). Quasi-experiments, that is, designs that compare groups created by some method other than random assignment, provide an alternative to true experiments. Despite their limitations, some of these designs can be quite powerful in their ability to eliminate alternative explanations for the relationship between an intervention and the outcomes in a study. Two examples of quasi-experimental designs are shown in Figures 21.11 and 21.12.

Quasi-Experiment With Pretest and Posttest Design, Comparison/Control Group, No Random Assignment. In the quasi-experiment illustrated in Figure 21.11, there is an experimental group and an attention control group both of which receive a treatment, but the subjects have not been randomly assigned to the two study groups, so the probability of equal study groups cannot be assured. Therefore, a pretest is administered so that it can be determined whether the two study groups are equal at baseline before the intervention is delivered. In quasi-experiments, pretesting is especially important to assess whether the subjects are similar at baseline on the variable(s) that will be used as the outcome(s) in the study. However, even with pretesting that shows no preintervention differences, a quasi-experiment is still not as strong as a true experiment that uses random assignment. Because the groups are preexisting or created by a means other than random assignment in a quasi-experiment, there could be other unexplored differences between them that might account for any differences found on the outcome variables. If only posttesting is conducted in a quasi-experimental design in which random assignment was not used, it would be very difficult to have confidence in the findings because it would not be known whether the study groups were similar on key variables at the beginning of the study. In contrast, when random assignment is used in true experimental designs, it is very likely that the study groups will be equivalent on pretest measures.

Interrupted Time Series Design. Another example of a quasi-experimental study is the interrupted time series design (Figure 21.12). In this study, there is no random assignment or comparison/attention control group. This design incorporates a long series of pretest observations, an intervention, and a long series of posttest observations.

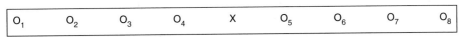

| O_1 | O_2 | O_3 | O_4 | X | O_5 | O_6 | O_7 | O_8 |

Figure 21.12: Time series design, which shows that the variable of interest is measured at intervals four times prior to the intervention and four times at intervals after the intervention is implemented.

The time series design is used most frequently in communities or agencies that maintain careful archival records. It can also be used with community survey data if the survey questions and sample remain constant over time. An intervention effect is evidenced if a stable pattern of observations over a long period of time is found, followed by a marked change at the point of the intervention, then a stable pattern again over a long time after the intervention. For example, adolescent truancy rates might be tracked over several years, followed by an intervention with the tracking of truancy rates for several additional years. If there is a marked drop in truancy rates at the point of the intervention, there is reasonable evidence for a program's effect. Even though this is a single-group design, this is often sufficient to rule out a variety of alternative explanations.

One frequent challenge to single-group designs is the threat of **history**, which involves the occurrence of some event or program unrelated to the intervention that might account for the change observed. History remains a viable alternate explanation for a change in the dependent variable only if the event happens at the same time point as the intervention. If the event occurs earlier or later than the experimental intervention, it cannot explain a change in outcome that occurs at or around the time of the intervention.

Another possible alternate explanation for observed changes in a single-group design is the **maturation** threat. Maturation is a developmental change that occurs even in the absence of the intervention. A true maturation effect will occur gradually throughout the pretest and posttest periods and thus could not account for sharp changes that occur at the point of the intervention.

Observed changes also might occur because of repeated testing or changes in instrumentation. Repeat testing of individuals typically influences their subsequent scores. In addition, performance on skills-based tests should increase over time simply because of practice. Finally, mortality as well as attrition or movement into and out of a community could also influence the outcome data, but they offer an alternate explanation only if it started at the point of treatment.

Pre-experimental Studies. **Pre-experiments** lack both random assignment and a comparison/attention control group (Figure 21.13). As such, they are very weak in internal validity and allow too many competing explanations for a study's findings.

Comparative Effectiveness Trials. **Comparative effectiveness trials (CETs)** are experimental studies that seek to determine which of at least two established healthcare interventions or treatments work better on selected outcomes. Other questions typically addressed in CETs are for whom as well as under what circumstances the interventions work best. Benefits and harms of the various treatments are typically addressed in these studies.

Other Important Experimental Design Factors. Methods to ensure quality and consistency in the delivery of the intervention (i.e., maintenance of integrity) are crucial for being able to determine whether and how well an intervention works. Pre-experimental designs are more appropriately used in early intervention development and pilot testing phases.

Integrity and Reproducibility. Frequently, investigators spend inordinate amounts of time paying particular attention to the dependent variable(s) or measure(s) to be used in a study and do not give sufficient time and attention to how an intervention is delivered. In addition, at the outset of an intervention study, it is critical to give thought to whether the intervention

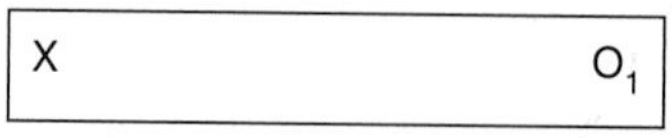

X	O_1

Figure 21.13: Pre-experiment in which there is no random assignment or no comparison/control group. X, intervention; O, observation.

will be able to be reproduced by others in real-world clinical settings. Reproducibility or **scalability** is critical if translation of the intervention into real-life practice settings is going to occur. As such, it is important to manualize or create standardized materials that specifically outline the content of the intervention so that others can replicate it and expect the same results in their practice settings. Use of videotapes, DVDs, or other types of reproducible materials to deliver an intervention ensures that each subject will receive all of the intervention content in exactly the same manner. However, this type of delivery is not always best suited to a particular clinical population. For example, groups may be the best strategy to deliver interventions to teens at high risk for STIs because they allow for the teaching of refusal skills through role-playing.

In a study conducted by Morrison-Beedy et al. (2012), several healthcare providers were used to deliver an information/motivation/behavioral skills training program in four 2-hour group sessions to urban minority female adolescents. The content of the program and necessary skills to be taught for each of the sessions were detailed in a written manual. However, before the actual study commenced, intensive training of the interventionists occurred (e.g., practice groups and role-playing) to ensure that each of them would deliver the content of the program and the teaching of behavioral skills in the same manner. Once the study started, sessions were audiotaped and reviewed by the investigators to ensure quality and completeness in the delivery of the educational information and behavioral skills.

If rigorous standards to ensure the integrity of an intervention do not occur in a study, it would be difficult to know whether the findings generated were the result of the intervention itself or other extraneous variables (Melnyk & Fineout-Overholt, 2015). When the integrity of an intervention is maintained, greater confidence can be placed in a study's findings.

Pilot Study. Before conducting a large experimental study, it is extremely beneficial to first conduct a pilot study, which is a preliminary study that is conducted with a small number of subjects (e.g., 30 to 40), versus a full-scale clinical trial with large numbers of subjects. A pilot study is critical in determining the feasibility of subject enrollment, the intervention, the protocol or data collection plan for the study, and the likelihood that subjects will complete follow-up measures. With the development and implementation of new study measures, it is also essential to pilot them before use in a full-scale study to determine their **validity** and reliability. Pilot work enables investigators to identify weaknesses in their study design so that they can be corrected for the full-scale study. Subjects used for the pilot study should match those individuals who will be participating in the full-scale clinical trial.

Pilot studies are frequently conducted by advanced practice nurses and other master's prepared clinicians and often lead the way to full-scale clinical trials. Working through the details for a large-scale intervention trial with a pilot study saves much time and energy and also prevents frustration as well as providing convincing evidence that a large-scale clinical trial is feasible and well worth the effort. Pilot studies can be used both to develop the intervention and to trial the intervention and control conditions in a smaller-scale version of the full-scale study.

Manipulation Checks. Manipulation checks are important assessments to determine whether the intervention was successfully conducted. For example, if an investigator was delivering an educational intervention intended to teach healthcare providers about a disease and its treatment in order to improve patient outcomes, a manipulation check might be a test given to the participants with a number of multiple-choice questions about the content of the intervention. Answering a certain percentage of these questions correctly would indicate that the subjects successfully processed the educational information. As another example, an investigator may be interested in the effects of a new aerobic exercise program on weight loss in young adults. Participants in the experimental group could be taught this program and

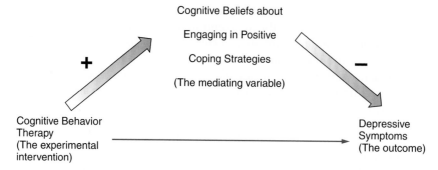

Figure 21.14: The proposed mediating effect of cognitive beliefs in explaining the effects of cognitive behavioral therapy on depressive symptoms.

instructed to complete the prescribed activities three times per week. A manipulation check to ensure that subjects actually adhered to the prescribed exercises may involve keeping a log that lists the dates and number of minutes spent following the program. These types of assessments are critical in order to verify that manipulation of the independent variable or completion of the treatment was achieved. If manipulation checks are not included in an experimental study and results indicate no differences between the experimental and attention control/comparison groups, it would be very difficult to explain whether it was a lack of intervention potency or the fact that subjects did not attend to or adhere to the intervention that was responsible for a lack of intervention effects.

Intervention Processes. When preparing to conduct an intervention study, it is important to think not only about the dependent variables or outcomes that the intervention might affect, but also about the process through which the intervention will exert its effects. The explanations about how an intervention works are important in facilitating its implementation into practice settings (Melnyk, Crean, Feinstein, & Alpert-Gillis, 2007). For example, an investigator proposes that a cognitive behavioral intervention (the independent variable) will reduce depressive symptoms (the dependent variable) in adults with low self-esteem. At the same time, however, the investigator proposes the mechanism of action (i.e., the mediating variable) through which the intervention will work. Therefore, it is hypothesized that the experimental intervention will enhance cognitive beliefs about one's ability to engage in positive coping strategies, which in turn will result in a decrease in depressive symptoms (Figure 21.14). Conceptualization of a well-defined theoretical framework at the outset of designing an intervention study will facilitate explanations of how an intervention program may influence a study's outcomes.

Control Strategies. When conducting experimental studies, it is critical to strategize about how to control for extraneous factors that may influence the outcome(s) so that the effects of the intervention itself can be determined. These extraneous factors include those internal or intrinsic to the individuals who participate in a study (e.g., fatigue and level of maturity) and those external to the participants (e.g., the environment in which the study is conducted).

As explained earlier, the best strategy to control for extraneous variables is randomization or random assignment. By randomly assigning subjects to study groups, there is a good probability that the subjects in the groups will be similar on important characteristics at the beginning of a study. When random assignment is not possible, other methods may be used to control extraneous or confounding variables. One of these strategies is **homogeneity**, or using subjects who are similar on the characteristics that may affect the outcome

AEROBIC EXERCISE

		Yes	No
MOTIVATION	High	High motivation and exercise	High motivation and no exercise
	Low	Low motivation and exercise	Low motivation and no exercise

Figure 21.15: A 2 × 2 randomized block design, blocking on motivation.

variable(s). For example, if a study were evaluating the effects of an intervention on parental stress during the critical care hospitalization of children, it may include only parents from intact marriages because divorced parents may have higher stress levels than nondivorced parents. In addition, very young mothers may have high stress levels. Therefore, this study's inclusion criteria may include only those parents who are from intact marriages as well as those who are older than 21 years. A limitation of this strategy is that at the end of the study, findings can be generalized only to married parents older than 21 years.

Another strategy to control intrinsic factors in a study is **blocking**. Blocking entails deliberately including a potential extraneous intrinsic or confounding variable in a study's design. For example, if there were a concern that level of motivation would affect the results of a study to determine the effects of aerobic exercise (i.e., the treatment) on weight loss in young adults, an investigator may choose to include motivation as another independent variable in the study, aside from the exercise program itself. In doing so, the effects of both motivation and exercise on weight loss could be studied in a 2 × 2 **randomized block design** (Figure 21.15) involving two independent variables with two levels: (a) exercise and no exercise and (b) high motivation and low motivation. The benefit of this type of design is that the interaction between motivation and exercise on weight loss could also be determined (i.e., Do individuals with high levels of motivation have greater weight loss than those with low motivation?).

Threats to Internal Validity. **Internal validity** is the extent to which it can be said that the independent variable (i.e., the intervention) causes a change in the dependent variable (i.e., outcome) and that the results are not attributable to other factors or alternative explanations. There are a number of major threats to the internal validity of a study that should be addressed in the planning process.

Attrition. The first threat to internal validity is **attrition**, or dropout of study participants, which may result in nonequivalent study groups (i.e., more individuals lost from the study in the attention control group than from the experimental group or more individuals with a certain characteristic withdrawing from participation). As a result of losing more subjects from the control group than from the experimental group or more subjects with a certain characteristic (e.g., high anxiety), the study findings may be different than they would be if those individuals had remained in the study. For example, if individuals with the poorest outcomes felt that they were not gaining any benefit from the study, which led them to drop out of a study, differences between the two study groups may not surface during statistical analyses.

One strategy for preventing differential attrition is not to overly persuade potential subjects to participate in a study. There is a fine line between encouraging a potential subject to participate in a study and overly persuading him or her to participate. If someone decides to participate only after much encouragement, there is an increased probability that he or she may drop out of the study.

Another strategy for preventing attrition is to offer research subjects a small honorarium for participating in a study. Some studies provide an honorarium during each time point that a subject completes a specific phase of a study protocol (e.g., completing a set of questionnaires or receiving an intervention), whereas others provide an honorarium when the subjects complete the entire study protocol. Providing an honorarium sends the message that an individual's time for participating in a study is valued.

If there will be substantial time between contacts in a study, it is important to maintain periodic communication through cards or telephone calls. Lengthy lapses in communication with subjects make it easier for them not to return phone calls and questionnaires as well as to miss follow-up appointments. To prevent attrition, another helpful strategy is to maintain consistency in who provides follow-up with the participants. One consistent person on the research team who follows a subject longitudinally over time will enhance the chances of successfully obtaining repeated follow-up data.

Finally, it is important to reduce subject burden to prevent attrition from a study. Participants can become easily overwhelmed if each contact involves the completion of several questionnaires that require a lot of time. An important question to ask for each proposed dependent variable is: How key is the measurement of this outcome, or is it just a nice additional piece of data to include in the study? As a general rule of thumb, the easier and less time consuming it is to participate in a study, the greater will be the probability of completion. It is also more valuable to have complete data on a few key variables than partial data on an extensive list of variables that are of interest.

Confounding Variables/Selection. The best strategy to control for or minimize the influence of confounding variables is to randomly assign subjects to study groups. Another strategy for controlling potential confounding variables is to establish thoughtful inclusion and exclusion criteria. Maintaining consistent study conditions for all participants is another strategy for controlling potential confounding variables. One way to ensure consistency is to establish clearly written study protocols so that every individual on the team understands the intricacies of when and how the interventions will be delivered, as well as the specific steps of data collection.

Nonadherence and Failure to Complete the Intervention Protocol. Designing a realistic intervention is important so that it will eventually be transportable to the real clinical practice world. There is a delicate balance between designing an intervention that will produce sustainable effects and one that will be easy to implement in practice. As such, much consideration should be given to the logistics of the intervention (e.g., feasibility and user-friendliness).

If there are multiple sessions with ongoing phases of the intervention, it is important to record which and how many sessions are attended and completed by study participants because this will facilitate the evaluation of whether a dose response exists (i.e., the greater the number of sessions one attends, the larger the effect of the intervention).

Measurement of Change in Outcome Variables. In intervention studies where it is important to demonstrate a change in key dependent variables that the treatment will impact, it is critical to use measures that are sensitive to change over time. For example, if a certain measure has high **test–retest reliability** (i.e., it is stable over time, such as an individual's personality), there will be little opportunity to effect a change in that measure. This is in contrast to other types of studies in which high test–retest reliabilities on certain measures are desirable (e.g., cohort studies that do not employ interventions in which you are following certain variables over time). For example, an individual's trait anxiety is the general predisposition to anxiety over time, which has been empirically shown to be a stable construct. In contrast, an individual's state anxiety fluctuates, depending on the situation. Therefore, an intervention would most likely affect state, not trait anxiety. Therefore, state anxiety would be a better outcome measure in an intervention study than would trait anxiety.

In conducting intervention studies, it is important to use the same measures longitudinally so that intervention effects over time can be determined. Carefully planning the timing of assessments is critical, especially if there is interest in both the short-term and long-term effects of an intervention. It is also important to use measures that assess variability and that have been tested in the population of interest to avoid **ceiling** and **floor** effects (i.e., participant scores that cluster toward the low-end or high-end score of a measure).

In addition to measuring the outcomes of interventions with quantitative scales, it is important to administer an evaluation questionnaire at the end of a study so that subjects can provide open-ended responses to whether and how they believed the intervention was helpful. These types of responses are especially important if, by chance, the quantitative measures in the study reveal no statistically significant differences between study groups on key outcome variables.

It is also important to assess both clinical meaningfulness and statistical significance when determining whether an intervention has been successful. For example, the greater the number of subjects that are included in a study, the more statistical *power* there will be to detect statistically significant differences between groups. In contrast, the smaller the sample size, the lower the power, and the more difficult it will be to detect statistically significant findings. For example, in one hypothetical study with 1,000 subjects, an investigator found that teens who were enrolled in an expensive smoking cessation program smoked two fewer cigarettes per day than did teens who did not receive the program. This finding was statistically significant at the 0.05 level. As a result of this significant finding, the costly smoking cessation program was widely implemented. Although the finding was statistically significant, the clinical meaningfulness of this finding is weak. In contrast, another investigator conducted the same study with 50 adolescents and found that the experimental group teens smoked 10 fewer cigarettes per day than did teens who did not receive the smoking cessation program. This difference, however, was not statistically significant because of a small number of subjects and low statistical power. Therefore, a decision was made not to implement the program routinely because there was not a statistically significant difference between the study groups. However, a 10-cigarette difference between groups is more clinically meaningful than a 2-cigarette difference. This is a good example of how faulty decisions can be made if only statistically significant findings are considered important and their clinical meaningfulness is ignored, and conversely if statistically and clinically relevant results cannot be assessed because the study was "underpowered."

History. History is another major threat to the internal validity of a study. This condition happens when external events take place concurrently with the treatment that may influence the outcome variables. For example, if a study were being conducted to determine the effects of a violence prevention intervention on anxiety in school-age children and a school shooting occurred that received extensive media attention during the course of the trial, children's anxiety levels at the end of the study could be high despite any positive effects of the intervention. The best way to minimize the threat of history is random assignment because at least both groups then should be equally affected by the external event.

Maturation. The passage of time alone can have an impact on the outcomes of a study. For example, when studying infants who are growing rapidly, an acceleration in cognitive development may occur, regardless of the effects of an intervention that is aimed at enhancing cognition. The best way to deal with the threat of maturation is to use random assignment to allocate subjects to experimental and control groups as well as to recognize it as a potential alternative explanation for a study's findings.

Testing. Completing measures repeatedly could influence an individual's responses the next time a measure is completed. For example, answering the same depression scale three or four times could program someone to respond in the same way on subsequent administrations of the scale.

On the other hand, lengthy lapses in the administration of an instrument may result in a failure to detect important changes over time. Therefore, the best way to deal with this threat to internal validity is to think very carefully about how many times subjects are being asked to complete study measures and provide a strong rationale for these decisions.

Step 7: Identify the Sample and Enhance External Validity

External validity addresses the **generalizability** of research results (i.e., our ability to apply what we learn from a study sample to the larger population from which the sample was drawn). Clearly, a great deal is learned from the samples we study. However, there is always interest in applying that knowledge to a broader population (e.g., to the next 100,000 patients, not just the 100 in a particular study).

The key to external validity is the degree to which the sample that is being studied is representative of the population from which it was drawn. Creating a representative sample is a complex and challenging task. Samples are rarely, if ever, perfectly representative of the populations of interest, but there can be reasonable approximations.

There are four steps to consider when building a sample (Trochim, Donnelly, & Arora, 2015):

1. Carefully define the theoretical population. The theoretical population is the population to which you wish to generalize your results (e.g., all 3-year-old children).
2. Describe the population to which you have access (i.e., the study population). Continuing with our example, this might include all 3-year-old children in the county in which you work, or perhaps in all of the counties in which your collaborators work. At this point, it is necessary to consider how similar the study population is to the theoretical population. Typically, if the county is large and diverse, it is reasonable to assume that the study population is an acceptable substitute for the theoretical population. However, if the focus of your work is strongly influenced by regional factors, such as climate, culture, or access to services, the choice of a study population could severely limit generalizability to the theoretical population.
3. Describe the method you will use to access the population; in other words, define the sampling frame. It is highly unlikely that there will be a single comprehensive list of all 3-year-old children living in any one region at a particular time. You must find some practical method of identifying eligible children; then assess how the available methods might introduce bias or nonrepresentativeness. One strategy might be to approach the day care programs in the region. This would certainly be efficient, but not all 3-year-olds attend day care, and those who do are unlikely to be fully representative of the study population. For example, children whose mothers do not work outside the home are less likely to attend day care. Another approach might be to contact all of the pediatric offices in the region and solicit their cooperation in identifying the 3-year-olds under their care. Certainly, all young children see a pediatrician or nurse practitioner from time to time, even if they do not regularly keep their well child appointments. However, not all children in the region may receive care at the local pediatric offices. Perhaps families at one or both ends of the socioeconomic spectrum travel outside of the region for their care; perhaps others avoid care because of a lack of insurance and use only the emergency department on an as-needed basis. Finally, the records at the pediatric offices

might be out of date. A child may have come in for a 2-year visit and then moved away. Each of these possible alternatives needs to be reviewed and evaluated. *The method that balances efficiency with representativeness will be the best choice.* If there are more sites (day care centers and pediatric offices) than one can efficiently work with, a mechanism to choose a portion of the sites must be selected. The options will be described in the next section, along with mechanisms for selecting actual subjects from the sampling frame.

4. Typically, the sampling frame will include many more potential subjects than are required for the study. Thus, the fourth step in the process is identifying a method to select those individuals who will be invited to participate. Once again, the method chosen should balance efficiency and representativeness.

Random Sampling

Randomly selecting both study sites (e.g., clinics or day care centers) and subjects within these sites is the method most likely to avoid bias. In **random sampling**, every potential subject has an equal chance of being selected. The most straightforward way to think about random sampling is to imagine taking the list of everyone in the sampling frame, cutting it into small pieces with one name on each piece, placing all the names in a bowl, and drawing from the bowl the number of names required for the study design. This might work for selecting 6 day care programs from a list of 25, but in practice, it is an inefficient way to draw a sample of 200 children from a sampling frame of 10,000. That is quite a bit of cutting!

A more efficient method is to assign everyone in the sampling frame a unique number, then, reading down the columns of a random number table or a list of random numbers generated by a computer algorithm, select those cases whose identifiers are included in the list of random numbers. If the entire sampling frame is available electronically, most computer database programs will draw random samples of cases of any specified number. A major limitation with random sampling is that the full list of members of a population (e.g., women with cervical cancer) rarely exists.

Random sampling is an efficient way in which to create a representative sample, but it does not guarantee representativeness. By definition, the process is random. However, it is possible, although quite unlikely, that a very atypical sample might emerge. In using random sampling to create a sample of 200 from 10,000 children, every possible sample of 200 has an equal chance of being drawn. It is possible, although very unlikely, that the sample drawn will contain 200 boys and no girls. More realistically, smaller (proportionately) subgroups might be underrepresented or entirely absent. If the research involves handedness or physical stature, it is possible that the selected sample will have no left-handed children or no children below or above a given height. To avoid this possibility, sampling procedures frequently incorporate **stratification**.

Stratified Sampling

Stratification involves dividing the study population into two or more subpopulations, then sampling separately from each. For example, if you would like to ensure that exactly 50% of the 200 children in the study sample are male, you would divide the study population into male and female groups and randomly sample 100 from each. This type of simple stratification works only if information about the stratification variable is included in the sampling frame data, that is, in the day care center or pediatric office records. It is unlikely that you would be able to stratify by handedness using this simple strategy. Similarly, it would be unlikely that you would be able to stratify on measures such as depression, self-esteem, or life stress because information about these variables is unlikely to be included in any accessible preexisting database.

A variation on this theme involves a second stage of information gathering and sampling. Once the initial sampling frame is identified, a brief survey is conducted with a large random sample. The survey includes questions about variables on which you would like to stratify. A second random sample can now be drawn from the sample of completed surveys. The second-stage sampling can be stratified based on this new information. Such sampling designs are somewhat more complex to analyze, but they do ensure that all of the subgroups of interest are included in adequate numbers.

Cluster (Area) Random Sampling

If the study population is spread over a wide geographical area, you can use another variation of two-stage sampling. First, you divide the large area into regions or clusters (e.g., counties or census tracts). From the full list of clusters, you can randomly sample a sufficiently manageable number of clusters. Then individual subjects from each cluster can be randomly sampled. Clearly, it is best to have the same sampling strategy and the same sampling frame within each cluster. Like the other two-stage strategies, this requires somewhat more complex approaches to data analysis, but it makes collecting data across large geographic regions economical. If, for example, your sample population is all women in a state and you randomly sample from that population (e.g., from state motor vehicle or telephone records), you then must drive all over the state to collect your data. If you divide the state into counties and randomly sample six counties, the logistics of data collection become manageable as long as you believe that these six counties fairly reflect the overall state profile.

Nonprobability or Purposive Samples

There are occasions when it is not feasible to use random sampling; in fact, random sampling is not feasible when conducting many studies in clinical settings. Nevertheless, you should make every effort to develop a representative sample and to employ a systematic approach that can be well described. This is purposive sampling. A good description of your sampling strategy, whether random or not, permits the readers of your work to judge for themselves the representativeness of your sample and the generalizability of your results. Simply characterizing the sampling strategy as one of "convenience" with no further discussion leaves the reader with the impression that no thought whatsoever was given to external validity and no judgment can be made about generalizability. The reader is left to believe that you are assuming that your findings are invariant across all people and all places.

Heterogeneity Sampling

With this approach, instead of sampling just the modal or typical case, you take care to sample heterogeneously (select a sample of people unlike each other) to ensure a broad spectrum of subjects. In the example involving counties described previously, rather than sampling just the modal rural counties, you would sample rural, urban, and suburban counties. With respect to schools, you might select comprehensive, magnet, and some specialized school programs. With respect to individual children, you might sample college-bound students, those in vocational programs, and perhaps even some who have dropped out or are about to drop out of school.

Snowball Sampling

Snowball sampling is helpful when assembling a sample of infrequent or hard-to-find cases. With snowball sampling, each subject is asked to recommend other potential subjects or to inform other possible subjects about the opportunity to participate in the study. For example, if one is studying older adults with relatively rare diseases or conditions, the spouses of one case will be likely to know or at least to have met other individuals whose spouses have the same condition. In snowball sampling, the investigator is less concerned with the broad representation of a large study population and more concerned with finding the relatively few members of that population who exist.

Respondent-Driven Sampling

When studying a population that is generally "hidden" or otherwise difficult to reach, respondent-driven sampling (RDS) can be employed to recruit individuals who might otherwise have been unobserved, such as prostitutes or drug users. RDS is derived from snowball sampling; once an individual is accepted into the study, he or she is given a set number of vouchers with unique serial numbers and is then incentivized to recruit additional persons with similar inclusion criteria. The original group of participants is recruited, generally, from locations that may be more accessible to researchers. For example, for a study on intravenous drug users, researchers could recruit their original cohort from locations where needles are exchanged. Nelson (2009) utilized RDS to recruit black adolescent mothers for his study on the influence of sexual partner type on condom-use decision making. The first participants were recruited from a sexual-health clinic or through response to marketing materials and were identified as the "seed." This seed group launched a growing chain of peer referrals, with participants from each subsequent group (or "wave") referring additional peers for recruitment waves. A visual representation of this process is illustrated in Figure 21.16.

Determination of Sample Size

Determining adequate sample size is a critical step and should be done early in the process of designing a study. It is important to remember that the sample size estimate should be calculated on how many subjects need to be enrolled at the last data collection period, not just enrolled at

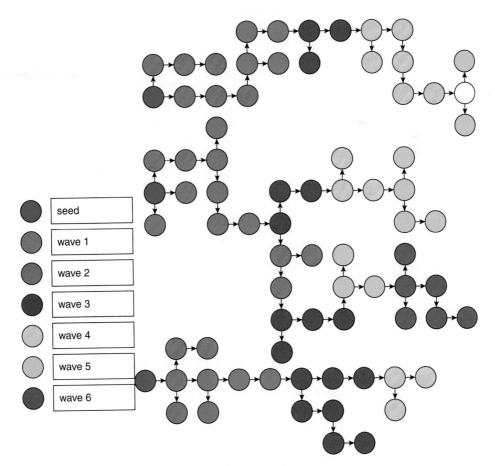

Figure 21.16: Respondent-driven sample network.

the start of the study. It is important to build in anticipated study attrition (the rate of dropout of participants) to determine the sample size needed. For some studies, 20% or greater attrition is not unexpected depending on the characteristics of the sample (e.g., children, the very ill) and what is required of participants to enroll in the study (e.g., multiple data collections, invasive procedures). Examining prior studies with similar participants or interventions should provide insight into approximate attrition rates that can be used in designing your study and estimating sample size. Too few subjects will result in low statistical power and the inability to detect significant findings in a study when they truly do exist (i.e., making a **type II error**, such as when an investigator accepts a false null hypothesis, which states there is no relationship between the independent and dependent variables). Many studies conducted in the health professions result in nonsignificant findings because of samples that are too small. On the other hand, enrolling more subjects than needed will result in greater costs to a study than necessary. When estimating sample size, it is important to obtain the statistics on the number of patients who would have met your study criteria who were available in the clinical setting during the prior year where the study will be conducted. These data will allow you to determine the feasibility of recruiting the necessary number of subjects during the course of your study.

Power analysis is a procedure used for determining the sample size needed for a study and helps to reduce type II errors (Polit & Beck, 2016). Readers are encouraged to refer to available resources to assist with the process of power analysis and calculation of sample size (Cohen, 1988, 1992; Jaccard & Becker, 2009).

Refusal to Participate and Study Attrition

The actual generalizability of the results depends not on who is approached to participate in a study but on who actually completes the study and is not lost to study attrition. Not everyone who is approached agrees to participate, and not everyone who agrees to participate completes the study. If the number of people who refuse or drop out is relatively small and there is no reason to believe that any subgroup of subjects was more likely to drop out than any other (i.e., the pattern of refusals and dropouts was random), the final sample will still be representative of the study population. Quite frequently, however, those who refuse to participate and those who drop out are not a random subset.

The best strategy to enhance external validity is to minimize refusal and dropout rates. To assess the potential impact of these threats, it is essential to have a clear sampling frame and to keep records of who is approached, who agrees to participate, who refuses, and ultimately who completes the study.

If anything is known about those who were approached and refused, the possibility of bias can be addressed by comparing those who refused with those who did not as well as those who dropped out with those who did not. Understanding the impact of refusal rates is not possible using convenience sampling in which advertisements are placed in the newspaper or signs are posted and only those who are interested are identified. Such strategies must assume that the findings of the study (e.g., the impact of the intervention or the beliefs of the participants) are invariant across people.

Strategies to Promote Participation

There are several strategies that encourage participation in a study.

Have Direct, Personal Contacts with Prospective Subjects. Avoid making potential participants take any action or demonstrate any initiative to enroll, such as requiring them to complete enrollment forms or make telephone calls. Be persistent but respectful when contacting prospective subjects. Send letters of introduction on official stationery introducing the study and stating who and when someone will call to explain the study further. Use high-powered mailings (e.g., special delivery and/or hand-addressed envelopes) because individuals are much more likely to open such mail. Have the letters come from the PI whose credentials lend credibility to the study. Finally, communicate that volunteering is normative, not unusual behavior. You do not want to start out by saying, "You are probably quite busy. . .." This conveys an expectation that the person will refuse and actually gives them a socially acceptable reason.

Make Participation As Easy As Possible.   Do what you can to remove any barriers, such as the cost of babysitting or transportation. If possible, have babysitting available at the study site. If that is not possible, provide a sufficient honorarium to cover the cost. Cover the cost of transportation or send a cab to transport individuals to the study site. Make the study as nonthreatening, stress free, and brief as possible, given the research design. Lengthy interviews covering a number of personal topics will burden the subjects. Be certain each section is essential. Train the recruiters and interviewers well. Make certain that they are comfortable with the recruitment protocol, script, and interview before working with actual subjects. Interviewers must be accepting and nonjudgmental. They must not appear shocked, awkward, or unprepared during any conversation or interview.

Make Participation Worthwhile.   Carefully and clearly explain the importance of the work and the manner in which the study results might improve care or services to patients and/ or families like theirs. Make participation sound interesting. Emphasize what the subjects might learn about themselves or their families. Tell them about any activities they might actually enjoy.

Step 8: Determine Measures

Selection of measures or instruments to assess or observe a study's variables is a critical step in designing a clinical study. As a rule, it is best to choose measures that yield the highest level of data (i.e., *interval* or *ratio data*, otherwise known as *continuous variables*) because these types of measures will allow fuller assessments of the study's variables as well as permit the use of more robust statistical tests. Examples of interval- or ratio-level data that have quantified intervals on an infinite scale of values are weight in pounds, number of glasses of beverages consumed a day, and age. **Ordinal data** are those that have ordered categories with intervals that cannot be quantified (e.g., none, a little, some, a lot, and very much so). Finally, **categorical data** have unordered categories in which one category is not considered higher or better than another (e.g., sex, gender, and race).

Measures should be both **valid** (i.e., they measure what they are intended to measure) and **reliable** (i.e., they consistently and accurately measure the construct of interest). If possible, it is best to use measures that have been used with similar samples as the study being planned, as well as those that are reported to have **reliability coefficients** of at least 0.70 or better instead of measures that have not been tested in prior work or have been tested with samples very different from the proposed study. It is very difficult to place confidence in a study's findings if the measures used did not have established validity or the **internal consistency reliability** of the measures was less than 0.70.

It is also important to recognize that obtaining two forms of assessment on a particular variable (e.g., self-report and observation) enhances the credibility of the findings when the data from these different sources converge. For example, if a parent reports that his or her child is high on externalizing behaviors (i.e., acting-out behaviors) on an instrument that measures these behaviors and if the child's teacher also completes a teacher version of the same instrument that yields high scores, the convergence of these findings produces a convincing case for the child being high on externalizing behaviors.

If observation data are being gathered, it is important to train observers on the instrument that will be used in a study so that there is an **interrater reliability** or agreement on the construct that is being observed (e.g., maternal–infant interaction) at least 90% of the time. In addition, for intervention studies, it is important that observers be blind to the study group (i.e., unaware as to whether the subjects are in the experimental or control groups) to avoid bias in their ratings.

Step 9: Outline Data Collection Plan

The data collection plan typically specifies when and where each phase of the study (e.g., subject enrollment, intervention sessions, and completion of measures) will be completed and exactly when all the measures will be obtained. Careful planning of these details is essential before the study commences. A timetable is often helpful to outline the study procedures so that each member of the team is aware of the specific plan for data collection (Table 21.1).

Step 10: Apply for Human Subjects Approval

Before the commencement of research, it is essential to have the study approved by an RSRB that will evaluate the study for protection of human subjects. Federal regulations (Code of Federal Regulations, 2016) now mandate that any research conducted be reviewed to ensure the following:

- Risks to subjects are minimized.
- Selection of subjects is equitable (e.g., women, children, and individuals of a certain race/ethnicity are not excluded).
- Informed consent is obtained and documented if indicated (see Appendix G, available on thePoint®, for an example of an approved consent form).

TABLE 21.1	*Timetable for a Study's Data Collection Plan*			
Year	2018	2018–2019	2019–2022	2022
Months	1–5	6–20	21–51	52–60
Setup/logistics	*			
Buy equipment	*			
Hire and train staff	*			
Meet with consultants	*			
Refine procedures	*			
Pilot group training (6/18)		*		
Recruit participants/pre-assessment (start 7/18)		*	*	
Intervention sessions		*	*	
Postassessment		*	*	
Data analysis (4/22)				*
Final reports				*
Prepare presentations and manuscripts (12/22)				*

- A data and safety monitoring plan is implemented when indicated (e.g., for clinical trials; see this book's companion website at http://thepoint.lww.com/melnyk4e for an example of a data safety and monitoring plan).

In addition, any individual involved in a study as an investigator, subinvestigator, study coordinator, or enroller of human subjects must pass a required test on the protection of human subjects, based on the Belmont Report. The Belmont Report was issued in 1978 by the National Commission of the Protection of Human Subjects of Biomedical and Behavioral Research and outlined three principles on which standards of ethical conduct in research are to be based:

1. Beneficence (i.e., no harm to subjects)
2. Respect for human dignity (e.g., the right to self-determination, as in providing voluntary consent to participate in a study)
3. Justice (e.g., fair treatment and nondiscriminatory selection of human subjects)

Guidelines for RSRB application and review should be obtained from the institution(s) in which the study will be conducted.

 See The Ohio State University's website at http://orrp.osu.edu/irb/ for one example of required guidelines and forms for submission of a research study for human subjects' review.

Step 11: Implement the Study

Once human subjects' approval for the study is obtained, data collection can begin. Particular detail and attention should be paid to the process of data collection for the first 5 to 10 subjects regarding the ease of enrollment and completion of study questionnaires.

These first 5 or 10 cases can be considered a pilot phase used to identify problems in the intervention, recruitment, or data gathering so that changes can be made if needed. This is a good time for the research team to work through any challenges encountered and to implement strategies to overcome them. Once the main study begins, no changes should be made. If changes are made, subjects evaluated before the changes cannot be analyzed along with subjects evaluated afterward.

During the conduct of the study, emphasis should be placed on the review of questionnaires after completion by the study participants to prevent missing data that pose challenges for data analysis as well as to determine whether subjects meet clinical criteria on sensitive measures or those that identify them as at risk for certain conditions (e.g., major depression, suicide). Weekly or biweekly team meetings are very beneficial for the research team to overcome challenges in data collection and to maintain cohesiveness during the conduct of the study.

Step 12: Prepare and Analyze Data

In the preparation phase of data analysis, it is important to assess study measures for completeness and to make determinations about what strategies will be used to handle missing data. For example, if less than 30% of the data are missing on a questionnaire, it is acceptable practice to impute the mean for the missing items. If, on the other hand, more than 30% of the data are missing on a questionnaire, investigators commonly eliminate them from data analysis. There is a growing body of literature on handling missing data, and researchers should document the details of the missing data and the methods for dealing with the missing values into their data analysis (Penny & Atkinson, 2012).

Creating a codebook regarding how certain responses will be translated into numerical form is important before data can be entered into a statistical program, such as Statistical Package for the Social Sciences (SPSS). For example, marital status could be coded as "1"—married, "2"—not married, "3"—divorced, or "4"—married for the second or third time. Verifying all entered data is also a critical step in preparing to analyze the data.

Multiple statistical tests can be conducted to answer research questions and to test hypotheses generated in quantitative studies, and readers are encouraged to consult a statistical resource for detailed information on these specific tests. For example, *Munro's Statistical Methods for Healthcare Research, 6th edition* (2012), is a user-friendly book that provides excellent information and examples of common statistical analyses for quantitative studies.

Step 13: Interpret the Results

Careful interpretation of the results of a study (i.e., explaining the study results) is important and should be based on the theoretical/conceptual framework that guided the study as well as prior work in the area. Alternative explanations for the findings should always be considered in the discussion. In addition, it is important to discuss findings from prior research that relate to the current study as well as the study's implications for clinical practice and/or policy.

Step 14: Disseminate the Findings

Once a study is completed, it is imperative to disseminate the findings to both researchers and clinicians who will use the evidence in guiding further research in the area or in making decisions about patient care. The vehicles for dissemination should include both conferences in the form of oral and/or poster presentations and publications (see Chapter 20 for helpful strategies on preparing oral and poster presentations, as well as writing for publication). In addition, the findings of a study should also be disseminated to the media, healthcare policy makers, and the public (see Chapter 20).

Step 15: Incorporate Findings into EBP and Evaluate Outcomes

Once evidence from a study is generated, it is important to factor that evidence into a decision regarding whether it should be incorporated into patient care. Studies should be critically appraised with respect to three key questions:

1. Are the findings valid (i.e., as close to the truth as possible)?
2. Are the findings important (e.g., strength and preciseness of the intervention)?
3. Are the findings applicable to your patients? (See Unit 2.)

Once a decision is made to incorporate the findings of a study into practice, an outcomes evaluation should be conducted to determine the impact of the change on the process or outcomes of clinical care (see Chapter 10).

Pragmatic Trials

The need for **pragmatic trials** arose because of concerns that RCTs impose too many controls that often are not realistic in real-world clinical settings and, therefore, do not adequately inform practice and policy (Ford & Norrie, 2016). Pragmatic trials, which are growing in number, are designed to evaluate the effectiveness of interventions in real-life routine practice conditions and show real-world effectiveness with broader patient groups. In contrast,

RCTs are considered explanatory trials that aim to test whether an intervention works under optimal situations and controlled settings (Patsopoulos, 2011). Pragmatic trials produce results that can be generalized and applied in routine practice settings.

QUALITATIVE RESEARCH

It is likely that most readers have an initial idea of what **qualitative research** is but little understanding of its rich underpinnings and purposes. This section provides an overview of qualitative research, including its philosophical and historical underpinnings. Suggestions regarding when a qualitative study may be the most appropriate approach for addressing a research question and the best way to add to knowledge to guide practice will be presented. In addition, this section also discusses how to judge the rigor of qualitative studies and how best to use findings from qualitative work to extend and advance science.

Overview of Qualitative Research

Qualitative research is an area of knowledge development that seeks to uncover, explore, describe, and understand human conditions from those who are experiencing or living a phenomenon. This approach to the human subjective view is in contrast to research that is conducted to test the researcher's view of the world, that is, quantitative research. Qualitative inquiry is done without reliance on measurement, numbers, and statistical analysis. Rather, the researcher seeks to learn what it is like for those experiencing the phenomenon. Qualitative research began in the social sciences and was brought to nursing in the 1970s by nurses who earned doctoral degrees in the social sciences, such as sociology and anthropology. These new researchers recognized that nurses were very interested in and needed to study health-related topics from the perspective of those having the health issues. Whether a researcher wants to learn what it is like for individuals experiencing a particular disease, or understand those dealing with a difficult treatment, or comprehend another's life within a different world or culture—these are all possible topics that can be explored through qualitative research.

Qualitative traditions, such as **phenomenology, ethnography, grounded theory**, and **participatory action research**, all hold a common belief that the best way to seek new knowledge is from those who are actually living what we are interested in. The qualitative researcher seeks out those who can tell them what the experience is really like—whether that be having a child die, experiencing horizontal violence in the workplace, or receiving suboptimal care for want of access to services, these are all questions that would benefit from qualitative approaches. Qualitative researchers are not seeking to find a single truth but multiple ones, without interfering with what they are studying, but rather observing it in its natural state. Often, it is through conversation—interviews, focus groups, the written word—that researchers hear the voices of those who, from personal experience, know what it is like to have a health crisis or what it is like to be who they are themselves. In qualitative approaches to research, there is no right or wrong, no one way to look at anything; rather, the goal is to gain understanding and description, not to test interventions or measure relationships.

Unlike quantitative research where the researcher tends to remain separate from the study participants and the data, the qualitative researcher is imbedded in the data collection and analysis process. Although it is important for the researcher to acknowledge one's own biases and perspectives, it is imperative that the investigator become immersed in the words and contexts of the participants so as to see patterns and language. The researcher is indeed an instrument of the research, and this is an essential part of the process. The researcher's role is to describe or interpret what he or she sees, hears, and reads from the researcher's informants (observations, individuals, texts).

This is done through inductive processes, moving from the specific, subjective perspective to a more general one. An example of this would be listening to a few parents' experiences of their child's hospitalization and then moving to a general sense of what it is like to have a child that is hospitalized. This is in sharp contrast to a quantitative deductive approach, moving from the broad general observation to specific conclusions. Using the same example of parents whose children are hospitalized, a quantitative study would start from a known theory, such as stress and coping, and seek to learn how parents use various coping mechanisms when their children are hospitalized.

Designing a Qualitative Study

Literature Review

In order to learn what is known about a topic, it is critical to determine what has been published about the topic of interest. This is accomplished by writing a PICOT (Population, Issue or Intervention of interest, Comparison of interest, Outcome and Time for intervention) question and searching the literature electronically using multiple databases. Key articles then need to be read and critically appraised; the study findings must then be synthesized in answer to the question "What do we know about this topic?" The introduction and background sections of an article generally present what is known about the problem and the significance of the issue. What is not known should also be clearly stated. Research is conducted because there is some aspect of knowledge that is missing. A study should be designed to fill the identified gap.

The length and depth of an evidence review may vary, depending on what is known on the topic of interest. Some qualitative approaches stress the need to start a study with minimal preconceived notions or the need to *bracket* previous assumptions. When this approach is used, the literature review may be truncated.

Purpose of the Study

The goal of a qualitative study can be written as the study purpose, specific aim, or research question. A research question is an interrogative statement that clarifies the focus of the study, population, setting, and approach to investigating a researchable problem. The question to be answered should fill a knowledge gap that was identified. Qualitative methodologies are appropriate when the purpose or research question focuses on human experience from the perspective of those living that experience, or on understanding textual data within context. Qualitative methodology might also be appropriate when little is known about a topic or there are no theories to guide our understanding of it. The purpose statement for a qualitative study would likely suggest: *This study seeks "to explore," "to describe," or "to understand" the phenomenon of interest in a certain setting and group of people.*

Methodological Approach

The approach to designing a qualitative study begins with the study purpose and then the identification of the tradition needed to guide the study. For example, if the purpose is to describe "the lived experience" of some people within a certain circumstance, it is likely that a phenomenological approach is appropriate. Likewise, when gaining knowledge about a culture or community is sought, **ethnography** is likely the best methodology. See Table 21.2 for an overview of these qualitative traditions and their respective roots.

Within each tradition, there are common methods of data collection and analysis. These need to be consistent with the purpose of the study and the chosen tradition. For example, ethnography generally requires prolonged engagement in a culture, and data are collected through multiple means, including observation, interviews, and artifacts. **Grounded theory**

TABLE 21.2	*Qualitative Approaches and Their Historical Roots*	
Tradition	**Description**	**Roots**
Phenomenology	The study of lived experience, from the perspective of the study participants. Can be descriptive or interpretive.	Philosophy underlying social sciences originated by Husserl and Heidegger professes that each individual has their own reality.
Ethnography	Seeking to describe knowledge of culture through prolonged engagement in the field, participant observation, exploration of artifacts outsider and insider perspectives.	Anthropologists and social scientists who sought to gain knowledge from the natives in a culture.
Grounded theory	An approach used to study social processes from which a substantive theory results.	Interpretive symbolic interactionism. Developed by Glaser and Strauss.
Participative action research	Social research brought to bear by a researcher and members of a group collaboratively in the process of social or group change. Not a single method.	Also known as community-based action research, cooperative inquiry. First came out of the work of Kurt Lewin, social psychologist and change theorist.

Sources: Polit, D. F., & Beck, C. T. (2016). *Nursing research: Generating and assessing evidence for nursing practice* (10th ed.). Philadelphia, PA: Wolters Kluwer; Streubert, H. J., & Carpenter, D. R. (2011). *Qualitative research in nursing: Advancing the humanistic imperative* (5th ed.). Philadelphia, PA: Wolters Kluwer/Lippincott Williams & Wilkin.

studies usually dictate the use of interviews as the primary data collection method, with purposive and theoretical sampling employed to locate key participants.

Sampling

Participants (also known as informants) can be recruited through convenience (those easy to find) and nonprobability sampling. However, purposive (or purposeful) sampling is commonly used in qualitative studies. This is where individuals with characteristics that can best inform the researcher are sought and handpicked. A specialized type of purposive sampling that is used in grounded theory is theoretical sampling. Seeking all the pieces of a theory likely requires further participant recruitment and data collection through *theoretical sampling*, which is seeking individuals who can shed light on unclear aspects of the theory being developed.

Whatever approach is selected for sampling, inclusion and exclusion criteria should be clearly stated, to define the population from which participants are sought.

In qualitative studies, sample sizes are generally small but are rarely completely determined at the start of a project. Each interview may reveal new details that require broadening the sample; the person conducting the study is similar to a detective with new details leading to new informants. The final sample size is determined by the researcher when she/he begins to hear the same thing over and over (this is known as saturation or redundancy), when nothing new is uncovered, or the theory that is discovered is complete. When critically appraising a study, a main question to be addressed about the sample is "Do these informants have the characteristics that provide adequate and appropriate information to answer the research question?"

Data Collection

Data are collected through interviews, observation, focus groups, or the examination of textual data or artifacts. These methods are conducted with individuals who share their experience with the topic, observing behaviors of those parts of a culture, or examining historical textual data. The investigator must have adequate *prolonged engagement* with the participants, in the field or when examining artifacts such as documents or texts. Extensive time in the field is also necessary when the development of trust and relationships with community members is critical to access and understanding. Notes on details of data collection are written in *fieldnotes*, and those notes are part of the database. Interviews and focus group conversations should be transcribed into a textual document. Data collection is complete when saturation is reached, the theory is fully clear, or community members agree that goals have been met.

Data Analysis

Data analysis is a lengthy process in qualitative research, and it begins during data collection. It is not completely preplanned because the researcher needs to be free to follow leads from what he or she hears and sees and to go where the data are pointing to. However, data analysis should be systematic, consistent and thorough. For example, during an interview, the researcher hears significant statements from the participant and perhaps the personal meaning behind the statement. The researcher would find it helpful to make notes, called *memos*, about his or her analytic thoughts while listening to or observing the participants.

The recognition of patterns within the data occurs through an iterative analysis process that begins during data collection, followed by reading and rereading of the transcripts. As familiarity with the data increases, the researchers become *immersed* in those data such that their thinking of the data evolves to new understanding. While coding the data, the investigators are beginning to *make sense of the data*; sorting and groupings of those data come to their minds. This is analogous to having many jigsaw puzzle pieces without having the puzzle picture to guide you; the investigator is seeking to understand the picture the pieces form. During data analysis, pieces of similar colors, patterns, or familiarity are grouped together; edge pieces and corners are sought to provide structure. Patterns emerge that are noted through *codes* about topics, processes, behaviors, assumptions, relationships, and social structures. These groups may be called *themes or categories; relationships between themes* might lead to a picture or schematic of those relationships. In the case of grounded theory, a theory slowly emerges through *constant comparative analysis* that seeks to explain the social processes under study. The collection of memos, methodological notes, and other analysis details is often housed in a research notebook, and reported as thick detail that provides an *audit trail* for the consumer of the research. In an article or monograph describing a study, there should be adequate details that allow the reader to follow the decisions that were made during data analysis.

Trustworthiness of the Study

Trustworthiness, or rigor, refers to the confidence one has in the worth, accuracy, and believability of the qualitative study findings. It answers the questions: Does this study reveal truth? Does it provide a new understanding of the personal perspective? Is the approach appropriate/reasonable given the purpose or research question being asked? Did they include the people who truly know the inside of this topic? If not, who or what is missing? (Lincoln & Guba, 1985).

The focus here is similar to the concepts of reliability and validity in quantitative research but speaks more to the question: "How does the reader know that what the researchers report is truly the way it is?" "Does this represent what the participants meant and intended?" While various concepts have been outlined, Lincoln and Guba's (1985) landmark four criteria for trustworthiness cover the critical areas for examining qualitative studies. These areas are credibility, dependability, confirmability, and transferability.

Credibility is the most important aspect of trustworthiness, that is, what was done to ensure that the investigators got it right; for credibility, prolonged engagement is a basic requirement. Did they spend enough time, talk with enough individuals to gain a comprehensive view of the phenomenon. "Did they get it right?" The use of direct quotes from the participants themselves is one way that the reader can hear some of the words actually spoken. Do these words match what the researchers are saying about the research topic? Credibility is increased when prolonged engagement, persistent observation, and triangulation of verification measures are used. Member checking, by returning to the study participants with the study findings, is one commonly used technique to build credibility.

There can be no credibility if there is no dependability. Dependability is increased by having more than a single person conducting the study. Communication between members of the research team while keeping independent inquiry should be reported in all reports and articles documenting a rich audit trail.

Confirmability is just as it sounds—the ability of the reader to confirm or follow the process used by the investigators. Triangulation and journaling can be used to increase confirmability. External readers deem or confirm its credibility from the thick description and audit trail provided by the authors about how the study was conducted.

The final criterion of transferability asks: Will these findings be useful or have meaning with others? This concept is comparable to generalizability but relates more to similarities of the participants in the study and the reader's population of interest. The thick description and audit trail are essential here as well to allow the consumer to make a judgment about his or her own context.

Results

The results from a qualitative study are most commonly presented as themes and categories, illustrated through several direct quotes of each. The quotes provide the exact words from the source and are verification of the original data. The themes should be consistent with the quotes. Relationships between and among themes, into categories, a theory, or steps taken by a community action group should also be presented if consistent with the research tradition. Collectively, the results should paint a picture of a new understanding of the phenomenon under investigation. Alternatively, results can be presented as a lengthy narrative of aspects of a culture, or steps taken within a community action group.

Application of Qualitative Research in Practice

Being able to take research results and apply them to a larger population, known as generalizability, is not a goal of qualitative research. Rather, qualitative research findings are useful in understanding experiences of some people under certain circumstances. They may provide a thick description that provides sensitivity and insight into the needs of patients in similar situations through the words of the participants. Or a new theory can be used or tested for applicability or predictability in new groups of patients. Results from an ethnographic study provide a context-rich description of cultures within which healthcare providers are situated.

The purpose of a qualitative study may be to describe the lived experience of individuals with various health issues or cultures. For example, what is the lived experience of a patient newly diagnosed with diabetes or of those who live and work within a military battlefield? Three exemplars are presented in Table 21.3 to illustrate qualitative approaches and clinical areas of investigation.

Qualitative research methods also provide a platform on which to build quantitative research investigations and can be useful for seeking empirical support for research hypotheses. The aim of this approach is to gain in-depth understanding of why the phenomenon occurs and details of how it is experienced. Through qualitative research, a new instrument to measure a concept can be developed; it can then subsequently be tested quantitatively. Ultimately, new knowledge garnered from qualitative investigations can change perceptions, understanding, and alter the focus of future care. Previously unrevealed information is now available to guide new practices or programs.

TABLE 21.3	*Exemplars of Qualitative Investigations*

"Have no regrets": Parents' experiences and developmental tasks in pregnancy with a lethal fetal diagnosis

Côté-Arsenault, D., & Denney-Koelsch, E. (2016). *Social Science and Medicine, 154*, 100–109.

Parents who learn during pregnancy that their unborn infant has a lethal fetal diagnosis sometimes choose to continue their pregnancy. For them, the pregnancy experience is greatly altered. The purpose of this study was to identify the altered developmental tasks of pregnancy for these parents as they adjust to their new reality and plan for the birth and death of their infant. Hermeneutic phenomenology guided this longitudinal study. Thirty parents (16 mothers, 13 fathers, 1 lesbian partner) were interviewed jointly and individually several times across pregnancy and up to 2 to 3 months postbirth. Data analysis began during data collection and continued iteratively through coding and theme identification. Parents' overall goal was to "Have no regrets" when all was said and done. Their experiences revealed 5 stages of pregnancy and 7 developmental tasks of pregnancy. The resulting developmental approach could sensitize care providers who care for parents anticipating their baby's death as to what is most important to parents across the rest of pregnancy and postpartum.

Counteracting ambivalence: Nurses who smoke and their health promotion role with patients who smoke

Radsma, J., & Bottorff, J. L. (2009). *Research in Nursing and Health, 32*, 443–452.

Smoking has been associated with morbidity and mortality. Nurses are responsible for identifying smoking as a risk factor in their patients and should counsel them to reduce and cease their smoking. However, a large number of nurses themselves smoke. This grounded theory study used principles and methods of Strauss and Corbin to identify the ways 23 nurses who were purposively sampled managed the ambivalence they felt when caring for patients who smoked. Countering ambivalence refers to the basic social process that was identified in these nurses' descriptions. They managed the contradictions they experienced in one of four ways: indifferent, evasive, engaged, and forced compliance. This resulting theory illustrates the challenges for nurses who need to address preventive antismoking recommendations in their patient care. The connection and relevance to clinical practice is straightforward. Nurses may have a bias toward patients who smoke that they are caring for; additionally, nurses who are smokers or former smokers were found to alter their approach to patients.

TABLE
21.3   *Exemplars of Qualitative Investigations* **(continued)**

Adolescent input on the development of an HIV risk reduction intervention

Morrison-Beedy, D., Carey, M, Aronowitz, T., Mkandawire, L., & Dyne, J. (2002). *Journal of the Association of Nurses in AIDS Care, 13*(1), 21–27.

To adapt an HIV-prevention intervention for use with adolescent girls, focus groups were conducted with thirty teens aged 11 to 17. The purpose of this formative study was to determine baseline levels of information, motivation, and behavioral skills related to HIV prevention and ascertain useful participant recruitment and retention strategies. Participants were primarily economically disadvantaged young women of color, and focus group sizes ranged from 9 to 11 girls. These groups were conducted at various community-based sites that served teens. Using a trained moderator and interview guide developed for the study, focus group guide questions included: (a) What information related to the transmission or prevention of HIV do your friends or other young women your age want to know? (b) Why do you think some women your age practice safer sex, whereas others do not? (c) What, if any, safer sex behaviors do young women your age practice? and (d) What ideas can you give us to encourage girls to attend intervention groups and to participate? Audio tapes of the groups were transcribed verbatim, and coding and theming followed for analysis. Content analysis was used to cluster similar data into our descriptive categories. The elicitation research helped us determine the target population's preintervention levels of HIV-related information, motivation, and behavioral skills as well as girl's risk behaviors. This study also identified misconceptions regarding prevention and transmission and developed recruitment and retention strategies for a longitudinal intervention study.

EBP FAST FACTS

- Descriptive and predictive studies lay the foundation for developing interventions.
- True experiments or RCTs are the strongest designs to support cause and effect (i.e., the independent variable or intervention causes a change in the dependent or outcome variable).
- Study feasibility addresses factors including adequate time and resources, access to participants, team member expertise, and ethical and legal constraints.
- Threats to internal validity (the ability to say that it was the intervention or treatment that caused a change in outcome) and external validity (generalizability) require a balanced approach because increasing strategies to lessen one usually decreases strategies to minimize the other.
- Success of transferring the evidence generated by a quantitative study depends largely on developing an innovative yet answerable research question that addresses a "so what" factor and measures outcomes that matter in real-world healthcare settings (e.g., patient complications, length of stay, rehospitalizations, cost).
- Pragmatic trials are designed to evaluate the effectiveness of interventions in real-life routine practice conditions and show real-world effectiveness with broader patient groups.
- Qualitative research is an area of knowledge development that seeks to uncover, explore, describe, and understand human conditions from those who are experiencing or living a phenomenon.

WANT TO KNOW MORE?

A variety of resources are available to enhance your learning and understanding of this chapter.

- Visit thePoint® to access:
  - Appendix G: Example of an Approved Consent Form for a Study
  - An example of a data safety and monitoring plan
  - Articles from the AJN EBP Step-By-Step Series
  - Journal articles
  - Checklists for rapid critical appraisal and more!
- Lippincott CoursePoint combines digital text content with video case studies and interactive modules for a fully integrated course solution that works the way you study and learn.

References

Campbell, D. T., & Stanley, J. C. (1963). *Experimental and quasi-experimental designs for research*. Chicago, IL: Rand McNally.

Code of Federal Regulations. (2016). *Protection of human subjects*. Washington, DC: Department of Health and Human Services. Retrieved from https://www.hhs.gov/ohrp/regulations-and-policy/regulations/common-rule/index.html

Cohen, J. (1988). *Statistical power analysis for the behavioral sciences* (2nd ed.). Mahwah, NJ: Lawrence Erlbaum.

Cohen, J. (1992). *A power primer: Psychological bulletin*. Washington, DC: American Psychological Association.

Ford, I., & Norrie, J. (2016). Pragmatic trials. *New England Journal of Medicine, 375*, 454–463.

Jaccard, J., & Becker, M. A. (2009). *Statistics for the behavioral sciences* (5th ed.). Belmont, CA: Wadsworth.

Johnson, J. E., Fieler, V. K., Jones, L. S., Wlasowicz, G. S., & Mitchell, M. L. (1997). *Self-regulation theory: Applying theory to your practice*. Pittsburgh, PA: Oncology Nursing Press.

Lincoln, Y. S., & Guba, E. G. (1985). *Naturalistic inquiry*. Newbury Park, CA: Sage.

Melnyk, B. M., Alpert-Gillis, L., Feinstein, N. F., Crean, H., Johnson, J., Fairbanks, E., . . . Corbo-Richert, B. (2004). Creating opportunities for parent empowerment (COPE): Program effects on the mental health/coping outcomes of critically ill young children and their mothers. *Pediatrics, 113*(6), e597–e606.

Melnyk, B. M., Crean, H. F., Feinstein, N. F., & Fairbanks, E. (2008). Maternal anxiety and depression following a premature infants' discharge from the NICU: Explanatory effects of the COPE program. *Nursing Research, 57*, 383–394.

Melnyk, B. M., Crean, H. F., Feinstein, N. F., & Alpert-Gillis, L. (2007). Testing the theoretical framework of the COPE program for mothers of critically ill children: An integrative model of young children's post-hospital adjustment behaviors. *Journal of Pediatric Psychology, 32*(4), 463–474.

Melnyk, B. M., Feinstein, N. F., Alpert-Gillis, L., Fairbanks, E., Crean, H. F., Sinkin, R., . . . Gross, S. J. (2006). Reducing premature infants' length of stay and improving parents' mental health outcomes with the COPE NICU program: A randomized clinical trial. *Pediatrics, 118*(5), 1414–1427.

Melnyk, B. M., & Fineout-Overholt, E. (2015). Evidence-based Practice in Nursing & Healthcare. *A Guide to Best Practice* (3rd ed.). Philadelphia, PA: Wolters Kluwer.

Melnyk, B. M., & Morrison-Beedy, D. (2012). Setting the stage for intervention research: The "so what" factor. In B. M. Melnyk & D. Morrison-Beedy (Eds.), *Intervention research: Designing, conducting, analyzing and funding*. New York, NY: Springer.

Morrison-Beedy, D., Jones, S., Xia, Y., Tu, X., Crean, H., & Carey, M. (2012). Reducing sexual risk behavior in adolescent girls: Results from a randomized controlled trial. *Journal of Adolescent Health, 52*(3), 314–321. doi:10.1016/j.jadohealth.2012.07.005

Munro, B. H. (2012). *Statistical methods for health care research* (6th ed.). Philadelphia, PA: Lippincott, Williams & Wilkins.

National Commission for the Protection of Human Subjects of Biomedical and Behavioral Research. (1978). *Belmont report: Ethical principles and guidelines for research involving human subjects*. Washington, DC: U.S. Government Printing Office.

Nelson, L. (2009). *Influence of sexual partner type on condom-use decision making by Black adolescent mothers* (ProQuest dissertations and theses 361-n/a). University of Rochester School of Nursing. Retrieved from http://search.proquest.com/docview/accountid=14745

Patsopoulos, N. (2011). A pragmatic view on pragmatic trials. *Dialogues in Clinical Neuroscience, 13*(2), 217–224.

Penny, K. I., & Atkinson, I. (2012). Approaches for dealing with missing data in health care studies. *Journal of Clinical Nursing, 21*(19/20), 2722–2729. doi:10.1111/j.1365-2702.2011.03854.x

Polit, D. F., & Beck, C. T. (2016). *Nursing research: Generating and assessing evidence for nursing practice* (10th ed.). Philadelphia, PA: Wolters Kluwer.

Powers, B. A., & Knapp, T. R. (2010). *A dictionary of nursing theory and research* (4th ed.). New York, NY: Springer.

Trochim, W. M., Donnelly, J. P., Arora, K. (2015). *Research Methods. The Essential Knowledge Base.* Boston, MA: Cengage Learning.

Whittemore, R., & Grey, M. (2002). The systematic development of nursing interventions. *Journal of Nursing Scholarship, 34*(2), 115–120.

22

Writing a Successful Grant Proposal to Fund Research and Evidence-Based Practice Implementation Projects

Bernadette Mazurek Melnyk and
Ellen Fineout-Overholt

> There's always a way if you are willing to pay the price of time, energy, or effort.
>
> —*Robert Schuller*

EBP Terms to Learn

Attention control group
Booster interventions
Construct validity
Content validity
Convenience sampling
Data and safety
  monitoring plan
External validity
Face validity
Generalizability
Internal consistency
  reliability
Interrater reliability
Manipulation checks
Observer drift

Random sampling
Reliability

"So what" factor
Theoretical framework

Learning Objectives

After studying this chapter, learners will be able to:

1. Describe key strategies for writing a successful grant proposal.

2. Identify the steps in writing a grant application.

3. Discuss strategies for resubmitting a grant proposal when not funded on the first attempt.

4. Identify funding agencies for research and evidence-based implementation/quality improvement projects.

Writing grants is often critical to obtain the funding that you need to conduct a study or project in order to make the impact that you want. Although grant writing can be "character-building," it is a worthwhile means to an end dream of being able to do something that is meaningful to you and one that can lead to substantial improvements in the quality of care and patient outcomes. Once a decision has been made to conduct a study to generate evidence that will guide clinical practice or to implement and evaluate a practice change as part of an evidence-based practice (EBP) implementation or outcomes management project, the feasibility of conducting such an initiative must be assessed. Although small pilot studies or outcomes management projects can be conducted with relatively few resources, most studies (e.g., randomized controlled trials [RCTs]) typically require funding to cover items such as research assistants, staff time, instruments to measure outcomes of interest, intervention materials, and data management and analyses. This chapter focuses on strategies for developing a successful grant proposal to fund research as well as EBP implementation or outcomes management projects. Many of these grant-writing strategies are similar, whether applying for large-scale grants from federal agencies, such as the National Institutes of Health (NIH), the Agency for Healthcare Research and Quality (AHRQ), the Patient Centered Outcomes Research Institute (PCORI), or more small-scale funding from professional organizations or foundations. Potential funding sources and key components of a project budget also are highlighted.

PRELIMINARY STRATEGIES FOR WRITING A GRANT PROPOSAL

A grant proposal is a written plan outlining the specific aims, background, significance, methods, and budget for a project requesting funding from sources such as professional organizations, federal agencies, or foundations. It is not uncommon for the process of planning, writing, and revising a rigorous detailed grant proposal for certain funding sources (e.g., NIH, AHRQ, the Centers for Disease Control and Prevention [CDC]) to take several months. In contrast, other sources (e.g., foundations and professional organizations) may require only the submission of a concise abstract or two- to three-page summary of the project for funding consideration.

The Five Ps

For writing a successful grant proposal, whether for a large or small project, there are five critical qualities that the writer must possess—the five "Ps": (1) passion; (2) planning; (3) persuasion; (4) persistence; and (5) patience.

The first quality is *passion* for the proposed initiative. Passion for the project is essential, especially because many character-building experiences (e.g., writing multiple drafts, resubmissions) will surface along the road to successful completion.

Second, detailed *planning* must begin. Every element of the project needs to be carefully considered, along with strategies for overcoming potential obstacles. Developing a strong team to carry out the project as well as plan and write the grant facilitates success.

The third element for successful grant writing is *persuasion*. The grant application needs to be written in a manner that excites the reviewers and creates a compelling case for why the project should be funded.

Finally, *persistence* and *patience* are indispensable qualities, especially because the grant application process is very competitive across federal agencies, professional organizations, and foundations. In many cases, repeated submissions are required to secure funding. Therefore, resubmitting applications and being patient and receptive to grant reviewers' feedback are crucial ingredients for success. One tip for success is to surround yourself with uplifting motivational quotes to inspire and encourage you through the writing process (Box 22.1).

First Impressions

Remember that you never get a second chance to make a great first impression. Paying attention to details and being as meticulous as possible for the first grant submission will be well worth the effort when your grant is reviewed.

Once the idea for a study project is generated, the literature searched and critically appraised, and a planning meeting conducted to determine the design and methods (see Chapters 19 and 20), it is time to search for potential funding sources.

BOX
22.1   *Motivational Quotes for Success With Grant Writing*

Failures are only temporary setbacks and
"character-building" experiences.
—Les Brown

Most people give up just when they're about to achieve success.
They quit on the one yard line. They give up at the last minute of
the game, one foot from a winning touchdown.
—H. Ross Perot

I do not think there is any other quality so essential to success
of any kind as the quality of perseverance. It overcomes
almost everything, even nature.
—John D. Rockefeller

Credentials

To obtain grants from most national federal funding agencies (e.g., NIH, AHRQ, PCORI, CDC), a Doctor of Philosophy (PhD) degree is usually the minimum qualification necessary for the principal or lead investigator (PI) on the project. However, many clinicians with master's degrees substantially contribute to federally funded studies as members of research teams that are spearheaded by clinicians with doctorates. For many professional organizations and foundation funding sources, a master's degree is usually sufficient to obtain grant funding, although it typically fares well in the peer review of the grant proposal to have a researcher with a PhD as part of the team.

Potential Funding Sources

Academic medical centers, schools within university settings, and healthcare organizations frequently have internal mechanisms available to fund small research projects (e.g., pilot and feasibility studies), often through a competitive grants program. External funding agencies, such as NIH and AHRQ; foundations, such as the W.T. Grant Foundation, the Robert Wood Johnson Foundation, or Josiah Macy Jr. Foundation; for-profit corporations, such as pharmaceutical companies; and professional organizations, such as the Society of Critical Care Medicine and the American Heart Association, often list priorities or areas that they are interested in supporting (e.g., palliative care, pain management for critically ill patients, symptom management, and HIV risk reduction).

Establishing a list of potential funding agencies whose priorities match the type of study or project that you are interested in conducting will enhance chances for success.

Grants.gov is an outstanding site that lists all current discretionary funding opportunities from 26 agencies of the U.S. Government, including NIH and the National Science Foundation along with all of the most important funders of research in the United States. Internet links to various potential funding agencies/organizations are listed in Table 22.1.

| TABLE 22.1 | *Internet Links to Various Potential Funding Agencies* |

Type	Organization	Internet Link
V	U.S. Department of Health and Human Services	http://www.grants.gov
M	National Institute of Mental Health	http://gopher.nimh.nih.gov/
V	National Institutes of Health	https://www.nih.gov/
M	National Alliance on Mental Illness	https://www.sigmanursing.org/ https://www.nami.org/
V	National Institute of Nursing Research	http://www.ninr.nih.gov/
N	American Nurses Foundation (American Nurses Association)	http://www.anfonline.org/
V	Sigma Theta Tau International	https://www.sigmanursing.org/
N	American Academy of Nursing	http://www.aannet.org/
V	Agency for Healthcare Research and Quality	http://www.ahrq.gov/fund/
V	Centers for Disease Control and Prevention	http://www.cdc.gov/
M	Substance Abuse and Mental Health Services Administration	http://www.samhsa.gov/
G	National Institute on Aging	http://www.nia.nih.gov/
M	National Institute on Drug Abuse	http://www.drugabuse.gov/funding
V	National Center for Complementary and Alternative Medicine	http://nccam.nih.gov/research/
M	Alzheimer's Association	http://www.alz.org/
M	American Academy of Child and Adolescent Psychiatry	http://www.aacap.org/
N	National League for Nursing	http://www.nln.org/researchgrants/index.htm
M	American Psychiatric Association	https://www.psychiatry.org/
V	Foundation Center	http://www.foundationcenter.org
V	Robert Wood Johnson Foundation	http://www.rwjf.org/
P	The Annie E. Casey Foundation	http://www.aecf.org/
O	Oncology Nursing Society	http://www.ons.org/
V	Patient Centered Outcomes Research Institute	https://www.pcori.org/
O	American Cancer Society	http://www.cancer.org/
P	National Association of Pediatric Nurse Practitioners	www.napnap.org

G, geriatric; M, mental health; N, nursing issues (e.g., recruitment/retention, competencies); O, oncology; P, pediatric; V, multi-type (nonspecific, general categories).

Additional helpful resources are databases that match a clinician's interests with federal and foundation research grant opportunities. Two databases that most universities have to provide this type of matching include the Sponsored Programs Information Network (SPIN), the world's largest database of sponsored funding opportunities, and Genius Smarts. With information from thousands of different sponsoring agencies, SPIN facilitates the identification of potential grants in an individual's area of interest, once specified in the database. Genius Smarts sends email messages to people registered in the SPIN database whenever there is a match between the identified areas of interest and potential funding opportunities.

Foundation Center is a website that assists individuals learn about and locate foundations that match their individual interests. The center's mission is to support and improve institutional philanthropic efforts by promoting public understanding of the field and assisting grant applicants to succeed. Helpful online education and tutorials on grant writing are also available at this website. Registration is free for Foundation Center.

 The Foundation Center can be found at http://foundationcenter.org

---

Application Criteria

Before proceeding with an application to a specific funding agency or organization, the criteria required to apply for a grant need to be identified. For example, to be eligible for a research grant from some professional organizations, membership in the organization is required. In addition, some foundations require that the grant applicant live in a particular geographical area to apply for funding. Obtaining this type of information as well as conducting a background investigation on a particular organization or foundation will save precious time and energy in that grant applications will be submitted only to sources that match your interest area and qualifications.

Some grant writers find it helpful to contact an individual from the agency or to write a letter of inquiry with an abstract of the proposed project before actually writing and submitting the full proposal for funding. The names and contact information for program officers (i.e., the program development/administration contact personnel for grant applicants) are typically listed on an agency's home page. Although some individuals prefer to write the grant abstract after the entire proposal is completed, others find it worthwhile to develop the abstract first and seek up-front consultation about the project's compatibility with a potential funding agency's interests.

Importance of the Abstract

The proposal's abstract is key to the success of the proposal and should create a compelling case for why the project needs to be funded. Important components of the abstract should include the following:

- Clinical significance of the project, including the **"so what?" factor** (i.e., the potential impact of the project) (Melnyk & Morrison-Beedy, 2012);
- Study's aims or hypotheses/study questions;
- Conceptual or **theoretical framework**;
- Design and methods, including sample and outcome variables to be measured, as well as the intervention if the study is a clinical trial;
- Approach to analyses.

Finding a Match

If the preconsultation indicates that the proposed work is not a good match for the potential funding agency, fight off discouragement. Much time and energy will be saved in developing a grant proposal for an agency that is interested in the project as opposed to one that is not. Because grant funding is very competitive, consider targeting several potential funding sources to which your proposal can be submitted simultaneously. However, first determine whether multiple submissions of essentially the same proposal to different funding agencies are allowed by carefully reading the guidelines for submission or asking the program officer from the funding source. Also, keep in mind that various agencies may be willing to fund specific parts of the overall project budget.

Once potential funding agencies are identified, it is extremely beneficial to obtain copies of successfully funded proposals if available. Review of these proposals for substantive quality as well as layout and formatting often strengthens the proposal, especially for first-time grant applicants. Federal agencies (e.g., NIH, AHRQ, PCORI, CDC) will provide copies of successfully funded proposals on request; however, the time to obtain them can be lengthy. A better approach is contacting the PI to ask for a copy of his or her funded grant.

Grant writing tip sheets are available at https://grants.nih.gov/grants/grant_tips.htm
In addition, abstracts of past and currently funded federal proposals are available at NIH RePORTER at https://projectreporter.nih.gov/reporter.cfm

For copies of grants funded by professional organizations and foundations, requests should be made directly to the investigator(s). Abstracts of currently funded projects from professional organizations and foundations are often available on their websites or publicized in their newsletters.

Guidelines for Submission

Before writing the proposal, guidelines for grant submission should be obtained from each potential funding source (e.g., length of the proposal, desired font, specifications on margins), reviewed carefully, and followed meticulously. Some funding agencies will return the grant proposals if all directions are not followed, which may delay their evaluation until the next review cycle. Also, be sure that the grant proposal looks pleasing aesthetically and does not contain grammatical and typographical errors. A well-organized proposal that is clear and free of errors indicates to reviewers that the actual project will be carried out with the same meticulous detail.

Criteria for Rating and Reviewing

In addition to obtaining the guidelines for grant submission, ask whether the funding agency provides grant applicants with the criteria on which grants are rated and reviewed.

The NIH publishes the review criteria on which grant applications are rated by reviewers at https://grants.nih.gov/grants/peer-review.htm

In addition to overall impact of the project, the following core criteria are fairly typical of rating systems used by multiple funding agencies:

- **Significance of the study:** Does the project address an important problem or a critical barrier to progress in the field? How will successful completion of the aims change the concepts, methods, technologies, treatments, services, or preventive interventions that drive this field?

- **Investigator(s):** Are the project directors (PDs)/PIs, collaborators, and other researchers well suited to the project?
- **Innovation:** Does the application challenge and seek to shift current research or clinical practice paradigms by using novel theoretical concepts, approaches or methodologies, instrumentation, or interventions?
- **Approach:** Are the overall strategy, methodology, and analyses well reasoned and appropriate to accomplish the specific aims of the project? Are potential problems, alternative strategies, and benchmarks for success presented?
- **Environment:** Will the scientific environment in which the work will be done contribute to the probability of success? Are the institutional support, equipment, and other physical resources available to the investigators adequate for the project proposed?

In addition, reviewers are typically asked to rate the overall impact of the study being proposed, specifically whether it will have a meaningful and sustained influence on the field. Other review criteria include (a) protection for human subjects and (b) inclusion of women, minorities, and children (National Institutes of Health, n.d.).

Develop the Outline

Before writing the proposal, it helps to develop an outline including each component of the grant application with a timeline and deadline for completion. If working within a team, the PI can then assign specific sections of the grant proposal to various team members. Team members should be informed that the document may require several revisions before the final product is ready for submission.

As a rule of thumb, it is important to avoid the "old and predictable." Grant reviewers look favorably on innovative projects. In addition, never assume that the reviewers will know what you mean when you are writing the grant. Writing with clarity and providing rationales for the decisions that you have made about your design and methods are instrumental in receiving a positive grant review.

At the same time, avoid promising too much or too little within the context of the grant. Thinking that it is advantageous to accomplish a multitude of goals within one study is a commonly held belief, but projects that are so ambitious in scope that feasibility is in question tend to fare poorly in review.

Any time your team lacks a particular expertise related to your project, it is important to obtain expert consultants who can provide guidance in needed areas. These individuals can critique the proposal to strengthen the application before it is submitted. Of additional benefit is a mock review in which successful grant writers and others with expertise in the project area are convened to critique the grant's strengths and limitations. With this type of feedback, you can strengthen the grant application before it is even submitted for funding consideration. Another strategy is to ask individuals with no expertise in the project area to read the grant proposal and provide feedback on its clarity.

Some individuals find it helpful to place a draft of the grant aside for a few days, and then read it again. A fresh perspective a few days later is often invaluable in making final revisions. Additionally, obtaining an editorial review of the grant proposal before submitting it is important to achieve the strongest possible product. See Box 22.2 for a summary of general strategies for successful grant writing.

SPECIFIC STEPS IN WRITING A SUCCESSFUL GRANT PROPOSAL

The typical components of a grant proposal are listed in Box 22.3. Although not all of these components may be required for every grant, it helps to consider each one when planning the project.

General Strategies for Writing and Funding Grant Proposals

- Possess the five Ps: (1) passion; (2) planning; (3) persuasion; (4) persistence; and (5) patience.
- Remember, you never get a second chance to make a great first impression. Submit a high-quality proposal the first time.
- Formulate a great team with the expertise needed to successfully conduct the project.
- Write a concise, compelling abstract of the project that addresses the **"so what" factor**.
- Identify potential funding sources that match your project.
- Obtain presubmission consultation from staff at the potential funding agency to determine whether the project is a good match with the agency's priorities.
- Obtain and meticulously follow the guidelines for grant submission from the potential funding agency.
- Review successfully funded proposals from the same funding agency.
- Obtain the criteria on which grants are rated if available from the funding agency.
- Develop a topical outline of the proposal with a timeline for when specific components will be completed.
- Be innovative; avoid the "old and predictable."
- Write with clarity and provide rationales for your decisions; always justify!
- Do not promise too much or too little.
- Conduct a mock review of the proposal in which both experts and nonexperts in the area can critique it.
- Make the document look aesthetically pleasing.
- Spell check and also personally review the document for grammatical and typographical errors.
- Obtain editorial review before the proposal is submitted.
- Celebrate successful completion of the grant!

Typical Components of a Grant Application

- Abstract
- Table of contents
- Budget
- Biosketches of investigators (usually a condensed two- to three-page curriculum vitae or resume)
- Specific aims
- Introduction to the problem
- Goals or objectives of the study
- Research hypotheses or research questions
- Background for the study, including background, impact, and innovation of the project
- Critical review and synthesis of the literature (consider the inclusion of a table that summarizes findings from prior studies)

> BOX
> **22.3**   *Typical Components of a Grant Application*
>   *(continued)*
>
> - Discussion on how the proposed work will fill a gap in prior work or extend what is known
> - Theoretical/conceptual framework
> - Prior research experience of the investigators
> - Inclusion of prior studies by the principal or lead investigator and research team as well as professional experience
> - Research methods
> - Design (e.g., experimental, nonexperimental)
> - Methods
> - Sample and setting (selection criteria, sampling design, plans for recruitment of subjects)
> - Intervention if applicable (detailed descriptions of experimental and control or comparison interventions)
> - Variables with measures (validity and reliability information for each measure)
> - Procedure for data collection
> - Approach to data analysis
> - Potential limitations with alternative strategies
> - Timetable for the proposed work
> - Human subjects and ethical considerations
> - Consultants
> - References
> - Appendix
> - Letters of support
> - Instruments
> - Resources available and environment
> - Prior publications

The Abstract

A large amount of time should be invested in developing a clear, compelling, comprehensive, and concise abstract of the project. Because it is a preview of what is to come, the abstract needs to pique the interest and excitement of the reviewers so that they will be compelled to thoroughly read the rest of the grant application. A poorly written abstract will immediately set the tone for the review and may bias the reviewers to judge the full proposal negatively or dissuade them from reading the rest of the proposal, given that reviewers typically review multiple grant applications simultaneously. See Box 22.4 for two examples of grant abstracts from funded grants that are clear and comprehensive as well as concise and compelling.

Table of Contents

The table of contents containing the components of the grant and corresponding page numbers must be completed accurately so that a reviewer who wants to refer back to a section of the grant can easily identify and access it.

BOX 22.4

Examples of Grant Abstracts From Two Funded Studies

Example #1: Functional Outcomes After Intensive Care Among Elders

Funded by the American Nurses Foundation (Principal investigator: Diane Mick, PhD, RN, CCNS, GNP; Total cost = $2,700).

Objective: Both age and probability of benefit have been suggested as criteria for allocation of healthcare resources. This study will evaluate elders' functional outcomes after intensive care in an effort to discern benefit or futility of interventions.
Methods: A descriptive correlational design will be used. Subjects who are 65 years of age will be identified as "elderly" or "frail elderly" on admission to the ICU, using Katz's Index of Activities of Daily Living scale. Illness severity will be quantified using the Acute Physiology and Chronic Health Evaluation II Scale. Functional status at admission and at discharge from the ICU, and at 1-month and 3-month post-ICU discharge intervals will be quantified with the Medical Outcomes Study 36-Item Short-Form Health Survey (SF-36). Significance of relationships among age, frailty, gender, illness severity, and functional outcomes will be determined, as well as which patient characteristics and clinical factors are predictive of high levels of physical functioning after ICU discharge.
Significance: Findings may be useful as an adjunct to clinical decision making. As the clinicians who are closest to critically ill elderly patients, nurses are positioned to facilitate dialogue about elderly patients' wishes and expectations.

Example #2: Cope/Healthy Lifestyles For Teens: A School-Based RCT

Funded by the NIH/National Institute of Nursing Research (Principal Investigator: Bernadette Mazurek Melnyk, PhD, RN, CPNP/PMHNP, FAANP, FNAP, FAAN; Coinvestigators: Diana Jacobson, PhD, RN, CPNP; Stephanie Kelly, PhD, RN, FNP; Michael Belyea, PhD; Gabriel Shaibi, PhD; Leigh Small, PhD, RN, FAANP, FAAN; Judith O'Haver, PhD, RN, CPNP; and Flavio F. Marsiglia, PhD. [R01NR012171]; Total cost = $2.3 million).

The prevention and treatment of obesity and mental health disorders in adolescents are two major public health problems in the United States today. The incidence of adolescents who are overweight or obese has increased dramatically over the past 20 years, with approximately 17.1% of teens now being overweight or obese. Furthermore, approximately 15 million children and adolescents (25%) in the United States have a mental health problem that is interfering with their functioning at home or at school, but less than 25% of those affected receive any treatment for these disorders. The prevalence rates of obesity and mental health problems are even higher in Hispanic teens, with studies suggesting that the two conditions often coexist in many youth. However, despite the rapidly increasing incidence of these two public health problems with their related health disparities and adverse health outcomes, there has been a paucity of theory-based intervention studies conducted with adolescents in high schools to improve their healthy lifestyle behaviors as well as their physical and mental health outcomes. Unfortunately, physical and mental health services continue to be largely separated instead of integrated in the nation's healthcare system, which often leads to inadequate identification and treatment of these significant adolescent health problems.

Therefore, the goal of the proposed RCT is to test the efficacy of the COPE/Healthy Lifestyles TEEN Program, an educational and cognitive-behavioral skills-building intervention guided by cognitive behavior theory, on the healthy lifestyle behaviors and depressive symptoms of 800 culturally diverse adolescents enrolled in Phoenix, Arizona high schools. The specific aims of the study are to (1) use a RCT to test the short- and more long-term efficacy of the COPE TEEN Program on key outcomes, including healthy

BOX 22.4

Examples of Grant Abstracts From Two Funded Studies (continued)

lifestyles behaviors, depressive symptoms, and body mass index percentage; (2) examine the role of cognitive beliefs and perceived difficulty in leading a healthy lifestyle in mediating the effects of COPE on healthy lifestyle behaviors and depressive symptoms; and (3) explore variables that may moderate the effects of the intervention on healthy lifestyle behaviors and depressive symptoms, including race/ethnicity, gender, SES, acculturation, and parental healthy lifestyle beliefs and behaviors. Six prior pilot studies support the need for this full-scale clinical trial and the use of cognitive-behavioral skills building in promoting healthy lifestyles beliefs, behaviors, and optimal mental health in teens.

This study is consistent with the NIH roadmap and goals of improving people's health and preventing the onset of disease and disability as well as promoting the highest level of health in a vulnerable population.

COPE, Creating Opportunities for Personal Empowerment; ICU, intensive care unit; NIH, National Institutes of Health; RCT, randomized controlled trial; SES, socioeconomic status; TEEN, Thinking, Feeling, Emotions, and Exercise.

Budget

Many hospitals and universities have research centers or offices with an administrator specifically skilled in developing budgets for grant proposals. It is helpful to seek the assistance of this person, if available, when developing the budget for your project, to avoid overestimating or underestimating costs. Knowing which expenses the funding organization will and will not cover is important before developing the budget. This information is often included in the potential funder's guidelines for grant submission.

Most budgets have two categories: personnel and non-personnel (e.g., travel, costs associated with purchasing instruments, honoraria for the subjects). Many professional organizations pay only for **direct costs** (i.e., those costs directly required to conduct the study, such as personnel, travel, photocopying, instruments, and subject fees) and not for **indirect costs** (i.e., those costs that are not directly related to the actual conduct of the study but are associated with the "overhead" in an organization, such as lights, telephones, office space). Reviewers will critically analyze whether there are appropriate and adequate personnel to carry out the study and whether the costs requested are allowable and reasonable. In applying for small grants from professional organizations and foundations, which may not provide enough funds to cover a portion of the salaries for the investigators/clinicians who will implement the project, it is important to negotiate release time with administrators during the preparation of the grant so that there will be ample time to successfully complete the project if funded. Typically, subscriptions to journals, professional organization memberships, and entertainment are examples of nonallowable costs. See Table 22.2 for an example of a grant application's proposed budget.

Biosketches of the Principal Investigator and Research Team Members

For the review panel to assess the qualifications of the research team so that it can judge the team's ability to conduct the proposed project, **biosketches** are typically required as part of the grant application. A biosketch is a condensed two- to four-page document, similar to a resume or brief curriculum vitae, which captures the individual's educational and professional work experience, honors, prior research grants, and publications.

TABLE
22.2

Example of a Grant Application's Proposed Budget

Principal Investigator	Mary Smith
Funding Agency	ANF
Submission Date	02-01-18
Earliest Start Date	09-01-18

Personnel	Role of project	First Year Type of Appointment	% of Effort	Base Salary ($)	Salary ($)	Benefit Rate (%)	Benefits ($)	Total Salary and Benefits ($)
Mary Smith	Principal investigator	12	5	68,000	3,400	28.50	969	4,369
Roberta Picarazzi	Coinvestigator	12	5	68,000	3,400	28.50	969	4,369
TBA (24 hours at $38/hr)	Research associate	12			912	28.50	260	1,172
TBA (49 hours at $18/hr)	Research assistant	12			882	31.00	273	1,155
					0		0	0
					8,594		2,471	11,065
Consultant costs								0
NA								
Equipment								0
NA								
Supplies								50
General office supplies	50							
Travel								0
Local								

(continued)

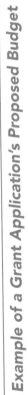

TABLE 22.2 *Example of a Grant Application's Proposed Budget (continued)*

Item				
Domestic				
Other expenses				4,350
Laboratory supplies		500		
Pharmacy setup fee				
Drug/material costs and labor	$15/d × 3 d	3,600	Sample size = 80	
Photocopying		50		
Instrument for data collection				
Patient satisfaction tool				
Human subjects				
Consent form				
Presentation materials (poster and slides)		200		
Subtotal direct costs for initial budget period				15,465
Consortium/contractual costs				
Direct costs				
Indirect costs				
Total direct costs for initial budget period				15,465
Less equipment costs				15,465
Indirect costs				—

NA, not applicable; TBA, to be announced.

Introduction and Specific Aims

The significance of the problem should be immediately introduced in the grant proposal so that the reviewers can make the judgment that the project is worth funding right from the beginning of the proposal. The **"so what?" factor**, which is a term used to describe the development and conduct of a study or project with high-impact potential, should be discussed in the introduction (Melnyk & Morrison-Beedy, 2012; see Chapter 21). Key questions that every individual needs to reflect on as they begin to develop a study or project include the following:

- "So what" is the prevalence of the problem?
- "So what" will be the end outcome of the study or project once completed?
- "So what" difference will the study or project make in improving health, education or healthcare quality, costs, and, most importantly, patient, family, or community outcomes? (Melnyk & Morrison-Beedy, 2012)

For example, the following introduction is quickly convincing of the "so what?" outcome factor and the need for more intervention studies with teenagers who use tobacco:

Approximately 3,000 adolescents become regular tobacco users every day. Evidence from prior studies indicates that teens who smoke are more likely to abuse other substances, such as alcohol and drugs, than teens who do not smoke. There also is accumulating evidence that morbidities associated with cigarette smoking include hypertension, hypocholesteremia, and lung and heart disease.

In the introduction to the grant, it is important to be clear about what the study will accomplish (i.e., the goals or objectives). For example, "This proposal will evaluate the effects of a conceptually driven, reproducible intervention program on smoking cessation in 15- to 18-year-old adolescents."

Background and Significance

In this section of the grant proposal, it is important to convince the reviewers that the problem being presented is worthy of study because the findings are likely to improve the clinical practice and/or health outcomes of a specific population. How the proposal will extend the science in the area or have a positive impact on clinical practice should be explicitly stated. In addition, a comprehensive but concise review of prior studies in the area should be presented along with a critical analysis of their major strengths and limitations, including the gaps of prior work. It is beneficial to use a table to summarize the sample, design, measures, outcomes, and major limitations of prior studies. The literature review must clearly provide justification for the proposed study's aims, hypotheses, and/or research questions.

The inclusion of a well-defined conceptual or theoretical framework is important in guiding the study and explaining findings of the study. If a separate section devoted to the conceptual or theoretical framework is not specified in the guidelines for grant submission, it is typically included in the background section of the proposal. When crafted appropriately, it is clear how the theoretical/conceptual framework is driving the study hypotheses, the intervention if applicable, the outcomes, and/or the relationship between the proposed study variables. This section of the grant should also include definitions of the constructs being measured along with a description of how the constructs to be studied relate to one another.

For example, if an individual is using a coping framework to study the effects of a stress-reduction intervention program with working women, it would be important in the theoretical framework to state that coping comprises two functions: emotional coping, which regulates emotional responses (e.g., anxiety and depression), and functional coping, which is the solving of problems (e.g., the ability to demonstrate high-quality work performance). Therefore, a study of working women that uses this coping framework should evaluate the effects of the stress-reduction program on the outcome measures of anxiety, depression, and work performance.

The background section should conclude with the study's **hypotheses**, which are statements about the predicted relationships between the **independent** and **dependent** or **outcome variables**. Hypotheses should be clear, testable, and plausible. The following is an example of a well-written hypothesis:

> *Family caregivers who receive the CARE program (i.e., the independent variable or treatment) will report less depressive symptoms (i.e., the dependent variable) than family caregivers who receive the comparison program at 2 months following their relative's discharge from the hospital.*

When there is not enough prior literature on which to formulate a hypothesis, the investigator may instead present a research question to be answered by the project. For example, if no prior intervention studies have been conducted with family caregivers of hospitalized older adults, instead of proposing a hypothesis, it would be more appropriate to ask the following research question: "What is the effect of an educational intervention on anxiety and depressive symptoms in family caregivers of hospitalized older adults?"

Prior Research Experience

A summary of professional experience and/or prior work conducted by the PI or project coordinator as well as the research team members should be included in the grant application. Inclusion of this type of information demonstrates that a solid foundation has been laid on which to conduct the proposed study and leaves the reviewers feeling confident that the research team will be able to complete the work that it is proposing.

Study Design and Methods

The design of the study should be clearly described. For example, "This is a **randomized controlled trial** with repeated measures at 3 and 6 months following discharge from the neonatal intensive care unit." Another example might be, "The purpose of this 6-month project is to determine the effect of implementing transdisciplinary rounds on care delivery and patient outcomes in the burn/trauma unit of a large tertiary hospital."

In discussing the study's methods, it is important to provide rationales for the selected methods so that the reviewers will know that you have critically thought about potential options and made the best decision, based on your critical analysis. Nothing should be left to the reviewers' imagination and all decisions should be justified.

If the proposed study is an intervention trial, it is very important to discuss the strategies that will be undertaken to strengthen the **internal validity** of the study (i.e., the ability to say that it was the independent variable or the treatment that caused a change in the dependent variable, not other extraneous factors). See Chapter 21 for a discussion of strategies to minimize threats to internal validity in **quantitative studies**.

The sample should be described in this section of the proposal, including its inclusion criteria (i.e., who will be included in the study) and exclusion criteria (i.e., who will be excluded from participation), as well as exactly how the subjects will be recruited into the study. The feasibility of recruiting the targeted number of subjects should also be discussed, and support letters confirming access to the sample should be included in the grant application's appendix. In addition, it is essential to have a description of how subjects from both genders as well as diverse cultural groups will be included. If people younger than 21 years will not be a part of the research sample, it is imperative to provide a strong rationale for their exclusion because Public Law 103–43 requires that women and children be included in studies funded by the federal government. In quantitative studies, a **power analysis** (i.e., a procedure for estimating sample size) should always be included (Cohen, 1992). This calculation is critical for the reviewers to know that there is an adequate sample size for the statistical analysis. Remember, **power** (i.e., the ability of a study to detect existing relationships among variables and thereby reject the null hypothesis that there is no relationship (Polit & Beck, 2016) in a study increases when sample size increases. Many clinical research studies do not obtain significant findings solely because the sample size is not large enough and the study does not have adequate power to detect significant relationships between variables.

Next, the sampling design (e.g., **random** or **convenience sampling**) should be described. When it is not possible to randomly sample subjects when conducting a study, strategies to increase representativeness of the sample and enhance **external validity** (i.e., **generalizability**) should be discussed. For example, the investigators might choose to recruit subjects from a second study site.

For intervention studies/clinical trials, all components of the intervention must be clearly described (Melnyk & Morrison-Beedy, 2012). Discussion about how the theoretical/conceptual framework guided the development of the intervention will help the reviewers see a clear connection between them. Issues of reproducibility and feasibility of the proposed intervention should also be discussed. In addition, it is important to include information about what the comparison or **attention control group** will receive throughout the study.

For intervention studies, it is important to provide details regarding how the integrity of the intervention will be maintained (i.e., how the intervention will be delivered in the same manner to all subjects), as well as assurance that the intervention will be culturally sensitive. Additionally, it is important to include a discussion about what type of **manipulation checks** (i.e., assessments to determine whether subjects actually processed the content of the intervention or followed through with the activities prescribed in the intervention program) will be used in the study. **"Booster" interventions** (i.e., additional interventions at timed intervals after the initial intervention) are a good idea to include in the study's design if long-term benefits of an intervention are desired.

It is important to include how outcomes of the study will be measured. If using formal instruments, describe each measure in the grant proposal, including **face**, **content**, and **construct validity** (i.e., does the instrument measure what it is intended to measure?) and **reliability** (i.e., does the instrument measure the construct consistently?). In addition, describe the scoring of each of the instruments along with their cultural sensitivity. Justification for why a certain measure was selected is important, especially if there are multiple valid and reliable instruments available that tap the same construct. If collecting patient outcomes, descriptions of how, when, and by whom the data will be collected should be included in the proposal. Incorporating outcomes in studies and projects that the current healthcare system is most concerned about (e.g., patient complications, rehospitalizations, length of stay, costs) is especially important to speed the translation at which findings are incorporated into real-world practice settings.

Internal consistency reliability (i.e., the degree to which all the subparts of an instrument are measuring the same attribute of an instrument [Polit & Beck, 2016]) should be at least 80%, whereas **interrater reliability** (i.e., the degree to which two different observers assign the same ratings to an attribute being measured or observed [Polit & Beck, 2016]) should be at least 90% and assessed routinely to correct for any **observer drift** (i.e., a decrease in interrater reliability; Melnyk & Morrison-Beedy, 2012). For intervention studies, it is important to include measures that are sensitive to change over time (i.e., those with low test–retest reliabilities) so that the intervention can demonstrate its ability to affect the study's outcome variables.

When conducting research, both self-report and nonbiased observation measures should be included whenever possible because convergence of both of these types of measures will increase the credibility of the study's findings. In addition, the use of valid and reliable instruments is preferred whenever possible over the use of instruments that are newly developed and lacking established validity and reliability.

The procedure or protocol for the study should be clearly described. Specific information about the timing of data collection for all measures should be discussed. Using a table helps summarize the study protocol in a concise snapshot so that reviewers can quickly grasp when the study's measures will be collected (Table 22.3).

TABLE
22.3   *Summary of a Study's Protocol*

Variables	Measures	Cronbach's Alphas	Times for Data Collection								
			1	2	3	4	5	6	7	8	9
Maternal Emotional Outcomes											
State anxiety	State anxiety inventory (A-state)	0.94–0.96	•	•	•	•		•	•	•	•
Negative mood state	POMS	0.92–0.96	•	•	•	•		•	•	•	•
Depression	Depression subscale, POMS	0.92–0.96	•	•	•	•	•	•	•	•	•
Stress related to PICU	PSS:PICU	0.90–0.91	•	•							
Posthospitalization stress	Posthospitalization stress index for parents	0.83–0.85	•	•	•	•					
Maternal Functional Outcomes											
Parent participation in care	Index of parent participation	0.85	•	•							
Other Key Maternal Variables											
Parental beliefs	Parental beliefs scale	0.91	•								
Manipulation checks evaluation	Manipulation checks self-report questionnaire	NA	•	•	•	•					
		NA	•	•	•	•					
Child Adjustment Outcomes											
Posthospitalization stress	Posthospitalization stress index for children	0.78–0.85	•	•	•	•					
Child behavior	Behavioral assessment scale for children	0.92–0.95	•	•	•	•	•				

Notes: Example of a study protocol for a randomized controlled trial to determine the effects of an intervention program on the coping outcomes of young critically ill children and their mothers. Time 1, phase I intervention (6 to 16 hours after PICU admission); Time 2, phase II intervention (16 to 30 hours after PICU admission); Time 3, phase III intervention (2 to 6 hours after transfer to pediatric unit); Time 4, observation contact (24 to 36 hours after transfer to pediatric unit); Time 5, phase III intervention (2 to 3 days following hospital discharge); Time 6, 1 month postdischarge follow-up (1 month following hospital discharge); Time 7, 3 months postdischarge follow-up (3 months following hospital discharge); Time 8, 6 months postdischarge follow-up (6 months following hospital discharge); Time 9, 12 months postdischarge follow-up (12 months following hospital discharge).

NA, not applicable; PICU, pediatric intensive care unit; POMS, profile of mood states; PSS, parental stressor scale.

The description of data analysis must include specific and clear explanations about how the data to answer each of the study hypotheses or research questions will be analyzed. Adding a statistical consultant to your study team to assist with the writing of the statistical section and the analysis of the study's data will fare favorably in the review process.

Even if the guidelines for the proposal do not call for it, it is very advantageous to include a section in the grant that discusses potential limitations of the proposal with alternative approaches. Doing so demonstrates to the reviewers that potential limitations of the study have been recognized, along with plans for alternative strategies that will be employed to overcome them. For example, inclusion of strategies to guard against study attrition (i.e., loss of subjects from your study) would be important to discuss in this section.

A timetable that indicates when specific components of the study will be started and completed should be included in the grant application (Figure 22.1). This projected timeline should be realistic and feasible.

Human Subjects

When writing a research proposal, it is essential to discuss the risks and benefits of study participation, protection against risks, and the importance of the knowledge to be gained from the study. The demographics of the sample that you intend to recruit into your study are also very important to describe in the proposal. In addition, the process through which informed consent will be obtained needs to be discussed, along with how confidentiality of the data will be maintained. Some funding agencies require the proposal to be reviewed and approved by an appropriate research subject review board, and others require proof of approval if funding is awarded before commencement of the project.

In addition, if a study is a clinical trial, federal agencies (e.g., NIH) require a **data and safety monitoring plan**, which outlines how adverse effects will be assessed and managed.

If applying to the NIH for funding, Public Law 103–43 requires that women and minorities be included in all studies unless there is acceptable scientific justification provided as to why their inclusion is not feasible or appropriate with regard to the health of the subjects or the purpose of the research. NIH also requires that children younger than 21 years be included in research unless there are ethical or scientific reasons for their exclusion.

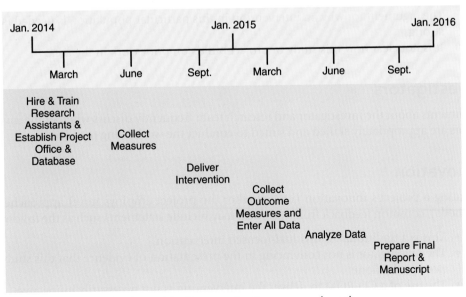

Figure 22.1: Sample timetable for a project's proposed work.

More specific information on the protection and inclusion of human subjects can be found in Chapter 23 and at http://grants.nih.gov/grants/frequent_questions.htm

Consultants, References, and Appendices

A section for consultants is often included in grant applications. The expertise and role of each consultant on the project should be described.

Each citation referenced in the grant proposal should be included in the reference list. All references should be accurate, complete, and formatted according to the guidelines for submission (e.g., American Psychological Association [APA] or American Medical Association [AMA] formatting).

Grant applications typically require or allow the investigator to include letters of support from consultants or study sites, copies of instruments that will be used in the study, lists of resources available, and publications of the research team that support the application. Support letters from consultants indicate to the reviewers that they are enthusiastic about the proposed study or project and that they are committed to their role on the project. Letters of support from study sites help indicate enthusiasm for the study and permission for subjects to be recruited from those sites.

COMMON FEEDBACK FROM GRANT REVIEWS

This section of the chapter describes typical feedback that you may receive from the individuals who review your grant. The feedback is often organized according to typical categories used for rating grant applications. It should help strengthen your proposed study and facilitate your professional growth.

Significance

Reviewers typically judge the significance of a project by whether the study addresses an important problem or extends what is known in the area. Common feedback in this category may include statements such as the following:

- The literature does not capture the entire body of information on the selected concepts.
- The argument for why an intervention in this particular population is needed is not strong.
- It is not clear how this study or project builds on prior work in the area.

Investigators

Comments about the investigator and research team frequently discuss whether the investigators are appropriately skilled and suited to conduct the work being proposed.

Innovation

In rating a project's innovation (i.e., whether the project employs novel approaches or methods), common feedback from reviewers may include statements such as the following:

- This is a traditional, individual-focused intervention.
- The investigator is not convincing in the presentation of evidence that this study needs to be done.
- The use of a CD-ROM to deliver the intervention is not necessarily innovative, given the wide array of media currently available.

Approach

Common feedback regarding a research study's approach (e.g., conceptual framework, design, methods, and analyses) typically includes statements such as the following:

- The conceptual/theoretical framework to guide the study is weak.
- The theory does not drive the proposed intervention or the selection of study variables.
- The study design is weak.
- Some of the details for the methods are unclear.
- The sample size is not adequate to test the hypotheses.
- The measures are not adequately described.
- The data analysis section needs a fuller discussion.
- The number of measures being used creates too much burden for the subjects.
- The project is too ambitious for the timetable proposed.

In addition, comments from reviewers about intervention studies typically focus on concerns about cross-contamination between the experimental and control groups (e.g., sharing of experimental information), reproducibility and feasibility of the intervention, and cultural sensitivity.

Environment

Reviewers typically comment on whether the environment is conducive to support the work being proposed (e.g., whether there is evidence of enough resources and institutional support for the project).

Major Pitfalls of Grant Proposals

There are numerous weaknesses in grant proposals that limit their ability to fare well during the review process. Box 22.5 outlines these common pitfalls.

BOX 22.5 *Major Pitfalls of Grant Proposals*

- Lack of new or original ideas
- Failure to acknowledge published relevant work
- Fatal flaws in the study design or methods
- Applications that are incomplete or do not contain enough detail about the methods
- Unrealistic amount of work
- Uncritical approach
- Human subjects concerns
- Absence of a theory or conceptual framework that guides the intervention and/or study variables
- Absence of links to current literature
- Lack of significance
- Inappropriate or weak data analysis plan
- Promising too much or too little

Major Characteristics of Funded Grant Proposals

Unlike proposals that are weak, strong proposals have characteristics that enhance their fundability. These characteristics include the following:

- Potential for high impact in the field;
- Innovation;
- High scientific quality;
- Clarity;
- Excellent technical quality (e.g., organized, easy to read, and free of grammatical and spelling errors);
- Greater depth in thinking about conceptual issues.

Successful grant proposals also include a thoughtful discussion about the limitations of the proposed work as well as strategies for dealing with potential problems without over-emphasizing these issues.

 Copies of successful grant applications funded by NIH are posted on the NIH website and various professional organization-funded applications may be able to be obtained on request. See https://nccih.nih.gov/grants/resources/grantwrite-advice.htm

A Nonfunded Grant: Strategies for Resubmission

Many individuals feel dejected when their proposals are not successful in securing funding. However, openness to constructive feedback, continued belief in one's ability to be successful, and persistence are often necessary to turn a nonfunded proposal into a funded one.

> **"**
> The only limit to our realization of tomorrow
> will be our doubts of today.
>
> **FRANKLIN DELANO ROOSEVELT**

> **"**
> If you believe you can, you probably can. If you believe you
> won't, you most assuredly won't. Belief is the ignition
> switch that gets you off the launching pad.
>
> **DR. DENNIS WAITLEY**

Even the most successful grant writers face rejection at times during their careers. When confronted with a rejected proposal, being able to seek the advice of a seasoned mentor who has faced and overcome grant rejections is invaluable in addressing how you will handle the revisions and further pursuit of funding.

Once a grant proposal is rejected, it is important to determine whether a resubmission will be allowed by the funding agency. If permitted, it is important to ask whether there are specific guidelines for resubmission and, if so, to obtain them. For example, the NIH allows one resubmission of a grant proposal. Individuals who are resubmitting are allowed a certain number of pages as an introduction to the revised proposal in which they specifically respond to how they have addressed the reviewers' concerns and suggestions.

If a resubmission is allowed, it is helpful to discuss the plans for addressing the reviewers' comments with the appropriate program officer or contact person at the funding agency. Individuals from the funding agency can often provide insights into the critique and suggest revisions.

After reading the reviewers' feedback, recognize that it is normal to feel sad, frustrated, and/or angry about the critique. It also is common to believe that the reviewers did not read your grant thoroughly or to feel that they did not understand your work and were overly critical of it. After reading the review comments, it is helpful to file them away for a week or two until you can come back to them with an open mind to begin the process of revising the proposal.

In the introduction to the revised application, first inform the review committee that its critique has assisted you in clarifying and strengthening your proposed work. It is critical to respond point by point to the major issues raised by the review panel, without a defensive posture. If you disagree with a recommendation from the review panel, do so gently and astutely. Be sure to include a good rationale, as in the following example:

> *We agree that cross-contamination is always a concern in clinical intervention studies and have given it thoughtful consideration. However, we believe that this potential problem can be minimized by taking several precautions. For example, we will administer the interventions to the subjects in a private room adjacent to the intensive care unit so that the staff nurses will not overhear the content of the interventions and begin to share it with the families.*

Finally, revise the text enough so that reviewers will note that you took their suggestions seriously, but do not completely rewrite the application as though it were new. Guidelines for resubmission will often inform applicants to use a boldface or italic font to identify the content that has been changed within the context of the grant proposal.

Unhelpful responses in the resubmission process include not taking the reviewers' critique seriously by ignoring their suggestions, as well as denigrating the review panel's criticisms. In addition, changing the research design in an attempt to please the review panel without critical thought and analysis will not fare well in the re-review of the grant proposal.

SPECIFIC CONSIDERATIONS IN SEEKING FUNDS FOR EBP IMPLEMENTATION OR OUTCOMES MANAGEMENT/ EVIDENCE-BASED QUALITY IMPROVEMENT PROJECTS

EBP implementation and outcomes management projects as well as evidence-based quality improvement initiatives that focus on improving practice performance, including changes in care delivery modalities (e.g., primary nursing versus team nursing), system supports for the healthcare team (e.g., electronic health record with clinical decision support system), and evaluation of the effect of a practice change on patient outcomes within a particular environment (e.g., how substance abusers respond to education about drug rehabilitation and the subsequent effect on the recurrence of abuse in a small county rehabilitation program), are usually not funded by federal agencies. Internal funding sources and foundations are typically the most viable places to obtain funding for these types of endeavors. The application process for a foundation can range in rigor from a one- to two-page abstract to a full-scale NIH-style grant proposal.

For internal sources of funding within one's institution (e.g., colleges/schools of nursing, academic health centers, hospitals), guidelines are usually available on request from the research office, if one exists, or from the department that handles professional, educational, or research affairs. As with other types of grant applications, obtaining and explicitly following the guidelines for submission are essential for success. In both cases, one of the primary tenets of securing funding is that the project reflects the mission and stated goals of the organization or foundation. Specifically, the grant application needs to be an excellent match, often between what the funding source desires and what can be provided. Generally, foundations are very clear about the specific areas in which they are willing to provide fiscal support. For example, a major funding area for the Kellogg Foundation is ensuring that children obtain the education they need to be successful in life.

 More specific information about the Kellogg Foundation and a list of recent grant awards can be found on their website at http://www.wkkf.org/

Many universities and medical centers have a foundation relations office that can assist individuals in locating a good foundation match and pursuing funding for their proposals. In fact, some universities and medical centers require that all requests for foundation funds be streamlined through their foundation relations office so that multiple applications from various departments are not submitted simultaneously to the same foundation.

One way to determine whether the foundation that you wish to query about funding is a good match with your project is to peruse projects that were recently funded, which can typically be found on the foundation's website. Scanning the list of these funded projects can provide a sense of the types of projects that are currently being funded. If few to no healthcare projects are funded, realize that this may not be a good match and that more inquiry is necessary before soliciting funding from that organization. If you determine that a foundation is a good match for your project, carefully study the requirements for proposal submission. Some foundations require that the first step in the application process include only an abstract of the proposed project. If the abstract matches the organization's goals and is reviewed favorably, the applicant may be asked to provide a more detailed proposal. However, some foundations or organizations may provide funding based on the abstract alone, especially if the budget request is small (e.g., less than $10,000). Other foundations require a full-scale proposal, including detailed budgets and biographical sketches for the PD and team members. By carefully following the guidelines provided by the organization, the chance of funding will increase.

Keep in mind that most foundations require that the sponsoring organization meet the regulations of the U.S. Internal Revenue Service as a 501c3 organization (i.e., tax exempt). When seeking foundation funding, be aware that many foundations seldom provide large funding relative in size to federal grants. In perusing foundation websites, you may note that, on average, most foundation grants range between $500 and $50,000.

An example of an organization that funds initiatives such as outcomes management or evidence-based quality improvement projects is the American Association of Critical-Care Nurses (AACN).

 Information about AACN's small grant opportunities along with specific requirements for submission can be found at http://www.aacn.org

FUNDING FOR EVIDENCE-BASED PRACTICE IMPLEMENTATION PROJECTS

EBP implementation projects are typically clinical projects that use research findings to improve clinical practice. They are usually conceived in response to an identified clinical problem. Unlike research studies that have a goal to generate new knowledge, EBP implementation projects are usually meant to solve clinical problems through the application of existing research-based knowledge (e.g., evidence-based clinical practice guidelines).

The application of the pain management guidelines developed by AHRQ to healthcare settings nationwide is a good example of an EBP implementation project in action. These guidelines were based on sound scientific evidence and developed by nationally known clinical experts. Managers, clinical specialists, and educators then implemented the published guidelines in their clinical settings, measuring clinical outcomes preimplementation and postimplementation.

Sources that fund EBP implementation projects, such as AACN's Small Project Grants, do not generally require the scientific rigor of a typical research proposal. Because this type of funding is small (i.e., usually $500 to $2,500), the timeline from funding to project implementation is short (usually less than 12 months), and the project usually involves the application of well-established research evidence (e.g., guidelines, procedures, and protocols). Thus, the application process is modified accordingly and typically includes the following:

- Cover letter
- Grant application form
- Timetable for the project
- **Budget:** Funding requested and justification for funding requested
- **Evidence of ethical review:** If an institutional review board is not available in the institution, a letter of approval from facility administration should be requested, indicating that they are aware of the project and its implications for their patients.
- **Participant consent:** All subjects in the project must give written consent, especially if the eventual publication of project results is anticipated. (Exception: Data abstraction from medical records with elimination of all patient-specific identifying data.)
- **Program questions:** Specific to each grant, these questions should be answered in detail. When describing the project, use the information outlined in the methods section of this chapter as a general guide.

Remember that many organizations require membership or registration on their websites to be eligible to apply for funding or to gain access to funding guidelines.

Foundations typically restrict their focus to certain populations or service areas (e.g., rural nursing homes). For example, the Washington Square Health Foundation focuses on funding grants to promote and maintain access to adequate healthcare for all people in the Chicagoland area regardless of race, sex, creed, or financial need. This foundation funds medical and nursing educational programs, medical research institutions, and direct healthcare services (e.g., outcomes management initiatives). General guidelines for submitting a grant proposal to the Washington Square Health Foundation include the following:

- Collected assessment data about the healthcare needs of high-risk, underserved, and/or disadvantaged populations in the service area;
- Implemented targeted activities to increase the accessibility of healthcare services to one or more high-risk, underserved, and/or disadvantaged populations;
- Designed and implemented with community involvement, new or expanded services to address the healthcare needs of one or more high-risk, underserved, and/or disadvantaged populations;
- Identified opportunities to increase assets of high-risk, underserved, and/or disadvantaged communities, such as by employing community members as staff in health programs, locating health service delivery sites in the community, and negotiating purchasing contracts with local businesses for health service–related products.

 The Washington Square Health Foundation can be found at http://www.wshf.org

Some foundations fund demonstration and evidence-based quality improvement projects as well as community initiatives versus research because of the desire to influence practice or healthcare improvements quickly. For example, the Fan Fox and Leslie R. Samuels Foundation has shifted the focus of its healthcare program from applied research to patient-based and social service activities that assist older adults in New York City. The refocused program is designed to improve the mechanism for health and social services to be delivered through support to organizations that reflect inventive, useful, competent, and thoughtful care to their patients. Requirements for a grant application to the Fan Fox and Leslie R. Samuels Foundation include the following:

- The program will improve the overall quality of life or healthcare service delivery to New York City's older adult population.
- The program has a realistic, achievable work plan and a rational, well-justified budget.
- The program staff members who will perform the work are experienced and highly qualified.
- The sponsoring organization is stable, competent, and committed.

To submit an abstract for funding to the Fan Fox and Leslie R. Samuels Foundation, applicants must compile a cover sheet with the following information: legal name, address, phone, fax, and email and website addresses (if available) of the institution or organization; the PD's name, address, phone, fax, and email (if available); the name and exact title of the organization's CEO; the program title and its duration; the total dollar amount requested; and a one-paragraph summary of the proposed program. In addition, a three-page letter (1-inch margins, 12-point font) that clearly states the following must be submitted:

- The general problems and issues being addressed and their importance;
- A brief description of the nature of the program and its significance, with clear goals and objectives;
- The recommended approach to care or services that represents an improvement over how services are delivered now; how the proposed program makes care or service provision better;
- A description of the anticipated benefit of the program to older adults, including the number of individuals who will be affected;
- The program's overall significance;
- A summary of the critical activities to be performed, the timeframe for the proposed program, and a brief breakdown of the projected budget;
- If successful, the likelihood that the program will be continued by the institution;
- The commitment of the sponsoring institution (e.g., contribution of salaries, space, overhead) during and after the grant term.

 The Fan Fox and Leslie R. Samuels Foundation can be found at http://www.samuels.org/

The pursuit of foundation funding is a good option to follow for EBP implementation or evidence-based quality improvement projects and outcomes management initiatives. Most requirements for foundation applications are readily available on the internet, which enhances the timeliness of application submission. As with any other funding endeavor, assuring that the foundation or organization's goals are a good match for your project, carefully following the supplied guidelines, and providing the clearest and most informative presentation of the project, whether that be only an abstract or a full proposal, will increase chances for successful funding.

The process of writing a grant proposal is a challenging but rewarding experience. Formulating a great team, judicious planning, careful attention to the detailed requirements of the grant application, and background homework on potential funding sources as well as prior work in the area will facilitate the writing of an innovative, compelling, clear proposal that is matched appropriately to the potential funding agency.

It is helpful to remember that the process of writing a grant proposal resembles the eating of a 2-ton chocolate elephant. If you sit on a stool in front of the elephant and look up, the whole elephant appears too large to consume. However, if you sit on the stool looking straight ahead and consume the part of the elephant that is directly in front of you, then move the stool to the next parts in sequential order and consume them one at a time, soon the whole chocolate elephant will be eaten! In addition, when writing a grant proposal, it is helpful to remember the following individuals who succeeded in their endeavors as the result of not being afraid to take risks in combination with strong belief in themselves and sheer persistence:

- *Babe Ruth struck out 1,330 times. In between his strikeouts, he hit 714 home runs.*
- *R. H. Macy failed in retailing seven times before his store in New York became a success.*
- *Abraham Lincoln failed twice in business and was defeated in six state and national elections before being elected president of the United States.*
- *Theodor S. Geisel wrote a children's book that was rejected by 23 publishers. The 24th publisher sold six million copies of it—the first "Dr. Seuss" book—and that book and its successors are still staples of every children's library (Kouzes & Posner, 2017).*

Remember, successful people often fail their way to success with enthusiasm. This also applies to the process of grant writing. Therefore, keep your dream of the impact that you want to make alive and focus on it every day, prepare well, believe in yourself and your team's ability to write a great grant proposal, seek mentorship and critique, and stay persistent through the "character-builders" to resubmit until your project is funded!

EBP FAST FACTS

- You never get a second chance to make a great impression, so make sure that your grant application follows directions precisely and is of high quality when submitted the first time.
- Comprise a great team that builds on each other's strengths for the project.
- Review grants funded by the organization or agency to which you intend to submit your grant application.
- Be meticulous about planning each component of the application.
- Write a clear compelling abstract that excites reviewers about the project.
- Obtain reviews of your grant from experts before it is officially submitted.
- Do Not Give Up! Persist through the character-builders until your project is funded.

WANT TO KNOW MORE?

A variety of resources is available to enhance your learning and understanding of this chapter.

- Visit thePoint' to access:
  - Articles from the AJN EBP Step-By-Step Series
  - Journal articles
  - Checklists for rapid critical appraisal and more!
- Lippincott CoursePoint combines digital text content with video case studies and interactive modules for a fully integrated course solution that works the way you study and learn.

References

Cohen, J. (1992). A power primer. *Psychological Bulletin, 112*(1), 155–159.

Kouzes, J. M., & Posner, B. Z. (2017). *The leadership challenge* (6th ed.). San Francisco, CA: Jossey-Bass.

Melnyk, B. M., & Morrison-Beedy, D. (2012). *Intervention research: Designing, conducting, analyzing and funding.* New York, NY: Springer Publishing.

National Institutes of Health. (n.d.). *Peer review.* Retrieved from https://grants.nih.gov/grants/peer-review.htm

Polit, D. F., & Beck, C. T. (2016). *Nursing research: Generating and assessing evidence for nursing practice* (10th ed.). Philadelphia, PA: Wolters Kluwer.

23

Ethical Considerations for Evidence Implementation and Evidence Generation

Dónal P. O'Mathúna

> In great affairs men show themselves as they wish to be seen; in small things they show themselves as they are.
>
> —*Nicholas Chamfort*

EBP Terms to Learn

Audit
Autonomy
Beneficence
Justice
Nonmaleficence
Principle of fidelity
Quality assurance

Learning Objectives

After studying this chapter, learners will be able to:

1. Describe the principles of ethics and how they are imperative for all of healthcare, from science to service.

2. Explain the importance of ethics to EBP.

3. Discuss the difference in ethical responsibilities of researchers and clinicians.

CONNECTING EVIDENCE-BASED PRACTICE AND ETHICS

Evidence-based practice (EBP) involves applying evidence to practice, which should lead to improved outcomes. The outcomes resulting from evidence implementation should be carefully evaluated; otherwise, our confidence in applying the evidence can be weak. The impetus for evaluating the implementation of evidence may arise from a commitment to EBP itself or from a commitment to ethical practice and improving outcomes. "How evidence and ethics interrelate is an often neglected and overlooked dimension of evidence-based approaches to health care" (Upshur, 2013, p. 86). Ethical principles influence both the importance of evaluating the impact of evidence on patients and the way those evaluations are conducted.

Ethical Principles

Ethics examines issues of right and wrong, good and bad, in any area of human interaction. Various sets of ethical principles have been articulated to guide healthcare practice. Beauchamp and Childress (2012) developed one widely used approach that focuses on four core ethical principles. **Beneficence** captures the importance of doing good for patients. **Nonmaleficence** addresses the importance of not harming patients. **Autonomy** acknowledges that patients have the right to make decisions about their health, lives, and bodies. **Justice** declares that resources should be distributed fairly among people and without prejudice. The **principle of fidelity** is often added to capture the importance of trust and honesty. Other ethical principles have been proposed to capture the diverse range of situations in which disagreements arise over the right thing to do or the right way to be (Box 23.1). Ethical decision making can be

23.1 Fifteen Ethical Principles of the Universal Declaration on Bioethics and Human Rights

1. Human dignity and human rights
2. Benefit and harm
3. Autonomy and individual responsibility
4. Consent
5. Persons without the capacity to consent
6. Respect for human vulnerability and personal integrity
7. Privacy and confidentiality
8. Equality, justice, and equity
9. Nondiscrimination and nonstigmatization
10. Respect for cultural diversity and pluralism
11. Solidarity and cooperation
12. Social responsibility and health
13. Sharing of benefits
14. Protecting future generations
15. Protection of the environment, the biosphere, and biodiversity

Source: Adapted from ten Have, H. A. M. J., Jean, M. S. (Eds.). (2009). *The UNESCO universal declaration on bioethics and human rights: Background, principles and application* (pp. 360–363). Paris, France: United Nations Educational, Scientific and Cultural Organization. © UNESCO 2009. Retrieved from http://unesdoc.unesco.org/images/0017/001798/179844e.pdf

seen as a method of balancing such principles when they conflict in the complex situations encountered in life and, particularly, in healthcare.

As with any area of healthcare, EBP raises ethical issues. Some of the motivations underlying the advancement of EBP are, at their core, ethical. Organizations in the United States, such as the National Academy of Medicine (NAM; formerly the Institute of Medicine; IOM) and the Agency for Healthcare Research and Quality (AHRQ), have found evidence of problems with the quality of American healthcare (Institute of Medicine [IOM], 2006). Important progress has been made in various areas in recent years (National Committee for Quality Assurance [NCQA], 2012), but more needs to be done in other areas. For example, a systematic review of health interventions for humanitarian settings found significant deficiencies in the available evidence, in spite of the imperative for collecting good data in such settings (Blanchet et al., 2017). The United States spends more per capita on healthcare than any other country in the world, yet performs poorly on many health outcomes (Papanicolas, Woskie, & Jha, 2018). These authors note that the reasons for this are complex but include the overuse of medical services, with various estimates attributing between 20% and 50% of U.S. health spending to overuse (Fred, 2016). This is both an ethical issue of using evidence appropriately and of using resources wisely and justly.

Other countries also report serious problems with their healthcare systems. A survey of primary care doctors in 10 developed countries (i.e., Australia, Canada, France, Germany, the Netherlands, New Zealand, Norway, Switzerland, the United Kingdom, and the United States) identified strengths and weaknesses in each system (Schoen et al., 2012). In another survey of eight developed countries, patients with chronic illnesses reported system-wide problems with their healthcare systems in the areas of access, safety, and care (Schoen, Osborn, How, Doty, & Peugh, 2009). These involve the ethical principles of justice, nonmaleficence, and beneficence.

The NAM has developed a conceptual framework to help understand healthcare quality and how it can be improved practically. It defines quality as "the degree to which health services for individuals and populations increase the likelihood of desired health outcomes and are consistent with current professional knowledge" (IOM, 2018). The core dimensions of quality, as articulated in several NAM reports, are safety, effectiveness, patient-centeredness, timeliness, equity, and efficiency (Baily, Bottrell, Lynn, & Jennings, 2006).

 To learn more about the NAM's Healthcare Quality Framework, visit https://www.ahrq .gov/professionals/quality-patient-safety/talkingquality/create/sixdomains.html

Each of these dimensions is underpinned by ethical principles (see Box 23.1). For example, the ethical principle of increasing benefit and reducing harm promotes safety. The ethical principle of equality, justice, and equity promotes the use of resources according to effectiveness in a timely, equitable fashion. The ethical principle of human dignity (i.e., respect for persons) promotes patient-centeredness and equity. Thus, promotion of healthcare quality can be seen as an ethical enterprise. EBP, as the backbone of all quality initiatives, is also underpinned by the same ethical principles. However, that does not mean that every approach to improving quality is necessarily ethical (or evidence based).

Ethics, Quality Improvement, and Research

Situations where evidence-based quality improvement (EBQI) initiatives (for more information on EBQI, see Chapter 10) could conflict with ethical principles include (a) attempts to improve quality for some patients that may inadvertently cause harm for others, for example, if people or resources are diverted away from them; (b) strategies intended to improve quality that may turn out to be ineffective or even lower the quality of care; and (c) activities declared to be quality improvement (QI) that may be more accurately described as clinical research or vice versa. The term *clinical research* will be used here, although *human subjects research* is also used, especially in regulatory contexts.

Clinical research is defined as research where investigators directly interact with human subjects or material of human origin (National Institutes of Health, 2017). If research activities are carried out without patient informed consent, they may be seen as an unethical use of patients as research subjects (Baily et al., 2006). Research participation is viewed as an optional activity, and informed consent is therefore required to respect the ethical principle of autonomy. In contrast, it may be seen as unethical to require patients to provide their consent for care that is known to provide them with better outcomes compared to their acceptance of mediocre care that does not have that guarantee. Despite these issues, if efforts are not made to improve quality, healthcare professionals may violate their ethical responsibility to promote beneficence and nonmaleficence by providing patients with the most safe and effective clinical care possible. When this violation happens, patients will continue to be put at risk from lower quality healthcare.

One approach to improving the quality of healthcare is referred to as performance improvement (PI) or QI. Such projects can be defined as "systematic, data-guided activities designed to bring about immediate improvements in healthcare delivery in particular settings" (Lynn et al., 2007, p. 667). These activities include an array of methods designed to solve practical clinical problems and to bring about and evaluate change, sometimes based on evidence. Some similarity between QI and EBP can be seen in the description of QI as an approach that "means encouraging people in the clinical care setting to use their daily experience to identify promising ways to improve care, implement changes on a small scale, collect data on the effects of those changes, and assess the results" (Baily et al., 2006, p. S5).

This is much like the EBP paradigm that requires clinicians to bring their expertise as well as empiric knowledge into innovative clinical decision making. However, the QI approach does not explicitly require the participation of the patient as does EBP.

Ethics and EBP Implementation

The EBP implementation approach can be centered on an issue arising in a unit, an institution, or a system. Evidence can be applied to bring about change for one patient, or it may be intended to effect change across a system or profession. Documenting the change is imperative. Here is where the EBP implementation approach is often confused with clinical research. These two enterprises involve human participants and sometimes use similar methods to evaluate outcomes. For some, EBP implementation activities are seen as a form of clinical research that should come under the same ethical and regulatory requirements, particularly the ethical requirement for informed consent. Others claim that some EBP implementation activities are sufficiently different that they should not be considered clinical research. In this view, they would fall within general clinical care and not require explicit informed consent; however, specific ethical principles still apply. One factor often used to distinguish these two approaches is the generalizability of their findings. Clinical research should be conducted with samples that are representative of the population of interest so that the findings can be applied to that population. The ethical principle of justice supports this approach because the group that takes on the additional risks of research participation also benefits from the results. In contrast, implementation of evidence in practice is the application of interventions, practices, or approaches that are known to produce outcomes with some degree of confidence; however, the people to whom the care is provided are not usually representative of the same population. Rather, they are the patients under that provider's care, no matter what the setting (e.g., hospital, community, primary care practice, or long-term care facility). This type of process often occurs when trying to improve the quality of care; however, the goal of EBP implementation is not to generalize the process or the findings (i.e., outcomes). Rather, the goal is to initiate and sustain meaningful change within the clinicians' practice and for particular patients or clients.

Controversy exists around the ethical issues with EBP implementation and how it compares and contrasts with clinical research. The formal processes often seem to be viewed differently by different institutional review boards (IRBs; otherwise known as research ethics committees). Some IRBs and regulators view the EBP implementation process as research based on descriptions of the deliberate application of an evidence-based protocol across all patients and the evaluation of outcomes. However, if clinicians withheld known beneficial treatment from patients, this could be considered unethical. In addition, collection of data, in and of itself, should not be viewed as clinical research. To follow that logic would require that daily intake and output values that are totaled and described would be considered research that produced generalizable knowledge. Research produces knowledge in such a way that it can be applied to a broader population than those from which it came. EBP implementation is applying research, with internal evidence, to improve care. To guard against this issue hindering best practice for patients and violating beneficence, clinicians and IRBs must use caution to ensure that unique ethical requirements for research are applied to research and that the ethical requirements fitting to EBP implementation are appropriately applied.

ETHICAL EXEMPLARS

This ethical debate has raged in the literature for a number of years. Given that the answers accepted will significantly impact efforts to improve the quality of healthcare, it is important to understand these ethical issues. Although much of the debate has been triggered by how these issues have been dealt with in the United States, the ethical issues have relevance for other jurisdictions. Two prominent cases that have triggered much ethical debate are presented in the following section to highlight the issues involved.

> ## It is not fair to ask of others
> ## what you are unwilling to do yourself.
>
> **ELEANOR ROOSEVELT**

An Ethical Exemplar: The Michigan ICU Study

In the United States, thousands of bloodstream infections related to catheters occur each year in intensive care units (ICUs), putting many patients at risk and leading to increased lengths of stay and costs (O'Horo, Maki, Krupp, & Safdar, 2014). Researchers continue to investigate interventions to reduce morbidity and costs (Gandra & Ellison, 2015). In 2004, clinicians from Johns Hopkins University coordinated a prospective cohort study to examine the impact of introducing evidence-based strategies to reduce infection rates in all ICUs in Michigan (to be referred to in this chapter as the Michigan ICU study). Just over 100 ICUs participated in the 18-month study (Pronovost et al., 2006). A large and sustained reduction in rates of catheter-related infections occurred (up to 66% reduction). The median number of infections per 1,000 catheter-days decreased from 2.7 at baseline to 0 during the final study period ($P < 0.002$).

The study involved a number of educational interventions targeted at ICU personnel to improve patient safety. This included designating one physician and one nurse as team leaders in each ICU. The researchers developed a checklist to promote clinicians' use of five evidence-based procedures recommended by the Centers for Disease Control and Prevention. These were (a) hand washing; (b) using full-barrier precautions during insertion of central venous catheters; (c) cleansing the skin with chlorhexidine prior to catheter insertion; (d) avoiding, where possible, the femoral site for catheter insertion; and (e) removing unnecessary catheters. Neither expensive technology nor additional ICU staff was required, although each hospital provided adequate staff to implement the educational intervention.

The study had limitations and, as with any study, required critical appraisal (Daley, 2007; Jenny-Avital, 2007). Nonetheless, the results were praised in *The New York Times* as "stunning" because of how the study saved more than 1,500 lives during its 18 months (Gawande, 2007). However, a few weeks after the study results were published, the Office for Human Research Protections (OHRP), the federal agency charged with protecting people involved in research in the United States, ordered an investigation into possible ethical violations in the study (Miller & Emanuel, 2008). In November 2007, the OHRP ruled that the project had violated ethics regulations and should be shut down, including planned expansions in other states (Gawande, 2007).

The OHRP held that the Michigan ICU study had violated two ethics regulations. The study was submitted to the Johns Hopkins University IRB, which deemed it exempt from review. The IRB viewed the project as an EBP implementation and QI initiative, not clinical research. The OHRP disagreed and held that it was research. Informed consent was not obtained in the project because it was considered exempt from IRB review (Pronovost et al., 2006). OHRP held that informed consent should not have been waived because of its assessment of the project as clinical research.

Wide application of OHRP's approach could mean that "whole swaths of critical work to ensure safe and effective care would either halt or shrink" (Gawande, 2007). In the resolution to the situation, both the parties agreed that the study was clinical research because an educational intervention of unknown efficacy was tested on clinicians (Miller & Emanuel, 2008). At the same time, the study most likely would have satisfied the regulations for expedited IRB review because it involved no more than minimal risks. The IRB review could also have determined that informed consent was not ethically required because the five infection-control guidelines were evidence based (i.e., their expected outcomes previously had been demonstrated through research) and patients were not being put at additional risks (Saginur, 2009). The protocol could have been introduced as part of standard clinical practice and covered by patients' general consent to treatment. Thus, their autonomy would still be respected even though explicit informed consent was not obtained. The OHRP also concluded that because the Michigan ICU study demonstrated the effectiveness of its interventions, future implementation and monitoring of the checklists would not be research but improving clinical care.

Spanish ICU Study

The importance of establishing whether a project is research or evidence implementation is revealed by another exemplar, this time in Spain. An educational program on compliance with evidence-based guidelines in patients with severe sepsis was prospectively evaluated for its impact on mortality (Ferrer et al., 2008). About 20% of Spain's ICUs participated. The authors concluded from the results that if the educational program was implemented in all Spanish hospitals, 490 lives might be saved each year. As with any project or study, this one had limitations and should be critically appraised, especially as its design falls at a lower level of evidence in the study hierarchy for interventions (Kahn & Bates, 2008). Such study designs make causation difficult to establish, but the project remains a good example of an educational program introduced to promote evidence-based guidelines on a national level while also including an objective evaluation of its impact. It would appear to be ethically sound based on its promotion of beneficence and nonmaleficence.

The project was subsequently criticized for ethical reasons similar to those of the Michigan ICU study. Based on viewing the Spanish project as clinical research, the project coordinators were criticized for not obtaining informed consent from the patients involved and thus not respecting their autonomy (Lemaire, 2008). The authors defended their decision on the grounds that the project was EBQI and thus part of good clinical care (Ferrer, Artigas, & Levy, 2008). They gave several reasons for not viewing their project as clinical research. Foremost among these was that the educational program taught previously established evidence-based guidelines and did not expose patients to test interventions. In particular, they noted that the project was reviewed by the research ethics committee at every participating hospital and in that way ensured that appropriate ethical standards were maintained.

> If the people who make the decisions are the people
> who will also bear the consequences of those decisions,
> perhaps better decisions will result.
>
> **JOHN ABRAMS**

Practical Consequences

Much controversy has revolved around establishing whether evidence implementation activities fall within the definition of clinical research. The focus of this chapter is on the ethical aspects of this distinction, which have important practical and regulatory implications. The OHRP can impose severe penalties on organizations found to be in violation of

U.S. regulations. The OHRP has regularly defined research very broadly and thereby often included QI activities within its oversight (Lynn et al., 2007). The 2017 Revised Common Rule acknowledged the problems and concerns about such inclusions but determined not to exclude any of those activities from its definition of research (Coleman, 2017). Similar regulatory uncertainty and confusion can exist in the United Kingdom (Hill & Small, 2006) and elsewhere in Europe (Lemaire, Ravoire, & Golinelli, 2008). Attempts to distinguish QI activities from research have focused on differences between methodologic rigor and generalizability of findings, but these are conceptually and practically difficult to support (Fiscella, Tobin, Carroll, He, & Ogedegbe, 2015).

Another practical consequence of the research/nonresearch distinction arises with publication of the findings from QI activities. Sometimes, clinicians conducting evidence implementation activities decide to pursue publication after their project is completed, and the findings are viewed as having broader interest (Hill & Small, 2006). However, many journals will not publish articles they deem to be clinical research if they have not already had IRB review (Lynn et al., 2007). If the QI activity was deemed not to require IRB approval, but the journal decides it was research requiring ethical approval, the clinicians may find it very difficult to get published. Some journals evaluate the ethics of a study or project themselves regardless of whether or not an ethics committee reviewed the original proposal, but not all take the time and effort this requires (Abbasi & Heath, 2005).

The more significant consequences relate to patients. Since responsibility for classifying a project or study as research currently rests with the investigators, inappropriate classification could avoid ethical review or lead to less intensive review and miss the opportunity to identify ethical or methodologic concerns (Abbasi & Heath, 2005). If projects are inappropriately classified as research, patients may be overburdened with unnecessary protective precautions, while projects viewed as nonresearch may underprotect patients for want of ethical oversight (Fiscella et al., 2015). If EBP project coordinators view an ethics application as an onerous, lengthy, and perhaps nonrelevant process, they may decide to forgo conducting important practice evaluations. Given that current practice can always be improved, this may leave practitioners unwilling to make evidence-based changes, putting patients at risk for continued lower quality care, or to promote the introduction of practice changes without monitoring their effects (Lynn et al., 2007). It is important that the ethical considerations that apply to EBP initiatives, such as protection of privacy, be addressed by project coordinators; however, other ethical safeguards designed for clinical research, such as individual informed consent, may not be feasible or appropriate for EBP implementation projects.

PIERS (Preeclampsia Integrated Estimate of RiSk) Project

Research ethics review itself is beginning to be empirically evaluated, leading to some evidence that applying research standards to QI projects can have detrimental effects. The PIERS project was a multicenter international study of a standardized assessment tool for women admitted to hospital with preeclampsia (Firoz, Magee, Payne, Menzies, & von Dadelszen, 2012). The tool was designed to monitor maternal and fetal predictors of adverse outcomes based on established evidence-based criteria. A project was designed to introduce the tool and evaluate its impact by examining the outcomes in patients' medical records. The project was submitted for ethical approval at all seven participating sites. Three ethics committees viewed it as continuous quality improvement (CQI) that did not require individual informed consent, while four viewed it as research requiring informed consent from the women to have their medical records examined by the researchers. The investigators found that when informed consent was required, those with more severe preeclampsia were less likely to enroll. This biased their sample and risked compromising the scientific validity at the research sites compared to the CQI sites where all women's data were analyzed. In addition, obtaining informed consent required additional time and resources, which sometimes were not available, leading to lower enrollment.

Informed consent should not be abandoned just because it restricts research or takes time. However, the type of informed consent required in clinical research may not always be necessary or appropriate for evidence-based QI. Different approaches to consent may be more appropriate with different types of studies or projects and forms of data collection and analysis (Hansson, 2010). Before examining this more closely, the ethically relevant differences between research and QI will be reviewed.

DISTINGUISHING RESEARCH, EVIDENCE IMPLEMENTATION, AND QUALITY IMPROVEMENT

Research can be viewed as generating the evidence upon which practice should be based, that is, the *why* of practice. Rigorous methodology is key to the conduct of a research study. Evidence-based implementation projects use the EBP process to bring about change in practice to improve patient outcomes. Attending rigorously to the EBP process is imperative for an evidence implementation project to be successful and ethical. Poorly designed research and EBP projects will waste valuable resources (violating the principle of justice) and may lead to practice that is neither effective nor beneficent. Through the EBP process, clinicians find, evaluate, apply, and reevaluate the impact of an evidence-based intervention on an outcome—the *what* of practice. In a complimentary fashion, clinicians use QI methods to know whether the processes they are employing are reliable for obtaining consistent outcomes. Two terms must be mentioned when discussing EBQI: *quality assurance* and *audit*. Both the terms are designed to assess how well current practice compares with best practice (Casarett, Karlawish, & Sugarman, 2000). Quality assurance involves planned, systematic processes, which should have been established using evidence—the *how* of practice. These processes are the core of QI and are designed to assure patients and providers that quality of care is addressed in a systematic and reliable manner. An audit evaluates whether or not current (or past) practice is based on the best available evidence. Different methods are also used within QI projects. EBQI includes a set of processes designed to align with the best available evidence; therefore, in this chapter, audit and quality assurance will be subsumed under the term EBQI (Casarett et al., 2000).

The Methodologic Spectrum

Evidence implementation and EBQI involve methodologies that are also used in clinical research, which is why distinctions can be difficult. A spectrum of methods is involved in these approaches to problem solving. Randomized controlled trials are on the clinical research end of the spectrum. These require specific protection of study participants from harm due to unknown outcomes. Across the spectrum, practitioners may use similar data collection methods to evaluate outcomes before and after they introduce something new to their practice; this generates internal evidence. In this instance, there are no comparison or control groups or sample sizes. For example, consider a group of practitioners caring for some middle-aged male patients who are not taking their blood pressure medication consistently. When the practitioners review the patients' current (baseline) blood pressures (i.e., internal evidence), they realize that some intervention is necessary to improve this parameter. To make a practice change and improve the quality of care, they discuss what they would recommend and conduct a preliminary search for evidence regarding other interventions that may impact blood pressure in middle-aged males. In our example, let's say the clinicians find a well-done systematic review of the benefits of exercise on multiple outcomes, including blood pressure. They consider how to introduce the intervention so that everyone in the clinic is aware of the outcomes of their plan as well as how to achieve them. They offer the exercise intervention to all middle-aged male patients with elevated blood pressure, collect data on how the intervention was used by the men, and record their blood pressures to evaluate whether the intervention achieved the expected outcome. As the clinicians review the data, they note some positive changes. As a result, they talk about how well the evidence-based exercise intervention worked, what adjustments they may make so that it might work better, and how they can incorporate the intervention into their routine clinical discussions with patients. An EBQI activity like this would lead to a higher quality of care for patients and produce evidence that this change led to better outcomes in practice.

Along this spectrum of EBQI and research are a range of activities. A practitioner might tell colleagues about an evidence-based change that improved care. They decide to introduce this change across the unit. Others hear about it and decide to evaluate the outcomes from units that applied the evidence and make comparisons with other units that did not implement the change. Someone then suggests that the activities should be written up and submitted for publication. When considered from an ethical viewpoint, the question arises whether at some point the project has become one that should be submitted for ethical approval because patient information is being used in a way for which it was not originally collected. However, for EBQI and evidence implementation projects, ethical review could be useful to ensure patient information is managed appropriately, for example, that all appropriate steps were being taken to protect patient privacy. The question then arises as to who should provide such ethical review, which is a matter we will consider later in the chapter.

EBQI and evidence implementation (the EBP process) meet only a portion of the U.S. regulatory definition of research as "a systematic investigation, including research development, testing and evaluation, designed to develop or contribute to generalizable knowledge" (Baily et al., 2006, p. S28). Although EBQI and the EBP process are systematic and involve evaluation and testing, only research methods contribute to generalizable knowledge. Nevertheless, the methods of research, QI and EBP can be similar, which triggers much of the ethical debate about these different approaches to problem solving. Bailey goes on to comment:

> QI uses the kind of reasoning that is inherent in the scientific method, it involves systematic investigations of working hypotheses about how a process might be improved, and it frequently employs qualitative and quantitative methods and analytic tools that are also used in research projects.
>
> (Baily et al., 2006, p. S11)

Since there are no established criteria for distinguishing these approaches unambiguously, people can review the same QI project and come to different conclusions as to whether it should be classified as research and require research ethics approval. Two articles by research ethicists came to opposite conclusions regarding whether the Michigan ICU study should have been regulated as clinical research and obtained informed consent from participants. Miller and Emanuel (2008) held that the project was research because it prospectively implemented a protocol, tested hypotheses, and had a goal of contributing to generalizable knowledge (inferred only from its publication). However, Baily (2008) concluded that it was not research because it was designed to promote clinicians' use of evidence-based procedures and placed patients at no additional risk than the original ethically reviewed studies.

Ethically Relevant Distinctions

Clear distinctions between research, EBQI, and the EBP process can be difficult to make. However, there are differences, and some of them are ethically significant, particularly regarding informed consent. When examining a study or project, these factors must be considered when determining what ethical issues may arise and how they should be addressed. From an ethical perspective, classifying a study or project as research, QI, or EBP is not the most important factor, as this can lead to an overly simplistic approach to ethics. The OHRP criticized Johns Hopkins University for its general conclusion that all EBQI or EBP projects were not clinical research and were therefore exempt from review (Miller & Emanuel, 2008). Instead, OHRP held that each project needed to be evaluated individually as to whether it warranted exemption. Several ethical issues must be addressed no matter how a project or study is classified. Overall, protecting and promoting the well-being of everyone involved (beneficence and nonmaleficence) in a project or a study, including how their personal data are protected (privacy and confidentiality), should be paramount. This suggests that some ethical evaluation of EBQI and EBP projects is important, regardless of whether they are classified as research (Flaming, 2017).

Research is focused on questions for which answers are not known. When we don't know whether intervention A is better than intervention B, research in the form of a randomized controlled trial may be conducted. When we don't know how diet influences the risk of cancer, epidemiologic research is conducted. When we don't know how patients experience and cope with a disability, qualitative research is carried out. Research is focused on *generating* evidence *for* practice, EBP is focused on *implementing* evidence *in* practice, and EBQI is focused on *evaluating* how well practice is working. Activities should be regarded as EBP when clinicians take a body of established evidence and use this to improve outcomes. In this way, the EBP process falls within good clinical management (Figure 23.1). Both EBP and EBQI seek to promote use of the best available evidence with the best processes so that practice outcomes are improved.

In evidence-based care, clinical practice relies on knowledge generated by research to provide best care; however, patients are not required to be involved in research projects to receive quality clinical care. Research may occur in clinical settings, and then patients are asked to volunteer to participate in research. Although exceptions may exist, the informed consent process aims to document their voluntary participation (Rebers, Aaronson, van Leeuwen, & Schmidt, 2016). "In contrast, QI is *an integral part of the ongoing management of the system for delivering clinical care*, not an independent, knowledge-seeking enterprise" (Baily et al., 2006, p. S12). EBP is integral to the ongoing improvement (versus management) of quality care. This distinction among research, EBP, and EBQI is crucial and will be discussed in more detail later in the chapter.

Research often carries risks for patient safety, which is one of the reasons for informed consent. Research on interventions involving risk is justified when researchers do not know which alternative is best. The risks may be side effects, known or unknown. Or the risks may

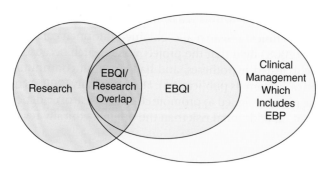

Figure 23.1: Distinguishing between research and evidence-based quality improvement (EBQI) projects. EBP, evidence-based practice.

be that a patient receives an intervention that turns out to be less effective. Because research is pursuing knowledge that is not known, risks are inherent. The risks with EBP, because it is based on previously reviewed research, are primarily in the area of patient information. EBQI activities are also usually associated with very low risks, such as revealing personal information in questionnaires or interviews. As patient information is collected for evaluation, privacy and confidentiality must be protected. Some EBQI activities may carry some risk of harm because there is insufficient external evidence to guide the project, and internal evidence becomes paramount, which must be evaluated when designing the project. However, sometimes the risks may be greater if the EBQI activities are *not* implemented and the old way of doing things remains in place or important outcomes are never reviewed (Hansson, 2010).

Researchers conducting studies are often not part of the clinical team caring for patients, whereas EBP and EBQI are almost always carried out by clinicians involved in caring for patients in the project. This supports the notion that EBP and EBQI are part of routine clinical practice and can foster a culture of continual improvement toward the highest quality care and outcomes. Another distinction between EBP, EBQI, and research is that the former two often use data that practitioners have regular access to in their clinical roles, whereas research data are usually distinct from clinical care and generated primarily for the study.

Funding for research is often generated externally, whereas EBP and EBQI projects are usually conducted using the resources available to the clinical team. External funding can generate conflicts of interest for researchers. The research study itself may put researchers' interests at odds with those of the participants (the patients), and this is one reason for IRB review. In contrast, EBP and EBQI projects, by their nature, are intended to improve the quality of care the patients receive.

Research, EBP, and EBQI have been distinguished on the basis of generalizability, but this may not be as clear-cut as desired (Fiscella et al., 2015). One perspective is that the goal of publication is an indicator of generalizability, but that is not necessarily the case. EBP and EBQI projects, just as case reports, are helpful to clinicians. As discussed in Chapter 5, case reports should not be considered generalizable information, but they remain valuable to practitioners. Case reports, and case series, describe clinical practice in a systematic way, yet they are reports of clinical practice, not research. They reflect on what has happened in clinical practice and help others to learn from those experiences.

In the same way, publication of EBP and EBQI projects provides opportunities for others to learn from those experiences. A desire to share the findings of these projects should be seen as part of the ethical commitment to help others improve patient outcomes, either by introducing the same evidence-based changes or by avoiding them if they turn out to be unhelpful. Publication of the results of these projects should not change the nature of the original EBP or EBQI activities. However, the context-dependent nature of these projects must be taken into account if others choose to consider implementing these processes elsewhere.

In research, publication is usually envisioned as one of the outcomes expected, if not required, for the project to be successful. For EBP and EBQI, this is not always the case, and publication is unlikely to be a strong motivation for the project. In some cases, publication may be preplanned, but in others "it is more likely that a successful project will prompt its instigators to tell others what they have done, [and] that there will be a retrospective decision to seek publication" (Hill & Small, 2006, p. 103). Although not a major motivator for an EBP or EBQI project, the final step in the EBP process is the dissemination of results, which can be viewed as an ethical obligation.

Overall, clinicians must carefully consider whether a project is best classified as clinical research, EBP, or EBQI. Figure 23.1 is an adaptation of a diagram used to represent the distinctions (Baily et al., 2006). This also offers the opportunity for some studies to be classified as overlapping research and EBQI. For example, a systematic QI investigation designed to bring about local clinical improvements may also develop generalizable knowledge as part of the evolution of the work (Baily et al., 2006). The Michigan ICU study and the Spanish sepsis project could be placed in this overlapping region, whereas the preeclampsia study was originally intended to be generalizable given its multicenter, international design.

This serves to emphasize that the important factor for ethical review is not how a project or study is classified, but whether the activity is ethically appropriate. EBP does not fall into this overlapping region because the basis for all EBP projects is an already ethically reviewed body of evidence that has been deemed safe for patients; however, the ethical responsibility to protect patients and their information still remains.

ETHICAL PRINCIPLES AS APPLIED TO RESEARCH, EBP, AND EBQI

Much has been written on research ethics (Emanuel et al., 2008). A set of seven ethical requirements have been proposed as the ethical foundations upon which clinical research should be based (Emanuel, Wendler, & Grady, 2000):

1. Social or scientific value
2. Scientific validity
3. Fair subject selection
4. Favorable risk–benefit ratio
5. Independent review
6. Respect for potential and enrolled subjects
7. Informed consent

They are summarized in the following sections as originally proposed for clinical research, and their relevance for EBQI activities is also described, where appropriate (Baily et al., 2006). All seven principles are ethically important and are not listed in any order of priority.

Social or Scientific Value

For research to be ethical, it should be worth doing. Appropriate use of resources is an ethical issue because of the principle of justice. Further research on questions that have been adequately answered by prior studies is ethically questionable. Exposing human subjects to any level of risk is unethical if the research does not have value to society or healthcare. This also places an ethical obligation on researchers to share their results and findings with others so that they can benefit from the new knowledge.

Similarly, EBP and EBQI activities are ethical only if they are worth doing. The value of the activity may initially be very local. Practitioners should identify significant clinical outcomes that could benefit from improvements. The value of different proposed activities may need to be compared to determine those that have the potential to improve care the most, which is the essence of EBP. After conducting a local project or study, its wider value may be noted. For example, the results of the Michigan ICU study were extremely valuable worldwide, and it would have been unethical not to disseminate them broadly.

Scientific Validity

To be ethical, a research project must be methodologically rigorous to ensure a well-done study that can produce generalizable, valid findings. Methodologic rigor has been used to distinguish research from QI processes, but this seems highly questionable (Fiscella et al., 2015). Nonadherence to appropriate methods in the EBP process or QI activities can result in poorly designed or implemented projects that waste resources and the time of those involved. The goal of EBQI is usually local improvement, not generalizable knowledge, so different methods may be used, but they should still be rigorously applied. Context and local factors are embedded in EBP and EBQI, whereas they are usually minimized in research by its methodologic rigor. Nevertheless, exposing people to any risk in a flawed study or project is unethical.

Fair Subject Selection

The selection of subjects for research studies should be fair so that risks and benefits are shared equally. Inclusion and exclusion criteria for recruiting study participants should be based on good scientific reasons, not convenience or vulnerability. People should not be selected *because* they are marginalized, powerless, or poor. Such groups may become human subjects or participants, but only if the research is relevant to people in those groups. Those groups that bear the risks and burdens of research should have the potential to benefit from the results.

The same criteria should apply in EBP and EBQI activities. Those involved in an EBP or EBQI project should be determined more by where the project is conducted and the population of patients than recruitment techniques aimed at representative sampling. If resources prevent improvement of care in all areas, decisions about where to focus should be made fairly and not based on people's status or other irrelevant factors. EBP and EBQI should be present across healthcare, including clinics or services that serve the underprivileged. Funding for services for the underprivileged should include resources for EBP and EBQI, just as they should for fee-paying or profitable services.

Favorable Risk–Benefit Ratio

Both research and EBQI should be committed to minimizing the risks and maximizing the gains of all studies and projects. Risks in research can range from very high to none, whereas risks in EBQI are usually low. Risks may be physical but can also include risks to privacy and respect. Wherever possible, the risk–benefit ratio should be improved as much as possible. This way both beneficence and nonmaleficence are promoted. With EBP, risks are known because of the body of evidence that guides practice and defines expected outcomes. No new risks should be associated with EBP when the fidelity (how the evidence is implemented) is high.

Independent Review

Independent review of research is ethically required because of the potential conflicts of interest. Research subjects are inherently used as means toward the goal of new knowledge. They may be placed at risk of harm for the good of others. In clinical contexts, the potential exists to exploit patients as research subjects because what is best for the research project may not be what is best for patients.

Different views exist on the nature of the review that EBP and EBQI activities ethically require. Increasingly, it is being recognized that different types of ethical review are best for different types of EBP and EBQI activities (Flaming, 2017). The reasons for this will be developed in the following sections and will be brought together in the chapter's conclusion.

Respect for Potential and Enrolled Subjects

Research has scientific goals, with respect for the participants involved in the research remaining paramount. As the Declaration of Helsinki states, "While the primary purpose of medical research is to generate new knowledge, this goal can never take precedence over the rights and interests of individual research subjects" (World Medical Association [WMA], 2013). This respect applies to those who are asked to participate in the research and decide not to do so. It includes protecting privacy and confidentiality, maintaining participants' welfare during the project, keeping them informed of significant changes during the research, and allowing them to withdraw from research.

In EBP and EBQI activities, respect for patients must also take precedence. Improving their outcomes is the goal of EBQI and inherent to the nature of the activities. As with research, it includes protecting privacy and confidentiality, maintaining welfare, and keeping patients informed. However, the issue of withdrawing from EBQI (i.e., initiatives designed to produce known improvement in outcomes) is tied up with informed consent, and its appropriateness to EBQI is discussed later in this chapter. The focus of EBP is best care for patients to achieve best outcomes. It does not seem logical or ethical to exclude patients from these projects or to allow them to remove themselves. However, refusal of treatment is always a right of patients and should be respected in these EBP projects as well.

Informed Consent

Informed consent is one of the bedrocks of clinical ethics and research ethics. Participating in research is viewed as voluntary, and this places an ethical obligation on researchers to provide information so that people can make informed decisions to enroll or not. This requirement is based on the importance of respecting an individual's autonomy over his or her body and health. Researchers must provide information about the risks and benefits of participation and help people understand this information. Informed consent is a process that often must be revisited as subjects engage in the research and understand its expectations and implications more fully.

The issue of informed consent for EBP and EBQI is one of the more widely debated ethical issues. Informed consent is not necessary for involvement in EBP because such projects fall within good clinical practice, are supported by a body of external evidence (i.e., research), and are covered by a patient's consent to clinical care. However, EBQI is driven usually by internal evidence and a small amount of external evidence, and therefore informed consent for EBQI will be examined in depth in the following section.

> The bravest thing you can do when you are not brave
> is to profess courage and act accordingly.
>
> **CORRA HARRIS**

INFORMED CONSENT AND EVIDENCE-BASED QUALITY IMPROVEMENT

One of the important issues debated within EBQI is whether informed consent is necessary. This was a central ethical issue in the two projects discussed in detail in this chapter. Part of the reason for informed consent is to protect patients, both from harm and from ways they might not be respected as persons. People who come to health services do not usually expect to become participants in research. Therefore, to respect them as individuals, they are offered the opportunity to participate or not in the research. If they agree, a *process* of informed consent will be initiated. From an ethical perspective, this process should not be simply one of getting an informed consent form signed but an ongoing dialogue between researcher and participant about the research study.

Many activities happen when patients are within the health services. These activities are designed to restore or maintain optimal health for those patients. Patients enter the healthcare system trusting that clinicians are there to assist them toward health and to minimize their risks while in their care. Therefore, obtaining informed consent for each individual action or intervention would not be practical. Collecting multiple informed consents likely would be unethical if this took away from the care patients received because so much time would be spent garnering informed consents. Consequently, separate informed consent is usually not expected when patients engage in what they might normally anticipate to be part of usual care. Furthermore, patients, whether in primary care or in acute care, sign a consent for treatment with the understanding that their best interest will be most important when decisions are made regarding what interventions are provided to them.

Debate over informed consent can be seen as a question of whether patients should expect EBQI and EBP to be seen as part of standard healthcare practice. Some argue that "much of QI is simply good clinical care combined with systematic, experiential learning. Individual practitioners are constantly learning by doing and taking steps to improve their own practice" (Baily et al., 2006, p. S8). The ethical commitment to care for and do good for patients (beneficence), coupled with an avoidance of harm (nonmaleficence), implies a commitment to improve clinical practice whenever possible. Taking steps to improve one's own practice includes evaluating whether or not improvement has occurred. This can be done through formal examinations, peer feedback, and other methods. A commitment to improve care more generally should similarly include steps to evaluate the quality of care (i.e., outcomes) in formal and informal ways. EBQI and EBP play a role in this, and as such, professionals and organizations have an ethical responsibility to conduct these types of projects to demonstrate whether or not change in process or implementation of evidence demonstrates sustainable improvement in outcomes.

This understanding of EBQI also places a responsibility on patients to participate in such activities. In that case, informed consent would not be necessary. This can be seen as similar to the responsibilities of teachers and students. If teachers have a responsibility to evaluate and improve their teaching, feedback from students is vital. This could be viewed as a mutual ethical responsibility, so students should provide feedback in response to the teaching. Certainly, protections need to be put in place, such as ensuring that the feedback is anonymous so that students who point out problems need not fear reprisal. Since students benefit from improved teaching, students have a responsibility to provide accurate information that will contribute to improved learning, and therefore signed informed consent is not necessary. In fact, it may be counterproductive, because such forms may be the only items that identify which students provided feedback and which did not.

This understanding of healthcare (and education) may not sit well with the current emphasis on autonomy and individualism. Individual rights should be valued in healthcare, but sometimes individual autonomy is prioritized over all other ethical principles. A culture can exist in which patients see themselves primarily as customers, purchasing the services they desire. This can foster an environment in which patients feel little or no obligation to the service or system that provides their care. They may feel they are paying for a service and can go elsewhere if they are not satisfied.

An individualistic paradigm brings a significant loss of the sense of a social commitment to improve the healthcare services that will be available to everyone. Viewing healthcare as primarily a business can have this same effect. Customers rightly feel little sense of responsibility to improve the quality of a local hardware store or the goods they buy from the store. The market is supposed to take care of that. But healthcare is not the same type of commodity as hardware.

In addition, such individualism is not realistic in healthcare and does not produce quality care or relevant research. Patients are part of a social network and benefit from the experiences of others who have participated in prior clinical research, EBP, and EBQI. What is needed is an appropriate balance between individual autonomy and group responsibility (Greaney & O'Mathúna, 2017). Patients should be able to see with gratitude how others have contributed to the care and service they receive and be willing to become involved in helping improve healthcare outcomes. We can all do this by accepting responsibility to participate in EBP and EBQI activities and managing our own health to maximize limited resources. Such a sense of moral obligation to the quality of our healthcare services is vital if the outcomes are to improve. Paradoxically, a commitment by everyone to improve the healthcare available for everyone should mean that we will each individually receive higher quality healthcare when we need to avail of those services and resources.

Such a view of healthcare places ethical responsibilities on healthcare organizations, professionals, and patients to participate in improving the quality of healthcare processes as well as outcomes. Patients may be unaware of this responsibility. For a long time, patients were afforded little opportunity to give feedback to healthcare professionals. In some cases, such feedback was overlooked, and in others, the feedback was actively rejected. The necessity of improving healthcare means that the voices of patients must be heard. One initiative taking this approach is the federally funded Patient-Centered Outcomes Research Institute (PCORI). This institute funds and promotes high-quality research that is guided by patients, caregivers, and the broader healthcare community (Frank, Basch, Selby, & Patient-Centered Outcomes Research Institute, 2014).

 To learn more about PCORI, visit https://www.pcori.org/about-us

---

Creating opportunities for patients to shape research agendas and other initiatives like PCORI points to the ethical responsibility patients have to engage in improvement processes. This type of partnership with patients requires strategies that inform the general public about opportunities for working in tandem with healthcare organizations to improve outcomes through daily implementation of evidence.

This means that someone seeking care from a healthcare organization cannot insist on the freedom to opt out completely from efforts to improve the quality of care in that organization without jeopardizing the very benefits he or she seeks. In fact, it is in the best interest of patients to cooperate with EBP and EBQI activities and even to seek out the healthcare organizations that are the most committed to improving processes and outcomes. As an ethical matter, the responsibility of patients to cooperate in healthcare improvement activities is justified by the benefits that each patient receives because of the cooperation of others in the collective enterprise (Baily et al., 2006).

REVIEWING RESEARCH, EBP, AND EBQI PROJECTS

Review of research studies by an IRB is imperative and safeguards people who are participating in research. Some ethical review activities involve an overlap between research and EBQI. These situations could continue to be sent to IRBs for review, but the IRB has an obligation to examine them with the distinctions between EBQI and research in mind. The majority of EBQI is low risk, and when no more than minimal risks are involved, such projects could be reviewed within clinical management and supervision structures, or another mechanism

(WHO, 2013). This can be justified on the basis that EBQI is part of normal healthcare activities and is thus "a systematic, data-guided form of the clinical and managerial innovation and adaptation that has always been an integral part of clinical and managerial practice" (Baily et al., 2006, p. S28). EBP projects should be ethically reviewed also to ensure that patient privacy is maintained.

Various practical structures could be put in place to facilitate an ethical review (Flaming, 2017). In some cases, external review may be necessary; for example, when projects involve more risk or seem to become more like research. Clinicians and ethical review boards need flexibility and knowledge of the purpose of the project or study. One benefit of keeping the review in the clinical setting would be that it could contribute to fostering a culture of evidence implementation in practice. This may also prevent ethical review from being seen as unwelcome scrutiny or a bureaucratic hurdle to be overcome (O'Mathúna & Siriwardhana, 2017). What is needed is

> . . . *a scrutiny process that can recognise when a light hand is needed. We have to be able to deconstruct projects, be they research audit or QI, such that appropriate scrutiny is imposed— to improve the proposed activities and to defend the interests of those subjected to them.*
>
> (Hill & Small, 2006, p. 105)

Bringing EBQI review into the normal routine of clinical management offers an opportunity to enhance quality, ethical care. It gives everyone the opportunity to become more familiar with the review of EBQI activities and how ethical standards can be upheld. This is also true of appropriate ethical review of EBP projects. These reviews require adequate knowledge and skills in critical appraisal and ethical reflection. Ethical reviews are also an opportunity to remind everyone of the importance of implementing evidence in practice, continual practice improvement, monitoring of change, and ethical practice. The idea of a one-size-fits-all ethical review does not apply to the current complex culture that incorporates EBP, EBQI, and generation of research (Flaming, 2017).

EBP FAST FACTS

- Research is focused on *generating* evidence *for* practice, EBP is focused on *implementing* evidence *in* practice, and EBQI is focused on *evaluating* how well practice is working.
- EBP and EBQI can be ethically justified by the intent to benefit patients and use resources wisely.
- EBQI has some similarities with research and may have unknown risks and should therefore be ethically reviewed and implemented. It also differs from research, and this should be taken into account in ethical review.
- The key ethical principles of good research are applicable and important for EBQI.
- Ethical considerations that apply to EBP initiatives, such as protection of privacy, are important to address; however, other ethical safeguards designed for clinical research, such as individual informed consent, are not explicitly appropriate or feasible for EBP implementation projects.
- Partnership among patients, caregivers, and clinicians to provide input into the design and conduct of EBP, EBQI, and research can keep projects patient centered and help identify and address ethical issues.
- What is most important is not how a study or project is classified but whether the activity is ethically appropriate.

> **WANT TO KNOW MORE?**
>
> A variety of resources are available to enhance your learning and understanding of this chapter.
>
> - Visit thePoint® to access:
>   - Articles from the AJN EBP Step-By-Step Series
>   - Journal articles
>   - Checklists for rapid critical appraisal and more!
> - Lippincott **CoursePoint** combines digital text content with video case studies and interactive modules for a fully integrated course solution that works the way you study and learn.

References

Abbasi, K., & Heath, I. (2005). Ethics review of research and audit. *British Medical Journal, 330,* 431–432.

Baily, M. A. (2008). Harming through protection? *New England Journal of Medicine, 358*(8), 768–769.

Baily, M. A., Bottrell, M., Lynn, J., & Jennings, B. (2006). The ethics of using QI methods to improve health care quality and safety. *Hastings Center Report, 36*(4), S1–S408.

Beauchamp, T. L., & Childress, J. F. (2012). *Principles of biomedical ethics* (7th ed.). New York, NY: Oxford University Press.

Blanchet, K., Ramesh, A., Frison, S., Warren, E., Hossain, M., Smith, J., . . . Roberts, B. (2017). Evidence on public health interventions in humanitarian crises. *The Lancet, 390*(10109), 2287–2296. doi:10.1016/S0140-6736(16)30768-1

Casarett, D., Karlawish, J. H. T., & Sugarman, J. (2000). Determining when quality improvement initiatives should be considered research: Proposed criteria and potential implications. *Journal of the American Medical Association, 283*(17), 2275–2280.

Coleman, C. H. (2017). Reining in IRB review in the Revised Common Rule. *IRB: Ethics & Human Research, 39*(6), 2–5.

Daley, M. R. (2007). Catheter-related bloodstream infections [letter]. *New England Journal of Medicine, 356*(12), 1267–1268.

Emanuel, E. J., Grady, C., Crouch, R. A., Lie, R., Miller, F., & Wendler, D. (Eds.). (2008). *The Oxford textbook of clinical research ethics.* New York, NY: Oxford University Press.

Emanuel, E. J., Wendler, D., & Grady, C. (2000). What makes clinical research ethical? *Journal of the American Medical Association, 283*(20), 2701–2711.

Ferrer, R., Artigas, A., & Levy, M. (2008). Informed consent and studies of a quality improvement program [letter]. *Journal of the American Medical Association, 300*(15), 1762–1763.

Ferrer, R., Artigas, A., Levy, M. M., Blanco, J., González-Díaz, G., Garnacho-Montero, J., . . . de la Torre-Prados, M. V. (2008). Improvement in process of care and outcome after a multicenter severe sepsis educational program in Spain. *Journal of the American Medical Association, 299*(19), 2294–2303.

Firoz, T., Magee, L. A., Payne, B. A., Menzies, J. M., & von Dadelszen, P. (2012). The PIERS experience: Research or quality improvement? *Journal of Obstetrics and Gynaecology Canada, 34*(4), 379–381.

Fiscella, K., Tobin, J. N., Carroll, J. K., He, H., & Ogedegbe, G. (2015). Ethical oversight in quality improvement and quality improvement research: New approaches to promote a learning health care system. *BMC Medical Ethics, 16*(1):63.

Flaming, D. (2017). Appropriate ethics review is required. *Healthcare Management Forum, 30*(1), 46–48.

Frank, L., Basch, E., Selby, J. V., for the Patient-Centered Outcomes Research Institute. (2014). The PCORI perspective on patient-centered outcomes research. *Journal of the American Medical Association, 312*(15), 1513–1514.

Fred, H. L. (2016). Cutting the cost of health care: The physician's role. *Texas Heart Institute Journal, 43*(1), 4–6.

Gandra, S., & Ellison III, R. T. (2015). Modern trends in infection control practices in intensive care units. *Journal of Intensive Care Medicine, 29*(6), 311–326.

Gawande, A. (2007). A lifesaving checklist. *The New York Times.* Retrieved from http://www.nytimes.com/2007/12/30/opinion/30gawande.html

Greaney, A.-M., & O'Mathúna, D. P. (2017). Patient autonomy in nursing and healthcare contexts. In P. A. Scott (Ed.), *Key concepts and issues in nursing ethics* (pp. 83–99). New York, NY: Springer International Publishing.

Hansson, M. G. (2010). Do we need a wider view of autonomy in epidemiological research? *British Medical Journal, 340,* 1172–1174.

Hill, S. L., & Small, N. (2006). Differentiating between research, audit and quality improvement: Governance implications. *Clinical Governance, 11*(2), 98–107.

Institute of Medicine. (2006). *Preventing medication errors.* Washington, DC: National Academy Press.

Institute of Medicine. (2018). *Crossing the quality chasm: The IOM health care quality initiative.* Retrieved from http://www.nationalacademies.org/hmd/Global/News%20Announcements/Crossing-the-Quality-Chasm-The-IOM-Health-Care-Quality-Initiative.aspx

Jenny-Avital, E. R. (2007). Catheter-related bloodstream infections [letter]. *New England Journal of Medicine, 356*(12), 1267.

Kahn, J. M., & Bates, D. W. (2008). Improving sepsis care: The road ahead. *Journal of the American Medical Association, 299*(19), 2322–2323.

Lemaire, F. (2008). Informed consent and studies of a quality improvement program [letter]. *Journal of the American Medical Association, 300*(15), 1762.

Lemaire, F., Ravoire, S., & Golinelli, D. (2008). Non-interventional research and usual care: Definition, regulatory aspects, difficulties and recommendations. *Thérapie, 63*(2), 103–106.

Lynn, J., Baily, M. A., Bottrell, M., Jennings, B., Levine, R. J., Davidoff, F., . . . James, B. (2007). The ethics of using quality improvement methods in health care. *Annals of Internal Medicine, 146*(9), 666–673.

Miller, F. G., & Emanuel, E. J. (2008). Quality-improvement research and informed consent. *New England Journal of Medicine, 358*(8), 765–767.

National Committee for Quality Assurance. (2012). *The state of health care quality report 2012.* Washington, DC: Author.

National Institutes of Health. (2017). *Glossary.* Retrieved from https://humansubjects.nih.gov/glossary

O'Horo, J. C., Maki, D. G., Krupp, A. E., & Safdar, N. (2014). Arterial catheters as a source of bloodstream infection: A systematic review and meta-analysis. *Critical Care Medicine, 42*(6), 1334–1339.

O'Mathúna, D., & Siriwardhana, C. (2017). Research ethics and evidence for humanitarian health. *The Lancet, 390*(10109), 2228–2229.

Papanicolas, I., Woskie, L. R., & Jha, A. K. (2018). Health care spending in the United States and other high-income countries. *Journal of the American Medical Association, 319*(10), 1024–1039.

Pronovost, P., Needham, D., Berenholtz, S., Sinopoli, D., Chu, H., Cosgrove, S., . . . Goeschel, C. (2006). An intervention to decrease catheter-related bloodstream infections in the ICU. *New England Journal of Medicine, 355*(26), 2725–2732.

Rebers, S., Aaronson, N. K., van Leeuwen, F. E., & Schmidt, M. K. (2016). Exceptions to the rule of informed consent for research with an intervention. *BMC Medical Ethics, 17,*9.

Saginur, R. (2009). Research ethics and infection control. *Clinical Infectious Diseases. 49*(8), 1254–1258.

Schoen, C., Osborn, R., How, S. K. H., Doty, M. M., & Peugh, J. (2009). In chronic condition: Experiences of patients with complex health care needs, in eight countries, 2008. *Health Affairs, 28*(1), w1–w16.

Schoen, C., Osborn, R., Squires, D., Doty, M., Rasmussen, P., Pierson, R., & Applebaum, S. (2012). A survey of primary care doctors in ten countries shows progress in use of health information technology, less in other areas. *Health Affairs, 31*(12), 2805–2816.

Upshur, R. E. (2013). A call to integrate ethics and evidence-based medicine. *Virtual Mentor, 15*(1), 86–89.

World Health Association. (2013a). *Ethical issues in patient safety research: Interpreting existing guidance.* Retrieved from http://www.who.int/patientsafety/research/ethical_issues/en/

World Medical Association. (2013b). *Declaration of Helsinki.* Retrieved from https://www.wma.net/policies-post/wma-declaration-of-helsinki-ethical-principles-for-medical-research-involving-human-subjects/

SELECTED EXCERPTS FROM A FUNDED GRANT APPLICATION

COPE/Healthy Lifestyles for Teens: A School-Based RCT

Bernadette Mazurek Melnyk, Principal Investigator
Co-Investigators: Diana Jacobson, Stephanie Kelly, Michael Belyea,
Gabriel Shaibi, Leigh Small, and Flavio Marsiglia
Funded by the NIH/National Institute of Nursing Research (#1R01NR012171)

The prevention and treatment of overweight/obesity and mental health disorders in adolescence are two major public health problems in the United States today [11, 12]. The incidence of adolescents who are overweight or obese has increased dramatically over the past 20 years, with approximately 17.1% of teens now being overweight (i.e., a gender- and age-specific body mass index [BMI] at or above the 85th percentile) or obese, which is defined as a gender- and age-specific body mass index at or above the 95th percentile [13, 14]. Furthermore, approximately 15 million children and adolescents in the United States have a mental health problem that is interfering with their functioning at home or at school, but less than 25% receive treatment for these disorders [21, 25]. Depression among adolescents is associated with disabling morbidity, significant mortality, and substantial healthcare costs [26, 27]. The prevalence rates of obesity and mental health problems are even higher in Hispanic teens, with the two conditions often coexisting [13, 32–35].

Despite the rapidly increasing incidence and adverse health outcomes associated with both overweight and mental health problems, very few theory-based intervention studies have been conducted with adolescents to improve both their healthy lifestyle behaviors and mental health outcomes [36]. Unfortunately, physical and mental health services continue to be largely separated instead of integrated in the nation's healthcare system, and this often leads to inadequate identification and treatment of these significant adolescent health problems. Furthermore, most obesity treatment and prevention trials have focused on school-age children [37–45].

Findings from our recent pilot studies of the feasibility and efficacy of the Creating Opportunities for Personal Empowerment (COPE)/Healthy Lifestyles Thinking, Emotions, Exercise, and Nutrition (TEEN) Program, a theory-driven, cognitive behavioral skills building (CBSB) healthy lifestyles intervention program, with overweight and normal weight culturally diverse adolescents, have indicated promising short-term positive physical and mental health outcomes (e.g., an increase in healthy lifestyle behaviors, decrease in weight, decrease in depressive symptoms) (see Preliminary Studies). Therefore, the primary goal of the proposed study is to test the short-term and more long-term efficacy of the COPE/Healthy Lifestyles TEEN Program on the healthy lifestyle behaviors and depressive symptoms of 800 culturally diverse teens enrolled in Phoenix, Arizona, high schools for the ultimate purpose of preventing overweight and mental health disorders.

Specific Aim 1

Use a randomized controlled trial (RCT) to test the short-term and more long-term efficacy of the COPE/Healthy Lifestyles TEEN Program to improve healthy lifestyle behaviors and depressive symptoms of 14- to 16-year-old culturally diverse adolescents enrolled in Phoenix, Arizona, high schools.

- **Hypothesis 1a** *(primary outcomes)*. Immediately following the COPE program and at 6 and 12 months postintervention, teens who receive the COPE program versus teens who receive an attention control program (i.e., Healthy Teens) will report:
- more healthy lifestyle behaviors
- less depressive symptoms
- **Hypothesis 1b** *(subgroup analysis: secondary outcome)*. Immediately following the COPE program and at 6 and 12 months postintervention, among teens with elevated depressive symptoms at baseline, those who receive the COPE program versus teens who receive the attention control program will have less depressive symptoms.
- **Hypothesis 1c** *(subgroup analysis: secondary outcome)*. Immediately following the intervention and at 6 and 12 months postintervention, overweight teens at baseline who receive the COPE program versus teens who receive an attention control program will have less weight gain.
- **Hypothesis 1d** *(subgroup analysis: secondary outcome)*. Fewer normal weight teens in COPE versus the attention control program will convert to *overweight* at 6 and 12 months postintervention.

Specific Aim 2

Examine the role of cognitive beliefs and perceived difficulty in leading a healthy lifestyle in mediating the effects of the COPE program on healthy lifestyle behaviors and depressive symptoms in 14- to 16-year-old adolescents.

- **Hypothesis 2** *(theory building exploratory)*. The effects of the COPE program on the teens' healthy lifestyle behaviors and depressive symptoms will be mediated by their beliefs about their ability to make healthy lifestyles choices and perceived difficulty in leading a healthy lifestyle.

Specific Aim 3

Explore variables that may moderate the effects of the intervention on healthy lifestyle behaviors and depressive/anxiety symptoms (e.g., race/ethnicity, gender, socioecomonic status, family composition, acculturation, structural barriers to activity, and parental healthy lifestyle beliefs and behaviors).

Background and Significance

The prevalence of unhealthy lifestyle behaviors leading to overweight and obesity as well as mental health problems in adolescents continues to be a significant public health concern. Data from the National Health and Nutrition Examination Survey (NHANES) from 2003 to 2004 indicate that, in all youth aged 12 to 19 years, 34.3% had a BMI percentile greater than or equal to the gender- and age-adjusted 85th percentile (overweight). For all adolescents, the prevalence of obesity (>95th percentile) was 17.4. Mental health/psychosocial problems, risk-taking behaviors, and injuries, many of which are preventable, currently cause more morbidity and mortality in the pediatric and adolescent population than do physical diseases and disorders [30]. Children and adolescents who are affected by depression often have lower self-esteem, underdeveloped social skills, and poor academic functioning [30]. Depression in adolescents also has been associated with risk-taking behaviors, such as alcohol and drug use, cutting behaviors, and high-risk sexual behaviors. Unfortunately, childhood and adolescent mental health is often underestimated as the foundation for adult health. Less than 25% of teens with a significant mental health disorder are seen by an appropriate mental health service provider [30, 60]. As most of the major mental health disorders begin in adolescence, intensified efforts must be placed on preventing and treating these disorders during this critical time in development [12].

Theoretical Framework for the Proposed Study

Driven by cognitive behavior theory (CBT), the COPE/Healthy Lifestyles TEEN Program is a series of 15 educational and CBSB sessions that focus on empowering teens to engage in healthy lifestyle behaviors (i.e., nutrition, physical activity, positive strategies to cope with stress, problem-solving, regulation of negative mood, and goal setting). It is designed to be easily integrated into high-school health education classes. Based on cognitive theory, we teach the teens how to cognitively restructure their thinking when negative events or inter-personal situations arise that tend to lead them into negative thought patterns and how to turn that thinking into a more positive interpretation of the situation or interpersonal inter-action so that they will emotionally feel better and behave in more healthy ways. Emphasis is placed on how patterns of thinking have an impact on behavior and emotions (i.e., the thinking, feeling, and behaving triangle). The program also includes educational content to increase teens' knowledge of how to lead a healthy lifestyle and homework activities to reinforce skills that are being learned in the classroom, *which assists them with putting into daily practice what they are learning in the educational sessions.* Brief bouts of physical activity (i.e., 15 to 20 minutes) are also incorporated into each of the 16 sessions to assist the teens in raising their beliefs or confidence in their ability to develop regular activity patterns (see the COPE Conceptual Model).

Conclusion, Significance, and Innovation of the Proposed Study

School is an ideal environment in which to test innovative interventions designed to increase healthy lifestyle behaviors and ultimately prevent or treat overweight/obesity as well as to enhance the highest level of mental health outcomes in adolescents. Preventive interventions that are implemented in schools need to be reproducible, teacher friendly, and inexpensive

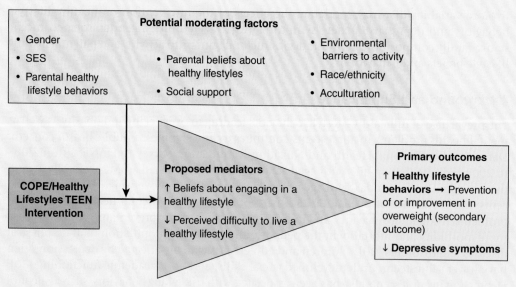

COPE conceptual model.

to implement. There is some evidence indicating that healthy lifestyle interventions that incorporate education, physical activity, and behavior modification may be the most promising strategies for preventing and treating overweight and obesity in teens; however, more long-term efficacy of these interventions is unknown [140]. Furthermore, the processes through which these interventions work are not known, and moderating variables that could shed light on circumstances under which or for whom the interventions work best have not been studied. Use of CBSB is a novel conceptual approach to targeting two of the most pressing public health problems in teens. Another innovative aspect of our proposed study is that we have powered it so that we have a large enough sample to study subgroups of the teens (i.e., those who are already overweight; those who are mildly to moderately depressed) where the effects of COPE may have the greatest impact.

Research Design and Methods

Overview of Design

This study is a prospective, blinded, randomized controlled test of the efficacy of the COPE/ Healthy Lifestyles TEEN Program and the mediational roles of cognitive beliefs and perceived difficulty in leading a healthy lifestyle in improving the healthy lifestyle behaviors and depressive symptoms of culturally diverse adolescents in high school. Participants ($N = 800$) will be recruited from teens, aged 14 to 16 years, who are freshmen and sophomores enrolled in health education courses at eight high schools in Phoenix, Arizona (i.e., four high schools in the Phoenix Union School District and four high schools in the Paradise Valley School District). Two of the four schools within each of the two school districts will be randomly assigned by a random number generator to receive either the COPE/Healthy Lifestyles TEEN Program or the Healthy Teens Program. All teens in the health education courses in the *eight* high schools will be invited to participate in the study. The teens in the health education courses will receive either: (1) an 8-week, 15-session (i.e., an average of two sessions per week) multicomponent educational and CBSB program with physical activity (i.e., COPE/Healthy Lifestyles) or (2) an 8-week, 15-session attention control program (Healthy Teens). In addition to baseline assessments, outcomes will be measured at three time points: (1) immediately following completion of the 8-week intervention, (2) 6 months following completion of the intervention, and (3) 12 months following completion of the intervention (see Table 1). **Rationale for Three Follow-Up Assessments (Postintervention, 6 Months, 12 Months)** Follow-up at three times is important to determine whether the effects of COPE can be sustained over time and to determine the appropriate timing of booster interventions, if needed, for future studies.

Intervention Conditions (Independent Variable)

COPE/Healthy Lifestyles TEEN Program: COPE is a manualized 15-session educational and cognitive behavioral skills building program guided by CBT with physical activity as a component of each session (see Appendix B). It was first developed by the primary investigator (PI) in 2002 and has been pilot tested three times with White, Hispanic, and African-American adolescents as a group intervention in high-school settings and once with 18- and 19-year-old college freshmen.

Each session of COPE contains 15 to 20 minutes of physical activity (e.g., walking, dancing), not as an exercise training program but rather to build beliefs/confidence in the teens that they can engage in and sustain some level of physical activity on a regular basis. Those healthy lifestyle intervention programs that have employed exercise interventions only have not led to sustained changes in healthy lifestyle behaviors. Our program is designed to enhance healthy lifestyle behaviors and sustain them because lifelong cognitive behavioral

			Baseline	Intervention	Postintervention	6-Month Follow-Up	12-Month Follow-Up
Phoenix Union High-School District	R	O1	X1	O2	O3	O4
	R	O1	X2	O2	O3	O4
Paradise Valley High-School District	R	O1	X1	O2	O3	O4
	R	O1	X2	O2	O3	O4

TABLE 1 **Study Design**

R, Random assignment of four high schools in the same school district to COPE or control for *a total of eight randomly assigned schools*; O, measurement times; X1, COPE program; X2, attention control (Healthy Teens Program).

skills are taught in the program. Because the COPE/Healthy Lifestyles TEEN Program is completely manualized for the teens and instructors, it can be easily implemented by health teachers in high-school settings. COPE sessions are detailed in Table 2.

Rationale for the Healthy Teens Attention Control Program: An attention control program that controls for the time spent with the adolescents in the COPE group is essential to determining the efficacy of the experimental program. The Healthy Teens Program will assist in ruling out alternative explanations of the mechanism by which the intervention works. It will be standardized like the COPE program to ensure that it can be evaluated. It will be administered in a format like that of the COPE intervention program and will include the same number and length of sessions but not include the theoretical active components of CBT or theoretical mechanisms to produce our hypothesized changes in outcomes. Teens in the attention control group also will receive the sessions in their required health class. The difference between the two programs will lie in the content of the sessions, with the Healthy Teens Program being focused on safety and common health topics/issues for teens (e.g., road safety, skin care, acne, sun safety). Workbook activities and homework assignments will focus on the topics being covered in class as well.

Assessment of Fidelity of the Intervention: Monitoring fidelity of the intervention program is essential to having greater confidence in the findings, being able to explain the results obtained, and in helping to ensure internal validity of the study.

Measures

Rationale for the Study Instruments: Instruments fall into four categories, including those administered: (1) to identify potential covariates/moderators, (2) to define outcomes, (3) to quantify proposed mediators, and (4) to evaluate the experimental process. Teens who participate in the program will complete outcome instruments on four occasions (weeks 0, 9, 34, and 58). Outcome and mediator instruments were chosen because they measure key components of the theoretical framework on which the intervention is based. Process instruments will be used to inform the design of future research and dissemination studies.

TABLE 2	COPE/Healthy Lifestyles TEEN Program Content[a]	

Session #	Session Content	Key Constructs From the Conceptual Model and COPE Intervention
1	Introduction of the COPE Healthy Lifestyles TEEN Program and goals.	
2	Healthy Lifestyles and the Thinking, Feeling, Behaving triangle.	*Cognitive behavioral skills building (CBSB)*
3	Self-esteem. Positive thinking/self-talk.	*CBSB*
4	Goal setting. Problem solving.	*CBSB*
5	Stress and coping.	*CBSB*
6	Emotional and behavioral regulation.	*CBSB*
7	Effective communication. Personality and communication styles.	*CBSB*
8	Barriers to goal progression and overcoming barriers. Energy balance. Ways to increase physical activity and associated benefits.	*CBSB and physical activity information*
9	Heart rate. Stretching.	*Physical activity information*
10	Food groups and a healthy body. Stoplight diet: Red, yellow, and green.	*Nutrition information*
11	Nutrients to build a healthy body. Reading labels. Effects of media and advertising on food choices.	*Nutrition information*
12	Portion sizes. "Super size." Influence of feelings on eating.	*Nutrition information*
13	Social eating. Strategies for eating during parties, holidays, and vacations.	*Nutrition information*
14	Snacks. Eating out.	*Nutrition information*
15	Integration of knowledge and skills to develop a healthy lifestyle plan; Putting it all together	*CBSB*

[a]Fifteen to twenty minutes of physical activity also is a component of each COPE session to build beliefs/confidence in the teens that they can engage in and sustain some level of physical activity on a regular basis.

Overview of Analysis Plan

Statistical analysis of data from this first full-scale test must serve several purposes beyond that of simply demonstrating the efficacy of COPE; for example, estimating effect sizes, mapping the trajectory of group differences over time, and identifying subgroup differences. Analysis will begin with careful characterization of the sample with descriptive statistics that identify (a) potential problems caused by skewed sampling, (b) differences between intervention and control groups that are evident at baseline despite randomization, and (c) differences between groups that appear at follow-up because of differential attrition.

The second phase of the analysis will use linear hierarchical models (also referred to as random coefficient and mixed models) to explore the effect of the intervention over time because these models incorporate random effects to reflect the correlation among observations from members of the same group [163, 164].

The entire grant application may be accessed at http://thepoint.lww.com/Melnyk3e.

Appendix A

Question Templates for Asking PICOT Questions

INTERVENTION

In _____ (P), how does _____ (I) compared to _____
(C) affect _____ (O) within _____ (T)?

ETIOLOGY

Are _____ (P) who have _____ (I) compared with those without
_____ (C) at _____ risk for/of _____ (O) over
_____ (T)?

DIAGNOSIS OR DIAGNOSTIC TEST

In _____ (P), are/is _____ (I) compared to _____ (C)
more accurate in diagnosing _____ (O)?

PROGNOSIS/PREDICTION

In (For) _____ (P), how does _____ (I) compared to
_____ (C) influence _____ (O) during/over _____ (T)?

MEANING

How do _____ (P) with _____ (I) perceive _____ (O)
during _____ (T)?

SHORT DEFINITIONS OF DIFFERENT TYPES OF QUESTIONS:

Intervention: Questions addressing the treatment of an illness or disability.
Etiology: Questions that address the causes or origin of disease, the factors that produce or predispose toward a certain disease or disorder.
Diagnosis: Questions addressing the act or process of identifying or determining the nature and cause of a disease or injury through evaluation.
Prognosis/Prediction: Questions addressing the prediction of the course of a disease.
Meaning: Questions addressing how one experiences a phenomenon.

SAMPLE QUESTIONS:

Intervention: In elderly patients in acute care facilities (P), how do fall prevention programs with risk assessment (I) compared to fall prevention programs without risk assessment (C) affect fall rates (O) within one quarter after intervention (T)?

Etiology: Are 50- to 60-year-old women (P) who have family history of obesity (I) compared with those without family history of obesity (C) at increased risk for increased body mass index (BMI) (O) during the first 3 years after hysterectomy or menopause (T)?

Diagnosis: In middle-aged males with suspected myocardial infarction (P), are serial 12-lead electrocardiograms (ECGs) (I) compared to one initial 12-lead ECG (C) more accurate in diagnosing an acute myocardial infarction (O)?

Prognosis/Prediction: (1) For patients 65 years and older (P), how does receiving the influenza vaccine (I) compared with not receiving the vaccine (C) influence the risk of developing pneumonia (O) during flu season (T)?

(2) In patients who have experienced an acute myocardial infarction (P), how does being a smoker (I) compared to being a nonsmoker (C) influence death and infarction rates (O) during the first 5 years after the myocardial infarction (T)?

Meaning: How do parents (P) of toddlers with a new diagnosis of a terminal disease (I) perceive their parenting role (O) during the first 3 months after diagnosis (T)?

Appendix B

Rapid Critical Appraisal Checklists

These rapid critical appraisal (RCA) checklists have been developed over several years and are designed to help you strive for mastery of the RCA phase of critical appraisal of evidence. The questions in the first section of the checklists are about what makes good research—and, therefore, contribute to determining the validity of a study. The second section of the checklists asks about information that helps establish study reliability within clinical practice. The third section of the RCA checklists contains questions about applicability of the study findings to patients. Becoming proficient at understanding the different aspects within the RCA checklists and consistently using them when appraising evidence will improve clinicians' understanding of various types of research methods, designs, statistical analyses, and translation of evidence into practice.

Caveat: Though these resources have been developed over several years, they don't get old. Thinking that requires everything to have the latest year on it is flawed thinking. These resources have been updated as the science of rigorous research methodology grows; however, their essence has not changed from the original intent of helping clinicians find the pearls within a study that demonstrate the validity, reliability, and applicability of research.

Note: These RCA checklists are also available in MS Word format on thePoint® for ease of use.

GENERAL APPRAISAL OVERVIEW FOR ALL STUDIES

Date:

Reviewer:

Article Citation (APA):

PICOT Question:

Overview/General Description of Study

- Purpose of Study:

- Study Design:
- General Description of Study:

Research Question(s) or Hypotheses:

Study Aims:

Sampling Technique, Sample Size, and Characteristics:

Major Variables Studies:

- Independent Variable(s):

- Dependent (outcome) Variable(s):

Variable Analysis Used (include whether appropriate to answer research questions/hypothesis or discover themes):

© Fineout-Overholt, 2010. This form was designed to help learners engage research as a fundamental tool in evidence-based decision-making. If you use this form for another use, please contact the author at ellen.fineout.overholt@gmail.com.

RAPID CRITICAL APPRAISAL QUESTIONS FOR SYSTEMATIC REVIEWS AND META-ANALYSES OF CLINICAL INTERVENTIONS QUESTION

VALIDITY

1. **Are the results of the review valid?**

a. Are the studies contained in the review randomized controlled trials (RCTs)?	Yes No Unknown
b. If not, were all relevant studies included in the review?	Yes No Unknown
c. Does the review include a detailed description of the search strategy to find all relevant studies?	Yes No Unknown
d. Does the review describe how validity of the individual studies was assessed (e.g., methodological quality, including the use of random assignment to study groups and complete follow-up of the participants)?	Yes No Unknown
e. Were the results consistent across studies?	Yes No Unknown
f. Were individual patient data or aggregate data used in the analysis?	Individual Aggregate
g. Does the review include a description of how studies were compared using statistical analysis?	Yes No Unknown

RELIABILITY

2. **What were the results?**

   a. How large is the intervention or treatment effect (OR, RR, effect size)?

   b. How precise is the intervention or treatment (CI)?

APPLICABILITY

3. **Will the results assist me in caring for my patients?**

a. Are my patients similar to the ones included in the review?	Yes No Unknown
b. Is it feasible to implement the findings in my practice setting?	Yes No Unknown
c. Do the pooled or combined results of the studies support the hospital's values and goals of service delivery? (i.e., Is it feasible to implement the findings in my practice setting?)	Yes No Unknown
d. Were all clinically important outcomes considered, including risks and benefits of the treatment?	Yes No Unknown
e. What is my clinical assessment of the patient and are there any contraindications or circumstances that would inhibit me from implementing the treatment?	Yes No Unknown
f. What are my patient's and his or her family's preferences and values about the treatment that is under consideration?	Yes No Unknown

Would you use the study results in your practice to make a difference in patient outcomes?

- If yes, how?
- If yes, why?
- If no, why not?

Additional Comments/Reflections:

Recommendation for article use within a body of evidence:

RAPID CRITICAL APPRAISAL QUESTIONS FOR RANDOMIZED CLINICAL TRIALS (RCTS)

VALIDITY

1. **Are the results of the study valid?**

a.	Were the participants randomly assigned to the experimental and control groups?	Yes	No	Unknown
b.	Was random assignment concealed from the individuals who were first enrolling participants into the study?	Yes	No	Unknown
c.	Were the participants and providers blind to the study group?	Yes	No	Unknown
d.	Were reasons given to explain why participants did not complete the study?	Yes	No	Unknown
e.	Were the follow-up assessments conducted long enough to fully study the effects of the intervention?	Yes	No	Unknown
f.	Were the participants analyzed in the group to which they were randomly assigned?	Yes	No	Unknown
g.	Was the control group appropriate?	Yes	No	Unknown
h.	Were the instruments used to measure the outcomes valid and reliable?	Yes	No	Unknown
i.	Were the participants in each of the groups similar on demographic and baseline clinical variables?	Yes	No	Unknown

RELIABILITY

2. **What are the results?**

a.	How large is the intervention or treatment effect (NNT, NNH, effect size?	_____
b.	How precise is the intervention or treatment (CI)?	_____

APPLICABILITY

3. **Will the results help me in caring for my patients?**

a.	Were all clinically important outcomes measured?	Yes	No	Unknown
b.	What are the risks and benefits of the treatment?	_____		
c.	Is the treatment feasible in my clinical setting?	Yes	No	Unknown
d.	What are my patient's/family's values and expectations for the outcome that is trying to be prevented and the treatment itself?	_____		

Would you use the study results in your practice to make a difference in patient outcomes?

- If yes, how?
- If yes, why?
- If no, why not?

Additional Comments/Reflections:

Recommendation for article use within a body of evidence:

RAPID CRITICAL APPRAISAL QUESTIONS FOR QUASI-EXPERIMENTAL STUDIES

Explain your answers and recommendation for use of this study in the body of evidence to answer your PICOT question.

VALIDITY

1. **Are the results of the study valid?**	Yes	No	Unknown	Rationale/Comment
• Study participants in intervention and comparison groups are similar.	1	2	3	
• The intervention is clearly identified.	1	2	3	
• There is a control group.	1	2	3	
• Participants in the comparison group(s) received a reasonable treatment/care to the exposure or intervention of interest given to the intervention group.	1	2	3	
• Follow-up between groups is adequately described and analyzed.	1	2	3	
• Appropriate statistical analysis was used for the data gathered.	1	2	3	
• Measurement of the outcome was obtained pre- and postintervention.	1	2	3	
• The outcomes are the same across all groups and were measured with the same instrument.	1	2	3	
• Outcomes were measured with valid and reliable instruments.	1	2	3	

RELIABILITY

2. **What are the results?**
   • What were the magnitude of the results?
   • What was the precision of the results?

APPLICABILITY

3. **Will the results help me in caring for my patients?**				
• Were the study patients similar to my own?	1	2	3	
• Will the results lead directly to selecting or avoiding therapy?	1	2	3	
• Are the results useful for reassuring or counseling patients?	1	2	3	

Would you use the study results in your practice to make a difference in patient outcomes?
• If yes, how?
• If yes, why?
• If no, why not?

Additional Comments/Reflections:

Recommendation for article use within a body of evidence:

RAPID CRITICAL APPRAISAL QUESTIONS FOR COHORT STUDIES

VALIDITY

1. Are the results of the study valid?

a. Was there a representative and well-defined sample of patients at a similar point in the course of the disease?	Yes	No	Unknown
b. Was follow-up sufficiently long and complete?	Yes	No	Unknown
c. Were objective and unbiased outcome criteria used?	Yes	No	Unknown
d. Did the analysis adjust for important prognostic risk factors and confounding variables?	Yes	No	Unknown

Comments

RELIABILITY

2. What are the results?

a. What is the magnitude of the relationship between predictors (i.e., prognostic indicators) and targeted outcome? _____

b. How likely is the outcome event(s) in a specified period of time? _____

c. How precise are the study estimates? _____

APPLICABILITY

3. Will the results help me in caring for my patients?

a. Were the study patients similar to my own?	Yes	No	Unknown
b. Will the results lead directly to selecting or avoiding therapy?	Yes	No	Unknown
c. Are the results useful for reassuring or counseling patients?	Yes	No	Unknown

Comments

Would you use the study results in your practice to make a difference in patient outcomes?

- If yes, how?
- If yes, why?
- If no, why not?

Additional Comments/Reflections:

Recommendation for article use within a body of evidence:

RAPID CRITICAL APPRAISAL QUESTIONS FOR DESCRIPTIVE STUDIES

VALIDITY

1. Are the results of the study valid?

• Were study/survey methods appropriate for the question?	Yes	No	Unknown
• Was sampling methods appropriate for the research question?	Yes	No	Unknown
• Were sample size implications on study results discussed?	Yes	No	Unknown
• Were variables studied appropriate for the question?	Yes	No	Unknown
• Dependent variables are:			
• Independent (outcome) variables are:			
• Were outcomes appropriate for the question?	Yes	No	Unknown
• Were valid and reliable instruments used to measure outcomes?	Yes	No	Unknown
• Were the chosen measures appropriate for study outcomes?	Yes	No	Unknown
• Were outcomes clearly described?	Yes	No	Unknown
• Did investigators and/or funding agencies declare freedom from conflict of interest?	Yes	No	Unknown

RELIABILITY

2. What are the results?

• What were the main results of the study?			
• Was there statistical significance? Explain.			
• Was there clinical significance? Explain.			
• Were safety concerns, including adverse events and risk/benefit described?	Yes	No	Unknown

APPLICABILITY

3. Will the results help me in caring for my patients?

• Are the results applicable to my patient population?	Yes	No	Unknown
• Will my patients' and families' values and beliefs be supported by the knowledge gained from the study?	Yes	No	Unknown

Would you use the study results in your practice to make a difference in patient outcomes?

- If yes, how?
- If yes, why?
- If no, why not?

Additional Comments/Reflections:

Recommendation for article use within a body of evidence:

RAPID CRITICAL APPRAISAL QUESTIONS FOR QUALITATIVE EVIDENCE

VALIDITY

1. **Are the results of the study valid (i.e., trustworthy and credible)?**

   a. How were study participants chosen?

   b. How were accuracy and completeness of data assured?

   c. How plausible/believable are the results?

i. Are implications of the research stated?	Yes	No	Unknown
1. May new insights increase sensitivity to others' needs?	Yes	No	Unknown
2. May understandings enhance situational competence?	Yes	No	Unknown

   d. What is the effect on the reader?

1. Are results plausible and believable?	Yes	No	Unknown
2. Is the reader imaginatively drawn into the experience?	Yes	No	Unknown

RELIABILITY

2. **What were the results?**

a. Does the research approach fit the purpose of the study?	Yes	No	Unknown
i. How does the researcher identify the study approach?	Yes	No	Unknown
1. Are language and concepts consistent with the approach?	Yes	No	Unknown
2. Are data collection and analysis techniques appropriate?	Yes	No	Unknown
ii. Is the significance/importance of the study explicit?	Yes	No	Unknown
1. Does review of the literature support a need for the study?	Yes	No	Unknown
2. What is the study's potential contribution?			
iii. Is the sampling strategy clear and guided by study needs?	Yes	No	Unknown
1. Does the researcher control selection of the sample?	Yes	No	Unknown
2. Do sample composition and size reflect study needs?	Yes	No	Unknown
b. Is the phenomenon (human experience) clearly identified?			
i. Are data collection procedures clear?	Yes	No	Unknown
1. Are sources and means of verifying data explicit?	Yes	No	Unknown
2. Are researcher roles and activities explained?	Yes	No	Unknown
ii. Are data analysis procedures described?	Yes	No	Unknown
1. Does analysis guide direction of sampling and when it ends?	Yes	No	Unknown
2. Are data management processes described?	Yes	No	Unknown
c. What are the reported results (description or interpretation)?			
i. How are specific findings presented?			
1. Is presentation logical, consistent, and easy to follow?	Yes	No	Unknown
2. Do quotes fit the findings they are intended to illustrate?	Yes	No	Unknown
ii. How are overall results presented?			
1. Are meanings derived from data described in context?	Yes	No	Unknown
2. Does the writing effectively promote understanding?	Yes	No	Unknown

(continued)

APPLICABILITY

3. **Will the results help me in caring for my patients?**

   a. Are the results relevant to persons in similar situations?   Yes   No   Unknown

   b. Are the results relevant to patient values and/or circumstances?   Yes   No   Unknown

   c. How may the results be applied in clinical practice?

Would you use the study results in your practice to make a difference in patient outcomes?

- If yes, how?
- If yes, why?
- If no, why not?

Additional Comments/Reflections:

Recommendation for article use within a body of evidence:

RAPID CRITICAL APPRAISAL QUESTIONS FOR EVIDENCE-BASED PRACTICE (EBP) IMPLEMENTATION OR QUALITY IMPROVEMENT (QI) PROJECTS

Indicate the extent to which the item is met in the published report of the EBP or QI project.

Validity of Evidence Synthesis (i.e., good methodology)	1 No	2 A Little	3 Somewhat	4 Quite a Bit	5 Very Much
1. The title of the publication identifies the report/project as an EBP implementation or QI project.					
2. The project report provides a structured summary that includes, as applicable, data to establish the existent and background of the clinical issue; inclusion and exclusion criteria and source(s) of evidence; evidence synthesis, objective(s), and setting of the EBP or QI project; project limitations; results/outcomes; and recommendation and implications for policy.					
3. Report includes existing internal evidence to adequately describe the clinical issue.					
4. Provides an explicit statement of the question being addressed with reference to participants or population/intervention/comparison/outcome (PICO).					
5. Explicitly describes the search method (i.e., was it systematic), inclusion and exclusion criteria, and rationale for search strategy limits.					
6. Describes multiple information sources (e.g., databases, contact with study authors to identify additional studies, or any other additional search strategies) included in the search strategy, and date.					
7. States the process for title, abstract, and article screening for selecting studies.					
8. Describes the method of data extraction (e.g., independently or process for validating data from multiple reviewers).					
9. Includes conceptual and operational definitions for all variables for which data were abstracted (e.g., define blood pressure as systolic blood pressure, diastolic blood pressure, ambulatory blood pressure, automatic cuff blood pressure, or arterial blood pressure).					
10. Describes methods used for assessing risk of bias of individual studies (including specification of whether this was done at the study or outcome level).					

(continued)

Validity of Evidence Synthesis (i.e., good methodology)	1 No	2 A Little	3 Somewhat	4 Quite a Bit	5 Very Much
11. States the principal summary measures (e.g., risk ratio, difference in means).					
12. Describes the method of combining results of studies, including quality, quantity, and consistency of evidence.					
13. Specifies assessment of risk of bias that may affect the cumulative evidence (e.g., publication bias, selective reporting within studies).					
14. Describes appraisal procedure and conflict resolution.					
15. Provides number of studies screened, assessed for eligibility, and included in the review, with reasons for exclusion at each stage, ideally with a flow diagram.					
16. For each study, presents characteristics for which data were extracted (e.g., study size, design, method, follow-up period) and provides citations.					
17. Presents data on risk of bias of each study and, if available, any outcome-level assessment.					
18. For all outcomes considered (benefit or harms), includes a table with summary data for each intervention group, effect estimates, and confidence intervals, ideally with a forest plot.					
19. Summarizes the main findings, including the strength of evidence for each main outcome; considering their relevance to key groups (i.e., healthcare providers, users, and policy makers).					
20. Discusses limitations at study and outcome levels (e.g., risk of bias) and at review level (e.g., incomplete retrieval of identified research, reporting bias).					
21. Provides a general interpretation of the results in the context of other evidence, and implications for further research, practice, or policy changes.					
Validity of Implementation (i.e., well-done project)					
1. Purpose of project flows from evidence synthesis					
2. Stakeholders (active and passive) are identified and communication with them is described					

	1 No	2 A Little	3 Somewhat	4 Quite a Bit	5 Very Much
3. Implementation protocol is congruent with evidence synthesis (fidelity of the intervention)					
4. Implementation protocol is sufficiently detailed to provide for replication among project participants					
5. Education of project participants and other stakeholders is clearly described					
6. Outcomes are measured with measures supported in the evidence synthesis					
Reliability of Implementation Project (i.e., I can learn from or implement project results)					
1. Data are collected with sufficient rigor to be reliable for like groups to those participants of the project					
2. Results are evidence implementation and are clinically meaningful (statistics are interpreted as such)					
Application of Implementation (i.e., this project is useful for my patients)					
1. How feasible is the project protocol?					
2. Have the project managers considered/included all outcomes that are important to my work?					
3. Is implementing the project safe (i.e., low risk of harm)?					
Summary Score					

Recommendations with consideration of this type of level IV intervention evidence:

- 32–64: consider evidence with extreme caution
- 65–128: consider evidence with caution
- 128–160: consider evidence with confidence

RAPID CRITICAL APPRAISAL QUESTIONS FOR CASE STUDIES

VALIDITY

1. Are the results of the study valid?

• Is the study question/issue clearly articulated?	Yes	No	Unknown
• Is the researcher's perspective clearly described and taken into account?	Yes	No	Unknown
• Are the methods for collecting data clearly described?	Yes	No	Unknown
• Are the methods for analyzing the data likely to be valid and reliable?	Yes	No	Unknown
• Are quality control measures used?	Yes	No	Unknown

Comments

RELIABILITY

2. What are the results?

• Are the results credible, and if so, are they relevant for practice?	Yes	No	Unknown

Comments

APPLICABILITY

3. Will the results help me in caring for my patients?

• Are the conclusions drawn justified by the results?	Yes	No	Unknown
• Are the findings of the study transferable to other settings?	Yes	No	Unknown

Comments

Would you use the study results in your practice to make a difference in patient outcomes?

- If yes, how?
- If yes, why?
- If no, why not?

Additional Comments/Reflections:

Recommendation for article use within a body of evidence:

RAPID CRITICAL APPRAISAL QUESTIONS FOR LITERATURE REVIEW (LEVEL VII)

VALIDITY

1. **Are the results of the review valid?**

A. Are the designs of the articles in the review identified?	Yes	No	Unknown
B. Does the review include a detailed description of the search strategy to find all relevant studies and was it systematic?	Yes	Yes	Unknown
C. Do the reviewers use standard criteria to describe the validity of the individual studies (e.g., criteria about methodological quality)?	Yes	No	Unknown
D. Were the results consistent across studies?	Yes	No	Unknown

RELIABILITY

2. **What were the results?**

A. Were the results described across the studies or were the findings described study by study? (Hint: Were there synthesis tables?)	Yes	No	Unknown
B. What are sources of bias within the report that make the literature review unreliable? (See validity questions above.)			
C. Does the bias within the literature review methodology make the results as described unusable? (if so, stop here.)	Yes	No	Unknown

APPLICABILITY

3. **Will the results assist me in caring for my patients?**

A. Are my patients similar to the ones included in the review?	Yes	No	Unknown
B. Is it feasible to implement the findings in my practice setting?	Yes	No	Unknown
C. Were all clinically important outcomes considered, including risks and benefits of the treatment?	Yes	No	Unknown
D. What is my clinical assessment of the patient and are there any contraindications or circumstances that would inhibit me from implementing the treatment?	Yes	No	Unknown
E. What are my patient's and his or her family's preferences and values about the treatment that is under consideration?			

Would you use the study results in your practice to make a difference in patient outcomes?

- If yes, how?
- If yes, why?
- If no, why not?

Additional Comments/Reflections:

Recommendation for article use within a body of evidence:

RAPID CRITICAL APPRAISAL QUESTIONS FOR EVIDENCE-BASED GUIDELINES

CREDIBILITY

1. Who were the guideline developers?			
2. Were the developers representative of key stakeholders in this specialty (interdisciplinary)?	Yes	No	Unknown
3. Who funded the guideline development?			
4. Were any of the guidelines developers funded researchers of the reviewed studies?	Yes	No	Unknown
5. Did the team have a valid development strategy?	Yes	No	Unknown
6. Was an explicit (how decisions were made), sensible, and impartial process used to identify, select, and combine evidence?	Yes	No	Unknown
7. Did the developers carry out a comprehensive, reproducible literature review within the past 12 months of its publication/revision?	Yes	No	Unknown
8. Were all important options and outcomes considered?	Yes	No	Unknown
9. Is each recommendation in the guideline tagged by the level/strength of evidence upon which it is based and linked with the scientific evidence?	Yes	No	Unknown
10. Do the guidelines make explicit recommendations (reflecting value judgments about outcomes)?	Yes	No	Unknown
11. Has the guideline been subjected to peer review and testing?	Yes	No	Unknown

APPLICABILITY/GENERALIZABILITY

12. Is the intent of use provided (e.g., national, regional, local)?	Yes	No	Unknown
13. Are the recommendations clinically relevant?	Yes	No	Unknown
14. Will the recommendations help me in caring for my patients?	Yes	No	Unknown
15. Are the recommendations practical/feasible (e.g., resources—people and equipment— available)?	Yes	No	Unknown
16. Are the recommendations a major variation from current practice?	Yes	No	Unknown
17. Can the outcomes be measured through standard care?	Yes	No	Unknown

Modified from Slutsky, J. (2005). Using evidence-based guidelines: Tools for improving practice. In B. M. Melnyk & E. Fineout-Overholt (Eds.), *Evidence-based practice in nursing & healthcare. A guide to best practice* (pp. 221–236). Philadelphia, PA: Lippincott, Williams & Wilkins. This form may be used for educational, practice change, and research purposes without permission.

Appendix C

Evaluation Table Template and Synthesis Table Examples for Critical Appraisal

EVALUATION TABLE TEMPLATE

Citation: Author, Date of Publication & Title	Purpose of Study	Conceptual Framework	Design/ Method	Sample/ Setting	Major Variables Studied and Their Definitions	Measurement of Major Variables	Data Analysis	Study Findings	Worth to Practice LOE Strengths/Weaknesses Feasibility Conclusion RECOMMENDATION

Here is where you list your abbreviations in alpha order. Example, LOE, level of evidence.

CAVEATS

1. *This is one table for ALL studies, not one table per study. The prompts below are offered to help you populate your table with the proper information for each column. Do not repeat the prompts in your evaluation table—only provide the information from your articles.*
2. *Parsimony is key, so keep all info succinct and clear. No complete sentences in any column, except for the final one under* **NOTES.**
3. Use abbreviations and create your own unique legend to help readers read your table.
4. Keep your desired outcome in mind and *put only relevant info into your table.* Extraneous, unrelated content can confuse and take away from your relevant content, discovery, and synthesis.

First author, year, title	Why the study was conducted. Could include the research question, hypothesis, or specific aims of the study?	Theoretical basis for the study	What research design was used and what was the study protocol (what was done)?	Number, characteristics, attrition rate and why?	Independent variables (e.g., IV1 = NAME—use abbreviations IV2 = same) Dependent variables (e.g., DV = NAME—use abbreviations)	What scales were used to measure the outcome variables (e.g., DV: variable abbreviation, name of scale, author, reliability info [e.g., Cronbach alphas])?	What stats were used to answer the clinical question (i.e., all stats do not need to be put into the table)? LIST ONLY THE NAME OF THE STAT	Statistical findings or qualitative findings (i.e., for every statistical test you have in the data analysis column, you should have the variable abbreviation and corresponding numerical finding; do not put increase or decrease etc. few to no words in this column)	• Level of evidence (LOE) • Strengths and limitations of the study • Risk or harm if study intervention or findings implemented • Feasibility of use in your practice • Conclusion from the study (YOURS not the researcher's) • Recommendation for use of evidence in practice (BSN, MSN, DNP) • Recommendation for further research (PhD) • Notes regarding gems or caveats about the article • Remember: level of evidence + quality of evidence = strength of evidence and confidence to act • Consider using grading criteria such as the USPSTF grading schema to compare across studies http://www.ahrq.gov/clinic/3rduspstf/ratings.htm

EVIDENCE SYNTHESIS TABLES

(e.g., Comparisons of Variable of Interest: Outcome, Intervention, Measurement, Definition of Variable, Levels of Evidence [design] Across Studies)

Example One: The table below is **one example** for how you could construct a synthesis table for interventions across studies.

	Studies	A	B	C	D	E	F
Interventions							
1		X	X			X	X
2				X	X		X
3				X	X		X

A, study author and year; B, study author and year; C, study author and year; etc.
X, presence of the intervention.

Example Two: The table below is **another example** of a synthesis table—this one is focused on design, sample, and outcome across studies.

Minimally, there should be three synthesis tables: One that reflects level of evidence, one that reflects variety of interventions used and one that both intervention and impact on outcome. (see Unit 2 EBP Exemplar)—there could be many more types of tables. Choose your information carefully that you will include in your syntheses tables. Create your **OWN** synthesis table—remember the studies are telling the story about your issue! Your studies should indicate what is important to put in the synthesis table.

Studies	Design	Sample		Outcome
A	RCT	$N = 450$ Age: 60–90	Ethnicity: 80% Asian 20% Caucasian	Falls ↓
B	Quasi-experimental, correlational	$N = 35$ Age: 75–85	Ethnicity: 73% Caucasian 10% African American 17% Hispanic	Falls ↓
C	EBP Implementation Project	$N = 50$ Age: 55–90	Ethnicity: 100% Caucasian	Falls ↓

Used with permission, © 2007 Fineout-Overholt. If you use this evaluation template or the synthesis information, please let Dr. EFO know how it worked for you by contacting her at ellen.fineout.overholt@gmail.com

Appendices Online

Visit thePoint* to view all Appendices available with this book:

- Appendix D: Walking the Walk and Talking the Talk: An Appraisal Guide for Qualitative Evidence
- Appendix E: Example of a Health Policy Brief
- Appendix F: Example of a Press Release
- Appendix G: Example of an Approved Consent Form for a Study
- Appendix H: System-Wide ARCC Model EEP Mentor Role Description

Appendix I

ARCC Model Timeline for an EBP Implementation Project

PICOT Question:		
Team Members:		
Evidence-Based Practice (EBP) Mentor and Contact Info:		
Preliminary Checkpoint A	• Describe the chosen EBP model(s) and how it/they will guide the implementation project	Notes:
Preliminary Checkpoint B	• Who are the stakeholders for your project? • Active (on the implementation team) and supportive (not on the team, but essential to success) • Identify project team roles and leadership • Begin acquisition of any necessary approvals for project implementation and dissemination (e.g., system leadership, unit leadership, ethics board [IRB]) • ***Consult with EBP mentor***	Notes and Progress:
Checkpoint One	• Hone PICOT question and assure team is prepared • Build EBP knowledge and skills • ***Consult with EBP mentor***	Notes and Progress:
Checkpoint Two	• Conduct literature search and retain studies that meet criteria for inclusion • Connect with librarian • Meet with implementation group—TEAM BUILD • ***Consult with EBP mentor***	Notes and Progress:
Checkpoint Three	• Critically appraise literature • Meet with group to discuss how completely evidence answers question; pose follow-up questions and re-review the literature as necessary • ***Consult with EBP mentor***	Notes and Progress:
Checkpoint Four	• Meet with group • Summarize evidence with focus on implications for practice and conduct interviews with content experts as necessary to benchmark • Begin formulating detailed plan for implementation of evidence • Include who must know about the project, when they will know, how they will know • ***Consult with EBP mentor***	Notes and Progress:

Checkpoint Five	• Define project purpose—connect the evidence and the project • Define baseline data collection source(s) (e.g., existing dataset, electronic health record), methods, and measures • Define postproject outcome indicators of a successful project • Gather outcome measures • Write data collection protocol • Write the project protocol (data collection fits in this document) • Finalize any necessary approvals for project implementation and dissemination (e.g., system leadership, unit leadership, IRB) • ***Consult with EBP mentor***	Notes and Progress:
Checkpoint Six (about midway)	• Meet with implementation group • Discuss known barriers and facilitators of project • Discuss strategies for minimizing barriers and maximizing facilitators • Finalize protocol for implementation of evidence • Identify resources (human, fiscal, and other) necessary to complete project • Supply EBP mentor with written IRB approval and managerial support • Begin work on poster for dissemination of initiation of project and progress to date to educate stakeholders about project—get help from support staff • Include specific plan for how evaluation will take place: who, what, when, where, and how and communication mechanisms to stakeholders • ***Consult with EBP mentor***	Notes and Progress:
Checkpoint Seven	• Meet with implementation group to review proposed poster • Make final adjustment to poster with support staff • Inform stakeholders of start date of implementation and poster presentation • Address any concerns or questions of stakeholders (active and supportive) • ***Consult with EBP mentor***	Notes and Progress:
Checkpoint Eight	• Poster presentation (preferred event is a system-wide recognition of quality, research, or innovation) • LAUNCH EBP implementation project • ***Consult with EBP mentor***	Notes and Progress:

(continued)

Checkpoint Nine	• Midproject meet with all key stakeholders to review progress and provide outcomes to date • Review issues, successes, aha's, and triumphs of project to date. • **Consult with EBP mentor**	Notes and Progress:
Checkpoint Ten	• Complete final data collection for project evaluation • Present project results via poster presentation—locally and nationally • **Celebrate with EBP mentor and agency leadership**	Notes and Progress:
Checkpoint Eleven	• Review project progress, lessons learned, new questions generated from process • **Consult with EBP mentor about new questions**	Notes, Progress, and Next Steps:

Appendix J

Sample Instruments to Evaluate EBP in Educational Settings

EBP BELIEFS SCALE FOR EDUCATORS (EBPB-E)

Below are 22 statements about evidence-based practice (EBP). Please circle the number that best describes your agreement or disagreement with each statement. There are no right or wrong answers.

	Strongly Disagree	Disagree	Neither Agree nor Disagree	Agree	Strongly Agree
1. I believe that EBP results in the best clinical care for patients.	1	2	3	4	5
2. I am clear about the steps of EBP.	1	2	3	4	5
3. I am sure that I can implement EBP.	1	2	3	4	5
4. I believe that critically appraising evidence is an important step in the EBP process.	1	2	3	4	5
5. I am sure that evidence-based guidelines can improve clinical care	1	2	3	4	5
6. I believe that I can search for the best evidence to answer clinical questions in a time-efficient way.	1	2	3	4	5
7. I am sure that I can teach how to search for the best evidence.	1	2	3	4	5
8. I believe that I can overcome barriers in implementing EBP.	1	2	3	4	5
9. I am sure that I can implement EBP in a time-efficient way.	1	2	3	4	5
10. I am sure that implementing EBP will improve the care that my students deliver to patients.	1	2	3	4	5
11. I am sure about how to measure the outcomes of clinical care.	1	2	3	4	5
12. I believe that EBP takes too much time.	1	2	3	4	5
13. I am sure that I can access the best resources in order to integrate EBP in the curriculum.	1	2	3	4	5
14. I believe EBP is difficult.	1	2	3	4	5

(continued)

	Strongly Disagree	Disagree	Neither Agree nor Disagree	Agree	Strongly Agree
15. I know how to implement EBP sufficiently enough to make curricular changes.	1	2	3	4	5
16. I am confident about my ability to implement EBP where I work.	1	2	3	4	5
17. I believe the care that I deliver is evidence based.	1	2	3	4	5
18. I am sure that I can teach EBP in a time-efficient way.	1	2	3	4	5
19. I am sure that integrating EBP into the curriculum will improve the care that students deliver to their patients.	1	2	3	4	5
20. I am sure that I can teach EBP.	1	2	3	4	5
21. I am sure that I can teach how to develop a PICOT question.	1	2	3	4	5
22. I know how to teach EBP sufficiently enough to impact students' practice.	1	2	3	4	5

EBP BELIEFS SCALE—STUDENT

Below are 20 statements about EBP. Please circle the number that best describes your agreement or disagreement with each statement. There are no right or wrong answers.

	Strongly Disagree	Disagree	Neither Agree nor Disagree	Agree	Strongly Agree
1. I believe that EBP results in the best clinical care for patients.	1	2	3	4	5
2. I am clear about the steps of EBP.	1	2	3	4	5
3. I am sure that I can implement EBP.	1	2	3	4	5
4. I believe that asking the PICOT question drives the systematic search for evidence to answer the question and is not a project.	1	2	3	4	5
5. I understand that the role of EBP is ensuring best practice and reliable outcomes for healthcare.	1	2	3	4	5
6. I know how to describe a clinical issue using data generated from practice (e.g., quality improvement data).	1	2	3	4	5
7. I believe that I can systematically search for the best evidence to answer clinical questions in a time-efficient way.	1	2	3	4	5
8. I understand the language of EBP (e.g., terms like research design, statistics, outcomes, clinical question).	1	2	3	4	5
9. I believe that learning how to critically appraise evidence is an important step in implementing the EBP process.	1	2	3	4	5
10. I believe that I can identify and overcome barriers to implementing EBP.	1	2	3	4	5
11. I am sure that evidence-based guidelines can improve clinical care.	1	2	3	4	5
12. I am sure that I can implement EBP in a time-efficient way.	1	2	3	4	5
13. I am sure that implementing EBP will improve the care that I deliver to my patients.	1	2	3	4	5
14. I am sure I know how to measure the outcomes of my care.	1	2	3	4	5
15. I believe that EBP takes too much time.	1	2	3	4	5

(continued)

	Strongly Disagree	Disagree	Neither Agree nor Disagree	Agree	Strongly Agree
16. I am sure that I can access the best resources in order to implement EBP.	1	2	3	4	5
17. I believe EBP is difficult.	1	2	3	4	5
18. I know how to implement EBP sufficiently enough to initiate practice changes.	1	2	3	4	5
19. I am confident about my ability to implement EBP within my clinical practicum settings.	1	2	3	4	5
20. I believe the care that I currently deliver is evidence based.	1	2	3	4	5

EBP IMPLEMENTATION SCALE FOR EDUCATORS (EBPI-E)

Below are 18 questions about EBP by educators. Some health professions educators do some of these things more often than other health professions educators. There is no certain frequency in which you should be performing these tasks. Please answer each question by circling the number that best describes **how often each item has applied to you in the past 8 weeks**.

In the **past 8 weeks**, I have:

	0 Times	1–3 Times	4–5 Times	6–8 Times	>8 Times
1. Used evidence to change my teaching	0	1	2	3	4
2. Critically appraised evidence from a research study	0	1	2	3	4
3. Generated a PICO question about my teaching/practice specialty	0	1	2	3	4
4. Informally discussed evidence from a research study with a colleague	0	1	2	3	4
5. Collected data on a clinical/educational issue	0	1	2	3	4
6. Shared evidence from a study or studies in the form of a report or presentation to more than two colleagues	0	1	2	3	4
7. Evaluated the outcomes of an educational change	0	1	2	3	4
8. Shared an evidence-based guideline with a colleague	0	1	2	3	4
9. Shared evidence from a research study with a student	0	1	2	3	4
10. Shared evidence from a research study with a multidisciplinary team member	0	1	2	3	4
11. Read and critically appraised a clinical research study	0	1	2	3	4
12. Accessed the Cochrane database of systematic reviews	0	1	2	3	4
13. Accessed the evidence-based guidelines	0	1	2	3	4
14. Used an evidence-based guideline or systematic review to change educational strategies where I work	0	1	2	3	4
15. Evaluated an educational initiative by collecting outcomes	0	1	2	3	4
16. Shared the outcome data collected with colleagues	0	1	2	3	4
17. Changed curricular policies/materials based on outcome data	0	1	2	3	4
18. Promoted the use of EBP to my colleagues	0	1	2	3	4

© Fineout-Overholt & Melnyk, 2010. Please DO NOT USE without permission. For further information about use, please contact Dr. EFO at ellen.fineout.overholt@gmail.com. Validity of this scale has been established and Cronbach's alphas have been ≥0.85 across various samples.

EBP IMPLEMENTATION SCALE—STUDENTS (EBPI-S)

Below are 18 questions about EBP. Some health professions students do some of these things more often than other health professions students. There is no certain frequency in which you should be performing these tasks. Please note that colleagues in this instance can be classmates, instructors, clinical preceptors, or other health professionals. Please answer each question by circling the number that best describes **how often each item has applied to you in the past 8 weeks**.

In the **past 8 weeks**, I have:

	0 Times	1–3 Times	4–5 Times	6–8 Times	>8 Times
1. Used evidence as the basis for my clinical decision making	0	1	2	3	4
2. Critically appraised evidence from a research study	0	1	2	3	4
3. Generated a PICOT question	0	1	2	3	4
4. Informally discussed evidence from a research study with a student colleague, faculty member, or clinical partner	0	1	2	3	4
5. Collected data of a patient problem, clinical issue, or clinical scenario (simulation)	0	1	2	3	4
6. Shared evidence from a study or studies in the form of a report or presentation to more than two students or clinical colleagues or faculty	0	1	2	3	4
7. Evaluated the outcomes of a clinical practice decision	0	1	2	3	4
8. Shared an evidence-based guideline with a student or clinical colleague or faculty member	0	1	2	3	4
9. Shared evidence from a research study with a patient/family member	0	1	2	3	4
10. Shared evidence from a research study with a multidisciplinary colleague	0	1	2	3	4
11. Read and critically appraised a clinical research study	0	1	2	3	4
12. Accessed the Cochrane database of systematic reviews	0	1	2	3	4
13. Accessed an evidence-based guideline	0	1	2	3	4
14. Used an evidence-based guideline or systematic review as the basis for a clinical decision	0	1	2	3	4
15. Evaluated a care initiative by collecting patient outcome data	0	1	2	3	4
16. Shared the outcome data collected with a student or clinical colleague or faculty member	0	1	2	3	4
17. Made a clinical decision about how to care for a patient based on patient outcome data	0	1	2	3	4
18. Promoted the use of EBP to my student or clinical colleagues	0	1	2	3	4

ORGANIZATIONAL CULTURE AND READINESS FOR SCHOOL-WIDE INTEGRATION OF EVIDENCE-BASED PRACTICE SURVEY—EDUCATORS (OCRSIEP-E)

Below are 19 questions about EBP. Please consider the state of your educational organization for the readiness of EBP and indicate which answer best describes your response to each question. There are no right or wrong answers.

Item	None at All	A Little	Somewhat	Moderately	Very Much
1. To what extent is EBP clearly described as central to the mission and philosophy of your educational agency?	1	2	3	4	5
2. To what extent do you believe that evidence-base education is practiced in your organization?	1	2	3	4	5
3. To what extent is the faculty with whom you work committed to EBP?	1	2	3	4	5
4. To what extent is the community partners with whom you work committed to EBP?	1	2	3	4	5
5. To what extent are there administrators within your organization committed to EBP (i.e., have planned for resources and support [e.g., time] to initiate EBP)?	1	2	3	4	5
6. In your organization, to what extent is there a critical mass of faculty who have strong EBP knowledge and skills?	1	2	3	4	5
7. To what extent is there ongoing research by nurse scientists (doctorally prepared researchers) in your organization to assist in generation of evidence when it does not exist?	1	2	3	4	5
8. In your organization, to what extent are there faculty who are EBP mentors?	1	2	3	4	5
9. To what extent do faculty model EBP in their educational and clinical settings?	1	2	3	4	5
10. To what extent do faculty have access to quality computers and access to electronic databases for searching for best evidence?	1	2	3	4	5
11. To what extent do faculty have proficient computer skills?	1	2	3	4	5

(continued)

Item	None at All	A Little	Somewhat	Moderately	Very Much
12. To what extent do librarians within your organization have EBP knowledge and skills?	1	2	3	4	5
13. To what extent are librarians used to search for evidence?	1	2	3	4	5
14. To what extent are fiscal resources used to support EBP (e.g., education—attending EBP conferences/workshops, computers, paid time for the EBP process, mentors)	1	2	3	4	5
15. To what extent are there EBP champions (i.e., those who will go the extra mile to advance EBP) in the environment among:					
a. Administrators?	1	2	3	4	5
b. Community partners?	1	2	3	4	5
c. Clinical faculty?	1	2	3	4	5
d. Junior faculty?	1	2	3	4	5
e. Senior faculty?	1	2	3	4	5
16. To what extent is the measurement and sharing of outcomes part of the culture of the organization in which you work?	1	2	3	4	5

Item	None	25%	50%	75%	100%
17. To what extent are decisions generated from:					
a. Faculty?	1	2	3	4	5
b. College administration?	1	2	3	4	5
c. University administration?	1	2	3	4	5

Item	Not ready	Getting Ready	Been Ready But Not Acting	Ready to Go	Past Ready and Onto Action
18. Overall, how would you rate your institution in readiness for EBP	1	2	3	4	5

Item	None at All	A Little	Somewhat	Moderately	Very Much
19. Compared to 6 months ago, how much movement in your educational organization has there been toward an EBP culture?	1	2	3	4	5

ORGANIZATIONAL CULTURE AND READINESS FOR SCHOOL-WIDE INTEGRATION OF EVIDENCE-BASED PRACTICE SURVEY—STUDENTS (OCRSIEP-ES)

Below are 19 questions about EBP in education. Please consider the culture of your educational organization and its readiness for EBP. Indicate which answer best describes your response to each question; there are no right or wrong answers.

Item	None at All	A Little	Somewhat	Moderately	Very Much
1. To what extent is EBP clearly described as central to the mission and philosophy of your educational agency?	1	2	3	4	5
2. To what extent do you believe that evidence-base education is practiced in your organization?	1	2	3	4	5
3. To what extent are the faculty who teach you committed to EBP?	1	2	3	4	5
4. To what extent are the community partners with whom you have clinical practicum committed to EBP?	1	2	3	4	5
5. To what extent are there administrators within your educational organization committed to EBP (i.e., have planned for resources and support [e.g., time] to teach EBP across your courses)?	1	2	3	4	5
6. In your educational organization, to what extent is there a critical mass of faculty who have strong EBP knowledge and skills?	1	2	3	4	5
7. To what extent is there ongoing research by nurse scientists (doctorally prepared researchers) in your educational organization to assist in generation of evidence when it does not exist?	1	2	3	4	5
8. In your educational organization, to what extent are there faculty who are EBP mentors?	1	2	3	4	5
9. To what extent do faculty model EBP in your didactic and clinical settings?	1	2	3	4	5
10. To what extent do students have access to quality computers and access to electronic databases for searching for best evidence?	1	2	3	4	5
11. To what extent do students have proficient computer skills?	1	2	3	4	5

(continued)

Item	None at All	A Little	Somewhat	Moderately	Very Much
12. To what extent do librarians within your educational organization have EBP knowledge and skills?	1	2	3	4	5
13. To what extent are librarians used to search for evidence?	1	2	3	4	5
14. To what extent are fiscal resources used to support EBP (e.g., education—attending EBP conferences/ workshops, computers, paid time for the EBP process, mentors)	1	2	3	4	5
15. To what extent are there EBP champions (i.e., those who will go the extra mile to advance EBP) in the environment among:					
a. Dean?	1	2	3	4	5
b. Associate deans?	1	2	3	4	5
c. Didactic course faculty?	1	2	3	4	5
d. Clinical course faculty?	1	2	3	4	5
e. Students?	1	2	3	4	5
16. To what extent is the measurement and sharing of outcomes part of the culture of your educational organization?	1	2	3	4	5

Item	None	25%	50%	75%	100%
17. To what extent are decisions generated from:					
a. Faculty?	1	2	3	4	5
b. Dean/Director?	1	2	3	4	5
c. Students?	1	2	3	4	5

Item	Not Ready	Getting Ready	Been Ready But Not Acting	Ready to Go	Past Ready and Onto Action
18. Overall, how would you rate your educational organization in readiness for EBP (how ready is it)?	1	2	3	4	5

Item	None at All	A Little	Somewhat	Moderately	Very Much
19. Compared to 6 months ago, how much movement in your educational organization has there been toward an EBP culture?	1	2	3	4	5

©Fineout-Overholt & Melnyk, 2011. Please DO NOT USE without permission. For further information about use, please contact Dr. EFO at ellen.fineout.overholt@gmail.com. Cronbach's alphas have been ≥0.85 across various samples.

Appendix K
Sample Instruments to Evaluate EBP in Clinical Settings

EBP BELIEFS SCALE

Below are 16 statements about evidence-based practice (EBP). Please circle the number that best describes your agreement or disagreement with each statement. There are no right or wrong answers.

	Strongly Disagree	Disagree	Neither Agree nor Disagree	Agree	Strongly Agree
1. I believe that EBP results in the best clinical care for patients.	1	2	3	4	5
2. I am clear about the steps of EBP.	1	2	3	4	5
3. I am sure that I can implement EBP.	1	2	3	4	5
4. I believe that critically appraising evidence is an important step in the EBP process.	1	2	3	4	5
5. I am sure that evidence-based guidelines can improve clinical care.	1	2	3	4	5
6. I believe that I can search for the best evidence to answer clinical questions in a time-efficient way.	1	2	3	4	5
7. I believe that I can overcome barriers in implementing EBP.	1	2	3	4	5
8. I am sure that I can implement EBP in a time-efficient way.	1	2	3	4	5
9. I am sure that implementing EBP will improve the care that I deliver to my patients.	1	2	3	4	5
10. I am sure about how to measure the outcomes of clinical care.	1	2	3	4	5
11. I believe that EBP takes too much time.	1	2	3	4	5
12. I am sure that I can access the best resources in order to implement EBP.	1	2	3	4	5

(continued)

	Strongly Disagree	Disagree	Neither Agree nor Disagree	Agree	Strongly Agree
13. I believe EBP is difficult.	1	2	3	4	5
14. I know how to implement EBP sufficiently enough to make practice changes.	1	2	3	4	5
15. I am confident about my ability to implement EBP where I work.	1	2	3	4	5
16. I believe the care that I deliver is evidence based.	1	2	3	4	5

© Melnyk & Fineout-Overholt, 2003. Please DO NOT USE this instrument without permission from the authors. For further information about use of this scale, please contact Bernadette Melnyk at bernmelnyk@gmail.com. Validity of this scale has been established and Cronbach's alphas have been ≥0.85 across various samples.

EBP IMPLEMENTATION SCALE

Below are 18 questions about EBP. Some healthcare providers do some of these things more often than other healthcare providers. There is no certain frequency in which you should be performing these tasks. Please answer each question by circling the number that best describes **how often each item has applied to you in the past 8 weeks**.

In the **past 8 weeks**, I have:

	0 Times	1–3 Times	4–5 Times	6–8 Times	>8 Times
1. Used evidence to change my teaching	0	1	2	3	4
2. Critically appraised evidence from a research study	0	1	2	3	4
3. Generated a PICO question about my teaching/practice specialty	0	1	2	3	4
4. Informally discussed evidence from a research study with a colleague	0	1	2	3	4
5. Collected data on a clinical/educational issue	0	1	2	3	4
6. Shared evidence from a study or studies in the form of a report or presentation to more than two colleagues	0	1	2	3	4
7. Evaluated the outcomes of an educational change	0	1	2	3	4
8. Shared an evidence-based guideline with a colleague	0	1	2	3	4
9. Shared evidence from a research study with a patient/family member	0	1	2	3	4
10. Shared evidence from a research study with a multidisciplinary team member	0	1	2	3	4
11. Read and critically appraised a clinical research study	0	1	2	3	4
12. Accessed the Cochrane database of systematic reviews	0	1	2	3	4
13. Accessed an evidence-based guideline	0	1	2	3	4
14. Used an evidence-based guideline or systematic review to change clinical practice where I work	0	1	2	3	4
15. Evaluated a care initiative by collecting patient outcome data	0	1	2	3	4
16. Shared the outcome data collected with colleagues	0	1	2	3	4
17. Changed practice based on patient outcome data	0	1	2	3	4
18. Promoted the use of EBP to my colleagues	0	1	2	3	4

ORGANIZATIONAL CULTURE AND READINESS FOR SYSTEM-WIDE INTEGRATION OF EBP SURVEY

Below are 19 questions about EBP. Please consider the state of your organization for the readiness of EBP and indicate which answer best describes your response to each question. There are no right or wrong answers.

Item	None at All	Less Than 1 Year ago	As Much as 1 Year Ago	More Than 1 Year Ago	A Great Deal More Than 1 Year Ago
1. To what extent is EBP clearly described as central to the mission and philosophy of your institution?	1	2	3	4	5
2. To what extent do you believe that EBP is practiced in your organization?	1	2	3	4	5
3. To what extent is the nursing staff with whom you work committed to EBP?	1	2	3	4	5
4. To what extent is the physician team with whom you work committed to EBP?	1	2	3	4	5
5. To what extent are there administrators within your organization committed to EBP (i.e., have planned for resources and support [e.g., time] to initiate EBP)?	1	2	3	4	5
6. In your organization, to what extent is there a critical mass of nurses who have strong EBP knowledge and skills?	1	2	3	4	5
7. To what extent are there nurse scientists (doctorally prepared researchers) in your organization to assist in generation of evidence when it does not exist?	1	2	3	4	5
8. In your organization, to what extent are there Advanced Practice Nurses (APNs) who are EBP mentors for staff nurses as well as other APNs?	1	2	3	4	5
9. To what extent do practitioners model EBP in their clinical settings?	1	2	3	4	5
10. To what extent do staff nurses have access to quality computers and to electronic databases for searching for best evidence?	1	2	3	4	5
11. To what extent do staff nurses have proficient computer skills?	1	2	3	4	5

(continued)

Item	None at All	Less Than 1 Year ago	As Much as 1 Year Ago	More Than 1 Year Ago	A Great Deal More Than 1 Year Ago
12. To what extent do librarians within your organization have EBP knowledge and skills?	1	2	3	4	5
13. To what extent are librarians used to search for evidence?	1	2	3	4	5
14. To what extent are fiscal resources used to support EBP (e.g., education—attending EBP conferences/workshops, computers, paid time for the EBP process, mentors)	1	2	3	4	5
15. To what extent are there EBP champions (i.e., those who will go the extra mile to advance EBP) in the environment among:					
a. Administrators?	1	2	3	4	5
b. Physicians?	1	2	3	4	5
c. Nurse educators?	1	2	3	4	5
d. Advance nurse practitioners?	1	2	3	4	5
e. Staff nurses?	1	2	3	4	5
16. To what extent is the measurement and sharing of outcomes part of the culture of the organization in which you work?	1	2	3	4	5

Item	None	25%	50%	75%	100%
17. To what extent are decisions generated from:					
a. Direct care providers?	1	2	3	4	5
b. Upper administration?	1	2	3	4	5
c. Physician or other healthcare provider groups?	1	2	3	4	5

Item	Not Ready	Getting Ready	Been Ready But Not Acting	Ready to Go	Past Ready and Onto Action
18. Overall, how would you rate your institution in readiness for EBP?	1	2	3	4	5
19. Compared to 6 months ago, how much movement in your educational organization has there been toward an EBP culture?	1	2	3	4	5

THE EBP COMPETENCIES SCALE

Copyright, Gallagher-Ford & Melnyk, 2017

Please use the following descriptors when deciding which category you align most closely with for each item on the self-assessment below:

- **Not Competent:** Does not possess essential knowledge, skills, or attitude to engage in EBP; needs significant guidance.
- **Needs Improvement:** Possesses some essential knowledge, skills, and attitude to engage in EBP, but needs guidance.
- **Competent:** Possesses essential knowledge, skills, and attitude to engage in EBP without guidance; is able to mentor and lead others.
- **Highly Competent:** Possesses advanced knowledge, skills, and attitude to engage in EBP without guidance, is able to mentor, teach, and lead others in EBP.

This scale is based on the EBP competencies developed by Melnyk, Gallagher-Ford, and Fineout-Overholt (2014).

THE EBP COMPETENCIES SCALE FOR PRACTICING REGISTERED PROFESSIONAL NURSES

Please identify your level of competence for each of the EBP competencies using the following 4-point Likert rating scale:
   (1=Not Competent | 2=Needs Improvement | 3=Competent | 4=Highly Competent)

Competency	1	2	3	4
Competency 1: Questions clinical practices for the purpose of improving the quality of care.	O	O	O	O
Competency 2: Describes clinical problems using internal evidence.*	O	O	O	O
Competency 3: Participates in the formulation of clinical questions using PICO(T)[†] format.	O	O	O	O
Competency 4: Searches for external evidence[‡] to answer focused clinical questions.	O	O	O	O
Competency 5: Participates in critical appraisal of preappraised evidence.**	O	O	O	O
Competency 6: Participates in critical appraisal of published research studies to determine their strength and applicability to clinical practice.	O	O	O	O
Competency 7: Participates in the evaluation and synthesis of a body of evidence gathered to determine its strength and applicability to clinical practice.	O	O	O	O
Competency 8: Collects practice data (e.g., individual patient data, quality improvement data) systematically as internal evidence for clinical decision making in the care of individuals, groups, and populations.	O	O	O	O
Competency 9: Integrates evidence gathered from external and internal sources in order to plan EBP changes.	O	O	O	O
Competency 10: Implements practice changes based on evidence, clinical expertise, and patient preferences to improve care processes and patient outcomes.	O	O	O	O
Competency 11: Evaluates outcomes of evidence-based decisions and practice changes for individuals, groups, and populations to determine best practices.	O	O	O	O
Competency 12: Disseminates best practices supported by evidence to improve quality of care and patient outcomes.	O	O	O	O
Competency 13: Participates in strategies to sustain an EBP culture.	O	O	O	O

*Evidence generated internally within a clinical setting, such as patient assessment, outcomes management, and quality improvement data.

[†]PICO(T), Patient population; Intervention or area of Interest; Comparison intervention or group; Outcome; Time.

[‡]Evidence generated from research.

**Preappraised evidence such as clinical guidelines, evidence-based policies and procedures, and evidence summaries and syntheses.

© Gallagher-Ford & Melnyk, 2017. For further information about use of this scale, please contact Lynn Gallagher-Ford at Gallagher-Ford.1@osu.edu or Bernadette Melnyk at bernmelnyk@gmail.com

THE EBP COMPETENCIES SCALE FOR PRACTICING ADVANCED PRACTICE NURSES

All competencies of registered professional nurses AND:

Please identify your level of competence for each of the EBP competencies using the following 4-point Likert rating scale:

(1=Not Competent | 2=Needs Improvement | 3=Competent | 4=Highly Competent)

Competency	1	2	3	4
Competency 14: Systematically conducts an exhaustive search for external evidence[‡] to answer clinical questions.	O	O	O	O
Competency 15: Critically appraises relevant preappraised evidence** and primary studies, including evaluation and synthesis.	O	O	O	O
Competency 16: Integrates a body of external evidence[‡] from allied health and related fields with internal evidence* in making decisions about patient care.	O	O	O	O
Competency 17: Leads transdisciplinary teams in applying synthesized evidence to initiate clinical decisions and practice changes to improve the health of individuals, groups, and populations.	O	O	O	O
Competency 18: Generates internal evidence through outcomes management and EBP implementation projects for the purpose of integrating best practices.	O	O	O	O
Competency 19: Measures processes and outcomes of evidence-based clinical decisions.	O	O	O	O
Competency 20: Formulates evidence-based policies and procedures.	O	O	O	O
Competency 21: Participates in the generation of external evidence with other healthcare professionals.	O	O	O	O
Competency 22: Mentors others in evidence-based decision making and the EBP process.	O	O	O	O
Competency 23: Implements strategies to sustain an EBP culture.	O	O	O	O
Competency 24: Communicates best evidence to individuals, groups, colleagues, and policy-makers.	O	O	O	O

improvement data.

[‡]Evidence generated from research.

**Preappraised evidence such as clinical guidelines, evidence-based policies and procedures, and evidence summaries and syntheses.

For further information about use of this scale, please contact Lynn Gallagher-Ford at Gallagher-Ford.1@osu.edu or Bernadette Melnyk at bernmelnyk@gmail.com

Glossary

A

Absolute risk increase (ARI): The absolute risk increase for an undesirable outcome is when the risk is more for the experimental/condition group than the control/comparison group.

Absolute risk reduction (ARR): The absolute risk reduction for an undesirable outcome is when the risk is less for the experimental/condition group than the control/comparison group.

Accountability (HIPAA) Act: The Health Insurance Portability and Accountability Act (HIPAA) was approved by the U.S. Congress in 1996 to protect the privacy of individuals. It enforces protections for works that improve portability and continuity of health insurance coverage.

Action research: A general term for a variety of approaches that aim to resolve social problems by improving existing conditions for oppressed groups or communities.

Adjacency searching: Using ADJ in advanced searching enables searchers to find words that are next to each other in a specified order or within *x* words of each other regardless of the order; for example, *evidence ADJ based* will yield results in which evidence is next too based. Adjacency searching is part of proximity searching.

Adoption of research evidence: A process that occurs across five stages of innovation (i.e., knowledge, persuasion, decision, implementation, and confirmation).

Aim statement: A well-written statement created prior to an implementation project or a study that provides clear direction for the work; the statement is *time specific*, *measurable*, and contains the *specific* population of patients involved.

Analysis: The process used to determine the findings in a study or project.

Analytic notes: Notes researchers write to themselves to record their thoughts, questions, and ideas as a process of simultaneous data collection and data analysis unfolds.

Applicability (of study findings): Whether or not the results of the study are appropriate for a particular patient situation.

Article synopsis: A summary of the content of a single article.

Atheoretical: Research conducted without a theoretical explanation of how variables should relate to one another; therefore, the study is without underpinnings for proposed relationships.

Attrition: When participants are lost from or drop their participation in a study (see loss of participants to follow-up).

Audit: To examine carefully and verify the findings from a study or project.

Authentic leadership: Leadership who are confident, hopeful, optimistic, resilient, transparent, and possess high moral character.

Author name: The name of the person who wrote a paper.

Autonomy: Patients' right to make decisions about their health, lives, and bodies.

Axial coding: A process used in grounded theory to relate categories of information using a coding paradigm with predetermined subcategories (Strauss & Corbin, 1990).

B

Background questions: Questions that need to be answered as a foundation for asking the searchable, answerable foreground question. They are questions that ask for general information about a clinical issue.

Balancing measures: Measures taken to improve implementation processes and outcomes when unanticipated results are noted and when a new practice is introduced.

Barriers to EBP implementation: Those factors that stymie evidence implementation, such as inadequate EBP knowledge and skills, weak beliefs about the value of EBP, lack of EBP mentors, social and organizational influences, or economic restrictions.

Basic research: The phase of research that explores and describes which variables may be amenable to intervention; the content, strength, and timing of interventions; and the outcome measures for a study.

Basic social process (BSP): The basis for theory generation—recurs frequently, links all the data together, and describes the pattern followed regardless of the variety of conditions under which the experience takes place and different ways in which persons go through it. There are two types of BSP: a basic social psychological process (BSPP) and a basic social structural process (BSSP).

Benchmarking: The process of looking outward to identify, understand, and adapt outstanding (best) practices and (high performance) to help improve performance.

Beneficence: Importance of doing good for patients.

Bias: Divergence of results from the true values or the process that leads to such divergence.

Bibliographic database: An indexed, electronic database of journal articles and other publications that can provide citations and abstracts, as well as articles in full text or links to full text, when available.

Biography: An approach that produces an in-depth report of a person's life. Life histories and oral histories also involve gathering of biographical information and recording of personal recollections of one or more individuals.

Biosketch: A two- to three-page document, similar to a resume or brief curriculum vitae, that captures an individual's educational and professional work experience, honors, prior research grants, and publications.

Blind review: A review process in which identification of the author/creator/researcher is removed and, likewise, the identity of the reviewers so that anonymity of both parties is assured.

Blocking: A strategy introduced into a study that entails deliberately including a potential extraneous intrinsic or confounding variable in a study's design in order to control its effects on the dependent or outcome variable.

Body of evidence: All relevant keeper studies, high and lower level evidence, retrieved by systematically searching all appropriate databases using keywords, subject headings, and titles, as necessary.

Boolean operator AND: Defines the relationships between words, phrases, or subject headings. The Boolean operator AND is used for narrowing a search by retrieving records containing all of the words it separates.

Boolean operator OR: Defines the relationships between words, phrases, or subject headings. The Boolean operator OR is used to broaden a search by retrieving records containing any of the words, phrases, or subject headings that are specified.

Booster interventions: Interventions that are delivered after the initial intervention or treatment in a study for the purpose of enhancing the effects of the intervention.

BOPPPS model: A template for creating a presentation that includes Bridge, Objectives, Pretest, Participatory learning, Posttest, and Summary.

Bracketing: Identifying and suspending previously acquired knowledge, beliefs, and opinions about a phenomenon.

C

Case–control study: A type of research that retrospectively compares characteristics of an individual who has a certain condition (e.g., hypertension) with one who does not (i.e., a matched control or similar person without hypertension); often conducted for the purpose of identifying variables that might predict the condition (e.g., stressful lifestyle, sodium intake).

Case reports: Reports that describe the history of a single patient, or a small group of patients, usually in the form of a story.

Case study: An intensive investigation of a case involving a person or small group of persons, an issue, or an event.

Categorical data/variables: Data that are classified into categories (e.g., gender, hair color) instead of being numerically ordered.

Ceiling effects: Participant scores that cluster toward the high end of a measure.

Citation: The mechanism used to inform readers the origin of designated material within a work (i.e., the source); included typically are author, work title, publisher, date of publication, and inclusive pages of the work.

Clinical decision support system: Computer programs with updated latest external evidence that interface with patient data from the electronic health record and through analysis assist healthcare providers in making clinical decisions.

Clinical expertise: Clinical expertise is more than the skills, knowledge, and experience of clinicians; rather it is expertise that develops from multiple observations of patients and how they react to certain interventions, with the central aspects of experiential learning and clinical judgment as main contributors and products.

Clinical inquiry: A process in which clinicians gather data together using narrowly defined clinical parameters; it allows for an appraisal of the available choices of treatment for the purpose of finding the most appropriate choice of action. Clinical inquiry in action includes problem identification and clinical judgment across time about the particular transitions of particular patient/family clinical situations. Four aspects of clinical inquiry in action are making qualitative distinctions, engaging in detective work, recognizing changing relevance, and developing clinical knowledge about specific patient populations.

Clinical practice guidelines: Systematically developed statements to assist clinicians and patients in making decisions about care; ideally, the guidelines consist of a systematic review of the literature, in conjunction with consensus of a group of expert decision makers, including administrators, policy makers, clinicians, and consumers who consider the evidence and make recommendations.

Clinical significance: Study findings that will directly influence clinical practice, whether they are statistically significant or not.

Clinical wisdom and judgment: Wisdom and judgment that comes from experiences and establishes clinicians as credible, thereby influencing how clinicians use supporting evidence, patients' preferences and values, and the context of the client–provider caring relationship.

Cochrane Central Register of Controlled Trials: A database of controlled trials identified by contributors to the Cochrane Collaboration and others.

Cochrane Database of Systematic Reviews: A database containing reviews that are highly structured and systematic with explicit inclusion and exclusion criteria to minimize bias.

Cochrane Methodology Register: Studies prepared by the Cochrane Empirical Methodological Studies Methods Group that examine the methods used in reviews and more general methodological studies that could be used by anyone conducting systematic reviews.

Cohort study: A longitudinal study that begins with the gathering of two groups of patients (the cohorts), one who received the exposure (e.g., to a disease) and one who does not, and then following these groups over time (prospective) to measure the development of different outcomes (diseases); an observational study.

Comparative effectiveness trial: Experimental studies designed to discover which of at least two established healthcare interventions works better to affect selected outcomes.

Competency: Performance (observable behavior) that is demonstrated in expected levels of integration of evidence-based knowledge, skills, abilities, and judgment.

Complexity science: A study of a system or issue using nonlinear thinking to explore theories and conceptual tools from a variety of disciplines to explain its dynamic complexity. These unpredictable, multifactorial systems and issues have interrelated relationships and parts.

Computer-assisted qualitative data analysis: An area of technological innovation that, in qualitative research, has resulted in uses of word processing and software packages to support data management.

Conceptual framework: A group of interrelated statements that provide a guide or direction for a study or project; sometimes referred to as a theoretical framework.

Confidence interval (CI): A measure of the precision of the estimate. The 95% CI is the range of values within which we can be 95% sure that the true value lies for the whole population of patients from whom the study patients were selected.

Confirmability: Demonstrated by providing substantiation that findings and interpretations are grounded in the data (i.e., links between researcher assertions and the data are clear and credible).

Confounding: Occurs when two factors are closely associated and the effects of one confuses or distorts the effects of the other factor on an outcome. The distorting factor is a confounding variable.

Confounding variables: Those factors that interfere with the relationship between the independent and dependent variables.

Constant comparison: A systematic approach to analysis that is a search for patterns in data as they are coded, sorted into categories, and examined in different contexts.

Construct validity: The degree to which an instrument measures the construct it is supposed to be measuring.

Contamination: The inadvertent and undesirable influence of an experimental intervention on another intervention.

Content analysis: In qualitative analysis, a term that refers to processes of breaking down narrative data (coding, comparing, contrasting, and categorizing bits of information) and reconstituting them in some new form (e.g., description, interpretation, theory).

Content validity: The degree to which the items in an instrument are tapping the content they are supposed to measure.

Context: The conditions in which something exists.

Context of caring: Client–healthcare provider relationships are uniquely represented in a caring context that recognizes and respects this important dyad.

Control group: A group of participants who do not receive the experimental intervention or treatment.

Controlled vocabulary or thesaurus: A hierarchical arrangement of descriptive terms that serve as mapping agents for searches; often unique to each database.

Convenience sampling: Drawing readily available participants to participate in a study.

Correlational descriptive study: A study that is conducted for the purpose of describing the relationship between two or more variables.

Correlational predictive study: A study that is conducted for the purpose of describing what variables predict a certain outcome.

Covariate: A variable that is controlled for in statistical analyses (e.g., analysis of covariance); the variable controlled is typically a confounding or extraneous variable that may influence the outcome.

Critical appraisal: The process of evaluating a study for its worth (i.e., validity, reliability, and applicability to clinical practice).

Critical inquiry: Theoretical perspectives that are ideologically oriented toward critique of and emancipation from oppressive social arrangements or false ideas.

Critical theory: A blend of ideology (based on a critical theory of society) and a form of social analysis and critique that aims to liberate people from unrecognized myths and oppression, in order to bring about enlightenment and radical social change.

Critical thinking: Thinking that uses skillful analysis, assessing, and reconstruction of subsequent thinking to impact process and outcomes; this thinking is generated, refined, and intentionally used by the person.

Critique: An in-depth analysis and critical evaluation of a study that identifies its strengths and limitations.

Cronbach's alpha: An estimate of internal consistency or homogeneity of an instrument that is comprised of several subparts or scales.

Cross-contamination: Diffusion of the treatment or intervention across study groups.

Cross-sectional study: A study designed to observe an outcome or a variable at a single point in time, usually for the purpose of inferring trends over time.

Culture: Shared knowledge and behavior of people who interact within distinct social settings and subsystems.

Cybernetic evidence–innovation dynamic: The closed loop interaction of evidence on innovation and innovation on evidence that creates their ongoing impact that perpetuates each other.

D

Data and safety monitoring plan: A detailed plan for how adverse effects will be assessed and managed.

Data driven: Refers to a process, activity, or decision founded on data versus tradition, intuition or personal experience; that is, hard empirical evidence versus speculation or "gut feel."

Database of Abstracts of Reviews of Effects (DARE): Database that includes abstracts of systematic reviews that have been critically appraised by reviewers at the NHS Centre for Reviews and Dissemination at the University of York, England.

Deep web: The part of the Internet that cannot be accessed by standard search engines. Search engines such as Google retrieve information from the surface web.

Delphi study: A research method (not a design) with expert participants who provide feedback through iteratively reviewing study content two or more times to arrive at a consensus.

Demographic: Characteristics of populations (i.e., age or income) used especially to identify particular subsets, such as samples or project participants.

Dependent or outcome variable: The variable or outcome that is influenced or caused by the independent variable.

Descriptive studies: Those studies that are conducted for the purpose of describing the characteristics of certain phenomena or selected variables.

Design: The overall plan for a study that includes strategies for controlling confounding variables, strategies for when the intervention will be delivered (in experimental studies), and how often and when the data will be collected.

Dialogical engagement: Thinking that is like a thoughtful dialog or conversation.

Direct costs: Actual costs required to conduct a study (e.g., personnel, subject honoraria, instruments).

Discourse analysis: A general term for approaches to analyzing recorded talk and patterns of communication.

Discussion board: A specific online mechanism designed for users to submit or read messages as they discuss a specific topic; often within a learning management system.

Dissemination: The process of distributing or circulating information widely.

E

EBP champion: Clinicians who hold expertise in EBP and are able to bring about evidence-based change, disseminate how they do their work, and improve the uptake of EBP within a culture; individual work focused.

EBP competencies: A set of 24 competencies, developed through expertise and verified through research, that are designed to establish the observable behaviors that demonstrate expected levels of integration of evidence-based knowledge, skills, abilities, and judgment required for actualizing the EBP process; there are basic and advanced competencies.

EBP mentor: Typically, an advanced practice clinician with in-depth knowledge and skills in EBP as well as in individual behavior and organizational change; organizational work focused.

EBP process: Seven-step process that must be followed rigorously to achieve best outcomes: (0) inquiry, (1) clinical question, (2) systematic search, (3) critical appraisal, (4) implementation of recommendations for synthesis of best available evidence, (5) evaluation of outcomes, and (6) dissemination of implementation results.

EBP vision (shared mental framework): A compelling and motivating image of desired changes that is shared across providers, resulting in excellence in clinical practice throughout the healthcare organization.

Educational prescription (EP): Two types of EPs. One is a reflective tool for *self-evaluation* of what one knows about EBP, what one needs to know, and how to fill the gaps, usually through a written plan. The other EP is used to address *educator-assessed learner needs* by providing focused guidance to dig deeper into specific steps of the EBP process. This EP usually contains each step of the EBP process with a primary focus on one or two steps, such as searching or critical appraisal.

Effect size: The strength of the effect of an intervention.

Effectiveness trial: Analysis of an intervention effect in clinical practice and clinical effectiveness is determined (establishing external validity/generalizability of a study).

Efficacy trials: Evaluation of an intervention in an ideal setting and clinical efficacy is determined (focus—internal validity or well-done methodology to determine whether an intervention works or not).

Electronic health record (EHR): An electronic record of client information designed to provide comprehensive information that can be shared among all clinicians involved in a patient's care. The purpose is to have information travel with the patient across settings and locations; note an electronic medical record is the digital version of the paper charts in the clinician's office.

Emergence: Glaser's (1992) term for conceptually driven ("discovery") versus procedurally driven ("forcing") theory development in his critique of Strauss and Corbin (1990).

Emic and etic: Contrasting "insider" views of informants (emic) and the researcher's "outsider" (etic) views.

Environment: Surroundings.

Epistemic justification: The right standing between personal beliefs and knowledge; whether the beliefs are more likely to be true or whether they are more likely to be knowledge, or whether personal beliefs are responsible.

Epistemologies: Ways of knowing and reasoning.

Essences: Internal meaning structures of a phenomenon grasped through the study of human lived experience.

Ethnographic studies: Studies of a social group's culture through time spent combining participant observation and in-depth interviews in the informants' natural setting.

Evaluation: An evaluation of worth.

Event rate: The rate at which a specific event occurs.

Evidence-based clinical practice guidelines: Specific practice recommendations that are based on a methodologically rigorous review of the best evidence on a specific topic.

Evidence-based clinical rounds: A small gathering of interprofessional or single discipline staff and leadership to present and discuss evidence to guide clinical practice changes, designed to meaningfully involve clinical staff in the decision-making process.

Evidence-based decision making: Healthcare and health decisions based on the integration of best research evidence with clinician expertise in the field (generating internal evidence) and other experiences; patient preferences and values; and cultural context—be they decisions about programs, practices, or policies.

Evidence-based interventions: Interventions that are based on the latest and best internal and external evidence.

Evidence-based practice (EBP): A paradigm and lifelong problem-solving approach to clinical decision making that involves the conscientious use of the best available evidence (including a systematic search for and critical appraisal of the most relevant evidence to answer a clinical question) with one's own clinical expertise and patient values and preferences to improve outcomes for individuals, groups, communities, and systems.

Evidence-based quality improvement (EBQI)/ evidence-based practice improvement: Systematic improvement of the quality of practice and performance processes through evidence implementation, combining the EBP process with quality improvement processes to impact process outcomes.

Evidence-based theories: A theory that has been tested and supported through the accumulation of evidence from several studies.

Evidence-informed Health Policy (EIHP): Combining the best available evidence with clinician expertise about a specific issue and stakeholder values and ethics as part of the discussion that informs healthcare providers and policy makers as they craft the best possible health policy.

Evidence summaries: Short summary of available evidence that generally provides recommendations for practice and research. Careful evaluation of how summaries are produced is warranted, ranging from comprehensive synthesis (e.g., systematic review) to simple listing of studies' findings.

Evidence user: Anyone who uses valid evidence to support or change practice; demonstrating skills in interpreting evidence, not generating evidence.

Evidentialism: What is required for clinicians to have credible information as the basis of clinical decisions, that is, the evidence it takes to justifiably believe/know what is required to improve practice.

Excerpta Medica Online: A major biomedical and pharmaceutical database.

Exclusion criteria: Investigator identified characteristics that are (a) possessed by individuals that would exclude them from participating in a study and (b) specified to exclude studies from a body of evidence.

Experiential learning: Experience requiring a turning around of preconceptions, expectations, sets, and routines or adding some new insights to a particular practical situation; a way of knowing that contributes to knowledge production; should influence the development of science.

Experimental design/experiment: A study whose purpose is to test the effects of an intervention or treatment on selected outcomes. This is the strongest design for testing cause-and-effect relationships.

Explode the subject heading: To include all the specific terms listed under a more general subject heading

External evidence: Evidence that is generated from rigorous research.

External validity: Generalizability; the ability to generalize the findings from a study to the larger population from which the sample was drawn.

Extraneous variables: Those factors that interfere with the relationship between the independent and dependent variables.

F

Face validity: The degree to which an instrument appears to be measuring (i.e., tapping) the construct it is intended to measure.

Facilitators: Those clinicians who can adjust their roles and styles to the different stages of an implementation project and the needs of those with whom they are working.

Factorial design: An experimental design that has two or more interventions or treatments.

False negative: A condition where the test indicates that the person does not have the outcome of interest when, in fact, the person does.

False positive: A condition where the test indicates that the person has the outcome of interest when, in fact, the person does not.

Feasibility: The ease of which a study can be conducted or project can be implemented within a real-world setting, including influencing factors such as time and resources required, participation issues, team member expertise, and approval, ethical, or legal issues.

Feminist epistemologies: A variety of views and practices inviting critical dialog about women's experiences in historical, cultural, and socioeconomic perspectives.

Fidelity of the evidence-based intervention: How well an intervention implemented in an evidence-based project follows what was described as the intervention delivery by the author(s) of the research study.

Field notes: Self-designed observational protocols for recording notes about field observations.

Field studies: Studies involving direct, firsthand observation and interviews in informants' natural settings.

Fieldwork: All research activities carried out in and in relation to the field (informants' natural settings).

Filters: A combination of search terms that helps eliminate unnecessary citations from the search yield; careful selection of filters helps with obtaining relevant articles; some databases have built-in filters, while others do not.

Fixed-effect model: Traditional assumption that the event rates are fixed in each of the control and treatment groups.

Floor effects: Participant scores that cluster toward the low end of a measure.

Focus groups: This type of group interview generates data on designated topics through discussion and interaction. Focus group research is a distinct type of study when used as the sole research strategy.

Foreground questions: Those questions that can be answered from scientific evidence about diagnosing, treating, or assisting patients with understanding their prognosis, focusing on specific knowledge.

Forest plot: Diagrammatic representation of the results (i.e., the effects or point estimates) of trials (i.e., squares) along with their CIs (i.e., straight lines through the squares).

Frequency: The number of occurrences in a given time period.

Full-text: Any print resource that is available electronically.

Funnel plot: The plotting of sample size against the effect size of studies included in a systematic review. The funnel should be inverted and symmetrical if a representative sample has been obtained.

G

Generalizability: The extent to which the findings from a study can be generalized or applied to the larger population (i.e., external validity).

Gold standard: An accepted and established reference standard or diagnostic test for a particular illness.

Grey literature: Refers to publications such as brochures and conference proceedings.

(Grounded) formal theory: A systematic explanation of an area of human/social experience derived through meta-analysis of substantive theory.

(Grounded) substantive theory: A systematic explanation of a situation-specific human experience/social phenomenon.

Grounded theory: Studies to generate theory about how people deal with life situations that is "grounded" in empirical data and describes the processes by which they move through experiences over time.

H

Handsearch: Screening for relevant materials that have been missed during the indexed-searching process (i.e., in databases) by manually reviewing predefined and selected journals, conference proceedings, and other publications.

Harm: When risks outweigh benefits.

Health policy: Written principles, procedures, and guidelines that underpin the decisions, plans, and actions within the healthcare community to achieve specific healthcare goals within a culture.

Health policy brief: A clearly written, summary with accessible, pertinent description of a particular health issue, potential related policy options, and recommendations for the best option—all of which are designed to inform policy makers, journalists, and others who influence healthcare-focused policy.

Health Technology Assessment Database: Database containing information on evaluation of medical procedures and technologies in healthcare.

Health topic summaries: Concise overviews of a health topic.

Hermeneutics: Philosophy, theories, and practices of interpretation.

Hierarchy of evidence (see levels of evidence): A mechanism for determining which study designs have the most power to predict cause and effect. The highest level of evidence is systematic reviews of randomized controlled trials (RCTs), and the lowest level of evidence is expert opinion and consensus statements.

History: The occurrence of some event or program unrelated to the intervention that might account for the change observed in the dependent variable.

Hits: Studies obtained from a search that contain the searched word.

Homogeneous study population/Homogeneity: When participants in a study are similar on the characteristics that may affect the outcome variable(s).

Hospital Consumer Assessment of Healthcare Providers and Systems (HCAHPS): Survey measuring patients' perceptions of their hospital experience, focused on satisfaction with care.

HSR queries: Health and safety regulation questions.

Hyperlink: A connection to organized information that is housed in cyberspace and usually relevant to the site on which it was found.

Hypotheses: Predictions about the relationships between variables (e.g., adults who receive cognitive behavioral therapy will report less depression than those who receive relaxation therapy).

I

Implementation science: The study of the methods and strategies use to foster the acceptance of interventions that have been shown to effectively influence daily practice for the purpose of improving population health outcomes.

Incidence: New occurrences of the outcome or disorder within the at-risk population in a specified time frame.

Inclusion criteria: Essential characteristics specified by investigator that (a) potential participants must possess in order to be considered for a study and (b) studies must meet to be included in a body of evidence.

Independent variable: The variable that is influencing the dependent variable or outcome; in experimental studies, it is the intervention or treatment.

Indirect costs: Costs that are not directly related to the actual conduct of a study but are associated with the "overhead" in an organization, such as lights, telephones, and office space.

Informatics: How data, information, knowledge, and wisdom are collected, stored, processed, communicated, and used to support the process of healthcare delivery to clients, providers, administrators, and organizations involved in healthcare delivery.

Innovation: The introduction of something new that promises to challenge existing concepts, practices, or products.

Innovative leadership: Leaders who create an infrastructure that weaves innovation into the DNA of their organization.

Institutional review board (IRB): A committee that approves, monitors, and reviews research involving human participants for the purpose of protecting the rights and welfare of research participants.

Integrative reviews: Systematic summaries of the accumulated state of knowledge about a concept, including highlights of important issues left unresolved.

Integrity of the intervention: The extent to which an intervention is delivered as intended.

Internal consistency reliability: The extent to which an instrument's subparts are measuring the same construct.

Internal evidence: Evidence generated within a clinical practice setting from initiatives such as quality improvement, outcomes management, or EBP implementation projects.

Internal validity: The extent to which it can be said that the independent variable (i.e., the intervention) causes a change in the dependent variable (i.e., outcome), and the results are not due to other factors or alternative explanations.

Interpretive ethnography: Loosely characterized, a movement within anthropology that generates many hybrid forms of ethnographic work as a result of crossing a variety of theoretical boundaries within social science.

Interprofessional collaboration: Cooperation within a team of healthcare providers from various disciplines that have a common goal of shared decision making to improve healthcare outcomes.

Interrater reliability: The degree to which two individuals agree on what they observe.

Interval data: Data that have quantified intervals and equal distances between points but without a meaningful zero point (e.g., temperature in degrees Fahrenheit); often referred to as continuous data.

Introspection: A process of recognizing and examining one's own inner state or feelings.

J

Journal club: A mechanism for disseminating best evidence, in which groups of clinicians—interprofessional or single discipline—gather in person or online, either asynchronous or synchronously, to discuss evidence upon which healthcare practice is based, including practice protocols and expected outcomes.

Journal title: The title of a journal.

Justice: Distribution of resources fairly among people and without prejudice.

K

Keeper studies: Studies relevant to the clinical question that are retained at the end of the systematic search and rapid critical appraisal to move through the entire critical appraisal process.

Key driver program: Graphical representation of the plan for structured process improvement that reflects project aims, what is required to accomplish the aims (i.e., key drivers) and how to achieve them (i.e., strategies, also known as secondary drivers).

Key informant: A select informant/assistant with extensive or specialized knowledge of his or her own culture.

Key stakeholder: An individual or institution that has an investment in a project.

Keyword: A word that is not a part of the database's controlled vocabulary/thesaurus. Keywords are sometimes searched only in titles and abstracts, so caution should be used when searching only with keywords. Sometimes called textwords.

L

Level of evidence: A ranking of evidence by the type of design or research methodology that would answer the question with the least number of error and provide the most reliable findings. Leveling of evidence, also called hierarchies, vary by type of question asked. An example is provided for intervention questions.

Level I evidence: Evidence that is generated from systematic reviews or meta-analyses of all relevant RCTs or evidence-based clinical practice guidelines based on systematic reviews of RCTs; the strongest level of evidence to guide clinical practice.

Level II evidence: Evidence generated from at least one well-designed randomized clinical trial (i.e., a true experiment).

Level III evidence: Evidence obtained from well-designed controlled trials without randomization.

Level IV evidence: Evidence from well-designed case–control and cohort studies.

Level V evidence: Evidence from systematic reviews of descriptive and qualitative studies.

Level VI evidence: Evidence from a single descriptive or qualitative study.

Level VII evidence: Evidence from the opinion of authorities and/or reports of expert committees.

Likelihood ratio: The likelihood that a given test result would be expected in patients with a disease compared to the likelihood that the same result would be expected in patients without that disease.

Limit: Mechanisms within databases that allow the search to be narrowed (reduce the yield);

search limits can be applied to keyword and title searches as well as subject heading searches.

LISTSERV: An electronic information-sharing application that typically is used to distribute messages to subscribers through e-mail; topic-specific information and announcements are discussed/shared. Originally, LISTSERV was the trademarked application, but the word, such as Kleenex, has come to have a generic meaning.

Lived experience: Everyday experience, not as it is conceptualized, but as it is lived (i.e., how it feels).

Loss of participants to follow-up: The proportion of people who started the study but do not complete the study, for whatever reason.

M

Macrolevel change versus macrolevel: Change at a large-scale level (e.g., nationwide systems or large institutions).

Magnitude of effect: Expressing the size of the relationship between two variables or difference between two groups on a given variable/outcome (i.e., the effect size).

Manipulation checks: Assessments verifying that participants have actually processed the experimental information that they have received or followed through with prescribed intervention activities.

Maturation: Developmental change that occurs, even in the absence of the intervention.

Mean: A measure of central tendency, derived by summing all scores and dividing by the number of participants.

Mediating variable: The variable or mechanism through which an intervention works to impact the outcome in a study.

Mediating variables and processes: The mechanisms through which an intervention produces the desired outcome(s).

MeSH: Medline's controlled vocabulary: Medical Subject Headings.

Meta-analysis: A process of using quantitative methods to summarize the results from the multiple studies, obtained and critically reviewed using a rigorous process (to minimize bias) for identifying, appraising, and synthesizing studies to answer a specific question and draw conclusions about the data gathered. The purpose of this process is to gain a summary statistic (i.e., a measure of a single effect) that represents the effect of the intervention across multiple studies.

Meta-synthesis: A rigorous process of analyzing findings across qualitative studies. The results address a specific research question and are obtained through the synthesis of qualitative studies. The process allows researchers to find greater meaning through interpreting the qualitative data.

Method: The theory of how a certain type of research should be carried out (i.e., strategy, approach, process/overall design, and logic of design). Researchers often subsume description of techniques under a discussion of method.

Microlevel change: Change at a small-scale level (e.g., units within a local healthcare organization or small groups of individuals).

Model for improvement: Model focused on accelerating process improvement by asking the following guiding questions—What are we trying to accomplish?; How will we know that a change is an improvement? and What change can we make that will result in improvement? Often, PDSA is used to jumpstart this model implementation.

N

Narrative analysis: A term that refers to distinct styles of generating, interpreting, and representing data as stories that provide insights into life experiences.

Narrative review: A summary of primary studies from which conclusions are drawn by the reviewer based on his or her own interpretations.

National Guidelines Clearinghouse: A comprehensive database of up-to-date English language evidence-based clinical practice guidelines developed in partnership with the American Medical Association, the American Association of Health Plans, and the Association for Healthcare Research and Quality.

Naturalistic research: Commitment to the study of phenomena in their naturally occurring settings (contexts).

News embargo: A restriction on the release of any media information about the findings from a study before they are published in a journal article.

NHS Economic Evaluation Database: A register of published economic evaluation of health interventions.

Nominated/snowball sample: A sample obtained with the help of informants already enrolled in the study.

Nonexperimental study design: A study design in which data are collected but whose purpose is not to test the effects of an intervention or treatment on selected outcomes.

Nonmaleficence: Importance of not harming patients.

Null hypothesis: There is no relationship between or among study variables.

Number needed to harm (NNH): The number of clients, who, if they received an intervention, would result in one additional person being harmed (i.e., having a bad outcome) compared to the clients in the control arm of a study.

Number needed to treat (NNT): The number of people who would need to receive the experimental therapy to prevent one bad outcome or cause one additional good outcome.

O

Observation: Facts learned from observing.

Observation continuum: A range of social roles encompassed by participant observation and ranging from complete observer to complete participant at the extremes.

Observer drift: A decrease in interrater reliability.

Odds ratio (OR): The odds of a case patient (i.e., someone in the intervention group) being exposed (a/b) divided by the odds of a control patient being exposed (c/d).

Open access: Choice for authors within the Cochrane Database beginning on February 1, 2013. Gold open access allows immediate access to the entire review if the authors agree to pay the publication charge fee. Green open access offers free access to the full review 12 months after publication.

Opinion leaders: Individuals who are typically highly knowledgeable and well respected in a system; as such, they are often able to influence change.

Ordinal data: Variables that have ordered categories with intervals that cannot be quantified (e.g., mild, moderate, or severe anxiety).

Organizational culture of EBP: Organization mores that reflect system-wide implementation of EBP across disciplines, leadership levels, and venues; reflected in clinician beliefs about the value of and ability to EBP as well as excellence in outcome.

Organizational policy: The guidelines, procedures, and principles within an organization that are intended to underpin the work and decisions therein, so that organizational goals, long and short term, can be achieved; these are usually easily available online or hardcopy.

Outcomes: A direct result of an intervention, strategy, implementation, or process.

Outcomes management: The use of process and outcomes data to coordinate and influence actions and processes of care that contribute to patient achievement of targeted behaviors or desired effects.

Outcomes measurement: A generic term used to describe the collection and reporting of information about an observed effect in relation to some care delivery process or health promotion action.

Outcomes of healthcare delivery: The outcomes that are influenced by the delivery of clinical care.

Outcomes research: The use of rigorous scientific methods to measure the effect of some intervention on some outcome(s).

P

Paradigm: A worldview or set of beliefs, assumptions, and values that guide clinicians' and researchers' thinking about their work, contributions and impact on health care outcomes; derived from such issues as the nature of reality (ontology) distinguishing justifiable belief from opinions (epistemology), use of language (rhetoric) and process (methodology).

Pareto chart: A bar graph designed to show the distribution of categorical data organized in descending order to demonstrate impact of each determinant (i.e., contributing factor).

Participant observation: Observation and participation in everyday activities in study of informants' natural settings.

Participatory action research (PAR): A form of action research that is participatory in nature (i.e., researchers and participants collaborate in problem definition, choice of methods, data analysis, and use of findings); democratic in principle; and reformatory in impulse (i.e., has as its objective the empowerment of persons through the process of constructing and using their own knowledge as a form of consciousness-raising with the potential for promoting social action).

Patient-centered quality care measures: Measures enacted to preserve the value patients and families place on the healthcare received; a result of actualization of the philosophy of care that views patients as equal partners rather than passive recipients of care.

Patient preferences/choices: Values the patient holds, concerns the patient has regarding the clinical decision/treatment/situation, and choices the patient has/prefers regarding the clinical decision/treatment/situation.

Peer-reviewed: A project or paper or study is reviewed by a person(s) who is a peer to the author and has expertise in the subject.

Phenomenological: Pertaining to the study of essences (i.e., meaning structures) intuited or grasped through descriptions of lived experience.

Phenomenological reduction: An intellectual process involving reflection, imagination, and intuition.

Phenomenology: The study of lived experience, from the perspective of the study participants. Can be descriptive or interactive.

PICOT format: A process in which clinical questions are phrased in a manner that yields the most relevant information from a search; P, Patient population; I, Intervention or issue of interest; C, Comparison intervention or status; O, Outcome; T, Time frame for (I) to achieve the (O).

Pilot research or project: Small-scale study or project. Study tests an intervention with a small number of participants to decide if a large-scale study is feasible. Project is launching an evidence-based initiative with one unit or smaller portion of the population to determine how best to make launch the project system or population wide. Both study and project pilots serve to offer insight into alternative strategies to address potential problems discovered in the pilot process.

Placebo: A sham medical intervention or inert pill; typically given to participants in experimental research studies to control for time and attention spent with participants getting the experimental intervention.

Plan-Do-Study-Act cycle: Rapid cycle improvement in healthcare settings in which changes are quickly made and studied.

Point-of-care clinicians: Clinicians who work directly with patients/clients—at the point of care.

Point-of-care resources: Resources to search for evidence, such as summaries, synopses, and systematic reviews.

Power: The ability of a study design to detect existing relationships between or among variables.

Power analysis: Procedure used for determining the sample size needed for a study.

Practice-based data/evidence: Data that are generated from clinical practice or a healthcare system.

Pragmatic trial: Quantitative studies designed to evaluate the effectiveness of interventions in real-life routine practice conditions and show real-world effectiveness with broader patient groups.

Pragmatism: A practical approach to solutions.

Pre-appraised evidence: A bucket of evidence that has been evaluated with a specific review process to establish its worth established through systematic review.

Pre-experiment: Quantitative studies that lack both random assignment and a comparison/attention control group, creating internal validity concerns.

Prevalence: Refers to the persons in the at-risk population who have the outcome or disorder in a given "snapshot in time."

Primary source: Provides direct evidence (primary studies) to answer a clinical question.

Principal investigator (PI): The lead person who is responsible and accountable for the scientific integrity of a study as well as the oversight of all elements in the conduct of that study.

Principle of fidelity: Importance of trust and honesty in ethics.

Process measures: What is done and how it is done.

Prognosis: The likelihood of a certain outcome.

Provider-skill mix: A method of combining or grouping staff based on different categories of workers.

Proximity searching: Searching for two or more words occurring close to one another—within a certain number of words—using what are called proximity operators (N or W) and a number (to specify a number of words; not more than 255).

Psychometric properties: The validity and reliability information on a scale or instrument.

Purposeful/theoretical sample: A sample intentionally selected in accordance with the needs of the study.

p **Value:** The statistical test of the assumption that there is no difference between an experimental intervention and a control. *p* Value indicates the probability of an event, given the assumption that there is no true difference. By convention, a *p* value of 0.05 is considered a statistically significant result.

Q

Quadruple aim: The triple aim was initiated in 2007 by the Institute for Healthcare Improvement and included improve health of populations, enhance individual's experience and outcomes of care, and reduce per capita healthcare cost. The quadruple aim (2014) extended these three to four with a focus either on (1) empowering clinicians to secure joy at work or (2) securing health equity.

Qualitative data analysis: A variety of techniques that are used to move back and forth between data and ideas throughout the course of the research.

Qualitative data management: The act of designing systems to organize, catalog, code, store, and retrieve data. System design influences, in turn, how the researcher approaches the task of analysis.

Qualitative description: Description that "entails a kind of interpretation that is low-inference (close to the 'facts'), or likely to result in easier consensus (about the 'facts') among researchers" (Sandelowski, 2000b, p. 335).

Qualitative evaluation: A general term covering a variety of approaches to evaluating programs, projects, policies, and so on using qualitative research techniques.

Qualitative research: Research that involves the collection of data in non-numeric form, such as personal interviews, usually with the intention of describing a phenomenon or experience seeking an in-depth understanding within a natural setting.

Quality assurance: The process of ensuring that initiatives or the care being delivered in an institution is of high quality.

Quality improvement data/outcomes: Data that are collected for the purpose of improving the quality of healthcare or patient outcomes.

Quality improvement projects: Initiatives with a goal to improve the processes or outcomes of the care being delivered.

Quantitative research: The investigation of phenomena using manipulation of numeric data with statistical analysis. Can be descriptive, predictive, or causal. This research emphasizes precise measurement of variables; often conducted in the form of rigorously controlled studies.

Quasi-experiments: A type of experimental design that tests the effects of an intervention or treatment but lacks one or more characteristics of a true experiment (e.g., random assignment; a control or comparison group).

R

Random assignment (also called randomization): The use of a strategy to randomly assign participants to the experimental or control groups (e.g., tossing a coin).

Random error: Measurement error that occurs without a pattern, purpose, or intent.

Random sampling: Selecting participants to participate in a study using a random strategy (e.g., tossing a coin); in this method of selecting participants, every subject has an equal chance of being selected.

Randomized block design: A type of control strategy used in an experimental design that places participants in equally distributed study groups based on certain characteristics (e.g., age) so that each study group will be similar prior to introduction of the intervention or treatment.

Randomized controlled trial (RCT): A true experiment (i.e., one that delivers an intervention or treatment in which participants are randomly assigned to control and experimental groups); the strongest design to support cause-and-effect relationships.

Rate of occurrence: The rate at which an event occurs.

Ratio-level data: The highest level of data; data that have quantified intervals on an infinite scale in which there are equal distances between points and a meaningful zero point (e.g., ounces of water, height); often referred to as continuous data.

Readmission rates: Readmission rates are generally referred to as patient admission to a hospital within 30 days after discharge from a prior hospital stay (CMS core measure).

Reference manager: Often referred to as citation managers/management, this software is designed to offer options that save, search, sort, share, and continuously add, delete, and organize promising citations.

Reference population: Those individuals in the past, present, and future to whom the study results can be generalized.

Reflection: The act of contemplating.

Relative risk (RR): Measures the strength of association and is the risk of the outcome in the exposed group (Re) divided by the risk of the outcome in the unexposed group (Ru). RR is used in prospective studies such as RCTs and cohort studies.

Relative risk reduction (RRR): Proportion of risk for bad outcomes in the intervention group compared to the unexposed control group.

Reliability: The consistency of an instrument in measuring the underlying construct.

Reliability coefficients: A measure of an instrument's reliability (e.g., often computed with a Cronbach's alpha).

Reliability of study findings: Whether or not the effects of a study have sufficient influence on practice, clinically and statistically; that is, the results can be counted on to make a difference when clinicians apply them to their practice.

Reliable measures: Those that consistently and accurately measure the construct of interest.

Representation: Part of the analytic process that raises the issue of providing a truthful portrayal of what the data represent (e.g., essence of an experience, cultural portrait) that will be meaningful to its intended audience.

Research design meeting: A planning meeting held for the purpose of designing a study and strategizing about potential funding as well as the roles of all investigators.

Research subjects review board (RSRB): Often referred to as an IRB; a group of individuals who review a study before it can be conducted to determine the benefits and risks of conducting the research to study participants.

Research utilization: The use of research knowledge, often based on a single study, in clinical practice.

Return on investment: A measure of performance that demonstrates the efficiency of an investment/intervention; includes but is not limited to financial benefits of an evidence-based intervention.

Risk: The probability that a person (currently free from a disease) will develop a disease at some point.

Risk ratio: See relative risk (RR).

Rules of evidence: Standard criteria for the evaluation of domains of evidence; these are applied to research evidence to assess its validity, the study findings, and its applicability to a patient/system situation.

Run chart: Graphical representation of data change over time using line charts.

S

Saturation: The point at which categories of data are full and data collection ceases to provide new information.

Saturation level: The level at which a searcher no longer finds any new references but, instead, is familiar and knowledgeable with the literature.

Scalability: The extent to which an intervention is translatable into real-life practice settings.

Science of improvement: Emphasizes innovation and rapid cycle testing using applied science with a focus on spread to facilitate learning about what/where/how/in what context improvement in outcomes occurs; generally uses a combination of interprofessional experts' subject knowledge and quality improvement methods/measures results in gestalt of clinical science, systems theory, psychology, and statistics.

SCOT analysis: Identifying and evaluating the strengths and challenges within an organization as well as the opportunities and threats outside the organization to the success of a specific initiative.

Search history: The recorded search strategy that is saved, printed, or screenshotted to enable the searcher or others to rerun the search strategy or to establish how the search was conducted.

Search strategy: A process used by a clinician or librarian to search a database. Involves identifying databases to search; keywords and subject headings searched along with combinations thereof; and inclusion/exclusion criteria.

Secondary sources: Evidence that describes, discusses, interprets, comments upon, analyzes, evaluates, summarizes, and processes primary sources of evidence.

Semiotics: The theory and study of signs and symbols applied to the analysis of systems of patterned communication.

Semi-structured interviews: Formal interviews that provide more interviewer control and question format structure but retain a conversational tone and allow informants to answer in their own ways.

Senior leadership: Corporate-suite (C-suite) leadership in an organization; typically includes chief executive officer (CEO), chief financial officer (CFO), chief operating officer (COO), and chief information officer (CIO). May also include chief nursing officer (CNO) and chief medical officer (CMO).

Sensitivity: The probability of a diagnostic test finding disease among those who have the disease or the proportion of people with disease who have a positive test result (true positive).

Servant leadership: Leadership in which leaders and followers share power. Leaders focus on follower growth and well-being to reach their full potential and performance.

Shared mental framework: See EBP vision.

SMART goals: Goals that are Specific (no extraneous information—only who, what, when, where, why), Measurable (observable outcomes using metrics), Achievable (can make it happen), Relevant (aligned with project/organizational/policy objectives), and Time-bound (target date for deliverables stated and reasonable).

SnNout: When a test has a high Sensitivity, a Negative result rules out the diagnosis.

Sociolinguistics: The study of the use of speech in social life.

Solomon four-group design: A type of experimental study design that uses a before–after design for the first two experimental groups and an after-only design for the second experimental and control groups so that it can separate the effects of pretesting the participants on the outcome measure(s).

"So what" factor in research/so what outcomes in EBP: The conduct of research or implementation of EBP process with high-impact potential to improve outcomes that the current healthcare system is focused on, such as patient complications, readmission rates, length of stay, or cost.

Specificity: The probability of a diagnostic test finding NO disease among those who do NOT have the disease or the proportion of people free of a disease who have a negative test (true negatives).

Spirit of inquiry: A persistent questioning about how to improve current practices; a sense of curiosity.

SpPin: When a test has a high Specificity, a Positive result rules in the diagnosis.

Standard error: An estimate due to sampling error of the deviation of the sample mean from the true population mean.

Statistical significance: The results of statistical analysis of data are unlikely to have been caused by chance, at a predetermined level of probability.

Strategic plan: A specific road map of carefully written goals that have specific implementation strategies or action tactics with a timeline and specific measureable outcomes, as well as process indicators of success (what shows that things are going well); a carefully outlined implementation strategy is required for each established goal.

Stratification: A strategy that divides the study population into two or more subpopulations and then samples separately from each.

Structure measures: Measures that capture components such as manpower, use of a specific specialty unit for patient management, and the availability of technology or highly specialized services.

Structured, open-ended interviews: Formal interviews with little flexibility in the way that questions are asked but with question formats that allow informants to respond on their own terms (e.g., "What does . . . mean to you?" "How do you feel/think about . . .?").

Subject heading: A set of terms or phrases (known as controlled vocabulary) that classify materials.

Symbolic interaction: Theoretical perspective on how social reality is created by human interaction through ongoing, taken-for-granted processes of symbolic communication.

Synthesis: The process of putting together parts to make a whole (e.g., integrating the results of several studies to tell a story about an entire body of evidence).

Systematic review: A summary of evidence, typically conducted by an expert or expert panel on a particular topic, that uses a rigorous process (to minimize bias) for identifying, appraising, and synthesizing studies to answer a specific clinical question and draw conclusions about the data gathered.

T

Taxonomy: The process of naming and classifying things.

Techniques: Tools or procedures used to generate or analyze data (e.g., interviewing, observation, standardized tests and measures, constant comparison, document analysis, content analysis, statistical analysis). Techniques are method neutral and may be used, as appropriate, in any research design—either qualitative or quantitative.

Test–retest reliability: A test of an instrument's stability over time assessed by repeated measurements over time.

Thematic analysis: Systematic description of recurring ideas or topics (themes) that represent different, yet related, aspects of a phenomenon.

Theoretic interest: A desire to know or understand better.

Theoretical framework: The basis upon which a study is guided; its purpose is to provide a context for selecting the study's variables, including how they relate to one another as well as to guide the development of an intervention in experimental studies.

Theoretical generalizability: See transferability.

Theoretical sampling: Decision making, while concurrently collecting and analyzing data, about what further data and data sources are needed to develop the emerging theory.

Theoretical sensitivity: A conceptual process to accompany techniques for generating grounded theory (Glaser, 1978).

Thick description: Description that does more than describe human experiences by beginning to interpret what they mean, involving detailed reports of what people say and do, incorporating the textures and feelings of the physical and social worlds in which people move, with reference to that context (i.e., an interpretation of what their words and actions mean).

Transferability: Demonstrated by information that is sufficient for a research consumer to determine whether the findings are meaningful to other people in similar situations (analytic or theoretical vs. statistical generalizability).

Transformational leadership: Leadership that foster leader and follower discovery of meaning and purpose in work through their relationship.

Translational research: This term has two definitions, and these definitions are sequential (2 follows 1): (1) from bench to bedside—translating basic science into research about new healthcare options for patients and (2) research that explores how evidence-based interventions can be best translated to real-world clinical settings.

Triggers: Issues in current practice that may be concerns about current knowledge (deficits or new availability of information) or identified clinical problems; both types of triggers must have data to demonstrate their existence.

True experiment: The strongest type of experimental design for testing cause-and-effect relationships; true experiments possess three characteristics: (a) a treatment or intervention, (b) a control or comparison group, and (c) a random assignment.

Truncation: The use of a symbol (e.g., * or ?) to shorten a word to its root. This results in additional words with the same root being found. For example, truncating child * will pick up the words child, childless, and children.

Type I error: Mistakenly rejecting the null hypothesis when it is actually true.

Type II error: Mistakenly accepting (not rejecting) the null hypothesis when it is false.

U

Unstructured, open-ended interviews: Informal conversations that allow informants the fullest range of possibilities to describe their experiences, thoughts, and feelings.

V

Valid measures: Those that measure the construct that they are intended to measure (e.g., an anxiety measure truly measures anxiety, not depression).

Validity (of study findings): Whether or not the results of the study were obtained via sound scientific methods.

Value-based purchasing (VBP): Purchasing practices based in quality and cost that are focused on improving the value of healthcare services. A helpful consideration is to think of value as quality divided by cost; consider that value increases as quality increases when costs are maintained.

Volunteer/convenience sample: A sample obtained by solicitation or advertising for participants who meet study criteria.

Y

Yield: The number of hits obtained by a literature search. This can be per database and/or total yield; there can be several levels of yield (e.g., first yield and final yield, that is, only those studies that were kept for review).

All Cochrane definitions came from http://www.update-software.com/cochrane/content .htm

Index

Note: Page numbers followed by "*b*" denote boxes; those followed by "*f*" denote figures; those followed by "*t*" denote tables.